DATE DUE

APR 1 4 2008	
AUG 1 4 2009	
Oct. 31, 2017	

BRODART, CO.   Cat. No. 23-221-003

HANDBOOK OF SOCIALIZATION

HANDBOOK OF SOCIALIZATION
Theory and Research

Edited by
JOAN E. GRUSEC
PAUL D. HASTINGS

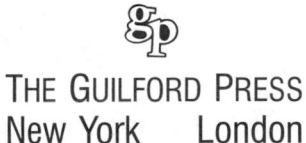

THE GUILFORD PRESS
New York   London

©2007 The Guilford Press
A Division of Guilford Publications, Inc.
72 Spring Street, New York, NY 10012
www.guilford.com

Printed in the United States of America

This book is printed on acid-free paper.

Last digit is print number: 9   8   7   6   5   4   3   2   1

Library of Congress Cataloging-in-Publication Data

Handbook of socialization : theory and research / edited by Joan E. Grusec, Paul D. Hastings.
    p. cm.
  Includes bibliographical references and indexes.
  ISBN-13: 978-1-59385-332-7 (hardcover : alk. paper)
  ISBN-10: 1-59385-332-7 (hardcover : alk. paper)
 1. Socialization. I. Grusec, Joan E. II. Hastings, Paul D. (Paul David), 1966–
HM686.H36 2006
303.3'2—dc22

                                        2006021486

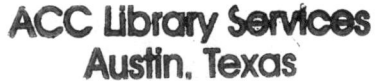

About the Editors

Joan E. Grusec, PhD, is Professor of Psychology at the University of Toronto. Her research interests focus on the impact of parenting on children's socialization as well as determinants of parenting practices. She is the author or editor of several books, including *Parenting and Children's Internalization of Values: A Handbook of Contemporary Theory* (coedited with Leon Kuczynski). She is a former Associate Editor of *Developmental Psychology.*

Paul D. Hastings, PhD, is Associate Professor of Psychology in the Centre for Research in Human Development at Concordia University in Montreal, Quebec. He completed his graduate studies at the University of Toronto and postdoctoral fellowships at the University of Waterloo and the National Institute of Mental Health. His research interests are focused on the joint contributions of socialization influences and physiological regulation to trajectories of adaptive and maladaptive development.

Contributors

Jeffrey Jensen Arnett, PhD, Department of Psychology, Clark University, Worcester, Massachusetts

Hideko H. Bassett, MS, Department of Psychology, George Mason University, Fairfax, Virginia

John E. Bates, PhD, Department of Psychological and Brain Sciences, Indiana University, Bloomington, Indiana

David A. Beaulieu, PhD candidate, Department of Psychology, University of California, Santa Barbara, Santa Barbara, California

John W. Berry, PhD, Department of Psychology, Queen's University, Kingston, Ontario, Canada

Mara Brendgen, PhD, Department of Psychology, University of Quebec at Montreal, Montreal, Quebec, Canada

Daphne Blunt Bugental, PhD, Department of Psychology, University of California, Santa Barbara, Santa Barbara, California

William M. Bukowski, PhD, Centre for Research in Human Development, Department of Psychology, Concordia University, Montreal, Quebec, Canada

Avshalom Caspi, PhD, Social, Genetic, and Developmental Psychiatry Research Centre, Institute of Psychiatry, King's College, London, United Kingdom; Department of Psychology, University of Wisconsin, Madison, Madison, Wisconsin

Timothy A. Cavell, PhD, Department of Psychology, University of Arkansas, Fayetteville, Arkansas

Pamela M. Cole, PhD, Department of Psychology, The Pennsylvania State University, University Park, Pennsylvania

Rand D. Conger, PhD, Family Research Group, Department of Human and Community Development, University of California, Davis, Davis, California

Maricela Correa-Chávez, PhD, Graduate School of Education, University of California, Los Angeles, Los Angeles, California

Maayan Davidov, PhD, Center for the Study of Child Development, University of Haifa, Mount Carmel, Haifa, Israel

Susanne A. Denham, PhD, Department of Psychology, George Mason University, Fairfax, Virginia

Amy Dexter, MS, Department of Psychology, University of California, Santa Cruz, Santa Cruz, California

Shannon J. Dogan, MS, Family Research Group, Department of Human and Community Development, University of California, Davis, Davis, California

Eric F. Dubow, PhD, Department of Psychology, Bowling Green State University, Bowling Green, Ohio

Judy Dunn, PhD, Social, Genetic, and Developmental Psychiatry Research Centre, Institute of Psychiatry, King's College, London, United Kingdom

Jacquelynne S. Eccles, PhD, Institute for Research on Women and Gender, University of Michigan, Ann Arbor, Michigan

Karen L. Fingerman, PhD, Child Development and Family Studies, Purdue University, West Lafayette, Indiana

Carly Kay Friedman, MS, Department of Psychology, University of California, Santa Cruz, Santa Cruz, California

Mary Gauvain, PhD, Department of Psychology, University of California, Riverside, Riverside, California

Dara Greenwood, PhD, Department of Communication Studies, University of Michigan, Ann Arbor, Michigan

Joan E. Grusec, PhD, Department of Psychology, University of Toronto, Toronto, Ontario, Canada

Paul D. Hastings, PhD, Centre for Research in Human Development, Department of Psychology, Concordia University, Montreal, Quebec, Canada

L. Rowell Huesmann, PhD, Institute for Social Research, University of Michigan, Ann Arbor, Michigan

Shelley Hymel, PhD, Department of Educational and Counseling Psychology, and Special Education, University of British Columbia, Vancouver, British Columbia, Canada

Leon Kuczynski, PhD, Department of Family Relations and Applied Nutrition, University of Guelph, Guelph, Ontario, Canada

Deborah Laible, PhD, Department of Psychology, Lehigh University, Bethlehem, Pennsylvania

Campbell Leaper, PhD, Department of Psychology, University of California, Santa Cruz, Santa Cruz, California

Lisa Looney, PhD, Department of Psychology, California State University, San Bernardino, California

Eleanor E. Maccoby, PhD, Department of Psychology, Stanford University, Stanford, California

Kenya T. Malcolm, MS, Department of Psychology, University of Arkansas, Fayetteville, Arkansas

Terrie E. Moffitt, PhD, Social, Genetic, and Developmental Psychiatry Research Centre, Institute of Psychiatry, King's College, London, United Kingdom; Department of Psychology, University of Wisconsin, Madison, Madison, Wisconsin

Leslie Moore, PhD, Department of Psychology, University of California, Santa Cruz, Santa Cruz, California

Behnosh Najafi, MA, Department of Psychology, University of California, Santa Cruz, Santa Cruz, California

C. Melanie Parkin, MSc, Department of Psychology, University of Guelph, Guelph, Ontario, Canada

Charlotte J. Patterson, PhD, Department of Psychology, University of Virginia, Charlottesville, Virginia

Susan M. Perez, PhD, Department of Psychology, University of North Florida, Jacksonville, Florida

Gregory S. Pettit, PhD, Department of Human Development and Family Studies, Auburn University, Auburn, Alabama

Lindsay Pitzer, BA, Child Development and Family Studies, Purdue University, West Lafayette, Indiana

Rena Repetti, PhD, Department of Psychology, University of California, Los Angeles, Los Angeles, California

Barbara Rogoff, PhD, Department of Psychology, University of California, Santa Cruz, Santa Cruz, California

Fred Rothbaum, PhD, Eliot-Pearson Department of Child Development, Tufts University, Medford, Massachusetts

Darby Saxbe, MA, Department of Psychology, University of California, Los Angeles, Los Angeles, California

Amy Seay, MS, Department of Psychology, University of Arkansas, Fayetteville, Arkansas

Jocelyn Solís, PhD (deceased), Department of Psychology, University of California, Santa Cruz, Santa Cruz, California

Caroline Sullivan, MA, Centre for Research in Human Development, Department of Psychology, Concordia University, Montreal, Quebec, Canada

Patricia Z. Tan, BS, Department of Psychology, The Pennsylvania State University, University Park, Pennsylvania

Shelley E. Taylor, PhD, Department of Psychology, University of California, Los Angeles, Los Angeles, California

Ross A. Thompson, PhD, Department of Psychology, University of California, Davis, Davis, California

Gisela Trommsdorff, PhD, Department of Psychology, University of Konstanz, Konstanz, Germany

William T. Utendale, MA, Centre for Research in Human Development, Department of Psychology, Concordia University, Montreal, Quebec, Canada

Frank Vitaro, PhD, Research Unit on Children's Psychosocial Maladjustment, School of Psychoeducation, University of Montreal, Montreal, Quebec, Canada

Kathryn R. Wentzel, PhD, Department of Human Development, University of Maryland, College Park, Maryland

Todd Wyatt, BA, Department of Psychology, George Mason University, Fairfax, Virginia

Acknowledgments

Many people were involved in the production of this handbook, and our gratitude for their contributions is deep. Our greatest debt is obviously owed to the book's contributors. We learned an incredible amount from working with them. The level of scholarship displayed in their chapters was impressively high, and we were proud to see the quality of work currently being conducted by socialization researchers. Each chapter went through a number of revisions in response to comments by both editors. We truly appreciated the contributors' patience as they responded to our questions and suggestions. Throughout the process, they remained even-tempered and gracious, and we hope that the final product reflects the frequently very interesting and informative exchanges that occurred. We also solicited valuable feedback from colleagues for our own chapters and offer our sincere thanks to Everett Waters and Carolyn Zahn-Waxler for their generosity and advice.

The idea for the book came from Seymour Weingarten, Editor-in-Chief at The Guilford Press. He has been available with wise advice and assistance whenever approached. Anna Nelson, Senior Production Editor, continued to add to the high level of professionalism we observed in all those with whom we have worked at Guilford.

Contents

Introduction

JOAN E. GRUSEC and PAUL D. HASTINGS

Across the diverse range of communities and cultures in which they live, human beings need to safely and harmoniously exist together as well as maintain their own well-being. Socialization encompasses the array of processes by which these needs are met. In this book we have tried to draw together information from a multitude of areas in order to shed light on how socialization is accomplished and what the mechanisms are that underlie that accomplishment. Each of the contributing authors has addressed socialization from a particular perspective. What has emerged is a comprehensive picture of how socialization is conceptualized by psychologists at the beginning of the 21st century.

DEFINITION AND OVERVIEW

How is socialization defined? In the broadest terms, it refers to the way in which individuals are assisted in becoming members of one or more social groups. The word "assist" is important because it infers that socialization is not a one-way street but that new members of the social group are active in the socialization process and selective in what they accept from older members of the social group. In addition, new members may attempt to socialize older members as well.

Socialization involves a variety of outcomes, including the acquisition of rules, roles, standards, and values across the social, emotional, cognitive, and personal domains. Some outcomes are deliberately hoped for on the part of agents of socialization while others may be unintended side effects of particular socialization practices (e.g., low self-esteem, anger and reactance, and aggression to peers as a function of harsh parenting). Socialization can also occur through many paths (e.g., discipline after deviation, modeling, proactive techniques, routines, rituals, and as a function of styles of interaction between the agent of socialization and the individual participating in the socialization process). Socialization is

1

ongoing throughout the life course and can be accomplished by a variety of individuals including parents, teachers, peers, and siblings, as well as by schools/daycare, the media, the Internet, and general cultural institutions. Finally, and most important, we note that socialization cannot be adequately understood without a consideration of how biological and sociocultural factors interact in a complex and intertwined manner.

The field of socialization research, always an important area in psychology, has made considerable advances in recent years. These advances are partially attributable to more sophisticated methodological, conceptual, and statistical tools, as well as to the inclusion of a wide variety of theoretical perspectives and approaches. For example, although evolutionary theory has been part of the thinking of socialization theorists, particularly attachment theorists, since at least the 1970s, it increasingly is having an impact on how socialization is conceptualized. Advances in behavior genetics are helping to shed light on the impact of environmental experiences on children, and new work on biological and hormonal regulatory systems is enriching analyses of socialization experiences and the nature of their impact on children. In a time where massive immigration is the norm and where global interconnections grow ever stronger, researchers have enlarged their focus of interest from middle-class participants of Western European extraction to people from all over the world. All of these exciting changes are represented in this *Handbook*.

What are some of the themes that emerge from contemporary research on socialization? The first has to do with the interdependence of biology and experience. As just noted, evolutionary, cultural, genetic, and biological approaches are currently prominent and one of the major tasks for future researchers will be to map the interrelationships among these various approaches to the socialization process. Another theme, which emerges in most of the chapters in this volume, has to do with the fact that socialization involves bidirectionality, with targets of socialization having an impact on how agents of socialization act. Indeed, the complexity of the interaction is underlined by the fact that it occurs in a developmental context—each member of the dyad is responding to the constantly changing behavior of the other members. A third theme has to do with the many contributing factors that interact to produce multiple socialization processes and pathways. The issue is raised in a number of different forms in many of the chapters. The impact of socialization experience is moderated by genetic predispositions and the child's temperament. Interactions between socialization strategies also occur as a function of a whole other host of variables including age, sex, and mood of child, the nature of the parent–child relationship, the domain of behavior under consideration, and the cultural context. Context gives meaning to much of what goes on during the socialization process, and as a result, socialization cannot be understood independent of that context.

THE STRUCTURE OF THE BOOK

The book is divided into seven parts. The order in which to present the parts caused us some concern. Certainly a chapter on history should go first. But should chapters describing biological approaches to socialization precede or follow those describing sociocultural approaches? Should those dealing with the family as an agent of socialization precede those focusing on other agents of socialization? If we put biological approaches before cultural ones, or discussions of the family before discussions of peers, schools, and the media, would readers think we considered these as somehow more important or basic or foundational? This was not an impression we wished to create. We do, in fact, believe that the central role of primary caregivers in socialization is undeniable, and that is no doubt reflected in the chapters we commissioned (although we certainly acknowledge that socialization agents other than parents have profound impacts on development across the lifespan). With respect to biology and culture, however, the evidence points to a constant interplay between them, such that it is impossible to untangle their interactions. Moreover, without sociocultural research it would not be possible for those with biological interests to know what kinds of questions they should be asking. The ordering of chapters, then, should be seen as relatively arbitrary. And, of course, the reader may read the chapters in any order desired.

Part I includes two chapters. Chapter 1 provides an historical overview of socialization research over the last century, written by one of the most influential individuals in the area, Eleanor E. Maccoby. Maccoby focuses on in-family socialization and processes of parenting, in part because, historically, this is where most research and theorizing has taken place. She also traces early work on socialization as the teaching of good habits and as the regulation of impulses through to current views of socialization as specific to domains, bidirectional in character, and occurring in the context of a relationship that changes over time. She concludes with the observation that a major question underlying modern parenting research is not whether parents should exercise their authority but, instead, how that authority can best be exercised so as to promote effective socialization. In Chapter 2 Cavell, Hymel, Malcolm, and Seay address the features of intervention programs in cases where appropriate socialization would seem to have failed, that is, with antisocial youth. In so doing they provide an introduction to the rest of the *Handbook* by focusing on the links between theory and practice and how the two can inform each other. Thus interventions, guided by theories about normative socialization, provide experimental evidence for these theories. Interestingly, Cavell et al. argue that behavior management approaches are not successful because they ignore the importance of the parent–child relationship and the ratio of positive to negative exchanges in the dyad. Thus parents of antisocial children are operating within a "quota system" where they may have to ignore some negative events in order to maintain a reasonable level of positivity in the relationship. This emphasis on the quality of the parent–child relationship is one that is continually echoed throughout the *Handbook*.

Part II considers socialization from a biological perspective. In Chapter 3, Beaulieu and Bugental present an evolutionary perspective on socialization, focusing on adaptations that have evolved across our ancestral past, and that continue to influence the impact of socialization experiences. They argue that socialization occurs in different domains, each with its own distinctive set of processes. These domains reflect different aspects of the relationship between the child and the agent of socialization and include protection, hierarchical power, coalition formation, and mutual reciprocity. In their discussion of the protection domain, Beaulieu and Bugental devote considerable space to parental investment theory as it reflects the time and effort spent in caring for progeny rather than in other activities. Chapter 4 moves from a concern with genetic features common to the species to individual differences in these genetic features. Thus Moffitt and Caspi describe some of the current work in behavior genetics that addresses the hotly debated issue of the extent to which child outcomes are mediated by socialization experiences and to which they are genetically mediated. Using aggression as the outcome variable, they ask and answer a variety of questions including whether parenting has an effect on children's aggressive development, after various genetic confounds are controlled. The bottom line for socialization researchers is that behavior genetics studies indicate that parents do have an impact on their children's aggression, and the importance of this impact is made even clearer when interactions between genes and socialization experiences are considered. In Chapter 5, Repetti, Taylor, and Saxbe describe the impact of parenting on biological regulatory systems. They introduce basic research paradigms and methods used in animal and human research and summarize what is known about the impact of early experience on brain structure and function, the major neuroendocrine stress-response systems, immune functioning, and growth and sexual development. They note that different experiences can lead to differently valenced short- and long-term adaptations of the body's biological systems and that, as a result, it is not possible to conclude that these experiences have either a positive or a negative impact on development. Finally, Repetti et al. call for researchers to chart the reciprocal connections among biological, social, emotional, and behavioral phenomena. This, of course, is the ultimate goal for socialization research. In the final chapter in this part, Bates and Pettit pick up the issue of gene-by-environment interactions in Chapter 6, as they discuss research on temperament, a genetically mediated feature of children's behavior, and socialization experiences. Their careful review of the relevant research indicates, again, that the most interesting avenue of research has to do with parenting by temperament interactions. As two examples, the nature of parenting matters more for children who are high in negative emotionality than for those who are less irritable, and challenging and directive parenting prevents the development of behavioral inhibition in children who are irritable, whereas harsh parenting increases the risk for externalizing behavior in these same children.

Part III takes a developmental perspective on socialization. Chapter 7 uses a relational framework to organize research on socialization processes operating during childhood. Thus Laible and Thompson describe broad aspects of the parent–child relationship that include warmth, security, and mutual responsiveness, as well as immediate aspects such as reinforcement, modeling, and sensitive responsiveness on the parent's part, developing understanding of the self and others on the child's part, and conversational exchanges that involve both parent and child. Once again, we see the emphasis on relationships as central in socialization. As well, we see once again the importance of moderation, in this case, the interaction between socialization strategies and the quality of the dyadic relationship. In Chapter 8, Arnett describes young people who are in the stage of emerging adulthood, no longer dependent on their families but not yet having assumed for themselves the responsibilities of marriage and parenthood. Parents are still important as they encourage financial and decision-making responsibility, as are experiences in the workplace. Peers and the media, on the other hand, assume a reduced role compared to that seen in the adolescent years. Chapter 9 deals with socialization in old age where instrumental dependence on others becomes necessary once again. Fingerman and Pitzer note some of the different foci of socialization at this point in the lifespan, among them a concern with the past and present rather than the future, adaptation to changes in health and social partners, and coping with losses in primary control. Agents of socialization change as health care workers promote or undermine feelings of self-efficacy and autonomy and on occasion socialize dependent behavior. Modeling is no longer a potent force for socialization, as few role models exist in present-day society where aging has become a distinctive process.

Part IV focuses on socialization by parents and siblings, as well as socialization in nontraditional families. The first chapter is a discussion of bidirectionality of influence, particularly as it pertains to parent–child relationships. Kuczynski and Parkin describe a variety of approaches to the topic in Chapter 10, including ones in which immediate reciprocal exchanges of behaviors between members of the dyad are seen to produce linear, incremental change, and ones in which a dialectical process is postulated in which parent and child construct meanings from each other's behavior and produce transformational change. They favor a social relational model, arguing, along with Laible and Thompson, that parent and child are influenced by the cognitive representations and expectations they have developed from a long history of interactions and by a desire to maintain a long-standing positive relationship with each other. In Chapter 11 Grusec and Davidov return to the notion of domains of socialization introduced by Beaulieu and Bugental. They argue for the primacy of parents as agents of socialization as well as for the thesis that socialization is situation specific, occurring either in the context of protection, control, a desire to be like other members of the group, or as part of a mutually compliant dyad. In the course of parent–child interactions different domains become activated and deactivated, depending on features of the situation as well as the characteristics, goals, and needs of both parent and child. The significant point is that socialization strategies that are effective in one domain may be counterproductive when a different domain is activated.

Families also contain siblings whose important impact on socialization is described by Dunn in Chapter 12. Sibling relationships have a strong emotional quality as well as being high in familiarity and intimacy, features that have significance for socialization processes. Also notable are the large individual differences in their quality, just as there is with parents. Dunn describes the impact of siblings on children's adjustment, pointing out their importance as models of antisocial or prosocial behavior as well as their impact on each other's self-esteem. Siblings can also be a source of support when children are faced with stressful experiences. In addition, siblings play an important role in children's development of social understanding, whereas their impact on the quality of relationships with peers outside the family is somewhat more ambiguous. In the final chapter in this part, Chapter 13, Patterson and Hastings look at socialization in families having a different structure from the traditional two-parent, heterosexual dyad. They begin by describing the essentials for successful parenting: adequate resources, good parenting, a positive and stable family climate, and supportive social networks. They then explore the relevant research on single-parent families, unmarried two-parent heterosexual families, families formed using reproductive technologies, lesbian- and gay-parented families, and custodial grandparent families. Their review suggests that families are more successful when they contain two parents and, possibly, two married parents. Genetic linkage, parent sexual orientation, and parent gender do not appear to matter for successful socialization.

Socialization begins in the home, and relationships with parents and other family members continue to be important influences on development across the lifespan. From a very early age, however, children also interact with nonfamilial agents of socialization, and the time spent with these sources of influence increases as children progress through adolescence.

In Part V, the contributions of peers, school experiences, and multiple forms of media to child and adolescent development are considered. In Chapter 14, Bukowski, Brendgen, and Vitaro describe how rejection by prosocial or conventional peers, particularly of children prone to aggression, can exacerbate affective and social cognitive biases that contribute to subsequent affiliation with deviant friends and delinquent peer groups.

These deviant peers, in turn, normalize, reinforce, and promote antisocial attitudes and behaviors. Highlighting the interconnectedness of youths' social realms, parents may decrease deviant peer exposure and affiliation through effective monitoring and maintenance of positive relationships with adolescents. In contrast to aggression, children's risk for internalizing problems appears more linked to their experiences of isolation, as lacking close friendships and being the target of bullying and victimization strongly erode personal resources and self-esteem. Wentzel and Looney also recognize the importance of peer relationships in Chapter 15, in which they examine the socialization in school settings of social competence: the motivation and ability to achieve personally relevant goals while integrating with the peer group and meeting the behavioral and academic requirements of teachers. Structural components of school settings, such as classroom size, have limited effects on children, and these effects are strongly shaped by children's family and sociodemographic conditions. In contrast, close, supportive and positive relationships with both teachers and peers appear to establish facilitative classroom and school contexts that promote well-being. The differential organization of elementary and high schools and the changing needs of children and adolescents contribute to declines in teacher influence and increases in peer influence with age, but across development, prosocial behavior in classrooms is expected, reinforced, and conducive to social competence. In Chapter 16, Dubow, Huesmann, and Greenwood examine the subtle and profound effects of television, radio, video games, and computers on child and adolescent development from a social-cognitive information-processing framework. Immediate reactions of imitation, arousal, and priming of cognitive schema contribute to more long-term effects of media through the unconscious or automatic processes of observational learning and activation and desensitization of emotional arousal, and the more conscious and effortful processes of deliberate teaching. Echoing a theme that recurs throughout this *Handbook,* media socialization needs to be understood as context bound, as media effects are moderated by children's characteristics and motivations, their relationships with parents, siblings and peers, and the broader social and cultural milieu.

Many of the contributors to the *Handbook* have emphasized the necessity of understanding socialization as a culturally bound phenomenon. Part VI includes five chapters that delve more deeply into this rapidly growing area of research, and in so doing, present a set of valuable frameworks for the understanding of culture and socialization. These frameworks begin in Chapter 17 with Conger and Dogan's examination of the probable mechanisms underlying the associations between social class, or socioeconomic status (SES), and children's development. They evaluate models of social causation, through both the adverse and stressful impacts of economic hardship on parenting efficacy and the beneficial influences of advantaged resources on parental investments in children, and social selection, whereby individuals' strengths and vulnerabilities have an impact on both their SES and parenting ability. These perspectives are then integrated into a lifespan developmental model that reflects a truly biopsychosocial framework for understanding the multiple and dynamic roles of SES in socialization. In Chapter 18, Rothbaum and Trommsdorff discuss the complex, and apparently often contradictory, within-culture and between-culture research in Western and non-Western countries on the socialization of autonomy and relatedness, or self-agency and belongingness. Cultural norms establish a context of parenting goals and practices for the care of infants and young children that facilitate children's successful integration with their broader social networks and community institutions. As a result, the nature of relatedness varies across cultures. Although sharing the conveyance of love and security, parenting in Western cultures promotes a sense of general trust in new relationships that is complementary to autonomy, whereas parenting in the non-Western majority of the world promotes assurance in the stability of relationships that supports cohesive and harmonious family and community groups. Rogoff, Moore, Najafi, Dexter, Correa-Chávez, and Solís consider the everyday routines of family and community life that implicitly and explicitly teach children the repertoires of their cultural practices in Chapter 19. Cultures vary in their use of three multidimensional traditions of learning, whereby (1) children observe adults performing tasks and gradually become integrated participants in the activities, (2) children are explicitly instructed by parents at home or by teachers in educational settings, and (3) children as novices are led by experts through memorization, rehearsal, and performance. These learning traditions form the foundation by which individuals process information about their experiences with new communities and traditions, thereby providing the grounds for active transformation of cultural beliefs and practices. In Chapter 20, Cole and Tan present an innovative perspective on the cultural socialization of emotional competence (which complements well the subsequent chapter on socialization of emotion by Denham and colleagues, in Part VII). Resonating with Rothbaum and Trommsdorff, their focus is on culture's shaping of parents' socialization goals, beliefs about child development, and normative socialization practices, and how these in turn establish patterns of communication and interaction that implicitly guide emotional development. Thus, there is variation across cultures in parents' expression of emotions during child-rearing, their encouragement of children's emotional expressiveness, and their discussions about emotional experience that all contribute to children's emotional understanding, regulation and comfort. In the final chapter of this part, Chapter 21, Berry examines the processes and qualities of acculturation, or the adaptations made by individuals and groups when ethnocultural communities with differing traditions and practices come into contact. Individual stress and health can be affected by the majority group's policies of multiculturalism, "melting pot," segregation, or exclusion, and the minority groups' experiences of integration, assimilation, separation, or marginalization. As contact, cohabitation, and, often, conflict between ethnocultures is steadily increasing within this era of globalization and constant immigration and emigration, Berry's chapter serves as a useful framework for understanding the acculturation experience and developing means of promoting intergroup acceptance and harmony.

Much of the *Handbook* is focused on mechanisms of socialization. But socialization is also broad with respect to the aspects of functioning that may be influenced. Depending upon exactly what content area is being considered, different agents or actions of socialization may be more influential. In Part VII, specific aspects of socialization in five content areas are discussed. The topics of gender, cognition, emotion, prosocial behavior, and achievement have been the focus of considerable empirical and theoretical attention and are likely to continue to be so. In Chapter 22, Leaper and Friedman examine links between multiple agents' socialization of gender and children's development of gender beliefs, social norms, play and athletics, academic motivation, and household labor. In so doing, they show that boys and girls often behave quite similarly when given the opportunity to do so. This has important implications for societal increases in gender equality, and the progression towards more egalitarian male and female potentials that has occurred in postindustrial societies. In Chapter 23, as with many of the other chapters in the Handbook, family, peer and school contexts are emphasized in Gauvain and Perez's examination of cognitive development as a social process. Given that relationships and social groups have formed the contexts for human evolution, the development of memory, problem solving, and planning must necessarily be directed toward promoting successful adaptation within these interpersonal settings. Their consideration of teaching, discourse, modeling, and everyday routines illustrates some of the commonalities in socialization processes that may connect diverse content areas. Denham, Bassett and Wyatt, in Chapter 24, identify three components of emotional competence that are especially likely to be shaped or influenced: Children's outward expression of emotion; their knowledge about emotions in themselves and others; and their ability to effectively regulate their emotional experiences. Three key socialization mechanisms may impact each of these: modeling of emotion, teaching about emotion, and contingent reactions to emotion. This heuristic model highlights valuable areas for future research, including greater attention to socialization by agents other than mothers, and socialization of emotion after the early childhood period. Hastings, Utendale, and Sullivan's chapter (Chapter 25) on the socialization of prosocial behavior is focused almost exclusively on longitudinal studies, in order to evaluate the evidence for socialization agents' lasting influences on the development of prosocial characteristics. They show that children's natural, nascent prosocial tendencies can be fostered—or undermined—through their interactions and relationships with parents, siblings, peers, teachers, and broader social institutions. How studying the socialization of prosocial development informs our understanding of both gender and antisocial behavior is given particular emphasis. Finally, in Chapter 26, Eccles considers the development of achievement motivation. Young people's perceptions of their competencies and goals, and therefore their decisions about where and when to strive for accomplishment, are shaped in their relationships at home and school. Thus, the doors to youths' future work, scholastic, and leisure activities may be opened or closed by the messages others convey. Eccles notes that understanding the person–environment fit appears key to supporting the effective skills-training that promotes a child's successful development.

THE FUTURE

Throughout the chapters of this *Handbook* the contributing authors have skillfully sifted information about socialization from bodies of theory and research that are vast and complicated. Although this information may at first seem daunting, the way in which it appears and reappears in different places, and in different guises, leads us to think that the field has been brought together in a meaningful way throughout the book.

Evolutionary history determines who humans are and how they respond to different socialization experiences. Individual variation in genetic makeup further alters the way in which socialization experiences manifest themselves, and socialization experiences, in turn, indicate how genetically directed tendencies reveal themselves. Individuals are active in their own socialization, eliciting specific patterns of reactions from others and seeking out environments that fit with their own dispositions.

Socially and genetically mediated events have both physiological as well as behavioral outcomes, and these outcomes are involved in a complex interplay and interaction. It is evident as well that the impact of any environmental event is determined by the physical and psychological context in which it takes place. Further complexity emerges from the fact that the targets of socialization are in a constant state of change and that different influences and content assume importance at different points during the life span. Although this may seem an overwhelming set of conditions to be considered in the study of socialization processes, it is also true that, once the orderliness of the complex process of socialization becomes evident, the task of studying it is simplified.

What does the future hold? Clearly, the themes of culture and biology and the delineation of their interactions must appear in any complete attempt to analyze the mechanisms underlying socialization. Psychological research as a whole is undergoing major changes in the way it is practiced, and the field of socialization brings together approaches and conceptualizations perhaps to a greater extent than any other area in psychology. We hope the present book both stimulates and guides ongoing efforts to understand this most essential feature of the human condition.

PART I

Historical and Methodological Perspectives on Socialization

CHAPTER 1

Historical Overview of Socialization Research and Theory

ELEANOR E. MACCOBY

The term "socialization" refers to processes whereby naïve individuals are taught the skills, behavior patterns, values, and motivations needed for competent functioning in the culture in which the child is growing up. Paramount among these are the social skills, social understandings, and emotional maturity needed for interaction with other individuals to fit in with the functioning of social dyads and larger groups. Socialization processes include all those whereby culture is transmitted from each generation to the next, including training for specific roles in specific occupations. To speak of cross-generational cultural transmission might imply that "culture" is something static, encapsulated, and that the new generation is being rubber-stamped in the image of its predecessors. But, of course, cultures can and do undergo rapid change under the impact of new technology, warfare, climate change, pestilence, and, in recent generations, contraception.

When new generations adopt social structures and modes of social behavior that are different from those of the parent generation, does this mean that socialization processes have failed? Yes and no. Certainly the transmission of specific patterns of behavior has been disrupted, as in the case of Japanese youth who no longer bow to elders as their parents did. But in the larger sense, individuals can be socialized to adapt to changing circumstances. Training regimes can have much broader objectives than teaching specific behavior patterns, as in the case of K–12 schools whose objective is to produce individuals who are broadly educated in ways that will help to fit them for participating in a wide range of social enterprises, including innovative ones. And then there is the broadest socialization of all: to instill "character" or the internalization of certain enduring social norms, which are presumably still relevant however social structures change, and however different from the parent generation's circumstances the new circumstances are in which a new generation must function. Through such socialization, the trainee is presumably led to behave responsibly toward, and refrain from injuring, a large variety of interaction partners the individual will encounter in a variety of social settings. Presumably, in times of rapid cultural change, the importance of broad socialization for adaptation increases.

While a deep and lasting socialization is often assumed to occur primarily in childhood, socialization does of course go on throughout the lifespan, as individuals enter new social settings where new patterns of social behavior may be needed. Many agents are involved in the socialization of an individual, but parents (and religious teachers in some societies) have been thought to be the primary agents responsible for the broad "moral" socialization of the growing child.

We can conceive of socialization, then, as a succession of processes occurring at successive stages of development, with the child's family of origin being the first, and in many cases the most enduring, socializing institution, joined by peer groups, schools, religious institutions, and, in adulthood, employers and intimate partners as sources of norms for social behavior. The reader will note that socialization, as I have described it so far, is a normative concept. A given child can be said to be either well or poorly socialized. Certain families can be described as well functioning, providing effective parenting, if the child emerging from the family adjusts well to the social requirements of major settings encountered later (e.g., the army, the workplace, marriage, and parenthood) while other families are "dysfunctional" in the sense that they fail to socialize the child to become able to take on these various adult roles, or to become a law-abiding citizen who is reasonably free of pathology.[1] For some time now, we have seen children as playing an active part in the construction of their own standards, so socialization should not be seen as the child's simply taking on the standards of others (Bugental & Goodnow, 1998; Bugental & Grusec, 2006). But I would urge that we can still apply some sort of normative yardstick to whatever standards children self-construct, as to how compatible they are with the likely future requirements of the social contexts in which children will live their lives. We cannot, and need not, take an entirely relativist position, or free the idea of socialization from its normative connotations.

In this chapter I focus primarily on in-family socialization and the processes of parenting. The nature of research on these processes underwent a number of deep changes during the 20th century—changes stemming from changes in the conceptual viewpoints guiding the research, as well as from some technological advances that expanded the menu of methods that could be used to study parenting and its effects. A number of historical reviews already exist in which the major viewpoints are described in detail (see Baldwin, 1955; Goslin, 1969; Maccoby & Martin, 1983; Maccoby, 1992; Grusec, 1997; Bugental & Goodnow, 1998; Parke & Buriel, 1998). This chapter does not go over in detail the ground already covered in these sources but traces a number of salient ideas concerning socialization, and the ways in which they have been modified or metamorphosed over time.

SOCIALIZATION AS THE TEACHING OF GOOD HABITS

A dominant point of view in the mid-20th century was that socialization is a process of instilling in a child a set of desired behavioral habits. Parents and other adults serve as teachers, the children as learners. Young children need to learn table manners, how to dress themselves, habits of personal hygiene, proper ways to speak to older people, and myriad other things—things that increase in complexity as children grow older. From the "socialization as habit-building" point of view, a well-socialized child is one who has accumulated a large store of the habits needed for acceptable social behavior and acceptable levels of skills, while not having acquired bad (antisocial or nonfunctional) habits. By making progress with the acquisition of good habits, the child is presumably enabled to become more and more self-reliant.

Skinnerian and Hullian learning theories placed *reinforcement* (i.e., learned connections between stimuli and responses) as the central process in the formation of habits. It was not always clear what could be considered a "response": Was it always a single action, or could it be something as global as a personality trait? In early work, the definition of responses was quite narrow. Initially, all stimulus–response (S–R) connections were thought to be equally easy to learn, but the possibility that certain connections might be "privileged" did begin to emerge as some of the work on "imprinting" by German ethologists became well known, and Chomsky's claims about innate processes in children's language acquisition (Chomsky, 1959) entered the discourse about learning processes in the 1960s. (Gewirtz, 1969).

S–R learning theories were progressively incorporated into thinking about parenting and its effects. Parents could "shape" their children's development by judiciously reinforcing desired behavior and punishing or withholding reward for undesired behaviors. Parents might, of course, unwittingly reinforce undesired behavior. In early writings it was noted that during the first year infants began to cling to their parents and protest separation from them. J. B. Watson, early in his career, said such "bad habits" could be avoided if parents would only refrain from kissing, cuddling, and holding their infants. Sears, Maccoby, and Levin (1957) regarded the development of "dependency" on mothers (i.e., clinging, following, and protesting separation) as inevitable because the reinforcing power of the mother herself becomes so great due to her role in feeding, comforting, and helping the child. However, the dependent behavior was thought to be "changeworthy," a habit appropriate only for early childhood, and one that must be weakened or eliminated through socialization pressures from the parents as the child grows older. Learned habits can be unlearned, and reinforcement theories did not assign any greater importance to habits learned early versus those learned at a later age. The theories were thus not developmental. They had little to say about any differences between younger and older children in what could be learned or in *how* learning occurred. However, early learned habits, such as using table utensils in a prescribed way, could persist for very long periods, indeed for a lifetime.

An important research program emerging during the 1970s from the behavioral perspective on parenting is the one organized and led by Gerald Patterson at the Oregon Social Learning Center (Patterson, 1982). This program continues actively to the present time. Patterson and colleagues focused on the families of aggressive children, comparing the interactive sequences between parent and child that occurred in these families to those in the families of nonaggressive children. They noted that parents could inadvertently build children's aggression by backing away from their control efforts when the child was aggressively defiant (they termed this process "negative reinforcement"). They stressed that parents needed to provide consequences (i.e., reward or punishment) for desired or undesired child behavior, and noted that in order to do so, parents needed to be vigilant

in detecting infractions and keeping track of whether children have complied with parental directives. Thus parental "monitoring" was a crucial element in parental management
of children—a variable that has since been adopted by many other researchers studying
parent–child interaction. The thinking by Patterson and his colleagues quickly moved beyond a simple Skinnerian paradigm in that it increasingly focused on dyads and two-way
influence rather than on a simple "shaping" of children by parents.

In the 1950s and 1960s, Skinnerian ideas were brought to bear on the treatment of
children with behavior problems (see summary in Alexander & Malouf, 1983), and behavioral therapy models based on reinforcement principles continue in active use to the
present day. In general, however, developmental psychologists began to turn away from
simple reinforcement accounts of parenting effects. Skinner's effort to explain language
acquisition in reinforcement terms was notably unsuccessful (Chomsky, 1959). The concept of reward itself proved to be problematic: Children differed in what parental responses they found rewarding. Customary (expected) levels of reward or praise were
adapted to, so that they lost their efficacy.

Perhaps the most powerful critique of reinforcement learning theory came from the
work on observational learning, initiated in the 1960s by Bandura, Mischel, and their
colleagues. Experimental evidence showed that children could learn without ever having
performed, or been reinforced for, the responses in question, merely by observing models
perform them. Bandura called this "no trial learning." He made a crucial distinction:
Performance, he claimed, was governed by reinforcement contingencies; learning was not
(Bandura, 1969).

SOCIALIZATION AS THE REGULATION OF IMPULSES

Pychodynamic views of socialization emerged concurrently with the "learned habits"
view described above. The two streams of thought were similar in that they were both
"drive" theories, but they differed in fundamental respects. Beginning with Freud,
psychodynamic theorists saw behavior in infancy and early childhood as the free expression of instinctual impulses, including aggressive and sexual impulses. Impulsive behavior
was not just elicited by external stimuli. Rather, it was driven by strong intrinsic energy.
The young child's impulses inevitably came into conflict with the requirements of social
living, and adults—especially parents—had the responsibility for curbing and directing
the child's impulsive behavior, channeling the energy according to what was allowed and
what was not allowed in the culture in which a child was growing up. These adult constraints inevitably generated resistance and anger on the part of the young child, and controlling this anger itself then necessarily became a focus of adult control. Freud's writings
were interpreted as meaning that harsh parental blocking of children's impulses would
carry long-term risks, and the roots of many forms of adult psychopathology were
thought to lie in the early childhood relationship of children with their parents and other
socialization agents (Whiting & Child, 1953). A basic psychodynamic tenet was that socialization moves from a process of external control by parents to self-control by the
child, and that self-control is achieved through a child's identifying with parents and internalizing their controls, thus developing a *superego* (i.e., conscience). The twin concepts
of "internalization" and "identification" have continued to influence socialization research over many decades, though some of the psychodynamic theories about the

psychosexual stages of early life have faded into what is, in my view, well-deserved oblivion. Unlike habit formation theories, psychodynamic theories were strongly developmental, with an early set of behavioral tendencies being transformed at a particular stage of development—around age 4 or 5, when the Oedipus complex was presumably being resolved—when great gains in children's self-control and social maturity would then became possible.

Beginning in the 1930s, an interdisciplinary group at Yale University asked whether it would be possible to bring Hullian learning theory to bear on psychoanalytic concepts. The Freudian concept of identification was operationally defined as imitation, and imitation was explained as a generalized habit of imitation, formed as a consequence of children's being reinforced so often for doing things as adults do them (Miller & Dollard, 1941). Anxieties acquired through punishment were conceptualized as learned motivational states whose reduction could then reinforce the learning of new habits.

In the 1950s, Robert Sears and colleagues (Sears, Whiting, Nowlis, & Sears, 1953; Sears et al., 1957; Sears, Rau, & Alpert, 1965) brought this line of thinking into the field of socialization research, studying childrearing practices and their relation to a set of children's personality traits. Their objective was to translate psychoanalytic hypotheses into the language of Hullian learning theory, and to develop a set of hypotheses that could be objectively assessed (see Grusec, 1997, for fuller exposition of some of these translations). Freudian theory held that children resolved their psychosexual conflicts with their parents by identifying with the same-sex parent. Successful identification would presumably bring about a coherent set of developments toward greater maturity. Although all children were thought to go through these developmental processes, individual children differed in how quickly and how successfully they would do so, and variations in parenting were thought to have a central role in determining how individual children would progress.

In this work, the choice of variables was governed largely by psychoanalytic theory, drawing on learning theory mainly in its relevance to punishment and anxiety. Thus parenting attributes such as severity of weaning and toilet training, punishment for aggression, permissiveness for dependency, and the use of withdrawal of love as a technique of discipline were chosen for assessment. The "outcome" variables for the children included sex typing, adult role taking, aggression, dependency, and manifestations of "conscience" (e.g., resistance to temptation and feelings of guilt over transgressions).

The results of these studies were disappointing. A major problem was that the set of child characteristics that were presumably all the outcomes of successful identification with the same-sex parent cohered only slightly (i.e., weakly for girls and not at all for boys; Sears et al., 1965). On the whole, these studies did not confirm the idea that children achieved self-controlling levels of maturity through identification with the same-sex parent. The measured variations in parenting were not found to be consistent predictors of the child attributes that were chosen for study. The weak results of these studies called for rethinking the theories that underlay them. Nevertheless, the work by Sears and colleagues was important in giving impetus to the empirical study of parenting, specifically to the ways in which variations in the quality of parenting might be related to children's developing attributes.

Some psychodynamic concepts received strong support in objective studies. Bandura, Mischel, and colleagues conducted several studies of imitation in which the hypotheses were drawn from the psychoanalytic concepts of anaclytic and defensive identification. They found that children were indeed more likely to imitate adult models who were shown to be nurturant and also to imitate powerful models (those in a position to dispense desired rewards), by comparison with models who did not have these characteristics (Mischel & Liebert, 1967; Bandura, Ross, & Ross, 1963). Because parents are typically both powerful and nurturant, their children would presumably be motivated to emulate them preferentially. Bandura and collegues, however, did not see imitation as a process of "taking over" whole personality qualities from models. Indeed, they stressed that children learn from many models, and the "final common path" of their behavior may involve a blending of what they have learned observationally from many sources. This formulation puts the child's own agency at center stage, involving a considerable degree of self-socialization on the part of the child (see, e.g., Bandura, 1986).

As we see later, the Freudian idea that successful socialization must involve children's coming to be able to control their own impulses—to self-regulate—is very much alive, and in fact has been receiving increasing emphasis in recent work. The processes that lead to self-regulation, however, have come to be seen very differently from the processes Freud proposed.

GOOD PARENTING AS DEMOCRACY

During the 1930s and early 1940s, a number of distinguished European intellectuals came as refugees to the United States and established research programs relevant to socialization. Else Frenkel-Brunswik came to Berkeley, bringing a strong psychoanalytic orientation; she joined with a group of colleagues (Adorno, Frenkel-Brunswik, Levinson, & Sanford, 1950) to study the roots of "authoritarian" personality structures. They concluded that harsh and threatening parenting was a key element in the formation of such personalities.

Kurt Lewin, also a refugee from Europe, brought a very different theoretical orientation. He was a "configurational" theorist, and his field theory, like Gestalt theories, emphasized holistic concepts such as the contextual and organizational properties of environments, rather than focusing on specific "stimuli." During the 1930s, Lewin joined with American colleagues in a set of studies on the effects of group atmospheres and leadership styles on the functioning of task-oriented groups. Most pertinent for developmental psychology was the study of groups of 10- and 11-year-old boys, who undertook a variety of tasks under the leadership of adult leaders who had been trained to create one of three different kinds of "group atmospheres": authoritarian, democratic, or laissez faire. (Lewin, Lippit, & White, 1939). They found, as expected, that when working under a democratic leadership regime, the boys became more involved in the tasks, more able to carry on with the work when the leader was out of the room, and more competent in accomplishing their tasks successfully, than boys in either the authoritarian or laissez-faire groups.

It was a natural step to apply these concepts to families, which could be seen as small groups with adult leaders, and to ask whether some families could be identified as having an authoritarian group atmosphere while others functioned more democratically. A further question was what effect such different atmospheres might have on the children growing up in these families. As it happened, Alfred Baldwin was a graduate student at

Harvard during the 1930s, at a time when Lewin came there as a visiting faculty member. Baldwin was greatly impressed by the work on group atmospheres. When he left Harvard to set up his own research enterprise at the Fels Institute, he organized a longitudinal study of parenting styles. He and his colleagues made successive visits to the homes of young children over a period of several years, interviewing the mothers and at the same time making detailed notes of the interaction of the mother and child. They were able to identify several different parenting styles, one of which corresponded closely to the democratic style Lewin had identified. They found it important, however, to distinguish "scientific democracy," which involved emotional detachment from the child, and "warm democracy," which entailed more affectionate behavior toward the child and more empathy for both the child's point of view and the child's emotional reactions to parental socializing efforts. Other parental patterns were labeled passive–neglectful, actively hostile, and possessive–indulgent. They reported that warm-democratic parenting was associated with stronger intellectual development in children, more spontaneity, and less anxiety than the other parenting styles. The warm-democratic parents allowed the child a great deal of freedom, and this was associated with many positive developments but also with more antisocial behavior on the part of the child (see Baldwin, 1955).[2]

Both the Baldwin work and the work of the Berkeley group on authoritarian personalities pointed to undesired outcomes of authoritarian childrearing, implying that parents should be less strict, less focused on getting obedience and deference from their children, and more willing to express unconditional acceptance and love toward their children. To many, this seemed to amount to recommending unconditional permissiveness.

There was a backlash. Diana Baumrind was convinced that both authoritarian and laissez-faire leadership styles were ineffective in promoting optimal functioning of groups, and became concerned about the ways in which the authoritarian personality findings were being interpreted. In the 1960s, she and her colleagues began studying parenting styles, and their connections with a variety of characteristics of pre-school-age children. As is now well known, she developed a three-part typology of parenting styles: an *authoritarian* style, a *permissive* style, and an *authoritative* style (Baumrind & Black, 1967). This latter style involved parents' making age-appropriate demands on children, and setting up firmly enforced rules for their behavior. At the same time, authoritative parents were responsive to their children's needs, willing to listen to them and take their viewpoint into account, involving them in decisions whenever possible. They used reasoning and gave children explanations for parental demands. They both assigned responsibilities and made room for children's autonomy. They were affectionate and supportive of the child's enterprises. This could be seen as a form of democratic parenting, but it was combined with a level of strictness not found in Baldwin's "warm democracy" group. Comparing the nursery school behavior of children from these three kinds of homes, Baumrind and colleagues reported that it was the children from authoritative households who were most mature and competent, being assertive in pursuing their own ends but also considerate toward other children and cooperative with teachers.

The Baumrind work was stronger conceptually than it was empirically. A considerable number of families could not be classified as belonging to any one of the three groups. The connections between parenting styles and child behaviors were not robust. And later studies showed that most parents employed all three styles at one time or another, depending on a variety of contextual factors, such as the nature of the child's infraction, the parents' socialization goal, and the child's current mood (Grusec &

Goodnow, 1994). The Baumrind work did call attention to the importance of parental authority as well as parental sensitivity, but more recent research has turned away from the goal of classifying parents according to some dominant parenting type, focusing instead on the nature of interactive relationships (see below).

SOCIALIZATION BY PARENTS AS A PRODUCT OF EVOLUTION

In 1969, a ground-breaking book was published. It was the first of a three-volume series, *Attachment and Loss*, by John Bowlby. It described the development of the emotional attachment of young infants and toddlers to their mothers (or other primary caregivers) as *instinctive* behavior.[3] Bowlby's perspective was strongly evolutionary. Drawing on the work of Tinbergen and Lorenz, he described the way in which, in some species of birds, newly hatched chicks imprinted on the first moving creature they saw (usually the maternal bird) but considered this to be only roughly analogous to attachment in human children because birds have been on a separate evolutionary track from mammals for a very long time. However, he was unequivocal about human kinship with other mammals, and particularly with nonhuman primates. He said: "Whatever behaviour is found in subhuman primates we can be confident is truly homologous with what obtains in man" (Bowlby, 1969, p. 183). He described in detail the early appearance of a primate mother's greater orientation toward her own infant than toward other infants, and the appearance of a matching own-mother bias in the infant. He described how attachment behavior in monkeys, and in several species of great apes, waxes and wanes during the early phases of development. He said that attachment behavior in the human infant develops more slowly than it does in other primates, but that the nature of the behavior, the conditions that elicit it, and its time course relative to species-specific maturity were remarkably similar across primate species. He noted that the caregiving behavior of primate mothers changed in synchrony with the developmental status of the infant, but that even when the young animal had become fairly independent, mother and offspring would quickly move toward one another in the presence of threat.

Work by Harry Harlow and colleagues in Wisconsin showed quite clearly that infant monkey's attachment to their mothers was not a by-product of feeding by her but should be seen as a separate behavioral system. The Harlows believed that the analogy to human infant attachment was clear (Harlow & Harlow, 1965). The bidirectional nature of the mother–infant attachment was underscored by stress-hormone work showing that in both monkeys and humans, stress levels in both mother and infant diminish when a separated pair are reunited. Bowlby (1969) saw attachment in primates as a reciprocal system in which evolution had equipped both child and mother with prepared readinesses to form a mutual bond.[4] He saw the bonding process as a *species* characteristic. That is, in both humans and other primates, some degree of attachment between mother and her own infant must occur if the infant is to survive. Individual differences would have to be seen within this larger framework. He noted, however, that at least in humans, there were striking individual differences among mother–child pairs in the nature and closeness of the bond that developed over the first year He thought that these differences stemmed partly from variations among the infants in their temperamental predispositions but also from variations in maternal involvement with, and responsiveness and sensitivity to, the infant. His work was important, too, in emphasizing the emotional as well as the behavioral components of socialization.

Suomi (2002) has summarized extensive observational data on the interactions of maternal monkeys with their infants, showing how the nature of mothering changes as the infant matures. He points to individual variations in maternal styles, ranging from highly protective and restrictive to more "laissez faire." These variations are related to the mother's social status, to the birth order of the infant, the size of the troupe in which the mother and infant live, and the occurrence of environmental perturbations. Naturally occurring variations in maternal style are associated with certain outcomes for the infants (e.g., their subsequent social status is affected).

The biological factors in the readiness of mothers and infants for bonding with one another begins much earlier than the appearance of attachment behaviors. Recent research has shown that the hormones of pregnancy and parturition contribute to mothers' close caregiving attention to their infants, and both mothers and infants appear to be predisposed for quick selective learning of their own partner's distinctive vocalizations and facial features (see review by Bugental & Grusec, 2006). Interestingly, fathers who are present during the pregnancy and involved in infant care also undergo some hormonal changes (though more limited than for mothers) that support bonding to infants.

Of course, attachment is not the only behavioral domain in which strong similarities have been noted between human children and the young of nonhuman primates. For example, these similarities exist with respect to many aspects of gender differentiation (Maccoby, 1998), social dominance and aggressive behavior, even sympathy and altruism (de Waal, 1996). These similarities serve to underscore the evolutionary roots of many aspects of human behavior and development, but they have also pointed to ways in which environmental inputs affect the ways in which evolved predispositions are overtly expressed.

SOCIALIZATION AS SUPPORT FOR CHILDREN'S CAPACITIES TO SELF-REGULATE

Research interest in the development of self-regulation has a long history, and increasingly, the development of self-regulatory abilities is seen as a building block, a necessary precursor, for a set of subsequent developmental achievements. Traditional learning theory had little to say about self-regulation. When children acquired and performed a habit, no intervening regulatory process between the stimulus and response was invoked, nor thought to be needed. Psychoanalytic theory, by contrast, was centrally concerned with self-regulation. We have already seen that, in psychoanalytic views, infants and young children have strong instinctive drives that impel them to impulsive behavior that must be curbed and directed by adults, but which eventually must come under the child's own control. I have selected three research programs on self-regulation to illustrate how self-regulation has been conceptualized and how socialization practices might affect self-regulatory development in children.

In psychoanalytic theory, two intrapsychic structures were thought to be involved in a child's controls: the *superego*, an internalized representation of the controlling parent, and the *ego*, a self-controlling entity which guides efforts to avoid fearful situations, deal with new circumstances, and regulate impulses. Beginning in the 1970s, Jack and Jeanne Block reformulated the psychoanalytic views of self-regulation. They distinguished between *ego control* (conceptualized as the degree of impulse control and modulation, ranging from undercontrol to overcontrol, with midscale scores representing an "appropriate" level of control) and *ego resiliency* (conceptualized as "the dynamic capacity of an individual to modify his/her modal level of ego-control, in either direction, as a function of the demand characteristics of the environmental context"; see Block & Block, 1980, p. 48). Working with a longitudinal sample, they traced distinctive developmental trajectories for children varying on their two dimensions.

Walter Mischel and his colleagues, beginning in the 1960s, mounted an extensive program of research on a different aspect of self-regulation, namely, *postponement of gratification* (Mischel & Metzner, 1962; Mischel & Grusec, 1967). In typical studies, a child would be offered a choice between obtaining a small or relatively unattractive reward immediately, or waiting some time in order to receive a larger or more desirable reward. The studies showed that the ability to postpone gratification varies with a number of conditions (e.g., the trustworthiness of the promise of future reward, the length of time the child has to wait, and the cognitive strategies the child brings to bear during the waiting period). Self-regulation of attention deployment was shown to be a central component of successful delay.

Another approach to the development of self-regulation came out of studies of temperament. In this tradition, the focus has been on attempts to identify distinctive dimensions of temperament, such as sociability or fearfulness, thought to be constitutionally based. Rothbart and colleagues, in studying the temperamental characteristics of infants and young children, identified a set of characteristics that cluster together into a single dimension that they labeled "effortful control." In infancy, this control is manifest primarily in the form of being able to inhibit a dominant response in order to perform a subdominant response, as in the Piagetian A-not-B task (Rothbart & Bates, 1998). As the child grows into toddlerhood and preschool age, a child's ability to detect his or her own errors and engage in planning becomes part of the "effortful control" cluster. Engaging in effortful control means that a child must exercise control over the deployment of attention—(i.e., maintain attentional focus and resist distraction) as well as inhibit impulsive behavior. Researchers have developed an impressive battery of measures for assessing children's ability to exercise effortful control (Posner & Rothbart, 1998; Kochanska, Murray, & Harlan, 2000), and have explored related aspects of brain function (Rothbart & Rueda, 2005).

Although these three streams of research have been conducted independently over many years, there have been some notable convergences. In all three, there is demonstrable stability of individual differences over a number of years. In all three, there are documented increases with age. Especially important is the fact that in all these research programs, self-regulatory abilities have been shown to presage the future development of a variety of "outcomes" which can be qualitatively quite distinct from, but conceptually linked with, self-regulation (Block & Block, 1980; Mischel, Shoda, & Peake, 1988; Shoda, Mischel, & Peake, 1990; Kochanska, Coy, & Murray, 2001).

For our present purposes, the important question is: What is the impact of parenting on the kind and degree of self-regulation children develop? Block (1971) was among the first to address this question. He reported that undercontrolled people came from chaotic, conflict-ridden households in which parents often neglected their teaching responsibilities. The mothers and fathers of ego-resilient children, by contrast, had good relations with one another and agreed on values, were both loving and fair in their dealings with their children, and encouraged free interchange concerning feelings and problems. At the same time they were concerned with firmly transmitting values. Above all, they were seriously committed to their parenting responsibilities and devoted sustained effort and attention to childrearing. We can see links between the parenting clusters described by the Blocks and the trio of clusters described by Baumrind.

With rare exceptions, researchers in the Mischel tradition have not focused on what the possible socialization antecedents of the individual differences in abilities to postpone gratification might be. But inferences can be made from the experimental conditions that have been shown to affect children's ability to postpone gratification. For example, children are more willing to wait if they have experience with an experimenter who has kept a promise to provide a larger reward later, as compared with an experimenter whose promise proved unreliable. (Mischel & Grusec, 1967). The implication for parenting would be that parents who follow though on their promises will support children's ability to postpone gratification.

Eisenberg, Smith, Sadovsky, and Spinrad (2004) have summarized a substantial research literature on the socialization of emotional self-regulation. They adopt Rothbart's term "effortful control" for the set of self-regulatory processes they review but define the term somewhat more broadly as the ability to "manage attention, motivation and behavior voluntarily," and they do not adopt the assumptions about primarily constitutional foundations that underlie the work on temperament. They report that children's development of strong self-regulatory capacities in early childhood is linked to parental responsiveness, parental warmth and emotional support, and a minimum of interference and intrusion into the child's autonomous activities, along with an absence of disciplinary practices that frighten the child unduly.

Students of moral development have noted that "moral" behavior involves the regulation of impulse (i.e., children must inhibit immediately-gratifying self-serving behavior to make way for more reasoned consideration of social obligations to others). Such self-regulation depends on a set of values with respect to which children evaluate and guide their own behavior. Grolnick, Deci, and Ryan (1997) say: "Whereas socializing agents can 'teach' their children the values and attitudes they hold dear, the important thing is having the children 'own' those attitudes and values." (p. 135)—in other words, to internalize them. In an influential chapter, Hoffman (1970) distinguished among several aspects of parental discipline, noting that while withdrawal of love did not appear to be an effective technique for building children's internalization of moral values, there was evidence for the importance of parental use of "induction" (explaining, and appealing to children's pride in being more grown up), and especially "other-oriented induction" (calling children's attention to the effects of their behavior on others). Hoffman also stressed the minimal use of parental power assertion as a factor in moral internalization.

SOCIALIZATION AS SPECIFIC TO CONTEXTS AND DOMAINS

In much of the socialization research done through the 1960s, 1970s, and 1980s, the primary interest was in the variation *between* parents, in terms of trait-like attributes that characterized their parenting. Many studies used factor analysis and other statistical techniques to try to identify major dimensions of parenting, and issues arose as to whether it was more productive to keep major dimensions separate in analyses, or combine them into Baumrind-like typologies (see review by Darling & Steinberg, 1993). But whether dimensions or typologies were used, the assumption was that individual parents, or individual children, could be characterized as having some degree of a fairly stable property or set of properties which they habitually manifested in their interactions with each other. Some researchers, although not dismissing these trait-like approaches as unimportant, began to find them to be too limited. Beginning in the early 1980s, Grusec began to produce evidence of considerable *within parent* variability. In their 1994 review paper, Grusec and Goodnow summarized the evidence, noting that the techniques parents typically use with their children depend on the nature and seriousness of the infraction and the context in which it has occurred, as well as the age and momentary emotional state of the child. And, Grusec and Goodnow claimed, the effect of a given kind of discipline would be different, depending on these same contextual conditions. They urged further that we have paid too little attention to the *content* of parental messages to children: their consistency and clarity, their "truth value" (i.e., there verifiability), and their direct relevance to the issue at hand. These things determine not only how well a parental message will be understood by the child but also the child's judgment about whether to believe and accept the message as being fair.

Building on the fact that individual parents do vary considerably from one context to another, Bugental and Goodnow (1998; Beaulieu & Bugental, Chapter 3, this volume) propose a domain-specific account of socialization. The domains they identify are (1) protective care, which encompasses attachment and nurturance; (2) coalitional groups, the avenue whereby a child acquires a sense of in-group belonging (more pertinent to the interactions in peer groups but still relevant to family membership); (3) hierarchical power, encompassing disciplinary encounters, and involving continuing renegotiation of power relationships as children mature; and (4) reciprocity/mutuality. Any given parent will function within each of these domains from time to time, depending on the issue or parental task involved. For each domain, they say, distinctive parenting patterns are called into play, and they argue that these have an evolutionary basis in both parent and child that prepare the dyad for interaction within a given domain. Sensitive parenting, then, means that a parent uses the parenting that is appropriate to the domain of interaction that is occurring at a given time. Thus if a child is distressed, a sensitive parent soothes, an insensitive one might try to initiate a game or become power assertive; at a moment when a child is angrily defiant, hierarchical power comes into play and power assertion is appropriate and should be seen as reflecting parent sensitivity, while soothing would be inappropriate to the domain.

CHILDREN AS AGENTS IN THEIR OWN SOCIALIZATION

We have already seen that children are active agents in observational learning, as they choose preferred models for imitation and deploy attention toward some kinds of modeled activities rather than others. But their agency is much broader than this: They can *elicit* or even control some of the directive, controlling, and nurturing activity that parents direct toward them, and select which parental directives they will give more credence to.

The role of children in their own socialization has been underscored in studies that emphasize the role of children's genetic predispositions in determining how they will be socialized. For many decades, psychologists have been aware of genetic influences on children's development. There were early intensive studies of maturation, which were seen as evidence that there is an inborn developmental timetable driving changes in the child. The implication was that socialization must be organized around this timetable, changing as the child changes. And twin and adoption studies were widely cited, pointing to genetically based individual differences in children's temperaments and abilities. As we have seen in the review so far, however, most of the early socialization research focused on the kind of impact parenting processes might have on the developing child, with little regard to any genetic characteristics individual children might bring to parent–child encounters. Researchers were looking for general laws governing parenting effects, and when they found connections between parenting methods and children's "outcomes," these were usually interpreted as showing that parents were influencing children in predictable ways.

There were voices warning about possible reverse effects (Bell & Harper, 1977). Some excellent studies followed showing how children's behavior could determine the way adults treated them (e.g., Grusec & Kuczynski, 1980; Bugental, Corporeal, & Shennum, 1980). Challenges to claims about strong parenting effects continue to the present day. For example, researchers studying adolescents have repeatedly found that weak, erratic monitoring by parents is associated with a number of problematic adolescent outcomes, including juvenile delinquency, drug use, and risky sexual activity (see Kerr & Stattin, 2003, for a review). These risky behaviors have been interpreted as "outcomes" of poor parental monitoring. Kerr and Stattin have strongly challenged this interpretation, arguing that parents can monitor effectively only if their adolescents are willing to talk to them openly about their activities, so that successful parental monitoring is driven by properties of the child (see review of this debate throughout this volume).

The strongest demand for reinterpretation of the direction of effects has come from behavior geneticists (see Moffitt, & Caspi, Chapter 4, this volume). What behavior geneticists reported in work appearing through the 1980s and early 1990s was sobering to people who had been stressing top-down effects from parent to child. Strong heritability coefficients, clustering around 50% or higher, were found with respect to many child characteristics. Especially startling was the claim that shared environmental effects were weak, indeed often close to zero (Plomin & Daniels, 1987), while *unshared* environmental effects were often substantial. The inference that was drawn from such findings was that variations in parenting could hardly be having much effect on children's development. These arguments were elaborated by Rowe (1994) and given a more popular treatment by Harris (1998). Sandra Scarr (1992), in her presidential address to the Society for Research in Child Development, argued that while extreme parental abuse or neglect could of course harm children, in the vast majority of families parenting was "good enough" to support children's development, and that other factors—children's genetics, nonfamilial environmental influences—were more important in determining individual differences in how children turned out. The extreme version of this point of view would be that parents hardly socialize their children at all—children socialize themselves, aided by a variety of nonparental influences. A more nuanced version would be that all parents do manage to socialize their children up to some base level regardless of their methods, but variations in parenting above this level account for very little variance in child outcomes.

There were strong reactions against these claims, and vigorous efforts to rebut them were mounted, along with presentations of studies with demonstrable parenting effects (see Collins, Maccoby, Steinberg, & Hetherington, 2000; Turkheimer, 2000; Maccoby, 2000; Borkowski, Ramey, & Bristol-Power, 2002). Several of the behavior geneticists' strongest points have been widely accepted (if sometimes reluctantly!) and have greatly influenced more recent socialization research. One is the simple fact that children's genetic endowments do have an influence on the kind of parent–child relationship that is likely to develop, so that in attempting to evaluate parenting influences, it is important to take into account children's initial variations in temperament and abilities and the influence these things may have on what parents do and what effects they can have. Another is that parenting researchers have often overclaimed for the strength of their effects. And a third is that siblings growing up together can be very different, and in fact usually are. Until the 1980s, socialization researchers almost always studied only one child per family. Now it is understood that given the importance of so-called unshared rather than shared environmental factors, it must be the case that parental influence is often not the same for different children in the same family, and indeed that parental influence probably rarely functions to make siblings more alike with respect to the outcomes that are commonly measured.

These things said, it must be noted that there have been widespread misinterpretations of some of the behavior geneticists' claims, and corrections have been called for. They define "shared environment" as any aspect of the environment that makes coresident children more alike. However, important parental influences that do not make children in the same family more alike can nevertheless serve to shape the development of individual children. It is important to note, too, that in interpreting behavior genetic studies, much depends on the magnitudes of the G, shared E, and nonshared E effects. All these, of course, depend on the original estimates of heritability, since E effects have been defined as the residual when heritability coefficients are subtracted from 100%. And these estimates of heritability turn out to be unstable (see Shonkoff & Phillips, 2001, for fuller exposition). In particular, they depend on the range of variation in G & E factors within the particular population studied, and they are highly responsive to data source. Comparisons of heritability estimates based on observational reports of mother–child interaction are almost always lower that such estimates based on parent report or child report, so that observational data allow more room for shared and unshared environmental effects to be shown. A recent example can be found in Neiderhiser et al. (2004), where the child's genetic contribution to mother's positivity is estimated at 48% from mother reports, 19% from child reports, and 0% from observer reports. Clearly, very large brackets must be put around any estimate of heritability, until the method variance in these estimates can be more fully understood.

To many researchers, the problem has remained one of trying to identify the causal contributions of each party in the parent–child dyad. And certainly if the larger agenda is to trace the ways in which parents pass culture on to the next generation of children, it would seem to make sense to focus on the kind and degree of influence parents can have, net of any contribution the child and nonparental environmental factors make to the process. Several methods have been pursued for covarying genetic and parenting variables so that their respective contributions can be independently assessed. These methods include (1) using longitudinal data, and assessing the connections of parenting at Time 1 with child behavior at Time 2 or 3, net of the child's initial Time 1 behavior—in other words, to study *change* in children's behavior as predicted from earlier parenting; (2) using measures of temperament as proxies for genetic variations, allowing researchers to control for these variations and identify independent parent effects; (3) adopting "genetically sensi-tive" research designs in which variations in the degree of genetic relatedness among fam-ily members is known, and entered into multivariate analyses along with parenting vari-ables; (4) ruling out genetic differences by studying pairs of identical twins, to assess the differences in parenting and estimating their effects; (5) cross-fostering experiments with animals in which littermates are placed for rearing with mothers differing in parenting behaviors; and (6) intervention studies, in which families are randomly assigned to parent-training or no-training groups—with randomization controlling for initial varia-tion in a large range of both genetic and environmental factors—and testing for the ef-fects of intervention-produced changes in parenting behavior (e.g., Martinez & Forgatch, 2001; Brody et al., 2004).

A detailed assessment of the strengths and weaknesses of these and other approaches to identifying the causal power of genetic and environmental risk factors can be found in Rutter, Pickles, Murray, and Eaves (2001). A number of these approaches permit the eval-uation of $G \times E$ interactions—something that was seldom done in the early behavior ge-netics research—and it has been shown that a given parental action can have a different effect on children of different temperament but be an important source of influence none-theless (e.g., Kochanska, 1995; Bates, Pettit, Dodge, & Ridge, 1988). Current work on molecular genetics stresses gene–environment interactions much more heavily than statis-tical behavior-genetic work has done (Moffitt, Caspi, & Rutter, 2006). There is now abundant evidence that from the moment of conception on, environmental inputs affect which genes will be activated at successive points in development. Some genes remain in-active unless triggered by specific environmental inputs. Environmental inputs help to guide brain development, and specifically the neuroendocrine system, in ways that will affect behavior. The usefulness of the "additive assumption" (that G and E effects, taken separately, add up to 100% of the forces controlling variance in any trait) is being widely challenged (Cairns, Elder, & Costello, 1996; Maccoby, 2000; Shonkoff & Phillips, 2000; Bugental & Grusec, 2006). It is now widely understood that feedback loops pervade parent–child interactions, so that whatever eliciting powers the genetic predispositions of parent or child might have had in initiating an interaction, these are quickly enmeshed in mutual influence. Within this bidirectional perspective, emphasis on the child's agency in the socialization process is now a central aspect of theory and research (e.g., Grolnick et al., 1997).

PARENTING AS A BIDIRECTIONAL, RECIPROCAL PROCESS

In 1951, Sears urged that parent and child be studied as a dyad in which each influenced the other. For a number of years this idea lay dormant, but from the publication of Bowlby's work and the early work of G. R. Patterson and colleagues, there has been in-creasing recognition of the reciprocal nature of parent–child interaction. But as this shift in focus occurred, researchers became increasingly aware of methodological issues that plagued the study of reciprocal interactions. While earlier research had relied heavily on parent interviews and questionnaires as the source of information about parenting, it be-came evident that parents were often not able to report accurately on some aspects of the dynamics of day-to-day interaction between parent and child. Researchers turned to a greater use of direct observation of parent–child interaction, and they were immediately struck by the way in which each responds to the other, and adapts his or her own behavior to that of the other. They encountered issues that were both methodological and conceptual: How could the behavior of each partner be coded in real time so that sequential dependencies could be detected? Should successive behaviors be separated into event units or time units? What is the optimum length of time units that will best capture the realities of a stream of interaction?

Methodological Advances

Technological developments helped to answer these questions. The Patterson research group in Oregon pioneered the recording of observed parent–child interaction in real time. They used an accordian-like keyboard that would allow the concurrent coding of parent and child behavior into predetermined categories. The growth of videotaping technology greatly enhanced the ability of researchers to code interaction reliably, and to re-examine interaction sessions for elements not originally selected for study. From videotapes it was possible to identify sequential dependencies of parents' and children's behavior on the other's prior actions, by coding the behavior of each in successive units of time. Or, more global ratings and behavioral scores could be derived from longer interaction segments.

A second major technological advance was in the computer processing of data. Beginning in the 1980s, computer programs were developed to carry out microanalytic analyses of sequential dependencies in real-time interaction data, and to compare several strategies for doing so (see Martin, Maccoby, Baran, & Jacklin, 1981). Enhanced computer power was especially important in handling the snowballing amounts of data accumulated in large longitudinal studies. Sophisticated structural modeling became feasible.

Micoanalytic studies of interactive sequences have been intended to reveal the extent to which the behavior of each participant is contingent upon the prior behavior of the partner. Studies with infants and toddlers have shown that mother and infant do indeed influence one another's moment-to-moment behavior (with mothers, early in the child's life, adapting more to the behavior of their infants than vice versa). And, importantly, the reciprocation of affect—with parent and young child responding in kind to the other's positive or negative emotional signals—emerged as ubiquitous during parent–child interaction. While microanalytic studies have thus produced useful information, students of socialization have generally been more interested in understanding the longer-term influences of parents and children on one another than in the moment-to-moment give and take between them. In the 1980s, a number of short-term longitudinal studies extended the logic of sequential analysis over longer periods, by using cross-lagged analyses with longitudinal data to trace effects of parent on child and child on parent over several months or even years. In more recent years, such analyses have largely been replaced by structural modeling.

Mutual Responsiveness

In their 1983 chapter on parent–child interaction, Maccoby and Martin noted that while the importance of parental responsiveness to children's bids had been extensively studied, much less attention had been paid to children's responsiveness to parental signals or demands. They distinguished between "receptive" compliance and "situational" compliance, the former occurring without coercion, the latter occurring with parental bribery or power assertion. "Receptive" compliance has since been called "willing" compliance, or "committed" compliance (Kochanska & Askan, 1995; Kochanska & Thompson, 1997). Regardless of the label chosen, the distinction between the two different motivations underlying compliance has continued to be recognized as an important one. Kochanska and colleagues note that willing compliance is associated with young children's readiness to imitate the mother: (i.e., with readiness to learn observationally from her), and they regard this "teachability" as another aspect of a child's receptive stance toward parental socialization (Forman & Kochanska, 2001).

Maccoby and Martin noted the mutuality of compliance, pointing to some suggestions in the literature that when a parent complied with a child, the likelihood of the child's complying to the parent increased. Following up on this theme, Parpal and Maccoby (1985) trained a group of mothers in responsive play. They showed that responsive maternal compliance with child directives did elevate the children's subsequent compliance with maternal directives. Lay, Waters, and Park (1989) showed that children's mood was elevated during mother-responsive play and showed further that experimentally elevating a child's mood would increase children's subsequent compliance, even in the absence of maternal responsive play. This work emphasizes once again the importance of affective reciprocity in mother–child interaction.

This theme also appears in the work of Martinez and Forgatch (2001), who report that children's willing compliance with parental directives improves when the mothers have been trained to engage in "positive parenting." Such parenting includes not only warmth, support, and concern for the child's interests but also *politeness*—in other words, a cluster of parenting features which imply some parental respect for the child's autonomy, as well as the creation of a pleasant family atmosphere. In this work, training in positive parenting proved to be even more important than training mothers not to yield to their children's coercion, although that too was important.

Maccoby and Martin proposed that if a state of positive mutual responsiveness prevails during much of infancy and early childhood, it will create a foundation for a well-functioning socialization relationship at a later time. Over a period of nearly two decades, Kochanska and colleagues have carried out a set of longitudinal studies of several cohorts of children, exploring the early dyadic relationship between mother–child pairs and looking to see what connections (if any) can be found between this relationship and the child's subsequent "internalized" compliance (i.e., ability to resist temptation and carry out a required task in the parent's absence) (see summary in Kochanska & Thompson, 1997). Among other findings, Kochanska and her colleagues have shown that measures of shared positive affect and mutual responsiveness taken at 33 months predict the child's ability, a year later, to persist in a task and resist temptation when the mother is out of the room. They have found, too, that willing face-to-face compliance by a young toddler or preschooler is a stepping-stone to a cluster of measures of "conscience" at a later age.

The reciprocity between parent and child was initially studied largely at the level of behavioral interaction, but as we have seen, reciprocity at the level of affect quickly emerged as a central feature of interaction. The study of reciprocity broadened further as it began to include the cognitive level. There is not space here to discuss the reciprocities that are made possible by the child's development of language. But several points emerging from socialization research in the 1980s and more recently deserve special notice: Parent and child develop expectancies about how the other will respond, based on the cumulating history of their interactions through time (see Lollis, 2003). Expectancies can become firmly established and embedded in automated, scripted interactive sequences. While such sequences can greatly smooth daily interaction, they can short-circuit needed communication when they run their course inflexibly, without regard to relevant contextual factors.

The success of parent and child in communicating with one another depends on the clarity of the messages each sends to the other, and on the openness of each to the other's messages. Grusec and Ungerer (2003) note that these things in turn frequently depend on emotional states. An angry child, or one who suffers from chronic anxiety or dysphoria (conditions which can stem from a history of dysfunctional interactions with parents), has difficulty taking in and digesting parental messages and indeed may fend them off defensively. Reciprocally, some parents tend to have distorted cognitions about their children's needs and to misinterpret their children's emotional cues, especially in ignoring or denying signs of children's negative affect These cognitive distortions are bound up with parental depression and a low sense of parental efficacy. By contrast, when parent and child have a history of good cognitive synchrony in their interactions, each partner's sense of efficacy is enhanced.

Clearly, there must be serious consequences for the self-concepts of one or both members of the dyad if either resists the influence of the other. Bugental (1992) has focused on the minority of parents who feel that their children have more control over parent–child interactions than the parents themselves do. She documents how dysfunctional parenting can become in such families. Feelings of inefficacy are closely associated with maternal depression, and maternal depression, in turn, is associated with poor outcomes for children (Byrne, 2003). The causal connections between these things are of course complex, but recent work suggests that in some families a dynamic sequence starts with a difficult child, leading to a maternal sense of lacking control, which induces or exacerbates maternal depression and deteriorating parenting, followed by increased child misbehavior. This sequence is suggested by longitudinal intervention work in which teaching the mother to deal with child misbehavior firmly but not harshly leads to improvements in the child's behavior, which is then followed by a lessening of maternal depression (DeGarmo, Patterson, & Forgatch, 2004). Of course, initially dysfunctional parents do not all benefit equally from such training—some cannot muster sufficient self-regulation to become effective regulators of children.

DEVELOPMENTAL CHANGE IN PARENT–CHILD INTERACTION

A theme emerging strongly from the mid-1980s through the 1990s was a focus on developmental change—that is, on in-family socialization as a sequential process in which the parent–child relationship changes dramatically as children grow older, with each new phase growing out of the parent–child relationship established earlier. Although for many years studies of attachment mainly considered attachment to be a property of the child (i.e., the child is described as being either securely or insecurely attached), it has been evident from the beginning that the mother is reciprocally attached to the child. Developmental changes in the nature of this reciprocal relationship became a focus for study. Sroufe and Fleeson (1986) said: "The infant-caretaker attachment relationship is the womb from which the incipient person emerges. The first organization is dyadic, and it is from that organization, and not from inborn characteristics of the infant, that personality emerges" (p. 67). In his 1996 book on early emotional development, Sroufe integrated the developmental changes in children's attachment behavior with reciprocal changes in parenting. In this book, he drew on the decades-long work on attachment and its sequelae that he and his colleagues carried out. He saw the development of ego controls as central to emotional development. He said: "The evolving attachment relationship is conceptualized as progressive changes in the dyadic regulation of emotions, with an in-creasingly active role for the infant at each phase" (p. 10). He saw the acquisition of ego controls (self-regulation) as emerging out of this dyadic regulation, and as being central to emotional development. Sroufe (1996) has offered a beautifully detailed timetable, showing the successive changes that occur in the role of the mother (or other primary caregiver) in supporting the child's development of self-regulation through infancy and toddlerhood. Following this, at preschool age, Sroufe said that the child must be centrally concerned with managing impulses and maintaining acceptable behavior outside the immediate control of adults, while learning to interact with other children. During this time, the parent shifts from direct and immediate controls—prohibitions, interventions, demonstrations—to more indirect controls and the encouragement of the child's internal-ization of standards. This involves transmission of values, increasingly through reasoning and persuasion.

In their recent review of earlier work on developmental change in parenting, Collins and Madsen (2003) note that as children grow older, there is a progressive decrease in the amount of time parent and child spend together; physical displays of affection lessen, as do the frequency of disciplinary encounters and the direct expressions of anger between parent and child. Furthermore, the actions of parent and child increasingly depend on how they interpret one another's intentions. As children grow older, parents are more and more likely to view misbehavior as knowing and intentional, responding accordingly (Dix, Ruble, Grusec, & Nixon, 1986). With the decrease in direct, face-to-face interac-tion, cognitive aspects of the parent–child relationship become central. Parent–child reci-procity increasingly takes the form of coordinating cognized plans and agendas, and such coordination depends on the flow of information between parent and child, and how each codes the other's messages.

In 1994, Grusec and Goodnow said that the success of intergenerational transmis-sion of values depended on two things: the accuracy of the child's perception of the par-ent's message, and the child's acceptance or rejection of the perceived message. With re-spect to the *accuracy* of children's understanding of parental messages, they note the importance of parents fitting their messages to the child's existing schemas. They note too that children's changing cognitive abilities affect what kind of parental reasoning they can digest, whether they can read the intent behind other' reactions, and whether they can interpret affective cues (especially when these are not consistent with what parents are saying). Children's *acceptance* depends on whether the child sees the parent's action as appropriate to the child's misdeed, whether the parent's message is believable (i.e., verifi-able), and whether threats to the child's autonomy are minimized.

Research on the changes in parent–child interaction as children enter adolescence has brought into central focus the issue of how well the parent and child synchronize their ideas about the child's autonomy. Early adolescence is a time when parents' and children's perspectives concerning the rights of each diverge most strongly. Breakdowns in communication exacerbate this disjunction. Kerr and Stattin (2003) describe families in which an adolescent is defiant and secretive at home—a stance sometimes stemming from a history in which parents have reacted badly to disclosures. The youth may have confided about negative things that have happened away from home, only to have the parents respond with ridicule, blame, or punishment, or use the confided information against the adolescent on future occasions. The young person becomes wary, no longer confiding in the parents; they, in turn, worry about what might be going on behind their backs, lose trust, and show diminished affection and support, leading the adolescent to become more and more closed to communication with the parent. Parents, for their part, become reluctant to start up a conflict and diminish their efforts at control. We may suspect that such a dysfunctional spiral did not spring into being *de novo* in adolescence but may be traceable in part to missed opportunities in early childhood for forming a mutually responsive orientation.

Presenting a picture of more functional interaction between parents and adolescents, Youniss and Smoller in their groundbreaking 1985 book stressed the point that adolescence need not be—and usually is not—a time of *sturm and drang*—at least not within the economically comfortable two-parent families included in their research. Youniss and Smoller found that adolescents typically continue to recognize parental authority, while parents grant increasing freedom in synchrony with their children's increasing competence, so that conflict need not escalate. They did note, however, that children discriminate between domains of decision making, appropriating some domains (e.g., choice of clothes, hairstyles, friends—the "personal" domain) more than others as belonging to their own proper sphere of influence, not their parents'.

SOCIALIZATION AS A FAMILY-SYSTEM FUNCTION

From the mid-1980s through the 1990s, as more and more researchers studied parent–child interaction longitudinally, there was a shift from a focus on the actions of individual parents and children—and on how each influenced the other—to a focus on their coaction and the nature of the relationship between them. At least from the time of Gestalt psychologists' early writings about development there have been claims about the holistic qualities of behaving organisms, with some thinking about how these change developmentally. From a family systems perspective, a family can be seen as composed of individuals, but also as a higher-level system with several dyadic subsystems, with systems and subsystems having properties of their own over and above the properties of the individuals making them up. In the 1980s, formulations from the work on adult close relationships began to percolate into developmental psychology, a landmark publication being Hartup and Rubin's (1986) *Relationships and Development*. This book began to bring thinking about the dynamic properties of within-family dyads into central focus, and research has burgeoned since that time (see Kuczynski, 2003).

An important aspect of dynamic systems theories as applied to family functioning is that systems are seen to be self-equilibrating. Parent and child both act in such a way as to keep the partner's behavior within acceptable boundaries. When one person in the system goes beyond the boundaries within which the family normally functions, the other members will react in such a way as to restore the balance. Though of course family dynamic systems can and do change over time, this self-corrective property of systems is a conservative force, serving to dampen change.

The Parent–Child Dyad

In the foregoing discussion of reciprocity we have already considered some dynamic properties of the parent–child subsystem within the family. Here we need only note that some researchers have studied properties of the dyad over and above the contributions to interaction that each participant makes. Kochanska and Aksan (1995) have used dyadic scores such as "shared positive affect," in which the score is not merely a sum of instances in which the child or the parent displays positive aspect but a count of the number of instances in which the interactive pair displayed positive affect *simultaneously*. Other researchers have noted that while the nature of the relationship between an interacting pair is partly accounted for by the individual characteristics of the two persons involved, there is a large interactive component not attributable to either participant but to the pair jointly (Coie et al., 1999). William Cook (2003), studying the relationships between parents and their young-adult children, notes that the flow of mutual influence is to a large degree unique to specific pairs, so that the relationships between a mother and child 1 may involve quite a different pattern of mutual influence than that between this mother and child 2, and this same child 1 may have a different reciprocal relation with the mother than with the father. A unique interaction resides in the dyad.

The Parental Dyad

Much of the research on the parental dyad has examined the nature of the emotional relationships between the two parents, and the effect that harmony or discord in the parental relationship has on children (see review by Parke & Buriel, 1998) and on the parenting behavior of each (see summary in Katz, Kramer, & Gottman, 1995), but the importance of the parental dyad goes much beyond these issues. Minuchin (1974) was among the first to call attention to the importance of what he called the "executive subsysterm" within the family (i.e., the importance of cooperation, communication, and coordination between two or more adults as they are involved in the joint rearing of a child). In recent years, a body of research has grown up on the functioning of the two as a coparental team (see review in McHale et al., 2002). These authors ask whether the quality of coparenting has effects on children's adjustment, over and above the effects of the conflict or harmony prevailing in the relation of the two parents to one another. Their review indicates that indeed there are real incremental effects of the way the two function as coparents.

A basic coparental issue has to do with the way in which child care and childrearing responsibilities shall be apportioned between the two parents. In early studies of childrearing, role differentiation between the parents in childrearing was a built-in feature of the different economic roles of the two parents, with fathers being the almost exclusive breadwinners and mothers responsible for child care and home management. Later studies included many more families in which the mothers worked, and the feminist movement that burgeoned in the 1970s energized wide-ranging research on the effects of mothers' outside employment on the childrearing responsibilities of the two parents and on the interparental relationships (see summary in Maccoby, 1998). In modern societies in which mothers commonly have been working outside the home, the birth of the first child makes the question of how child-care responsibilities will be divided between mother and father a major one. Through a program of research beginning in the mid-1980s, Phillip and Carolyn Cowan have shown how these issues are renegotiated after the birth of the first child, with mothers usually assuming a considerably larger proportion of the child care (and housework) than had been planned by the couple, with the fathers in many families increasing their hours of out-of-home work to compensate for losses of the mother's earnings (Cowan et al., 1985).

As McHale and colleagues note, a family's executive subsystem can vary in the quality of its functioning quite independently of how much division of labor there is between the parents; that is, a family can function effectively whether or not the two parents have equal and similar roles in daily childrearing. There are multiple ways in which parents can cooperate. A traditional mode is for one parent to specialize in providing economic support while the other cares for the children on a daily basis. But the less involved parent can nevertheless step in to defuse tensions between a child and the other parent, take over child-care responsibilities when the other parent is tired or ill, or back up the other's authority. And most parents, regardless of their division of labor, discuss their childrearing objectives and practices in an effort to achieve consistency. Belsky, Crnic, and Gable (1995) have documented ways in which parents of a toddler son support or undermine one another's parenting activities. They note that a high level of daily hassles can amplify elements of dysfunctional coparenting that are otherwise minor in degree.

The quality of coparenting may depend on the gender of the parent or that of the child or both. McHale (1995) notes, in observations of mother and father jointly interacting with their infant, that when the two parents have a conflicted relationships with one another, the father tends to engage in hostile undermining of the mother's interaction with an infant son, while he tends to withdraw if the infant is a girl. Other studies have found different pathways from coparenting to child outcomes for mothers than for fathers (see summary in Cowan & McHale, 1996). But in most observational studies of coparenting, samples have been too small to analyze fully for gender effects, so the findings to date remain only suggestive.

Issues of coparenting come to the fore in families in which the parents have divorced but continue to share responsibility for raising the children. Some work has focused on the interparental transactions that must occur when parents share custody of the children or when regular visitation occurs (Hetherington, Cox, & Cox, 1982; Maccoby & Mnookin, 1992). These studies have shown that if divorced parents are able to coodinate rules between the two households, avoid open conflict with one another, and communicate with one another about the children, the children benefit. However, these kinds of coparental cooperation diminish over time. Divorced parents become progressively more disengaged from each other even if the children continue to spend time in both households, especially if either parent has a new partner.

The Whole-Family System

A number of the coparenting studies discussed above have involved observations of two parents who were both present and interacting with their child—for example, studies of the parent–parent–child *triad* (see monograph edited by Cowan & McHale, 1996). Several aspects of all-family atmospheres or modes of interaction that might affect children's development have also been studied. These include family "climate," family paradigms, family coordinated practices, and family myths and rituals (see review by Parke & Buriel, 1998). *Residential stability* and *level of household organization* have emerged as important family-level characteristics (Hetherington, Cox, & Cox, 1982; Adam, 2004; Buchanan,

Maccoby, & Dornbusch, 1996; Weisner, Matheson, Coots, & Bernheimer, 2004). Both have been linked to children's achievement and positive adjustment. Asbury, Dunn, Pike, and Plomin (2003) have shown that the more chaotic a household is, the greater the connection between harsh parenting and children's maladjustment.

To date, research on family systems and subsystems is culturally limited. The work on coparenting and family triads of necessity deals almost exclusively with two-parent families, and these studies along with those on family atmospheres and household organization have included mainly middle-class families in industrialized Western societies. Thus we do not know how closely the research described above applies in families in which a broader kinship network is involved in childrearing.

WHERE WE STAND

Clearly, there have been great changes in the way we think about and carry out research on in-family socialization. Evolutionary thinking has been incorporated into accounts of parent–child roles and relationships. The early emphases on reinforcement, impulse control, and democratic and "authoritative" parenting have not been lost; they have simply been reconceptualized. For example, no one doubts that children's behavior is greatly influenced by the consequences of certain actions, through directly experiencing reward or discipline for these actions or observing these consequences experienced by others. But this is no longer thought of as a process of reinforcement whereby the habit strength of specific responses to specific stimuli is increased. Rather, a child's knowledge about the probability of receiving reward or punishment for certain actions in a specific context is now thought to enter into the child's moment-to-moment weighing of many possible short-term and long-term risks, benefits, and goals.

"Democratic" parenting has morphed into reciprocal responsiveness and has been incorporated into analyses of interactive processes between parents and children. "Internalization" continues to be a central process for study, but it is no longer seen as a product mainly of identification with parents. Rather, it is increasingly conceptualized as the development of self-regulation. There has been a shift away from the earlier almost exclusive focus on the *behavior* of parent and child to a greater concern with the ways in which each cognizes the other, and with the emotional valence that pervades parent–child interaction (i.e., with the balance between positive and negative affect in their encounters).

There has been a shift, too, away from the earlier studies of parental "traits," with greater recognition of situational variability in parent practices. Although certain parental traits such as "warmth," "responsiveness," or "power-assertiveness" have continued to hold up as useful concepts for describing individual differences among parents, our understanding of them has been greatly augmented by seeing them as reciprocal properties of parent–child dyads. This shift is part of the more general change from the top-down perspective of early behaviorist and psychoanalytic theories to interactive viewpoints which place increasing emphasis on the agency of the child as well as the parent in socialization processes.

There has been increasing interest in the sequential properties of socialization—in the way parenting must change with the development of the child, and the way in which early interactive processes undergird the later phases of parent–child relationships. Evidence has been accumulating for the importance of establishing a "good socializing relationship" with a child early in life. A major element in such a relationship appears to be the young child's growing willingness to be guided by parent directives and to accept parental values—something which is itself fostered by a parent's emotional reciprocity and positive affect. There is now increasing reason to believe that such an early relationship does facilitate the successful negotiation by parent and child of the issues concerning control and autonomy that pervade later childhood and adolescence. What is not known is how firm a foundation this is—how vulnerable it is to the vicissitudes of later episodes in family interaction, or to the pressures of the free-wheeling and highly commercialized adolescent culture the child encounters outside the family.

Theorizing about parental authority is perhaps the arena in which the most interesting and subtle shifts have taken place. Early studies pointed to deleterious effects of authoritarian childrearing, and a strong body of evidence grew up concerning the undesired side effects of parental power assertion. Yet, at the same time, there was increasing evidence for the benefits of parental "firm control." Several writers have noted that the parent–child relationship is intrinsically a hierarchical one, in that parents do have the responsibility for teaching and directing their children and reining in their impulsive or destructive behavior. Parents who do not succeed in these managerial functions begin to lose their sense of parenting efficacy, and in a negative feedback loop this further undermines their parental control functions (Patterson & Forgatch, 1990; DeGarmo et al., 2004).

How then do parental firm control and parental power assertion differ? How can their opposing effects be reconciled? Research has dealt with this issue in a number of ways. In rejecting authoritarian parenting, Baumrind offered instead a parenting pattern which combined responsive, supportive parenting with "firmness" (i.e., holding children to rules and standards). In the work of G. R. Patterson and colleagues, there has been an unwavering emphasis on rule-setting, monitoring, and following up infractions with discipline, but in recent years there has been increasing emphasis on the importance of balancing these parental control functions with "positive parenting" (i.e., warmth, humor, responsiveness, and politeness to children). In the studies by Grusec and colleagues on disciplinary strategies (Grusec, 1997), effective parents are seen to maintain their management goals while adapting their strategies to constantly changing contexts. Kochanska and colleagues have never doubted that parents must be able to induce their children to comply with parental directives; however, they have shown that it matters whether the children can be led to do so willingly or only under coercion, in that children's willingness allows parents to exercise control benignly rather than coercively. Barber and Olson (1997) distinguish between parental *regulation* of their children's behavior (setting fair and consistent limits) and parents' exercising *psychological control* (not permitting children to experience, value and express their own thoughts and emotions). Barber and colleagues report that the highest levels of adjustment and competence are found in children coming from families that combine strong parental regulation with rare use of psychological control, along with a relationship of close emotional connectedness between parent and child.

The question underlying much modern parenting research, then, is not *whether* parents should exercise authority and children should comply but, rather, *how* parental control can best be exercised so as to support children's growing competence and self-management. Thus it is increasingly understood that strong parent agency and strong child agency are not incompatible. Both can be maintained within a system of mutually understood realms of legitimate authority, though this understanding must be progressively renegotiated as children grow older. The agency of both parties can be encompassed within the bidirectional perspective that is now so widely accepted.

NOTES

1. A child who is "well socialized" is not necessarily synonymous with one who is "well adjusted," but both are normative ideas that are central to distinguishing "good" parenting (or "good enough" parenting) from generally unsuccessful parenting.
2. It is worth noting that although the Baldwin work was going on at the same time as the studies of authoritarian personalities at Berkeley, the two groups did not cite each other and seemed to be entirely independent of one another.
3. Bowlby rejected any simple antithesis between "innate" and "acquired" behavior, noting that situational variations determined whether an instinctive system would be activated (see summary in Maccoby & Masters, 1970).
4. Recent work with animals (Hofer, 2006) has separated the concept of attachment or mother–infant bond into several elements, each infant component being regulated by a distinct feature of maternal contact.

REFERENCES

Adam, E. K. (2004). Beyond quality: Parental and residential stability and children's adjustment. *Current Directions in Psychological Science, 13*, 210–213.

Adorno, T. Frenkel-Brunswik, E., Levinson, D., & Sanford, R. (1950). *The authoritarian personality*. New York: Harper.

Alexander, J. F., & Malouf, R. E. (1983). Intervention with children experiencing problems in personality and social development. In P. H. Mussen, & E. M. Hetherington (Eds.), *Handbook of child psychology* (4th ed., Vol. 4, pp. 913–981). New York: Wiley.

Asbury, K., Dunn, J. F., Pike, & A., Plomin, R. (2003). Nonshared environmental influences on individual differences in early behavioral development: A monozygotic twin differences study. *Child Development, 74*, 933–943.

Baldwin, A. L. (1955). *Behavior and development in childhood*. New York: Dryden Press.

Bandura, A. (1969). Social-learning theory of identificatory processes. In D.A. Goslin (Ed.), *Handbook of socialization theory and research* (pp. 213–262). Chicago: Rand McNally.

Bandura, A. (1986). *Social foundations of thought and action: A social-cognitive theory*. Englewood Cliffs, NJ: Prentice-Hall.

Bandura, A., Ross, D., & Ross, S. A. (1963). A comparative test of the status-envy, social power and secondary reinforcement theories of identificatory learning. *Journal of Abnormal and Social Psychology, 67*, 527–534.

Barber, B. K., & Olsen, J. A. (1997). Socialization in context: Connection, regulation and autonomy in the family, school, and neighborhood, and with peers. *Journal of Adolescent Research, 12*, 287–315.

Bates, J., Pettit, G., Dodge, K., & Ridge, B. (1998). Interaction of temperamental resistance to control and restrictive parenting in the development of externalizing behavior. *Developmental Psychology, 34*, 982–995.

Baumrind, D., & Black, A. E. (1967). Socialization practices associated with dimension of competence in preschool boys and girls. *Child Development, 38*, 291–327.

Bell, R. Q. & Harper, L. V. (1977). *Child effects on adults*. Hillsdale, NJ: Erlbaum.

Belsky, J., Crnic, K., & Gable, S. (1995). The determinants of coparenting in families with toddler boys: Spousal differences and daily hassles. *Child Development, 66*, 629–642.

Black, J. (1971). *Lives through time*. Berkeley, CA: Bancroft Books.

Block, J. H., & Block, J. (1980). The role of ego-control and ego-resiliency in the organization of behavior. In W. Andrew Collins (Ed.), *Development of cognitions, affect, and social relations (Vol. 13).* Hillsdale, NJ: Erlbaum.

Borkowski, J. G., Ramey, S. L., & Bristol-Power, M. (Eds.). (2002) *Parenting and the child's world: Influences on academic, intellectual and social-emotional development.* Mahwah NJ: Erlbaum.

Bowlby, J. (1969) *Attachment and loss, Vol. 1. Attachment.* New York: Basic Books.

Brody, G. H., Murry, V. M., Gerard, M., Gibbons, F.X., Molgaard, V., McNair, L, (2004). The strong African-American family program: Translating research into prevention programming. *Child Development, 75,* 900–917.

Buchanan, C. M., Maccoby, E. E., & Dornbusch, S. M. (1996). *Adolescents after divorce.* Cambridge, MA: Harvard University Press.

Bugental, D. B. (1992). Effective and cognitive processes within threat-oriented family systems. In I. E. Sigel, A. McGielicuddy-DiLise & Goodnow, (Eds.), *Parental relief systems: The psychological consequences for children* (pp. 219–248). Hillsdale, NJ: Erlbaum.

Bugental, D. B., Corporael, L., & Shennum, W. A. (1980). Experimentally induced child uncontrollability: Effects on the potency of adult communication patterns. *Child Development, 51,* 520–528.

Bugental, D. B., & Goodnow, J. J. (1998) Socialization processes. In W. Damon & N. Eisenberg (Eds.), *Handbook of child psychology* (5th ed., Vol. 3, pp. 389–462). New York: Wiley.

Bugental, D. B., & Grusec, J. E. (2006). Socialization processes. In N. Eisenberg (Vol. Ed.), *Handbook of child psychology* (6th ed., Vol. 3, pp. 366–428). Hoboken, NJ: Wiley.

Byrne, C. (2003). Parental agency and mental health: Construction and proaction in families with a depressed parent. In L. Kuczynski (Ed.), *Handbook of dynamics in parent–child relations* (pp. 229–244). Thousand Oaks, CA: Sage.

Cairns, R. B., Elder, G. H., & Costello, E. J. (Eds.). (1996). *Developmental science.* Cambridge, UK: Cambridge University Press.

Chomsky, N. (1959) Verbal behavior (Review of *Verbal behavior* by B. F. Skinner). *Language, 35,* 26–58.

Coie, J. D., Cillessen, A. H. N., Dodge, K. A., Hubbard, J.A., Schwartz, D., Lemarise, A., et al. (1999). It takes two to fight: A test of relational factors and a method for assessing aggressive dyads. *Developmental Psychology, 35,* 1179–1188.

Collins, W. A., Maccoby, E. E., Steinberg, L., & Hetherington, E. M. (2000). Contemporary research on parenting: The case for nature *and* nurture. *American Psychologist, 55,* 218–232.

Collins, W. A., & Madsen, S. D. (2003). Developmental change in parenting interactions. In L. Kuczynski (Ed.), *Handbook of dynamics in parent–child relations* (pp. 49–66). Thousand Oaks, CA: Sage.

Cook, W. L. (2003). Quantitative methods for deductive (theory-testing) research on parent–child dynamics. In L. Kuczynski (Ed.), *Handbook of dynamics in parent–child relations.* Thousand Oaks, CA: Sage.

Cowan, C. P., Cowan, P. A., Heming, G., Garrett, E., Coysh, W. S., Curtis-Boles, H., et al. (1985). Transitions to parenthood. *Journal of Family Issues, 6,* 451–481.

Cowan, P. A., & McHale, J. P. (1996). Coparenting in a family context: Emerging achievements, current dilemmas, and future directions. In J. P. McHale & P. A. Cowan (Eds.), *Understanding how family-level dynamics affect children's development.* (No. 77 of *New Directions for Child Development*). San Francisco: Jossey Bass.

Darling, N., & Steinberg, L. (1993). Parenting style as context: An integrative model. *Psychology Bulletin, 113,* 487–496.

DeGarmo, D. S., Patterson, G. R., & Forgatch, M. S. (2004). How do outcomes in a specified parent-training intervention maintain or wane over time? *Prevention Science, 5,* 73–89.

De Waal, F. (1996). *Good natured: The origins of right and wrong in humans and other animals.* Cambridge, MA: Harvard University Press.

Dix, T., Ruble, D. N., Grusec, J. E., & Nixon, S. (1986). Social cognitions in parents: Inferential and affective reactions to children of three age levels. *Child Development, 57,* 879–894.

Eisenberg, N., Smith, C. L., Sadovsky, A., & Spinrad, T. L. (2004). Effortful control: Relations with emotion regulation, adjustment, and socialization in childhood. In R. R. Baumeister & K. D. Vohs (Eds.), *Handbook of self-regulation: Research, theory, and applications* (pp. 259–282). New York: Guilford Press.

Forman, D. R., & Kochanska, G. (2001). Viewing imitation as child responsiveness: A link between the teaching and discipline dimensions of socialization. *Developmental Psychology, 37,* 198–206.

Gewirtz, J. L. (1969) Mechanisms of social learning: Some roles of stimulation and behavior in human development. In D. A. Goslin, (Ed.), *Handbook of socialization theory and research* (pp. 57–213). Chicago: Rand McNally.

Goslin, D. A. (Ed.). (1969). *Handbook of socialization theory and research.* Chicago: Rand McNally.

Grolnick, W. S., Deci, E. L., & Ryan, R. M. (1997). Internalization within the family: The self-Determination theory perspective. In J. E. Grusec & L. Kiczynski (Eds.), *Parenting and children's internalization of values* (pp. 135–161). New York: Wiley.

Grusec, J. E. (1997). A history of research on parenting strategies and children's internalization of values. In J. E. Grusec & L. Kuczynski (Eds.), *Parenting and children's internalization of values* (pp. 3–22). New York: Wiley.

Grusec, J. E., & Goodnow, J. J. (1994). Impact of parental discipline on the child's internalization of values: A reconceptualization of current points of view. *Developmental Psychology, 30,* 4–13.

Grusec, J. E., & Kuczynski, L. (1980). Direction of effects in socialization: A comparison of the Parent's versus the child's behavior as determinants of disciplinary techniques. *Developmental Psychology, 16,* 1–9.

Grusec, J. E., & Ungerer, J. (2003). Effective socialization as problem solving and the role of parenting cognitions. In L. Kuczynski (Ed.), *Handbook of dynamics in parent–child relations* (p. 211–228). Thousand Oaks, CA: Sage.

Harlow, H. F., & Harlow, M. K. (1965). The affectional systems. In A. M. Schrier, H. F. Harlow, & F. Stollnitz (Eds.), *Behavior of non-human primates, Vol. 2.* New York: Academic Press.

Harris, J. R. (1998). *The nurture assumption: Why children turn out the way they do.* New York: Free Press.

Hartup, W. W., & Rubin, Z. (1986). *Relationships and development.* Hillsdale, NJ: Erlbaum.

Hetherington, E. M., Cox, M., & Cox, R. (1982). Effects of divorce on parents and children. In M. Lamb (Ed.), *Nontraditional families: Parenting and child development* (pp. 233–288). Hillsdale, NJ: Erlbaum.

Hofer, M. A. (2006). Psychobiological roots of early attachment. *Current Directions in Psychological Science, 15,* 84–88.

Hoffman, M. L. (1970). Moral development. In P. H. Mussen (Ed.), *Carmichael's manual of child psychology* (Vol. 2, pp. 261–359). New York: Wiley.

Katz, L. F., Kramer, L., & Gottman, J. M. (1995). Conflict and emotions in marital, sibling and peer relationships. In C. U. Shantz & W. W. Hartup (Eds.), *Conflict in child and adolescent development* (p. 142–149). Cambridge, UK: Cambridge University Press.

Kerr, M., & Stattin, H. (2003). Parenting of adolescents: Action or reaction? In A. C. Crouter & A. Booth (Eds.), *Children's influence on family dynamics* (pp. 121–152). Mahwah, NJ: Erlbaum.

Kochanska, G. (1995). Children's temperament, mothers' discipline, and security of attachment: Multiple pathways to emerging internalization. *Child Development, 66,* 597–615.

Kochanska, G., & Aksan, N. (1995). Mother–child mutually positive affect, the quality of child compliance to requests and prohibitions, and maternal control as correlates of early internalization. *Child Development, 66,* 236–254.

Kochanska, G., Coy, K. C., & Murray, K. T. (2001). The development of self-regulation in the first four years of life. *Child Development, 72,* 1091–1111.

Kochanska, G., Murray, K. T., & Harlan, E.T. (2000). Effortful control in early childhood: Continuity and change, antecedents, and implications for social development. *Developmental Psychology, 36,* 220–232.

Kochanska, G., & Thompson, R. A. (1997). The emergence and development of conscience in toddlerhood and early childhood. In J. Grusec & L. Kuczynski (Eds.), *Parenting and children's internalization of values* (pp. 53–77).

Kuczynski, L. (2003). *Handbook of dynamics in parent–child relations. Thousand Oaks, CA: Sage.*

Lay, K., Waters, E., & Park, K. A. (1989). Maternal responsiveness and child compliance: The role of mood as a mediator. *Child Development, 60,* 1405–1411.

Lewin, K., Lippitt, R., & White, R. K. (1939). Patterns of aggressive behavior in experimentally created "social climates." *Journal of Social Psychology, 10,* 271–299.

Lollis, S. (2003). Conceptualizing the influence of the past and the future in parent–child relationships. In L. Kuczynski (Ed.), *Handbook of dynamics in parent–child relations* (pp. 67–88). Thousand Oaks, CA: Sage.

Maccoby, E. E. (1992). The role of parents in the socialization of children: An historical overview. *Developmental Psychology, 28,* 1006–1017.

Maccoby, E. E. (1998). *The two sexes: Growing up apart, coming together.* Cambridge, MA: Harvard University Press.

Maccoby, E. E. (2000). Parenting and its effects on children. *Annual Review of Psychology, 51,* 1–27.

Maccoby, E. E., & Martin, J. A. (1983). Socialization in the context of the family: Parent–child interaction. In P. H. Mussen, & E. M. Hetherington (Eds.), *Handbook of child psychology* (4th ed., Vol. 4., pp. 1–102). New York: Wiley.

Maccoby, E. E., & Masters, J. C. (1970). Attachment and dependency. In P. H. Mussen (Ed.), *Carmichael's manual of child psychology* (4th ed., Vol. 2, pp. 73–158). New York: Wiley.

Maccoby, E. E., & Mnookin, R. H. (1992). *Dividing the child: Social and legal dilemmas of custody.* Cambridge, MA: Harvard University Press.

Martin, J. A., Maccoby, E. E., Baran, K., & Jacklin, C. N. (1981). Sequential analysis of mother–child interaction at 18 months: A comparison of microanalytic methods. *Developmental Psychology, 17,* 146–157.

Martinez, C. R., & Forgatch, M. S. (2001). Preventing problems with boys' noncompliance: Effects of a parent training intervention for divorcing mothers. *Journal of Consulting and Clinical Psychology, 69,* 416–428.

McHale, J. (1995). Co-parenting and triadic interactions during infancy: The roles of marital distress and child gender. *Developmental Psychology, 31,* 985–996.

McHale, J., Khazan, I., Erera, P., Rotman, T. DeCourcey, W., & McConnell, M. (2002). Coparenting in diverse family systems. In Marc H. Bornstein (Ed.), *Handbook of parenting* (2nd ed., Vol. 3, pp. 75–108). Mahwah NJ: Erlbaum.

Miller, N. E., & Dollard, J. (1941). *Social learning and imitation,* New Haven, CT: Yale University Press.

Minuchin, S. (1974). *Families and family therapy.* Cambridge, MA: Harvard University Press.

Mischel, W., & Grusec, J. (1967). Waiting for rewards and punishments: Effects of time and probability on choice. *Journal of Personality and Social Psychology, 5,* 24–31.

Mischel, W., & Liebert, R. M. (1967). The role of power in the adoption of self-reward patterns. *Child Development, 38,* 673–684.

Mischel, W., & Metzner, R. (1962). Preference for delayed reward as a function of age, intelligence, and length of delay interval. *Journal of Abnormal and Social Psychology, 64,* 425–431.

Mischel, W., Shoda, Y., & Peake, P. (1988). The nature of adolescent competencies predicted by preschool delay of gratification. *Journal of Personality and Social Psychology, 54,* 687–696.

Moffett, T. E., Caspi, A., & Rutter, M. (2006). Measured gene-environment interactions in psychopathology: Concepts, research strategies, and implications for research, intervention and public understanding of genetics. In *Perspectives in Psychology Science, 1,* 5–27.

Neiderhiser, J. M., Reiss, D., Pedersen, N. L., Lichenstein, P., Spotts, E. L., Hansson, K., et al. (2004). Genetic and environmental influences on mothering of adolescents: A comparison of two samples. *Developmental Psychology, 40,* 335–351.

Parke, R. D., & Buriel, R. (1998). Socialization in the family: Ethnic and ecological perspectives. In W. Damon & N. Eisenberg (Eds.), *Handbook of child psychology* (5th ed., Vol. 3, pp. 463–552). New York; Wiley.

Parpal, M., & Maccoby, E. E. (1985). Maternal responsiveness and subsequent child compliance. *Child Development, 56,* 1326–1324.

Patterson, G. R. (1982). *Coercive family process,* Eugene, OR: Castalia.

Patterson, G. R., & Forgatch, M. S. (1990). Initiation and maintenance of processes disrupting single-mother families. In G. R. Patterson (Ed.), *Depression and aggression in family interaction* (pp. 209–245). Hillsdale, NJ: Erlbaum.

Plomin, R., & Daniels, D. (1987). Why are children in the same family so different from each other? *Behaviorall and Brain Sciences, 10,* 1–16.

Posner, M. L., & Rothbart, M. K. (1998). Attention, self-regulation and consciousness. *Philosophical Transactions of the Royal Society of London, B., 353,* 1915–1927.

Rothbart, M. K., & Bates, J. E. (1998). Temperament. In W. Damon & N. Eisenberg (Eds.), *Handbook of child psychology* (5th ed., Vol. 3, pp. 105–176). New York: Wiley.

Rothbart, M. K., & Rueda, M. R. (2005). The development of effortful control. In U. Mayr, E. Awh, & S. W. Keele (Eds.), *Developing individuality in the human brain: A festschrift honoring Michael I. Posner—May, 2003* (pp. 167–188). Washington DC: American Psychological Association Press.

Rowe, D. C. (1994). *The limits of family influence: Genes, experience, and behavior.* New York: Guilford Press.

Rutter, M., Pickles, A., Murray, R., & Eaves, L. (2001). Testing hypotheses on specific environmental causal effects on behavior. *Psychological Bulletin, 127,* 291–324.

Scarr, S. (1992). Developmental theories for the 1990's: Development and individual differences. *Child Development, 63,* 1–19.

Sears, R. R. (1951). A theoretical framework for personality and social behavior. *American Psychologist, 6,* 476–483.

Sears, R. R., Maccoby, E. E., & Levin, H. (1957). *Patterns of child rearing.* Evanston, IL: Row, Peterson.

Sears, R. R., Rau, L., & Alpert, R. (1965). *Identification and child rearing,* Stanford, CA: Stanford University Press.

Sears, R. R., Whiting, J. W. M., Nowlis, V., & Sears, P. S. (1953). Some child-rearing antecedents of aggression and dependency in young children. *Genetic Psychology Mongraphs, 47,* 135–234.

Shoda, Y., Mischel, W., & Peake, P. (1990). Predicting adolescent cognitive and self-regulatory competencies from preschool delay of gratification: Identifying diagnostic conditions. *Developmental Psychology, 26,* 978–986.

Shonkoff, J. P., & Phillips, D. A.(Eds.). (2001). *From neurons to neighborhoods: The science of early childhood development.* Washington, DC: National Academy Press.

Sroufe, L. A. (1996). *Emotional development.* Cambridge, UK: Cambridge University Press.

Sroufe, L. A., & Fleeson, J. (1986). Attachment and the construction of relationships. In W. Hartup & Z Rubin (Eds.), *Relationships and development* (pp. 51–71). Hillsdale, NJ: Erlbaum.

Suomi, S. J. (2002). Parents, peers, and processes of socialization in primates. In J. G. Borkowski, S. L. Ramey, & M. Bristol-Power (Eds.), *Parenting and the child's world* (pp. 265–282). Mahwah, NJ: Erlbaum.

Turkheimer, E. (2000). Three laws of behavior genetics and what they mean. *Current Directions in Psychological Science, 9,* 160–164.

Weisner, T. S., Matheson, C., Coots, J., & Bernheimer, L. P. (2004). Sustainability of daily routines as a family outcome. In A. Maynard & M. Martini (Eds.), *Learning in cultural context: Family, peers and school.* New York: Kluwer/Plenum.

Whiting, J. W. M., & Child, I. L., (1953). *Child training and personality.* New Haven, CT: Yale University Press.

Youniss, J. & Smollar, J. (1985). *Adolescent relations with mothers, fathers and friends.* Chicago: University of Chicago Press.

CHAPTER 2

Socialization and Interventions for Antisocial Youth

TIMOTHY A. CAVELL, SHELLEY HYMEL, KENYA T. MALCOLM, and AMY SEAY

Scholars have long been drawn to the question of why some children develop into solid, law-abiding citizens whereas others become juvenile delinquents or even career criminals. When youth behave in antisocial ways, the results are negative and noteworthy: Others get hurt and the direct costs to victims can be considerable. In the United States, Cohen (1998) estimates that each youth who becomes a career criminal costs society $1.3–$1.5 million over a lifetime (e.g., lost wages, medical expenses, stolen property, and costs of incarceration). Antisocial behavior also significantly affects its young perpetrators. The adjustment problems of antisocial youth can be extensive, at times leaving a legacy of dysfunction that lasts for generations.

Antisocial youth are often considered socialization failures—clear examples of what can go wrong when the job of inculcating society's younger members is left undone or poorly done (Patterson, Reid, & Dishion, 1992; Tremblay, 2003). What can be learned about socialization from attempts to alter directly the developmental trajectories of antisocial youth? Ideally, the link between theory and practice is bidirectional and mutually beneficial: Research on normative socialization processes informs the design of interventions for antisocial youth, and well-implemented intervention studies test experimentally the role of causal mechanisms considered essential to socialization (see Cavell & Hughes, 2000; Lochman & Wells, 2002). We begin our chapter by noting common misconceptions about antisocial behavior and its interventions. Next, we review research assessing the long-term outcomes of existing interventions and discuss the implications of this research for reducing antisocial behavior. We conclude our chapter with recommendations for future intervention studies.

MYTHS ABOUT CHILD AND ADOLESCENT ANTISOCIAL BEHAVIOR

The term "antisocial behavior" (ASB) refers to a broad spectrum of behavior that includes coercion, various forms of aggression, and a range of delinquent acts (e.g., Coie & Dodge, 1998; Tolan, Guerra, & Kendall, 1995). There is value in studying the developmental course of specific antisocial behaviors such as physical aggression (Tremblay, 2000, 2003), but interventionists are often concerned with a broad class of ASB, one marked by developmental heterotopy and range of maladaptive outcomes. For a small minority of youth, labeled "early starters" (Patterson et al., 1992) or "life-course-persistent offenders" (Moffitt, 1993), ASB begins in early childhood, is maintained at high levels in adolescence, and is associated with greater violence. For a larger percentage of youth, involvement in ASB is "adolescent limited" and thought to be rooted in teenage rebellion and a desire for greater autonomy (Moffitt, 1993, 2003). The distinction between child and adolescent onset, now codified in the *Diagnostic and Statistical Manual of Mental Disorders* (DSM; American Psychiatric Association, 1994), suggests divergent developmental processes, perhaps requiring differing approaches to intervention. Despite such advances in our understanding of ASB, there continue to be misconceptions about antisocial youth and the strategies needed to alter their negative trajectory.

- *Myth 1: It is impossible to treat delinquent, antisocial youth.* In years past, it was not uncommon for researchers and practitioners to lament the lackluster performance of treatments for delinquent youth (Hazelrigg, Cooper, & Borduin, 1987; Lipsey, 1992). Traditional psychotherapy was clearly ineffective, and alternative treatments (Hoefler & Bornstein, 1975; Minuchin, 1974) generated more excitement than robust outcome data (e.g., Bank, Marlowe, Reid, Patterson, & Weinrott, 1991). Today, the outlook for treating delinquent youth is more positive (Chamberlain & Rosicky, 1995; Tate, Reppucci, & Mulvey, 1995). Newer treatment approaches, capitalizing on lessons learned from previous treatment failures and building on increased knowledge about the multiple causes of ASB, have yielded impressive results (e.g., Alexander, Robbins, & Sexton, 2000; Chamberlain & Reid, 1998; Henggeler, Schoenwald, Borduin, Rowland, & Cunningham, 1998; Szapocznik & Williams, 2000).

Particularly impressive are findings in support of multisystemic therapy (MST; Borduin et al., 1995; Henggeler et al., 1998) and multidimensional treatment foster care (MTFC; Chamberlain & Reid, 1998; Eddy & Chamberlain, 2000). In MST, therapists custom-fit treatment plans to families' strengths and modify them as needed. MST therapists target a range of contexts (family, school, peer) and take their intervention to settings (e.g., homes, playgrounds, and job sites) rarely visited by conventional therapists. MST therapists have small case loads, are highly mobile and accessible, and are compensated in part based on their treatment successes (Henggeler, 2003). In Chamberlain's (2003) MTFC program, delinquent youth are removed from settings that support ASB (e.g., chaotic homes and violent neighborhoods) and placed with specially trained foster parents who provide consistent rewards for prosocial behavior and strict limits on associations with deviant peers. Also targeted is the quality of parenting in the home, with the goal of eventually returning youth to improved family contexts (Eddy & Chamberlain, 2000).

Despite promising treatments such as MST and MTFC, important questions remain, including the important question of which youth are benefiting. In general, treatment studies involving adjudicated youth rarely distinguish between late- and early-onset ASB trajectories and few target seriously delinquent youth (cf. Chamberlain & Reid, 1998; Borduin et al., 1995). More common is for investigators to focus on first-time offenders or milder forms of ASB, such as substance abuse (e.g., Elliot, Orr, Watson, & Jackson, 2005). A second issue is the lack of long-term, follow-up evaluations. Woolfenden, Williams, and Peat (2002) found that parent- or family-focused interventions led generally to lower recidivism 1 to 3 years posttreatment, but the findings were based on only eight randomized clinical trials. The most compelling long-term findings were reported by Schaeffer and Borduin (2005), who found that delinquent youths receiving MST 14 years earlier had significantly lower recidivism than youth who participated in individual therapy (50% vs. 81%, respectively). Collectively, these reports, despite some limitations, indicate that treating delinquent youth is no longer an exercise in futility.

• *Myth 2: Delinquency is easily preventable through the use of evidence-based programs.* There is a growing body of empirical research on interventions designed to prevent the negative developmental course of ASB. Some scholars argue that several programs have shown their worth and all that remains for effective prevention is disseminating those programs on a broader scale (e.g., Taylor, Eddy, & Biglan, 1999; Webster-Stratton & Taylor, 2001). The value of adopting programs with a proven track record is seen in the proliferation of lists of evidence-based programs (e.g., www.casel.org and www.colorado.edi/cspv/blueprints). But the moniker of "evidence based" can be applied too loosely by those seeking an easy solution to the complex problem of preventing delinquency and serious ASB. For example, volunteer mentoring is currently touted as a proven method of delinquency prevention (Dortch, 2000) based in part on a widely publicized report that mentored children are less likely to hit others or to use alcohol or drugs (Grossman & Tierney, 1998). Currently, a major initiative of the U.S. Office of Juvenile Justice and Delinquency Prevention is to pair mentors with delinquent youth and children of incarcerated parents. However, carefully conducted meta-analytic studies reveal that reductions in ASB are rare outcomes in youth mentoring (e.g., DuBois, Holloway, Valentine, & Cooper, 2002). Prevention programmers must be careful to rely on accepted, scientific criteria when selecting for dissemination programs designed to prevent ASB (Biglan, Mrazek, Carnine, & Flay, 2003; Greenberg, 2004).

Studies that investigate the dissemination of evidence-based practices are critical to a science of prevention (Coie et al., 1993; Pettit & Dodge, 2003), but basic questions of efficacy (Dodge & Pettit, 2003; Moffitt, 2005; Rutter, 2003a; Strand & Cavell, 2005) and effectiveness still remain (Wandersman & Florin, 2003; Weisz, Weiss, Han, Granger, & Morton, 1995). Needed are studies that evaluate whether preventive interventions are effective over time, across diverse populations, and in real-world settings (Hinshaw, 2002; Kazdin, 2005). Also needed are studies that identify specific mechanisms of change, without which the goal of broad and efficient dissemination will be delayed (Kazdin, 2005; Rutter, 2003b). Most prevention programs are constructed from models of risk and resilience, but passive, longitudinal designs can leave unspecified which variables are causal *and* malleable (Moffitt, 2005; Tremblay, 2003). Finally, the emphasis on dissemination does not preclude the development of new interventions; it merely underscores the need to evaluate critically any promise of innovation.

PREVENTING DELINQUENCY: FOUR TYPES OF INTERVENTIONS

Published studies of delinquency prevention suggest four types of interventions that vary with respect to children's age (e.g., infants, preschoolers, schoolchildren, and teens), the form of ASB addressed, the level of risk or dysfunction currently experienced, and whether the goal is universal or selective prevention. Selective prevention programs target populations known to be at risk for later problems, whereas universal prevention programs are delivered to whole schools or communities (Coie et al., 1993).

One approach to prevention selects children based on risk variables far removed from the long-term goal of reduced delinquency. Such programs often target infants and toddlers whose mothers are at risk for rearing children with behavior problems. A prime example is the nurse visitation program developed by Olds and colleagues (Eckenrode et al., 2001; Olds, 2002). Reported benefits from nurses' support and information include reductions in maternal substance use (particularly tobacco) during pregnancy, child maltreatment, family size, and closely spaced pregnancies. Follow-up evaluations conducted when children were 15 years old also showed a moderated intervention effect: Child maltreatment and early-onset behavior problems were linked, but only for children who did not have the benefit of a nurse visitor (Eckenrode et al., 2001). Olds (2002) also reported fewer arrests and convictions and less substance use and promiscuous sexual activity among teens who participated as infants in the nurse visitation program. A similar program is Johnson's (1989) Houston Parent–Child Development Center, which targeted low-income, Mexican American families with 1-year-old children. Its primary goal was to promote children's intellectual and social competence, although lower rates of child problem behavior were noted 5 to 8 years following intervention (Johnson, 1989). Unfortunately, subsequent assessments (6–13 years postintervention) revealed few intervention effects (Johnson & Blumenthal, 2004).

A second type of selective prevention program targets preschoolers who exhibit conduct problems or are at risk for later conduct problems because of poverty, parental divorce, or other environmental factors (DeGarmo & Forgatch, 2005; Forgatch & DeGarmo, 1999; Webster-Stratton, 1998; Webster-Stratton, Reid, & Hammond, 2001, 2004). The goal of these programs is to catch relatively early the pattern of coercive processes that can lead to more ingrained patterns of ASB (Webster-Stratton & Taylor, 2001). Most involve clinic-based parent management training (PMT) programs (e.g., Eyberg, 1988; Forehand & McMahon, 1981), although more recent PMT efforts involve partnerships with Head Start centers or additional components designed specifically for teachers (Webster-Stratton et al., 2001, 2004). Despite strong evidence for the short-term efficacy of these programs (Brestan & Eyberg, 1998; Kazdin, 2005), long-term gains are less evident, in part because few studies report follow-up data beyond 1 year (Serketich & Dumas, 1996). An exception is the study by Webster-Stratton (1990) in which participants were assessed 3 years after intervention. Her results indicated that 30–50% of treated families showed little or no improvement at follow-up. Other parent training studies report long-term outcomes but lack the control group used in the Webster-Stratton (1990) study. Hood and Eyberg (2003) found that gains from parent training were maintained for 3 to 6 years, and Long, Forehand, Wierson, and Morgan (1994) reported that adolescents whose parents participated in parent training 14 years earlier were comparable to a matched community sample on measures of psychosocial functioning. Of course, the lack of data on untreated or control participants makes it difficult to interpret these findings. Other long-term studies suffer from differential dropout rates (e.g., see Forehand & Long, 1991; Long et al., 1994) or reveal that initial gains were not maintained over time. The latter is more common among low-income families and parents who are socially isolated and emotionally distressed (Serketich & Dumas, 1996). It is also possible for sizable numbers of hard-to-manage preschoolers to improve with little or no intervention. Pierce, Ewing, and Campbell (1999) found that only 41% of difficult 3-year-olds met diagnostic criteria for oppositional defiant disorder or conduct disorder at age 13.

A third type of prevention program targets school-age children whose aggressive behavior indicates the possibility of early-onset ASB. In these programs, eligible families are actively recruited and key intervention components (e.g., parent training and child skills training) are often conducted in the school. To date, school-based prevention programs that target aggressive, elementary children have yielded more modest gains than clinic-based interventions for younger, less antisocial preschoolers (Barkley, 2000; Cavell & Strand, 2003). The most ambitious of these programs is FAST Track, a multisite trial targeting aggressive children at school entry. The intervention included both universal and selective components, some of which lasted into high school (Conduct Problems Prevention Research Group, 2002, 2004). Outcomes assessed in grades 4 and 5 revealed significant, albeit modest treatment effects on measures of social competence, social cognition, and involvement with deviant peers. There was no evidence that intervention made a significant impact on children's aggression at school. Similar findings have been reported for other, smaller-scale interventions (e.g., August, Lee, Bloomquist, Realmuto, & Hektner, 2004; Cavell & Hughes, 2000; Hughes, Cavell, Meehan, Zhang, & Collie, 2005; Kazdin, Siegel, & Bass, 1992; Lochman, 1992; Prinz, Blechman, & Dumas, 1994). Thus, despite increased sophistication in school-based prevention programs targeting children with early-onset ASB, questions remain about the long-term benefits of such programs.

The last type of prevention program is universally administered to classrooms, schools, or communities with the goal of reducing the overall incidence and prevalence of problem behavior. Most target adolescents' use or abuse of alcohol, tobacco, or illicit drugs (e.g., Botvin, Griffin, & Diaz, 2000; Mason, Kosterman, Hawkins, Haggerty, & Spoth, 2003), although some are designed to prevent emerging ASB (Herrenkohl et al., 2003; Dishion & Kavanagh, 2000; Ialongo, Werthamer, Brown, Kellam, & Wai, 1999). In programs involving parents or families, it is not uncommon to provide participants with a multitiered menu of intervention options that vary in intensity and time demands (Dishion & Kavanagh, 2000; Sanders, Markie-Dadds, Tully, & Bor, 2000). In other programs, all participants receive the same intervention (e.g., Herrenkohl et al., 2003; Ialango et al., 1999; Olweus, 1993). The goals and strategies of these universal prevention programs fit well a public health perspective in which success is measured in terms of the relative costs and benefits to society (Birckmayer, Holder, Yacoubian, & Friend, 2004; Foster, Dodge, & Jones, 2003; Wandersman & Florin, 2003). A potential downside to universal prevention programs is the risk that chronic and seriously antisocial youth will not benefit despite substantial reductions in the overall rate of ASB. On the other hand, a universal program that can reduce normative beliefs in support of ASB could be a useful complement to selective intervention programs (e.g., Conduct Problems Prevention Research Group, 2004).

SOCIALIZATION AND REDUCTIONS IN ANTISOCIAL BEHAVIOR

Current research on the prevention of serious ASB reveals continued uncertainty about the most effective ways to promote the long-term socialization of high-risk children. Reducing ASB requires an appreciation for individual differences in crime proneness (Krueger et al., 1994; Moffitt, 1993) and for the interdependence of multiple socialization contexts (Harris, 1995, 1998; Parke et al., 2002; Vaillancourt & Hymel, 2004) in the development of ASB (Patterson et al., 1992; Snyder & Patterson, 1995). An integrated *life course–social learning* model fits well the premise that human development is a recurring process of nature interacting with nurture and that children contribute substantially to that process (Collins, Maccoby, Steinberg, Hetherington, & Bornstein, 2000, 2001; Moffitt, 2005). Much of what has been written about socialization and children's capacity for agency has sought to correct a consistent overemphasis on the role of shared environmental influence, those experiences that children share with siblings (Scarr, 1992; Scarr & Deater-Deckard, 1997). Twin and adoption studies show that children's developmental outcomes, including their involvement in ASB, are due largely to genetic endowment and nonshared environment influences (Rhee & Waldman, 2002). Socialization researchers who long viewed parents as the primary contributors to children's development eventually conceded that the case for shared environmental influence had been overstated and underspecified (Collins et al., 2000, 2001). Other scholars have asserted that nonparental socialization forces, including peers, schools, and other extrafamilial institutions, had not been adequately considered as determinants of children' development (Harris, 1995, 1998). Still others have argued for the interdependence of family and peer social systems, both of which interact with children's genetic and biological predispositions (Parke et al., 2002). These trends underscore recent interventions that go beyond parenting factors and consider linkages to other key socialization contexts. For example, evaluating a 2-year prevention program, Vitaro, Brendgen, and Tremblay (2001) found that reductions in delinquency 7 years after treatment were mediated by increased parental supervision *and* greater association with nondeviant peers, underscoring the multiple factors contributing to delinquent behavior.

Both children and adults are active agents in the process of socialization, despite the fact that their roles and goals are quite distinct. For children and adolescents, *socialization* involves the process of actively seeking, routinely accessing, and effectively participating in contexts that provide greater and more reliable benefits than other, competing contexts. Children are active players in their own development and they seek, access, and invest in environmental niches that capitalize on specific genetic endowments (Scarr, 1992). Individual differences and early experiences also affect children's success in various social contexts and codetermine their choice of future social contexts. Simply put, children invest time and energy in contexts that offer greater and more reliable payoffs than other contexts. Thus, for the developing child, socialization is not a process where outcomes are inherently prosocial or antisocial; instead, the moral valence of those outcomes is largely a reflection of the values and behaviors rewarded by the contexts in which children and adolescents are actively engaged. Philosophically, one can debate the existence of moral absolutes, but the science of socialization cannot afford to ignore the obdurateness and the appeal of those aspects of society considered by some to be deviant or immoral (Berger & Luckman, 1966). For parents and other stakeholders, *socialization* is the process of promoting children's access to and success in prosocial contexts while limiting their access to contexts that encourage or condone ASB. The family, often considered the fundamental crucible of socialization, is but one context among many that competes for the opportunity to influence developing youth. A case can be made for the unique role of the parent–child relationship in children's socialization (Maccoby, 1992), but parents and other adults also function as social managers and supervisors (Parke et al., 2002) who codetermine where and with whom children and adolescents spend their time.

Current efforts to explain how social contexts and contingencies shape individual growth in ASB cannot rely on Thorndike's simple law of effect (Cavell & Strand, 2003; Conger & Simons, 1997). Needed are recent applications of the "matching law," which holds that the probability of an individual performing a response tends to match the probability of being reinforced for the response relative to other, competing responses (McDowell, 1982, 1988). This conceptualization is more informational than mechanical: "Responses are selected rather than strengthened" (Snyder, Edwards, McGraw, Kilgore, & Holton, 1994, p. 319). Equally important for understanding the role of context is the "time allocation" component of the matching law, which posits that "time spent in an environment will also be relative to the rate of reinforcement provided by that environment" (Conger & Simons, 1997, p. 62). The distribution of reinforcing contingencies *within* a given context influences whether children perform ASB, but it is the distribution of reinforcing contingencies *across* social contexts that influences whether children spend time and energy in contexts that support ASB (Conger & Simons, 1997; Snyder et al., 1994). Accordingly, it becomes critical to consider the competing value of social contexts that differentially support prosocial versus antisocial activities.

The notion that children coconstruct their developmental experiences (Bell, 1968; Patterson, 1976; Shaw, Bell, & Gilliom, 2000) and selectively move in and out of various social niches is well documented, especially for antisocial youth (Dishion, Capaldi, Spracklen, & Li, 1995). Lagging behind are efforts to integrate fully the implications of these phenomena into models of socialization generally (Kuczynski, 2003) and ASB specifically (Cavell & Strand, 2003) and to use this information to enhance intervention outcomes. By definition, antisocial youth are a poor fit with prosocial contexts; they tend to find greater success in more deviant contexts. Most available interventions operate from frameworks that tend to underestimate the confluence of (1) children's individual differences, (2) their learning histories, and (3) the quality of available social contexts. Especially lacking are interventions that consider children's active pursuit of contexts that are both rewarding and deviant, or that recognize the difficulty of sustaining prosocial contexts that are both appealing and rewarding to antisocial youth. It might take a village to raise a child, but both need reason to keep at it or the two will soon part ways.

- *Short-term reductions in ASB are possible when antisocial youth actively participate in prosocial contexts.* Short-term reductions in ASB should follow directly from positive changes in the contexts in which children and adolescents participate. In line with the matching law, reductions in ASB are to be expected when children and adolescents spend more time and energy in contexts in which the rewards for acting in prosocial ways are greater than the rewards for using ASB. There are several ways to create such contextual changes.

Some changes in context are the result of formal intervention efforts. For example, it is not uncommon for troubled youth to be placed in facilities designed to be therapeutic and prosocial, including inpatient psychiatric hospitals, long-term residential treatment facilities, and therapeutic foster homes. There is the risk, of course, that antisocial youth will use these settings to engage in deviancy training (Dishion, McCord, & Poulin, 1999), but programs that effectively block youths' access to deviant contexts and that control available reinforcers should produce significant, short-term reductions in ASB (e.g., Hoefler & Bornstein, 1975). Parents can also create positive changes in context when they move families to a neighborhood or city that affords greater prosocial opportunities. Little is known about the benefits of such moves on youths' level of ASB. Studies have examined court-mandated placements in treatment foster care (e.g., Farmer, Wagner, Burns, & Richards, 2003) and the effects of children of teenage mothers living with other relatives (Holtan, Ronning, Handegard, & Sourander, 2005). However, with few exceptions (e.g., Eddy & Chamberlain, 2000), these studies have not involved children and teens placed in others' homes *because* of their ASB. What happens to troubled youth placed with a caring relative or neighbor? What happens to antisocial youth who emancipate or simply leave home, often to live with other disenfranchised youth? Informal changes in living arrangements are to be expected when family members feel frustrated and hopeless in the face of chronic ASB, but clinical researchers have lacked conceptual models that would prompt the study of such events.

Instead of moving children to a different context, a less restrictive intervention strategy is to alter the contexts in which children and adolescents typically participate (i.e., homes and schools). The most commonly used and frequently evaluated of these interventions is PMT, in which parents are taught to alter the contingencies that follow children's misbehavior (Kazdin, 2005). Studies find that PMT leads generally to significant *short-term* reductions in ASB (Brestan & Eyberg, 1998) and that enhanced parenting often predicts the level of treatment gains (Patterson, 2005; Patterson, DeGarmo, & Forgatch, 2004). Other home-based interventions target the entire family and assume that system-wide changes are needed (Minuchin, 1974; Nichols & Schwartz, 2004). Unclear at this point is whether the immediate positive outcomes from parent- and family-based interventions are due to improvements in parent-imposed contingencies, to changes in family-wide beliefs, to greater cohesion among family members, to structural changes in family hierarchy, or to other unrecognized factors (Nichols & Schwartz, 2004; Patterson, 2005; Strand & Cavell, 2005). Tests of hypothesized mediators are uncommon; rarer still are studies that test competing mediating mechanisms (Kazdin, 2005). From a matching law perspective, short-term reductions in ASB could simply reflect increases in the *overall* level of reinforcement in the home (Cavell, 2000; Hagopian, Crockett, van Stone, DeLeon, & Bowman, 2000). When the rate of reinforcement is low, children will use a range of behaviors—including verbal and physical aggression—to extract available reinforcers from the environment (McDowell, 1982, 1988). But when parents increase the total level of reinforcement in the home, they indirectly lower the relative value of coercive behavior. Recent studies also suggest that increased reinforcement would not have to be contingent upon children's use of "good" or "bad" behaviors to have this positive effect (e.g., Hagopian et al., 2000).

Another common intervention strategy is to alter the school or classroom context of difficult, antisocial students. Typically these interventions are implemented by teachers, school counselors, or school psychologists. An excellent example is the Good Behavior Game (GBG; Barrish, Suanders, & Wolf, 1969), an intervention that directly targets group contingencies that function to reward misbehavior. Instead of being rein-forced by peers for misbehavior, students are assigned to teams that earn rewards (e.g., free time, class party, and extra recess) when the collective behavior of team members meets certain criteria (Embry, 2002). Kellam, Ialongo, and colleagues (e.g., Ialongo et al., 1999) have documented the efficacy of the GBG in reducing the aggressive behav-ior of high-risk children. From a matching law perspective (Embry, 2002), the GBG re-duces the relative value of disruptive behavior in the classroom and increases the value of conforming to class rules. There are also empirically supported interventions that seek to modify the entire school context. For example, school-wide antibullying pro-grams have been found to reduce reported bullying and victimization (see Olweus, 1993; Smith, Pepler, & Rigby, 2004). Although programs vary, emphasis is generally placed on changing the contingencies that function to maintain bullying (e.g., raising awareness and consistently applying rules against bullying such behavior). Parents can also change a child's school context by requesting a transfer to a different classroom, grade, or school. There is a body of research that examines the effect of school changes on children's academic or social outcomes (e.g., Akos & Galassi, 2004), but less con-sideration has been given to the impact on students' involvement in ASB. One excep-tion is research suggesting that elementary students' ASB tends to rise or fall, depend-ing on the quality of the teacher–student relationship (Hughes, Cavell, & Willson, 2001), a finding that appears to be particularly true for disadvantaged, minority stu-dents (Meehan, Hughes, & Cavell, 2003).

Strategies for reducing ASB via changes in context appear to offer documented suc-cess as well as unexplored potential. Studies are needed that reflect an expanded view of the variety of contexts that promote ASB and that examine the malleability of those con-texts and the mechanisms accounting for their influence. Should practitioners encourage parents to move to communities that provide greater support for prosocial behavior? Can practitioners reliably predict when changes in community, neighborhood, or school con-texts will lead to reductions in ASB? Therapeutic folklore tends to dismiss the value of "geographical cures," casting such efforts as a denial of the "real" source of dysfunction (Chamberlain & Jew, 2003). However, such arguments are usually based on the notion that recurring patterns of problem behavior are due to forces within the individual and not to forces operating in the contexts in which he or she lives.

Two factors constrain the potential benefit of contextual changes on future ASB: dif-ficulties in sustaining extraordinary contextual changes and difficulties in sustaining anti-social youths' success in prosocial contexts. Treatment gains are typically lost when anti-social youth end their active participation in prosocial, therapeutic contexts (e.g., Kirigin, Braukmann, & Atwater, 1982); moreover, inpatient facilities typically offer short-term care, the composition of school classrooms changes every year, and intervention pro-grams that support struggling parents are often subject to funding constraints. There is also reason to question whether antisocial youth can effectively participate in prosocial contexts over an extended period of time. Succeeding in prosocial contexts is not deter-mined unilaterally (Snyder, Reid, & Patterson, 2003). A different school, the next grade, and a new community are all rich with potential, but children with little history of success in prosocial contexts and ample deficiencies in self-regulatory skills can be ill-equipped to take advantage of these opportunities. Studies assessing aggressive children's interactions with unfamiliar peers (Dodge, 1983) or unrelated adults (Dumas & LaFreniere, 1993) document how quickly these children recreate negative patterns of relating even when placed in new, more benign contexts. Youth with ASB could also experience waning enthusiasm for available rewards, growing fatigue from the pursuit of those rewards, or emotional and relational costs if they were to rely on long-standing coercive strategies to influence others. Parents, teachers, counselors, employers, and probation officers all bear witness to opportunities missed or "spoiled" by antisocial youth given a second chance in a new setting. So if special treatments and costly interventions are merely short-term solutions, is there hope for long-term reductions in ASB?

• *Long-term reductions in ASB are possible when antisocial children and adolescents (1) experience sustained success in prosocial contexts and (2) invest in systems of shared, prosocial commerce.* Achieving long-term reductions in ASB is essentially an exercise in socializing antisocial youth into systems that are based on shared, prosocial commerce (Richters & Waters, 1991). Unless antisocial youth invest time and energy in prosocial contexts, socialization attempts will fail or have only short-lived results. Youth engaged in late-onset ASB, by virtue of their previous successes in prosocial contexts, are more likely to benefit from and invest in prosocial contexts. If they can manage to avoid the "snares" of their adolescent foray into ASB (Moffitt, 1993, 2003), one would expect them to reengage in the workings of prosocial commerce. Early-onset antisocial youth, on the other hand, are less likely to seek, access, and effectively participate in contexts that are prosocial; their future is more foreboding. Nevertheless, intervention research shows that if they experience sustained success in prosocial contexts and buy into the assumptions that underlie prosocial systems, their chance of avoiding a chronic antisocial lifestyle is greatly enhanced (e.g., Vitaro et al., 2001).

Maintaining antisocial youths' active involvement in prosocial contexts requires practical and effective strategies for overcoming a number of obstacles. For example, antisocial youth are often drawn to contexts that actively promote (via peer reinforcement) or passively condone (via modeling) ASB, and monitoring youths' involvement in those contexts presumes accurate disclosure of their whereabouts (Kerr & Stattin, 2000). Restricting their access to deviant contexts is also difficult, particularly if youth are engaged in covert forms of ASB, (Snyder et al., 2003). Early-starting antisocial youth present additional challenges: They are hard to manage and hard to like. They struggle in settings that require prosocial commerce and interacting with them on a daily basis can be costly emotionally, physically, and financially (Cavell, 2000). Those who live or work with antisocial youth suffer the weight of their coercive actions. Over time, the task of sustaining a prosocial context becomes increasingly difficult and the adults "in charge" are likely to feel frustrated, fatigued, and hopeless. When this happens, emotional tension rises and the overall level of available reinforcement drops (McDowell, 1988; Patterson et al., 1992). The danger is that each participant will begin to rely on strategies that optimize his or her own, immediate outcomes, instead of investing in long-term outcomes that benefit the greater good. Thus it is reasonable to ask, "Are there stakeholders who could resist this tendency and persist in the task of socializing an antisocial child or adolescent?"

From an evolutionary standpoint, parents carry the greatest investment in their offspring's future (Clutton-Brock, 1991). It is not surprising, therefore, that effective and committed parents are considered a critical protective factor in the face of emergent ASB (Masten, 2001). Even parents who seem hopeless and defeated are still the principal stakeholders in their child's socialization. They have the burden of ensuring that children with early-onset ASB can readily access and benefit from their participation in prosocial contexts. Parents also have the challenge of restricting children's use of ASB and their involvement in contexts that promote ASB. Performing either task can be difficult, but doing both tasks more or less simultaneously for a period of 18+ years can be almost impossible (Cavell, 2000; Cavell & Strand, 2003). Accordingly, it becomes critical to provide parents with strategies that offer a reasonable chance of helping their antisocial child become a law-abiding citizen.

As discussed earlier, PMT programs that teach parents to alter the contingencies for child behavior are the most widely used and empirically supported interventions for aggressive and antisocial children (Kazdin, 2005). Developed in the late 1960s (e.g., Hanf, 1969), the PMT curriculum has gone relatively unchanged despite significant advances in our understanding of ASB (Cavell, 2000, 2001; Cavell & Strand, 2003) and despite concerns about the generalizability and durability of PMT's outcomes (see earlier discussion of PMT in the context of preventing delinquency). Limiting PMT is a heavy focus on the short-term management of children's misbehavior rather than their long-term socialization. A second limitation is that teaching parents to respond contingently to specific misbehaviors can ignore at times the overall quality of the parent–child relationship in which those misbehaviors occur (e.g., Christopherson & Mortweet, 2001). Stated differently, PMT has underemphasized the parent–child relationship as a useful vehicle for socializing antisocial children. These limitations have created a gap between what is known about the development of ASB and what is typically offered to parents. In response to this gap, Cavell (2000, 2001; Cavell & Strand, 2003) has called for an updated and expanded approach to parent-based interventions. His responsive parent therapy (RPT) model integrates empirically supported PMT treatment strategies with expanded knowledge about aggressive children and the challenges parents face. Central to the RPT model is a long-term, relationship-based view of socialization. From this perspective, parents' response to child misbehavior is not evaluated apart from the overall quality and sustainability of the parent–child relationship (Baumrind, 1971; Cavell, 2000, 2001; Dumas, 1996; Kuczynski & Hildebrant, 1997; Richters & Waters, 1991; Strand, 2000), a point underscored by recent links between childhood aggression and the quality of parent–child attachments (Moretti, DaSilva, & Holland, 2004). The RPT model is guided by 10 principles (Cavell & Strand, 2003):

1. The long-term socialization of ASB takes precedence over short-term behavior management.
2. The parent–child relationship is a useful vehicle for socializing antisocial children.
3. Socializing relationships provide antisocial children, over time, with emotional acceptance, behavioral containment, and prosocial values.
4. The ratio of emotional acceptance to behavioral containment is a key parameter of the socializing relationship.
5. Characteristics of the parent, the child, and the ecology surrounding the parent–child relationship affect the degree to which socializing relationships are established and maintained.
6. The primary goal of parent-based interventions for antisocial children is helping parents establish and sustain a socializing relationship.
7. Behavioral containment begins with strict limits on aggressive, antisocial behavior.
8. Emotional acceptance begins with an implicit message of belonging.

9. Prosocial values begin with explicit norms against antisocial behavior.
10. Effective parent-based interventions for antisocial children are multisystemic.

The parent–child relationship is a particular kind of social context. It involves biological connections, recurring interactions, enduring social roles, culturally laden meanings, and strong emotional investments. All things being equal, these attributes give the parent–child relationship distinct advantages in its competition with other, possibly deviant contexts (Maccoby, 1992) and contributes to the potential protective function of parenting, especially for ASB (see Masten, 2001). A long-term, relationship-based model of socialization also has advantages over models that emphasize the short-term management of child misbehavior and give a "time dimension" to parent–child interactions (Kuczynski & Hildebrandt, 1997). Many factors determine the outcome of a given parent–child interaction, and not all are present immediately before, during, or after the interaction. Parents and children have overlapping histories as well as shared expectations that can affect their future interactions. For children with early-onset ASB, the parent–child relationship is only one of many available contexts, but it remains a unique resource in the campaign to promote their integration into society.

RECOMMENDATIONS FOR FUTURE INTERVENTION STUDIES

Figure 2.1 illustrates key aspects of an integrated life course–social learning model on the relation between socialization and ASB. Highlighted is the role of context as well as the potential interactions between biogenetic and environmental risk factors. In this model, self-regulatory skills and the availability of prosocial as well as deviant contexts

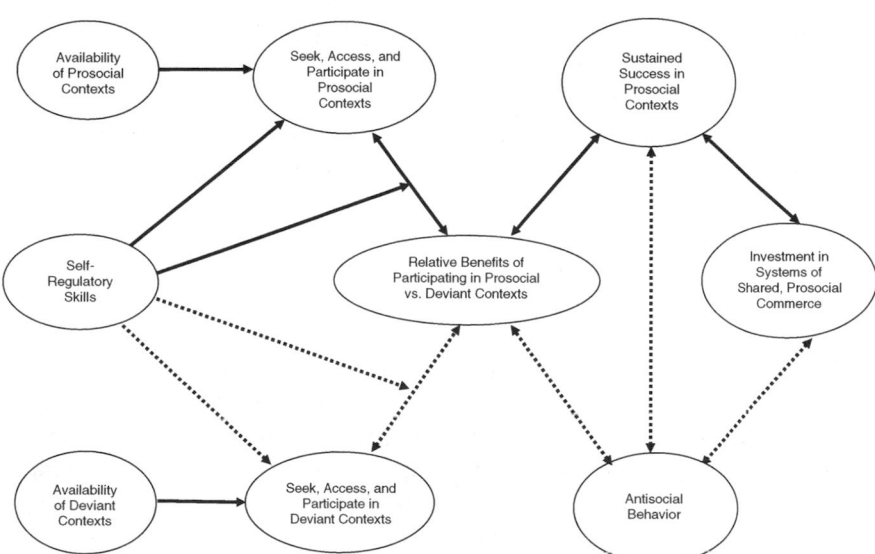

FIGURE 2.1. Integrated life course–social learning model depicting the relation between socialization processes and the development of antisocial behavior (ASB). Moderator effects are indicated by arrows pointing to a structural path rather than to a construct. Dotted lines indicate inverse relations.

codetermine the degree to which children seek, access, and participate in those contexts. Figure 2.1 also depicts the *interaction* between self-regulatory skills and children's participation in prosocial contexts—an interaction that determines the degree to which they benefit from more conventional contexts. In keeping with a matching law interpretation of environmental contingencies, benefits derived from prosocial contexts are only meaningful when considered relative to the benefits accruing from deviant contexts. Deficits in self-regulatory skills are thought to amplify the degree to which children find greater success in more deviant contexts, and children fitting this pattern are likely to be early starters on the path to chronic ASB. The extent to which children benefit from prosocial contexts (relative to deviant contexts) should affect their level of ASB. However, children's use of ASB is also a function of their sustained success in prosocial contexts and the degree to which they invest in systems of shared, prosocial commerce.

The heuristic value of this model lies in its ability to generate testable hypotheses and novel interventions. It should also reflect the existing literature on evidence-based practices. For example, interventions that promote and reward prosocial interactions among family members and classmates fit easily within the present model, as do family-based interventions that encourage parents to monitor and limit youths' associations with deviant peers. There is some support in this model for traditional skills-based interventions that teach troubled youth adaptive interpersonal and social cognitive skills, with the caveat that skill enhancement will be inadequate unless there are contexts to support the use of those skills. Moreover, children who lack basic self-regulatory skills will have more difficulty transporting targeted skills to prosocial contexts. This model also dovetails with research on newer, more promising interventions. For example, attempts by MST therapists (Henggeler et al., 1998) to intervene actively and directly in multiple social contexts could be seen by some as interesting but nonessential add-ons; under the current model, those efforts are cast as critical to altering ASB in delinquent youth. Also supported are efforts to remove delinquent youth from an established web of deviant activities and place them in therapeutic foster homes (e.g., Chamberlain, 2003). This strategy directly addresses concerns about availability of and access to prosocial versus deviant contexts. It also avoids the risks of iatrogenic effects stemming from the aggregation of deviant youth in a single treatment setting (Leve & Chamberlain, 2005). The model depicted in Figure 2.1 would question, however, the extent to which transitioning youth back into their original homes can be successful.

Are there newer, innovative interventions suggested by the points of emphasis in this model? Offered here is a sample of the possibilities.

• *Enhance children's self-regulatory skills via positive relationship experiences during infancy and toddlerhood.* Although children's self-regulatory skills are rooted in biogenetic processes, positive interactions with primary attachment figures could partially protect vulnerable infants from recurring problems with emotional dysregulation (Lyons-Ruth, 1996). For example, Lyons-Ruth (2004) considers parent–infant psychotherapy a strategy that could lessen attachment-related problems in high-risk mother–child dyads, and Tremblay (2003) has suggested that rough-and-tumble play and parent–child pretend play could equip high-risk children with the ability to experience, in a more controlled fashion, strong negative emotions. Similar notions have prompted Shaw, Dishion, and colleagues (Shaw, Gardner, Dishion, Supplee, & Wilson, 2005) to begin a multisite prevention trial targeting low-income mothers in families at risk for ASB. Based on studies demonstrating an inverse relation between mother–child joint play and later conduct problems (Gardner, Ward, Brown, & Wilson, 2003), their program emphasizes promoting mothers' capacity to participate effectively and frequently in joint play activities.

• *Increase availability of, access to, and success in prosocial contexts through the use of mentor-coaches.* For too many antisocial youth, access to prosocial contexts is limited because of economic or social impediments. Social disadvantage and prejudice conspire with mutual distrust and fear to keep many youth away from settings and opportunities that could enrich their developmental experiences. Also looming is the very real possibility that prosocial contexts will overwhelm children whose genetic endowment, learning history, and emerging social cognitions support a trajectory of early-onset ASB. The challenge is to develop strategies that can effectively overcome these obstacles. Cavell and Hughes (2004) proposed a strategy that integrates developmental psychopathology and positive youth development (PYD). The former helps explain the cumulative and transactional nature of children's risk profiles (Cicchetti & Toth, 1992), whereas the latter views problem behavior as "the absence of engagement in a positive life trajectory" (Larson, 2000, p. 170). Prevention scientists have begun to look to PYD for insights about protecting children against risk and promoting their healthy development (Catalano, Berglund, Ryan, Lonczak, & Hawkins, 1998; Larson, 2000). For example, Larson (2000) suggested that children's participation in structured voluntary activities is a particularly powerful determinant of their sense of initiative. He has also heralded the natural advantages that accrue when youth participate in "collaborative agency" with prosocial adults and peers.

Support for the role of PYD in prevention science comes primarily from data suggesting that positive developmental outcomes and problem behaviors share similar risk and protective factors (Catalano et al., 1998). Though logical, this notion rests on two untested assumptions: (1) that the frequency and quality of children's positive developmental achievements are alterable, and (2) that gains in positive development are functionally linked to negative developmental outcomes. These assumptions are fairly tenable when the focus is *universal* prevention and the majority of children or adolescents can readily access the benefits of positive socialization contexts. But these assumptions are more tenuous when the task is one of *selective* prevention and the target population is aggressive children or antisocial youth (Hughes et al., 2005). Cavell and Hughes (2004) proposed using a specialized mentoring program in which adult mentors are trained to shepherd and support antisocial children into prosocial settings that would otherwise be inaccessible and problematic (see also Herrera, 1999; Rhodes, Haight, & Briggs, 1999). Mentors could also coach children as they pursue the goals of a carefully chosen *personal project.* Cavell and Hughes used the term "purposeful collaborations" to describe this particular type of mentoring relationship. They proposed that support from mentor-coaches could directly enhance the degree to which target children achieve transactional success over the course of the intervention period and, in turn, develop more positive outcome expectancies about their ability to function in prosocial contexts. Transactional success and more benign outcome expectancies, coupled with active participation in purposeful collaborations, should also reduce children's involvement with deviant peers. The benefits of incorporating a PYD perspective into mentoring programs for high-risk children await empirical testing, but the approach proposed by Cavell and Hughes illustrates the value of rethinking traditional intervention models.

• *Enhance the quality of available prosocial contexts by yoking the twin tasks of restricting ASB and rewarding prosocial behavior.* Many are familiar with Baumrind's (1971) observation that authoritative parents use a style that is both responsive and demanding. Also familiar is the tendency for PMT programs to target both positive and disciplinary aspects of parenting (Eyberg, 1988; Forehand & McMahon, 1981; Webster-Stratton, 1990). However, the model of parenting that is implied (if not explicitly presented) in PMT is one that treats positive parenting and discipline practices in a piecemeal fashion. Parents are expected to use both, but rarely considered is the challenge of performing both tasks more or less simultaneously over time. The temporal and practical separation of these two parenting tasks can be particularly problematic for parents whose child is aggressive and antisocial. They struggle to restrict their child's use of coercion while not resorting to coercion themselves (Patterson et al., 1992).

As one solution to this dilemma, Cavell (2000, 2001; Cavell & Strand, 2003) suggested that parents yoke their disciplinary efforts to the level of positive emotional exchanges in the parent–child relationship. This recommendation is based, in part, on findings indicating that relationships are more stable and more adaptive when the proportion of positive emotional experiences consistently exceeds the proportion of negative emotional experiences (e.g., Dumas, 1996; Wahler, Herring, & Edwards, 2001). For example, Dumas (1996) found that mothers of nondisruptive children expressed positive affect toward their children about 80% of the time (a 4:1 ratio), whereas mothers of disruptive children expressed positive affect only 30% of the time. From a matching law perspective, a positive interaction ratio provides dyadic partners with an overall level of reinforcement that is sufficient enough to diminish the relative payoffs for aversive behavior (Hagopian et al., 2002; McDowell, 1982). The task of providing this kind of interaction ratio is conceptually similar to the task of providing a context in which the payoffs for acting in cooperative, prosocial ways is greater than the benefits of acting coercively.

Assuming the validity of such a ratio, it would appear that parents of antisocial children are operating within a kind of "quota system" in which efforts to manage child misbehavior are constrained by the need to maintain a proper balance of positive to negative exchanges. The notion that all parents are under the same quota system is likely to go unappreciated in families in which children are cooperative and high achieving and parents are characteristically even-tempered and deliberate. In those families, parents set high expectations, children meet those expectations, and the parent–child relationship is none the worse. But families whose high-risk children are vulnerable to early-onset ASB operate under a different set of childrearing conditions. The children are often uncooperative and coercive and parents tend to be inconsistent and emotionally reactive (Patterson et al., 1992). Typically added to this mix are economic stress, marital strife, poor schools, and neighborhood violence. Little wonder that frequent and extended chains of mutual coercion are common occurrences in these homes (Patterson, 1982). Empirically supported behavior management techniques will not eliminate entirely the tendency for antisocial children to display noncompliant and coercive behavior (Webster-Stratton, 1990). Needed, therefore, is a parenting approach that is forceful enough to contain the child's ASB but not so forceful that it spoils the affective quality of the parent–child relationship (see Cavell, 2000 and 2001 for possible strategies).

Strategies for maintaining a positive interactional balance could also be used by adults (e.g., teachers, coaches, and mentors) in other contexts. The GBG (Embry, 2002), for example, is an efficient way for teachers to establish and maintain a classroom context in which the payoffs for acting appropriately are explicitly and consistently greater than the benefits of being disruptive. Similarly, Friman, Jones, Smith, Daly, and Larzelere (1997) found that asking staff in a residential treatment facility to maintain a positive interactional ratio resulted in decreased disruptive behavior among adolescent residents. The notion that antisocial children can benefit from contexts in which discipline is yoked to the level of positive exchanges is intriguing, but further investigation is needed before practitioners can know if and when they should pursue such a goal.

• *Promote sustained success in prosocial contexts through enduring adult–child relationships.* For parents who are challenged by antisocial children, establishing an effective mix of disciplinary control and mutually positive exchanges will not be easy. Even more difficult is sustaining that mix over a period of years as children move through adolescence and into adulthood. Are there effective parenting strategies for parents of antisocial children that are practical and sustainable? Cavell (2000, 2001; Cavell & Strand, 2003) has recast this question as follows: "Under what conditions can a given parent and child live peaceably together over time with strict limits on ASB?" Drawing from a relationship-based view of parental influence (Kuczynski & Hildebrandt, 1997), Cavell recommends *minimal coverage* but *maximum sustainability* of the conditions necessary for a socializing relationship. It might be necessary, for example, for parents to adopt a disciplinary strategy that focuses very narrowly on containing aggression and other forms of coercion. This strategy is likely to be more realistic and developmentally relevant than the oft-recommended practice of punishing children's general noncompliance (Cavell, 2001). Because parents in high-risk families often have their own interpersonal and emotional difficulties (Patterson, 1997), they can also struggle with recommendations to interact more positively with their children. Rather than pushing these parents to engage in potentially positive interactions with their children, it might be better to promote the use of strategies that convey *implicit* messages of parental acceptance or belonging (Baumeister & Leary, 1995). For example, parents who sit rather quietly as their child watches a favorite TV show may not be seen as warm and involved, but they will also avoid being "harsh or rejecting." There might also be value in having parents schedule and script a limited number of activities or rituals that virtually guarantee a net positive exchange among family members (Cavell, 2000). Cavell (2000) has also suggested that sustaining a socializing relationship with an antisocial child is unlikely if parents do not engage in regular self-care. Regularly scheduled breaks from the job of parenting could prove to be a necessity for overwhelmed and struggling parents. Parents who combine all three strategies, very narrow disciplinary focus, implicit messages of belonging, and regularly scheduled self-care, might still have an atypical parent–child relationship, but they would also have a workable and sustainable plan for enhancing the socializing influence of the family context.

It would be unusual for adults who are *not* parents or guardians to commit to the goal of providing antisocial youth with a long-term, prosocial relationship. The few adults who would fill this role are typically paid for their services. For example, some long-term residential facilities offer supportive relationships with "therapeutic parents" (Shealy, 1995). A more recent phenomenon is the use of paid mentors for at-risk children (Friends of the Children, 2003). These mentors earn a salary commensurate with that of beginning school teachers for mentoring a small group of children from kindergarten till the end of 12th grade. The program has shown promise, despite its costs. Of course, a teacher's salary is no guarantee of continuity if the mentoring relationship is emotionally trying and the costs of leaving it are minimal. Even short-term mentoring relationships with mildly troubled youth are vulnerable to premature terminations. Rhodes, Grossman, and Resche (2000) found that 40% of mentoring relationships with children from single-parent homes ended prematurely (i.e., before the promised 1-year period). This finding is significant given that youth mentoring can actually be harmful when it ends early (Grossman & Rhodes, 2002) or when mentors' attendance is inconsistent (Karcher, 2005). Cavell and Hughes (2000) were able to reduce such risks by awarding college students academic credit when they finished the task of mentoring aggressive, high-risk children over a period of 18 months.

• Increase investment in systems of shared, prosocial commerce through activities that promote social bonding and interdependence. The benefits of sustained success in prosocial contexts are not limited to reductions in ASB. Also accompanying sustained success in prosocial contexts is greater investment in social networks and interpersonal relationships that are marked by mutual dependency and the valuing of prosocial exchange. This level of investment or initiative (Larson, 2000) can be observed behaviorally in the kinds of activities pursued (as well as in those avoided). Investment in prosocial commerce is also manifested in various social cognitive phenomena that likely contribute to recurring patterns of prosocial behavior. Included here are expectations for benign versus hostile interactions with others (Crick & Dodge, 1994), a sense of bonding to larger social institutions (Herrenkohl et al., 2003), and a social identity in which prosocial beliefs and values are clearly defined and internalized (Erikson, 1968; Larson, 2000). Typically these constructs are measured during childhood or adolescence, before the transition to adulthood. Scholars have recently expanded their developmental lens and begun to assess prosocial beliefs and identities in young adults, some of whom have a history of ASB during childhood or adolescence. For example, Kosterman et al. (2005) developed measures of constructive engagement, financial responsibility, and honesty, all negative correlates of crime and substance use. Measurement of these constructs was seen as a necessary step in building a science of social capital, citizenship, and positive adult development.

Informative are recent longitudinal studies predicting effective transitions to adulthood (Schulenberg, Sameroff, & Cicchetti, 2004). Not all researchers measure positive adult outcome variables, but commitment to prosocial pursuits (e.g., sustained romantic relationships, academic achievement, continuous employment, and occupational success) appears to be associated with desisting from previous involvement in ASB and with continued minimal involvement in ASB (e.g., Roisman, Aguilar, & Egeland, 2004; Schulenberg, Bryant, & O'Malley, 2004; Stouthamer-Loeber, Wei, Loeber, & Masten, 2004). There is even evidence that young adults with a history of early-onset ASB benefit from investing in systems of prosocial commerce, in particular work and romantic relationships between the ages of 21 and 23 (Roisman et al., 2004). Conversely, heavy involvement in deviant pursuits (e.g., substance abuse) during adolescence is generally predictive of maladaptive outcomes in early adulthood (e.g., Hussong, Curran, Moffitt, Caspi, & Carrig, 2004; Lahey, Loeber, Burke, & Applegate, 2005; Roisman et al., 2004; Stouthamer-Loeber et al., 2004). In keeping with the notion that long-term desistance from ASB requires fully investing in systems of shared, prosocial commerce, Lahey et al. (2005) found that youth who engaged in primarily *covert* forms of ASB were more likely as adults to have an antisocial personality disorder.

Research on successful transitions to adulthood focuses attention on positive developmental outcomes and broadens our thinking about the varied pathways that troubled youth follow once they take on new adult roles (Schulenberg et al., 2004). Ideally, this area of study will also lead prevention scientists to develop innovative strategies for promoting antisocial youths' investment in systems of shared, prosocial commerce. This will be difficult for antisocial youth who have little or no history of investing in prosocial relationships, activities, and organizations. Complicating the goal of building enduring connections and commitments to prosocial others is the fact that current interventions for antisocial youth often entail communing with other deviant youth—a strategy that risks iatrogenic outcomes (Dishion et al., 1999). But not all group interventions or treatment facilities are centers for deviancy training. Some long-term residential facilities, such as Boys and Girls Town (Handwerk, Field, & Friman, 2000), are capable of creating prosocial communities in which group contingencies support social cohesion, interdependence, and prosocial values. Boys and Girls Town also tries to maintain residents' investment in the community long after they graduate (www.girlsandboystown.org). Through various alumni association activities (e.g., newsletter, website, and reunion), graduates remain connected to one of the few prosocial contexts in which they enjoyed sustained success and enduring supportive relationships. Unfortunately, too many other youths in our society will search in vain for that same sense of community and interdependence (Slater, 1990).

Summary

The value of our proposed model is not in the success of these few recommendations; rather, it is in broadening how interventionists construe potential intervention targets and possible strategies for change. Parents are a primary socialization force and a critical protective factor for youth at risk for chronic ASB (Masten, 2001). But parents are not the only force, and it is imperative that researchers and prevention programmers consider the role of other socialization agents (e.g., teachers and mentors) and the power and allure of competing social contexts (e.g., peers and media). Fortunately, most children are not easily discouraged by the demands of prosocial contexts or strongly attracted to the thrill of deviant activities. For them, socialization involves moving with the social current and gathering momentum as they move forward developmentally toward good citizenship. Their parents are lucky, but this could change if their son or daughter becomes trapped by the snares of adolescent ASB (e.g., addiction, arrest, or sexually transmitted diseases).

Over a decade ago, Kazdin (1993) challenged interventionists to build innovative treatment models that were not tethered to outdated assumptions about the cause and course of ASB. Since then, the field has witnessed a number of impressive attempts to expand and improve interventions for antisocial youth. There is a risk, however, in becoming complacent about these recent gains. As discussed at the outset, there are misconceptions about what can and cannot be achieved by interventionists and too often those misconceptions become policy-related myths. Mindful of those risks, prevention scientists can further the goal of disseminating evidence-based programs while also clarifying the relation between socialization and ASB and explicating more fully and accurately the mechanisms that alter the serious risk trajectory of antisocial youth.

ACKNOWLEDGMENT

Support in preparing this chapter was provided to Shelley Hymel by the Canadian Institutes for Health Research.

REFERENCES

Akos, P., & Galassi, J. P. (2004). Middle and high school transitions as viewed by students, parents, and teachers. *Professional School Counseling, 7*(4), 212–221.

Alexander, J. F., Robbins, M. S., & Sexton, T. L. (2000). Family-based interventions with older at-risk youth: From promise to proof to practice. *Journal of Primary Prevention, 21,* 185–205.

American Psychiatric Association. (1994). *Diagnostic and statistical manual of mental disorders* (4th ed.). Washington DC: Author.

August, G. J., Lee, S. S., Bloomquist, M. L., Realmuto, G. M., & Hektner, J. M. (2004). Maintenance effects of an evidence-based prevention innovation for aggressive children living in culturally diverse urban neighborhoods: The Early Risers effectiveness study. *Journal of Emotional and Behavioral Disorders, 12*(4), 194–205.

Bank, L., Marlowe, J. H., Reid, J. B., Patterson, G. R., & Weinrott, M. A. (1991). Comparative evaluation of parent training for families of chronic delinquents. *Journal of Abnormal Child Psychology, 19,* 15–33.

Barkley, R. A. (2000). Commentary: Issues in training parents to manage children with behavior problems. *Journal of American Academy of Child and Adolescent Psychiatry, 39*(8), 1004–1007.

Barrish, H. H., Saunders, M., & Wolf, M. M. (1969). Good behavior game: Effects of individual contingencies for group consequences on disruptive behavior in a classroom. *Journal of Applied Behavior Analysis, 2,* 119–124.

Baumeister, R. T., & Leary, M. R. (1995). The need to belong: Desire for interpersonal attachments as a fundamental human motivation. *Psychological Bulletin, 117,* 497–529.

Baumrind, D. (1971). Current patterns of parental authority. *Developmental Psychology Monographs, 4,* 1–103.

Bell, R. Q. (1968). A reinterpretation of the direction of effects in studies of socialization. *Psychological Review, 75,* 81–95.

Berger, P., & Luckman, T. (1966). *The social construction of reality: A treatise in the sociology of knowledge.* Garden City, NY: Doubleday.

Biglan, A., Mrazek, P. J., Carnine, D., & Flay, B. R. (2003). The integration of research and practice in the prevention of youth problem behaviors. *American Psychologist, 58*(6–7), 433–440.

Birckmayer, J. D., Holder, H. D., Yacoubian, G. S., & Friend, K. B. (2004). A general causal model to guide alcohol, tobacco, and illicit drug prevention: Assessing the research evidence. *Journal of Drug Education, 34*(2), 121–153.

Borduin, C. M., Mann, B. J., Cone, L. T., Henggeler, S. W., Fucci, B. R., Blaske, D. M., et al. (1995). Multisystemic treatment of serious juvenile offenders: Long-term prevention of criminality and violence. *Journal of Consulting and Clinical Psychology, 63,* 569–578.

Botvin, G., Griffin, K., & Diaz, T. (2000). Preventing illicit drug use in adolescents: Long-term follow-up data from a randomized control trial of a school population. *Addictive Behaviors, 25,* 769–774.

Brestan, E. V., & Eyberg, S. M. (1998). Effective psychosocial treatments of conduct-disordered children and adolescents: 29 years, 82 studies, and 5,272 kids. *Journal of Clinical Child Psychology, 27,* 180–189.

Catalano, R. F., Berglund, M. L., Ryan, J. A. M., Lonczak, H. C., & Hawkins, J. D. (1998). *Positive youth development: Research findings on evaluations of positive youth development programs* (Technical report). Washington, DC: U.S. Department of Health and Human Services, National Institute for Child Health and Human Development.

Cavell, T. A. (2000). *Working with parents of aggressive children: A practitioner's guide.* Washington, DC: American Psychological Association.

Cavell, T. A. (2001). Updating our approach to parent training. I: The case against targeting noncompliance. *Clinical Psychology: Science and Practice, 8,* 299–318.

Cavell, T. A., & Hughes, J. N. (2000). Secondary prevention as context for assessing change processes in aggressive children. *Journal of School Psychology, 38,* 199–235.

Cavell, T. A., & Hughes, J. N. (2004). *Preventing substance abuse in antisocial 6th graders.* Unpublished manuscript, University of Arkansas.

Cavell, T. A., & Strand, P. S. (2003). Parent-based interventions for aggressive, antisocial children: Adapting to a bilateral lens. In L. Kuczynski (Ed.), *Handbook of dynamics in parent–child relations.* Thousand Oaks, CA: Sage.

Chamberlain, L., & Jew, C. (2003). Family assessment of drug and alcohol problems. In J. Karin (Ed.), *Handbook of couple and family assessment* (pp. 221–239). Hauppauge, NY: Nova Science.

Chamberlain, P. (2003). The Oregon Multidimensional Treatment Foster Care model: Features, outcomes, and progress in dissemination. *Cognitive and Behavioral Practice, 10*(4), 303–312.

Chamberlain, P., & Reid, J. B. (1998). Comparison of two community alternatives to incarceration for chronic juvenile offenders. *Journal of Consulting and Clinical Psychology, 66,* 624–633.

Chamberlain, P., & Rosicky, J. G. (1995). The effectiveness of family therapy in the treatment of adolescents with conduct disorders and delinquency. *Journal of Marital and Family Therapy, 21,* 441–459.

Christophersen, E. R., & Mortweet, S. L. (2001). *Treatments that work with children: Empirically supported strategies for managing childhood problems.* Washington, DC: American Psychological Association.

Cicchetti, D., & Toth, S. L. (1992). The role of developmental theory in prevention and intervention. *Development and Psychopathology, 4,* 489–493.

Clutton-Brock, T. H. (1991). *The evolution of parental care.* Princeton, NJ: Princeton University Press.

Cohen, A. (1998). The monetary value of saving a high-risk youth. *Journal of Quantitative Criminology, 14*(1), 5–33.

Coie, J. D., & Dodge, K. A. (1998). Aggression and antisocial behavior. In W. Damon & N. Eisenberg (Eds.), *Handbook of child psychology* (5th ed.): *Vol 3. Social, emotional, and personality development* (pp. 779–862). New York: Wiley.

Coie, J. D., Watt, N. F., West, S. G., Hawkins, J. D., Asarnow, J. R., Markman, H. J., et al. (1993). The science of prevention: A conceptual framework and some directions for a national research program. *American Psychologist, 48,* 1013–1022.

Collins, W. A., Maccoby, E., Steinberg, L., Hetherington, E. M., & Bornstein, M. (2000). Contemporary research on parenting: The case for nature *and* nurture. *American Psychologist, 55,* 218–232.

Collins, W. A., Maccoby, E., Steinberg, L., Hetherington, E. M., & Bornstein, M. H. (2001). Toward nature WITH nurture. *American Psychologist, 56,* 171–173.

Conduct Problems Prevention Research Group. (2002). The implementation of the Fast Track Program: An example of a large-scale prevention science efficacy trial. *Journal of Abnormal Child Psychology, 30,* 1–17.

Conduct Problems Prevention Research Group. (2004). The effects of the fast track program on serious problem outcomes at the end of elementary school. *Journal of Clinical Child and Adolescent Psychology, 33,* 650–661.

Conger, R. D., & Simons, R. L. (1997). Life-course contingencies in the development of adolescent antisocial behavior: A matching law approach. In T. P. Thornberry (Ed.), *Advances in criminological theory* (pp. 55–99). New York: Aldine.

Crick, N. R., & Dodge, K. A. (1994). A review and reformulation of social information-processing mechanisms in children's social adjustment. *Psychological Bulletin, 115,* 74–101.

DeGarmo, D., & Forgatch, M. S. (2005). Early development of delinquency in divorced families: Evaluating a randomized preventive intervention trial. *Developmental Science, 8,* 229–239.

Dishion, T. J., Capaldi, D., Spracklen, K. M., & Li, F. (1995). Peer ecology of male adolescent drug use. *Development and Psychopathology, 7,* 803–824.

Dishion, T. J., & Kavanagh, K. (2000). A multilevel approach to family-centered prevention in schools: Process and outcome. *Addictive Behaviors, 25*(6), 899–911.

Dishion, T. J., McCord, J., & Poulin, F. (1999). When interventions harm: Peer groups and problem behavior. *American Psychologist, 54,* 755–764.

Dodge, K. (1983). Behavioral antecedents of peer social status. *Child Development, 53,* 1386–1399.

Dodge, K. A., & Pettit, G. S. (2003). A biopsychosocial model of the development of chronic conduct problems in adolescence. *Developmental Psychology, 39,* 349–371.

Dortch, T. (2000). *The miracles of mentoring: The joy of investing in our future.* New York: Doubleday.

DuBois, D. L., Holloway, B. E., Valentine, J. C., & Cooper, H. (2002). Effectiveness of mentoring programs for youth: A meta-analytic review. *American Journal of Community Psychology, 30,* 157–197.

Dumas, J. (1996). Why was this child referred? Interactional correlates of referral status in families of children with disruptive behavior problems. *Journal of Clinical Child Psychology, 25,* 106–115.

Dumas, J. E., & LaFreniere, P. J. (1993). Mother–child relationships as sources of support or stress: A comparison of competent, average, aggressive, and anxious dyads. *Child Development, 64,* 1732–1754.

Eckenrode, J., Zielinski, D., Smith, E., Marcynyszyn, L., Henderson, C., Kitzman, H., et al. (2001). Child maltreatment and the early onset of problem behaviors: Can a program of nurse home visitation break the link? *Development and Psychopathology, 13,* 873–890.

Eddy, J. M., & Chamberlain, P. (2000). Family management and deviant peer association as mediators of the impact of treatment condition on youth antisocial behavior. *Journal of Consulting and Clinical Psychology, 68,* 857–863.

Elliott, L., Orr, L., Watson, L., & Jackson, A. (2005). Secondary prevention interventions for young drug users: A systematic review of the evidence. *Adolescence, 40* (157), 1–22.

Embry, D. D. (2002). The Good Behavior Game: A best practice candidate as a universal behavioral vaccine. *Clinical Child and Family Psychology Review, 5*(4), 273– 297.

Erikson, E. H. (1968). *Identity: Youth and crisis.* New York: Norton.

Eyberg, S. (1988). Parent child interaction therapy: Integration of traditional and behavioral concerns. *Child and Family Behavior Therapy, 10*(1), 33–45.

Farmer, E. M. Z., Wagner, H. R., Burns, B. J., & Richards, J. T. (2003). Treatment foster care in a system of care: Sequences and correlated of residential placements. *Journal of Child and Family Studies, 12,* 11–25.

Forehand, R., & Long, N. (1991). Prevention of aggression and other behavior problems in the early adolescent years. In D.J. Pepler & K.H. Rubin (Eds.), *Development and treatment of childhood aggression* (pp. 317–330). Hillsdale, NJ: Erlbaum.

Forehand, R. L., & McMahon, R. J. (1981). *Helping the noncompliant child: A clinician's guide to present training.* New York: Guilford Press.

Forgatch, M. S., & DeGarmo, D. S. (1999). Parenting through change: An effective prevention program for single mothers. *Journal of Consulting and Clinical Psychology, 67*(5), 711–724.

Foster, E. M., Dodge, K. A., & Jones, D. (2003). Issues in the economic evaluation of prevention programs. *Applied Developmental Science, 7*(2), 76–86.

Friends of the Children. (2003). *Northwest Professional Consortium (NPC) 2002–2003 annual evaluation report on Friends of the Children—Portland.* Portland, OR: Author.

Friman, P. C., Jones, M., Smith, G., Daly, D. L., & Larzelere, R. (1997). Decreasing disruptive behavior by adolescent boys in residential care by increasing their positive to negative interactional ratios. *Behavior Modification, 21,* 470–486.

Gardner, F., Ward, S., Brown, J., & Wilson, C. (2003). The role of mother-child joint play in the early development of children's conduct problems: A longitudinal observational study. *Social Development, 12,* 361–378.

Greenberg, M. T. (2004). Current and future challenges in school-based prevention: The researcher perspective. *Prevention Science, 5*(1), 5–13.

Grossman, J. B., & Rhodes, J.E. (2002). The test of time: Predictors and effects of duration in youth mentoring programs. *American Journal of Community Psychology, 30,* 199–219.

Grossman, J. B., & Tierney, J. P. (1998). Does mentoring work?: An impact of the Big Brothers/Big Sisters program. *Evaluation Review, 22,* 403–426.

Hagopian, L., Crockett, J., van Stone, M., DeLeon, I., & Bowman, L. (2000). Effects of noncontingent reinforcement on problem behavior and stimulus engagement: The role of satiation, extinction, and alternative reinforcement. *Journal of Applied Behavior Analysis, 33,* 433–449.

Handwerk, M. L., Field, C. E., Friman, P. C. (2000). The iatrogenic effects of group intervention for antisocial youth: Premature extrapolations? *Journal of Behavioral Education. 10,* 223–238.

Hanf, C. (1969). *A two stage program for modifying maternal controlling during mother–child (M–C) interaction.* Paper presented at the meeting of the Western Psychological Association, Vancouver, British Columbia.

Harris, J. R. (1995). Where is the child's environment? A group socialization theory of development. *Psychological Review, 102,* 458–489.

Harris, J. (1998). *The nurture assumption.* New York: Free Press.

Hazelrigg, M. D., Cooper, H. M., & Borduin, C. M. (1987). Evaluating the effectiveness of family therapies: An integrative review and analysis. *Psychological Bulletin, 101*(3), 428–442.

Henggeler, S. W. (2003). Advantages and disadvantages of multisystemic therapy and other evidence-based practices for treating juvenile offenders. *Journal of Forensic Psychology Practice, 3,* 53–59.

Henggeler, S. W., Schoenwald, S. K., Borduin, C. M., Rowland, M. D., & Cunningham, P. B. (1998). *Multisystemic treatment of antisocial behavior in children and adolescents.* Pacific Grove, CA: Brooks/Cole.

Herrenkohl, T. I., Hill, K. G., Chung, I., Guo, J., Abbott, R. D., & Hawkins, J. D. (2003). Protective factors against serious violent behavior in adolescence: A prospective study of aggressive children. *Social Work Research, 27*(3), 179–191.

Herrera, C. (1999). *School-based mentoring: A first look into its potential.* Philadelphia: Public/Private Ventures.

Hinshaw, S. P. (2002). Process, mechanism, and explanation related to externalizing behavior in developmental psychology. *Journal of Abnormal Child Psychology, 30,* 431–446.

Hoefler, S., & Bornstein, P. (1975). Achievement place: An evaluative review. *Criminal Justice and Behavior, 2*(2), 146–168.

Holtan, A., Ronning, J., Handegard, B., & Sourander, A. (2005). A comparison of mental health problems in kinship and nonkinship foster care. *European Child and Adolescent Psychiatry, 14,* 200–207.

Hood, K. K., & Eyberg, S. M. (2003). Outcomes of parent–child interaction therapy: Mothers' reports of maintenance three to six years after treatment. *Journal of Clinical Child and Adolescent Psychology, 32*(3), 419–429.

Hughes, J. N., Cavell, T. A., Meehan, B. T., Zhang, D., & Collie, C. (2005). Adverse school context moderates the outcomes of selective interventions for aggressive children. *Journal of Consulting and Clinical Psychology, 73*(4), 731–736.

Hughes, J. N., Cavell, T. A., & Willson, V. (2001). Further evidence of the developmental significance of the teacher-student relationship. *Journal of School Psychology, 39,* 289–302.

Hussong, A., Curran, P., Moffitt, T., Caspi, A., & Carrig, M. (2004). Substance abuse hinders desistance in young adults' antisocial behavior. *Development and Psychopathology, 16,* 1029–1046.

Ialongo, N., Werthamer, L., Brown, H. B., Kellam, S., & Wai, S. B. (1999). The effects of two first grade preventive interventions on the early risk behaviors of poor achievement and aggressive and shy behaviors. *American Journal of Community Psychology, 27,* 599–642.

Johnson, D. L. (1989). The Houston Parent–Child Development Center project: Disseminating a viable program for enhancing at-risk families. *Prevention in Human Services, 7*(1), 89–108.

Johnson, D. L., & Blumenthal, J. (2004). The parent–child development centers and school achievement: A follow-up. *Journal of Primary Prevention, 25*(2), 195–209.

Karcher, M. J. (2005). The effects of school-based developmental mentoring and mentors' attendance on mentees' self-esteem, behavior, and connectedness. *Psychology in the Schools, 42.* 65–77.

Kazdin, A. E. (1993). Treatment of conduct disorder: Progress and directions in psychotherapy research. *Development and Psychopathology, 5,* 277–310.

Kazdin, A. E. (2005). *Parent Management Training: Treatment for oppositional, aggressive, and antisocial behavior in children and adolescents.* London: Oxford University Press.

Kazdin, A. E., Siegel, T. C., & Bass, D. (1992). Cognitive problem-solving skills training and parent management training in the treatment of antisocial behavior in children. *Journal of Consulting and Clinical Psychology, 60,* 733–747.

Kerr, M. & Stattin, H. (2000). What parents know, how they know it, and several forms of adolescent adjustment: Further support for a reinterpretation of monitoring. *Developmental Psychology, 36*(3), 366–380.

Kirigin, K. A., Braukmann, C. J., & Atwater, J. D. (1982). An evaluation of teaching-family (achievement place) group homes for juvenile offenders. *Journal of Applied Behavior Analysis, 15*(1), 1–16.

Kosterman, R., Hawkins, J. D., Abbott, R. D., Hill, K. G., Herrenkohl, T. I., & Catalano, R. F. (2005). Measures of positive adult behavior and their relationship to crime and substance use. *Prevention Science, 6,* 21–33.

Krueger, R. F., Schmutte, P. S., Caspi, A., Moffitt, T. E., Campbell, K., & Silva, P. A. (1994). Personality traits are linked to crime among men and women: Evidence from a birth cohort. *Journal of Abnormal Psychology, 103,* 328–338.

Kuczynski, L. (2003). Beyond bidirectionality: Bilateral conceptual frameworks for understanding dynamics in parent–child relations. In L. Kuczynski (Ed.), *Handbook of dynamics in parent–child relations* (pp. 1–24). Thousand Oaks CA: Sage.

Kuczynski, L., & Hildebrandt, N. (1997). Models of conformity and resistance in socialization theory. In J. E., Grusec & L. Kuczynski (Eds.), *Parenting and the internalization of values: A handbook of contemporary theory* (pp. 227–256). New York: Wiley.

Lahey, B. B., Loeber, R., Burke, J. D., & Applegate, B. (2005). Predicting future antisocial personality disorder in males from a clinical assessment in childhood. *Journal of Consulting and Clinical Psychology, 73*(3), 389–399.

Larson, R. W. (2000). Toward a psychology of positive youth development. *American Psychologist, 55,* 170–183.

Leve, L. D., & Chamberlain, P. (2005). Association with delinquent peers: Intervention effects for youth in the juvenile justice system. *Journal of Abnormal Child Psychology, 33*(3), 339–347.

Lipsey, M. W. (1992). The effect of treatment on juvenile delinquents: Results from meta-analysis. In F. Lösel, D. Bender, & T. Bliesener (Eds.), *Psychology and law: International perspectives.* (pp. 131–143). Oxford: Walter De Gruyter.

Lochman, J. E. (1992). Cognitive behavioral intervention with aggressive boys: Three-year follow-up and preventive effects. *Journal of Consulting and Clinical Psychology, 60*(3), 426–432.

Lochman, J. E., & Wells, K. C. (2002). Contextual social-cognitive mediators and child outcome: A test of the theoretical model in the Coping Power Program. *Development and Psychopathology, 14,* 971–993.

Long, P., Forehand, R., & Wierson, M., & Morgan, A. (1994). Does parent training with young noncompliant children have long-term effects? *Behaviour Research and Therapy, 32*(1), 101–107.

Lyons–Ruth, K. (1996). Attachment relationships among children with aggressive behavior problems: The role of disorganized early attachment patterns. *Journal of Consulting and Clinical Psychology, 64*(1), 64–73.

Lyons-Ruth, K. (2004). Disorganized infant attachment strategies for helpless-fearful profiles of parenting: Integrating attachment research with clinical intervention. *Infant Mental Health Journal, 25*(4), 318–336.

Maccoby, E. E. (1992). The role of parents in the socialization of children: An historical overview. *Developmental Psychology, 28,* 1006–1017.

Mason, W. A., Kosterman, R., Hawkins, J. D., Haggerty, K. P., & Spoth, R. L. (2003). Reducing adolescents' growth in substance use and delinquency: Randomized trial effects of a parent-training prevention intervention. *Prevention Science, 4*(3), 203–212.

Masten, A. S. (2001). Ordinary magic: Resilience processes in development. *American Psychologist, 56,* 227–238.

McDowell, J. (1982). The importance of Herrnstein's mathematical statement of the law of effect for behavior therapy. *American Psychologist, 37,* 771–779.

McDowell, J. (1988). Matching theory in natural human environments. *Behavior Analyst, 11,* 95–109.

Meehan, B., Hughes, J., & Cavell, T. (2003). Teacher–student relationships as compensatory resources for aggressive children. *Child Development, 74*(4), 1145–1157.

Minuchin, S. (1974). *Families and family therapy.* Cambridge, MA: Harvard University Press.

Moffitt, T. E. (1993). Adolescence-limited and life-course-persistent antisocial behavior: A developmental taxonomy. *Psychology Review, 100,* 674–701.

Moffitt, T. E. (2003). Life-course-persistent and adolescence-limited antisocial behavior: A 10-year research review and a research agenda. In B. B. Lahey, T. E. Moffitt, & A. Caspi (Eds.), *Causes of conduct disorder and juvenile delinquency* (pp. 49–75). New York: Guilford Press.

Moffitt, T. E. (2005). The new look of behavioral genetics in developmental psychopathology: Gene–environment interplay in antisocial behavior. *Psychological Bulletin, 131*(4), 533–554.

Moretti, M., DaSilva, K., & Holland, R. (2004). Aggression from an attachment perspective. In M. Moretti, C. Ogders, & M. Jackson (Eds.), *Girls and aggression: Contributing factors and intervention principles* (pp. 41–56). New York: Kluwer Academic.

Nichols, M. P., & Schwartz, R. C. (2004). *Family therapy: Concepts and methods* (6th ed.). Boston: Allyn & Bacon.

Olds, D. L. (2002). Prenatal and infancy home visiting by nurses: From randomized trials to community replication. *Prevention Science, 3*(3), 153–172.

Olweus, D. (1993). *Bullying at school: What we know and what we can do.* Malden, MA: Blackwell.

Parke, R., Simpkins, S., McDowell, D., Kim, M., Killian, C., Dennis, J., et al. (2002). Relative contributions of families and peers to children's social development. In P. Smith & C. Hart (Eds.), *Blackwell handbook of childhood social development* (pp. 156–177). Oxford, UK: Blackwell.

Patterson, G. R. (1976). The aggressive child: Victim and architect of a coercive system. In E. Mash, L. Hamerlynck, & L. Handy (Eds.), *Behavior modifications and families* (pp. 267–316). New York: Brunner/Mazel.

Patterson, G. R. (1982). *Coercive family process*. Eugene, OR: Castalia.

Patterson, G. R. (1997). Performance models of parenting: A social interactional perspective. In J. E. Grusec & L. Kuczynski (Eds.), *Parenting and children's internalization of values* (pp. 193–226). New York: Wiley.

Patterson, G. (2005). The next generation of PMTO models. *The Behavior Therapist, 28*, 27–33.

Patterson, G. R., DeGarmo, D., & Forgatch, M. S. (2004). Systematic changes in families following prevention trials. *Journal of Abnormal Child Psychology, 32*, 621–633.

Patterson, G. R., Reid, J. B., & Dishion, T. J. (1992). *Antisocial boys: A social interactional approach*. Eugene, OR: Castalia.

Pettit, G. S., & Dodge, K. A. (2003). Violent children: Bridging development, intervention, and public policy. *Developmental Psychology. 39*, 187–188.

Pierce, E., Ewing, L. J., & Campbell, S. B. (1999). Diagnostic status and symptomatic behavior of hard-to-manage preschool children in middle childhood and early adolescence. *Journal of Clinical Child Psychology, 28*, 44–57.

Prinz, R.J., Blechman, E.A., & Dumas, J. E. (1994). An evaluation of peer coping-skills training for childhood aggression. *Journal of Clinical Child Psychology, 23*(2), 193–203.

Rhee, S. H., & Waldman, I. D. (2002). Genetic and environmental influences on antisocial behavior: A meta-analysis of twin and adoption studies. *Psychological Bulletin, 128*(3), 490–529.

Rhodes, J. E., Grossman, J. B., & Resche, N. L. (2000). Agents of change: Pathways through which mentoring relationships influence adolescents' academic adjustment. *Child Development, 71*, 1662–1671.

Rhodes, J. E., Haight, W. L., & Briggs, E. C. (1999). The influence of mentoring on the peer relationships of foster youth in relative and nonrelative care. *Journal of Research on Adolescence, 9*, 185–201.

Richters, J. E., & Waters, E. (1991). Attachment and socialization: The positive side of social influence. In M. Lewis & S. Feinman (Eds.), *Social influences and socialization in infancy* (pp. 185–214). New York: Plenum Press.

Roisman, G. I., Aguilar, B., & Egeland, B. (2004). Antisocial behavior in the transition to adulthood: The independent and interactive roles of developmental history and emerging developmental tasks. *Development and Psychopathology, 16*, 857–871.

Rutter, M. (2003a). Commentary: Causal processes leading to antisocial behavior. *Developmental Psychology, 39*, 372–378.

Rutter, M. (2003b). Crucial paths from risk indicator to causal mechanism. In B. B. Lahey, T. E. Moffitt, & A. Caspi (Eds.), *Causes of conduct disorder and juvenile delinquency* (pp. 3–24). New York: Guilford Press.

Sanders, M. R., Markie-Dadds, C., Tully, L. A., & Bor, W. (2000). The Triple P-Positive Parenting Program: A comparison of enhanced, standard, and self-directed behavioral family intervention for parents of children with early onset conduct problems. *Journal of Consulting and Clinical Psychology, 68*(4), 624–640.

Scarr, S. (1992). Developmental theories for the 1990s: Development and individual differences. *Child Development, 63*, 1–19.

Scarr, S., & Deater-Deckard, K. (1997). Family effects on individual differences in development. In S. S. Luthar, J. A. Burack, D. Cicchetti, & J. R. Weisz (Eds.), *Developmental psychopathology* (pp. 115–136). Cambridge, UK: Cambridge University Press.

Schaeffer, C. M., & Borduin, C. M. (2005). Long-term follow-up to a randomized clinical trial of Multisystemic Therapy with serious and violent juvenile offenders. *Journal of Consulting and Clinical Psychology, 73*(3), 445–453.

Schulenberg, J. E., Bryant, A. L., & O'Malley, P. M. (2004). Taking hold of some kind of life: How developmental tasks relate to trajectories of well-being during the transition to adulthood. *Development and Psychopathology, 16*, 1119–1140.

Schulenberg, J. E., Sameroff, A. J., & Cicchetti, D. (2004). The transition to adulthood as a critical juncture in the course of psychopathology and mental health. *Development and Psychopathology, 16*, 799–806.

Serketich, W. J., & Dumas, J. E. (1996). The effectiveness of behavioral parent training to modify antisocial behavior in children: A meta-analysis. *Behavior Therapy, 27*(2), 171–186.

Shaw, D. S., Bell, R. Q., & Gilliom, M. (2000). A truly early starter model of antisocial behavior revisited. *Clinical Child and Family Psychology Review, 3,* 155–172.

Shaw, D. S., Gardner, F., Dishion, T. J., Supplee, L., & Wilson, M. (2005). *A family based preventive intervention for toddlers at-risk for early conduct problems.* Paper presented at the Conference for the Society for Research on Child Development, Atlanta, GA.

Shealy, C. N. (1995). Outcomes of residential treatment: A study of the adolescent clients of Girls and Boys Town. *American Psychologist, 50,* 565–580.

Slater, P. (1990). *The pursuit of loneliness.* Boston: Beacon Press.

Smith, P. K., Pepler, D., & Rigby, K. (Eds.). (2004). *Bullying in schools: How successful can interventions be?* New York: Cambridge University Press.

Snyder J. J., Edwards, P., McGraw, K., Kilgore, K., & Holton, A. (1994). Escalation and reinforcement in mother-child conflict: Social processes associated with the development of physical aggression. *Development and Psychopathology, 6,* 305–321.

Snyder, J. J., & Patterson, G. R. (1995). Individual differences in social aggression: A test of a reinforcement model of socialization in the natural environment. *Behavior Therapy, 26,* 371–391.

Snyder, J., Reid, J., & Patterson, G. R. (2003). A social learning model of child and adolescent antisocial behavior. In B. B. Lahey, T. E. Moffitt, & A. Caspi (Eds.), *Causes of conduct disorder and juvenile delinquency* (pp. 27–48). New York: Guilford Press.

Stouthamer-Loeber, M., Wei, E., Loeber, R., & Masten, A. (2004). Desistance from persistent serious delinquency in the transition to adulthood. *Development and Psychopathology, 16,* 799–806.

Strand, P. S. (2000). Responsive parenting and child socialization: Integrating two contexts of family life. *Journal of Child and Family Studies, 9,* 269–281.

Strand, P. S., & Cavell, T. A. (2005). *Interrupting and preventing mindless parenting: An organizing theme for parent-based interventions for aggressive children.* Manuscript under review.

Szapocznik, J., & Williams, R. A. (2000). Brief Strategic Family Therapy: Twenty-five years of interplay among theory, research and practice in adolescent behavior problems and drug abuse. *Clinical Child and Family Psychology Review, 3,* 117–134.

Tate, D. C., Reppucci, N. D., & Mulvey, E. P. (1995). Violent juvenile delinquents: Treatment effectiveness and implications for future action. *American Psychologist, 50*(9), 777–781.

Taylor, T. K., Eddy, J. M., & Biglan, A. (1999). Interpersonal skills training to reduce aggressive and delinquent behavior: Limited evidence and the need for an evidence-based system of care. *Clinical Child and Family Psychology Review, 2,* 169–182.

Tolan, P. H., Guerra, N. G., & Kendall, P. C. (1995). A developmental-ecological perspective on antisocial behavior in children and adolescents: Toward a unified risk and intervention framework. *Journal of Consulting and Clinical Psychology, 63*(4), 579–584.

Tremblay, R. E. (2000). The development of aggressive behaviour during childhood: What have we learned in the past century? *International Journal of Behavioral Development, 24*(2), 129–141.

Tremblay, R. E. (2003). Why socialization fails: The case of chronic physical aggression. In B. B. Lahey, T. E. Moffitt, & A. Caspi (Eds.), *Causes of conduct disorder and juvenile delinquency* (pp. 182–224). New York: Guilford Press.

Vaillancourt, T., & Hymel, S. (2004). The social context of children aggression. In M. M. Moretti, C. L. Odgers, & M. A. Jackson (Eds.), *Girls and aggression: Contributing factors and intervention principles* (pp. 57–73). New York: Kluwer Academic.

Vitaro, F., Brendgen, M., & Tremblay, R. E. (2001). Preventive intervention: Assessing its effects on the trajectories of delinquency and testing for mediational processes. *Applied Developmental Science, 5*(4), 201–213.

Wahler, R. G., Herring, M., & Edwards, M. (2001). Co-regulation of balance between children's prosocial approaches and acts of compliance: A pathway to mother–child cooperation? *Journal of Clinical Child Psychology, 30,* 473–478.

Wandersman, A., & Florin, P. (2003). Community interventions and effective prevention. *American Psychologist, 58*(6–7), 441–448.

Webster-Stratton, C. (1990). Long-term follow-up of families with young conduct problem children: From preschool to grade school. *Journal of Clinical Child Psychology, 19,* 144–149.

Webster-Stratton, C. (1998). Preventing conduct problems in Head Start children: Strengthening parenting competencies. *Journal of Consulting and Clinical Psychology, 66*, 715–730.

Webster-Stratton, C., Reid, M. J., & Hammond, M. (2001). Preventing conduct problems, promoting social competence: A parent and teacher partnership in Head Start. *Journal of Clinical Child Psychology, 30*(3), 283–302.

Webster-Stratton, C., Reid, M. J., & Hammond, M. (2004). Treating children with early-onset conduct problems: Intervention outcomes for parent, child, and teacher training. *Journal of Clinical Child and Adolescent Psychology, 33*(1), 105–124.

Webster-Stratton, C., & Taylor, T. (2001). Nipping early risk factors in the bud: Preventing substance abuse, delinquency, and violence in adolescence through interventions targeted at young children (0 to 8 Years). *Prevention Science, 2*, 165–192.

Weisz, J. R., Weiss, B., Han, S. S., Granger, D. A., & Morton, T. (1995). Effects of psychotherapy with children and adolescents revisited: A meta-analysis of treatment outcome studies. *Psychological Bulletin, 117*, 450–468.

Woolfenden, S. R., Williams, K., & Peat, J. K. (2002). Family and parenting interventions for conduct disorder and delinquency: a meta-analysis of randomized controlled trials. *Archives of Disease in Childhood, 86*(4), 251–256.

PART II

Socialization within Biological Frameworks

CHAPTER 3

An Evolutionary Approach to Socialization

DAVID A. BEAULIEU and DAPHNE BLUNT BUGENTAL

Consideration of the outcomes of children as a function of their social history has traditionally made use of a standard socialization model—a perspective that draws from social learning theory, social cognition theory, and attachment theory. Within a largely independent literature, evolutionary psychologists have investigated social influence by emphasizing the role of evolved adaptations in creating the platform and pathways for social influence.

In this chapter, we begin by discussing the basic formulations of evolutionary psychology. We then go on to explain how those formulations have been (or may be) employed in accounting for social influence processes within the different domains of social life. In doing so, we focus on the evolutionary factors that contribute to the basic *design* (or biological platform) of socializing relationships—from the standpoint of both those who are the recipients and those who are the purveyors of socializing influences. We then consider the ways in which evolutionary forces serve to channel the outcomes of socialization efforts. On the one hand, children show high sensitivity to early social experience and often manifest *privileged learning* (i.e., acquiring particular kinds of information with exceptional ease). On the other hand, children may show high resistance to other kinds of social influence—resistance that often makes little sense in terms of their outcomes in the present world but which may be understood as adaptive in our evolutionary past. Finally, we argue for the advantages of integrating the standard socialization and evolutionary approaches in providing a more complete account of the processes that occur within the socialization of the young.

FORMULATIONS OF EVOLUTIONARY PSYCHOLOGY

Before turning to the application of evolutionary theory to socialization processes, it may be useful to consider some of the basic concepts of evolutionary psychology, along with the terminology employed therein.

Proximate versus Ultimate Causation

An important distinction between standard socialization theory and evolutionary approaches to socialization involves the different levels of causal analysis they employ. Standard socialization theory focuses on proximate causation (including both immediate causation within socializing transactions and causal influences that have occurred across the course of development). In contrast, evolutionary theory gives greater attention to ultimate causation (i.e., adaptations that evolved across our ancestral past).

Proximate explanations focus on ontogeny. Such explanations focus on the ways in which observed responses can be accounted for by socialization, development, or genetic factors. In contrast, ultimate explanations focus on how observed behavior can be explained by forces in our evolutionary past. In utilizing evolutionary explanations, social scientists are concerned with both (1) the phylogenetic history of a response pattern (exploring patterns shown both across and within species) and (2) the adaptive advantage of that response pattern within the organism's evolutionary past. Joint consideration of proximate explanations and ultimate explanations affords the possibility of a more complete explanation of human processes (Dewsbury, 1999).

The Principles of Evolutionary Psychology

Within evolutionary psychology, the ultimate causation that drives all other processes is that of reproductive success. This concept is definitional in nature (the terminology should not be misunderstood as implying a "goal"). That is, any genetic change that appears within one generation will only be passed on to future generations if the carriers of that change mate successfully and have progeny who themselves mate and bear healthy offspring (and thus allow the replication of those altered genes). In some cases, a change will emerge as an *adaptation*. An adaptation is the evolutionary selection of genetic variation(s) that demonstrate better ways of *solving* a problem associated with survival and/or reproduction. For instance, in solving problems associated with avoiding predators, these "better solutions" may involve an altered structural feature (e.g., a change in coloration that leads to better camouflage) or an altered behavior (e.g., enhanced sensitivity to the gaze of others which leads to a greater ability to predict the actions of one's adversary). When the carriers of this change go on to successfully leave descendants (more successfully than those who do not carry this change), the altered gene is passed along—and thus we speak of *reproductive success*.

It is important to point out that not all changes that persist represent adaptations. In earlier times, there was a tendency to draw the conclusion that any observed change must have served an adaptive function. However, some changes occur simply as a by-product of some other adaptive process (e.g., the residual belly button that appears as a by-product of the placenta) or as "genetic noise" (e.g., random variations in the size or shape of belly buttons).

Evolutionary Trade-Offs

Adaptations and the implementation of adaptations involve trade-offs (e.g., Dawkins, 1982). In our evolutionary past, individuals, in order to have been *reproductively successful* (i.e., pass on their genes), would have needed to divide their energies, time, and resources among many competing problems. Although all such efforts served the same basic ultimate function (i.e., survival and reproduction), the immediate function would have varied (selecting food, avoiding predators, etc.) (e.g., Symons, 1992). The reproductively successful individual would have constantly balanced his or her allocation of time, effort, and resources in solving the competing problems that were continuously faced across their life history. There would have been no "absolute solutions"—only a series of optimal solutions within different times and contexts. The individual's task would have been to strategically manage the trade-offs faced in directing time, effort, and resources in solving one problem as opposed to solving another problem. The allocation of exceptionally high efforts to self-maintenance and self-protection would have limited the ability to allocate effort to reproductive activity. Likewise, the allocation of exceptionally high effort in mating activity would have limited the availability of efforts for either self-maintenance or care of the young.

Although adaptations must always be understood as applicable to our evolutionary past, evolutionarily minded research remains important because those adaptations continue to strongly influence our cognitions, emotions, and actions today. As an example, most Western parents discover (to their dismay) that their very young children strongly resist nighttime separation from parents, in particular in a room by themselves. They are in actual fact perfectly safe under these circumstances in present times. However, in our evolutionary past, even brief separations were life-threatening by virtue of the constant threat from predators. Therefore, it was essential that infants and young children vigorously signal their parents in ways that strongly motivated the maintenance of continuous contact. As such, natural selection selected an *evolutionary design* (the term used to describe mechanisms that are effective in solving specific adaptive problems) that would ensure the safety of young throughout the night.

Common Misconceptions Concerning Evolutionary Psychology

It is a common belief that evolutionary psychology must necessarily rely on post hoc interpretations of observed actions. If this were indeed true, any of the explanations offered by evolutionary psychology could be written off as unfalsifiable. However, as noted by Ketelaar and Ellis (2000) in a review of this position, evolutionary psychology clearly adheres to the Lakatosian philosophy of science. That is, it demonstrates the ability to explain anomalies and generate novel predictions and explanations. In contemporary evolutionary psychology, predictions are typically made for commonly observed behaviors or beliefs that seem counterintuitive and that cannot easily be explained by rival predictions drawn from other theoretical perspectives. Those predictions may then be subjected to experimental tests. Evidence is provided when individuals show a unique and predicted response to a problem for which there is believed to be a specialized adaptation—a response that is not explainable by competing theoretical positions.

Another misunderstanding about evolutionary thought is that it is deterministic (i.e., that it implies genetically controlled evolutionary designs that cannot be overcome). This argument is flawed on several levels. At the most basic level, it fails to recognize that contemporary evolutionary psychology is concerned not with single designs for solving adaptive problems but with alternative designs for solving adaptive problems in different ecologies (i.e., environmental variations that have occurred repeatedly across our evolutionary history). That is, contemporary evolutionary theory proposes that organisms are designed for accommodation to different environments. From this perspective, social decisions (e.g., the care of the young) are based on evolved mechanisms that make use of environmental information from the broader ecology (e.g., presence of resources) and the individual's immediate social environment (e.g., the presence of supportive others). At a second level, the argument that evolutionary psychology implies genetic determinism is flawed in that it fails to note that learning processes themselves represent important adaptations. Evolutionary psychologists believe that the child comes into the world "prepared to learn"; however, they also maintain that some kinds of information are acquired more easily than others. Language acquisition represents a classic example (Chomsky, 1965). That is, children are "prepared" to learn whatever language they are exposed to as they grow up. This acquisition process occurs easily as a spontaneous outcome of social interaction and is not influenced by the principles of association or reinforcement. In contrast, there is no evolutionary design for reading (a relatively recent development); that is, children are not "prepared" to read. Literacy is acquired with considerable difficulty and as a result of the specific tuitional efforts of others. In both cases, however, the child's behavior changes as a result of experience.

Development is conceptualized (from an evolutionary perspective) as involving bidirectional relationships between biological and experiential factors (e.g., Bjorklund, Yunger, & Pellegrini, 2002). This process is not only important in understanding the child's behavior, it is also important in understanding changes at the level of the brain. Thus, the brain is designed to be "experience-expectant" in its initial design (i.e., showing a specialized sensitivity to particular types of experience) and "experience-dependent" (i.e., alterable as a function of particular types of life experiences). As a simple example, infants are designed to "expect" protective care. In actual fact, the levels of protective care they receive will be variable. Although most mothers may be highly responsive to the attention bids of the young, others will be less responsive (e.g., mothers who are depressed). In the latter case, children show exceptionally high levels of cortisol production (Bugental, Martorell, & Barraza, 2003), along with heightened levels of fearfulness (Pauli-Pott, Mertesacker, & Beckman, 2004). Although the child's reaction may represent a conditional adaptation (i.e., an optimal strategy for receiving care within a particular environment), their experiences also act back to influence the developing brain (as a manifestation of the "experience-dependent" brain). Although the focus of attention has primarily been on the design of the brain to "expect" events that have commonly occurred across our evolutionary history, it should also be understood that the brain (through selective gene expression, i.e., the transcription of information encoded in DNA into RNA, and subsequently translated into messenger RNA) is responsive to relevant events that actually occur within the individual's lifetime (Bruer & Greenough, 2001).

When this feature of evolutionary design is recognized, it can be seen that evolutionary thought is compatible with efforts to improve the life experiences of the young. One of the best ways to design remedial programs is to consider how changes can be produced in ways that are consistent with our evolutionary design. We return to this point when we talk about young children's sensitivity to social context.

EVOLUTIONARY DESIGN: PREPARATION FOR
AND REGULATION OF SOCIALIZATION

Consistent with its focus on ultimate causation, evolutionary psychology has been concerned with the ways in which our evolutionary history has prepared us for those social interactions that may be thought of as the medium for socialization. Across our evolutionary history, humans (and other species) have faced adaptive problems—problems that were ultimately solved through the evolutionary selection of specific adaptations. The implementation of these adaptations may be thought of as involving systematic variations in algorithms. Increasing attention has been given to the ways in which such algorithms or computational processes serve to organize various types of human relationships.

In this section, we consider the various notions that have been proposed in conceptualizing human relationships as involving distinctive domains. We then go on to describe some of the evolutionary processes that appear to influence the basic design of such domains, that is, the ways in which our shared genetic history prepares us for receptivity to the many facets of the social world. In doing so, we organize the available evidence in terms of the domains that are most relevant for socialization processes (protective care relationships; reciprocal/mutual relationships; coalitional relationships; and hierarchical power relationships).

Social Domains

As a definitional statement, social domains have been conceptualized as representing bodies of knowledge that act as guides to partitioning the world and that facilitate the solving of recurring problems faced by organisms within that world (Hirschfeld & Gelman, 1994). The greatest significance of this general approach for socialization theory is the implied need for different types of social receptivity, cognitive representation, emotional/motivation processes, and behaviors within different social domains.

The five domains that have most consistently been proposed are:

1. *Protective care:* Interaction within this domain is organized by mechanisms (e.g., proximity–maintenance) that provide for the safety and feeding of dependent offspring.
2. *Hierarchical power:* Interaction within this domain involves the management of control between individuals who differ in social dominance and resource holding potential.
3. *Coalition formation:* Interaction within this domain is organized to facilitate the establishment and maintenance of shared benefits within an in-group, and shared defense against threat from outsiders.
4. *Reciprocity/mutuality:* Interaction within this domain involves the regulation of matched benefits between functional equals.
5. *Mating:* Interaction within this domain serves to facilitate the selection and protection of access to high-value sexual partners.

The exact nature of social domains has been conceptualized in somewhat different ways by different theorists. For example, Fiske (1992) conceptualized domains in terms of domain-specific grammars or scripts and as representing natural categories. He also proposed that computational processes within different domains make use of different scaling systems. For example, he suggests that authority-ranked relationships (referred to here as hierarchical power) make use of an ordinal scale. Relationships that are "equality-matched" (referred to here as relationships based on reciprocity/mutuality) make use of equal-interval scales. Relationships that involve communal sharing (encompassing the domains of protective care and coalitional groups identified here) make use of nominal scales. Fiske proposed that different domains come online at different points in the course of development. Thus, communal sharing emerges very early, authority-ranked processes emerge next, and equality-matched relationships appear still later. The concepts and evidence provided by Fiske draw both from social cognition theory and anthropology, as well as more tangentially from evolutionary psychology.

Bugental (2000) proposed that the domains of social life are managed by distinctive algorithms. In addition, she suggested that there are distinctive developmental and (suites of) neurohormonal processes across domains. For example, preparation for some domains begins prenatally (and is organized through the involvement of prenatal hormones) whereas other domains are not fully instantiated until middle childhood (and are regulated by the changing hormones during this time period). In addition, she proposed that the functioning of different domains can be modified (within limits) as a result of (1) the characteristics of the particular environment, (2) the schematic representation of relationships acquired as a result of early experience within different social domains, and (3) socialization. In short, the social brain (as an organizer of domains) is both experience-expectant and experience-dependent. Thus the model draws from social cognition theory, socialization theory, and behavioral neuroscience as well as evolutionary psychology.

Kenrick, Li, and Butner (2003) have proposed that there are qualitatively different decision rules in domains organized around different social goals. In doing so, they integrated concepts from dynamical systems theory (which involves the study of complex, multicomponent systems) and evolutionary psychology. They suggested that the decision processes within different domains are expressed through a dynamic interplay between decision mechanisms and the decisions of others who occupy their social network. Ultimately, new patterns of social behavior emerge from the combined functioning of all the components within the system. Unlike other theorists concerned with domains, they proposed different domains for acquisition processes (e.g., formation of coalitional groups and mate selection) and maintenance processes (e.g., maintenance of coalitional groups and mate retention).

Panksepp and his colleagues (e.g., Panksepp, Nelson, & Bekkedal, 1997) have approached the topic of social domains from a behavioral neuroscience perspective. Within their system, attention is directed to the neurohormonal responses that are associated with the regulation of interpersonal responses in the domains of juvenile play, panic/acceptance (which combine within attachment relationships), lust, and social dominance. Although the empirical work of these investigators makes use of nonhuman models, their intended application is to human processes.

Across these approaches, social relationships can be seen as contingent upon the particular tasks to be accomplished at a particular time in a particular setting. In short, domain-specific processes operate according to "if/then" contingencies rather than as constant factors (consistent with the thinking of Mischel & Shoda, 1995). Relationships between the same individuals may operate according to different "rules" if the nature of the relationship or the context changes. For example, socialization processes between a given parent and child may be governed by protective care mechanisms when the child is highly dependent (a condition that occurs frequently in infancy but may recur at later times of stress). In contrast, the conflicts that emerge between the parent and the same child as a toddler (or early adolescent) may more typically invoke mechanisms from the hierarchical power domain; that is, the control previously held by parents must be renegotiated as the child acquires increasing resources, dominance, or capacity for autonomous action. Alternatively, when parents are involved in collaborative work or play, they may—for that time period—act as functional equals and coordinate their actions in a mutual, reciprocal manner. At other times, the parent–child interaction may be based on the dyad's shared identity as a family or community member. In this case, socialization may revolve around the young child's intrinsic motivation to acquire the rules and procedures of group life and the parent's motivation to prepare them for group life.

Across models, there is a shared concern with "default" mechanisms in computing information relevant to different social tasks and responding to that information at a behavioral, physiological, and decision-making level. This reflects the notion that we are "designed" by our evolutionary history for certain kinds of social interactions. At the same time, we are also designed for adaptive variations to environments that have occurred repeatedly across our evolutionary history. We focus here on the four social domains that are most relevant to socialization (protective care, hierarchical power, coalition formation, and reciprocity/mutuality). Although socialization processes ultimately come to influence mating relationships, concern with such effects is a growing area of research.

Protective Care Domain

Evolutionary psychology has directed primary attention to one particular domain of social life: protective care. As evolutionary formulations are best developed and empirical evidence is greatest within this domain, we focus our primary attention here on processes that operate within this type of relationship.

Attachment Theory

The earliest thoughts with respect to the evolutionary origins of protective care were put forward by Bowlby (1969, 1973, 1980). Together with the formulations and research of Ainsworth (e.g., Ainsworth, Blehar, Waters, & Wall, 1978) and Harlow (e.g., Harlow & Harlow, 1965), Bowlby's ideas challenged prevailing views regarding the nature of early relationships between parents and the young. That is, a challenge was offered to the view that children show a special attraction to their parents as a direct result of the benefits those parents provide (explainable either in terms of learning theory notions of "secondary reinforcement" or the psychoanalytic concept of cathexis). From this standpoint, children would not be attracted to parents who were poor providers of sustenance. The combined work of these investigators demonstrated that this was indeed not the case. Instead, the infant's attachment to the primary caregiver was explainable in terms of the child's attraction to the stimulus features of the mother rather than her provision of sustenance. This view was more consistent with an evolutionary position suggesting that infants respond selectively to stimulus features that are normally associated with their biological mother, the individual most likely to provide for their needs.

For humans, the basic adaptive problem to be solved by the attachment relationship was the provisioning of protection and care for highly dependent offspring (i.e., offspring who are relatively more dependent than the offspring of other primate mothers). With the evolution of upright posture (and the resultant freeing of the arms for weight-bearing), there were associated constraints in the design of the human torso that led to a relatively small birth canal. This in combination with the relatively large brains of *Homo sapiens* led to the evolutionary selection of progeny who were born with relatively small heads and *immature* brains. As a result, the young would be born in a state of dependence which exceeds that of most other primates (Bogin & Smith, 2000). To solve this adaptive problem a two-person algorithm was needed in which the young sought care and safety from their biological mother, and the mother in turn was motivated to provide care and safety to her biological offspring. The attachment process has been found to be regulated by relevant social cues (the specific appearance, touch, smell, etc., of the other individual in the dyad) and operating primarily in the service of safety (e.g., Goldberg, Grusec, & Jenkins, 1999). At the same time, the attachment relationship also affords benefits in terms of facilitated access to sustenance and acquisition of social skills and understanding. Attachment theory has historically fallen outside the purview of socialization theory (e.g., as reflected in the separate consideration given to attachment theory and socialization theory in the 1983 *Handbook of Child Psychology* [Hetherington, 1983] as well as the comment by Maccoby and Martin [1983], "A major change that occurs in the second year of life is a qualitative one: the onset of socialization pressure" [p. 36]). Nevertheless, attachment represents a social domain in which the child acquires a working model of caregiving relationships—a model that typically comes to influence the child's own actions when he or she becomes a caregiver (e.g., Waters, Merrick, Treboux, Crowell, & Albersheim, 2000). Thus, the experiences associated with attachment can be understood as influencing the child's long-term outcomes.

Design for Sensitivity to Protective Care

Children may be thought of as designed by their evolutionary history to "expect" social interaction as a whole and parental care in particular. On the first day of life, infants show a heightened interest in facial patterns that are species-specific (eyes, nose, and mouth in a particular arrangement; Goren, Sarty, & Wu, 1975; Maurer & Salapatek, 1976). In addition, they quickly come to recognize (even prenatally) the vocal properties of their parents in a manner that involves "privileged learning" (i.e., an unusual facility in acquiring this kind of information; DeCasper & Fifer, 1987). Across infancy, they operate in a manner that is synchronized with their changing needs. For example, at about the age they would ordinarily begin to crawl (and thus move away from the safe haven offered by the mother), they become increasingly wary of strangers and respond with increasing physiological and psychological distress, which is ultimately reflected in their distress signals.

Evolutionary theorists have proposed that very young children show a unique sensitivity to their early environment. Boyce and Ellis (2005) suggested that the context sensitivity shown by young children allows for the manifestation of "conditional adaptations," that is, adaptations that evolved as a means of calibrating the developing stress response system of the young to match the characteristics of the environment.

This context sensitivity may lead to vigilance to the possibility of threat (in a dangerous world) or to sensitivity to positive social support (in environments that provide protection).

Boyce and Ellis went on to consider the processes that may mediate and moderate the child's future outcomes. They suggested that if children experience chronic levels of early adversity (which includes harsh parenting), they are more likely to show chronic upregulation of their stress response systems. They also predicted that exposure to supportive early environments upregulates sensitivity to the social benefits of those environments. Ellis, Essex, and Boyce (2005) have obtained preliminary support for the prediction that the highest levels of reactivity (as measured in this study by cardiovascular reactivity to laboratory challenges) are shown by children who experience either highly stressful or highly protective early environments.

Belsky, Steinberg, and Draper (1991) have suggested that children make use of cues from their environment (without awareness) in ways that influence their later development. That is, the child's early life history may be seen as diagnostic with respect to the nature of the world that they may anticipate as adults. If, for example, children are reared without a father, the absence of protection might suggest the possibility that the world is dangerous and poses many hazards. In this case, their reproductive success (in our evolutionary past) would have best been achieved by following short-term strategies in their relationships with others, including their mating strategies (a strategy that may lead to a high level of mating activity and early parenting but does not ensure high-quality care of the young). Although there has been rather consistent evidence that children reared under high threat conditions do reach sexual maturity at a younger age than children who receive greater protective care, the hormonal route through which this process occurs is unclear. In addition, it has been suggested that there is better evidence for the role of supportive parental care as a predictor of delayed puberty than for the role of a harsh environment as a predictor of early puberty (Ellis, McFadyen-Ketchum, Dodge, Pettit, & Bates, 1999). In short, these theoretical notions are still in need of further empirical investigation before the processes involved can be fully understood.

Parental Investment Theory

Early evolutionary views of the attachment relationship between caregivers and the young were later expanded to include notions of parental investment. Parental investment as a whole consists of the amount of time and effort that is expended in the care of progeny (in comparison with the time and effort expended in other competing interests). As the most basic feature, it involves the provision of shelter and sustenance. Beyond this, there are many other ways in which mothers (in particular) may manifest their investment in the young. For example, Keller (2000) proposed that investment may include body contact and carrying, stimulus provision, and face-to-face contact. In modern industrial societies, cultural processes build on the basic features of parental investment. For example, at older ages, parental investment extends to other kinds of involvement with the child (e.g., reading, expressing concern and emotional support; monitoring the child's activities; and providing guidance in social values; Burgess & Drais, 1999) as well as the management of the child's social and educational opportunities (Parke & Buriel, 2006).

SEX DIFFERENCES IN INVESTMENT

An initial concern of evolutionary psychologists was the different ways that males and females (in our evolutionary past) would have best served their own reproductive success in their investment decisions (Buss, 1994; Trivers, 1972). It was pointed out that there are differential trade-offs for males and females in making investment decisions. To reproduce, males are obligated to invest only their sperm and the amount of time need to engage in copulation; females on the other hand must invest a very large amount of time and energy (e.g., 9 months of gestation). As such, the road leading from copulation to reproductive success is cheaper for males than females. Also the potential benefits of multiple partners (or focusing on mating effort rather than parenting effort) are greater for males than females. Males, unlike females, can optimize their reproductive success by mating with many partners. As such, male investment in care of the young occurs at the cost of missed mating opportunities. From an evolutionary perspective it is not surprising that in many species fathers provide less parental care than mothers (e.g., Buss, 1999).

BIOLOGICAL RELATEDNESS

Empirical evidence has shown that parents are more likely to invest in children to whom they are biologically related. In support of this, it has been shown that parents are more likely to abuse their stepchildren than their biological children (e.g., Daly & Wilson, 1984, 1988; Lightcap, Kurland, & Burgess, 1982). This relationship between abuse and biological relatedness remains even when one controls for potential confounds such as socioeconomic status, maternal age, and family size (Daly & Wilson, 1988). In addition, parents show lower levels of investment (e.g., amount of financial resources and amount of contact time) in their stepchildren than in their biological children (Anderson, Kaplan, Lam, & Lancaster, 1999; Anderson, Kaplan, & Lancaster, 1999; Zwoch, 1999). Again, the relationship between direct investment and biological relatedness remains even when controlling for number of familial dependents and socioeconomic status (Anderson, Kaplan, & Lancaster, 1999).

Paternity Uncertainty and Male Parental Investment. Male efforts to ensure the biological relatedness of the young before investing in parental care is a particular topic of concern for theories of paternal investment (Geary, 2000). For women, doubts concerning biological relatedness are nonexistent. However, males can never be 100% certain of the biological relatedness of subsequent offspring. Indeed, empirical evidence has emerged showing that males are more influenced than females by cues of biological relatedness. For instance, men, more than women, were found to be influenced by facial resemblance in their response to infant faces (e.g., feelings of parental care) in a hypothetical child adoption task (Volk & Quinsey, 2002). As a second test of this hypothesis, Platek, Burch, Penyavin, Wasserman, and Gallup (2002) asked adults to judge the faces of children for attractiveness, for their adoptive preferences, for the child they would most like to spend time with, for the child they would be willing to spend money on, and for the child they would least resent paying child support for. Judgments (unbeknownst to the judges) were based on photographs of children that were morphed either with the judge's own face or with the face of a stranger. Males expressed more willingness to invest in a child whose face had been morphed with their own face. Women were less influenced by facial resemblance. This observed difference between the sexes is an example of a process that is more easily explained by evolutionary theory than by learning theory.

PARENTAL RESOURCES

As the notion of parental investment developed within evolutionary psychology and evolutionary biology, systematic attention was given to other variables that influence the extent to which parents invest in the care of the young. As one parameter, interest turned to the differential investment of parents under different circumstances. For example, parental investment changed as a function of the resources available in caring for the young. Decisions were based on the answers to such questions as: How available is food? How available are other people to share in the caregiving process? Might there be greater resources in the future?

Parental resources take many forms. At the most basic level they include the ability of the parent to provide for the basic needs of the young (e.g., provision of sustenance). In contemporary times, economic resources serve as a basic marker of access to many kinds of resources important for the caregiving process. In addition, the availability of supportive others represents an important resource for parents. This may involve an extended network of supportive others who provide assistance at a social–emotional level as well as at the level of assistance in direct care of the young. Indeed it has been suggested that the family itself evolved as a means of facilitating the shared reproductive success of kin (MacDonald, 1988). As noted earlier, it has also been suggested that the sensitivity of the young to their early social context (primarily the family) evolved as an adaptation (Boyce & Ellis, 2005).

Resources also come in other forms. For example, analytic and decision-making skills, along with information acquisition, can be thought of as representing cognitive resources. That is, parents differ in the extent to which they have the knowledge or problem-solving skills to cope effectively with the demands of parenting.

Extensive observations have been made of the differential patterns of investment made by parents who differ in their resources. For example, parental lack of resources was identified in Belsky's (1993) review of the literature as an important contributor to physical abuse and neglect. It is well known that maltreatment of children is more likely to occur at lower socioeconomic levels (e.g., Gelles, 1992). In addition, parents living in poverty may respond with reduced investment patterns as a function of the high level of instability (i.e., lack of access to stable resources) and powerlessness (i.e., overall inability to acquire resources). As noted earlier, evolutionary design prepares the individual for changing responses (including changing parental investment) in response to changing ecologies.

Although the weight of correlational evidence with respect to the possible effects of parental resources is impressive, causal inferences cannot be safely drawn. Therefore, it is important to consider whether these findings are also supported by experimental evidence. Intervention programs offer an opportunity for assessing such effects when changing experiences are introduced experimentally. As an example of this type of effort, Bugental et al. (2002) conducted a community-based program directed to reducing child abuse and enhancing child health within an at-risk population. Most of the parents were recent immigrants from Mexico and lacked resources of many different types (access to jobs, language, support networks, etc.). Parents were identified during the mother's third trimester of pregnancy and randomly assigned to a "cognitive" condition or control conditions. In the cognitive condition (in comparison with control conditions), parents were assisted in acquiring what may be thought of as "cognitive resources." That is, they were assisted in developing relevant problem-solving skills in resolving caregiving problems as well as finding ways to gain access to needed resources within the community.

Analyses were conducted (Bugental et al., 2002) to determine the effects of the cognitive intervention on child outcomes. Children's outcomes were assessed at age 1 in terms of their levels of physical health (as well as their exposure to maltreatment). Parents within the cognitive condition (in comparison with the other two conditions, including a standard home visitation condition in which parents received the same number of home visits as those in the cognitive condition) showed higher levels of investment in their child. In addition, children showed better outcomes as a result of parental participation in the cognitive intervention. That is, they experienced higher levels of physical health as well as lower levels of abuse or harsh parenting (Bugental et al., 2002). These findings suggest the ways in which gains in parental resources reduce childhood morbidity and mortality and increase the likelihood that children will themselves grow up to become parents.

REPRODUCTIVE VALUE OF THE YOUNG

As another area of interest in parental investment theory, attention has been given to the characteristics of the young themselves. Across our evolutionary history, children have provided early cues to their health and thus the likelihood that they would survive to become parents themselves. Reference is made to child "value" in the sense that children vary in the probability that they would have enhanced the reproductive success of their parents in our ancestral past. Whereas some children demonstrated cues indicating high health and the higher probability of future reproductive benefits, other children provided cues that suggested that they would pose a cost (or relatively small benefit) to parents' reproductive success (e.g., Daly & Wilson, 1984). Thus from an evolutionary perspective, parents would be expected to show differential investment in children based on early indicators of their potential costs and benefits.

There is an extensive body of research on nonhumans that has demonstrated the circumstances under which the young are less likely to receive parental care. In this case, absence of parental care typically refers to the abandonment of the young. One of the circumstances that influence parental investment among some non-human species involves brood size or numerosity. For example, a brood or litter is more likely to be abandoned if it is small (Mock & Parker, 1986). Documenting the causal effects of size, broods that are experimentally reduced by human intervention are also more likely to be abandoned (Armstrong & Robertson, 1988).

In the same way, considerable attention has been given to differing patterns of parental investment of human parents, based on offspring cues. Particular attention has been given to the reduced parental investment that is typically shown in children who manifest some kind of physical or medical anomaly or health problem early in life. In addition, children who show cry anomalies (e.g., anomalous pitch properties) provide cues to their health (Boukydis & Lester, 1998); that is, cry quality provides honest cues to the infant's fitness. Children who have visible (or audible) indications of abnormalities early in life provide cues to high reproductive costs for their parents. Costs may be at many different levels. That is, the child could be expected to be less likely to survive, and even if he or she did survive, the child would require greater care than other children (thus posing a threat to the parents' ability to care for other existing or possible progeny). As summarized by Hagen (1999), even mild birth disorders (e.g., prematurity) are, in actual fact, predictors of later morbidity and mortality—in particular within countries that lack economic and medical resources to provide appropriate care for such children.

Historical accounts provide evidence that infanticide of children with physical abnormalities has been common across the history of Western civilization (Moseley, 1986). Daly and Wilson (1984) gave attention to the kinds of children in today's world that are more likely to be abandoned or killed at birth. They pointed out that children who demonstrate some type of physical abnormality or health problem at birth are at high risk for abandonment or infanticide in many traditional cultures. They also went on to document the prevalence of such outcomes (including infanticide) even in modern countries with strict laws against infanticide and child maltreatment. Furthermore, there is a substantial literature providing evidence for the higher levels of abuse and neglect experienced by children in industrialized countries who manifest medical, learning, or physical disorders (e.g. Bugental, 2003; Sullivan & Knutson, 2000). Amniocentesis often serves the same function in that the identified presence of abnormalities may lead to parental decisions for an abortion (Erikson, 2003).

An example that captures the nature of parental responses to such children is provided by a research program conducted by Weiss (1994, 1998). Within this program, a comparison was made of the children given up at birth for adoption based on their potential medical problems. Some of the children had problems that had visible components (e.g., microcephaly and spina bifida) whereas others were just as medically severe but did not have visible components (e.g., heart problems). Parents were found to base their decisions (keeping the child or relinquishing the child for adoption) on the visibility of the child's disorder rather than the actual severity of the child's disorder (and thus reflected perceptually based cues to risk rather than medically indicated risk). Whereas only 7% of children with medical problems that had no visible components were relinquished for adoption, two-thirds of children with visible medical conditions were relinquished. Such children were sometimes viewed as "monsters" (Weiss, 1994, p. 476). In addition, they were seen as a source of stigma and shame for their family.

Why should the visibility of a medical condition hold so much importance in making such parenting decisions? As pointed out earlier, parenting decisions evolved to take into consideration offspring cues that would have been reliably associated with reproductive success. However, the evolutionary design for sensitivity to child cues has its origins in our ancestral past, at a time when medical knowledge was not available as a basis for predicting the child's later outcomes. Thus, from an evolutionary standpoint, visible cues to health would be expected to carry more weight than medical predictions.

Finally, the same child may have a different value for a parent based on that parent's options. Thus, a mother may easily invest in even a very high-risk child if she is unlikely to bear any other children (due to the impending advent of menopause). Supporting this position, older mothers are much less likely to neglect, abuse, or kill their infants than are younger mothers (Daly & Wilson, 1988; Lee & George, 1999). This relationship between maternal age and infanticide remains even when one controls for the confounding variable of marital status (a marker of one's access to resources) (Daly & Wilson, 1988).

INTERACTIVE EFFECTS OF PARENTAL RESOURCES AND CHILD VALUE

Relatively recently, attention has turned not only to the independent factors that serve to influence the probability of parental investment in a high risk (or costly) child but also to the combination of factors that increase the probability of parental investment in such a child (Mann, 1992; Bugental & Beaulieu, 2003). When parents have low resources, higher levels of parental investment can be expected in high-value (rather than low-value) offspring—an intuitive prediction. In this case, parents maximize their outcomes by investing in the child most likely to survive. However, among parents with high resources—somewhat counterintuitively—higher levels of parental investment can be expected in low-value (rather than high-value) offspring. In this case, less healthy (low value) children are provided with the extra investment that is needed for their survival—without any loss to healthy (high value) children, who are also guaranteed sufficient parental resources. The net effect is that all children survive.

Evidence from Nonhuman Models. As an important step in providing evidence for an interactional model, Davis and Todd (1999) conducted a computer simulation study in which they assessed the ultimate size of a surviving brood of birds, based on the differential feeding strategies shown with high-value (large) versus low-value (small) chicks under different conditions of food accessibility (a key resource). As anticipated, the success of feeding strategies was contingent upon the availability of food. When food was scarce, the best strategy (i.e., the strategy that led to the greatest number of surviving chicks) was to feed the largest chick first. In contrast, the best strategy when food was plentiful was to feed the smallest chick first (i.e., the low-value chick). Naturalistic observations of the feeding pattern of birds have produced supportive evidence for this interactive pattern (e.g., Gottlander, 1987). The utility of research based on nonhumans follows from the fact that differential investment processes appear in the absence of the capability for reflective appraisal processes.

Evidence from Humans. The question then becomes: What do we know about humans with respect to the interactive influences of offspring value and parental resources? Belsky (1993) suggested that when resources are scarce, parents are more likely to show preferential investment in children based on their reproductive potential; thus, those children who show lower potential are more likely to be subjected to maltreatment than are those with higher potential. In similar fashion, Mann (1992) suggested that parents who lack resources must be selective in their allocation of scarce resources and thus may be particularly likely to selectively invest in offspring with high reproductive potential. In support of this notion, parents in high poverty areas are more likely than parents in more affluent areas to remove investment from sickly children (Schepher-Hughes, 1985).

Bugental and Beaulieu (2003) expanded on previous research by investigating further the interactive effects of parental resources and child value. They applied this proposed interactional approach to parental responses to medically at-risk children (e.g., infants born prematurely). Such children may be thought of as posing a potential reproductive cost by virtue of the fact that they are more likely than other children to have later medical problems (e.g., Gross, Spiker, & Haymes, 1997; Picard, Del Dotto, & Breslau, 2000; Schmitz & Reif, 1994). Bugental and Beaulieu spelled out the circumstances under which parents would be more likely to invest in high-risk children than low-risk children (as well as those under which parents would be more likely to invest in low-risk than high-risk children). As suggested by others, parents with low resources cannot "afford" to invest in high-risk children. On the other side of the picture, however, parents with high resources can "afford" to invest in a high-risk child without any threat to their ability to simultaneously provide high-quality care to other offspring or potential offspring. For such parents, reproductive success in our evolutionary past might have been highest when they invested disproportionately in a high-risk child.

Supportive evidence for these predictions has been found in both longitudinal and experimental investigations. For example, a study was conducted that assessed maternal responses to high-risk versus low-risk infants as a function of the caregiving attributions made by mothers prior to the birth of their children (Bugental & Happaney, 2004). As noted earlier, parental attributions (high vs. low perceived control over caregiving outcomes) may be thought of as reflecting a type of cognitive resource. Mothers with low perceived power as caregivers were found to show lower levels of safety maintenance for their medically at-risk infants than for their low-risk infants. In contrast, mothers with higher levels of perceived power showed equal levels of safety maintenance with both high- and low-risk infants. Thus, partial support for the interactive effects of parental resources and child value has been demonstrated longitudinally.

In addition, experimental support has been offered based on the outcomes of Bugental et al.'s (2002) intervention program. As noted earlier, children of mothers who participated in the cognitively based home visitation program—as a whole—demonstrated greater benefits than did the children of mothers in control conditions. However, these benefits were greater for at-risk children than for other children. Although high-risk children in the control conditions showed the lowest level of physical health during their first year of life, the same grouping of children showed the *highest* level of physical health in families participating in the cognitive condition. Their level of health even exceeded that shown by low-risk children in the cognitive condition (Bugental & Beaulieu, 2003).

The question then arises: Did mothers show a differential pattern of investment that was sensitive to both their resources (in this case, problem-solving skills and higher levels of perceived power in caregiving relationships) and child cost (in this case, medical risk)? Investment was measured by parents' willingness to spend a day (in the company of a familiar worker from the community who provided transportation) coming to an unfamiliar location in a neighboring community to obtain additional information about their child (Bugental & Beaulieu, 2003). As can be seen in Figure 3.1, parents who had participated in an "empowerment" intervention were more likely to show a positive investment in a high-risk than a low-risk child whereas parents in the control condition were more likely to show a positive investment in a low-risk child than a high-risk child. This observed pattern supports the prediction that parents show conditional investment patterns in high- versus low-risk children based on access to resources.

It could be argued that nonhuman parents may use a computational process that is not based on cognitions whereas humans may resolve the same adaptive problem by cognitive means. At the same time, it should be recognized that the same adaptations that operate automatically for nonhuman species may involve aware cognitions for humans. For example, differential responses to a high-cost child may be represented cognitively in notions of threat versus challenge (e.g., Blascovich & Mendes, 2001); that is, a costly child may be seen as a positive challenge (rather than a threat) for parents who have resources that allow them to cope with this situation. However, humans are often aware of

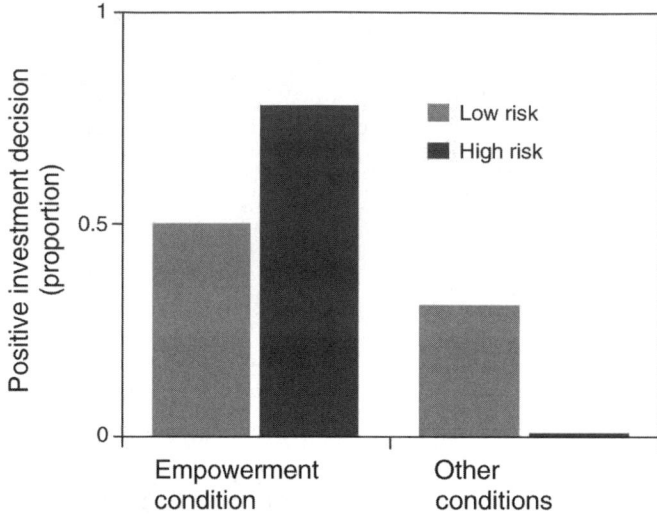

FIGURE 3.1. Positive parental investment, as measured by willingness to exert effort to obtain information on their child. Adapted from Bugental and Beaulieu (2003, p. 353). Copyright 2003 by Elsevier. Adapted by permission.

and influenced by preferences that reflect evolved adaptations. Mate preferences are a case in point. In our evolutionary past, there were evolutionary advantages for mating with a partner who showed cues to health. Thus, such cues are seen as "attractive" among humans. As a result, humans devote considerable attention and appraisal efforts to their own attractiveness and the attractiveness of potential partners in the "mating game." In the same way, infants who show cues to health are seen as attractive and are the object of positive attention.

HOW DOES PARENTAL INVESTMENT SERVE TO INFLUENCE REPRODUCTIVE OUTCOMES?

A final (but often overlooked) step in these formulations involves the means by which parental care would have produced its effect on parents' reproductive success. The key questions are as follows: How do parental actions potentially serve to buffer against these experiences? Can children, as a result of parental responses, show an enhanced capacity to cope with future stress? The primary focus in this area of research has been on parental responses that facilitate resilience among such children (e.g., Masten, 2001; Rutter & O'Connor, 2004). However, there are emerging indications that parental responses may also facilitate the child's enhanced capacity to cope with future stress. Employing the concept of "thriving," researchers are beginning to learn that those who experience early adversity—under some circumstances—show an exceptional ability to habituate (physiologically as well as psychologically) to repeated stresses that occur at later times in their lives (Epel, McEwen, & Ickovics, 1998; Bugental et al., 2004). That is, their experience with early adversity may foster actual benefits in that their capacity to habituate to future stress exceeds that of individuals who have not experienced early adversity. Most notably, the combination of early stress and high parental support (an indicator of parental investment) promotes the highest levels of habituation in coping with future stress.

Hierarchical Power Domain

The Adaptive Problem

The adaptive problem to be solved within the hierarchical power domain involves the regulation of relationships based on unequal dominance/resources. In our ancestral past, the individual's reproductive interests were served by high rank (and thus access to resources); at the same time, those interests are also served by use of dominance or resources to produce benefits for the young (as well as others with whom they share reproductive interests).

A power-based relationship between parents and their children typically begins in the toddler years when children are able to move away from their parents. At this point, their safety must be maintained at a distance—requiring that parents have some means of regulating their actions, for example, the "prohibition" calls described by Fernald (1993).

Sensitivity of Children to Power Cues

Across species, the young show a general sensitivity to cues to the power or dominance of others (Cheney & Seyfarth, 1985). This sensitivity protects the young in two ways. First, their sensitivity to the warning or prohibition calls of parents (and subsequent inhibition of actions) protected them from harm. Second, their sensitivity to the combined cues of dominance and novelty (e.g., the presence of unfamiliar males, who in our evolutionary past posed an actual source of threat) leads them to be wary and seek protection. In support of the ultimate as opposed to the proximate causes of such responses, it is important to note that the response patterns of the young are universal and occur at the time at which infants become mobile, moving away from the direct protection of their mothers; at the same time, these response patterns occur without any relevant learning history (actual threat from unfamiliar males).

Although early parental power assertion is generally successful in influencing the young, children also show variability in their susceptibility to parental control. Belsky (2005) reviewed the literature to document the fact that there is indeed very high variability in the extent to which children are susceptible to the influence attempts of their parents. The question arises: Why should such variability continue to exist in view of the seeming maladaptiveness of a child's lack of susceptibility to socializing influences? Why wasn't it eliminated through the process of natural selection? We typically think in terms of the negative life outcomes of such children—as mediated by the more conflictual relationships they have with parents (as well as others). Children with attention-deficit/ hyperactivity disorder (ADHD) are a good case in point. Such children are responded to more negatively by both parents and peers (Mash & Johnston, 1983; Whalen, Henker, Castro, & Granger, 1987). Belsky (2005) offers an evolutionary argument concerning the circumstances under which such children may fare better than other children. Ordinarily, children who are responsive to parental socialization are better able to cope with the world they typically face as adults. However, this benefit relies on the premise of a relatively stable environment. The potential advantage of children with ADHD in unstable environments has been suggested by Jensen et al. (1997). In such environments, the typical characteristics of such children may be conceptualized as involving "response readiness," as manifested in exploration of the environment for both threats and opportunities, hypervigilance for signs of danger, and fast responses to environmental change. In a physically threatening environment, such an individual may be better able to avoid harm and acquire benefits. Thus, the genes that contribute to ADHD stay within the gene pool as a function of the success they produced in earlier (and harsher) times, despite their current maladaptiveness.

Socialization of Power

There are sex differences in the biological preparation of the young for power-based interactions. For example, young males, based on the presence of prenatal androgens, are more likely than young females to engage in playful competitive interactions (rough-and-tumble play) (e.g., Breedlove, 1992; Mazur & Booth, 1996). These biologically prepared differences can be expected to lead to sex differences in receptivity to the socializing influences of parents and peers. For example, fathers and male peers are more likely (than mothers or female peers) to facilitate (or socialize) the involvement of young boys in rough-and-tumble play. Such experiences facilitate boys' later involvement in more serious types of rank-related competition at older ages. This early experience allows practice without risk of actual harm. In addition, such interactions are regulated in ways that maintain a 50–50 status of outcomes, thus ensuring experience in both wins and losses (Pellis, 2002). When boys reach pubescence (and associated increases in testosterone and muscle mass create risk of real harm), involvement in rough-and-tumble play essentially ceases (Panksepp, 1993). That is, the activation and deactivation of rough-and-tumble play follows a biologically set clock that facilitates its adaptiveness.

Coalitional Alliances

The Adaptive Problem

A third adaptive problem that has significance for socialization involves the creation and maintenance of coalitional alliances. On the one hand, clear benefits follow from collaboration with others in securing and protecting resources (from outsiders). To ensure such benefits, however, it is necessary that all members of the coalition contribute to the joint welfare of the group and are easily identified as a coalition member. Group sanctions or exclusion occurs in response to "free riders" (Price, Cosmides, & Tooby, 2002) or to those who fail to conform to group norms (Wenegrat, Castill-Yee, & Abrams, 1996).

Children's Sensitivity to Coalitional Alliances

Children's sensitivity to coalitional alliances appears at later ages than their sensitivity to the algorithms of the protective care or hierarchical power domains. One of the most striking age-related changes involves the emergent awareness of and compliance to group norms in early childhood, a process that focuses on receptivity to intragroup processes. By around 2 years of age, children show an emergent awareness of sensitivity to the conventional routines that are shared within groups (e.g., Dunn & Munn, 1985). Between the ages of 3 and 4 years, children continue to show a heightened receptivity and positive responsiveness to knowledge of social conventions and procedures and now follow those "rules" with a rigidity that borders on obsession (Emde, Biringen, Clyman, & Oppenheim, 1991). In addition, they show an increasing affinity for and cohesion with their own group (including their own family). These processes appear to reflect evolutionary design in that they manifest sensitive periods, occur without tuition or reinforcement, and are very easily acquired (i.e., they involve privileged learning).

In middle childhood, there is a shift to awareness of differences between groups (Aboud, 2003; Hirschfeld, 1996). Children now show an awareness of (often arbitrary) differences between groups and show a strong favoritism for their own group and derogation or hostility to outgroups. In addition, children manifest privileged learning of intergroup identity; that is, they easily come to distinguish groupings (and show a preference for their "own group") based on such simple visual markers as color of shirt (Bigler, Brown, & Markell, 2001).

Socialization of Coalitional Alliances

Early socialization of intragroup processes (cohesion and shared routines and norms) may involve a variety of sources. Such processes often involve mothers in Western society (e.g., Dunn & Munn, 1985) but just as easily involve other children in more communal societies (Harris, 1995). However, there is a striking shift away from parental influence in the socialization of intergroup processes. As observed by Aboud and Doyle (1996), children's views of outgroup members are not significantly influenced by their parents and instead are instantiated in response to the influence of other children within their group.

Reciprocal/Mutual Relationships

The Adaptive Problem

The adaptive problem to be solved within the reciprocity/mutuality domain involves the creation of dyadic relationships between nonkin that facilitate the reproductive success of both individuals. Although the provision of benefits to kin carries a personal benefit (in terms of the replication of one's own genes as kin reproduce), the provision of benefits to nonkin may carry a cost; that is, resources are shared in ways that may act to one's own disadvantage. The adaptation(s) that evolved to solve this problem involved the creation of a reciprocal relationship in which benefits are exchanged. As a feature of this type of relationship, a mechanism has evolved to ensure the continuing presence of matched benefits. Specifically, Cosmides and Tooby (1992) have demonstrated that when a logical problem is framed as a "social contract," judges show an exceptional ability to identify instances of rule violation ("cheating"). Socialization within this domain becomes important as a function of the early preparation and practice in such exchange-based relationships with others.

Children's Sensitivity to the Reciprocity/Mutuality Domain

The sensitivity to reciprocal relationships begins in early infancy. It has been suggested that humans are born ready to reciprocate interactions with others (Trevarthen, Kokkinski, & Flamenghi, 1999). This sensitivity begins with the affective responses shown to interpersonally contingent or noncontingent response patterns. Early research on this topic demonstrated the pleasure that even young infants take in contingency experiences (Watson & Ramey, 1987). More recently, Bigelow and Birch (1999), within a short-term longitudinal study, showed that 4- and 5-month old infants manifested preferences for interaction with others (strangers) with whom they had contingent experiences, in comparison with those with whom they had noncontingent experiences. During an initial interaction, the two strangers did the same things—but either in a way that was contingently or noncontingently responsive to the infant. The simple awareness of contingency may represent an early form of the "keep track" mechanism proposed to account for the management of reciprocal relationships (relationships that may be thought of as involving an implicit social contract; Cosmides & Tooby, 1992). Mutually beneficial relationships are maintained with others (whether or not they are kin) when reciprocal benefits are provided. At older ages, this sensitivity is manifested in the form of social exchange processes (e.g., Laursen & Hartup, 2002). Harris, Nunez, and Brett (2001) found that young children (ages 3 to 7) are sensitive to the obligations that follow from an exchange agreement. In addition, they understand that the victim of "cheating" on an agreement to swap will be upset, and completion of a swap leads both individuals to be happy.

Socialization of the Reciprocity/Mutuality Domain

The socialization of reciprocity involves interactions that may be initially introduced by parents or by older children (and subsequently maintained in interaction with peers). Most of the observations made during infancy have focused on mother–infant interaction in Western countries. Within that constraint, it appears that mothers set the stage for the child's later involvements in reciprocal relationships that involve a synchronization of actions at a single point in time, or a matching of benefits over time. An early manifestation is the turn-taking that takes places (as orchestrated by the mother) in early vocal dialogues (Papousek & Papousek, 1989). Such competencies are further developed by engagement of the infant in ritualized turn-taking games, which, in turn, prepare the child for more complex reciprocal processes (Parrot & Gletiman, 1989). Ultimately, this early experience serves to facilitate the child's competence in play interactions with peers (e.g., Lindsey, Mize, & Pettit, 1997). The long-term benefits of reciprocal relationships come in many different forms: reductions in level of stress (e.g., Field et al., 1992); protection against bullying (e.g., Schwartz, Dodge, Pettit, & Bates, 2000); and greater social skills and social understanding (e.g., Lindsey, 2002; Vaughn, Colfin, Azriak, Caya, & Krzik, 2001; Peterson & Siegal, 2002).

CONCLUSIONS

In this chapter, we have argued that the predictions made by evolutionary theory typically expand rather than compete with standard socialization models. Evolutionary psychology has focused on ultimate causation in terms of adaptations that have evolved to solve recurrent problems within our evolutionary history. As such, it is concerned with the "design" of the experience-expectant brain (as the means by which evolutionary design is implemented). In contrast, standard socialization theory has been concerned with proximate causation across the life course.

Evolutionary thought was described as offering unique advantages of three types. First, it provides a framework for understanding the biological design or blueprints for socialization—in terms of both children's receptivity and the facilitative efforts typically offered by caregivers (or other agents of socialization). Second, it provides a premise for the privileged learning that children (across cultures) show for acquiring particular kinds of knowledge or skills at particular ages and in particular settings. The biological basis of privileged learning is often supported by associated changes or variations in neurohormonal regulators—as, for example, has been found with sexually dimorphic differences in privileged learning. Third, evolutionary psychology offers an organized account of the ways in which and the times at which children are resistant to or uninfluenced by certain kinds of socialization efforts (e.g., toddler resistance to parents' efforts to maintain nighttime separation, resistance to efforts to integrate boys and girls during middle childhood, and children's high susceptibility to peer influence and low susceptibility to parental influence in connection with the identification of and response to outgroups).

Both evolutionary and standard socialization theories have been concerned with the differences that occur in different kinds of relationships—described in terms of "domains" within evolutionary thought and "contexts" within standard socialization theory. It was suggested here that evolutionary thought offers an advantage in that it provides a more complete account of the processes that occur within protective care relationships (including attachment relationships). The evolutionary account has extended the field of attachment to include a concern with parental investment. Up to this point, parental investment theory has been more concerned with the reasons for and effects of parental failure to invest in their children. We hope to have shown that it also represents a new way of thinking about the ways parents act to enhance the life outcomes of the young.

When added to the picture, developmental neuroscience provides guidance on the ways in which socialization processes are mediated. Finally, behavior genetics (through gene expression) provides the means by which the child's experiences feed back to influence the developing brain. The integration of these fields (evolutionary psychology, standard socialization theory, developmental neuroscience, and behavior genetics) is increasingly understood as providing the most complete picture of the developing child (Boyce & Ellis, 2005; Bugental & Grusec, 2006; Burgess & Drais, 1999). As a concluding point, we believe that it is time to bring evolutionary thought into the mainstream of socialization theory.

REFERENCES

Aboud, F. E. (2003). The formation of in-group favoritism and out-group prejudice in young children: Are they distinct attitudes? *Developmental Psychology, 39*, 48–60.

Aboud, F. E., & Doyle, A. B. (1996). Parental and peer influences on children's racial attitudes. *International Journal of Intercultural Relations, 20*, 371–383.

Ainsworth, M. D. S., Blehar, M. C., Waters, E., & Wall, S. (1978). *Patterns of attachment: A psychological study of the strange situation.* Hillsdale, NJ: Erlbaum.

Anderson, K. G., Kaplan, H., Lam, D., & Lancaster, J. (1999). Paternal care by genetic fathers and stepfathers II: Reports by Xhosa high school students. *Evolution and Human Behavior, 20*, 433–451.

Anderson, K. G., Kaplan, H., & Lancaster, J. (1999). Paternal care by genetic fathers and stepfathers. I: Reports from Albuquerque men. *Evolution and Human Behavior, 20*, 405–431.

Armstrong, T., & Robertson, R. J. (1988). Parental involvement based on clutch value. Nest desertion in response to partial clutch loss in dabbling ducks. *Animal Behaviour, 36*, 941–943.

Belsky, J. (1993). Etiology of child maltreatment: A developmental-ecological analysis. *Psychological Bulletin, 114*, 413–434.

Belsky, J. (2005). Differential susceptibility to rearing influence: An evolutionary hypothesis and some evidence. In B. J. Ellis & D. F. Bjorklund (Eds.), *Origins of the social mind: Evolutionary psychology and child development* (pp. 139–163). New York: Guilford Press.

Belsky, J., Steinberg, L., & Draper, P. (1991). Childhood experience, interpersonal development, and reproductive strategy: An evolutionary theory of socialization. *Child Development, 62,* 647–670.

Bigelow, A. E., & Birch, S. A. J. (1999). The effects of contingency in previous interactions on infants' preferences for social partners. *Infant Behavior and Development, 22,* 367–382.

Bigler, R. S., Brown, C. S., & Markell, M. (2001). When groups are not created equal: Effects of group status on the formation of intergroup attitudes in children. *Child Development, 72,* 1151–1162.

Bjorklund, D. F., Yunger, J. L., & Pellegrini, A. D. (2002). The evolution of parenting and evoloutionary approaches to childrearing. In M. H. Bornstein (Ed.), *Handbook of parenting. Volume 2. Biology and ecology of parenting* (pp. 3–30). Mahwah, NJ: Erlbaum.

Blascovich, J., & Mendes, W. B. (2001). Challenge and threat appraisals: The role of affective cues In J. P. Forgas (Ed.), *Feeling and thinking: The role of affect in social cognition* (pp. 59–82). New York: Cambridge University Press.

Bogin, B. & Smith, B. H. (2000). Evolution of the human life cycle. In S. Stinson, B. Bogin, R. Huss-Ashmore, & D. Orourke (Eds.), *Human biology: An evolutionary and biocultural approach* (pp. 377–424). New York: Wiley.

Boukydis, C. F. Z., & Lester, B. M. (1998). Infant crying, risk status and social support in families of preterm and term infants. *Early Development and Parenting, 7,* 31–40.

Bowlby, J. (1969). *Attachment and loss (Vol. I. Attachment).* New York: Basic Books.

Bowlby, J. (1973). *Attachment and loss (Vol. II. Separation).* New York: Basic Books.

Bowlby, J. (1980). *Attachment and loss (Vol. III. Loss).* New York: Basic Books

Boyce, W. T., & Ellis, B. J. (2005). Biological sensitivity to context: I. An evolutionary–developmental theory of the origins and functions of stress reactivity. *Development and Psychopathology, 17,* 271–301.

Breedlove, S. (1992). Sexual differentiation of the brain and behavior. In J. Becker, S. Breedlove, & D. Crews (Eds.), *Behavioral endocrinology* (pp. 39–68). Cambridge, MA: MIT Press.

Bruer, J. T., & Greenough, W. T. (2001). The subtle science of how experience affects the brain. In D. B Bailey, J. T. Bruer, F. J. Symons, & J. W. Lichtman (Eds.), *Critical thinking about critical periods* (pp. 209–232). Baltimore: Brookes.

Bugental, D. B. (2000). Acquisition of the algorithms of social life: A domain-based approach. *Psychological Bulletin, 26,* 187–209.

Bugental, D. B. (2003). *Thriving in the face of childhood adversity.* New York: Psychology Press.

Bugental, D. B., & Beaulieu, D. A. (2003). A bio-social-cognitive approach to understanding and promoting the outcomes of children with medical and physical disorders. In R. Kail (Ed.), *Advances in child development and behavior* (Vol. 31, pp. 329–361). New York: Academic Press.

Bugental, D. B., Beaulieu, D., Cayan, L., Fowler, E., O'Brien, E., & Kokotay, S. (2004). *Stress immunization in young adults: The role of early medical adversity and supportive parenting.* Unpublished paper.

Bugental, D. B., Ellerson, P. C., Lin, E. K., Rainey, B., Kokotovic, A., & O'Hara, N. (2002). A cognitive approach to child abuse prevention. *Journal of Family Psychology, 16,* 243–258.

Bugental, D. B., & Grusec, J. (2006). Socialization processes. In N. Eisenberg (Vol. Ed.), *Handbook of child psychology: Vol. 3. Social, emotional, and personality development* (6th ed., pp. 366–428). Hoboken, NJ: Wiley.

Bugental, D. B., & Happaney, K. (2004). Predicting infant maltreatment in low-income families: The interactive effects of maternal attributions and child status at birth. *Developmental Psychology, 40,* 234–243.

Bugental, D. B., Martorell, G. A., & Barraza, V. (2003). The hormonal costs of subtle forms of infant maltreatment. *Hormones and Behavior 43,* 237–244.

Burgess, R. L. & Drais, A. A. (1999) Beyond the "Cinderella effect": Life history theory and child maltreatment. *Human Nature, 10,* 373–398

Buss, D. M. (1994). *The evolution of desire.* New York: Basic Books.

Buss, D. M. (1999). *Evolutionary psychology: The new science of the mind.* Boston: Allyn & Bacon.

Cheney, D. L., & Seyfarth, R. M. (1985). Social and nonsocial knowledge in vervet monkeys. *Philosophical Transactions of the Royal Society of London, 308,* 187–201.

Chomsky, N. (1965). *Syntactic structures.* The Hague, The Netherlands: Mouton.

Cosmides, L., & Tooby, J. (1992). Cognitive adaptations for social exchange. In J. H. Barkow, L. Cosmides, & J. Tooby (Eds.), *The adapted mind: Evolutionary psychology and the generation of culture* (pp. 163–228). London: Oxford University Press.

Daly, M., & Wilson, M. (1984). A sociobiological analysis of human infanticide. In G. Hausfater & S. B. Hrdy (Eds.), *Infanticide: Comparative and evolutionary perspectives* (pp. 4887–5020). New York: Aldine.

Daly, M., & Wilson, M. (1988). *Homicide.* New York: Aldine de Gruyter.

Davis, J. N., & Todd, P. M. (1999). Parental investment by simple decision rules. In G. Gigerenzer & P. M. Todd (Eds.) *Simple heuristics that make us smart* (pp. 309–326). New York: Oxford University Press.

Dawkins, R. (1982). *The extended phenotype.* San Francisco: Freeman.

DeCasper, A. J., & Fifer, W. P. (1987). Of human bonding: Newborns prefer their mothers' voices. In J. Oates & S. Sheldon (Eds.), *Cognitive development in infancy* (pp. 111–118). Hillsdale, NJ: Erlbaum.

Dewsbury, D. A. (1999). The proximate and the ultimate: Past, present and future. *Behavioural Processes, 46,* 189–199.

Dunn, J., & Munn., P. (1985). Becoming a family member: Family conflict and the development of understanding. *Child Development, 56,* 480–492.

Ellis, B. J., Essex, M. J., & Boyce, W. T. (2005). Biological sensitivity to context: II. Empirical explorations of an evolutionary–developmental theory. *Development and Psychopathology. 17,* 303–328.

Ellis, B. J., McFadyen-Ketchum, S., Dodge, K. A., Pettit, G. S., & Bates, J. E. (1999). Quality of early family relationships and individual differences in the timing of pubertal maturation in girls: A longitudinal test of an evolutionary model. *Journal of Personality and Social Psychology, 77,* 387–401.

Emde, R. N., Biringen, Z., Clyman, R. B., & Oppenheim, D. (1991). The moral self of infancy. Affective core and procedural knowledge. *Developmental Review, 11,* 251–270.

Epel, E. S., McEwen, B. S., & Ickovics, J. R. (1998). Embodying psychological thriving: Physical thriving in response to stress. *Journal of Social Issues, 54,* 301–322.

Erikson, S. L. (2003). Post-diagnostic abortion in Germany: Reproduction gone awry, again? *Social Science Medicine, 56,* 1987–2001.

Fernald, A. (1993). Approval and disapproval: Infant responsiveness to vocal affect in familiar and unfamiliar languages. *Child Development, 64,* 657–674.

Field, T., Greenwald, P., Morrow, C. J., Healy, B. T., Foster, T., Guthertz, M., et al. (1992). Behavior state matching during interactions of preadolescent friends versus acquaintances. *Developmental Psychology, 28,* 242–250.

Fiske, A. P. (1992). The four elementary forms of sociality: Framework for a unified theory of social relations. *Psychological Review, 99,* 689–723.

Geary, D. C. (2000). Evolution and proximate expression of human parental investment. *Psychological Bulletin, 126,* 55–77.

Gelles, R. J. (1992). Poverty and violence toward children. *American Behavioral Scientist, 35,* 258–274.

Goldberg, S., Grusec, J. E., & Jenkins, J. M. (1999). Confidence in protection: Arguments for a narrow definition of attachment. *Journal of Family Psychology, 13,* 475–483.

Goren, C. C., Sarty, M., & Wu, P. Y. (1975). Visual following and pattern discrimination of face-like stimuli by new born infants. *Pediatrics, 56,* 544–549.

Gottlander, K. (1987). Parental feeding behavior and sibling competition in the pied flycatcher. Ficedula . *Ornis Scandanavica, 18,* 269–276.

Gross, R. T., Spiker, D., & Haymes, C. W. (1997). *Helping low birth weight, premature babies: The Infant Health and Development Program.* Palo Alto, CA: Stanford University Press.

Hagen, E. H. (1999). The functions of postpartum depression. *Evolution and Human Behavior, 20,* 325–359.

Harlow, H., & Harlow, M. (1965). The affectional system. In A. Schrier, H. F. Harlow, & F. Stolnitz (Eds.). *Behavior of nonhuman primates.* (Vol. 2, pp. 287–334). New York: Academic Press.

Harris, J. R. (1995). Where is the child's environment? A group socialization theory of development. *Psychological Review, 102,* 458–489.

Harris, P. I., Nunez, M., & Brett, C. (2001). Let's swap: Early understanding of social exchange by British and Nepali children. *Memory and Cognition, 29,* 757–764.

Hetherington, E. M. (Ed.). (1983). *Socialization, personality, and social development: Handbook of child psychology* (Vol. 4). New York: Wiley.

Hirschfeld, L. A. (1996). *Race in the making: Cognition, culture, and child's construction of human kinds.* Cambridge, MA: MIT Press.

Hirschfeld, L. A., & Gelman, S. A. (1994). Toward a topography of mind: An introduction to domain specificity. In L. A. Hirschfeld & S. A. Gelman (Eds.), *Mapping the mind* (pp. 3–36). Cambridge, UK: Cambridge University Press.

Jensen, P. S., Mirazek, D., Knapp, P. K., Steinberg, L., Pfeffer, C., Schowalter, J., et al. (1997). Evolution and revolution in child psychiatry: ADHD as a disorder of adaptation. *Journal of the American Academy of Child and Adolescent Psychiatry, 36*, 1672–1681.

Keller, H. (2000). Human parent–child relationships from an evolutionary standpoint. *American Behavioral Scientist, 43*, 957–969.

Kenrick, D. T., Li., N. P., & Butner, J. (2003). Dynamical evolutionary psychology: Individual decision rules and emergent social norms. *Psychological Review, 110*, 3–28.

Ketelaar, T., & Ellis, B. J. (2000). Are evolutionary explanations unfalsifiable? Evolutionary psychology and Lakatosian philosophy of science. *Psychological Inquiry, 11*, 1–21.

Laursen, B., & Hartup, W. W. (2002). The origins of reciprocity and social exchange in friendships. In B. Laursen, & W. G. Graziano (Eds.), *Social exchange in development. New directions for child and adolescent development* (pp. 27–40). San Francisco: Jossey-Bass.

Lee, B. J., & George, R. M. (1999). Poverty, early childbearing and child maltreatment: A multinomial study. *Child and Youth Services Review, 21*, 755–780.

Lightcap, J. L., Kurland, J. A., & Burgess, R. L. (1982). Child abuse: A test of some predictions from evolutionary theory. *Ethology and Sociobiology, 3*, 61–67.

Lindsey, E. W. (2002). Preschool children's friendships and peer acceptance: Links to social competence. *Child Study Journal, 32*, 145–156.

Lindsey, E. W., Mize, J., & Pettit, G. S. (1997). Mutuality in parent–child play: Consequences for children's peer competence. *Journal of Social and Personal Relationships, 14*, 523–538.

Maccoby, E. E., & Martin, J. A. (1983). Socialization in the context of the family: Parent-child interaction. In E. M. Hetherington (Ed.), *Socialization, personality, and social development: Handbook of child psychology* (Vol. 4, pp. 1–102). New York: Wiley.

MacDonald, K. B. (1988). *Social and personality development: An evolutionary synthesis.* New York: Plenum Press.

Mann, J. (1992). Nurturance or negligence: maternal psychology and behavioral preference among preterm twins. In J. H. Barkow, L. Cosmides, & J. Tooby (Eds.), *The adapted mind: Evolutionary psychology and the generation of culture* (pp. 367–390). Oxford, UK: Oxford University Press.

Mash, E. J., & Johnston, C. (1983). Parental perceptions of child behavior problems, parenting self-esteem, and mothers' reported stress in younger and older hyperactive and normal children. *Journal of Consulting and Clinical Psychology, 51*, 86–99.

Masten, A. S. (2001). Ordinary magic: Resilience processes in development. *American Psychologist, 56*, 227–238.

Maurer, D., & Salapatek, P. (1976). Developmental changes in the scanning of faces in young infants. *Child Development, 47*, 523–527.

Mazur, A., & Booth, A. (1996). Testosterone and dominance in men. *Behavioral and Brain Sciences, 21*, 353–391.

Mischel, W., & Shoda, Y. (1995). A cognitive-affective-system theory of personality: Reconceptualizing situations, dispositions, dynamics, and invariance in personality structure. *Psychological Review, 102*, 246–268.

Mock, D. W., & Parker, G. A. (1986). Advantages and disadvantages of egret and heron brood reduction. *Evolution, 40*, 459–470.

Moseley, K. L. (1986). The history of infanticide in Western society. *Issues in Law and Medicine, 1*, 345–361.

Panksepp, J. (1993). Rough and tumble play: A fundamental brain process. In K MacDonald (Ed.), *Parent–child play: Descriptions and implications* (pp. 147–184). New York: State University of New York Press.

Panksepp, J., Nelson, E., & Bekkedal, M. (1997). Brain systems for the mediation of functional domain specificity of social separation–distress and social-reward. *Annals of the New York Academy of Sciences, 807*, 78–100.

Papousek, H., & Papousek, M. (1989). Intuitive parenting: Aspects related to educational psychology. *European Journal of Psychology and Education. [Special Issue: Infancy and education: Psychological considerations], 4*, 201–210.

Parke, R. D., & Buriel, R. (2006). Socialization in the family: Ethnic and ecological perspectives. In N. Eisenberg (Vol. Ed.), *Handbook of child psychology: Vol. 3. Social, emotional, and personality development* (pp. 429–504). Hoboken, NJ: Wiley.

Parrot, G. W., & Gleitman, H. (1989). Infants' expectations in play: The joy of peek-a-boo *Cognition and Emotion*, 3, 291–311.

Pauli-Pott, U., Mertesacker, B., & Beckmann, D. (2004). Predicting the development of infant emotionality from maternal characteristics. *Development and Psychopathology*, 16, 19–42.

Pellis, S. M. (2002). Keep in touch: Play fighting and social knowledge. In M. Bekoff, C. Allen, & G. M. Burghardt (Eds.), *The cognitive animal* (pp. 421–427). London: MIT Press.

Peterson, C. C., & Siegal, M. (2002). Mindreading and moral awareness in popular and rejected preschoolers. *British Journal of Developmental Psychology*, 20, 205–224.

Picard, E. M., Del Dotto, J. E., & Breslau, N. (2000). Prematurity and low birthweight. In K. O. Yeates, M. D. Ris, & H. G. Taylor (Eds.), *Pediatric neuropsychology: Research, theory, and practice* (pp. 237–251). New York: Guilford Press.

Platek, S. M., Burch, R. L., Panyavin, I. B., Wasserman, B. H., & Gallup, G. G., Jr. (2002). Reactions to children's faces: Resemblance affects males more than females. *Evolution and Human Behavior*, 23, 159–166.

Price, M. E., Cosmides, L., & Tooby, J. (2002). Punitive sentiment as an anti-free rider psychological device. *Evolution and Human Behavior*, 23, 203–231.

Rutter, M., & O'Connor, T. G. (2004). Are there biological programming effects for psychological development? Findings from a study of Romanian adoptees. *Developmental Psychology*, 40, 81–94.

Schepher-Hughes, N. (1985). Culture, scarcity, and maternal thinking: Maternal detachment and infant survival in a Brazilian shantytown. *Ethos*, 13, 291–317.

Schmitz, K., & Reif, L. (1994). Reducing prenatal risk and improving birth outcomes: The public health nursing role. *Public Health Nursing*, 11, 174–180.

Schwartz, D., Dodge, K. A., Pettit, G. S., & Bates, J. E. (2000). Friendship as a moderating factor in the pathway between early harsh home environment and later victimization in the peer group. *Developmental Psychology*, 36, 646–662.

Sullivan, P. M., & Knutson, J. F. (2000). Maltreatment and disabilities: A population-based epidemiological study. *Child Abuse and Neglect*, 24, 1257–1273.

Symons, D. (1992). On the use of misuse of Darwinism in the study of human behavior. In J. H. Barkow, L. Cosmides, & J. Tooby, (Eds.), *The adapted mind: Evolutionary psychology and the generation of culture* (pp. 367–390). Oxford, UK: Oxford University Press.

Trevarthen, C., Kokkinski, T., & Flamenghi, G. A., Jr. (1999). In J. Nadel & G. Butterworth (Eds.), *Imitation in infancy. Cambridge studies in cognitive perceptual development* (pp. 127–185). New York: Cambridge Unversity Press.

Trivers, R. (1972). Parental investment and sexual selection. In B. Campbell (Ed.), Sexual selection and the descent of man (pp. 136–179). Chicago: Aldine.

Vaughn, B. E., Colvin, T. N., Azria, M. R., Caya, L. & Krzysik, L. (2001). Dyadic analyses of friendship in a sample of preschool-age children attending Head Start: Correspondence between measures and implications for social competence. *Child Development*, 72, 862–878.

Volk, A., & Quinsey, V. L. (2002). The influence of infant facial cues on adoption preferences. *Human Nature*, 13, 437–455.

Waters, E., Merrick, S., Treboux, D., Crowell, J., & Albersheim, L. (2000). Attachment security in infancy and early adulthood: A twenty-year longitudinal study. *Child Development*, 71, 684–689.

Watson, J. S., & Ramey, C. T. (1987). Reactions to response-contingent stimulation in early infancy. In J. Oates & S. Sheldon (Eds.), *Cognitive development in infancy* (pp. 77–85). Hillsdale, NJ: Erlbaum.

Weiss, M. (1994). Nonperson and nonhome: Territorial seclusion of appearance-impaired children. *Journal of Contemporary Ethnography*, 22, 463–487.

Weiss, M. (1998). Parents' rejection of their appearance-impaired newborns: Some critical observations regarding the social myth of bonding. *Marriage and Family Review*, 27, 191–209.

Wenegrat, B., Castillo-Yee, E., & Abrams, L. (1996). Social norm compliance as a signaling system: II. Studies of fitness-related attributions consequent on a group norm violation. *Ethology and Sociobiology*, 17, 417–429.

Whalen, D. K., Henker, B., Castro, J., & Granger, D. (1987). Peer perception of hyperactivity and medication effects. *Child Development*, 58, 816–828.

Zwoch, K. (1999). Family type and investment in education: A comparison of genetic and stepparent families. *Evolution and Human Behavior*, 20, 453–464.

CHAPTER 4

Evidence from Behavioral Genetics for Environmental Contributions to Antisocial Conduct

TERRIE E. MOFFITT and AVSHALOM CASPI

Despite assiduous efforts to eliminate it, antisocial behavior is still a problem. Approximately 20% of people in the developed world experience victimization by perpetrators of violent and nonviolent illegal behavior each year (U.S. Bureau of Justice Statistics, 2002; World Health Organization, 2002). Behavioral science needs to achieve a more complete understanding of the causes of antisocial behavior to provide an evidence base for effectively controlling and preventing antisocial behavior. A new wave of intervention research in the last decade has demonstrated clear success for a number of programs designed to prevent antisocial behavior (www.preventingcrime.org; Heinrich, Brown & Aber, 1999; Sherman et al., 1999; Weissberg, Kumpfer, & Seligman, 2003). Nevertheless, the reduction in antisocial behavior brought about by even the best prevention programs is, on average, modest (Dodge, 2003; Wasserman & Miller, 1998; Olds et al., 1998; Heinrich et al., 1999; Wandersman & Florin, 2003; Wilson, Gottfredson, & Najaka, 2001). The best-designed intervention programs reduce serious juvenile offenders' recidivism only by about 12% (Lipsey & Wilson, 1998). This modest success of interventions that were theory-driven, well designed, and amply funded sends a clear message that we do not yet understand the causes of antisocial behavior well enough to prevent it.

Simultaneous with the new wave of research evaluating interventions is a wave of research pointing to the concentration of antisocial behavior in families. In the 1970s, the astounding discovery that fewer than 10% of individuals perpetrate more than 50% of crimes (Wolfgang, Figlio, & Sellin, 1972) prompted researchers to investigate individual career criminals (Blumstein & Cohen, 1987) and examine the childhood origins of such persistent reoffenders (Moffitt, 1993). This research constructed the evidence base supporting the new wave of preventive intervention trials (Yoshikawa, 1994). Recently journalists have drawn public attention to certain families that across several generations seem to contain far more than their share of criminal family members (Butterfield, 1996, 2002). This familial concentration of crime has been confirmed as a characteristic of the general population (Farrington, Barnes, & Lambert, 1996; Farrington, Jolliffe, Loeber, Stouthamer-Loeber, & Kalb, 2001; Rowe, & Farrington, 1997). In general, fewer than 10% of the families in any community account for more than 50% of that community's criminal offenses. The family concentration of antisocial behavior could be explained by a genetic influence on antisocial behavior, but it could just as easily be explained by nongenetic social transmission of antisocial behavior within families. Again, causation is not well understood. Studies that cannot disentangle genetic and environmental influences cannot help.

ANTISOCIAL BEHAVIOR RESEARCH IS STUCK IN THE RISK-FACTOR STAGE

Influential reviewers have concluded that the study of antisocial behavior has been stuck in the "risk-factor" stage (Farrington, 1988, 2003; Hinshaw, 2002; Rutter, 2003a, 2003b) because so few studies have used designs that are able to document causality (Rutter, Pickles, Murray, & Eaves, 2001). A variable is called a risk factor if it has a documented predictive relation with antisocial outcomes, whether or not the association is causal. The causal status of most risk factors is unknown; we know what statistically predicts psychopathology outcomes but not how or why (Kraemer, 2003; Kraemer et al., 1997). There are consequences to the field's failure to push beyond the risk factor stage to achieve an understanding of causal processes. Valuable resources have been wasted because intervention programs have proceeded on the basis of risk factors, without sufficient research to understand causal processes.

A central barrier to interpreting an association between an alleged environmental risk factor and antisocial outcome as a cause–effect association is, of course, the old bugbear that correlation is not causation. Some unknown third variable may account for the association, and that third variable may well be heritable. During the 1990s, the assumption that "nurture" influences behavior came under fire. Traditional socialization studies of antisocial behavior, which could not separate environmental influences from their correlated genes, were challenged by four important empirical discoveries: (1) ostensible environmental measures are influenced by genetic factors (Plomin & Bergeman, 1991); (2) parents' heritable traits influence the environments they provide for their children (Kendler, 1996; Plomin, 1994); (3) people's genes influence the environments they encounter (Kendler, 1996; Plomin, DeFries, & Loehlin, 1977); and (4) environmental influences did not seem to account for the similarity among persons growing up in the same family (Rowe, 1994). It was said that although non-behavioral-genetic studies might show that certain rearing experiences predict young people's antisocial outcomes, theories of causation based on findings from such designs were guilty of a fundamental logical error: mistaking correlation for causation (Scarr, 1992). These challenges culminated in admonishments that so far the evidence for genetic influences outweighed the evidence for environmental influences within the family (Harris, 1998; Rowe, 1994). Many social scientists responded to this claim, reasserting evidence for environmental influences (Collins, Maccoby, Steinberg, Hetherington, & Bornstein, 2000; Reid, Patterson, & Snyder, 2002; Vandell, 2000). However, the reason there is all this controversy about the importance of the family environment in the first place is that the evidence base was not decisive enough to compel both camps. The best way forward to resolve the debate is to use research designs that can provide leverage to test environmental causation.

Ordinary studies cannot test whether a risk factor is causal, and it would be unethical to assign children to experimental conditions expected to induce aggression. Fortunately, researchers can use three other methods for testing causation: natural-experiment studies of within-individual change (Cicchetti, 2003; Costello, Compton, Keeler, & Angold, 2003), treatment experiments (Howe, Reiss, & Yuh, 2002), and the focus of this review: behavioral-genetic designs (Moffitt, 2005). None of the three alone can provide decisive proof of causation, but if all supply corroborative evidence by ruling out alternative noncausal explanations about a risk factor, then a strong case for causation can be made.

TESTING HYPOTHESES ABOUT ENVIRONMENTAL CAUSATION

Inference from Different Types of Behavioral-Genetic Designs

Antisocial behavior has been studied in twins reared together, adoptees, and twins reared apart. Behavioral-genetics research is not limited to exotic samples; researchers also examine ordinary families whose members vary in genetic relatedness (e.g., full siblings, half-siblings, step-siblings, cousins, and unrelated children reared in the same family) (Rowe, Almeida, & Jacobson, 1999). This variety of research designs offers a special advantage for inference, because comparing their estimates tells us that the environmental effect sizes for antisocial behavior are robust across different designs; they are not biased by the limitations and flaws peculiar to one design.

A number of potential flaws are unique to adoption studies. First, adoption agencies could attempt to maximize similarity between the adoptee's biological and adoptive families to increase the child's chance of fitting in with the new family ("selective placement"). Relatedly, biological mothers who intend to give their baby away may neglect prenatal care and continue to abuse substances during pregnancy, and many unwanted babies experience institutionalization before they are adopted. If adoptive homes, prenatal care, and institutional care were selectively worse for the babies given up by antisocial biological mothers, this could bias estimates of heritability upward and estimates of environment effects downward, by misattributing the criminogenic influences of these three unmeasured nongenetic factors to a criminogenic influence of genes (Mednick, Moffitt, Gabrielli, & Hutchings, 1986). Second, both adoptees and twins reared apart are likely to be reared in home environments that are unusually good for children because adoptive parents are carefully screened. Adoption breaks up the association between genetic risk and environmental risk naturally occurring in ordinary families by removing genetically at-risk children from damaging homes and placing them in salutary homes. As a result, interactions between environmental adversity and genetic vulnerability that exacerbate behavioral problems in ordinary children (and twins) are uncommon among adoptees (Stoolmiller, 1999). The restricted range of rearing environments resulting from screening of adoptive parents could suppress estimates of environmental effects and thus bias heritability estimates upward (Fergusson, Lynskey, & Horwood, 1995; Stoolmiller,

1999). However, this flaw of adoption studies is offset by studies of national twin registers (e.g., Cloninger & Gottesman, 1987) or stratified high-risk twin samples (e.g., Moffitt & E-risk Study Team, 2002), because such sampling frames represent the complete population range of environmental and genetic backgrounds.

Studies of twins avoid the potential flaws of adoption studies, but they suffer several potential flaws of their own. First, the logic of the twin design assumes that all the greater similarity between monozygotic (MZ) compared to dizygotic (DZ) twins can safely be ascribed to MZ twins' greater genetic similarity. This "equal environments assumption" requires that MZ twins are not treated more alike than DZ twins on the causes of antisocial behavior (Kendler, Neale, Kessler, Heath, & Eaves, 1994). Because MZ twins look identical, they might be treated more similarly than DZ twins in some way that promotes antisocial behavior, and as a result, estimates of heritability from studies of twins reared together could be biased upward, and estimates of environmental effects could be biased downward, relative to the correct population value (DiLalla, 2002). However, studies of adoptees do not suffer this flaw, and neither do studies of twins reared apart, because MZ twins reared apart do not share environments (unless their genetically influenced behaviors evoke similar reactions from caregivers in their separate rearing environments, which is a genetic effect). Second, in studies of twins, MZ twins differ more than DZ twins in prenatal factors affecting intrauterine growth; for example, MZ twins sharing the same chorion appear to suffer more fetal competition for nutrients. These intrauterine factors also violate the assumption that environments are equal for MZ and DZ twins, but intrauterine differences tend to make MZ twins less alike than their genotypes and thus would bias heritability estimates downward and environmental effects upward (Rutter, 2002). Third, genomic factors that make some MZ twin pairs' genotypes less than perfectly identical (such as random inactivation of genes on one of each girl's two X chromosomes; Jorgensen et al., 1992) could in theory affect twin-study estimates, but so far no evidence shows that these processes influence behavior. Fourth, parental assortative mating can bias heritability estimates. Coupled partners are known to share similarly high or low levels of antisocial behaviors (Galbaud du Fort, Boothroyd, Bland, Newman, & Kakuma, 2002; Krueger, Moffitt, Caspi, Bleske, & Silva, 1998). When parents of twins mate for similarity, it should increase the genetic similarity of DZ twins, but MZ twins' genetic similarity cannot increase beyond its original 100%, and as a result heritability estimates will be biased downward and environmental estimates upward, relative to the correct population value. The implication of biological-parent assortative mating for adoption studies is the opposite; biological-parent similarity for antisocial behaviors would bias adoptees' heritability upward relative to the correct population value (because adoptee/biological-parent correlations would represent a double dose of parental genes). Fifth, twin studies using adult reports to measure behavior sometimes suffer from rater artifacts; for example, adults may mix up or conflate the behavior of MZ twins and they may exaggerate differences between DZ twins. Such a rater artifact does not afflict adoption studies (nor twin studies using the twins' self-reports, as twins do not confuse themselves).

In any case, comparisons between designs have revealed that studies of twins reared together yield estimates that are more similar than different to the estimates from studies of twins reared apart or of adoptees (Rhee & Waldman, 2002). On the one hand, this is because any bias arising from factors such as selective adoptee placement, violations of the equal-environment assumption, intrauterine twin differences, or assortative mating, is only very small (Miles & Carey, 1997; Rutter, 2002). On the other hand, these factors bias estimates upward as often as they bias them downward, canceling each other out. The bottom line is that it is important for tests of environmental risk to exploit a variety of behavioral-genetics designs, as well as experimental designs and studies of within-individual change.

Behavioral-Genetic Studies of Parenting Effects on Children's Aggression

To illustrate how behavioral-genetic designs are helping to move the study of antisocial behaviors from the risk factor stage to causal understanding, we next review research investigating one risk factor, parents' "bad parenting" of their children, and one antisocial outcome, "children's aggression." Of course, behavioral-genetics studies address other socializing agents (e.g., siblings, peers, teachers, communities, and historical periods) and other behavioral outcomes (e.g. depression, anxiety, prosocial behaviors, cognitive abilities, and personality) but we focus on studies of parenting and aggression as our example, because that is the most developed body of literature.

We have construed bad parenting broadly; this review includes risk factors from mothers' smoking heavily during pregnancy to inconsistent or unskilled discipline to frank child neglect and abuse. The outcome, "children's physical aggression," includes hitting, fighting, bullying, cruelty, and so forth. It is already known that "bad parenting" statistically predicts children's aggression, and bad parenting plays a central causal role in leading theories of antisocial behavior (Lahey, Moffitt, & Caspi, 2003; Thornberry, 1996). The aim of the research reviewed here is to determine whether the relation between bad parenting and children's aggression is a true cause–effect relation.

Our research review systematically tackles six questions:

1. Is there evidence that children's aggression cannot be wholly explained by genetic factors, and must have non-genetic environmental causes as well?
2. Do parents' genes influence bad parenting?
3. Does a genetic effect on parents' bad parenting confound a cause-effect interpretation of the association between bad parenting and children's aggression?
4. Does a genetic "child effect" evoke bad parenting to further confound a cause–effect interpretation of the association between bad parenting and children's aggression?
5. After genetic confounds are controlled, does bad parenting have an environmentally mediated causal effect on children's aggression?
6. Does bad parenting interact with genetic risk, such that the effects of bad parenting are even stronger among genetically vulnerable children?

We address each question in a separate section, first describing research designs that can answer each question and then reviewing findings so far. The research designs covered here are not intended to be exhaustive but to illustrate what kinds of studies could be done, using the logic of behavioral-genetic methods.

1. Is Children's Aggression Wholly Accounted for by Genetic Factors, or Does It Have Nongenetic Causes as Well?

More than 100 twin, adoption, and sibling studies have been carried out to answer this question. This work has revealed that genetic causal processes account for only about half of the population variation in antisocial behavior, thereby unequivocally proving that environmental influences account for the other half. This fact constitutes a remarkable contribution to the understanding of causation (Plomin, 1994). In addition, it is now recognized that the heritability coefficient indexes not only the direct effects of genes but also the effects of interactions between genes and family-wide environments (Purcell 2002; Rutter & Silberg, 2002). In such interactions the effect of an environmental risk may be even larger than previously reported, among the subgroup of individuals having a vulnerable genotype. This is likely to be the case for antisocial behaviors.

One useful feature of behavioral-genetics research designs is that they offer two powerful methods for documenting the importance of environmental effects (Plomin, DeFries, McClearn, & McGuffin, 2001). One of these methods of detecting environmental influence tests whether any of the family members in a study sample are more similar than can be explained by the proportion of genes they share. For instance, MZ twins' genetic similarity is twice that of DZ twins, and therefore, if nothing but genes influenced antisocial behavior, MZ twins' behavior ought to be at least twice as similar as DZ twins'. If not, then something environmental has influenced the twins and enhanced their similarity. For almost all human behavioral traits studied so far, environmental factors shared by family members (variously labeled the "family-wide," "common," or "shared" environment) have not been found to make family members similar. In other words, the estimated influence of shared environment has been found to be almost nil for most human behavioral traits (Rowe, 1994). Antisocial behavior is a marked exception. A comparison of shared-environment effects across 10 psychiatric disorders revealed that such effects were stronger for antisocial personality and conduct disorder than for affective, anxiety, or substance disorders (Kendler, Prescott, Myers, & Neale, 2003). Estimates of shared-environment effects on population variation in antisocial behavior are about 15–20% as reported by meta-analyses and reviews (Miles & Carey, 1997; Rhee & Waldman, 2002). The small size of this shared-environment estimate should not be too surprising, because the twin-study coefficient indexing the shared environment does not include environmental effects involved in gene–environment interactions. We can think of the shared-environment coefficient as the residual effects of shared environments that remain, after controlling for gene–environment interactions. As most human behavior involves nature–nurture interplay, it is remarkable that as much as 20% of the population variation in antisocial behavior can be attributed to direct environmental effects not conditional on genetic vulnerability.

The second method of detecting the presence of environmental influence is to test whether any family members are less similar than expected from the proportion of genes they share (Plomin & Daniels, 1987). For instance, if a pair of MZ twins, despite sharing all their genes, are not perfectly identical in antisocial behavior, this indicates that experience has reduced their behavioral similarity. After estimates of the influences of heritability (50%) and shared family environment (20%) on antisocial behavior are calculated, the remainder of population variation, 30%, is assumed to reflect environmental influences not shared by family members (variously labeled "unique," "person-specific," or "nonshared" experiences). These experiences might include criminogenic experiences unique to the individual and not shared with his or her sibling, such as a head injury, being the unique target of sexual abuse, living with an antisocial spouse, or serving a prison sentence. There are two caveats about estimates of the effect of nonshared environments. First, measurement error inflates these estimates because random mistakes in measuring behavior will result in scores that look different for twins in an MZ pair, and it is not easy to differentiate such faux MZ differences from true MZ differences caused by the twins' nonshared experiences. The second caveat is that the coefficient for nonshared environmental effects indexes not only the direct effects of nonshared experiences but also the effects of interactions between nonshared environments and genes (Purcell, 2002; Rutter & Silberg, 2002). Thus, some portion of the nonshared environment effect may be attributable to error or genes, and the size of this portion is unknown.

In sum, behavioral-genetics studies have shown that the answer to question 1, "Does children's aggression have any nongenetic causes?," is a definite yes; there is strong evidence that environmental causes must exist.

2. Do Parents' Genes Influence Bad Parenting?

It is important to know the size of the contribution of parents' genotypes to their bad parenting, because if parenting is substantially influenced by parents' genotype, then its correlation with children's aggression cannot be confidently interpreted as a cause–effect relation. But how much do people's genes influence their parenting? Answering this question requires researchers to treat parenting as a phenotype in behavioral-genetics research.

What Research Designs Can Be Used to Answer This Question?

We can study *adoptions* to test if biological parents' bad parenting (of the children they did not give up for adoption) predicts that their adopted-away child will also engage in bad parenting when she becomes a parent. This study would show that bad parenting is genetically transmitted, in the absence of social transmission. However, this study has not been conducted, because of the difficulty of obtaining parenting data from two generations of adults separated by adoption.

We can study *adult MZ twins reared apart* to test whether they are similar in using bad parenting on their children. The Swedish Adoption Twin Study of Aging carried out this design, by asking 50 pairs of adult MZ twins reared apart to report their own parenting styles using the Moos Family Environment Scale (Plomin, McClearn, Pederson, Nesselroade, & Bergeman, 1989). Results indicated that 25% of the variation in parenting was genetically influenced.

We can study *adult twin parents* to ascertain how much variation in their bad parenting is attributable to genetic versus environmental sources. The aforementioned Swedish twin study carried out this design, studying 386 adult twin pairs, and again results indicated that 25% of the variation in the Family Environment Scale was genetically influenced (Plomin et al., 1989). In another study, 1,117 pairs of midlife twin volunteers who had on average reared three children reported their own parenting styles. The heritability estimate for an overall measure of parenting, called care, was 34% (Perusse, Neale, Heath, & Eaves, 1994). A Virginia sample of 262 pairs of adult twin mothers reported their own parenting styles, and the heritability estimates were 21% for "physical discipline," 27% for "limit-setting," and 38% for "warmth" (Kendler, 1996; Wade & Kendler, 2000). An Oregon sample of 186 pairs of adult twin mothers and adoptee mothers reported their own parenting styles, and the heritability estimates ranged from 60% for "positive support" to 24% for "control" (Losoya, Callor, Rowe, & Goldsmith, 1997). These findings were echoed by a study of 236 pairs of adult twin mothers reporting their own parenting, in which genetic effects were found for "positivity" and "monitoring" (Towers, Spotts, & Neiderhiser, 2001; Neiderhiser et al., 2004). Finally, a study of 1,034 adult twin mothers found a heritability estimate of more than 50% for self-reported smoking during pregnancy, which is a known prenatal parenting risk factor for children's aggression (D'Onofrio et al., 2003).

What Research Is Needed?

This very small literature is a good beginning, but a number of limitations need to be overcome. First, the studies have relied on the twin design, and twin-design weaknesses ought to be complemented by the strengths of the adoption design (see Deater-Deckard, Fulker, & Plomin, 1999). Second, measurement has relied on parents' self reports, and thus the findings are a mix between genetic influences on actual parenting behavior and genetic influences on self-perception and self-presentation (Kendler, 1996; Plomin, 1994). As a third limitation, studies have tended to focus on mothers and excluded fathers, for the obvious reason that fathers' nonparticipation in research disproportionately characterizes families of aggressive children. However, fathers' antisocial behavior in the home is a central aspect of bad parenting that predicts children's aggression (Jaffee, Moffitt, Caspi, & Taylor, 2003). Fourth, and most serious for our purposes of investigating antisocial behavior, the samples underrepresent families at serious risk, and the parenting measures do not address the most powerful bad-parenting risk factors for children's aggression, such as exposure to domestic violence, child neglect, maternal rejection, and child abuse. These serious forms of bad parenting themselves constitute antisocial acts, and as a result we should anticipate that the influence of parents' genes on them is much stronger than the genetic influences found for parenting styles within the normative range, such as spanking, monitoring, or limit-setting. Because serious bad parenting is antisocial, it is not unreasonable to expect genetic influence on serious bad parenting to resemble genetic influence on other antisocial behaviors (50%).

The answer to question 2, "Do parent's genes influence bad parenting?," seems to be "probably." It may be surprising that so little research has been done on the question of a genetic contribution to bad parenting. The question has been neglected because parenting has not often been viewed by behavioral-genetics researchers as a phenotypical outcome variable. Moreover, developmental researchers who are interested in parenting as an outcome almost never adopt behavioral-genetics research methods. It is quite likely that bad parenting is under some amount of genetic influence because parenting styles are known to be associated with parents' personality traits (Belsky & Barends, 2002; Spinath & O'Connor, 2003) and personality traits are known to be under genetic influence (Plomin & Caspi, 1999). Bad parenting should be treated as a phenotype in future behavioral-genetics research (McGuire, 2003).

3. Does an Effect of Parents' Genes on Bad Parenting Confound a Cause–Effect Interpretation of the Association between Bad Parenting and Children's Aggression?

The technical term for this question is "passive" correlation between genotype and an environmental measure, often abbreviated as "rGE" (Plomin et al., 1977). A passive rGE confound occurs when a child's behavior and the environment his or her parents provide are correlated because they have the same origins in his parents' genotype (i.e., not because bad parenting itself causes children's aggression).

It is important to note that the mere evidence that bad parenting is under influence of parents' genes (question 2) is not sufficient to conclude that this genetic influence goes on to mediate the connection between bad parenting and children's aggression. Rutter and Silberg (2002) make this point, explaining that genes influence which mothers have low-birthweight babies but babies' birthweights are wholly determined by environmental conditions, not by any genes inherited from their mothers. For this reason it is important to disentangle (1) the genetic origins of bad parenting from (2) the genetic and environmental mechanisms by which bad parenting produces children's aggression.

What Research Designs Can Be Used to Answer This Question?

There are at least four appropriate research designs, but to our knowledge none of them has been carried out. We can study *adoptions* to test if the biological parents' bad parenting predicts the adopted-away children's aggression, even if parent and child never have contact. This study has not been conducted, because of the difficulty of obtaining parenting data from adopted children's biological parents. We can compare correlations between bad parenting and children's aggression in *natural families versus adoptive families*. If the correlation is stronger in natural families (which have both genetic and environmental processes of transmission) than in adoptive families (which have only environmental transmission), then genetic transmission is taking place (Plomin, 1994). However, this design is biased toward finding evidence of an rGE confound, because there is more variation in bad parenting among natural than adoptive families, which could produce larger correlations with children's aggression in natural families (Stoolmiller, 1999). To avoid such bias, we can conduct a study *within adoptive families* to test if rearing parents' bad parenting is more strongly correlated with their natural children's aggression than with their adoptive child's aggression. The within-family design holds constant the variation in bad parenting across natural versus adoptive parent–child pairs but requires a sample of families having both an adopted and a natural child, not too far apart in age. We are not aware of a study that has compared the correlations between bad parenting and natural children's aggression versus adoptive children's aggression. However, a study was conducted of 667 adoptive families, which found adoptive parents' reports of "family functioning" were more strongly correlated with self-reported antisocial behavior in their natural child than their adopted child (McGue, Sharma, & Benson, 1996).

A promising method studies *the families of adult MZ twins who are mothers* to test if MZ aunts' bad parenting predicts their nephews' aggression. In this twin-mothers design, both MZ sisters are genetic mothers to each others' birth children. However, the MZ aunt does not provide the rearing environment for her nieces and nephews; only the children's birth mother is an environmental mother to them. If the MZ aunts' and the MZ mothers' parenting predicts the children's aggression to the same extent, this would be strong evidence of a complete rGE confound. But, if the MZ mother's parenting predicts the children's aggression better than does the MZ aunt's parenting, this would show that bad parenting has an environmental effect. This design offers the capacity to disentangle sources of bad parenting from mechanisms of risk for the children of bad parents, particularly when DZ twin mothers as well as MZ twin mothers are sampled (D'Onofrio et al., 2003; Silberg & Eaves, 2004). This children-of-twins design is newly being applied to the question of causes of children's aggression by Silberg (2002), but findings were not available at the time of this writing.

The aforementioned methods test the hypothesis that genetic transmission explains the observed association between bad parenting and child aggression by looking for an effect of parenting on behavior over and above genetic influence on behavior. Another method is to *compare the effect size of the association between bad parenting and children's aggression before versus after genetic influences are controlled.* Any shrinkage estimates the extent to which the association is mediated by genetic transmission. In their meta-analysis of studies of differential treatment of siblings, Turkheimer and Waldron (2000, Table 3) showed that the effect sizes for associations between risk factors and behavior outcomes tended to shrink by at least half when genetic confounds were controlled. However, this meta-analysis compared effect sizes across two groups of studies, those with versus without genetic designs, and the groups of studies differed on design features such as sample composition or sample size. Comparisons of the effect sizes for bad parenting predicting children's aggression before and after genetic controls within the same sample would be more informative.

What Research Is Needed?

A close reading of the literature reveals that researchers have neglected two questions: whether genes contribute to bad parenting, and whether genetic transmission confounds environmental interpretations of the link between bad parenting and children's aggression. The field seems to have presupposed affirmative answers to these questions but not to have built a conclusive evidence base. As such, research applying any of the designs described here to parenting is needed. However, a comparison of effect sizes in studies with versus without genetic controls suggests genetic transmission might explain as much as half the connection. The answer to question 3, "Are cause–effect interpretations of the connection between bad parenting and children's aggression confounded by genetic transmission?," seems to be "probably."

4. Does a Genetic "Child Effect" Evoke Bad Parenting to Confound a Cause–Effect Interpretation of the Association between Bad Parenting and Children's Aggression?

The technical term for this question is "evocative" correlation between genotype and an environmental measure, and it is also abbreviated as "rGE" (Plomin et al., 1977). Evocative rGE occurs when a child's behavior and the parenting he receives are correlated because they have the same origins in his own genotype (i.e., not because bad parenting itself causes children's aggression).

What Research Designs Can Be Used to Answer This Question?

A large number of studies has ascertained *twins' recollections of how they were treated by their parents* during childhood, and found that MZ twins' ratings of their parents' childrearing are more similar than DZ twins' ratings, suggesting an influence of childrens' genotype on parents' parenting (Hur & Bouchard, 1995; Rowe, 1983; Kendler, 1996). There is a basic difficulty with this literature, however. Although it seems reasonable to interpret the findings as evidence for a child effect on bad parenting, studies of twins' self-reports about their parents' treatment of them do not rule out the alternate interpretation of a genetic effect on perceptual bias, according to which MZ twins are more alike than DZ twins in how they interpret their parents' treatment or how they revise their childhood memories (Krueger, Markon, & Bouchard, 2003). Nonetheless, the body of studies is generally interpreted as evidence for genetic child effects on parenting because several other studies have shown genetic child effects using adoption and sibling family designs instead of twins, and by using observational or multi-informant measures of parenting instead of twins' self-reports (Braungart, Plomin, & Fulker, 1992; Deater-Deckard et al., 1999; Neiderhiser et al., 2004; O'Connor, Hetherington, Reiss, & Plomin, 1995, Reiss, Neiderhiser, Hetherington, & Plomin, 2000; Rende, Slomkowski, Stocker, Fulker, & Plomin, 1992). These numerous studies decidedly demonstrated that a genetic child effect on parenting exists, but they did not demonstrate what it is that children do to provoke bad parenting. In other words, these studies did not include children's aggression as a measured variable.

Another research design is to study *adoptions*, to test whether adoptees' aggression predicts their adoptive parents' bad parenting while establishing that the adoptees' aggression has a genetic basis (i.e., that it is predicted by their biological parents' antisocial behavior). Three studies have used this compelling design (Ge et al., 1996; O'Connor, Deater-Deckard, Fulker, Rutter, & Plomin, 1998; Riggins-Caspers, Cadoret, Knutson, & Langbehn, 2003). All three studies reported that adoptees who are at high genetic risk for psychopathology receive more discipline and control from their adoptive parents than adoptees who are at low genetic risk. Furthermore, unlike prior research, the three studies demonstrated that the link from a child's genetic risk to adoptive parent's parenting is mediated by the child's genetically influenced aggressive behavior problems. Individual studies in this threesome were limited by a small sample, or by single-source retrospective data, but as a set the three studies provide robust evidence for a genetically mediated child effect in which the causal arrow runs from children's aggression to parenting.

A third design for testing genetic child effects is to study *twin children*, asking whether twin A's aggression predicts the bad parenting received by twin B, and vice versa. This is an application of bivariate twin modeling. Its basic logic is that if the correlation between twin A's aggression and twin B's experience of bad parenting is higher among MZ pairs than DZ pairs, it would indicate that the same set of genetic influences causes children's aggression and provokes bad parenting. Bad parenting must be measured separately for each twin, so that it can be used as a phenotype, like each twin's aggression. Two studies of several hundred sibling pairs taking part in the study of Nonshared Environment in Adolescent Development (NEAD) have applied variations of this bivariate approach, using multisource measures of adolescents' and parents' behavior. A genetic-child effect accounted for most of the correlation between adolescents' antisocial behavior and parents' negativity assessed cross-sectionally (Pike, McGuire, Hetherington, Reiss, & Plomin, 1996) and longitudinally after accounting for the continuity of adolescent antisocial behavior (Neiderhiser, Reiss, Hetherington, & Plomin, 1999).

It is important to know whether the genetic-child effect for ordinary parenting (as indicated by previous adoption studies and the NEAD study) also applies to extreme forms of bad parenting associated with serious, persistent antisocial behavior. We applied the bivariate modeling approach to this question in our Environmental Risk ("E-risk") longitudinal study of 1,116 British families with young twins (Jaffee, Caspi, Moffitt, Polo-

Tomas, Price, & Taylor, 2004). To do this, the E-risk study incorporated two innovations (Moffitt & Erisk Study Team, 2002). First, it assessed a birth cohort in which one-third of families were selected to oversample families that were at high risk (findings are weighted back to represent the population of British families having babies in the 1990s). Second, the study interviewed mothers about parenting that was beyond normal limits (physical maltreatment: neglectful or abusive care resulting in injury, sexual abuse, registry with child protection services) as well as about parenting in the normative range (frequency of corporal punishment: grabbing, shaking, spanking). Children's genes influenced which children received corporal punishment, explaining 24% of the variation in the cohort, but children's genes were unrelated to becoming a victim of maltreatment. Bivariate twin modeling of the cross-twin, cross-phenotype correlations revealed that children's genes accounted for almost all the correlation between corporal punishment and children's aggression, indicating that most of the observed association between this form of parenting and children's aggression is a genetic child effect. However, children's genes did not account for the correlation between physical maltreatment and children's aggression, indicating that extreme, serious bad parenting causes children's aggression for reasons that are not genetic. Although difficult children can and do provoke their parents to use frequent corporal punishment in the normal range, factors leading to injurious maltreatment lie not within the child but within the family environment or the adult abuser. There are limits to child effects.

What Research Is Needed?

Taken together, the adoption and twin studies reviewed in this section provide evidence to answer question 4: Yes, the observed association between normative parenting and child aggression is in large part a spurious artifact of a third variable that causes both: the child's genotype. A provocative deduction from the research to date is that Scarr (1991) might have been correct when she argued that improving parenting in the normal range of environments will not produce significant changes in children's antisocial psychopathology because the associations between ordinary parenting and child outcome are not causal: "There is no evidence that family environments, except the worst, have any significant effect on the development of conduct disorders, psychopathy, or other common behavior disorders" (Scarr, 1991, p. 403). Scarr (1992) further argued that damaging environmental conditions outside the expected range will have causal influences on children quite apart from genetic influences, and in keeping with this notion, one study showed maltreatment makes children aggressive apart from any influence of their genotypes. This distinction between normative versus extreme forms of parenting has implications for future research. Most of the genetically informative studies to date have assessed parenting using omnibus measures (e.g., "family functioning," "negativism," and "control") because the goal was to ascertain whether or not genetic child effects existed at all. However, parenting intervention programs try to change specific well-defined forms of parental behavior. To inform these interventions, research is needed to query genetic versus environmental mediation of specific features of parenting. Furthermore, the aspects of parenting that correlate with children's aggression are probably quite different in early childhood, later childhood, and adolescence. Genetically informative studies of samples at different ages are needed to inform parenting interventions tailored to developmental stages.

We have looked here at the specific question of whether children's genotype evokes bad parenting, but it is useful to note that the evocative type of rGE is a subset of a larger class referred to as active rGE. Active rGE encompasses at least three different processes, when people's genetically influenced behavior leads them to "(1) create, (2) seek, or (3) otherwise end up in environments that match their genotypes" (Rutter & Silberg, 2002, p. 473). Antisocial behavior can bring about each of these three processes at any point in the life course (Scarr & McCartney, 1983). These active rGE processes are of enormous importance in understanding the continuity of antisocial behavior across the entire life course (Caspi & Moffitt, 1995; Laub & Sampson, 2003). Once genetically influenced behavior has brought a person into contact with an environment, the environment may have unique causal effects of its own, cutting off opportunities to develop alternative prosocial behaviors, promoting the persistence of antisocial behavior, and exacerbating its seriousness (Moffitt, 1993). Research is needed to test for active rGE processes involved in antisocial behavior at developmental stages across the life course.

5. After Both Genetic Confounds Are Controlled, Does Bad Parenting Have Any Environmentally Mediated Effect on Children's Aggression?

The new generation of research designs that can evaluate whether a risk factor has an environmentally mediated effect on children's aggression has three key features. First, the studies must employ a genetically sensitive design to control for the confounding effects of parents' genes or children's genes on putative environmental measures. Second, the genetically informative samples must accurately represent the full range of families' environmental circumstances. Many behavioral-genetics samples suffer substantial biases in recruitment and attrition, inadvertently restricting their range of participating families to primarily the middle class. The third key feature is that designs must employ an actual measure of the construct alleged to have environmental effects on children; in the case here, bad parenting. Traditional behavioral-genetics studies have reported latent environmental variance components (i.e., these studies report statistical inferences derived from the relative similarity of twins) but not direct measures. This has been problematic because even very large twin studies are underpowered to detect environmental influence on twin similarity as a latent variance component, whereas statistical power to detect such influence is increased if a putative environmental variable is measured so its effects can be estimated empirically (Kendler, 1993). In keeping with this, significant effects for a measured variable have been found even despite the presence of a nonsignificant shared-environment variance component (Kendler, Neale, Kessler, Heath, & Eaves, 1992). In this section we abandon the distinction between "shared" and "nonshared" environmental variance components because shared and nonshared effects are not features of a measured environmental risk; one form of bad parenting, such as maltreatment, can exert either shared or nonshared effects, or both (Rutter & Silberg, 2002; Turkheimer & Waldron, 2000).

What Research Designs Can Be Used to Answer This Question?

Four basic behavioral-genetics methods can be used to rule out gene–environment correlation confounds while testing causation by putative environmental risk factors. As mentioned before, natural experiments and intervention experiments can also assess environmental causation, but here we focus on genetically sensitive designs.

We can study *adoptions* to test if the adoptive parents' bad parenting increases adoptees' aggression, over and above the genetic influence from the biological parents' aggression. The large adoption studies of antisocial behavior that emerged from Scandinavia and the United States in the 1970s and 1980s were primarily cited for their innovation of demonstrating genetic influences; they showed that adoptees' criminal offending was significantly associated with the antisocial behavior of their biological parents, although these parents did not rear the adoptees. However, some of these same studies asked whether adoptees' criminal offending was also associated with the antisocial behavior of the adoptive parents who did rear them (Bohman, Cloninger, Sigverdsson, & von Knorring, 1982; Cadoret, Cain, & Crowe, 1983; Mednick & Christiansen, 1977; vanDusen, Mednick, Gabrielli, & Hutchings, 1983). Rates of antisocial behavior in adoptive parents were extremely low (because of adoption agency screening), and the adoptive-parent effects were very small and often nonsignificant, but these studies constituted the first real empirical attempts to test if bad parental behavior exerts a nongenetic effect on children's aggression.

We can study the *children of adult MZ twin mothers*. As described earlier, in this children-of-twin mothers design the MZ aunt constitutes a genetic mother to the child but not an environmental mother (Silberg & Eaves, 2004). Thus, if an MZ mother–son correlation is larger than its companion MZ aunt–nephew correlation, this provides evidence that environmental mothering influences children, over and above genes. Such research is under way (D'Onofrio et al., 2003; Silberg, 2002).

We can study *twin children* to test if the shared experience of bad parenting makes children more similar on aggression than could be predicted based on their degree of genetic relationship. A basic approach is to conduct ordinary behavior-genetics modeling that apportions genetic versus environmental effects on child behavior (denoted ACE), and then add a measured putative environmental risk factor (denoted M-ACE) to test if the children's shared experience of that risk factor can account for any of the shared environmental variation in their behavioral phenotype. The first twin study to apply this approach to problem behavior reported that living in a deprived neighborhood explained a significant 5% of the shared environmental variation in 2-year-olds' behavior problems (Caspi, Taylor, Moffitt, & Plomin, 2000). Another study applied this approach to examine 5-year-olds' exposure to their mothers' experience of domestic violence (Jaffee, Moffitt, Caspi, Taylor, & Arseneault, 2002). Exposure to domestic violence over the first 5 years of their lives was particularly relevant for children who developed both externalizing and internalizing problems simultaneously; such co-occurring problems are associated with poor prognosis. Domestic violence exposure explained a significant 13.5% of the shared-environment variance in children's comorbid outcome. A third, unpublished study reports that measured parental monitoring accounted for 15% of the shared-environment variance in behavior problems in a large sample of 11- to 12-year-old Finnish twins (described in Dick & Rose, 2002). A caveat about this approach is in order. Inference of environmental causation is compromised if parent and child share genes that simultaneously influence both the measure of parenting and the measure of child aggression.

The basic twin design can be improved on by adding indicators of mothers' and fathers' behavioral phenotype to the usual indicators of twin behavior. This approach, the "extended twin-family design" (Kendler, 1993), estimates the effect of the putative environmental risk factor on child behavior while controlling for genetic effects on both parents and children. An assumption of the design is that the parental phenotype measures carry genetic information parallel to that in the child phenotype measures. (Although this assumption is seldom fulfilled perfectly it seems not unreasonable for antisocial behavior, which has strong childhood-to-adulthood continuity.) The first twin study to apply this approach assessed antisocial conduct problems among adolescent twins and their parents (Meyer et al., 2000). The measured parenting variables were called marital discord and family adaptability. No effect was found for marital discord, but measured family adaptability accounted for 4% of the variance in adolescents' conduct problems.

A complementary approach to testing whether a risk factor has a causal (vs. noncausal) role in the origins of antisocial behavior has been used by studies that rule out passive rGE through statistical controls for parental antisocial behavior. This approach does not differentiate whether the risk factor is influenced at the genotype versus phenotype level of parental antisocial behavior. However, it does offer the advantage that it can be employed in nontwin samples, if phenotypical data are collected for all family members. In the aforementioned E-risk longitudinal twin study of 1,116 families, we examined the effects of fathers' bad parenting on young children's aggression (Jaffee et al., 2003). Mothers' antisocial behavior was statistically controlled, to make clear that the findings applied specifically to fathers' behavior. As expected from the literature on single mothers, a prosocial father's absence statistically predicted more aggression by his children. But the study revealed a new finding: An antisocial father's *presence* predicted more aggression by his children, and this harmful effect was exacerbated the more years a father lived with the family and the more time each week he spent taking care of the children. Inference of environmental causation was supported because the finding for conventional fathers (less involvement predicts more child aggression) was opposite that for antisocial fathers (more involvement predicts more child aggression), and the latter association held after ruling out passive rGE by statistically controlling for both parents' antisocial histories. Obtaining data from fathers is challenging (Caspi et al., 2001), but because fathers are often a target of social policies, a better evidence base about their parenting is needed.

In another report, the E-risk study evaluated the hypothesis that maternal depression promotes children's aggression (Kim-Cohen, Moffitt, Taylor, Pawlby, & Caspi, 2005). Research has shown that the children of depressed mothers are likely to develop conduct problems. However, it has not been clear that this correlation represents environmental transmission, because women's depression is under genetic influence (Kendler et al., 1992), it often co-occurs with a girlhood history of antisocial conduct, which is also under genetic influence (Moffitt, Caspi, Rutter, & Silva, 2001), and depressed women often mate assortatively with antisocial men (Moffitt, Caspi, Rutter, & Silva, 2001). We controlled for antisocial behavior in the twins' biological father, and for the mothers' own antisocial history. Although the connection between mothers' depression and children's conduct problems decreased after this stringent control for familial liability, it remained statistically significant. It concerned us that depressed women might exaggerate ratings of their children's problem behaviors, but the pattern of findings remained the same when teachers' ratings of child behavior were substituted as the outcome measure. A temporal analysis showed that the effect of maternal depression on children's aggression depended on the timing of the depression episodes (a type of natural experiment design). If E-risk mothers experienced depression, but only before their children's birth and not after, the children were not unusually aggressive. In contrast, only if mothers suffered depression while rearing their children were the children likely to develop aggression. Finally, the possibility that a child effect (in which children's aggression provoked mothers' depression) explained the association was ruled out by documenting within-individual change. After controlling for each child's aggression up to age 5, the children exposed to an episode of maternal depression between ages 5 and 7 became more aggressive by the age 7 assessment. Taken together, these four results are not consistent with a genetic account of the association between maternal depression and children's aggression.

The E-risk study also examined the effects of physical maltreatment on young children's aggression (Jaffee, Caspi, Moffitt, & Taylor, 2004), using twin-specific reports of maltreatment. This study satisfied six conditions that together supported the hypothesis that physical maltreatment has an environmentally mediated causal influence on children's aggression: (1) children's maltreatment history prospectively predicted aggression; (2) the severity of maltreatment bore a dose–response relation to aggression; (3) the experience of maltreatment was followed by increases in aggression from prior levels, within individual children; (4) there was no child effect provoking maltreatment; (5) maltreatment predicted aggression while mothers' and fathers' antisocial behavior were statistically controlled; and (6) modest but significant effects of maltreatment on aggression remained present after controlling for genetic transmission of liability to aggression in the family. A similar analytic approach using twin-specific measures of risk was taken by the Minnesota Twin Family Study (Burt, Krueger, McGue, & Iacono, 2003), which studied 808 11-year-old twin pairs. Models revealed that measured parent–child conflict accounted for 12% of the variance in the externalizing syndrome of oppositional, conduct, and attention-deficit/hyperactivity disorders (23% of the common environment variation in this syndrome).

As a final design, we can study *MZ twin children* to test if differences between siblings in their exposure to bad parenting makes them different on aggression. The fact that MZ twins are not perfectly concordant for aggression opens a window of opportunity to uncover if a nongenetic cause specific to one twin has produced the behavioral difference. A number of studies have tested if differential parental treatment can account for antisocial behavior differences between siblings and cousins within a family (e.g., Conger & Conger, 1994; Reiss et al., 2000; Rodgers, Rowe, & Li, 1994). Most of these studies have already been reviewed by Turkheimer and Waldron (2000). However, comparing the parenting experiences of discordant MZ twins allows the least ambiguous interpretation of results. Three studies have reported that MZ twin differences in bad parenting are correlated with MZ twin differences in antisocial behavior (Asbury, Dunn, Pike, & Plomin, 2003; Caspi et al., 2004; Pike, Reiss, Hetherington, & Plomin, 1996).

The E-risk study reported that within 600 MZ twin pairs, the twin who received relatively more maternal negativity and less maternal warmth developed more antisocial behavior problems (Caspi et al., 2004). Negativity and warmth were measured by coding voice tone and speech content in mothers' audiotaped speech about each of their twins separately, according to the well-known "expressed emotion" paradigm. This study provided the strongest evidence to date that the effect of mothers' emotional treatment of children causes aggression, by ruling out five alternative explanations of the finding.

1. Using MZ twin pairs ruled out the possibility that a genetically transmitted liability explained both the mother's emotion and her child's antisocial behavior.
2. Using MZ twins also ruled out the possibility that a genetic child effect provoking maternal emotion accounted for the finding.
3. The study used the longitudinal natural experiment approach to rule out that any non-genetic child effect provoking maternal emotion accounted for the finding, by controlling for prior behavior that could have provoked maternal negative emotion and showing that individual children whose mothers were negative toward them at age 5 evidenced a subsequent increase of antisocial behavior between age 5 and age 7.
4. The study controlled for twin differences in birthweight in an effort to rule out the possibility that twins with neurodevelopmental difficulties had more behavior problems and elicited more negative emotion from mothers.
5. The study measured the children's behavior using teacher reports to rule out the possibility that a mother's negativity toward a child led her to exaggerate her report of the child's behavior problems.

Effect sizes for the influence of maternal emotion on children's aggression ranged from large ($r = .53$) to small ($r = .10$), depending on how many controls were applied.

Not All Tests of Putative Environmental Risk Factors Confirm Environmental Effects

Lest readers assume that application of behavioral-genetics methods to a putative environmental risk factor will necessarily affirm that its effects are environmentally mediated, it is useful to mention that some known risk factors do not appear to be causal. First, as noted previously, we found that children's genes accounted for virtually all the association between their corporal punishment (i.e., spanking) and their conduct problems. This indicated a "child effect," in which children's bad conduct provokes their parents to use more corporal punishment, rather than the reverse (Jaffee, Caspi, Moffit, Polo-Tomas, et al., 2004).

Second, studies have reported that mothers' smoking during pregnancy is correlated with children's conduct problems, but pregnancy smoking is known to be concentrated among mothers who are antisocial, have mental health problems, mate with antisocial men, and rear children in conditions of social deprivation. When the family liability for transmission of psychopathology from parents to children was controlled through statistical controls for the parents' antisocial behavior, mental health, and social deprivation, the effect of even heavy smoking during pregnancy disappeared. This study suggests that although pregnancy smoking undoubtedly has undesirable effects on outcomes such as infant birthweight, it is probably not a cause of conduct problems (Maughan, Taylor, Caspi, & Moffitt, 2004).

A third finding of nil environmental influence concerned father absence. In families having absent fathers, the children are known to have more conduct problems. However, absent fathers are more antisocial on average than fathers who stay with their children, and antisocial behavior can be genetically transmitted. When we controlled for mother's and father's antisocial history, we found that the association between father absence and children's conduct problems disappeared. This suggests that father absence is not a direct cause of conduct problems but, rather, is a proxy indicator for familial liability to antisocial behavior (Jaffee et al., 2003).

What Research Is Needed?

To date, question 5, "Does bad parenting have an environmentally mediated causal effect on children's aggression?," has been answered in the affirmative by behavioral-genetics reports from several twin samples, finding such effects for family adaptability, parent–child conflict, parental monitoring, bad fathering, maternal depression, physical maltreatment, and mothers' negative expressed emotions. These studies share an Achilles' heel; because different forms of parenting risk are concentrated in the same families, the particular parenting measure targeted in a study may be a proxy for some other, correlated risk factor. Research is needed that isolates the effects of one risk factor from its correlates. Nevertheless, whatever the most influential parenting behaviors are, the studies attest that parents can have environmentally mediated effects.

It may surprise some developmentalists to learn that when familial liability and child effects are controlled, parenting influences on children drop to small effect sizes. However, small effects ought to be expected, for three reasons. First, it must be remembered that these small effects reflect true environmental associations after they have been purged of the confounding influences that inflate effect sizes in nongenetic studies. Associations between risk factors and behavior outcomes tend to shrink by at least half when genetic confounds are controlled (Turkheimer & Waldron, 2000). This shrinkage suggests that the risk–outcome correlations that social scientists are accustomed to seeing are inflated to about double their true size. Second, small effects for any particular risk factor make sense, in view of evidence that clear risk for antisocial behavior accrues only when a person accumulates a large number of risks (Rutter, Giller, & Hagell, 1998), each of which may individually have only a small effect (Daniels & Plomin, 1985).

A third reason why small effects should not be too surprising is that they represent the main effects of measured environments, apart from any environmental effects involved in gene–environment (G × E) interactions. Recall that adoption studies found no effects of bad adoptive parenting in the absence of genetic liability, but bad adoptive parenting was associated with elevated antisocial outcomes for adoptees at genetic risk (Cadoret, Yates, Troughton, Woodworth, & Stewart, 1995; Mednick, Gabrielli, & Hutchings, 1984). In twin designs, when testing whether the shared experience of bad parenting enhances twin similarity in aggression over and above genetic influences on similarity, G × E interactions are controlled along with other genetic influences. In twin designs testing whether differential experiences of bad parenting are associated with MZ twin differences in aggression, differential outcomes arising from G × E interactions are ruled out by the twins' identical genotypes. In contrast, genetic risk and bad parenting are not usually disentangled in real life as they are in behavioral-genetics studies. In ordinary lives, genetic and environmental risks often coincide. It is possible in theory that environmental effects conditional on genetic vulnerability could be quite large. We next turn to the question of G × E interactions influencing antisocial behavior.

6. Testing the Hypothesis of Interaction between Genes and Environments

The study of G × E interaction entails substantial methodological challenges. It requires measured environments that are truly environmental, measured genetic influence, some means of separating them from each other, and enough statistical power for a sensitive test of interaction (Rutter & Silberg, 2002). Despite the challenges, theory-driven hypotheses of G × E interaction are well worth testing, because where measured G × E is found to influence behavior disorders, both specific genes and specific environmental risks can conceivably have moderate-to-large effects, as opposed to the very small effects expected from prior quantitative genetic research. Specific genes revealed to be stronger in the presence of environmental risk would guide strategic research into those genes' expression, possibly leading to genetic diagnostics and improved pharmacological interventions (Evans & Relling, 1999). Specific environmental effects revealed to be stronger in the presence of genetic risk would prompt a new impetus for specific environmental prevention efforts, and would help to identify who needs the prevention programs most. The study of G × E is especially exciting in antisocial behavior research, where investigations have pioneered the way for all behavioral disorders. Studies of antisocial behavior were first to report evidence of interaction between latent genetic and latent environmental risks ascertained in adoption studies, and also first to report evidence of an interaction between a measured genetic polymorphism and a measured environmental risk. Four research designs have been used.

Adoption Studies of Latent G × E

The first evidence that genetic and environmental risks influence antisocial behavior in a synergistic way came from adoption studies. Among the 6,000 families of male adoptees in the Danish Adoption Study, 14% of adoptees were convicted of crime though neither their biological nor their adoptive parents had been convicted, whereas 15% were convicted if their adoptive parent alone was convicted, 20% were convicted if their biological parent alone was convicted, and 25% were convicted if both biological and adoptive parents were convicted, although there were only 143 such cases (Mednick & Christiansen, 1977). This pattern of percentages did not represent a statistically significant cross-over interaction term, but it did illustrate clearly that the effects of genetic and environmental risk acting together were greater than the effects of either factor acting alone. The finding was buttressed by two studies from American and Swedish adoption registers completed about the same time (Cadoret et al., 1983; Cloninger, Sigvardsson, Bohman, & von Knorring, 1982).

Adoption Studies of Latent G × Measured E

In a pool of 500 adoptees from the Iowa and Missouri adoption studies, adoptees had the most elevated antisocial behaviors when they experienced "adverse circumstances" in their adoptive homes as well as having birth mothers with antisocial personality problems or alcoholism (Cadoret et al., 1983). This landmark study documented that the interaction was statistically significant and replicated across two independent samples. This finding was replicated and extended in another Iowa adoption cohort of 200 families (Cadoret, et al., 1995). Adoptive parents' adversity was defined according to the presence of marital problems, legal problems, substance abuse, or mental disorder, and it interacted significantly with biological parents' antisocial personality disorder to predict elevated rates of childhood aggression, adolescent aggression, and diagnosed conduct disorder in the adoptees. This same Iowa adoption study was creatively analyzed to demonstrate that adversity in the adoptive home can moderate the genetic child effect in which children's aggression provokes bad parenting (Riggins-Caspers et al., 2003). Adoptees' genetic liability for antisocial behavior (defined as biological parents' psychopathology) provoked more harsh discipline from the adoptive parents in homes in which the adoptive parents suffered adversity (marital, legal, substance, or psychopathology problems). There is one problem with studying G × E in adoption designs, and it is that adoption itself breaks up the naturally occurring processes of rGE that characterize the nonadopted majority population, thereby precluding the possibility of G × E. This separation allows the empirical study of G × E, but paradoxically, it probably results in an underestimate of the influence of G × E on antisocial outcomes in the general population. For this reason, adoption G × E studies should be complemented with twin studies.

A Twin Study of Latent G × Measured E

Our E-risk twin study also yielded evidence that genetic and environmental risks interact (Jaffee et al., 2005). Because we already knew that conduct problems were highly heritable in the E-risk twin sample at age 5 years (Arseneault et al., 2003), we were able to estimate each child's personal genetic risk for conduct problems by considering whether his or her co-twin had already been diagnosed with conduct disorder, and whether he or she shared 100% versus 50% of genes with that diagnosed co-twin. This method's usefulness had been demonstrated previously in a landmark G × E study showing that the risk of depression following life-event stress depends on genetic vulnerability (Kendler et al., 1995). For example, an individual's genetic risk is highest if his or her co-twin sibling already has a diagnosis of disorder and the pair is monozygotic. Likewise, an individual's genetic risk is lowest if his or her co-twin has been free from disorder and the pair is monozygotic. Individuals in DZ twin pairs fall between the high and low genetic risk groups. In our study an interaction was obtained such that the effect of maltreatment on conduct problem symptoms was significantly stronger among children at high genetic risk than among children at low genetic risk. (Because there was no genetic child effect provoking maltreatment, the genetic risk groups did not differ on concordance for maltreatment or the severity of maltreatment.) In addition, the experience of maltreatment was associated with an increase of 24% in the probability of diagnosable conduct disorder among children at high genetic risk, but an increase of only 2% among children at low risk.

Studies of Measured G × Measured E: Testing a Measured Gene

The aforementioned adoption and twin studies established that genotype does interact with bad parenting in the etiological processes leading to antisocial behavior. However, the studies did not implicate any particular genes. We conducted one study to test the hypothesis of G × E interaction using a measured environmental risk, child maltreatment, and an identified gene, the monoamine oxidase A(MAOA) polymorphism (Caspi et al., 2002). We selected the MAOA gene as the candidate gene for our study for four reasons (supporting research is cited in Caspi et al., 2002). First, the gene encodes the MAOA enzyme, which metabolizes the neurotransmitters linked to maltreatment victimization and aggressive behavior by previous research. Second, drugs inhibiting the action of the MAO enzyme have been shown to prevent animals from habituating to chronic stressors analogous to maltreatment and to dispose animals toward hyperreactivity to threat. Third, in studies of mice having the MAOA gene deleted, increased levels of neurotransmitters and aggressive behavior were observed, and aggression was normalized by restoring MAOA gene expression. Fourth, an extremely rare mutation causing a null allele at the MAOA locus was associated with aggressive psychopathology among some men in a Dutch family pedigree, although no relation between MAOA genotype and aggression had been detected for people in the general population.

We selected maltreatment for this study for four reasons (supporting research is cited in Caspi et al., 2002). First, childhood maltreatment is a known predictor of antisocial outcomes. Second, not all maltreated children become antisocial, suggesting that vulnerability to maltreatment is influenced by heretofore unstudied individual characteristics. Third, our abovementioned twin research had established that maltreatment's effect on children's aggression is environmentally mediated (i.e., the association is not an artifact of a genetic child effect provoking maltreatment or of transmission of aggression-prone genes from parents). As such, maltreatment can serve as the environmental variable in a test of G × E interaction. Fourth, animal and human studies suggest that maltreatment in early life alters neurotransmitter systems in ways that can persist into adulthood and can influence aggressive behavior.

Based on this logic to support our hypothesis of G × E, we measured childhood maltreatment history (8% severe, 28% probable, 64% not maltreated) and MAOA genotype (37% low-activity risk allele, 63% high-activity allele) in the 442 caucasian males of the longitudinal Dunedin Multidisciplinary Health and Development Study. We found that maltreatment history and genotype interacted to predict four different measures of antisocial outcome: an adolescent diagnosis of conduct disorder, an age-26 personality assessment of aggression, symptoms of adult antisocial personality disorder reported by informants who knew the study members well, and court conviction for violent crime up to age 26, the latest age of follow-up. Among boys having the combination of the low-MAOA-activity allele and severe maltreatment, 85% developed some form of antisocial outcome. Males having the combination of the low-activity allele and severe-to-probable maltreatment were only 12% of the male birth cohort, but they accounted for 44% of the cohort's violent convictions, because they offended at a higher rate on average than other violent offenders in the cohort.

Replication of this study was of utmost importance, because the study reported the first instance of interaction between a measured gene and a measured environment in the behavioral sciences, and because reports of connections between measured genes and disorders are notorious for their poor replication record (Hamer, 2002). One initial positive replication and extension has emerged from the Virginia Twin Study for Adolescent Behavioral Development (Foley et al., 2004). This team studied 514 caucasian male twins and measured environmental risk using an adversity index comprised of parental neglect, interparental violence, and inconsistent discipline. MAOA genotype and adversity interacted significantly such that 15% of boys having adversity but the high-MAOA-activity allele developed conduct disorder, in comparison to 35% of boys having adversity plus the low-activity allele. This study went a step further, controlling for maternal antisocial personality disorder to rule out the possibility that passive rGE might have resulted in the co-occurrence of environmental and genetic risk. This study thus replicated the original G × E between the MAOA polymorphism and maltreatment, extended it to other forms of parental treatment, and showed that it is not an artifact of passive rGE. Another study has tested the MAOA G × E effect, and although the pattern of findings was consistent with the interaction, it did not attain statistical significance (Haberstick et al., 2005).

Genes as Protective Factors Promoting Resilience

An intriguing finding from the two MAOA G × E studies was that, in contrast to the G × E interaction's marked effects on antisocial outcomes, the unique effects of maltreatment apart from its role in the G × E interaction were very modest. Maltreatment initially predicted antisocial outcomes in the full cohorts, but within the high-MAOA-activity genotype group its effects were reduced by more than half (Caspi et al., 2002; Foley et al., 2004). This pattern is in keeping with the findings from adoption and twin studies cited earlier in this section, all of which found that measured bad parenting had relatively little effect on children who were at low genetic risk (Cadoret et al., 1983; Cadoret et al., 1995; Cloninger et al., 1982; Jaffee et al., 2005; Mednick et al., 1984). Taken together, these findings suggest the novel notion that genotype can be a protective factor against adversity. Some people respond poorly to adversity while others are resilient to it, and the reason for this variation has been a holy grail in developmental research. The search for sources of resilience has tended to focus on social experiences thought to protect children, overlooking a potential protective role of genes (but see Kim-Cohen, Moffitt, Caspi, & Taylor, 2004). The potential protective effect of genes deserves more attention (Insel & Collins, 2003).

CONCLUSION

In this chapter we reviewed the first studies in a new generation of research that exploits behavioral-genetics designs to address the interplay between measured environmental risks and genetic risks in the origins of antisocial behavior. This work has only recently accelerated, and more of it is needed before drawing conclusions (Dick & Rose, 2002; Kendler, 2001). However, even the few studies so far counteract prior claims that associations between family risk factors and child antisocial outcome might be nothing more than a spurious artifact of familial genetic transmission. This argument can be subjected to empirical test, and such tests need to address both child effects on environments (involving children's genes) and gene–environment correlations (involving parents' genes). Further, although the "residual main effects" of environmental risk factors may appear small after controlling for genetic transmission, that is not the whole story. Emerging evidence about G × E interactions suggests that environmental risks can affect people more strongly than previously appreciated, in genetically vulnerable segments of the population. Although this chapter has argued that twin and adoption studies together can provide a good evidence base, the most compelling information about gene–environment interplay will come from converging findings from behavioral-genetics designs, treatment experiments, and longitudinal natural experiments showing within-individual change.

ACKNOWLEDGMENTS

Work on this chapter was supported by grants from the U.S. National Institute of Mental Health (Nos. MH45070 and MH49414) and the U.K. Medical Research Council (Nos. G9806489 and G0100527), and by a Royal Society–Wolfson Research Merit Award.

REFERENCES

Arseneault, L., Moffitt, T. E., Caspi, A., Taylor, A., Rijsdijk, F. V., Jaffee, S., et al. (2003). Strong genetic effects on cross-situational antisocial behaviour among 5-year-old children according to mothers, teachers, examiner-observers, and twins' self-reports. *Journal of Child Psychology and Psychiatry, 44,* 832–848.

Asbury, K., Dunn, J., Pike, A., & Plomin, R. (2003). Nonshared environmental influences on individual differences in early behavioral development: A monozygotic twin differences study. *Child Development, 74,* 933–943.

Belsky, J., & Barends, N. (2002). Personality and parenting. In M.H. Bornstein (Ed.), *Handbook of parenting: Vol. 3. Being and becoming a parent* (2nd ed., pp. 415–438). Mahwah, NJ: Erlbaum.

Blumstein, A., & Cohen, J. (1987). Characterizing criminal careers. *Science, 237,* 985–991.

Bohman, M., Cloninger, R., Sigvardsson, S., & von Knorring, A.L. (1982). Predisposition to petty criminality in Swedish adpotees. I. Genetic and environmental heterogeneity. *Archives of General Psychiatry, 39,* 1233–1241.

Braungart, J. M., Plomin, R., & Fulker, D. W. (1992). Genetic mediation of the home environment during infancy: A sibling adoption study of the HOME. *Developmental Psychology, 28,* 1048–1055.

Burt, A. S., Krueger, R. F., McGue, M., & Iacono, W. (2003). Parent–child conflict and the comorbidity among childhood externalizing disorders. *Archives of General Psychiatry, 60,* 505–513.

Butterfield, F. (1996). *All God's children: The Bosket family and the American tradition of violence.* New York: Avon.

Butterfield, F. (2002, August 21). Father steals best: Crime in an American family. *The New York Times* [Online]. Available: www.nytimes.com/2002/08/21/national/21FAMI.html.

Cadoret, R. J., Cain, C. A., & Crowe, R. R. (1983). Evidence for gene–environment interaction in the development of adolescent antisocial behavior. *Behavior Genetics, 13,* 301–310.

Cadoret, R. J., Yates, W. R., Troughton, E., Woodworth, G., & Stewart, M. A. S. (1995). Genetic–environmental interaction in the genesis of aggressivity and conduct disorders. *Archives of General Psychiatry, 52,* 916–924.

Caspi, A., McClay, J, Moffitt, T. E., Mill, J., Martin, J., Craig, I., et al. (2002). Role of genotype in the cycle of violence in maltreated children. *Science, 297,* 851–854.

Caspi, A., & Moffitt, T. E. (1995). The continuity of maladaptive behavior. In D. Cicchetti & D. Cohen (Eds.), *Manual of developmental psychopathology* (Vol. 2, pp. 472–511). New York: Wiley.

Caspi, A., Moffitt, T., Morgan, J., Rutter, M., Taylor, A., Arseneault, L., et al. (2004). Maternal expressed emotion predicts children's antisocial behavior problems: Using MZ-twin differences to identify environmental effects on behavioral development. *Developmental Psychology, 40(2)* 149–161.

Caspi, A., Taylor, A., Moffitt, T. E., & Plomin, R. (2000). Neighborhood deprivation affects children's mental health: Environmental risks identified using a genetic design. *Psychological Science, 11,* 338–342.

Caspi, A., Taylor, A., Smart, M. A., Jackson, J., Tagami, S., & Moffitt, T. E. (2001). Can women provide reliable information about their children's fathers? Cross-informant agreement about men's antisocial behaviour. *Journal of Child Psychology and Psychiatry, 42,* 915–920.

Cichetti, D. (2003). Experiments of nature: Contributions to developmental theory. *Development and Psychopathology, 15,* 833–835.

Cloninger, C. R., & Gottesman I. I. (1987). Genetic and environmental factors in antisocial behavior disorders. In S. A. Mednick, T. E. Moffitt, & S. A. Stack (Eds.), *The causes of crime: New biological approaches* (pp. 92–109). New York: Cambridge University Press.

Cloninger, C. R., Sigvardsson, S., Bohman, M., & von Knorring, A. L. (1982). Predisposition to petty criminality in Swedish adoptees. II. Cross-fostering analysis of gene-environment interaction. *Archives of General Psychiatry, 39,* 1242–1247.

Collins, W. A., Maccoby, E. E., Steinberg, L., Hetherington, E. M., & Bornstein, M. H. (2000). Contemporary research on parenting. *American Psychologist, 55,* 218–232.

Conger, K. J., & Conger, R. D. (1994). Differential parenting and change in sibling differences in delinquency. *Journal of Family Psychology, 8,* 287–302.

Costello, E. J., Compton, S. N., Keeler, G., & Angold, A. (2003). Relationships between poverty and psychopathology: A natural experiment. *Journal of the American Medical Association, 290,* 2023–2029.

Daniels, D., & Plomin, R. (1985). Differential experience of siblings in the same family. *Developmental Psychology, 21,* 747–760.

Deater-Deckard, K., Fulker, D. W., & Plomin, R. (1999). A genetic study of the family environment in the transition to early adolescence. *Journal of Child Psychology and Psychiatry, 40,* 769–775.

Dick, D. M., & Rose, R. J. (2002). Behavior genetics: What's new? What's next? *Current Directions in Psychological Science, 11,* 70–74.

DiLalla, L. F. (2002). Behavior genetics of aggression in children: Review and future directions. *Developmental Review, 22,* 593–622.

Dodge, K. A. (2003). Investing in the prevention of youth violence. *International Society for the Study of Behavioral Development Newsletter, 2,* 8–10.

D'Onofrio, B. M., Turkheimer, E. N., Eaves, L. J., Corey, L. A., Berg, K., Solaas, M. H., et al. (2003). The role of the children of twins design in elucidating causal relations between parent characteristics and child outcomes. *Journal of Child Psychiatry and Psychology, 44,* 1130–1144.

Evans, W. E., & Relling, M. V. (1999). Pharmacogenetics: Translating functional genomics into rational therapeutics. *Science, 286,* 487–491.

Farrington, D. P. (1988). Studying changes within individuals: The causes of offending. In M. Rutter (Ed.) *Studies of psychosocial risk: The power of longitudinal data* (pp. 158–183). Cambridge, UK: Cambridge University Press.

Farrington, D. P. (2003) Developmental and life-course criminology. *Criminology, 41,* 221–255.

Farrington, D. P., Barnes, G. C., & Lambert, S. (1996). The concentration of offending in families. *Legal and Criminological Psychology, 1,* 47–63.

Farrington, D. P., Jolliffe, D., Loeber, R., Stouthamer-Loeber, M., & Kalb, L. (2001). The concentration of offenders in families, and family criminality in the prediction of boys' delinquency. *Journal of Adolescence, 24,* 579–596.

Fergusson, D. M., Lynskey, M., & Horwood, L. J. (1995). The adolescent outcomes of adoption: A 16-year longitudinal study. *Journal of Child Psychology and Psychiatry, 36,* 597–615.

Foley, D., Eaves, L., Wormley, B., Silberg, J., Maes, H., Hewitt, J., et al. (2004). Childhood adversity, MAOA genotype, and risk for conduct disorder. *Archives of General Psychiatry, 61,* 738–744.

Galbaud du Fort, G., Boothroyd, L. J., Bland, R. C., Newman, S. C., & Kakuma, R. (2002). Spouse similarity for antisocial behaviour in the general population. *Psychological Medicine, 32,* 1407–1416.

Ge, X., Conger, R. D., Cadoret, R. J., Neiderhiser, J.M., Yates, W., Troughton, E., et al. (1996). The developmental interface between nature and nurture: A mutual influence model of childhood antisocial behavior and parent behavior. *Developmental Psychology, 32,* 574–589.

Haberstick, B. C., Lessem, M., Hopfer, C. J., Smolen, A., Ehringer, M.A., Timberlake, D., et al. (2005). Monoamine oxidase A (MAOA) and antisocial behaviors in the presence of childhood and adolescent maltreatment. *American Journal of Medical Genetics: Neuropsychiatric Genetics, 135B,* 59–64.

Hamer, D. (2002). Rethinking behavior genetics. *Science, 298,* 71–72.

Harris, J.R. (1998). *The nurture assumption.* New York: Free Press.

Heinrich, C. C., Brown, J. L., & Aber, J. L. (1999). *Evaluating the effectiveness of school-based violence prevention: Developmental approaches* (Society for Research in Child Development Social Policy Report, XIII, No. 3, pp. 1–18). Ann Arbor, MI: SRCD Executive Office.

Hinshaw, S. P. (2002). Intervention research, theoretical mechanisms, and causal processes related to externalizing behavior patterns. *Development and Psychopathology, 14,* 789–818.

Howe, G. W., Reiss, D., & Yuh, J. (2002). Can prevention trials test theories of etiology? *Development and Psychopathology, 14,* 673–694.

Hur, Y., & Bouchard, T. J. Jr. (1995). Genetic influences on perceptions of childhood family environment: A reared-apart twin study. *Child Development, 66,* 330–345.

Insel, T. R., & Collins, F. S. (2003). Psychiatry in the genomics era. *American Journal of Psychiatry, 160,* 616–620.

Jaffee, S. R., Caspi, A., Moffitt, T. E., Dodge, K., Rutter, M., & Taylor, A., et al. (2005). Nature × nurture: Genetic vulnerabilities interact with physical maltreatment to promote behavior problems. *Development and Psychopathology, 17,* 67–84.

Jaffee, S. R, Caspi, A., Moffitt, T. E., Polo-Tomas, M., Price, T., & Taylor, A. (2004). The limits of child effects: Evidence for genetically mediated child effects on corporal punishment, but not on physical maltreatment. *Developmental Psychology, 40,* 1047–1058.

Jaffee, S. R., Caspi, A., Moffitt, T. E., & Taylor, A. (2004). Physical maltreatment victim to antisocial child: Evidence of an environmentally-mediated process. *Journal of Abnormal Psychology, 113(1),* 44–55.

Jaffee, S. R., Moffitt, T. E., Caspi, A., & Taylor, A. (2003). Life with (or without) father: The benefits of living with two biological parents depend on the father's antisocial behavior. *Child Development, 74,* 109–126.

Jaffee, S. R., Moffitt, T. E., Caspi, A., Taylor, A., & Arseneault, L. (2002). The influence of adult domestic violence on children's internalizing and externalizing problems: An environmentally-informative twin study. *Journal of the American Academy of Child and Adolescent Psychiatry, 41,* 1095–1103.

Jorgensen, A. L., Phillip, J., Raskind, W. H., Matsushita, M., Christensen, B., Dreyer, V., et al. (1992). Different patterns of X inactivation in MZ twins discordant for red-green color vision deficiency. *American Journal of Human Genetics, 51,* 291–298.

Kendler, K. S. (1993). Twin studies of psychiatric illness. *Archives of General Psychiatry, 50,* 905–915.

Kendler, K. S. (1996). Parenting: A genetic epidemiologic perspective. *American Journal of Psychiatry, 153,* 11–20.

Kendler, K. S. (2001). Twin studies of psychiatric illness: An update. *Archives of General Psychiatry, 58,* 1005–1014.

Kendler, K. S., Kessler, R. C., Walters, E. E., MacLean, C., Neale, M. C., Heath, A. C., et al. (1995). Stressful life events, genetic liability and onset of an episode of major depression in women. *American Journal of Psychiatry, 152,* 833–842.

Kendler, K. S., Neale, M. C., Kessler, R. C., Heath, A. C., & Eaves, L. J. (1992). Childhood parental loss and adult psychopathology in women: A twin study perspective. *Archives of General Psychiatry, 49,* 109–116.

Kendler, K. S., Neale, M. C., Kessler, R. C., Heath, A. C., & Eaves, L. J. (1994). Parental treatment and the equal environments assumption in twin studies of psychiatric illness. *Psychological Medicine, 24,* 579–590.

Kendler, K. S., Prescott, C. A., Myers, J., & Neale, M. C. (2003). The structure of genetic and environmental risk factors for common psychiatric and substance use disorders in men and women. *Archives of General Psychiatry, 60,* 929–937.

Kim-Cohen, J., Moffitt, T. E., Caspi, A., & Taylor, A. (2004). Genetic and environmental processes in young children's resilience and vulnerability to socio-economic deprivation. *Child Development, 75(3),* 651–668.

Kim-Cohen, J., Moffitt, T. E., Taylor, A., Pawlby, S. J., & Caspi, A. (2005). Maternal Depression and children's antisocial behavior: Nature and nurture effects. *Archives of General Psychiatry, 62,* 173–181.

Kraemer, H. C. (2003). Current concepts of risk in psychiatric disorders. *Current Opinion in Psychiatry, 16,* 421–430.

Kraemer, H. C, Kazdin, A. E., Offord, D. R., Kessler, R. C., Jensen, P. S., & Kupfer, D. J. (1997). Coming to terms with the terms of risk. *Archives of General Psychiatry, 54,* 337–343.

Krueger R. F., Markon K. E., Bouchard T. J. (2003). The extended genotype: The heritability of personality accounts for the heritability of recalled family environments in twins reared apart. *Journal of Personality, 71,* 809–833.

Krueger, R. F., Moffitt, T. E., Caspi, A., Bleske, A., & Silva, P. A. (1998). Assortative mating for antisocial behavior: Developmental and methodological implications. *Behavior Genetics, 28,* 173–186.

Lahey, B. B., Moffitt, T. E., & Caspi, A. (Eds.). (2003). *Causes of conduct disorder and juvenile delinquency.* New York: Guilford Press.

Laub, J. H., & Sampson, R. J. (2003). *Shared beginnings, divergent lives: Delinquent boys to age 70.* Cambridge, MA: Harvard University Press.

Lipsey, M. W., & Wilson, D. B. (1998). Effective intervention for serious and violent juvenile offenders: Synthesis of research. In R. Loeber & D. P. Farrington (Eds.), *Serious and violent juvenile offenders* (pp. 313–345). Thousand Oaks, CA: Sage.

Losoya, S. H., Callor, S., Rowe, D. C., & Goldsmith, H. H. (1997). Origins of familial similarity in parenting: A study of twins and adoptive siblings. *Developmental Psychology, 33,* 1012–1023.

Maughan, B., Taylor, A., Caspi, A., & Moffitt, T. E. (2004). Prenatal smoking and child conduct problems: testing genetic and environmental explanation of the association. *Archives of General Psychiatry, 61,* 836–843.

McGue, M., Sharma, A., & Benson, P. (1996). The effect of common rearing on adolescent adjustment: Evidence from a U.S. adoption cohort. *Developmental Psychology, 32,* 604–613.

McGuire, S. (2003). The heritability of parenting. *Parenting: Science and Practice, 3,* 73–94.

Mednick, S. A., & Christiansen, K. O. (1977). *Biosocial bases of criminal behavior.* New York: Gardner Press.

Mednick, S. A., Gabrielli, W. F., & Hutchings, B. (1984). Genetic factors in criminal behavior: Evidence from an adoption cohort. *Science, 224,* 891–893.

Mednick, S. A., Moffitt, T. E., Gabrielli, W. F., & Hutchings, B. (1986). Genetic factors in criminal behavior: A review. In J. Block, D. Olweus, & M. R. Yarrow (Eds.), *The development of antisocial and prosocial behavior* (pp. 33–50). New York: Academic Press.

Meyer, J. M., Rutter, M., Silberg, J. L., Maes, H., Simonoff, E., Shillady, L. L., et al. (2000). Familial aggregation for conduct disorder symptomatology: The role of genes, marital discord, and family adaptability. *Psychological Medicine, 30,* 759–774.

Miles, D. R., & Carey, G. (1997). Genetic and environmental architecture of human aggression. *Journal of Personality and Social Psychology, 72,* 207–217.

Moffitt, T. E. (1993). "Life-course-persistent" and "adolescence-limited" antisocial behavior: A developmental taxonomy. *Psychological Review, 100,* 674–701.

Moffitt, T. E. (2005). The new look of behavioral-genetics in developmental psychopathology. *Psychological Bulletin, 131,* 533–554.

Moffitt, T. E., Caspi, A., Rutter, M., & Silva, P. A. (2001). *Sex differences in antisocial behaviour: Conduct disorder, delinquency, and violence in the Dunedin longitudinal study.* Cambridge, UK: Cambridge University Press.

Moffitt, T. E., & E-risk Study Team (2002). Teen-aged mothers in contemporary Britain. *Journal of Child Psychology and Psychiatry, 43,* 1–16.

Neiderhiser, J. M., Reiss, D., Hetherington, E. M., & Plomin, R. (1999). Relationships between parenting and adolescent adjustment over time: Genetic and environmental contributions. *Developmental Psychology, 35,* 680–692.

Neiderhiser, J. M., Reiss, D., Pederson, N., Lichtenstein, P., Spotts, E. L., Hansson, K., et al. (2004). Genetic and environmental influences on mothering of adolescents: A comparison of two samples. *Developmental Psychology, 40,* 335–351.

O'Connor, T. G., Deater-Deckard, K., Fulker, D., Rutter, M., & Plomin, R. (1998). Genotype–environment correlations in late childhood and early adolescence: Antisocial behavioral problems in coercive parenting. *Developmental Psychology, 34,* 970–981.

O'Connor, T. G., Heatherington, E. M., Reiss, D., & Plomin, R. (1995). A twin-sibling study of observed parent-adolescent relations. *Child Development, 66,* 812–829.

Olds, D., Henderson, C. R. Jr., Cole, R., Eckenrode, J., Kitzman, H., Luckey, D., et al. (1998). Long-term effects of nurse home visitation on children's criminal and antisocial behavior: 15-year follow-up of a randomized trial. *Journal of the American Medical Association, 280,* 1238–1244.

Perusse, D., Neale, M. C., Heath, A. C., & Eaves, L. J. (1994). Human parental behavior: Evidence for genetic influence and potential implications for gene-culture transmission. *Behavior Genetics, 24,* 327–336.

Pike, A., McGuire, S., Hetherington, E. M., Reiss, D., & Plomin, R. (1996). Family environment and adolescent depressive symptoms and antisocial behavior: A multivariate genetic analysis. *Developmental Psychology, 32,* 590–603.

Pike, A., Reiss, D., Hetherington, E. M., & Plomin, R. (1996). Using MZ differences in the search for nonshared environmental effects. *Journal of Child Psychology and Psychiatry, 37,* 695–704.

Plomin, R. (1994). *Genetics and experience: The interplay between nature and nurture.* Thousand Oaks, CA: Sage.

Plomin, R., & Bergeman, C. S. (1991). The nature of nurture: Genetic influences on "environmental" measures. *Behavioral and Brain Sciences, 14,* 373–427.

Plomin, R., & Caspi, A. (1999). Behavior genetics and personality. In L. A. Pervin & O. P. John (Eds.), *Handbook of personality* (2nd ed., pp. 251–276). New York: Guilford Press.

Plomin, R., & Daniels, D. (1987). Why are children in the same family so different from each other? *Behavioral and Brain Sciences, 10,* 1–16.

Plomin, R., DeFries, J. C., & Loehlin, J. C. (1977). Genotype-environment interaction and correlation in the analysis of human behavior. *Psychological Bulletin, 84,* 309–322.

Plomin, R., DeFries, J. C., McClearn, G. E., & McGuffin, P. (2001). *Behavioral genetics,* (4th ed.). New York: Freeman.

Plomin, R., McClearn, G. E., Pederson, N. L., Nesselroade, J. R., & Bergeman, C. S. (1989). Genetic influence on adults' ratings of their current family environment. *Journal of Marriage and the Family, 51,* 791–803.

Purcell, S. (2002). Variance components models for gene–environment interaction in twin analysis. *Twin Research, 5,* 554–571.

Reid, J., Patterson G. R., & Snyder J. (2002). *Antisocial behavior in children and adolescents.* Washington, DC: American Psychological Association.

Reiss, D., Neiderhiser, J. M., Hetherington, E. M., & Plomin, R. (2000). *The relationship code: Deciphering genetic and social influences on adolescent development.* Cambridge, MA: Harvard University Press.

Rende, R. D., Slomkowski, C. L., Stocker, C., Fulker, D. W., & Plomin, R. (1992). Genetic and environmental influences on maternal and sibling interaction in middle childhood: A sibling adoption study. *Developmental Psychology, 28,* 484–490.

Rhee, S. H., & Waldman, I. D. (2002). Genetic and environmental influences on antisocial behavior: A meta-analysis of twin and adoption studies. *Psychological Bulletin, 128,* 490–529.

Riggins-Caspers, K. M., Cadoret, R. J., Knutson, J. F., & Langbehn, D. (2003). Biology–environment interaction and evocative biology–environment correlation: Contributions of harsh discipline and parental psychopathology to problem adolescent behaviors. *Behavior Genetics, 33,* 205–220.

Rodgers, J. L., Rowe, D. C., & Li, C. (1994). Beyond nature versus nurture: DF analysis of nonshared influences on problem behaviors. *Developmental Psychology, 30,* 374–384.

Rowe, D. C. (1983). A biometric analysis of perceptions of family environment. *Child Development, 54,* 416–423.

Rowe, D. C. (1994). *The limits of family influence: Genes, experience, and behavior.* New York: Guilford Press.

Rowe, D. C., Almeida, D. M., & Jacobson, K. C. (1999). School context and genetic influences on aggression in adolescence. *Psychological Science, 10,* 277–280.

Rowe, D. C., & Farrington, D. P. (1997). The familial transmission of criminal convictions. *Criminology, 35,* 177–201.

Rutter, M. (2002). Nature, nurture, and development: From evangelism through science toward policy and practice. *Child Development, 73,* 1–21.

Rutter, M. (2003a). Commentary: Causal processes leading to antisocial behavior. *Developmental Psychology* [Special issue], *39,* 372–378.

Rutter, M. (2003b). Crucial paths from risk indicator to causal mechanism. In B. B. Lahey, T. E. Moffitt, & A. Caspi (Eds.), *Causes of conduct disorder and juvenile delinquency* (pp. 3–24). New York: Guilford Press.

Rutter, M., Giller, H., & Hagell, A. (1998). *Antisocial behaviour by young people.* Cambridge, UK: Cambridge University Press.

Rutter, M., Pickles, A., Murray, R., & Eaves, L. (2001). Testing hypotheses on specific environmental causal effects on behavior. *Psychological Bulletin, 127,* 291–324.

Rutter, M., & Silberg, J. (2002). Gene–environment interplay in relation to emotional and behavioral disturbance. *Annual Review of Psychology, 53,* 463–490.

Scarr, S. (1991). The construction of the family reality. *Behavioral and Brain Sciences, 14,* 403–404.

Scarr, S. (1992). Developmental theories for the 1990's: Development and individual differences. *Child Development, 63,* 1–19.

Scarr, S., & McCartney, K. (1983). How people make their own environments. *Child Development, 54,* 424–435.

Sherman, L. W., Gottfredson, D. C., MacKenzie, D. L, Eck, J., Reuter, P., & Bushway, S. D. (1999). *Preventing crime: What works, what doesn't, what's promising.* New York: Russell Sage Foundation (also available from the U.S. Department of Justice, www.ojp.usdoj.gov/nij).

Silberg, J. L. (2002*). Parental effects on depression and disruptive behavior in the children of twins: A proposal to the US National Institute of Mental Health.* Richmond: Medical College of Virginia.

Silberg, J. L., & Eaves, L. J. (2004). Analysing the contributions of genes and parent–child interaction to childhood behavioural and emotional problems: A model for the children of twins. *Psychological Medicine, 34,* 1–10.

Spinath, F. M., & O'Connor, T. G. (2003). A behavioral genetic study of the overlap between personality and parenting. *Journal of Personality, 71,* 785–808.

Stoolmiller, M. (1999). Implications of the restricted range of family environments for estimates of heritability and nonshared environment in behavior–genetic adoption studies. *Psychological Bulletin, 125,* 392–409.

Thornberry, T.P. (Ed.). (1996*). Advances in criminological theory: Developmental theories of crime and delinquency.* London: Transactions.

Towers, H., Spotts, E. L., & Neiderhiser, J. (2001). Genetic and environmental influences on parenting and marital relationships: Current findings and future directions. *Marriage and Family Review, 33,* 11–29.

Turkheimer, E., & Waldron, M. (2000). Nonshared environment: A theoretical, methodological, and quantitative review. *Psychological Bulletin, 126,* 78–108.

U.S. Bureau of Justice Statistics. (2002). *Criminal victimization 2001* (NCJ Report 194610). Washington, DC: U.S. Department of Justice (Available: www.ojp.usdof.gov/bjs).

Vandell, D. L. (2000). Parents, peer groups, and other socializing influences. *Developmental Psychology, 36,* 699–710.

vanDusen, K., Mednick, S. A., Gabrielli, W. F., & Hutchings, B. (1983). Social class and crime in an adoption cohort. *Journal of Criminal Law and Criminology, 74,* 249–269.

Wade, T. D., & Kendler, K. S. (2000). The genetic epidemiology of parental discipline, *Psychological Medicine, 30,* 1303–1313.

Wandersman, A., & Florin, P. (2003). Community interventions and effective prevention. *American Psychologist, 58,* 441–448.

Wasserman, G. A., & Miller, L. S. (1998). The prevention of serious and violent juvenile offending. In R. Loeber & D. P. Farrington (Eds.), *Serious and violent juvenile offenders* (pp. 197–247). Thousand Oaks, CA: Sage.

Weissberg, R. P., Kumpfer, K. L., & Seligman, M. E. P. (2003). Prevention that works for children and youth. *American Psychologist, 58,* 425–432.

Wilson, D. B., Gottfredson, D. C., & Najaka, S. S. (2001). School–based prevention of problem behaviors: A meta-analysis. *Journal of Quantitative Criminology, 17,* 247–272.

Wolfgang, M. E., Figlio, R. M., & Sellin, T. (1972). *Delinquency in a birth cohort.* Chicago: University of Chicago Press.

World Health Organization. (2002). *World report on violence and health.* Geneva: Author.

Yoshikawa, H. (1994). Prevention as cumulative protection. *Psychological Bulletin, 115,* 28–54.

CHAPTER 5

The Influence of Early Socialization Experiences on the Development of Biological Systems

RENA REPETTI, SHELLEY E. TAYLOR, and DARBY SAXBE

Most psychologists who study socialization assess how those experiences shape social, emotional, cognitive, or health outcomes in children. Our chapter considers the effects that early experiences may have on biological systems during infancy and childhood—a perspective that may inform the developmental outcomes discussed in other chapters in this handbook. We present an overview of a wide range of animal and human studies that investigate how early rearing experiences help to guide the functioning and development of the central nervous system (CNS) and endocrine and immune systems of offspring.

Nursing offers one of the clearest examples of how mothers can act as external regulators of basic biological functions in infancy in the short term and play an important role in long-term biological development. In addition to providing nourishment, maternal cells in breast milk boost the infant's immune system, supplying some of the protection from infection and disease that the offspring's immature system is not yet able to provide. Nursing also promotes skin-to-skin contact between mothers and their infant, which leads to immediate reductions in some stress response indicators (Mooncey, Giannakoulopoulos, Glover, Acolet, & Modi, 1997). In the long term, skin-to-skin contact can speed the maturation of vagal tone and sleep cycles (Feldman & Eidelman, 2003), and research suggests that tactile stimulation may enhance growth and behavioral development in human infants (Kuhn & Schanberg, 1991). Other evidence indicates that in some mammals ventral contact between mother and offspring and maternal licking and grooming behaviors lead to an immediate reduction in biological stress responses in their young (Gunnar, Gonazalez, Goodlin, & Levine, 1981; Liu et al, 1997; Mendoza, Smotherman,

Miner, Kaplan, & Levine, 1978). In the case of rats, licking and grooming behaviors may also help to shape the long-term ability of offspring to prepare for and react to stress on their own (Cirulli, Berry, & Alleva, 2003). Even while the effects of early parenting experiences on biological development are being uncovered, investigators are beginning to dig deeper to discover the mechanisms by which parenting helps to craft those biological systems. For example, research discussed herein shows that early experiences can induce changes in the expression of genes that are required for neuronal development.

If physical contact with a mother and maternal behaviors such as licking and grooming play a role in shaping infant biological systems, how does the developing organism respond without the reliable presence of a sensitive parent? The chronic activation of biological stress-response systems may play a role in this process. This notion is consistent with a model of the long-term mental and physical health consequences of growing up in families characterized by conflict and aggression or by relationships that are cold, unsupportive, and neglectful. Repetti, Taylor, and Seeman's (2002) risky families model proposed that these early rearing environments can set in motion a cascade of risk reflected in disturbances in physiological and neuroendocrine system regulation, as well as deficits in the control and expression of emotion and in social competence. According to this model, the early disruptions in biological, emotional, and social development have cumulative, long-term effects in adolescence and adulthood, leading to a wide variety of physical and mental health problems.

The risky families model draws on the concept of allostatic load (McEwen, 1998; McEwen & Stellar, 1993). Allostasis is the process of activating neural, neuroendocrine, and neuroendocrine-immune mechanisms to adapt physiologically in the face of potentially stressful challenges. According to the allostatic load model, a period of recovery following physiological arousal is essential for the proper functioning of biological regulatory processes in the body; allostatic load can result when regulatory systems are overstimulated. Repetti et al. (2002) argued that the repeated activation of allostatic systems in risky family environments can disrupt the child's ability to mount a modulated physiologic/neuroendocrine response to stress and to quickly recover from that response. Chronic allostatic load, which can lead to disease over long periods, can result in maintenance of neuroendocrine activation following exposure to a stressful situation as indicated in poor recovery from stress. Long-term effects may include a flattening of the circadian rhythm of cortisol output, an indicator of hypothalamic–pituitary–adrenocortical (HPA) activity. We propose that consistent and sensitive parenting helps to control the frequency and timing of social challenges in the early rearing environment and to facilitate development of appropriate patterns of physiological regulatory processes when the young are confronted with potentially stressful situations. The links that researchers are beginning to uncover between physiological and emotional responses to stress in childhood (El-Sheikh, Cummings, & Goetsch, 1989) suggest that patterns of biological stress responding laid down in childhood may be tied to social and emotional development as well.

Although the focus of our chapter is clearly ontological, we recognize that phylogenetic questions about the evolutionary processes that may have resulted in these developmental trajectories are critical. Some of the biological responses to early negative experiences discussed in this chapter may represent adaptations. The functions of those responses (i.e., the evolutionary benefits that led to their selection) require explication. By investigating the potential short-term benefits of what appear to be adverse outcomes in the long run, we may come to understand some of the adaptive trade-offs that organisms make in harsh rearing environments (Simpson & Gangestad, 2001). For example, some of the evidence reviewed in our chapter may point to a quickened pace of maturation as one such trade-off. Among nonhuman primates, some of the immediate biological reactions to maternal separation include increased release of growth hormone (Laudenslager et al., 1995) and an early enhanced immune response (Coe, Lubach, Ershler, & Klopp, 1989). In the longer term, these reactions may set the stage for an acceleration of aging processes. The later outcomes of stressful early rearing conditions include earlier pubertal timing in humans (Surbey, 1990) and an increased and early vulnerability to disease in both human and nonhuman primates (Repetti et al., 2002). Because of the possibility of adaptations that maximize short-term survival benefits, even at the expense of long-term outcomes, the assignation of a "positive" or "negative" label to biological outcomes discussed in this chapter is not always possible, nor desirable. Therefore, readers who are accustomed to thinking about socialization with respect to "good" and "poor" developmental outcomes may find that the descriptions of research findings in this chapter at times seem incomplete.

Any research review must reflect the state of the field, and as should already be obvious, ours will rely heavily on studies of nonhuman mammals, particularly rats and monkeys. The rate of ontogeny of the animals commonly used in these studies and the experimental designs and invasive procedures that are possible have greatly advanced our understanding of how early rearing experiences can influence the biology of mammalian offspring. As psychologists interested in socialization, we believe it is critical to understand the concepts and findings in these fields. One of the goals of this chapter is to introduce basic research paradigms, methods, and results to socialization researchers who might not be familiar with this literature. The complexities of the biological and behavioral systems under investigation, compounded by differences among species, conspire to make this a difficult task. Nonetheless, we strive to summarize human and animal research while keeping in mind the unique socialization demands placed on human mothers and fathers.

Given the interdependence of the biological processes discussed here, the echoes of both short-term and long-term changes in one biological system should be observed throughout the organism. Indeed, the animal and human research summarized in this chapter suggests that the impact of early rearing experiences on development can be pervasive, influencing the offspring's CNS, endocrine, and immune systems. For the purposes of organizing our review of the research literature, we separate "biological systems" into different subsections of the chapter. However, these distinctions are clearly artificial when it comes to the functioning of those systems and the development of offspring.

Our chapter begins with the CNS. We present research on the effects that early experiences can have on brain structure and function, in particular neuronal activity. The second section discusses evidence from both animal and human studies that childhood family environments and other early rearing experiences influence the development of the major neuroendocrine stress-response systems, the HPA axis, and the sympathetic and parasympathetic branches of the peripheral nervous system. The third section summarizes research on the impact that early social deprivation, particularly maternal separation, has on immune functioning. The final literature review section presents research findings that link early rearing conditions to growth and sexual development in human and nonhuman primates. We close with conclusions, comments about the current state of research, and suggestions for future research directions.

CENTRAL NERVOUS SYSTEM RESPONSES TO SOCIALIZATION EXPERIENCES

Research indicates that parenting behavior has enduring effects on the development and functioning of the mammalian brain. Here we summarize findings from research literatures that relate early experiences to neurotransmitter regulation, in particular the "diffuse modulatory systems," as well as brain plasticity, neuronal density and viability, the expression of genes involved in neuronal development, and electroencephalogram (EEG) patterns.

Brain activity consists of an orderly set of chemical reactions. The chemicals that regulate the transmission of neural impulses in the brain are neurotransmitters, which are released by presynaptic elements upon stimulation and activate postsynaptic receptors. There are a large number of neurotransmitter systems in the mammalian brain, each one consisting of the transmitter molecule as well as the structures and processes involved in its synthesis, storage, action, reuptake, and degradation. Many of the regulatory functions of the brain are controlled by three neurotransmitter systems: norepinephrine, dopamine, and serotonin. These monoamines comprise "diffuse modulatory systems." These systems have numerous projections that are widely dispersed in the brain and they mediate broad protracted actions involving level of arousal and mood, and individual systems appear to be essential for aspects of motor control, memory, motivation, and metabolic state. For instance, in addition to their role in the peripheral nervous system, norepinephrine-containing neurons are found in the locus ceruleus in the pons from which they fan out to almost every part of the brain. These cells seem to be involved in the regulation of attention, arousal, sleep–wake cycles, learning, memory, anxiety, pain, mood, and brain metabolism. Serotonin-containing neurons are mostly clustered in the dorsal raphe nuclei and project to different regions of the brain. They are involved in the control of sleep–wake cycles, and in the different stages of sleep and have been implicated in the control of mood and certain types of emotional behavior, including aggressive behavior and clinical depression. Although there are dopamine-containing neurons scattered throughout the brain, there are two main projections from the midbrain. One group of dopaminergic cells arises in the substantia nigra and projects axons to the striatum (i.e., the caudate nucleus and the putamen); these cells facilitate the initiation of voluntary movement. The origin of the other group of cells is in the ventral tegmental area of the midbrain with axons that innervate an area that includes the frontal cortex and the limbic system. This projection is somehow involved in reward systems and emotion (Bear, Connors, & Paradiso, 1996).

Experimental evidence shows that early rearing conditions can influence the development of each of these important modulatory systems, as well as gamma aminobutyric acid (GABA), the major inhibitory neurotransmitter in the CNS. Many psychoactive drugs affect these neurotransmitter systems, and, because of that, the systems play a very important role in current thinking and research on the biological basis of certain psychiatric disorders. However, because the exact functions of these systems in the brain are not understood, we have only a limited understanding of the possible behavioral or functional significance of the changes in those systems that result from the early environmental inputs described in this section. Absent a mapping of the developmental consequences of observed changes in neurotransmitter systems, it is not possible to label individual research findings as contributing to beneficial or detrimental outcomes for the developing mammal.

Animal Studies

The animal research reviewed here focuses on the effects that early rearing experiences such as maternal separation, human handling, and social isolation have on the developing CNS in rodents and nonhuman primates. We know that maternal deprivation has an impact on the developing serotonin and dopamine systems of the infant rat. For example, postsynaptic serotonin receptors in the cortex and the hippocampus increased in number after infant rats were separated from their mothers for 24 hours (Vazquez, Lopez, Van Hoers, Watson, & Levine, 2000). Because the limbic–HPA axis is capable of modulating the serotonin system, modifications in the serotonin system in response to maternal separations are likely tied to the hyperresponsiveness of the limbic–HPA axis that also results from maternal deprivation (as discussed in the next section). There also appears to be a broad role for mesolimbic dopamine neurotransmitter systems in responses to social isolation, including maternal deprivation, although the specific effects may differ at different ages. For example, maternally deprived rats show enhanced release of dopamine in response to an amphetamine challenge (Hall, Wilkinson, Humby, & Robbins, 1999; Kehoe, Shoemaker, Arons, Triano, & Suresh, 1998). The dopaminergic pathways are critical to the brain's control of movement, and changes in the dopamine system are thought to play a role in the altered locomotive activity that is associated with early isolation experiences in rats.

Human handling of rat pups induces changes in maternal behavior; mothers of recently handled pups exhibit increased licking/grooming and arched-back nursing[1] (Liu et al., 1997). Research suggests that these forms of maternal stimulation mediate the human handling effects observed in rodents (though perhaps not the handling effects observed in other mammals, such as rabbits) (Denenberg, 1999). The impact of both handling and maternal deprivation on the rat brain extends to the major inhibitory neurotransmitter system. Rat pups subjected to handling showed higher $GABA_A$ and benzodiazepine receptor bindings as adults. This contrasts with the alterations observed in adult rats subjected to repeated separations from their mothers during the first 3 weeks of life; they showed reduced $GABA_A$ and benzodiazepine receptor bindings (Caldji, Francis, Sharma, Plotsky, & Meaney, 2000; Francis, Caldji, Champagne, Plotsky, & Meaney, 1999). These changes may partially mediate some of the behavioral responses to early rearing conditions that are observed in adult rats, such as decreased expression of fear-related behaviors in response to early handling and enhanced fearfulness among those exposed to early maternal separations.[2]

The handling of infant rat pups by humans also appears to improve the efficiency of synaptic connections in the rat brain and enable long-term learning through long-term potentiation. Long-term potentiation is a process that makes the links between certain synapses more powerful over time; when one synapse repeatedly triggers the firing of another, that second synapse eventually becomes more sensitive and responsive to the first. Early handling of rats seems to increase the amplitude of long-term potentiation in the hippocampus, suggesting that early handling and enhanced maternal care may bolster the offspring's eventual ability to learn (Cirulli et al., 2003).

Early maternal separation seems to affect the expression of neurotrophins in rats. Neurotrophins, such as nerve growth factor, are proteins that help establish connectivity in the nervous system and promote the density, viability, and differentiation of neurons. As such, they play an important role in brain plasticity. One study found that a 1-hour maternal separation increased the expression of nerve growth factor in the hippocampus of 3-day-old rats, while a follow-up study using a longer separation time found increased nerve growth factor expression in the hypothalamus, hippocampus, and other CNS regions (Cirulli, Alleva, Antonelli, & Aloe, 2000). Maternal licking has also been shown to increase nerve growth factor. In addition to their function as neurotransmitters, monoamines have been shown to act as neurotrophic factors during cortical development. Given the effects of maternal separation and licking on monoamine systems and neurotrophins, it is not surprising that these early maternal experiences have been linked to the growth of nerve fibers in the rat brain (e.g., Braun, Lange, Metzger, & Poeggel, 2000).

Some of the research discussed in this chapter examines early environmental influences on gene expression in the rat brain (Caldji et al., 2000; Cirulli et al., 2000; Plotsky & Meaney, 1993; Vazquez et al., 2000). Gene expression can be studied by examining the amount of messenger RNA (mRNA) in a tissue sample. Messenger RNA molecules are the "templates" that encode the manufacturing instructions for proteins from strands of DNA. The amount of mRNA for a particular protein present in a tissue sample indicates the rate at which the gene for that protein was transcribed. For example, in one study researchers were interested in RC3 (neurogranin), a postsynaptic protein kinase C substrate that is expressed in the dendritic spines of some neurons. They found that rats exposed to an experimental condition comprised of moderate amounts of both maternal separation and handling showed elevated RC3 mRNA expression in the hippocampus when compared to rats that either were not separated from their mothers (no handling) or were exposed to briefer periods of separation and handling (McNamara, Huot, Lenox, & Plotsky, 2002). By showing that environmental factors, such as maternal separation and handling, may induce changes in the expression of genes that are required for the development of circuitry in the rat brain, this research is beginning to point to the mechanisms by which early experiences shape the development and functioning of the CNS.

Investigations involving nonhuman primates similarly point to an effect of early rearing conditions on developing neurotransmitter systems. This line of research grows out of observations of the behavioral and social deficits that some primate species show when reared in total or partial social isolation. For example, rhesus monkeys reared under conditions of social deprivation display numerous social deficits in affiliation (social responsiveness, sexual and maternal behavior, communication) as well as in feeding and drinking, exploratory behavior, and learning ability (Lewis, Gluck, Beauchamp, Keresztury, & Mailman, 1990). They also exhibit high rates of stereotyped and self-injurious behaviors, such as rocking, self-biting, and self-hitting. Studies of the neurobiological mechanisms that mediate these extreme and unusual behavioral deficits focus on the role of the monoamine neurotransmitter systems described earlier: norepinephrine, serotonin, and dopamine. In these studies, concentrations of neurotransmitter metabolites, obtained from samples of cerebrospinal fluid, are used as indicators of the activity of that neuronal system in the brain.

In one experiment, rhesus monkeys were raised under one of three conditions during the first month of life: mother-reared, mother-deprived, and "reared" by a terry-cloth-covered surrogate mother. When samples of the monkeys' cerebrospinal fluid were tested, the surrogate-mother reared and mother-deprived monkeys had lower concentrations of norepinephrine compared to the mother-reared monkeys. However, there were no differences in the levels of dopamine and serotonin metabolites (Kraemer, Ebert, Schmidt, & McKinney, 1991). Other studies, however, have found that rhesus monkeys deprived of experience with a mother and critical aspects of peer interaction during the first 15 months of life had higher levels of metabolites of serotonin as well as lower concentrations of norepinephrine in cerebrospinal fluid (Kraemer & Clarke, 1990).

Concentrations of monoamine metabolites in cerebrospinal fluid do not provide a complete picture of the functioning of that neurotransmitter system. Therefore, it can be difficult to interpret the significance of increases or decreases of a neurotransmitter metabolite in cerebrospinal fluid. This is illustrated by the findings from a study of older adult rhesus monkeys (Lewis et al., 1990). Monkeys reared in total social isolation during the first 9 months of life were compared to monkeys that had been reared with peer and maternal contact. There were no differences in the concentrations of dopamine, serotonin, and norepinephrine metabolites in the cerebrospinal fluid taken from the two groups of monkeys. However, when a dopamine agonist (apomorphine) was administered to assess changes in dopamine receptors in the brain, the isolated monkeys had a much higher frequency of spontaneous eye blinking.[3] Because the monkeys were tested in older adulthood (all older than 14 years), these findings suggest that early, prolonged social isolation results in long-term alterations in the functioning of dopamine receptors in the brain.

Another research paradigm manipulates the monkey rearing environment by altering the availability of food. The increased demands of a "variable foraging" environment, in which food is sometimes plentiful and easily obtained and sometimes not, appear to reduce maternal responsivity (Andrews & Rosenblum, 1991). Squirrel monkey mothers in high demand conditions have been observed to spend 60% more time foraging for food and stopped carrying their infants at earlier ages (Lyons & Schatzberg, 2003). In one study, bonnet macaques were reared by their mothers under two conditions. Some lived in laboratory breeding groups under stable *ad libitum* conditions and others experienced adverse variable foraging demands (mothers were sometimes required to dig through wood chips to obtain food) for a few months during their early life. Cerebrospinal fluid was sampled when the monkeys reached an age comparable to the peripubertal–young adult phases of human development. In this study, monkeys reared under the stressful foraging conditions had higher cerebrospinal fluid concentrations of all three monoamines that were tested: serotonin, dopamine, and norepinephrine (Coplan et al., 1998). Another study of bonnet macaques reared under the same two conditions examined the behavioral effects of probes of two neurotransmitter systems.[4] The subjects who had been reared under variable foraging conditions were hyperresponsive to a probe of the norepinephrine system (yohimbine, an alpha-2 antagonist), but were hyporesponsive to a serotonin agonist (*m*CPP). Their behavioral reactions to the probes indicated that norepinephrine responses were exaggerated and serotonin responses were blunted compared to offspring reared by mothers under less stressful conditions (Rosenblum et al., 1994).

Studies by Suomi and associates suggest a role of maternal behavior in moderating genetic risk for serotonergic dysfunction. One study compared monkeys with two forms of the 5-HTT allele, a gene related to serotonin transport; the short form of the gene confers low serotonin reuptake efficiency, whereas the long form is associated with normal serotonin reuptake efficiency (Suomi, 1997). In addition, some of the monkeys were raised by their mothers and some were raised by peers. Being raised by peers is a risk factor for the development of a reactive, impulsive temperament and other deficits in social behavior, including more aggressive exchanges and less grooming. Monkeys with the short 5-HTT allele who were raised by peers showed lower concentrations of the primary central serotonin metabolite (5-HIAA) than was true for monkeys with the long allele. But for monkeys raised by their mothers, primary serotonin metabolite concentrations were identical for monkeys with either allele. This pattern clearly suggests a protective effect of maternal behavior on expression of genetic risk for low levels of serotonin. A promising direction for future research is the investigation of possible connections between early socialization experiences, serotonin functioning, and social behavior in monkeys.

Evidence also suggests that early adverse parenting experiences may cause neuronal metabolic impairments and affect neuronal density and integrity. Bonnet macaque infants reared by mothers exposed to variable foraging demand conditions for several months were studied 10 years later using proton magnetic resonance spectroscopic imaging, a method of detecting brain activity at the cellular level (Mathew et al., 2003). Compared to a matched control group, variable foraging demand monkeys displayed significantly decreased N-acetylaspartate (NAA)/Creatine (Cr) and increased glutamate-glutamine-aminobutyric acid (Glx)/Cr ratios in the anterior cingulate. NAA is typically used as a marker to assess neuron density and viability, so this result would suggest decreased neuronal viability. The finding of a lower NAA/Cr ratio in the anterior cingulate in the variable foraging demand group mirrors a previous finding in human teenagers with posttraumatic stress disorder (De Bellis, Keshavan, Spencer, & Hall, 2000), and other reports on adult posttraumatic stress disorder have found reductions in NAA in hippocampal or medial temporal lobe regions (Schuff et al., 1997). The investigators also argue that because heightened glutamate neurotransmission in the prefrontal cortex may partially mediate HPA activation, the GLx findings (showing increased glutamate functioning in the variable foraging demand group) may be an indication of heightened HPA activity in those subjects.

The impact of the social environment on neurotransmitter systems is not limited to early rearing experiences. In golden hamsters, for example, social subjugation during puberty in the form of daily exposure to aggressive adults resulted in increased serotonin innervation of the anterior hypothalamus (as well as a decrease in vasopressin levels). In addition, subjugated animals were more likely to attack younger and weaker animals but were less likely to attack animals of similar age and size (Delville, Melloni, & Ferris, 1998).

Although it may be too soon to say how each of the CNS alterations reported in animals might affect subsequent behavior and functioning, we can safely conclude at this point that there is an association between social experiences during development and neurobiological changes in several diffuse modulatory systems in the brains of rats and nonhuman primates.

Studies of Human Infants and Children

Human research is much more limited than the studies summarized previously both because of the invasiveness of procedures to assess neurotransmitter functioning and because of the need to use nonexperimental designs in socialization studies. However, findings are consistent with the animal literature in linking adverse early socialization experiences with differences in the developing neurotransmitter profiles of children. For example, one study compared infants of mothers who, on the basis of a 3-minute play interaction, had been classified as "intrusive" (rough tickling, poking and tugging, tense or fake facial expressions) or "withdrawn" (flat affect, rare touching and vocalizing, disengaged behaviors). Offspring of the intrusive mothers showed higher levels of monoamines (dopamine, epinephrine, and norepinephrine) in urine collected at 6 months of age, compared to infants whose mothers were withdrawn (Jones et al., 1997). The absence of a normal control group in this study makes it difficult to interpret these findings. Moreover, the long-term significance of the neurotransmitter profiles that were observed is not known. However, dysregulation of these neurotransmitters is associated with behavioral problems and psychopathology, including aggression, depression, and anxiety (Berman, Kavoussi, & Coccaro, 1997; Micallef & Blin, 2001; Thase, Jindal, & Howland, 2002).

Because the serotonergic nervous system appears to play a role in aggression, a few researchers have focused on the link between serotonin and abusive or aggressive family environments. An indirect approach to assessing central serotonergic activity in humans is the examination of responses to a serotonin challenge. An increase in serotonin activity in the brain stimulates a rise in prolactin measured in blood samples. The magnitude of the increase in peripheral prolactin is treated as an index of the increase in serotonergic activity in the CNS. An example of this approach is found in research indicating dysregulation in the serotonergic system of children who have been maltreated and abused. One study compared depressed–abused children to two groups of nonabused children; one group included depressed children and the other group consisted of nondepressed, control children (Kaufman et al., 1998). The majority of the abused children had experienced multiple forms of maltreatment, such as physical or sexual abuse, and half were living under adverse conditions, including homes in which there was ongoing spousal and emotional abuse. In response to a serotonergic challenge (intravenous administration of a serotonin precursor, L-5-HTP), the abused children secreted significantly more prolactin, indicating increased sertonergic activity. Moreover, this indicator of central serotonergic functioning (total prolactin post-L-5-HTP) was significantly correlated with ratings of aggressive behavior. The precise nature of the association between aggression and serotonin is not known. However, there is some support for a causal role of dysregulated serotonin functioning in the aggressive behavior of psychiatric patients (Berman et al., 1997).

Another study examined prolactin responses to fenfluramine hydrochloride, which increases the level of serotonin in CNS synapses (through release of serotonin from nerve terminals and by inhibiting the process of reuptake). In a sample of younger brothers of convicted delinquents, all of whose families were impoverished, less maternal regulation of child behavior was associated with a larger prolactin response to the challenge. Lower scores on the "encouragement of maturity" subscale of the HOME (Home Observation and Measurement of the Environment Inventory), which is based on observers' ratings of the degree of parental limit setting, were associated with larger increases in the boys' central serotonergic activity. A stronger prolactin response was also linked to greater aggression in this sample of prepubertal boys (Pine et al., 1997). In another report, based on the same study, an inverse relationship was found between harsh parenting and the density of 5-HT$_{2A}$ receptors on platelets (a peripheral index of CNS serotonin profile) (Pine et al., 1996). Lower receptor density was linked to mother–child relationships characterized by greater parental anger, use of physical punishment, and emotional upset. Together with the study by Kaufman and colleagues described earlier, this line of research suggests that there is an association between parenting and the activity of the serotonin neurotransmitter system, at least in high-risk samples of children.

Electroencephalographic Studies

Neurotransmitters regulate the transmission of electrical charges across neurons. The EEG uses scalp recordings to measure the resulting pattern of electrical activity in the brain. EEG studies have found differences in relative right- and left-hemisphere activation that seem to correlate with temperament, early childhood experiences, and genetic propensity. Davidson (1995, 1998) and Fox (1994) have suggested that affective styles connected with emotion regulation, such as approach and withdrawal behaviors, can be related to both state-dependent and more stable individual differences in cerebral asymmetry. The left frontal region typically appears activated during the expression of approach emotions like curiosity and joy, while the right frontal region activates during distress, fear, and other withdrawal emotions.

Several studies suggest a relationship between maternal psychopathology and infants' EEG patterns, although it is unclear whether this relationship derives from genes, maternal interaction style, or both. A study of 159 mother–infant pairs found that compared with a control group, the 13–15-month-old children of mothers diagnosed with depression were less likely to show relative left-hemisphere activation and more likely to show relative right-hemisphere activation (Dawson & Ashman, 2000). Insensitive mothering—both intrusive and withdrawn behaviors—partially mediated the association between depression and infant EEG in all mothers and fully mediated this association in the mothers who became depressed only after birth, providing support for the idea that parenting style influences infant EEG. In the study of withdrawn and intrusive mothering mentioned previously, Jones et al. (1997) found that the children of withdrawn mothers showed greater relative right frontal asymmetry than infants of intrusive mothers, whose EEG patterns showed greater relative left frontal EEG asymmetry. In a subsequent study, infants of withdrawn mothers, in comparison to infants of intrusive mothers, showed greater relative right frontal asymmetry. When a stranger modeled surprised and sad expressions, however, the infants of intrusive mothers shifted toward greater relative right frontal EEG asymmetry (Diego et al., 2002). While parenting style may influence EEG patterns, it remains unclear whether individual differences in EEG asymmetry stem from early experience or from genetic inheritance. When further elaborated, this body of research may eventually provide another line of evidence suggesting that early childhood experiences shape the brain's functioning and development.

Both animal and human research point to early rearing experiences playing a role in the development and functioning of neurons and neurotransmitter systems. However, the precise nature of the effects of socialization are difficult to interpret with currently available data. It is challenging to integrate findings from studies that are based on different species, focus on different kinds of early rearing conditions, and use a variety of strategies to assess multiple neurotransmitter systems and the activity of neurons in different parts of the brain. Moreover, because neuroscientists do not yet understand precisely how the diffuse modulatory systems function in the brain, we do not yet know what the implications are for behavior, adjustment, or development when neuron and neurotransmitter differences are observed under various rearing conditions. The different stages of development at which subjects are studied adds another layer of complexity to the picture. Nonetheless, the research does indicate that the development and activity of neurons and neurotransmitter systems in the mammalian brain are affected by a wide variety of rearing conditions, ranging from various degrees of maternal deprivation, to rearing by mothers under high demand, to human parenting that is intrusive, abusive, harsh, and unregulated. These socialization experiences appear to change the development and functioning of the CNS in ways that may be linked to behavioral deficits later in life.

STRESS-RESPONSE SYSTEMS

An important task of the CNS is to regulate biological responses to stress. Evidence suggests that the development and functioning of the main stress-responsive systems, namely the HPA axis and the sympathetic and parasympathetic nervous system are influenced by early socialization.

Hypothalamic–Pituitary–Adrenocortical Axis

There is manifold evidence from animal and human studies to suggest an important role of early family environment in the development of the HPA axis and its engagement in response to stress. So well established are these relations that depriving a young offspring of contact with its mother through maternal separation is the most commonly employed paradigm in animal studies for understanding the impact of early stress on development (e.g., Laudenslager et al., 1995; Kuhn & Schanberg, 1998). Moreover, it is now evident that changes due to a chronically stressful early environment can have permanent effects on stress responses across an offspring's lifetime. Although most of this evidence comes from animal studies, studies of human families reveal similar patterns. We begin this section with a brief description of the functions of the HPA axis and then describe the evidence relating early family environment, especially maternal-offspring ties, to HPA axis functioning.

The HPA axis plays a central role in managing threat. Corticotropin-releasing hormone, produced in the paraventricular nuclei of the hypothalamus, stimulates the secretion of adrenocorticotropic hormone by the anterior pituitary, resulting in the release of glucocorticoids from the adrenal glands (e.g., cortisol in humans and corticosterone in rats). Glucocorticoids serve an important function at low basal levels by permitting or restoring processes that prime homeostatic defense mechanisms (Munck & Naray-Fejes-Toth, 1994). This integrated pattern of HPA axis activation modulates a wide range of somatic functions including energy release, immune activity, mental activity, growth, and reproductive function. At low basal levels, glucocorticoids promote mental and physical health as well as normal development (Gunnar, 2000).

However, larger, more frequent, and more long-lasting elevations in glucocorticoids, as occur in chronically or recurrently stressful environments, can compromise HPA axis functioning and, ultimately, health. For example, a hyperresponsive HPA axis influences the development of hypertension and cardiovascular disease, immune suppression, hyperinsulimia, and insulin resistance, enhancing risk for diabetes. Glucocorticoids are also implicated in age-related decreases in immune competence and cognitive functioning.

Hyperactivity of the HPA axis is also thought to contribute to anxiety disorders and depression, as well as to growth retardation and developmental delay. As this analysis suggests, the HPA axis interacts with other systems, including the autonomic nervous system and the immune system, such that changes in the HPA axis functioning will affect these and other systems as well. Hyporesponsiveness of the HPA axis can also have deleterious effects on health and development. It can be associated with chronic fatigue and susceptibility to autoimmune and inflammatory diseases, including rheumatoid arthritis and asthma (Gunnar, 2000).

The question arises as to the relationship between hyperresponsive and hyporesponsiveness of the HPA axis. One theory is that stressful conditions early in life lead first to hypercortisolism, as children react intensely to chronic or recurring problems, such as family conflict. Over time, however, with repeated activation, the HPA axis may lose some of its resiliency, manifested in chronically elevated basal cortisol levels, a flattened diurnal cortisol rhythm, and/or weak cortisol responses to acute stress (see Gunnar & Vazquez, 2001; McEwen, 1998, for further discussion of this issue). At present, these sequential changes in HPA axis functioning in response to chronic stress represent a hypothesis rather than a definitive conclusion, and not all empirical evidence fits this hypothesized sequence (Gunnar & Vasquez, 2001; Heim et al., 2000). Linking these changes to socioemotional functioning will also be revealing. For example, heightened HPA responses to stress may be associated with anxious responses to stress, whereas an elevated flat cortisol trajectory may be associated with psychic numbing and/or coping through withdrawal instead.

Animal Studies

Research with rodents and nonhuman primates has demonstrated conclusively that maternal behavior affects an offspring's developing HPA axis as well as HPA responses to stress. For example, studies of rhesus monkeys have found that ventral contact between offspring and mother following a threatening event promotes rapid decreases in HPA axis activity (Gunnar et al., 1981; Mendoza et al., 1978). Meaney and associates have shown that the immediate effect of maternal licking and grooming and arched-back nursing is a reduction in corticosterone responses and sympathetic activity in offspring and mother alike (Liu et al., 1997; Francis, Diorio, Liu, & Meaney, 1999). These researchers have compared the offspring of mothers who are high versus low in licking and grooming and cross-fostered offspring of high or low licking-and-grooming mothers, to demonstrate experimentally the impact of these nurturant behaviors. The rats reared by mothers who engage in more licking and grooming during the first 10 days of life show reduced plasma adrenocorticotropic hormone and corticosterone responses to acute stress, increased hippocampal glucocorticoid receptor messenger RNA expression, enhanced glucocorticoid feedback sensitivity, and decreased levels of hypothalamic corticotropin-releasing hormone messenger RNA (Cirulli et al., 2003). Through these processes, early maternal nurturant behaviors appear to shape the infant's ability to prepare for and react to stress (Champagne, Francis, Mar, & Meaney, 2003).

The long-term effects of these maternal nurturant behaviors are evident as well. Offspring who are the recipients of early maternal attention also get lifelong protection against stress. Specifically, as adults, rat pups who received nurturant maternal care early in life had reduced plasma adrenocorticotropic hormone and smaller corticosterone re-

sponses to acute stress. As they matured, the offspring also showed more open-field exploration, suggesting less anxiety in novel situations, and as adults, they were less likely
to show age-related onset of HPA axis dysregulation in response to challenge and age-
related cognitive dysfunction. (Francis, Diorio, et al., 1999; Liu et al., 1999). Using a variety of correlational and experimental methods, Meaney and colleagues (Weaver et al.,
2004) showed that these changes occur via alteration of the offspring epigenome at a
glucocorticoid gene promoter in the hippocampus via changes in DNA methylation.
Thus, early nurturant maternal care can alter the expression of genes related to HPA responses to stress in ways that persist across the lifespan.

Similarly, Rosenblum, Coplan, and colleagues (Coplan et al., 1996) manipulated the
environments in which mother macaque monkeys raised their offspring through the variable foraging demand (VFD) paradigm described previously. In an environment with easily
obtainable food, and also in an environment in which finding food required more effort,
the mother monkeys were attentive to their offspring, whose development proceeded normally. In the VFD condition, however, the mothers became more inconsistent in their
mothering. The offspring of these mothers showed elevated cortisol responses to stress,
coupled with fearful and socially maladaptive behavior. We interpret these and related
findings as indicating that maternal nurturance, or its absence, helps to shape the HPA
axis. When maternal responses are nurturant, the offspring's HPA axis operates efficiently and returns to baseline quickly following a stressful encounter; these effects persist
across an offspring's lifespan. In contrast, those animals that receive less nurturant maternal behavior develop a "hair-trigger" HPA axis response to stress. Their glucocorticoid
responses to stressful events are strong and persistent and eventually carry health consequences (see Newport, Stowe, & Nemeroff, 2002, for a review).

Studies of Human Infants and Children

A broad array of evidence in humans likewise suggests that the cortisol response, reflecting HPA axis functioning, may be altered in the offspring of risky families. Indirect evidence for the role of early maternal nurturance is found in the elevated cortisol levels observed among children whose mothers suffer from psychological disorders that may
affect their ability to provide consistent nurturing. For example, infants of mothers with
panic disorder showed high salivary cortisol levels as well as disturbed sleep, although
their behavior was not otherwise adversely reflective of their mothers' panic disorder
(Warren et al., 2003). Essex, Klein, Cho, and Kalin (2002) reported that maternal depression was a significant predictor of children's cortisol levels beginning in infancy through
first grade and predicted symptoms of psychological distress at this last time point. However, the extent to which altered parenting behavior associated with panic disorder and
depression accounted for the differences in the children's cortisol levels and whether
cortisol mediates subsequent symptoms of emotional distress are not yet clear; shared genetic inheritance may have played a role in these associations.

Harsh parenting behavior may also be linked to HPA axis functioning. A study of
264 infants, children, and adolescents found an association between abnormal cortisol
profiles, diminished immunity, and frequent illnesses with a family environment characterized by few positive affectionate interactions and a high level of negative interactions,
including irrational punishment and unavailable or erratic attention from parents (Flinn
& England, 1997). Bugental, Martorell, and Barazza (2003) found that infants who re-

ceived corporal punishment showed high cortisol reactivity to stress; in addition, infants who experienced their mother's frequent emotional withdrawal demonstrated elevated basal levels of cortisol. Granger et al. (1998) reported that children's basal cortisol levels prior to a conflict-oriented mother–child task were associated with a family environment high in aggression, anger, and conflict, the child's internalizing behavior problems, the mother's childhood levels of socially withdrawn behavior (a potential indicator of a genetic contribution to this pattern), and current psychosocial problems. Spangler, Schieche, Ilg, Maier, and Ackermann (1994) found that a mother's insensitivity to her child during play predicted an increase in the child's cortisol during free play; infants of highly insensitive mothers also exhibited more negative emotional behavior during play as well. Abuse can also affect HPA axis functioning. In one study, children who had been physically abused in their families had somewhat elevated afternoon cortisol concentrations; maltreated children who were also depressed had lower morning cortisol concentrations compared to nondepressed maltreated children and were more likely to show a rise, rather than the expected decrease in cortisol, from morning to afternoon (Hart, Gunnar, & Cicchetti, 1996). In a review of the evidence, Chorpita and Barlow (1998) noted that in families characterized by low levels of warmth and high levels of restrictive, controlling parenting, HPA axis functioning may be disrupted in response to stress, leading to increased corticotrophin-releasing hormone and hypercortisolism (see also Gunnar & Donzella, 2002). These changes have been linked to a heightened risk for anxiety and depression (e.g., Chorpita & Barlow, 1998), although the causal connection between these sets of findings is not yet known.

A child's attachment to his or her parents appears to moderate cortisol responses to novel or potentially threatening conditions. For example, children with disorganized/disoriented attachment patterns are more likely to exhibit higher cortisol levels to situations that other children take in stride (Hertsgaard, Gunnar, Erickson, & Nachmias, 1995). In a series of studies, Gunnar and associates found that attachment patterns moderated cortisol responses of babies in stressful circumstances (Gunnar, Brodersen, Nachmias, Buss, & Rigatuso, 1996; Nachmias, Gunnar, Mangelsdorf, Parritz, & Buss, 1996). For example, Ahnert, Gunnar, Lamb, and Barthel (2004) examined cortisol levels in children at home before starting child care, during an adaptation phase in which their parents accompanied them, during a separation phase, and 5 months later. In the separation phase, cortisol responses rose for all children, and attachment security was unrelated to these levels, but during the adaptation phase, secure infants had significantly lower cortisol levels than insecure children did. The implications of these patterns for socioemotional development, if any, are not yet known.

The protective effects of a secure attachment relationship appear to be especially evident for socially fearful or inhibited children and children otherwise at risk. Gunnar and associates argued that temperamentally fearful children are especially vulnerable to stress, and an insecure attachment is implicated in their elevated cortisol responses to new situations, serving both as a marker of the parent–infant relationship and as a potential predictor of later anxiety disorders (Gunnar & Donzella, 2002). Children with other preexisting risk factors may also be especially vulnerable to the effects of parenting. Bugental (2004) tracked outcomes experienced by children born with medical or physical disorders and found that at-risk children who also experienced harsh parenting showed elevated cortisol and low habituation to potentially stressful events. In contrast, those at-risk children who experienced supportive parenting showed normal cortisol responses and normal habituation to stress. Unlike the research reviewed earlier, in this study the stress re-activity of children not at risk was unaffected by parenting style. This finding underscores the interactive role that parenting style may play with other risk factors, including genetic risks, in the etiology of biological and psychological stress responses.

Paralleling the animal studies, a number of findings suggest that effects of early environment on HPA axis functioning in children persist into adulthood. Several retrospective studies report that alterations in HPA axis functioning associated with a risky family environment continue to appear in young adulthood. In one study, poor family relationships, assessed by college students' ratings of their early family environment, were associated with elevated cortisol responses to a laboratory challenge (Luecken, 1998). In a second study, women who reported having been abused in childhood showed greater HPA responses to laboratory stress than did women without such histories; these responses were greater for abused women who also had symptoms of anxiety and depression (Heim et al., 2000; see also Kaufman, Plotsky, Nemeroff, & Charney, 2000). Taylor, Lerner, Sage, Lehman, and Seeman (2004) found that young adults who reported an early environment marked by conflict, by cold, unaffectionate behavior, or by neglect showed elevated baseline cortisol levels prior to a laboratory stress challenge, although responses to the challenge itself were not influenced by family background. A study of 6–12-year-old children reared in Romanian orphanages 6½ years after they had been adopted examined diurnal cortisol patterns. Most of the children raised in the orphanages had significantly higher cortisol levels over the daytime hours than did comparison adopted samples and nonadopted children. These effects were attributed to the risky early environment in which these children were raised, which included gross neglect of basic needs and chronic exposure to infectious agents (Gunnar, Morison, Chisholm, & Schuder, 2001). Thus, the evidence clearly suggests that HPA functioning can be potentially permanently altered in response to early stressful environments.

The impact of day care on children's diurnal cortisol responses may also reflect an effect of chronic stress on HPA axis activity. Watamura Sebanc, and Gunnar (2001) reported a rise in cortisol across the day among children in full-day child care. Although the cause of this pattern is not fully understood, factors involving the interactional demands of group settings during this developmental period may be implicated. A second study (Watamura, Donzella, Alwin, & Gunnar, 2003) reported that children who were socially fearful were more likely to demonstrate this cortisol increase, whereas those children who played more with peers exhibited lower cortisol levels. Possibly, these results may be understood as gene–environment interactions whereby the highly stimulating social environment interacted to produce heightened HPA axis activity primarily in children with some initial proclivity to social fearfulness.

Although research relates qualities of the early family environment to offspring's HPA axis development and functioning, several important issues remain. A first issue concerns how the HPA axis changes over time in response to long-term stress. A working hypothesis is that initial reactions to a risky family environment are marked by elevated HPA responses to stress which yield over time to the development of elevated basal cortisol levels and a muted HPA response to stress. More research is needed on this issue, however, especially on potential implications of flattened HPA stress responses for socioemotional functioning. A second issue concerns the role of shared genetic factors in explaining some of the relations between a harsh family environment and clinical outcomes, such as anxiety, depression, and certain diseases that have genetic bases. Although animal studies in which early environment is manipulated show definitively that maternal behavior can, in and of itself, affect HPA axis development and functioning, the degree to which genetic contributions figure into these relations in human offspring merits examination. A third issue concerns the fact that many different types of early adverse experience appear to affect HPA axis functioning in similar ways. As one of the primary stress systems of the body, the HPA axis is responsive to numerous insults, ranging from the harsh parenting described here to physical stressors such as malnutrition or exposure to drugs *in utero*. As such, the HPA axis may represent a general pathway to multiple mental and physical health outcomes. This hypothesis bears continued scrutiny, however, as specific effects on biological systems associated with specific types of stressors are being uncovered. This issue raises the more general point that research can now begin to examine ways in which particular stressors (such as abuse vs. neglect) may differentially shape the HPA axis and/or its interactions with other biological systems, a specificity that has largely been lacking in research findings to date.

Sympathetic and Parasympathetic Functioning

The sympathetic adrenal medullary system is also involved in the management of threat or challenge. The actions of the sympathetic system are mediated primarily by norepinephrine and epinephrine. These catecholamines exert effects on adrenergic receptors in the target tissues to produce, among other changes, increases in heart rate and blood pressure, dilation of the airways, and enhanced availability of glucose and fatty acids for energy. These coordinated responses facilitate short-term mobilization of an organism's resources for the rapid, intense physical activity involved in the "fight-or-flight" response.

A few studies with human infants and children indicate that the early family environment can have an impact on the immediate and long-term functioning of the autonomic nervous system. Although most children show increases in arousal in response to familial stress (El-Sheikh et al., 1989), children in families marked by chronic conflict experience this physiological activation on a recurrent basis. One study found that boys but not girls from families characterized as unsupportive by parents had stronger heart rate responses to laboratory stressors, compared with boys from more supportive families (Woodall & Matthews, 1989). It is unclear whether elevated autonomic reactivity to stress results from chronic exposure to family conflict, or whether shared genetic heritage plays a role as well (Ballard, Cummings, & Larkin, 1993; Ewart, 1991). Moreover, because much of this research measures heart rate and blood pressure, the studies do not enable one to identify which aspects of autonomic functioning (sympathetic changes, parasympathetic changes, or a combination) are responsive to a risky family environment.

Research on young adults suggests that the early family environment has long-term effects on sympathetic nervous system functioning and on risk factors for coronary heart disease as well as related metabolic disorders. Luecken (1998) reported that college students who reported poor family relationships in childhood had higher blood pressure both at resting levels and in response to a laboratory challenge. These family characteristics were also associated with elevated anger and hostility, suggesting that these factors may contribute to stronger sympathetic responses to stress. Taylor et al. (2004) found that young adult males, but not females, showed elevated heart rate and blood pressure responses to stress, if they were from families characterized by conflict or a cold, nonnurturant parenting style.

The research evidence suggests that these heightened sympathetic nervous system re-sponses to stress may have long-term consequences, as elevated sympathetic reactivity has been tied to risk factors for coronary heart disease. For example, heightened cardiovascu-lar reactivity to stress among boys 8–10 years old has been tied to increased left ventricu-lar mass, a risk factor for coronary heart disease (Allen, Matthews, & Sherman, 1997). Using evidence from 3,225 adults participating in the CARDIA study, Lehman, Taylor, Kiefe, and Seeman (2005) related reports of a risky family environment in childhood to adult metabolic function, which is a predictor of heart disease, diabetes, and other disor-ders. They found that individuals from families characterized by conflict, neglect, or cold, nonnurturant parenting were more likely to have dysregulations in metabolic functioning in adulthood, relations that were mediated by negative emotions and a lack of social sup-port.

Vagal Tone

The parasympathetic branch of the peripheral nervous system, and its main nerve, the vagus, is also implicated in reactivity to stress. The vagus, the 10th cranial nerve, commu-nicates bidirectionally between the viscera and the brain, influencing heart rate, intestinal movement, gastic acid secretion, and other important regulatory functions. The vagus is connected to the sinoatrial node, considered to be heart's pacemaker, and acts as a brake to decrease heart rate. This "vagal brake" allows individuals to regulate their responses, to engage and disengage from environmental stimuli, and to recover from arousal. In ad-dition, the vagal system plays a role in social behaviors such as facial expression, vocal-ization, and head turning. Polyvagal theory (Porges, 1995) proposes that cardiac vagal tone is an index of physiological regulatory capacity in infants, given the vagus's impact on a host of relevant systems. Indeed, vagal tone and heart rate variability have been linked to emotion regulation, social competence, and temperament in infants and children (Doussard-Roosevelt, Porges, Scanlon, Alemi, & Scanlon, 1997, Doussard-Roosevelt, McClenny, & Porges, 2001). Vagal tone also appears to be coordinated with the HPA axis, such that individuals who respond to a laboratory task with an increase in cortisol show a decreased vagal tone response to the task and vice versa (Porges, 2001).

Vagal tone may be influenced by prenatal or genetic factors: The newborns of women categorized as experiencing high anxiety during the second trimester of preg-nancy had lower vagal tone when tested on the first day of life, and their vagal tone ap-peared to be correlated with other markers such as sleep organization and alertness (Field et al., 2003). Vagal tone may also be affected by the quality of early care. A study of pre-mature infants found that those who received more kangaroo care (i.e., protracted mother–infant skin-to-skin contact) showed greater maturation of vagal tone between 32 and 37 weeks gestational age (Feldman & Eidelman, 2003). Kangaroo-care infants also spent more time in quiet sleep or alert wakefulness and less time in active sleep and also appeared more competent than non-kangaroo-care infants on neurodevelopmental tasks such as habituation and orientation. Another study assessed first-time mothers and their 6-month-old infants and found that infants' cardiac vagal tone correlated positively to the symmetry of mother–infant communication patterns (Porter, 2003). In other words, infants with attentive and attuned mothers tended to have higher vagal tone.

More research is warranted into the specific processes influencing the maturation and mylenization of the vagal nerve. While it is possible that infants develop high vagal tone as a result of sensitive caregiving, prenatal conditions and genetics may also play a role, as studies of neonates would suggest. Also, high vagal tone might be the cause, rather than the result, of symmetrical mother–infant communication. Children adept at emotional regulation may be more capable of remaining engaged in mother–infant communications and may prompt more reciprocal attentiveness in their mothers. A study that assessed vagal tone at 2 and 4 years of age found evidence for the stability of both vagal tone and mothers' parenting practices over that timespan (Kennedy, Rubin, Hastings, & Maisel, 2004). In addition, vagal tone at age 2 predicted parenting practices at age 4; for example, low vagal tone predicted harsher parenting, while high vagal tone was associated with more supportive parenting. Exposure to marital conflict also appears to be linked to lower vagal tone in 6-month-olds (Porter, Wouden-Miller, & Porter, 2003). Again, however, the direction of influence remains unclear. Not only does marital conflict seem to impact offspring vagal tone, but vagal tone also appears to influence children's reactions to intraparental conflict. In a group of 8- to 12-year-olds, higher vagal tone appeared to buffer children exposed to marital conflict against externalizing, internalizing, and health problems as a result of that conflict (El-Sheikh, Harger, & Whitson, 2001).

As with research on the HPA axis, research on the sympathetic and parasympathetic systems has associated early childhood stress with possible impairments in the functioning of these systems. These deficits appear to manifest themselves mainly in terms of heightened reactivity—for example, exaggerated blood pressure responses to a laboratory stressor—and in terms of compromised self-regulation (e.g., low vagal tone). However, much more work remains to be done on the specific causes and consequences of sympathetic and parasympathetic dysfunctions. For example, the possible genetic bases of these systems remains poorly understood. It is also unclear precisely which types of stressors, administered at what age, might have the greatest impact on the development of the sympathetic and parasympathetic systems.

IMMUNE FUNCTIONING

Given the influence of autonomic and endocrine activity on immune responses, it is not surprising that early experiences, such as maternal separation, have been found to have an impact on immune response (Worlein & Laudenslager, 2001). In particular, glucocorticoids, which are secreted as part of the HPA response to stress, are known to have immunosuppressive effects. Much of the immunological research has been conducted on monkeys. For example, rearing without exposure to a mother, as found in isolation rearing (without maternal or peer interactions) and peer socialization paradigms, has a long-lasting impact on monkey immune development (Coe et al., 1989; Coe, Lubach, Schneider, Dierschke, & Ershler, 1992; Lubach, Coe, & Ershler, 1995). As described below, experimental disruptions of the mother–infant bond produces evidence of both suppression and enhancement of immune responses in monkeys. Although an *enhanced* immune response was not initially expected, researchers have speculated that the absence of appropriate maternal stimulation could activate certain immune responses or alter the rate of maturation of the immune system (Coe et al., 1989). It is likely that the absence of breast feeding among the mother-deprived monkeys is also involved in this process. Breast milk can directly influence immune responses in the infant by the passage of maternal cells thereby altering the vulnerability of the young infant to infectious agents. Increased exposure to disease processes in the monkeys deprived of breast milk could affect the development of the maturing immune system (Coe et al., 1989; Lubach et al., 1995).

Two common *in vitro* measures of immune function in this literature are proliferative response and natural cytotoxicity.[5] Disruptions of the mother–infant bond, through various separation paradigms, produce complex alterations in immune responses in the monkey as assessed by these measures, with the effects sometimes lingering for years (Laudenslager, Capitanio, & Reite, 1985; Worlein & Laudenslager, 2001). The long-term alterations can include an enhanced immune functioning, suggested by increased natural cytotoxicity of lymphocytes, but also indications of a suppressed immune response, such as reduced B- and T- cell proliferative responses to mitogens. Interestingly, the effects of chronic stress on humans include both an enhancement and a suppression of immune responses, which contribute to immune dysregulation (Robles, Glaser, & Kiecolt-Glaser, 2005).

Although the changes in immune functioning are not yet fully understood, researchers speculate that any lasting effects of early separation experiences on immune responses are probably related to long-term changes in the mother–infant relationship that follow reunion. Similar to the rat mothers described earlier, who increase nurturing behaviors following reunion with their pups, pigtail macaque mothers tend to be more attentive and more restrictive when reunited with their infants and evidence suggests that there is a lasting impact of the separation–reunion experience on maternal behavior. Previously separated mothers wean their infants at a later age and maintain greater control over their infants' physical proximity when observed at 15 months of age (Worlein & Laudenslager, 2001). It is thought that these maternal behaviors may play a role in the long-term alterations in immune responses that have been observed in monkeys who experienced early disruptions of the mother–infant bond. It is possible that lasting changes in the primate mother–infant relationship mediate long-term changes in other biological systems following separation.

The effects of maternal separation on bonnet macaques' immune system can be ameliorated by the presence of a preferred peer partner (Boccia et al., 1997). Bonnet macaques who were separated from their mothers and their social group showed an initial suppressed immune response, but those changes were not observed in the infants who had a preferred peer partner present during the 2 weeks of separation.[6] Among the monkeys with a peer present, the magnitude of the immunological changes was related to the juvenile friend's affiliative behaviors. Infants who had more social behaviors, such as cradling, playing, and grooming, directed toward them during the separation period showed greater cytotoxicity and increased lymphocyte proliferation in response to two mitogens. This research suggests that alternative social attachments during separation can ameliorate the infant's immune response to maternal loss.

In the Boccia et al. (1997) study, the infants with friends present also showed less behavioral evidence of depression when separated from their mothers. This pattern is intriguing because of research suggesting that depression in humans is associated with compromised immune functioning (Cohen & Herbert, 1996). In fact, monkeys who show the greatest behavioral response to maternal separation (e.g, distress vocalizations, time spent in huddled, and withdrawn postures) also are the most likely to show declines in lymphocyte activation. Because the mother–infant relationship prior to the separation is known to impact behavioral responses, it may also play a role in the immune response (Worlein & Laudenslager, 2001).

Although the functional significance of the immunological changes observed in the monkey studies is not known, immune responses to abnormal rearing conditions early in life, even those that indicate enhanced immune activity, may set the stage for an increased vulnerability to disease later in life, when there is a natural decline in immunity (Lubach et al., 1995). As indicated previously, the impact of experiences like maternal separation on immune functioning can only be understood in the context of other biological responses to early stress, in particular changes in the HPA system.

GROWTH AND SEXUAL DEVELOPMENT

Research suggests that early rearing experiences can impact the secretion of growth hormone and the observed physical growth of offspring. Pubertal timing also appears to be influenced by the quality of family relationships and the presence of fathers in the home.

Growth and Growth Hormone

Growth hormone plays a role in growth, development, and immunoregulation. Appropriate maternal behavior is a stimulus for growth hormone secretion in nonhuman primates and in human infants (Kuhn & Schanberg, 1998), and growth hormone levels change in response to stress in nonhuman primates and rats (Laudenslager et al., 1995). In rat pups, maternal separation elicits a fall in serum growth hormone and a loss of tissue responsivity to exogenous growth hormone. Interestingly, stroking the pup with a paint brush restores serum growth hormone to control values, suggesting that the loss of tactile stimulation from the dam may account for the effects of separation on growth hormone (Kuhn & Schanberg, 1991). Research with human infants indicates that tactile stimulation can stimulate both somatic growth and behavioral development (Kuhn & Schanberg, 1991).

In contrast to the rat pups' response to separation, there is evidence in some monkey species that short-term responses to maternal separation may include a short-term *increase* in secretion of growth hormone. One study reported a slowly developing increase in plasma growth hormone in pigtail monkey infants in response to a 2-week maternal separation. Increases in growth hormone during the second week of separation were associated with a behavioral sign of distress, time spent in slouched huddled postures, suggesting that individual change in endocrine functioning was tied to the stressfulness of the separation for the monkey (Laudenslager et al., 1995). Although growth hormone secretion returned to baseline levels within a week following the pigtails' reunions with their mothers, frequent and prolonged repetition of reactions can be deleterious.

As in all the research discussed in this chapter, there are important distinctions between short-term responses to stressful experiences and the long-term consequences of chronically stressful early rearing experiences. For example, brief interruptions of growth hormone secretion in neonatal rats may be of little consequence. However, prolonged suppression of growth hormone reduces growth in all mammals (Kuhn & Schanberg, 1998). Early studies of human children exposed to inadequate caretaking identified consequences such as "deprivation dwarfism" and failure to thrive (Gardner, 1972; Glaser, Heagary, Bullard, & Pivchik, 1968). Contemporary research on the effects of institutionalization, particularly in Romanian orphanages, suggests that early deprivation experiences result in impairments across a wide range of domains, including cognitive and social development as well as physical growth (Zeanah et al., 2003). The findings also point to the remarkable resilience of human development to early insult, as cognitive and physical gains have been observed following adoption (O'Connor et al., 2000). However, the children in these studies spent the early months or years of their lives in grossly depriving conditions that included severe malnourishment. It is therefore impossible to discern how the social deprivation that these children experienced (e.g., most of their time was spent in individual cribs and they had very limited face-to-face interactions with caregivers) contributed to their impairments. Research on stressful, though less extreme, rearing environments has also found evidence of growth retardation. For example, in one longitudinal study, growing up in a difficult and conflictual family was associated with less height attainment in assessments made at age 7 and in adulthood (Montgomery, Bartley, & Wilkinson, 1997). Another study found that infants with less sensitive mothers were not growing as well (lower weight for age) as other infants (Valenzuela, 1997). The mechanisms underlying growth retardation in children growing up in risky environments are not yet understood. Behavioral processes, such as feeding and eating, as well as altered endocrine functioning, particularly growth hormone secretion, may be implicated.

Pubertal Timing

Early socioemotional stress seems to accelerate puberty in girls. A survey of over 1,100 girls related early puberty to the number of stressful life events and to family structure, specifically father absence (Surbey, 1990). In another study, better family relationships, fewer internalizing and externalizing problems, and lower levels of depressive affect were associated with later age at menarche in girls ages 10–14 (Graber, Brooks-Gunn, & Warren, 1995). These findings held even after controlling for the effects of pubertal development on family relationships and life stress. Early puberty in girls has been linked with a number of negative outcomes, from elevated breast cancer risk to weight gain to greater promiscuity and teenage pregnancy. Early-maturing girls also report more emotional problems, like depression, and more risk-taking behavior, like alcohol consumption (Ellis & Garber, 2000).

Because the HPA axis and hypothalamic–pituitary–gonadal axis regulate pubertal development, these axes may be pathways that link family stress to pubertal maturation. As the preceding sections have indicated, HPA axis overactivation characterizes children in stressful environments, and this activation may trigger the early development of the hypothalamic–pituitary–gonadal system. Research in this area appears inconclusive and even contradictory, however (Graber et al., 1995), perhaps because genes, body fat, and athletic activity also influence pubertal timing and may be linked to HPA axis functioning as well. Therefore, it is difficult to tease out the specific impact of psychosocial stress on pubertal maturation.

Father absence seems to have a separate, specific influence on girls' pubertal timing, above and beyond general familial stress (Romans, Martin, Gendall, & Herbison, 2003, Ellis & Garber, 2000). For example, the 1995 National Survey of Family Growth found that women whose parents separated in early childhood had twice the risk of early menarche, a fourfold risk of early sexual intercourse, and more than twice the risk for early pregnancy as women who lived with both parents during childhood (Quinlan, 2003). According to an evolutionary model, early experiences shape girls' eventual reproductive strategies (Belsky, Steinberg, & Draper, 1991). From this perspective, one could argue that girls in unstable families headed by single mothers may unconsciously abandon the search for a supportive mate and shift to a quantity-oriented rather than quality-oriented reproductive strategy, making earlier sexual maturation an adaptive phenomenon.

The research literature on pubertal timing in boys is much less substantial than the literature on girls' pubertal development. As with girls, boys reared in father-absent homes appear to reach puberty sooner, and boys raised without fathers show higher testosterone levels and more aggressive behavior (Granger et al., 2003). Perhaps the best illustration of older males' impact on younger males' pubertal timing comes from the animal kingdom. In the early 1990s, the rangers at Pilanesberg National Park in South Africa ended a series of elephant attacks on white rhinoceroses by introducing six older males to the park's elephant population (Slotow, Van Dyk, Poole, Page, & Klocke, 2000). After the older elephants arrived, the young males' testosterone levels dropped, suggesting that the mere presence of higher-ranking males exerts regulatory effects on sex hormones.

CONCLUSION

Physiological and behavioral adaptations that optimize maturation and survival are species-specific. Therefore, any general account of the role of parenting behaviors, or the behavioral and biological strategies observed in offspring in response to early rearing conditions, must include some oversimplification. With this caution in mind, we highlight patterns that emerge in our review of data from human and animal studies. The protective effects of parental nurturing behaviors extend to numerous aspects of biological functioning in mammals. Some of the behaviors that signal sensitive and responsive parenting appear, in the short run, to influence regulatory processes in immature biological systems and, in the long run, to facilitate the development of stress response systems. In the animal literature, maternal separation is often treated as a stressor. Our analysis suggests that a maternal separation stressor is unique in that it also removes an external regulator from the infant's environment—an individual who, under normal circumstance, helps to regulate the infant's response to environmental challenges. It is therefore not surprising that disruptions of the parent–child bond (especially the mother–child bond) through prolonged separation, parental stress, or poor parenting behavior can result in health outcomes that have been associated with biological dysfunction and dysregulation. Investigations are beginning to show how those changes may be mediated through gene expression. In some cases, early activation of stress-response systems seems to lead to early maturation of biological systems and subsequent evidence of accelerated aging and disease process.

In addition to understanding the implications for physical health, a critical next step is to address how the biological responses to early rearing conditions described in this chapter may relate to behavior over the course of development. In humans, the same stressful family environments that have been linked to children's neurotransmitter profiles and to their HPA axis and autonomic functioning also appear, in the longer term, to interfere with social and emotional development in childhood, promote risky behaviors in adolescence, and lead to poor mental health outcomes in adulthood (Repetti et al., 2002). The time is right for socialization researchers to begin to link these scientific literatures. Biological, social, emotional, and behavioral development are intertwined through reciprocal connections. Therefore, causal pathways will not necessarily always lead from socialization experiences to biological processes to social–emotional developmental outcomes. For example, biological systems are also influenced by individual emotional or social factors, as seen in the impact that negative affect and depression have on immune functioning.

Unfortunately, any effort to investigate the biological underpinnings of socialization effects on social and emotional development is limited by a paucity of human research. We found little research addressing human parenting effects on the development of offspring CNS, endocrine, and immune systems. Attempts to generalize experimental findings from other species to human development are fraught with the potential for inaccuracy. For example, the animal literature emphasizes the impact of very early rearing experiences, particularly in contrast to the length of time over which human parenting is distributed. On the one hand, because children are dependent on their parents for a much longer period of time, human parents influence offspring biological development long past infancy. On the other hand, parenting effects may be much greater during neonatal development in some of the animal species discussed in this chapter. For example, some aspects of development that occur in the neonatal rat, and are therefore vulnerable to changes in mother–infant interactions, occur prenatally in humans and may be less influenced by maternal behavior after birth (Kuhn & Schanberg, 1998). Another limitation of the experimental animal literature is the practice of keeping subjects in highly controlled environments during the intervening period between the early experience under study and the assessment of the biological outcome. As Gottlieb and Lickliter (2004) have pointed out, the animals are not exposed to naturally occurring variations in social experience that may play a corrective or remedial role. They note, for example, that the effects of handling on rat pups are enhanced by subsequent rearing under social conditions. Thus, findings from the animal early rearing literature may be misinterpreted as reflecting unalterable early programming on development.

One of the most pressing questions is how positive, nurturing socialization experiences shape the development of human biological systems. Most of the research reviewed in this chapter focuses on the impact of stressful early experiences such as social deprivation (e.g., maternal separation) and harsh or abusive parenting. For example, we know that adverse rearing conditions can affect the development of important neurotransmitter systems in the mammalian brain. However, we currently have much less comparable information about how sensitive and nurturant rearing influences the development of these systems. Yet we know that nurturant behaviors observed in mammals, such as licking, grooming, and other forms of physical contact, play a role in the functioning of immature biological systems (e.g., by helping babies to recover more quickly from stress responses). In the long term, the same behaviors also promote the development of vagal tone, sleep cycles, and the HPA axis. Researchers can build on this foundation to investigate how other sensitive and responsive parenting behaviors shape the development of the CNS and other biological systems. Knowledge about these biological connections will advance current socialization models in exciting directions.

Models will also be enhanced by research on socialization provided by fathers. Our search for research beyond the mother–child dyad yielded little outside the impact of father absence. Whether studying mothers or fathers, researchers need to take special care to correctly identify the source of correlations between socialization experiences provided by a parent and offspring biological outcomes. Without the experimental designs that are used with other species, it is critical that correlational investigations of human parenting avoid incorrectly attributing environmental influences to genetic ones.

Many socialization researchers seek to understand how parenting behaviors and family environments shape critical developmental outcomes such as learning, emotion regulation, social competence, and mental health. Although most current models focus on behavioral and cognitive mediators, many of the outcomes may also be shaped by the kinds of biological changes hinted at in this chapter. For that reason, we believe that human socialization research will be advanced as we learn more about the effects that early rearing experiences and parenting have on the development and functioning of the biological systems discussed here. An important next turn in the road ahead will be an integration of what we are learning about biological responses to early rearing conditions with the social and emotional developmental processes that are the primary focus of this volume.

ACKNOWLEDGMENTS

We would like to thank Carlos Grijalva, Joan Grusek, Paul Hastings, Teresa Seeman, Joan Silk, Cindy Yee-Bradbury, and participants in the Repetti research seminar at UCLA for their helpful comments on an earlier draft of this chapter.

NOTES

1. Dams assume several different nursing positions, even during the same nursing bout; licking and grooming are most likely to take place during nursing while the mother is in the arched-back position.
2. The handling and separation paradigms are distinct. Over the course of a normal day, dams are routinely off their nests and away from the pups for more than the 15 minutes that is required for the handling manipulation. In contrast, the maternal-separation procedure involves separations that are typically longer-lasting (e.g., 180 minutes per day) and extended over several days (Francis, Caldji, et al., 1999).
3. Because the spontaneous eye blink is at least partially controlled by dopamine neurons in the basal ganglia, the measure of spontaneous blink rates provides a method of assessing dopamine function.
4. Probes are drugs that target a neurotransmitter system. Biological or behavioral responses to the drug are observed; abnormal responses are thought to reflect abnormal neurotransmitter functioning.
5. The proliferative response can be assessed in the lab by using mitogens (antigens) to stimulate proliferation of cell populations that have been isolated from a sample of peripheral blood. The cytotoxicity, or destructive power, of an isolated population of lymphocytes is measured by their ability to lyse (rupture) a sample of target tumor cells.
6. Infants who did not have a juvenile friend with them during the separation showed less B- and T-cell proliferative response to mitogens, and an initial decrease in the natural cytotoxicity of peripheral blood lymphocytes, which gradually returned to normal by the end of the first week of separation.

REFERENCES

Ahnert, L., Gunnar, M. R., Lamb, M. E., & Barthel, M. (2004). Transition to child care: Associations with infant–mother attachment, infant negative emotion, and cortisol elevations. *Child Development, 75*, 639–650.

Allen, M. T., Matthews, K. A., & Sherman, F. S. (1997). Cardiovascular reactivity to stress and left ventricular mass in youth. *Hypertension, 30*, 782–787.

Andrews, M. W., & Rosenblum, L. A. (1991). Attachment in monkey infants raised in variable- and low-demand environments. *Child Development, 62,* 686–693.

Ballard, M., Cummings, E. M., & Larkin, K. (1993). Emotional and cardiovascular responses to adults' angry behavior and to challenging tasks in children of hypertensive and normotensive parents. *Child Development, 64,* 500–515.

Bear, M. F., Connors, B. W., & Paradiso, M. A. (1996). *Neuroscience: Exploring the brain.* Baltimore: Williams & Wilkins.

Belsky, J., Steinberg, L., & Draper, P. (1991). Childhood experience, interpersonal development, and reproductive strategy: An evolutionary theory of socialization. *Child Development, 62,* 647–670.

Berman, M. E., Kavoussi, R. J., & Coccaro, E. F. (1997). Neurotransmitter correlates of human aggression. In D. M. Stoff, J. Breiling, & J. D. Maser (Eds.), *Handbook of antisocial behavior* (pp. 305–313). New York: Wiley.

Boccia, M. L., Scanlan, J. M., Laudenslager, M. L., Berger, C. L., Hijazi, A. S., & Reite, M. L. (1997). Juvenile friends, behavior, and immune responses to separation in bonnet macaque infants. *Physiology and Behavior, 61*(2), 191–198.

Braun, K., Lange, E., Metzger, M., & Poeggel, G. (1999). Maternal separation followed by early social deprivation affects the development of monoaminergic fiber systems in the medial prefrontal cortex of *Octodon degus. Neuroscience, 95,* 309–318.

Bugental, D. B. (2004). Thriving in the face of early adversity. *Journal of Social Issues, 60*(1), 219–235.

Bugental, D. B., Martorell, G. A., & Barraza, V. (2003). The hormonal costs of subtle forms of infant maltreatment. *Hormones and behavior, 43,* 237–244.

Caldji, C., Francis, D., Sharma, S., Plotsky, P. M., & Meaney, M. J. (2000). The effects of early rearing environment on the development of GABA and central benzodiazepine receptor levels and novelty-induced fearfulness in the rat. *Neuropsychopharmacology, 22*(3), 219–229.

Champagne, F. A., Francis D. D., Mar, A., & Meaney, M.J. (2003). Variations in maternal care in the rat as a mediating influence for the effects of environment on development. *Physiology and Behavior, 79,* 359–371.

Chorpita, B. F., & Barlow, D. H. (1998). The development of anxiety: The role of control in the early environment. *Psychological Bulletin, 124,* 3–21.

Cirulli, F., Alleva, E., Antonelli, A., & Aloe, L. (2000). NGF expression in the developing rat brain: Effects of maternal separation. *Developmental Brain Research, 123*(2), 129–134.

Cirulli, F., Berry, A., & Alleva, E. (2003). Early disruption of the mother–infant relationship: Effects on brain plasticity and implications for psychopathology. *Neuroscience and Biobehavioral Reviews 27*(1–2), 73–82.

Coe, C. L., Lubach, G. R., Ershler, W. B., & Klopp, R. G. (1989). Influence of early rearing on lymphocyte proliferation responses in juvenile rhesus monkeys. *Brain, Behavior, and Immunity, 3,* 47–60.

Coe, C. L., Lubach, G. R., Schneider, M. L., Dierschke, D. J., & Ershler, W. B. (1992). Early rearing conditions alter immune responses in the developing infant primate. *Pediatrics, 90,* 505–509.

Cohen, S., & Herbert, T. B. (1996). Health psychology: Psychological factors and physical disease from the perspective of human psychoneuroimmunology. *Annual Review of Psychology, 47,* 113–142.

Coplan, J. D., Andrews, M. W., Rosenblum, L. A., Owens, M. J., Friedman, S., Gorman, J. M., et al. (1996). Persistent elevations of cerebrospinal fluid concentrations of corticotropin-releasing factor in adult nonhuman primates exposed to early-life stressors: Implications for the pathophysiology of mood and anxiety disorders. *Proceedings of the National Academy of Sciences, 93,* 1619–1623.

Coplan, J. D., Trost, R. C., Owens, M. J., Cooper, T. B., Gorman, J. M., Nemeroff, C. B., et al. (1998). Cerebrospinal flud concentrations of somatostatin and biogenic amines in grown primates reared by mothers exposed to manipulated foraging conditions. *Archives of General Psychiatry, 55,* 473–477.

Davidson, R. J. (1995). Cerebral asymmetry, emotion, and affective style. In R. J. Davidson & K. Hugdahl (Eds.), *Brain asymmetry* (pp. 361–366). Cambridge, MA: MIT Press.

Davidson, R. J. (1998). Affective style and affective disorders: Perspectives from affective neuroscience. *Cognition and Emotion, 12*(3), 307–330.

Dawson, G., & Ashman, S. B. (2000). On the origins of a vulnerability to depression: The influence of the early social environment on the development of psychobiological systems related to risk for affective disorder. In C. A. Nelson (Ed.), *Minnesota symposia on child psychology: Vol. 31. The effects of early adversity on neurobehavioral development.* (pp. 245–279). Mahwah, NJ: Erlbaum.

De Bellis, M. D., Keshavan, M. S., Spencer, S., & Hall, J. (2000). *N*-acetylaspartate concentration in the anterior cingulate of maltreated children and adolescents with PTSD. *American Journal of Psychiatry, 157*, 1175–1177.

Delville, Y., Melloni, R. H., & Ferris, C. F. (1998). Behavioral and neurobiological consequences of social subjugation during puberty in golden hamsters. *Journal of Neuroscience, 18*(7), 2667–2672.

Denenberg, V. H. (1999). Commentary: Is maternal stimulation the mediator of the handling effect in infancy? *Developmental Psychobiology, 34*, 1–3.

Diego, M. A., Field, T., Hart, S., Hernandez-Reif, M., Jones, N., Cullen, C., et al. (2002). Facial expressions and EEG in infants of intrusive and withdrawn mothers with depressive symptoms. *Depression and Anxiety, 15*(10–17).

Doussard-Roosevelt, J. A., McClenny, B. D., & Porges, S. W. (2001) Neonatal cardiac vagal tone and school-age developmental outcome in very low birth weight infants. *Developmental Psychobiology, 38*, 56–66.

Doussard-Roosevelt, J. A., Porges, S. W., Scanlon, J. W., Alemi, B., & Scanlon, K. (1997). Vagal regulation of heart rate in the prediction of developmental outcome for very low birthweight preterm infants. *Child Development, 68*, 173–186.

El-Sheikh, M., Cummings, E. M., & Goetsch, V. L. (1989). Coping with adults' angry behavior: Behavioral, physiological, and verbal responses in preschoolers. *Developmental Psychology, 25*, 490–498.

El-Sheikh, M., Harger, J., & Whitson, S. M. (2001). Exposure to interparental conflict and children's adjustment and physical health: The moderating role of vagal tone. *Child Development, 72*(6), 1617–1636.

Ellis, B. J., & Garber, J. (2000). Psychosocial antecedents of variation in girls' pubertal timing: Maternal depression, stepfather presence, and marital and family stress. *Child Development, 71*(2), 485–501.

Essex, M. J., Klein, M. H., Cho, E., & Kalin, N. H. (2002). Maternal stress beginning in infancy may sensitize children to later stress exposure: Effects on cortisol and behavior. *Biological Psychiatry, 52*, 776–784.

Ewart, C. K. (1991). Familial transmission of essential hypertension: Genes, environments, and chronic anger. *Annals of Behavioral Medicine, 13*, 40–47.

Feldman, R., & Eidelman, A. I. (2003). Skin-to-skin contact (Kangaroo Care) accelerates autonomic and neurobehavioural maturation in preterm infants. *Developmental Medicine and Child Neurology, 45*(4), 274–281.

Field, T., Diego, M., Hernandez-Reif, M., Schanberg, S., Kuhn, C., Yando, R., et al. (2003). Pregnancy anxiety and comorbid depression and anger: Effects on the fetus and neonate. *Depression and Anxiety, 17*(3), 140–151.

Flinn, M. V., & England, B. G. (1997). Social economics of childhood glucocorticoid stress responses and health. *American Journal of Physical Anthropology, 102*, 33–53.

Fox, N. A. (1994). Dynamic cerebral processes underlying emotion regulation. *Monographs of the Society for Research on Child Development, 59*, 152–166.

Francis, D. D., Caldji, C., Champagne, F., Plotsky, P. M., & Meaney, M. J. (1999). The role of corticotropin-releasing factor-norepinephrine systems in mediating the effects of early experience on the development of behavioral and endocrine responses to stress. *Biological Psychiatry, 46*, 1153–1166.

Francis, D., Diorio, J., Liu, D., & Meaney, M. J. (1999). Nongenomic transmission across generations of maternal behavior and stress responses in the rat. *Science, 286*, 1155–1158.

Gardner, L. I. (1972). Deprivation dwarfism. *Scientific American, 227*, 76–83.

Glaser, H. H., Heagarty, M. C., Bullard, D. M., & Pivchik, E. C. (1968). Physical and psychological development of children with early failure to thrive. *Journal of Pediatrics, 73*, 690–698.

Gottlieb, G. & Lickliter, R. (2004). The various roles of animal models in understanding human development. *Social Development, 13*, 311–325.

Graber, J. A., Brooks-Gunn, J, & Warren, M. P. (1995). The antecedents of menarcheal age heredity, family environment, and stressful life events. *Child Development, 66*, 346–359.

Granger, D. A., Serbin, L. A., Schwartzman, A., Lehoux, P., Cooperman, J., & Ikeda, S. (1998). Children's salivary cortisol, internalising behavior problems, and family environment: Results from the concordia longitudinal risk project. *International Journal of Behavioral Development, 22*(4), 707–728.

Granger, D. A., Shirtcliff, E. A., Zahn-Waxler, C., Usher, B. A., Klimes-Dougan B., & Hastings, P. D. (2003). Salivary testosterone diurnal variation and psychopathology in adolescent males and females: Individual differences and developmental effects. *Development and Psychopathology, 15*(2), 431–449.

Gunnar, M. R. (2000). Early adversity and the development of stress reactivity and regulation. In C. A. Nelson (Ed.), *Minnesota symposia on child psychology: Vol 31. The effects of early adversity on neurobehavioral development* (pp. 163–200). Mahwah, NJ: Erlbaum.

Gunnar, M. R., Brodersen, L., Nachmias, M., Buss, K., & Rigatuso, J. (1996). Stress reactivity and attachment security. *Developmental Psychobiology, 29*, 191–204.

Gunnar, M. R., & Donzella, B. (2002). Social regulation of the cortisol levels in early human development. *Psychoneuroendocrinology, 27*, 199–220.

Gunnar, M. R., Gonazalez, C. A., Goodlin, B. L., & Levine, S. (1981). Behavioral and pituitary–adrenal responses during a prolonged separation period in rhesus monkeys. *Psychoneuroendocrinology, 6*, 65–75.

Gunnar, M. R., Morison, S. J., Chisholm, K., & Schuder, M. (2001). Salivary cortisol levels in children adopted from Romanian orphanages. *Development and Psychopathology, 13*, 611–628.

Gunnar, M. R., & Vazquez, D. M. (2001). Low cortisol and a flattening of expected daytime rhythm: Potential indices of risk in human development. *Development and Psychopathology, 13*, 515–538.

Hall, F. S., Wilkinson, L. S., Humby, T., & Robbins, T. W. (1999). Maternal deprivation of neonatal rats produces enduring changes in dopamine functioning. *Synapse, 32*, 37–43.

Hart, J., Gunnar, M., & Cicchetti, D. (1996). Altered neuroendocrine activity in maltreated children related to symptoms of depression. *Development and Psychopathology, 34*, 687–697.

Heim, C., Newport, D. J., Heit, S., Graham, Y. P., Wilcox, M., Bonsall, R., et al. (2000). Pituitary adrenal and autonomic responses to stress in women after sexual and physical abuse in childhood. *Journal of the American Medical Association, 284*, 592–597.

Hertsgaard, L. G., Gunnar, M. R., Erickson, M. R., & Nachmias, M. (1995). Adrenocortical responses to the strange situation in infants with disorganized/disoriented attachment relationships. *Child Development, 66*, 1100–1106.

Jones, N., Field, T., Fox, N. A., Davalos, M., Malphurs, J., Carraway, K., et al. (1997). Infants of intrusive and withdrawn mothers. *Infant Behavior and Development, 20*(2), 175–186.

Kaufman, J., Birmaher, B., Perel, J., Stull, S., Brent, D., Trubnick, L., et al. (1998). Serotonergic functioning in depressed abused children: Clinical and familial correlates. *Biological Psychology, 44*, 973–981.

Kaufman, J., Plotsky, P. M., Nemeroff, C. B., & Charney, D. S. (2000). Effects of early adverse experiences on brain structure and function: Clinical implications. *Society of Biological Psychiatry, 48*, 778–790.

Kehoe, P., Shoemaker, W., Arons, C., Triano, L., & Suresh, G. (1998). Repeated isolation stress in the neonatal rat: Relation to brain dopamine systems in the 10-day old rat. *Behavioral Neuroscience, 112*, 1466–1474.

Kennedy, A. E., Rubin, K. H., Hastings, P. D., & Maisel, B. A. (2004). The longitudinal relations between child vagal tone and parenting behavior: 2 to 4 years. *Developmental Psychobiology, 45*, 10–21.

Kraemer, G., & Clarke, A. (1990). The behavioral neurobiology of self injurious behavior in rhesus monkeys. *Progress in Neuro-Psychopharmacology and Biological Psychiatry, 14*, 5141–5168.

Kraemer, G. W., Ebert, M. H., Schmidt, D. E., & McKinney, W. T. (1991). Strangers in a strange land: A psychobiological study of infant monkeys before and after separation from real or inanimate mothers. *Child Development, 62*, 548–566.

Kuhn, C. M., & Schanberg, S. M. (1991). Stimulation in infancy and brain development. In B. J. Carroll & J. E. Barrett (Eds.), *Psychopathology and the brain* (pp. 97–111). New York: Raven Press.

Kuhn, C. M., & Schanberg, S. M. (1998). Responses to maternal separation: Mechanisms and mediators. *Developmental Neuroscience, 16*(3/4), 261–270.

Laudenslager, M. L., Boccia, M. L., Berger, C. L., Gennaro-Ruggles, M. M., McFerran, B., & Reite, M. L. (1995). Total cortisol, free cortisol, and growth hormone associated with brief social separation experiences in young macaques. *Developmental Psychobiology, 28*(4), 199–211.

Laudenslager, M. L., Capitanio, J. P., & Reite, M. (1985). Possible effects of early separation experiences on subsequent immune function in adult macaque monkeys. *American Journal of Psychiatry, 142*(7), 862–864.

Lehman, B. J., Taylor, S. E., Kiefe, C. I., & Seeman, T. E. (2005). Relation of childhood socioeconomic status and family environment to adult metabolic functioning in the CARDIA study. *Psychosomatic Medicine, 67*(6), 846–854.

Lewis, M. H., Gluck, J. P., Beauchamp, A. J., Keresztury, M. F., & Mailman, R. B. (1990). Long-term effects of early social isolation in Macaca mulatta: Changes in dopamine receptor function following apomorphine challenge. *Brain Research, 513*, 67–73.

Liu, D., Diorio, J., Tannenbaum, B., Caldji, C., Francis, D., Freedman, A., et al. (1997). Maternal care, hippocampal glucocorticoid receptors, and hypothalamic–pituitary–adrenal responses to stress. *Science*, 277, 1659–1662.

Lubach, G. R., Coe, C. L., & Ershler, W. B. (1995). Effects of early rearing environment on immune responses of infant rhesus monkeys. *Brain, Behavior, and Immunity*, 9, 31–46.

Luecken, L. J. (1998). Childhood attachment and loss experiences affect adult cardiovascular and cortisol function. *Psychosomatic Medicine*, 60, 765–772.

Lyons, D. M., & Schatzberg, A. F. (2003). Early maternal availability and prefrontal correlates of reward-related memory. *Neurobiology of Learning and Memory*, 80, 97–104.

Mathew, S. J., Shungu, D. C., Mao, X., Smith, E. L. P., Perera, G. M, Kegeles, L. S., et al. (2003). A magnetic resonance spectroscopic imaging study of adult nonhuman primates exposed to early-life stressors. *Biological Psychiatry*, 54(7), 727–735.

McEwen, B. S. (1998). Stress, adaptation, and disease. *Annals of the New York Academy of Sciences*, 84, 33–44.

McEwen, B. S., & Stellar, E. (1993). Stress and the individual: Mechanisms leading to disease. *Archives of Internal Medicine*, 153, 2093–2101.

McNamara, R. K., Huot, R. L., Lenox, R. H., & Plotsky, P. M. (2002). Postnatal maternal separation elevates the expression of the postsynaptic protein kinase C substrate RC3, but not presynaptic GAP-43, in the developing rat hippocampus. *Developmental Neuroscience*, 24, 485–494.

Mendoza, S. P., Smotherman, W. P., Miner, M., Kaplan, J., & Levine, S. (1978). Pituitary-adrenal response to separation in mother and infant squirrel monkeys. *Developmental Psychobiology*, 11, 169–175.

Micallef, J., & Blin, O. (2001). Neurobiology and clinical pharamacology of obsessive–compulsive disorder. *Clinical Neuropharmacology*, 24, 191–207.

Montgomery, S. M., Bartley, M. J., & Wilkinson, R. G. (1997). Family conflict and slow growth. *Archives of Disease in Childhood*, 77, 326–330.

Mooncey, S., Giannakoulopoulos, X., Glover, V., Acolet, D., & Modi, N. (1997). The effect of mother–infant skin-to-skin contact on plasma cortisol and β-endorphin concentrations in preterm newborns. *Infant Behavior and Development*, 20(4), 553–557.

Munck, A., & Naray-Fejes-Toth, A. (1994). Glucocorticoids and stress: permissive and suppressive actions. *Academic Science*, 746, 115–133.

Nachmias, M., Gunnar, M., Mangelsdorf, S., Parritz, R. H., & Buss, K. (1996). Behavioral inhibition and stress reactivity: The moderating role of attachment security. *Child Development*, 67, 508–522.

Newport, D. J., Stowe, Z. N., & Nemeroff, C. B. (2002). Parental depression: Animal models of an adverse life event. *American Journal of Psychiatry*, 159, 1265–1283.

O'Connor, T. G., Rutter, M., Beckett, C., Keaveney, L., Kreppner, J. M., & English and Romanian Adoptees Study Team. (2000). The effects of global severe privation on cognitive competence: Extension and longitudinal follow-up. *Child Development*, 71(2), 376–390.

Pine, D. S., Coplan, J. D., Wasserman, G., Miller, L. S., Fried, J. A., Davies, M., et al. (1997). Neuroendocrine response to d,1-fenfluramine challenge in boys: Associations with aggressive behavior and adverse rearing. *Archives of General Psychiatry*, 54, 839–846.

Pine, D. S., Wasserman, G., Coplan, J., Fried, J. A., Huang, Y., Kassir, S., et al. (1996). Associations between platelet serotonin-2A receptor characteristics and parenting factors for boys at risk for delinquency. *American Journal of Psychiatry*, 153, 538–544.

Plotsky, P., & Meaney, M. (1993). Early postnatal experience alters hypothalamic corticotropin-releasing factor (CRF) mRNA, median eminence CRF content, and stress-induced release in adult rats. *Molecular Brain Research*, 18, 195–200.

Porges, S. W. (1995). Orienting in a defensive world: Mammalian modifications of our evolutionary heritage. A polyvagal theory. *Psychophysiology*, 32, 301–318.

Porges, S. W. (2001). The polyvagal theory: Phylogenetic substrates of a social nervous system. *International Journal of Psychophysiology*, 42(2), 123–146.

Porter, C. L. (2003). Coregulation in mother–infant dyads: Links to infants' cardiac vagal tone. Psychological Reports, 92(1), 307–319.

Porter, C. L., Wouden-Miller, M., Silva, S. S., & Porter, A. E. (2003). Marital harmony and conflict: Linked to infants' emotional regulation and cardiac vagal tone. *Infancy*, 4(2), 297–307.

Quinlan, R. J. (2003). Father absence, parental care, and female reproductive development. *Evolution and Human Behavior*, 24(6), 376–390.

Repetti, R. L., Taylor, S. E., & Seeman, T. E. (2002). Risky families: Family social environments and the mental and physical health of offspring. *Psychological Bulletin, 128*, 330–366.

Robles, T. F., Glaser, R., & Kiecolt-Glaser, J. K. (2005). Out of balance: A new look at chronic stress, depression, and immunity. *Current Directions in Psychological Science, 14*(2), 111–115.

Romans, S. E., Martin, M., Gendall, K., & Herbison, G. P. (2003). Age of menarche: The role of some psychosocial factors. *Psychological Medicine, 33*(5), 933–939.

Rosenblum, L., Coplan, J., Friedman, S., Bassoff, T., Gorman, J., & Andrews, M. (1994). Adverse early experiences affect noradrenergic and serotonergic functioning in adult primates. *Biological Psychiatry, 35*, 221–227.

Schuff, N., Marmar, C. R., Weiss, D. S., Neylan, T. C., Schoenfeld, F., Fein, G., et al. (1997). Reduced hippocampal volume and N-acetyl aspartate in posttraumatic stress disorder. *Annals of the New York Academy of Science, 821*, 516–520.

Simpson, J. A., & Gangestad, S. W. (2001). Evolution and relationships: A call for integration. *Personal Relationships, 8*, 341–355.

Slotow, R., Van Dyk, G., Poole, J., Page, B., & Klocke, A. (2000). Older bull elephants control young males. *Nature, 408*(6811), 425–426.

Spangler, G., Schieche, M., Ilg, U., Maier, U., & Ackermann, C. (1994). Maternal sensitivity as an external organizer for biobehavioral regulation in infancy. *Developmental Psychobiology, 27*(7), 425–437.

Suomi, S. J. (1997). Early determinants of behaviour: Evidence from primate studies. *British Medical Bulletin, 53*, 170–180.

Surbey, M. K. (1990). Family composition, stress, and the timing of human menarche. In T. E. Ziegler, & F. B. Bercovitch (Eds.), *Socioendocrinology of primate reproduction. Monographs in primatology, 13*, 11–32. New York: Wiley-Liss.

Taylor, S. E., Lerner, J. S., Sage, R. M., Lehman, B. J., & Seeman, T. E. (2004). Early environment, emotions, responses to stress, and health. *Journal of Personality, 72*, 1365–1393.

Thase, M. E., Jindal, R., & Howland, R. H. (2002). Biological aspects of depression. In I.H. Gotlib & C. L. Hammen (Eds.), *Handbook of depression* (pp. 192–218). New York: Guilford Press.

Valenzuela, M. (1997). Maternal sensitivity in a developing society: The context of urban poverty and infant chronic undernutrition. *Developmental Psychology, 33*, 845–855.

Vazquez, D. M., Lopez, J. F., Van Hoers, H., Watson, S. J., & Levine, S. (2000). Maternal deprivation regulates serotonin 1A and 2A receptors in the infant rat. *Brain Research, 855*, 76–82.

Warren, S. L., Gunnar, M. R., Kagan, J., Anders, T. F., Simmens, S. J., Rones, M., et al. (2003). Maternal panic disorder: Infant temperament, neurophysiology, and parenting behaviors. *Journal of the American Academy of Child and Adolescent Psychiatry, 42*(7), 814–825.

Watamura, S. E., Donzella, B., Alwin, J., & Gunnar, M. R. (2003). Morning-to-afternoon increases in cortisol concentrations for infants and toddlers at child care: Age differences and behavioral correlates. *Child Development, 74*, 1006–1020.

Watamura, S. E., Sebanc, A. M., & Gunnar, M. R. (2001). Rising cortisol at childcare: Relations with nap, rest, and temperament. *Developmental Psychobiology, 40*, 33–42.

Weaver, I. C., Cervoni, N., Champagne, F. A., D'Alessio, A. C., Sharma, S., Seckl, J. R., et al. (2004). Epigenetic programming by maternal behavior. *Nature Neuroscience, 7*, 847–854.

Woodall, K. L., & Matthews, K. A. (1989). Familial environment associated with Type A behaviors and psychophysiological responses to stress in children. *Health Psychology, 8*, 403–426.

Worlein, J., & Laudenslager, M. L. (2001). Effects of early rearing experiences and social interactions on immune function in nonhuman primates. In R. Ader, D. L. Felten & N. Cohen (Eds.) *Psychoneuroimmunology* (pp.73–85). New York: Academic Press.

Zeanah, C. H., Nelson, C. A., Fox, N. A., Smyke, A. T., Marshall, P., Parker, S.W., et al. (2003). Designing research to study the effects of institutionalization on brain and behavioral development: The Bucharest Early Intervention Project. *Development and Psychopathology, 15*, 885–907.

CHAPTER 6

Temperament, Parenting, and Socialization

JOHN E. BATES and GREGORY S. PETTIT

Theoretical accounts of socialization emphasize influences from the social environment, especially parenting, but also postulate complementary influences emanating from the individual child (Collins, Maccoby, Steinberg, Hetherington, & Bornstein, 2000). Child characteristics operate in two, main ways. First, they can bias a child's developmental trajectory of social adaptation. For example, children with a strong disposition to respond fearfully have some likelihood of developing anxiety problems, whereas fearless children continue to be more extraverted (Kagan, 1998; Rothbart & Bates, 1998). Second, child characteristics can operate in transaction with the environment, either creating experiences that support the basic bias stemming from the child's disposition or altering the implications of qualities of the social environment. For example, an outgoing child might be more likely than a fearful child to elicit friendly, fun behaviors from others and thus to reinforce the basic tendency. Or, for example, social disapproval might have little inhibitory meaning for an outgoing child, whereas an introverted child might find such feedback highly significant. Adjustment outcomes are important not only for the individual children but also for their families, peer groups, and classrooms. This chapter discusses convergences between temperament and parenting, with special emphasis on processes relating to children's behavioral adjustment, a major product of socialization and the major focus of research on the role of temperament.

TEMPERAMENT CONCEPTS

Most generally, temperament traits concern relatively early-appearing and relatively stable differences in responses to emotionally significant stimuli and in self-regulation of those re-

153

sponses (Rothbart & Bates, 1998). We say relatively early appearing because it has become clear that traits that make sense as temperament are not fully evident at birth. For example, effortful control of attention is an important dimension of individual difference that can be assessed only after the relevant brain structures, in the anterior attention system, have sufficiently developed, starting late in the second year (Rothbart, Derryberry, & Posner, 1994). Similarly, we define temperament as only relatively stable. For the sake of a tidy theory one would ideally like temperament traits to be constants. However, it appears likely that temperament traits show some development, not only at the level of observable behavior but also perhaps at the level of the neural structures and perhaps even the genes controlling neural development (Bates, 1989; Bates, Wachs, & Emde, 1994; Rothbart & Bates, 1998; Wachs & Bates, 2001). To an extent prenatally, and certainly from the earliest days after birth, infants' temperament dispositions are in transaction with the social environment. As with any personality trait, temperament traits have meaning as a descriptor of social interactions. How, then, do temperament and parenting complement one another?

What specific dimensions of temperament shall we consider? On the basis of rational considerations of relevant brain systems and factor analyses, including analyses of items and scales in the Thomas–Chess tradition (Thomas, Chess, & Birch, 1968; Chess & Thomas, 1984), the following dimensions seem most useful at the current time: (1) positive emotionality, which also includes activity level and extraversion, and is sometimes referred to as surgency; (2) irritable distress, which is often described as general negative emotionality; (3) fearful distress, sometimes called novelty distress or behavioral inhibition; (4) effortful control, which concerns attention and emotion regulation and task persistence; and (5) adaptability or agreeableness, which may pertain to affiliative tendencies. Each of these relatively broad dimensions of individual differences can be found in multiple measures of temperament describing children at different stages of development, each has analogs in other species, and each corresponds to reasonably well-described neural circuits (Rothbart & Bates, 2006). It also appears likely that these dimensions map onto the three- and five-factor models of adult (and child) personality that have become so widely employed (Costa & MacRae, 1988; Tellegen, 1985; Shiner & Caspi, 2003). For example, positive emotionality temperament dimensions map onto Extraversion and temperamental fearful distress maps onto Neuroticism.

Temperament in the Context of Parenting

Measures of parent–child relationships have been important since the beginning of modern temperament research. Parents provide the social context within which child behaviors have some of their most important meanings. Young children's temperamental emotional reactions and self-regulation are seen mainly against the background of parentally guided routines and social stimuli. Moreover, because parents are often the leading experts on individual children, seeing them in rare, but possibly key situations, researchers have often employed parents to describe their children. This brings up the question of how temperament is assessed.

MEASUREMENT ISSUES

Temperament constructs, like most conceptual tools used in the historically young field of social development research, are best seen as works in progress—continually undergoing validation and refinement. A detailed review of measurement issues is beyond the scope of this chapter, but it is worthwhile to consider a few points.

First, we find it useful to keep in mind that temperament is spoken of on multiple levels of definition. At the most basic level, there are genes coding for elements of emotional and attentional systems in the brain. It is reassuring that behavior genetics research has been demonstrating heritability for temperament traits (Goldsmith, Buss, & Lemery, 1997; Goldsmith, Lemery, Buss, & Campos, 1999). And it is exciting to see the emergence of research that identifies specific genes associated with production of temperament-relevant neurotransmission processes (Caspi et al., 2003). However, behavioral traits are very complex, influenced by multiple genes. Genes represent starting values in transactional processes with the environment rather than autonomous, deterministic mechanisms. We are a long way from being able to define temperament constructs strictly in terms of specific genes. Similarly, at the next higher level of complexity, neural bases of temperament traits, much is known about the basic functioning of the systems (e.g., circuits centering on the amygdala involved in fear, or the role of dopamine in proactive aggression) (Rothbart & Bates, 2006). However, much less is known about individual differences in these highly complex systems. As Zuckerman (1991) has argued, it is important to study temperament not only from the bottom up, from the genetic and neural levels, but also from the top down, with continued attention to the phenotypical behavioral patterns themselves. In most research, temperament constructs are defined on the basis of the observable phenotype, as we see in this chapter, but there is usually at least an implicit reference to the lower, constitutional levels of definition.

Second, the study of patterns of behavior requires attention to the principles of psychological assessment. The main question here is how temperament is to be operationally defined—what kinds of measures should be used? Some scientists distrust parental report measures of child temperament, preferring instead structured laboratory observation measures or, less often, naturalistic measures. It is argued that parent reports are too susceptible to personal biases to be valid (e.g., Kagan, 1998). However, we think of validity as an analog property of a measure rather than a digital, yes–no property. And we recognize that there are validity problems with all measures of temperament, not just parent reports (Rothbart & Bates, 1998). Nevertheless, a substantial body of research shows that parents' reports of child temperament converge, to a moderate extent, with other kinds of measures of temperament, such as observers' ratings. Therefore, establishing a standard "true" measure of temperament seems less important at this time than evaluating convergence between different kinds of temperament measure. It also seems important to learn how different kinds of temperament measure show parallel relations with other constructs, such as parenting and child behavioral adjustment measures.

Measurement of parenting also has validity concerns. As with assessment of temperament, we do not take a position on what the most valid measures of parenting are. However, we do note that self-reports of parenting may have the same kinds of subjective components that parental temperament ratings do, and also, the same kinds of objective factors. Although some of the relevant studies have employed self-reported parenting, there are strong traditions of naturalistic and structured observation in research on parenting, so many of the studies we refer to here involve observational measures. Observational measures do not necessarily provide an ideal sample of the relevant parenting, because they may fail to sample infrequent, but developmentally key situations, such as response to major child distress. But even so, they are especially helpful in interpreting studies using parent reports of temperament, because they obviate attributions of statistical relations to common source biases.

In summary, temperament can be thought of as biologically based individual differences, but it is good to keep in mind that actual measures of temperament are usually of phenotypical behavior patterns, not of the biological traits directly. Whatever the measure of a temperament behavior pattern, whether parent rating, observer rating, or objectively coded behavior in a structured laboratory task, there are limits to the measure's validity. We advocate a triangulation approach, in which different kinds of measures of temperament are compared to one another, both within and across studies. In what follows we identify the source of the measure of temperament where it seems important in the interpretation of the findings. In most of the studies reviewed, parent reports are the source. We try to be as clear as possible about the specific temperament construct, although a given scale might actually signify more than one of the major temperament dimensions listed earlier. With this brief consideration of the concepts and measurement of temperament, we now turn to the main topics of the chapter, how temperament and parenting are related, and how temperament and parenting combine in shaping children's social development.

RELATIONS BETWEEN TEMPERAMENT AND PARENTING

How Does Child Temperament Affect Parenting?

First we consider associations between temperament and parenting variables that are considered to be important in child socialization. Research suggests that relations between child temperament and parenting may depend on other variables, especially the child's age, the family's socioeconomic context, and the parent's personality. Most of the relevant research concerns the effects of child negative emotionality traits, but a few studies consider the effects of other kinds of temperament traits, too.

Effects of Age of Child

INFANT

Younger infants' negative emotionality most often has no significant negative effect on parenting and sometimes is associated with elevated levels of nurturance (Bates, 1989; Crockenberg, 1986; Putnam, Sanson, & Rothbart, 2002; Sanson, Hemphill, & Smart, 2004; Wachs & Gruen, 1982), but there are some negative effects. One such exception was found by Calkins, Hungerford, and Dedmon (2004): The 85 most easily frustrated 6-month-old infants (of 346), compared to the 77 who were low in frustration, received more intrusiveness and less physical stimulation, and, to a nonsignificant degree, less sensitive behavior from their mothers. Another exception is the finding that infant temperamental anger (in laboratory situations) did not predict parental behavior per se, but more angry infants did have fewer occasions of shared positive emotion with their mothers (Kochanska, Friesenborg, Lange, & Martel, 2004). Kochanska et al. also found that more joyful infants received more responsive mothering and visual tracking, even controlling for mother personality.

TODDLER

Most of the negative effects that have been reported are with samples of older infants or toddlers (Crockenberg, 1986; Wachs & Gruen, 1982). In one longitudinal study, at both age 6 months (Bates, Olson, Pettit, & Bayles, 1982) and age 13 months (Pettit & Bates, 1984), there were modest, positive effects of difficult temperament on mothers' nurturance. However, by 24 months, there were some negative effects of difficultness in mother–toddler interactions (Lee & Bates, 1985), and these effects were not only related to the concurrent measure of difficult temperament but also to measures from ages 6 and 13 months. Perhaps because of changes in parents' expectations for self-regulation in toddlerhood and cultural pressures toward stricter parental discipline, negative emotionality is less tolerated and more likely to lead to social conflict as children leave the infancy era (Bates, 1989; Crockenberg, 1986; Wachs & Gruen, 1982). However, even in toddlerhood, the direct links between child negative emotionality and parenting are not extremely robust (e.g., see Crockenberg, 1987), and there could also be links to positive parenting such as providing more cognitive stimulation (Putnam et al., 2002). Laible (2004) found that mothers elaborated more in conversations with preschoolers they described as higher in negative reactivity. Laible also observed more maternal elaboration with children who were higher in effortful control and those lower in extraversion. Rubin and his colleagues found that child shyness at age 2 forecasted reduced parental encouragement of independence at age 4 (Rubin, Nelson, Hastings, & Asendorpf, 1999), and that higher vagal tone—indexing a form of self regulation—predicted decreased parental restrictiveness (Kennedy, Rubin, Hastings, & Maisel, 2004).

Specific kinds of negative emotionality, irritable versus fearful characteristics, might have differential effects on the parent–child relationship. Gauvain and Fagot (1995) found that more difficult children, defined in a way that merges irritable and fearful traits, by a combination of negative mood, intensity, withdrawal, slow adaptability, and lack of rhythmicity, received both more cognitive assistance and more disapproval from their mothers during problem-solving tasks at about 33 months of age. Gauvain and Fagot (1995) primarily interpreted their correlations between child difficult temperament and more mother control during problem solving as indicating that, because of their emotional dysregulation, difficult children were getting less opportunity for self-directed cognitive growth. However, Frankel and Bates (1990) did not find a clear pattern of predictions from temperament to mother–child interactions in problem-solving tasks at age 24 months. They did find that boys with more difficult temperament at 6 months, defined by irritable, not fearful negative emotionality, paradoxically had less discordant problem solving interactions with their mothers at age 24 months. The two studies' discrepancy could be due to differences in the tasks and the ages of the children. However, a more interesting difference might be the definition of temperamental difficultness. In a second study, Gauvain and Fagot (1995) found that approach/withdrawal and adaptability (to new situations) were the only scales of their difficult temperament composite that correlated with mother behavior. Citing the Frankel and Bates (1990) finding that unadaptable (to new situations) toddlers, especially boys, were more dependent than adaptable toddlers in the problem-solving tasks, Gauvain and Fagot suggested that "difficult" children in their first study may actually have been less cognitively advanced and thus likely to elicit the mothers' extra assistance. Differences in cognitive development are not usually considered to be temperament, but discomfort with novelty is a temperament trait that may pertain to cognitive development. A shy child may underperform in situations of cognitive challenge, a cognitively slow child may not adapt quickly to a new situation, and shyness may impede the acquisition of information from experience (Bates, 1989). In support of this linkage, Miceli, Whitman, Borkowski, Braungart-Rieker, and Mitchell (1998) found that the mothers of 4-month-olds who were less efficient in processing information (on a test of attention to simple novel stimuli) tended to be more active and involved in toy play with them than the mothers of infants who were more efficient in processing information.

Effects of Socioeconomic Status

Socioeconomic status (SES) may be a second kind of moderator of relations between child temperament and parenting (Putnam et al., 2002). Prior, Sanson, Carroll, and Oberklaid (1989) suggested that higher SES mothers might respond more to their child's characteristics than lower SES mothers. Our reading of their Table 1, however, is that there were 9 significant correlations (of a possible 42) between self-reported parenting and temperament variables in the high SES group and 7 significant correlations in the low SES group, which does not clearly show a moderating effect for SES. However, although research has not yet established SES as a moderator, there are hints that it may be established someday: Studies that find less positive parenting with negatively reactive or difficult infants tend to do so in a lower SES sample (Owens, Shaw, & Vondra, 1998). For example, although not directly testing the moderating effect of social class, van den Boom (1989) found in a lower SES sample that mothers of highly irritable infants (based on observations in the first few weeks after birth) were relatively unresponsive to their infants' distress compared to mothers of nonirritable infants. And ultimately, the irritable babies were quite likely to be insecurely attached, unless their mothers were taught to be more sensitively responsive (van den Boom, 1994, 1995).

Parental Personality

One might suppose that parents' own personality and adjustment may moderate responses to child temperament. Evidence is mixed. Calkins et al. (2004) did not find that maternal self-reported adjustment interacted with high- versus low- infant frustration group to predict parenting behavior. Teti and Gelfand (1991) found that infant difficultness was associated with lower feelings of mothering self-efficacy for depressed but not for nondepressed mothers. However, mothers' depressed versus nondepressed classification did not interact with either perceived difficult temperament or maternal self-efficacy in predicting observed competent mothering. Boivin et al. (2004) replicated Teti and Gelfand (1991) in finding that maternal feelings of low self-efficacy were associated with high infant difficultness, and they also found that the same was true for fathers. Boivin et al. did not evaluate the possible interaction between maternal depression and infant difficultness. However, they did consider other interesting questions. Mothers' self-rated hostile-reactive behavior toward the infant was associated with the infants' difficultness, even when fathers provided the difficultness rating. How does this effect occur? Boivin et al. (2004) found in a sample of twins that mothers' self-rated hostile-reactive parenting was more similar toward their two twins if the twins were identical rather than fraternal, and a substantial portion of this genetic effect was explained specifically by the greater genetic similarities of identical twins in father-rated difficultness. Thus, the infants' difficultness may have evoked maternal irritation. Or, as the fact of a genetic effect reminds us, the mother and infant may share the genes for irritability.

More clear support for the notion that parents' personality moderates the effects of child temperament on parent behavior was provided by Clark, Kochanska, and Ready (2000), who found that mothers who were high in self-reported empathy when infants were 8–10 months were observed to be low in power assertive behavior 5 months later, no matter how high the infants were on negative emotionality observed in structured situations at 8–10 months. However, mothers who were low in empathy were higher in power assertion with more negative infants than with less negative infants. Clark et al. found the same pattern for maternal extraversion, too—with infant negative emotionality apparently eliciting more power assertion from extraverted rather than nonextraverted mothers.

Summary

One would assume that parenting responds to child temperament, but there have been relatively few relevant studies, and those studies reveal complex rather than simple relations. The largest part of the evidence concerns the effects of children's negative emotionality. Some studies find that parents behave more negatively with young infants high in negative emotionality; others studies do not. There may be a greater likelihood of a negative effect of difficult infant temperament when parents are low in empathy, depressed, or economically stressed than otherwise, but research has not resolved this yet. Negative parenting in response to difficult children has been more often found with older infants and toddlers than with young infants, perhaps because of maturation-related changes in roles and expectations. However, it is important to realize that even here, the effects are not universal. Nonfindings also can be noted. For example, Belsky, Hsieh, and Crnic (1998) found no evidence that infant negativity predicted parenting in toddlerhood. There are also a few hints in the literature that infants' challenging temperament qualities may also elicit positive parenting, such as greater warmth in response to negative emotionality and greater cognitive stimulation in response to novelty fear. And, finally, there are a few findings of positive temperament being associated with more positive parenting.

How Does Parenting Affect Child Temperament?

It is a theoretically interesting question whether and how parenting affects the development of children's temperament. If one thinks of temperament as a fixed quality in a child, then one would assume no effect. However, if one thinks of temperament as an emergent property of the child-environment system, at least at the level of the child's observable behavior (Rothbart & Bates, 1998), there should be some impact of parenting. The kind of study that would best answer the question would be transactional and longitudinal, and the measures of temperament and parenting would be both rich and sensitive to change. In one clearly transactional study, Rubin and his colleagues (Rubin et al., 1999; Kennedy et al., 2004) considered the possible impact of parenting upon temperament in a longitudinal path analysis but did not detect effects of parenting at age 2 upon child temperament at age 4. In another, Lengua and Kovacs (2005) found that maternal inconsistent discipline predicted child fearfulness and irritability in middle childhood in a

1-year follow-up, controlling for initial levels of parenting and temperament. Lengua and Kovacs also found some child temperament effects in the same models (e.g., irritability predicting increased inconsistent discipline). There has not been a great deal of work on the effects of child temperament on parenting, and there has been even less on the complementary process. It should also be recognized that most of the studies that we cited in the previous section as possible examples of child temperament affecting parenting, could, because they were cross-sectional or did not control for the effects of prior parenting, be seen as examples of parenting affecting child temperament. There have been too few longitudinal models like those of Rubin and his colleagues or Lengua and Kovacs. Most of the relations we have interpreted as effects of child temperament upon variations in parenting could actually be due to some quality of the parents that is reflected in their parenting and in their child's temperament, whether via passive gene–environment correlation or an active process of parent behavior shaping child behavior that operationally defines child temperament.

To summarize the research on direct relations between measures of parenting and child temperament, the literature does provide some examples of the kinds of relations that might be expected, such as between negative emotionality or difficultness and parental hostile control. However, the cumulative weight of the findings is not impressive. Relatively little research has been done. Further work, with more sensitive measures and powerful designs, may well discover patterns we are not seeing today.

PARENTING AND TEMPERAMENT IN CHILDREN'S ADJUSTMENT

Now we consider how parenting and child temperament are involved in the development of children's differences in adjustment, a key product of socialization processes. We use the term "adjustment" because we wish to consider a variety of adaptations, not just psychopathology. In most relevant studies, problem traits, such as aggressiveness and anxiety, are considered, but some studies consider positive traits, such as empathy and peer competence. Negative and positive adjustment are conceptually different on the surface, but in fact, there are as yet essentially no clear empirical distinctions (i.e., demonstrations of statistical independence). Until such distinctions are found, we can treat negative and positive adjustment as two sides of the same coin. Some have noted possible conceptual overlap between temperament and adjustment. For reasons described in Rothbart and Bates (2006), we do not see this possible overlap as a major concern, especially in longitudinal studies. We first discuss direct linkage findings and processes and then more indirect effects, with special emphasis on temperament × parenting interaction effects.

Parenting and Temperament as Additive Predictors

It is well established that both the presence of negative parenting (e.g., hostility) and the absence of positive parenting (e.g., warmth) are associated with child adjustment problems (Coie & Dodge, 1998; Patterson, Reid, & Dishion, 1992; Rothbaum & Weisz, 1994). Given the possibility that child problems could elicit negative parenting and suppress positive parenting (Bell, 1968), it is especially helpful to have longitudinal studies that show prediction of later problems from earlier parenting and control for earlier child behavior problems. For example, findings from the Child Development Project (Pettit, Bates, Dodge, & Meece; 1999; Pettit, Laird, Bates, Dodge, & Criss, 2001) have shown that low levels of parental monitoring in early adolescence are predictive of adolescent delinquent behavior problems, as rated by mothers and teens, independently of ratings of behavior problems in middle childhood. Others have presented evidence consistent with these findings (e.g., Ge, Best, Conger, & Simons, 1996; Kilgore, Snyder, & Lentz, 2000). In general, hostile, harsh, uninvolved, and inconsistent forms of negative parenting tend to be associated with both externalizing problems, such as aggression and rule-breaking, as well as with internalizing problems, such as anxiety and depression. This may pertain to the fact that there are often substantial correlations between externalizing and internalizing problems.

It is also well established that child temperament variables are concurrently associated with and longitudinally predictive of child adjustment (Bates, 1989; Rothbart & Bates, 1998, 2006). Interestingly, externalizing and internalizing problems are linked to different temperament variables. The main differential linkage pattern, not perfectly replicated but often found, is that temperamental fearfulness predicts internalizing problems more strongly than it predicts externalizing problems, temperamental unmanageability predicts externalizing problems more strongly than internalizing problems, and temperamental negative emotionality predicts both kinds of adjustment problem.

Given the modest overlap between parenting and child temperament described earlier and the fact that both parenting variables and temperament variables have been found in separate studies to predict child adjustment, one might expect parenting and temperament to increment one another's predictions in a multivariate analysis. A few studies with young children do confirm this expectation, but the array of findings is not as large and consistent as might have been expected. Bates and Bayles (1988) found that low maternal affection and child difficult temperament additively predicted externalizing behavior for boys but not girls; Kyrios and Prior (1990) found that parental punitiveness and difficult/unmanageable temperament additively predicted total behavior problem scores; and Rubin, Hastings, Chen, Stewart, and McNichol (1998) found that emotional dysregulation (which we view as temperament-based) and maternal intrusive dominance additively predicted concurrent behavior problems, although not problems at a later age (Rubin, Burgess, Dwyer, & Hastings, 2003). Diener and Kim (2004), on the other hand, found that neither child temperament nor parenting predicted prosocial or externalizing behavior. Likewise, Russell, Hart, Robinson, and Olsen (2003) found that preschoolers' prosocial and aggressive behaviors were associated with mother-rated temperament, but in general, self-rated parenting did not predict adjustment over and beyond the temperament scores.

A few studies have also shown additive effects in older children. Brody and Ge (2001) found that both nurturant–responsive parenting and low conflicted-harsh parenting and youths' self-regulation were independently predictive of adolescents' later high self-esteem and low depression and hostility. Self-regulation also predicted low teen alcohol use, but parenting variables did not add significantly to this prediction. Buckner, Mezzacappa, and Beardslee (2003) found that youth self-regulation and parental monitoring of the youth independently predicted the youths' current adaptive functioning in family, school, and peer settings and lack of mental health problems.

Another way temperament and parenting might combine is through mediating processes. There are few examples of such models (Rothbart & Bates, 1998), but it does seem possible that the impact of early temperament is mediated by subsequent life experience, including parenting (Dodge & Pettit, 2003), and that later temperament, such as self-regulation, mediates the impact of early parenting (Brody & Ge, 2001).

To summarize, there are substantial bodies of research showing that both temperament and parenting predict children's adjustment. There is some research showing that temperament and parenting independently combine as main or direct effects in the prediction of adjustment; however, the evidence for their additive prediction is not as impressive as the evidence for each considered separately. This mixed pattern may be due to unresolved issues in the research to date, such as the extent to which temperament and parenting do or do not correlate. However, it may also be that additive main effects or direct relations are not the most interesting avenue for research at this time, as has been argued by Wachs (2000). To understand individual children's developmental processes, it may be more important to consider how their temperamental characteristics fit to their social environment (Thomas et al., 1968). Individual parents can respond differently to a particular kind of child temperament, just as children with different temperaments can respond differently to a particular style of parenting. And those responses might shape socialization processes. Research on temperament by parenting interaction has shown remarkable growth in recent years.

Parenting × Temperament → Adjustment

There was some work on the theoretically vital topic of temperament and environment as interactive factors in children's adjustment by the late 1980s (Bates, 1989) and a little more by the late 1990s (Rothbart & Bates, 1998), but since then, the output of such work has sharply accelerated, as can be seen in recent reviews (Bates & McFadyen-Ketchum, 2000; Gallagher, 2002; Putnam et al., 2002; Rothbart & Bates, 2006; Sanson et al., 2004; Wills, Sandy, Yaeger, & Shinar, 2001). Here, we consider how temperament and parenting practices moderate one another's effects in the development of children's and adolescents' adjustment. Some studies focus on how a temperament trait moderates the effects of a parenting characteristic, such as children's temperamental self-regulation affecting the implications of mothers' emotional expressivity for child adjustment. Other studies focus on how parenting characteristics moderate a temperament trait's implications, such as parental discipline efforts moderating the prediction from child self-regulation to externalizing behavior problem outcomes. These reflect conceptually different questions, but analytically, they are equivalent. In many instances, the analysis suggesting an interaction effect involves a multiplication of a temperament variable and a parenting variable to create a predictor term in a multiple regression analysis. The researcher typically interprets significant interaction terms from one perspective, but either perspective could be meaningful. Sometimes the answers to the two questions are not exactly the same, but based on our own data-analytic explorations, it seems likely that answers would fundamentally converge most of the time, if researchers were to ask both questions. Therefore, we do not organize our review primarily by the particular framework within which the interaction question was posed, because this is fairly arbitrary, but rather by the substantive temperament and parenting dimensions.

The bigger issue is finding an interaction effect in the first place. Social development studies use predictor and moderator variables that are correlated, not independent as in a random-assignment experiment, so they often have problems in the joint distributions of variables and deficiencies in statistical power for detecting an interaction effect (McClelland & Judd, 1993; Stoolmiller, 2001; Wachs & Plomin, 1991). Because of the likelihood that some moderator effects might actually exist but not be found by conventional tests of statistical significance and the complementary likelihood that some interaction effects that do pass the significance test are spurious, we attend especially to interaction effects that have been even approximately replicated. We also give precedence to patterns over strict statistical considerations about the best ways to demonstrate an interaction effect (see Bates, 1989, and Bates & McFadyen-Ketchum, 2000, for more detailed discussion of some of these statistical issues in this area). At the rate that results are accumulating, it may be quite productive in a few years to apply methodological filters to the literature. For now, we feel that it makes more sense to emphasize substantive concepts. However, we also mention important methodological features, such as whether the study is longitudinal or cross-sectional or what kind of measure is used.

In reviewing the temperament × parenting interaction literature on development of adjustment, we consider the three temperament topics with the most relevant studies: (1) novelty distress, fearfulness, or unadaptability; (2) negative emotional reactivity, often referred to as difficult temperament; and (3) dysregulation traits, which include unmanageability, effortful control, and resistance to control. This is a useful way to organize the emerging findings, but we mention two possible concerns. First, the actual measure used in a given study may vary in how well it represents the "ideal" of the temperament construct. For example, for some researchers, the difficult temperament measure that we provisionally categorize as a negative emotionality measure also includes variables relevant to self-regulation and unadaptability. Second, even with relatively tightly defined constructs, it is quite possible that a given measure contains hidden influences from other dimensions, too. For example, what is measured as a young child's self-regulation may also reflect the child's fearfulness. A toddler who is afraid in a potentially exciting situation may appear to be higher on self-control than an equally self-regulated toddler who is less fearful. These issues, like a number of other methodological issues, are mentioned here but will have to be considered in more detail in future reviews.

Temperamental Fearfulness × Parenting Interactions

Temperamental fearfulness refers to initial withdrawal and slow adaptation to novel or potentially risky situations or behavioral inhibition (Kagan, 1998). Gray (1991) describes a set of brain structures underlying fearfulness, the Behavioral Inhibition System, which processes information concerning potential punishment and nonreward. A number of studies show that children high in early fearfulness are at elevated risk for the development of internalizing disorders, such as anxiety and depression (Rothbart & Bates, 1998). In general, fearfulness constructs used in moderator studies have been relatively pure, but a measure showing high behavioral inhibition or fear also could reflect, to some degree, a low level of approach motivation (the temperamental dimension of positive emotionality) and high self-regulation tendencies.

The most important example in the domain of temperamental fearfulness × parenting interaction is the widely cited study of Kochanska (1991). In this study, highly fearful 8–10-year-olds showed more signs of conscience when their mothers used gentle rather than harsh control. Gentle control, however, did not make a difference for the more fearless children. Theoretically, this pattern resulted from fearful children becoming too anxious in harsh discipline encounters to cognitively process the discipline information in an effective way. This pattern was essentially replicated by Colder, Lochman, and Wells (1997), who found that fearful children with harsh parents were more aggressive at school than either fearful children with mild parents or fearless children with harsh parents. Kochanska (1995) herself also replicated the finding with younger children. She also extended it: Not only was gentle discipline more strongly associated with self-control for high-fear toddlers than for low-fear toddlers, but a positive and warm mother–child relationship, measured by an attachment Q-sort, was more strongly associated with self-control for low-fear toddlers than the high-fear ones. Thus, which of the two different methods for teaching social values—discipline or a warm relationship—was more important depended on the level of child fearfulness. Kochanska (1997) followed these toddlers (average age 33 months) at about 46 and 60 months. She found that the toddler-age pattern replicated in predictions of conscience (self-control) measures at 46 months, using temperament and parenting measures from the toddler age. However, at 60 months, the pattern was not clearly replicated.

Independent replications of the Kochanska (1991, 1997) pattern were attempted by van der Mark, Bakermans-Kranenburg, and van IJzendoorn (2002) and van der Mark, van IJzendoorn, and Bakermans-Kranenburg (2002). These attempts were in a study of only girls and at ages younger than Kochanska used, ages 16 and 22 months, and a relatively high SES sample. Due to these differences or perhaps other methodological differences, the findings did not replicate the Kochanska pattern. Although we note nonreplications of the Kochanska pattern, we place more weight on the replications and conclude that the fear × parenting effect is supported. Nevertheless, given the pattern's importance, further studies are needed, both to solidly establish the basic pattern and, ultimately, to describe the processes that mediate the moderator effect.

There are also some studies of interactions between family environment and fearful temperament in the prediction of internalizing and externalizing behavior problems. Two studies are similar in providing a pattern in which children with fearful tendencies were less likely to develop internalizing symptoms when their families were *more*, rather than less, challenging. Theoretically, this may have something to do with how such a child learns to manage emotions, as described later. First, Tschann, Kaiser, Chesney, Alkon, and Boyce (1996) measured preschoolers' fearfulness with low scores on the approach scale of Keogh, Pullis, and Caldwell's (1982) Teacher Temperament Questionnaire and family qualities with mother reports of family conflict. Children low on approach were more likely to be observed to be socially withdrawn when their families were low in conflict, whereas those high on approach were more likely to be withdrawn when their families were high in conflict. Second, preliminary findings from two longitudinal samples partly converge with this effect: Bates (2003) measured fearful temperament with mother reports on the Unadaptable scale of the Infant Characteristics Questionnaire (ICQ)(Bates, Freeland, & Lounsbury, 1979; Bates & Bayles, 1984) and family qualities with observations of directive and restrictive control. In both samples, children's unadaptable temperament in early childhood showed a stronger relation with mother-rated internalizing problems across middle childhood in families where the mothers had been observed to be low in control rather than high in control.

These findings, suggesting that fearful children's internalizing problems may be moderated by a more directive and challenging family environment, conceptually converge with some additional important findings, which are described here, even though they would perhaps fit more properly under the temperament category of negative emotionality. The findings also suggest that parenting behaviors that would typically be classed as negative can sometimes produce desirable effects. Belsky et al. (1998) reported that for temperamentally negative infants (parent Infant Behavior Questionnaire [IBQ; Rothbart, 1986]) ratings + lab observations of both fear and frustration), fathers' intrusive and negative behavior predicted less inhibited child behavior in the laboratory at age 3 years, and for infants who were low in negative emotionality, father behavior was not associated with later inhibition. Similarly, but from the perspective of parenting as the moderator of implications of infant temperament, Arcus (2001) found that infants who were high in negative emotional reactivity in the lab were less likely to show behavioral inhibition later, at age 14 months, if their mothers were observed to be high in limit-setting. It is recognized that the limit-setting measured in the Arcus study is not necessarily the same as the intrusive and negative behavior measured in the Belsky et al. study, but a resemblance is quite possible, because what is called limit-setting with toddlers is often perceived as negative, and sometimes as intrusive control. Arcus (2001) also found that even beyond the effect of maternal limit-setting, when negatively reactive infants had boisterous and annoying siblings, they were less likely to show behavioral inhibition. Arcus interpreted these effects as mild frustrations and challenges augmenting development of emotionally reactive infants' self-regulatory abilities and thus preventing behavioral inhibition. Although it appears that fearful children may benefit in some ways from a degree of parental negativity, neither of the studies cited here suggest that fearful children would develop best with extreme levels of stress and harsh parenting.

A different pattern was reported by Rubin, Burgess, and Hastings (2002). In families in which mothers were high in psychological control, defined as intrusive affection or help and derisive comments in a laboratory task at age 2, the child's observed inhibition with a peer at age 2 predicted social reticence with unfamiliar peers at age 4, but in families in which mothers were low in psychological control, early inhibition was not predictive of later social reticence. This pattern may appear to conflict with findings reviewed previously. However, the Rubin et al. (2002) parenting variables do not clearly fit the Arcus concept of optimal challenge. Perhaps psychologically controlling parents undermine fearful children's confidence and thus make it more likely that they will continue to withdraw, whereas parents who are less psychologically controlling do the opposite, especially if they offer mild challenges. As Chess and Thomas (1984) noted, withdrawing children developed best when parents steadily demanded that children deal with novelty, but not when the parents were either highly forceful or overprotective.

In summary, studies suggest that the implications of early fearful tendencies for development of later adjustment problems depend on qualities of parenting. If a fearful child receives harsh discipline, conscience development will be slower, at least in the preschool years. If such a child receives optimal challenges and direction, the likelihood of later internalizing symptoms may be reduced, and it is also possible, for the same kind of child, that overnegative and intrusive parenting may increase the likelihood of internalizing symptoms. As a sidelight, Pettit et al. (2001) found that when youths had shown high levels of anxiety in preadolescence, maternal psychological control was positively and significantly associated with anxiety in adolescence, but not when they had shown low levels of anxiety in preadolescence. Although the studies we have described represent major progress in the study of social development, the patterns we have described are suggestive rather than definitive. More studies are needed.

Negative Emotionality × Parenting Interactions

Negative emotional reactivity or irritability, regarded as the core of "difficult" temperament (Bates, 1980), involves several kinds of reaction, especially beyond the early infancy period, including reactions to somatic discomfort, overstimulation, and frustration. Some researchers also include components of distress to novelty and poor self-regulation, instead of measuring these components separately. Nevertheless, negative emotionality has sufficient status as an independent dimension that it is worth separate treatment (Rothbart & Bates, 2006). Negative emotionality predicts both internalizing and externalizing kinds of behavior problems (Rothbart & Bates, 1998).

As mentioned earlier, the study by Arcus (2001) showed that early negative emotional reactivity was more predictive of later behavioral inhibition when parenting was observed to be less, rather than more restrictive, and Belsky et al. (1998) showed the converse—that less restrictive parenting predicted later inhibition more for highly reactive infants. In addition, however, the Belsky et al. (1998) study also showed that among highly reactive toddlers, mothers' and fathers' intrusive and negatively affective behavior during toddlerhood were more predictive of externalizing behavior at age 3 than among toddlers low in negative emotionality. Thus, despite findings that internalizing and externalizing behavior problems often covary and that they are both preceded by difficult temperament (Bates, 1989), Belsky et al. provide evidence that they may arise from different parent–child relationship processes. Feldman, Greenbaum, and Yirmiya (1999) found that an analog to maternal insensitivity, low synchrony in mother–infant play in the first year, was more predictive of observed noncompliance to the mother at age 2 for infants who were high on negative emotionality (mother ICQ + lab observations) than for those who were low on emotionality. A high level of noncompliance is typically regarded as a symptom of externalizing problems. Also considering temperament as the moderator, Pauli-Pott, Mertesacker, and Beckman (2004) found that maternal insensitivity at age 4 months more strongly predicted stranger distress at age 12 months for infants who were high in negative emotionality in the lab at 4 months than for infants who were low in negative emotionality. Of course, stranger distress at age 12 months may actually not represent an adjustment outcome like high levels of noncompliance or internalizing problems. Overall, it is encouraging that there is some consistency in the tendencies for more positive parenting to buffer against emotionally reactive children's externalizing problems and less positive parenting to buffer against reactive children's internalizing problems.

Three cross-sectional studies show stronger associations between parenting and behavior problems for high- versus low-irritable children. Morris et al. (2002) showed that child-rated maternal overt hostility was more strongly associated with teacher-rated child externalizing behavior among high-irritable children, defined by mother Child Behavior Questionnaire (CBQ; Rothbart, Ahadi, Hershey, & Fisher, 2001) reports of anger–frustration. Morris et al. also found perceived covert hostility and intrusive control of the child's feelings to be more strongly related to children's teacher-rated internalizing symptoms for more irritable than less irritable children. Tschann et al. (1996) showed a similar effect with a temperamental composite of negative emotionality and dysregulation as rated by preschool teachers, mother-reported family conflict, and teacher-rated internalizing and externalizing symptoms. Finally, Kilmer, Cowan, and Wyman (2001) did not actually test the interaction but did find that, among children living in high-stress environments, those who were well adjusted, despite being at risk for problems, were lower in difficult temperament than those who were poorly adjusted.

A similar longitudinal study, but using the parenting as moderator and temperament as predictor, was done by Gilliom, Shaw, Beck, Shonberg, and Lukon (2002). When mothers had been observed to be high rather than low in negative control and low rather than high in warmth, toddlers' negative emotionality (ICQ difficultness) was more predictive, 2 years later, of their ineffective self-regulation while waiting for a gift. Crockenberg (1987) found that infants' slow soothability, observed at age 3 months, was predictive of angry and noncompliant behavior at age 24 months, but only when the infants' adolescent mothers were angry and punitive. In a study of older children, Lengua, Wolchik, Sandler, and West (2000) did not find an interaction between negative emotionality as indexed by mother and child reports on the EAS (Buss & Plomin, 1984) and parenting in predicting adjustment (mother + child rating). However, Lengua et al. did find that maternal rejection (mother + child rating) was more strongly associated with child externalizing behavior and depression when the child was rated low rather than high in positive emotionality. Positive emotionality is conceptually unrelated to negative emotionality (Rothbart & Bates, 2006), but we mention this interaction finding because it is one of very few that has been reported for positive emotionality.

Owens and Shaw (2003) reported a different kind of rare finding. Their "outcome" was the slope of externalizing behavior from age 2 to 6. One would expect the average child's externalizing behavior problems at home to decline from early childhood across middle childhood (Keiley, Bates, Dodge, & Pettit, 2000). Owens and Shaw found slower declines in externalizing behavior for children with high negative emotionality (observed at 18 months) and depressed mothers (a proxy for disturbances in parenting) than for children with low negative emotionality and depressed mothers. Furthermore, in families with mothers low in depression, high negative children showed a faster decline in externalizing behavior than low negative children.

In one of the earlier examples of temperament × parenting interactions, Maziade et al. (1990) found that children rated as extremely difficult were more likely to show large numbers of externalizing symptoms and meet criteria for a diagnosed disorder (especially oppositional defiant disorder and attention-deficit/hyperactivity disorder) at age 12 and to show more self-reported symptoms at age 17 if their parents described themselves as inconsistent in their discipline than if discipline was more consistent. The general pattern, child negative emotionality moderating the effects of parenting, or the converse, has also been found in some studies considering substance use by adolescents (Mun, Fitzgerald, Von Eye, Putler, & Zucker, 2001; Stice & Gonzales, 1998; Wills et al., 2001).

To summarize, although explicit replications are lacking, the research does suggest a general pattern in which child negative emotionality appears to amplify the effects of negative parenting on the development of behavior problems or, conversely, negative parenting amplifies the effects of child negative emotionality. It seems possible that a child with tendencies toward negative emotionality might more readily engage in coercive cycles with hostile or ineffectual parents, and this might ultimately result in habitual, externalizing behavior problems. This is consistent with coercive family process theory (Patterson et al., 1992). Another pattern suggested by the literature is for controlling, somewhat negative parenting, as long as it is not too negative, to make child negative emotionality less likely to develop into internalizing problems. Here, as Arcus has argued, the process may be that moderate challenges by the parents require the child to develop adaptive means of emotion regulation, rather than relying on withdrawal. As in the fearful temperament × parenting domain, much research remains to be done, in providing clear replications of the most interesting effects, in clarifying the operative temperament and parenting dimensions and in detailing the processes mediating the moderator effects. A number of processes could explain how the interactions between child disposition to negative emotionality and parenting variables result in child adjustment outcomes. For example, to explain the Arcus (2001) effect in which parental limit-setting moderated the impact of infant negative emotionality on later behavioral inhibition, one could assume that the child's negative emotion signifies fear more than anger, and that there is a conditioning process in which the child is exposed to and not allowed to withdraw from novelty and thus extinguishes fear responses to novel stimuli. This is the effective ingredient of treatments for anxiety disorders (Thorpe & Olson, 1997). Or, one could assume a more operant conditioning process in which the child's assertive responses are shaped through modeling and reinforcement by assertive parents. Or, finally, one might assume genetic resemblance between the child and parent, in which early negative emotionality of restrictive, challenging parents is simply a marker of the trait of approach-oriented frustration and not of risk for future novelty fear.

Self-Regulation × Parenting Interactions

As mentioned, temperamental self-regulation traits (e.g., impulsivity, unmanageability, or resistance to control) probably involve effortful control systems (Rothbart & Bates, 1998), especially relatively late-developing frontal cortex brain structures that allow effortful control of attention. However, the phenotypical behaviors of this domain likely involve other systems, especially behavioral approach or positive emotionality. Temperamental unmanageability is more strongly predictive of externalizing behavior problems than internalizing problems (Bates, 1989; Rothbart & Bates, 1998). An accumulating body of research has documented interactions between self-regulation traits and parenting in the development of adjustment. We emphasize two main patterns here.

First, similar to findings in the negative emotionality domain, several studies show dysregulation tendencies in children to be more likely related to concurrent or subsequent externalizing behavior problems when parents are negative in their behavior. Rubin et al. (2003) found that children with poor self-regulation at age 2 (lab tasks + mother report on the Toddler Behavior Assessment Questionnaire [TBAQ; Goldsmith & Rothbart, 1991]) showed high levels of mother-reported externalizing behavior at age 4 to a greater extent when their mothers were intrusive and hostile (observed in lab + self-report) than when their mothers were not intrusive/hostile. Rubin et al. (1998) found a concurrent version of this pattern in this same sample at age 2, but only for boys.

Other cross-sectional examples of this general pattern include the following studies, most of which selected child temperament as the moderator. Bates, Viken, and Williams (2003) found in a mostly Head Start sample that the absence of positive parenting (self-report + home interviewer impressions) was more strongly associated with teacher-rated, poor adjustment in the preschool for children high on temperamental resistance to control than for more temperamentally manageable children. Morris et al. (2002) found a stronger relation between child-rated maternal hostility and teacher-rated child externalizing problems among children low in effortful control (on the CBQ) than children higher in effortful control. In a sample of children who had experienced parental divorce, Lengua et al. (2000) discovered that mothers' inconsistent discipline (mother + child report) was more strongly related to conduct problems and depression for children with impulsive temperament (mother + child report on the CBQ) than for children with nonimpulsive temperament. In a cross-sectional study based on adolescents' ratings, Stice and Gonzales (1998) found that high levels of parental support and control were more strongly associated with low levels of adolescent antisocial behavior for highly impulsive youths than for nonimpulsive youths. Prinzie et al. (2003) reported that parents' angry discipline was more closely related to children's self-rated externalizing problems when the children also described themselves as low rather than high in agreeableness, a dimension that is the inverse of unmanageability. This pattern was essentially replicated by Van Leeuwen, Mervielde, Braet, and Bosmans (2004).

Along these lines, but from the perspective of parenting as the moderator, Paterson and Sanson (1999) found that children's temperamental inflexibility (mother-rated resistance to demands and negative emotionality) was more strongly associated with mother-rated externalizing behavior when mothers used more harsh punishment (self-report) than when they used less harsh punishment. In a short-term longitudinal follow-up, Calkins (2002) found a very similar pattern. Children high on a composite of resistance and distress (observed in frustrating situations in the lab) at 18 months tended to be high on angry and aggressive behavior in the lab at 24 months if their mothers were observed to be low in positive parenting in structured play and teaching tasks, but not when their mothers were high in positive parenting.

Valiente et al. (2004) extended the general pattern to prosocial behavior, children's sympathetic responses, and a different kind of parenting variable. They found that parents' expressivity of negative emotion (self-rated + observed) was positively associated with children's sympathetic responses (self-reported), but only when the child was high in effortful control (parent and teacher ratings on the CBQ + observation).

In a study using a nonconventional measure of children's self-regulation, El-Sheikh, Harger, and Whitson (2001) measured self-regulation by vagal tone, which indexes parasympathetic nervous system functioning and may pertain to attentional self-regulation. They found that children who were exposed to frequent marital quarrels were less likely to develop externalizing and internalizing behavior and health problems if they had high vagal tone. This study essentially confirms a previous finding by Katz and Gottman (1995), in which there was a higher correlation between marital hostility and child behavior problems for children who were low rather than high in vagal tone, even though the Katz and Gottman interaction effect was not significant.

In addition to the general pattern of children's dysregulation tendencies predicting more antisocial behavior when parents are more negative, findings also suggest a quite different pattern. As described previously, some studies have suggested that parental negative control may prevent development of internalizing problems in negatively emotional or fearful young children. Some related findings suggest that parenting behaviors involving control may actually be effective in socializing children, especially children with temperamental tendencies toward dysregulation. Bates, Pettit, Dodge, and Ridge (1998) found in two separate, longitudinal studies that children's resistance to control (mother report on the ICQ) was more likely to predict later externalizing behavior problems (mother or teacher reports) if the mother had been observed at home to be low rather than high in control. This may seem to be the opposite of the general effect in other studies reviewed here, but we suggest that the parental control observed in these studies may have been somewhat different than the negative parenting measured in the other studies. Parental control in the Bates et al. studies involved the mothers' responses to child misbehavior. These reactions were sometimes hostile, such as scolding, but not always, and almost never truly harsh discipline, such as spanking. So, although the literature clearly suggests that hostile and cold parenting may increase the likelihood of children's dysregulated temperament tendencies becoming externalizing behavior problems, the findings of Bates et al. (1998) also raise the possibility that for some children parental control may serve to promote good development, too, moderating the evolution of unmanageable early temperament into symptoms of behavior problems. Bates et al. also found that high levels of maternal control with highly manageable youngsters predicted higher levels of externalizing problems than would have been predicted by the children's temperament alone. Thus, excessive control might impair social development in basically cooperative children. Our speculations on qualities of different studies' parenting measures suggest similar speculations on differences in temperament measures and ultimately demand specific, empirical comparisons.

In summary, there is now substantial support for one pattern of interaction between child self-regulation traits and parenting: Compared to well-regulated children, children with lower self-regulation are more susceptible to developing behavior problems, especially externalizing problems, when exposed to negative parenting and the absence of positive parenting. Research also suggests, however, that some forms of restrictive parenting may serve to prevent later problems in children with early tendencies to be unmanageable. In further research, we need to learn more about the particular parenting factors that interact with particular temperamental self-regulation factors, and we need to learn more about the developmental processes by which the combination of parent– child relationship and child temperament lead, over time, to socially significant differences in child adjustment.

CONCLUSION

Contemporary theories of socialization generally agree that children's temperament and their experiences with parents are major factors in individual differences in social and behavioral adjustment. These theories receive some support from research we have reviewed. However, as is typical for any area, research on temperament and parenting raises new questions, too. Theoretically, one would expect that children's temperament would affect parenting, and the literature does provide examples consistent with this (e.g., child negative emotionality being associated with more parental negative behavior). However, direct temperament–parenting relations are not as numerous or as strong as we had initially expected on the basis of a relatively simple child-effects model, and it appears that child negative emotionality is associated with both more supportive and more negative parenting. There are hints in the literature that whether there is a temperament– parenting relation and whether it reflects a negative reciprocity (negative child, negative parent) or compensatory response (negative child, warm parent) may be a function of other variables in the family system, such as the developmental stage of the child, parental psychological adjustment, or socioecological factors. Further research is needed to clarify these moderator effects. Further research may also be needed to evaluate parenting responses to child characteristics that are more subtle or complex than the kinds of behavior evaluated to date. Genetically informative designs would be helpful in evaluating responses to child temperament while controlling for genetic similarities between parents and children, as would longitudinal studies. Theoretically, one might also expect to see some influence of parenting upon the developing temperament of the child, at least at the level of the phenotype. However, work in this area is not yet substantial enough to draw even tentative conclusions. Again, longitudinal and genetically informative designs would be of considerable help in considering how children's basic personalities may be shaped by experience with their parents. Ultimately, as suggested by transactional models, there may be a dynamic interplay of child temperament and parenting, in which the effects of early temperament may be partially accounted for by parenting, and parenting may lead to changes in temperament or its manifestations.

A major way of talking about individual differences in social development is in terms of children's adjustment. Large bodies of research consider temperament and parenting separately as predictors of child adjustment. We did not review this work in depth but, rather, focused on combinations of temperament and parenting. First, we considered additive combinations. There is some evidence that temperament and parenting add to one another in prediction of adjustment. However, the evidence for this is not strong enough for specific conclusions. More longitudinal studies are needed on temperament and parenting as complementary versus overlapping predictors of adjustment.

Next, we considered how nonadditive, interactive combinations of temperament and parenting might predict adjustment. When we first seriously asked this question (Bates, 1989), there were very few relevant studies. Now, however, there are so many that we are able to discern some general patterns. The patterns do not meet the full standards of replication, except in a few instances, but there is enough convergence that we were able to offer some general conclusions. As one example, preschool children with fearful temperaments appear to develop signs of conscience earlier when their mothers are gentle rather than harsh in their control, whereas fearless children's development is more related to a positive, warm relationship with mothers. As another example, parenting qualities matter more for the future adjustment of children who are high in negative emotionality than for children who are not so irritable. In one variant on this, more challenging and directive parenting prevents the development of behavioral inhibition in irritable children, and in another variant, harsh or insensitive parenting appears to amplify risk for externalizing behavior problems in the same kind of child. And as a final example, children who are low in early self-regulatory traits may be less likely to develop externalizing behavior problems when their mothers are relatively controlling. The findings represent encouraging growth in the field. However, even the best-established patterns are more suggestive than solid at this point.

Further research is needed to replicate the important patterns and then to move toward describing the ways in which the interaction effects operate in development. What processes mediate a moderator effect? To take one example, assuming sufficient replications of the Kochanska (1997) interaction between parental harshness or warmth and child fearfulness or fearlessness in the development of conscience, the question becomes whether we can measure theoretically key processes that explain this effect. Is it the case, as has been suggested, that fearful children are more likely to fail to cognitively process harsh discipline encounters and that cognitive processing then explains a significant portion of the variance due to the interaction of temperamental fearfulness and harsh discipline in the prediction of later conscience?

Another step is to consider profiles of temperament dimensions in interaction with profiles of parenting dimensions. There has been a little research on how two different temperament variables may interact in the development of adjustment, but not a lot (Rothbart & Bates, 1998, 2006). The leading example is that high negative emotionality matters more in the context of low self-regulation than in the context of high self-regulation (Eisenberg, Fabes, Guthrie, & Reiser, 2000). Perhaps a parenting profile, such as harsh parenting in the context of low positive involvement, would have different child adjustment implications depending on the temperament profile of the child, such as fearfulness in the context of good versus poor self-regulation. We are not aware of any such research, which is not surprising given the statistical power demands of such a study. However, this kind of research may ultimately be required for a proper understanding of social development.

In conclusion, socialization is a complex, dynamic process. For nearly four decades, at least since Bell's (1968) seminal review, it has been thought that child characteristics and parenting must both play roles in socialization. However, in the past 10 years or so, research has begun to describe specific ways in which these factors interact. Now, with the exciting advances of recent years, we can ask questions that are far more complex than we could have asked even 10 years ago.

REFERENCES

Arcus, D. (2001). Inhibited and uninhibited children: Biology in the social context. In T. D. Wachs & G. A. Kohnstamm (Ed.), *Temperament in context* (pp. 43–60). Mahwah, NJ: Erlbaum.

Barber, B. K. (Ed.). (2002). *Intrusive parenting: How psychological control affects children and adolescents.* Washington, DC: American Psychological Association.

Bates, J. E. (1980). The concept of difficult temperament. *Merrill-Palmer Quarterly, 26,* 299–319.

Bates, J. E. (1989). Applications of temperament concepts. In G. A. Kohnstamm, J. E. Bates, & M. K. Rothbart (Ed.), *Temperament in childhood* (pp. 321–355). Chichester, UK: Wiley.

Bates, J. E. (2003). *Temperamental unadaptability and later internalizing problems as moderated by mothers' restrictive control.* Paper presented at the meeting of the Society for Research in Child Development, Tampa, FL.

Bates, J. E., & Bayles, K. (1984). Objective and subjective components in mothers' perceptions of their children from age 6 months to 3 years. *Merrill-Palmer Quarterly, 30,* 111–130.

Bates, J. E., & Bayles, K. (1988). Attachment and the development of behavior problems. In J. Belsky & T. Nezworski (Ed.), *Clinical implications of attachment* (pp. 253–299). Hillsdale, NJ: Erlbaum.

Bates, J. E., Freeland, C. B., & Lounsbury, M. L. (1979). Measurement of infant difficultness. *Child Development, 50,* 794–803.

Bates, J. E., & McFadyen-Ketchum, S. (2000). Temperament and parent–child relations as interacting factors in children's behavioral adjustment. In V. J. Molfese & Molfese D. L. (Ed.), *Temperament and personality across the life span* (pp. 141–176). Mahwah, NJ: Erlbaum.

Bates, J. E., Olson, S. L., Pettit, G. S., & Bayles, K. (1982). Dimensions of individuality in the mother–infant relationship at six months of age. *Child Development, 53,* 446–461.

Bates, J. E., Pettit, G. S., Dodge, K. A., & Ridge, B. (1998). Interaction of temperamental resistance to control and restrictive parenting in the development of externalizing behavior. *Developmental Psychology, 34*(5), 982–995.

Bates, J. E., Viken, R. J., & Williams, N. (2003). *Temperament as a moderator of the linkage between sleep and preschool adjustment.* Paper presented at the meeting of the Society for Research in Child Development. Tampa, FL.

Bates, J. E., Wachs, T. D., & Emde, R. N. (1994). Toward practical uses for biological concepts of temperament. In J. E. Bates & T. D. Wachs (Eds.), *Temperament: Individual differences at the interface of biology and behavior* (pp. 275–306.). Washington, DC: American Psychological Association Press.

Bell, R. Q. (1968). A reinterpretation of the direction of effects in studies of socialization. *Psychological Review, 75,* 81–95.

Belsky, J., Hsieh, K., & Crnic, K. (1998). Mothering, fathering, and infant negativity as antecedents of boys' externalizing problems and inhibition at age 3 years: Differential susceptibility to rearing experience? *Development and Psychopathology, 10,* 301–319.

Boivin, M., Perusse, D., Dionne, G., Saysset, V., Zoccolillo, M., Trabulsy, G., et al. (2005). The genetic–environmental etiology of parent's perceptions and self-assessed behaviours toward their 5-months-old infants in a large twin and singleton sample. *Journal of Child Psychology and Psychiatry, 46*(6), 612–630.

Brody, G. H., & Ge, X. (2001). Linking parenting processes and self-regulation to psychological functioning and alcohol use during early adolescence. *Journal of Family Psychology, 15*(1), 82–94.

Buckner, J. C., Mezzacappa, E., & Beardslee, W. R. (2003). Characteristics of resilient youths living in poverty: The role of self-regulatory processes. *Development and Psychopathology, 15,* 139–162.

Buss, A. H., & Plomin, R. (1984). *Temperament: Early developing personality traits.* Hillsdale, NJ: Erlbaum.

Calkins, S. D. (2002). Does aversive behavior during toddlerhood matter? The effects of difficult temperament on maternal perceptions and behavior. *Infant Mental Health Journal, 23*(4), 381–402.

Calkins, S. D., Hungerford, A., & Dedmon, S. E. (2004). Mothers' interactions with temperamentally frustrated infants. *Infant Mental Health Journal, 25*(3), 219–239.

Caspi, A., Sugden, K., Moffitt, T. E., Taylor, A., Craig, I. W., Harrington, H., et al. (2003). Influence of life stress on depression: Moderation by a polymorphism in the 5-HTT gene. *Science, 301,* 386–389.

Chess, S., & Thomas, A. (1984). *Origins and evolution of behavior disorders: from infancy to early adult life.* New York: Brunner/Mazel.

Clark, L. A., Kochanska, G., & Ready, R. (2000). Mothers' personality and its interaction with child temperament as predictors of parenting behavior. *Journal of Personality and Social Psychology, 79*(2), 274–285.

Coie, J. D., & Dodge, K. A. (1998). Aggression and antisocial behavior. In W. Damon (Series Ed.) & N. Eisenberg (Vol. Ed.), *Handbook of child psychology: Vol. 3, Social emotional and personality development* (5th ed., pp. 779–862). New York: Wiley.

Colder, C. R., Lochman, J. E., & Wells, K. C. (1997). The moderating effects of children's fear and activity level on relations between parenting practices and childhood symptomatology. *Journal of Abnormal Child Psychology, 25,* 251–263.

Collins, W. A., Maccoby, E. E., Steinberg, L., Hetherington, E. M., & Bornstein, M. H. (2000). Contemporary research on parenting: The case for nature and nurture. *American Psychologist, 55*(2), 218–232.

Costa, P. T., Jr., & McCrae, R. R. (1988). From catalog to classification: Murray's needs and the five-factor model. *Journal of Personality and Social Psychology, 55,* 258–265.

Crockenberg, S. (1986). Are temperamental differences in babies associated with predictable differences in care giving? In J. V. Lerner & R. M. Lerner (Ed.), *Temperament and social interaction during infancy and childhood: New directions for child development* (Vol. 31, pp. 53–73). San Francisco: Jossey-Bass.

Crockenberg, S. (1987). Predictors and correlates of anger toward and punitive control of toddlers by adolescent mothers. *Child Development, 58,* 964–975.

Diener, M. L., & Kim, D.-Y. (2004). Maternal and child predictors of preschool children's social competence. *Applied Developmental Psychology, 25,* 3–24.

Dodge, K. A., & Pettit, G. S. (2003). A biopsychosocial model of the development of chronic conduct problems in adolescence. *Developmental Psychology, 39,* 349–371.

Eisenberg, N., Fabes, R. A., Guthrie, I. K., & Reiser, M. (2000). Dispositional emotionality and regulation: Their role in predicting quality of social functioning. *Journal of Personality and Social Psychology, 78,* 136–157.

El-Sheikh, M., Harger, J., & Whitson, S. M. (2001). Exposure to interparental conflict and children's adjustment and physical health: The moderating role of vagal tone. *Child Development, 72*(6), 1617–1636.

Feldman, R., Greenbaum, C. W., & Yirmiya, N. (1999). Mother–infant affect synchrony as an antecedent of the emergence of self-control. *Developmental Psychology, 35*(5), 223–231.

Frankel, K. A., & Bates., J. E. (1990). Mother-toddler problem-solving: Antecedents in attachment, home behavior, and temperament. *Child Development, 61,* 810–819.

Fullard, W., McDevitt, S.C., & Carey, W.B. (1984). Assessing temperament in one- to three-year-old children. *Journal of Pediatric Psychology, 9*(2), 205–217.

Gallagher, K. C. (2002). Does child temperament moderate the influence of parenting on adjustment? *Developmental Review, 22,* 623–643.

Gauvain, M., & Fagot, B. (1995). Child temperament as a mediator of mother–toddler problem solving. *Social Development, 4*(3), 257–276.

Ge, X., Best, K. M., Conger, R. D., & Simons, R. L. (1996). Parenting behaviors and the occurrence and co-occurrence of adolescent depressive symptoms and conduct problems. *Developmental Psychology, 32,* 717–731.

Gilliom, M., Shaw, D. S., Beck, J. E., Schonberg, M. A., & Lukon, J. L. (2002). Anger regulation in disadvantaged preschool boys: Strategies, antecedents, and the development of self-control. *Developmental Psychology, 38*(2), 222–235.

Goldsmith, H. H., Buss, K. A., & Lemery, K. S. (1997). Toddler and childhood temperament: Expanded content, stronger genetic evidence, new evidence for the importance of environment. *Developmental Psychology, 33,* 891–905.

Goldsmith, H. H., Lemery, K. S., Buss, K. A., & Campos, J. J. (1999). Genetic analyses of focal aspects of infant temperament. *Developmental Psychology, 35,* 972–985.

Goldsmith, H. H., & Rothbart, M. K. (1991). Contemporary instruments for assessing early temperament by questionnaire and in the laboratory. In A. Angleitner & J. Strelau (Eds.), *Explorations in temperament: International perspectives on theory and measurement* (pp. 249–272). New York: Plenum Press.

Gray, J. A. (1991). The neuropsychology of temperament. In A. Angleitner & J. Strelau (Eds.), *Explorations in temperament: International perspectives on theory and measurement* (pp. 105–128). New York: Plenum Press.

Kagan, J. (1998). Biology and the child. In W. Damon (Series Ed.) & N. Eisenberg (Vol. Ed.), *Handbook of child psychology: Vol. 3. Social, emotional and personality development* (5th ed., pp. 177–235). New York: Wiley.

Katz, L. F., & Gottman, J. M. (1995). Vagal tone protects children from marital conflict. *Development and Psychopathology, 7,* 83–92.

Keiley, M. K., Bates, J. E., Dodge, K. A., & Pettit, G. S. (2000). A cross-domain growth analysis: Externalizing and internalizing behaviors during 8 years of childhood. *Journal of Abnormal Child Psychology, 28*(2), 161–179.

Kennedy, A. E., Rubin, K. H., Hastings, P. D., & Maisel, B. (2004). Longitudinal relations between child vagal tone and parenting behavior: 2 to 4 years. *Developmental Psychobiology, 45,* 10–21.

Keogh, B., Pullis, M. E., & Caldwell, J. (1982). A short form of the Teacher Temperament Questionnaire. *Journal of Educational Measurement, 19,* 323–329.

Kilgore, K., Snyder, J., & Lentz, C. (2000). The contribution of parental discipline, parental monitoring, and school risk to early-onset conduct problems in African American boys and girls. *Developmental Psychology, 36,* 835–845.

Kilmer, R. P., Cowen, E. L., & Wyman, P. A. (2001). A micro-level analysis of developmental, parenting, and family milieu variables that differentiate stress-resilient and stress-affected children. *Journal of Community Psychology, 29*(4), 391–416.

Kochanska, G. (1991). Socialization and temperament in the development of guilt and conscience. *Child Development, 62,* 1379–1392.

Kochanska, G. (1995). Children's temperament, mothers' discipline, and security of attachment: Multiple pathways to emerging internalization. *Child Development, 66,* 597–615.

Kochanska, G. (1997). Multiple pathways to conscience for children with different temperaments: From toddlerhood to age 5. *Developmental Psychology, 33*(2), 228–240.

Kochanska, G., Friesenborg, A. E., Lange, L. A., & Martel, M. M. (2004). Parents' personality and infants' temperament as contributors to their emerging relationship. *Journal of Personality and Social Psychology, 86*(5), 744–759.

Kyrios, M., & Prior, M. (1990). Temperament, stress and family factors in behavioral adjustment of 3–5-year-old children. *International Journal of Behavioral Development, 13,* 67–93.

Laible, D. (2004). Mother–child discourse in two contexts: Links with child temperament, attachment security, and socioemotional competence. *Developmental Psychology, 40*(6), 979–992.

Lee, C. L., & Bates, J. E. (1985). Mother–child interaction at age two years and perceived difficult temperament. *Child Development, 56,* 1314–1325.

Lengua, L. J., & Kovacs, E. A. (2005). Bidirectional associations between temperament and parenting and the prediction of adjustment problems in middle childhood. *Applied Developmental Psychology, 26,* 21–38.

Lengua, L. J., Wolchik, S. A., Sandler, I. N., & West, S. G. (2000). The additive and interactive effects of parenting and temperament in predicting adjustment problems of children of divorce. *Journal of Clinical Child Psychology, 29*(2), 232–244.

Maziade, M., Caron, C., Cote, R., Merette, C., Bernier, H., Laplante, B., et al. (1990). Psychiatric status of adolescents who had extreme temperaments at age 7. *American Journal of Psychiatry, 147*(11), 1531–1536.

McClelland, G. H., & Judd, C. M. (1993). Statistical difficulties of detecting interactions and moderator effects. *Psychological Bulletin, 114,* 376–390.

Miceli, P. J., Whitman, T. L., Borkowski, J. G., Braungart-Rieker, J., & Mitchell, D. W. (1998). Individual differences in infant information processing: The role of temperamental and maternal factors. *Infant Behavior and Development, 21*(1), 119–136.

Morris, A. S., Silk, J. S., Steinberg, L., Sessa, F. M., Avenevoli, S., & Essex, M. J. (2002). Temperamental vulnerability and negative parenting as interacting predictors of child adjustment. *Journal of Marriage and Family, 64,* 461–471.

Mun, E. Y., Fitzgerald, H. E., Von Eye, A., Puttler, L. I., & Zucker, R.A. (2001). Temperamental characteristics as predictors of externalizing and internalizing child behavior problems in the contexts of high and low parental psychopathology. *Infant Mental Health Journal, 22*(3), 393–415.

Owens, E. B., & Shaw, D. S. (2003). Predicting growth curves of externalizing behavior across the preschool years. *Journal of Abnormal Child Psychology, 31*(6), 575–590.

Owens, E. B., Shaw, D. S., & Vondra, J. I. (1998). Relations between infant irritability and maternal responsiveness in low-income families. *Infant Behavior and Development, 21,* 761–778.

Patterson, G. R., Reid, J. B., & Dishion, T. J. (1992). *Antisocial boys.* Eugene, OR: Castalia.

Paterson, G., & Sanson, A. (1999). The association of behavioural adjustment to temperament, parenting and family characteristics among 5-year old children. *Social Development, 8*(3), 293–309.

Pauli-Pott, U., Mertesacker, B., & Beckman, D. (2004). Predicting the development of infant emotionality from maternal characteristics. *Development and Psychopathology, 16,* 19–42.

Pettit, G. S., & Bates, J. E. (1984). Continuity of individual differences in the mother-infant relationship from 6 to 13 months. *Child Development, 55,* 729–739.

Pettit, G. S., Bates, J. E., Dodge, K. A., & Meece, D. W. (1999). The impact of after-school peer contact on early adolescent externalizing problems is moderated by parental monitoring, perceived neighborhood safety, and prior adjustment. *Child Development, 70,* 768–778.

Pettit, G. S., Laird, R. D., Bates, J. E., Dodge, K. A., & Criss, M. M. (2001). Antecedents and behavior-problem outcomes of parental monitoring and psychological control in early adolescence. *Child Development, 72,* 583–598.

Prinzie, P., Onghena, P., Hellinckx, W., Grietens, H., Ghesquiere, P., & Colpin, H. (2003). The additive and interactive effects of parenting and children's personality on externalizing behaviour. *European Journal of Personality, 17,* 95–117.

Prior, M., Sanson, A., Carroll, R., & Oberklaid, F. (1989). Social class differences in temperament ratings by mothers of preschool children. *Merrill-Palmer Quarterly, 35*(2), 239–248.

Putnam, S. P., Sanson, A.V., & Rothbart, M.K. (2002). Child temperament and parenting. In M. Bornstein (Ed.), *Handbook of parenting* (2nd ed., pp. 255–277). Mahwah, NJ: Erlbaum.

Rothbart, M. K. (1986). Longitudinal observation of infant temperament. *Developmental Psychology, 22,* 356–365.

Rothbart, M. K., Ahadi, S. A., Hershey, K. L., & Fisher, P. (2001). Investigations of temperament at three to seven years: The Children's Behavior Questionnaire. *Child Development, 72,* 1394–1408.

Rothbart, M. K., & Bates, J. E. (1998). Temperament. In W. Damon (Series Ed.) & N. Eisenberg (Vol. Ed.), *Handbook of child psychology: Vol. 3, Social, emotional and personality development* (5th ed., pp. 105–176.). New York: Wiley.

Rothbart, M. K., & Bates, J. E. (2006). Temperament. In N. Eisenberg (Ed.), *Handbook of child psychology* (6th ed., Vol. 3, pp. 99–106). Hoboken, NJ: Wiley.

Rothbart, M. K., Derryberry, D., & Posner, M. I. (1994). A psychobiological approach to the development of temperament. In J. E. Bates & T. D. Wachs (Eds.), *Temperament: Individual differences at the interface of biology and behavior* (pp. 83–116). Washington, DC: American Psychological Association.

Rothbaum, F., & Weisz, J. R. (1994). Parental caregiving and child externalizing behavior in nonclinical samples: A meta-analysis. *Psychological Bulletin, 116,* 55–74.

Rubin, K. H., Burgess, K. B., Dwyer, K. M., & Hastings, P. D. (2003). Predicting preschoolers' externalizing behaviors from toddler temperament, conflict, and maternal negativity. *Developmental Psychology, 39*(1), 164–176.

Rubin, K. H., Burgess, K. B., & Hastings, P. D. (2002). Stability and social-behavioral consequences of toddlers' inhibited temperament and parenting behaviors. *Child Development, 73*(2), 483–495.

Rubin, K. H., Hastings, P., Chen, X., Stewart, S., & McNichol, K. (1998). Intrapersonal and maternal correlates of aggression, conflict, and externalizing problems in toddlers. *Child Development, 69*(6), 1614–1629.

Rubin, K. H., Nelson, L. J., Hastings, P., & Asendorpf, J. (1999). The transaction between parents' perceptions of their children's shyness and their parenting styles. *International Journal of Behavioral Development, 23*(4), 937–957.

Russell, A., Hart, C. H., Robinson, C. C., & Olsen, S. F. (2003). Children's sociable and aggressive behaviour with peers: A comparison of the US and Australia, and contributions of temperament and parenting styles. *International Journal of Behavioral Development, 27*(1), 74–86.

Sanson, A., Hemphill, S. A., & Smart, D. (2004). Connections between temperament and social development: A review. *Social Development, 13*(1), 142–170.

Shiner, R., & Caspi, A. (2003). Personality differences in childhood and adolescence: Measurement, development, and consequences. *Journal of Child Psychology and Psychiatry, 44*, 2–32.

Stice, E., & Gonzales, N. (1998). Adolescent temperament moderates the relation of parenting to antisocial behavior and substance use. *Journal of Adolescent Research, 13*(1), 5–31.

Stoolmiller, M. (2001). Synergistic interaction of child manageability problems and parent-discipline tactics in predicting future growth in externalizing behavior for boys. *Developmental Psychology, 37*(6), 814–825.

Tellegen, A. (1985). Structures of mood and personality and their relevance to assessing anxiety, with an emphasis on self-report. In A. H. Tuma & J. D. Maser (Ed.), *Anxiety and the anxiety disorders* (pp. 681–706). Hillsdale, NJ: Erlbaum.

Teti, D. M., & Gelfand, D. M. (1991). Behavioral competence among mothers of infants in the first year: The mediational role of maternal self-efficacy. *Child Development, 62*, 918–929.

Thomas, A., Chess, S., & Birch, H. G. (1968). *Temperament and behavior disorders in children.* New York: New York University Press.

Thorpe, G. L., & Olson, S. L. (1997). *Behavior therapy: Concepts, procedures, and applications.* Boston: Allyn & Bacon.

Tschann, J. M., Kaiser, P., Chesney, M.A., Alkon, A., & Boyce, W. T. (1996). Resilience and vulnerability among preschool children: Family functioning, temperament, and behavior problems. *Journal of the American Academy of Child and Adolescent Psychiatry, 35*(2), 184–192.

Valiente, C., Eisenberg, N., Fabes, R. A., Shepard, S. A., Cumberland, A., & Losoya, S. (2004). Prediction of children's empathy-related responding from their effortful control and parents' expressivity. *Developmental Psychology, 40*(6), 911–926.

van den Boom, D.C. (1989). Neonatal irritability and the development of attachment. In G. A. Kohnstamm, J. E. Bates, & M. K. Rothbart (Eds.), *Temperament in childhood* (pp. 299–318). Chichester, UK: Wiley.

van den Boom, D. C. (1994). The influence of temperament and mothering on attachment and exploration: An experimental manipulation of sensitive responsiveness among lower-class mothers with irritable infants. *Child Development, 65*(5), 1457–1477.

van den Boom, D. C. (1995). Do first-year intervention effects endure? Follow-up during toddlerhood of a sample of Dutch irritable infants. *Child Development, 66*(6), 1798–1816.

van der Mark, I. L., Bakermans-Kranenburg, M. J., & van IJzendoorn, M. H. (2002). The role of parenting, attachment, and temperamental fearfulness in the prediction of compliance in toddler girls. *British Journal of Developmental Psychology, 20*, 361–378.

van der Mark, I. L., van IJzendoorn, M. H., & Bakermans-Kranenburg, M. J. (2002). Development of empathy in girls during the second year of life: Associations with parenting, attachment, and temperament. *Social Development, 11*(4), 451–468.

Van Leeuwen, K. G., Mervielde, I., Braet, C., & Bosmans, G. (2004). Child personality and parental behavior as moderators of problem behavior: Variable- and person-centered approaches. *Developmental Psychology, 40*(6), 1028–1046.

Wachs, T. D. (2000). *Necessary but not sufficient: The respective roles of single and multiple influences on individual development.* Washington, DC: American Psychological Association.

Wachs, T. D., & Bates, J.E. (2001). Temperament. In G. Bremner & A. Fogel (Eds.), *Blackwell handbook of infant development* (pp. 465–501). Oxford, UK: Blackwell.

Wachs, T. D., & Gruen, G. (1982). *Early experience and human development*. New York: Plenum Press.

Wachs, T. D., & Plomin, R. (1991). *Conceptualization and measurement of organism-environment interactions*. Washington, DC: American Psychological Association.

Wills, T. A., Sandy, J. M., Yaeger, A., & Shinar, O. (2001). Family risk factors and adolescent substance use: Moderation effects for temperament dimensions. *Developmental Psychology, 37*(3), 283–297.

Zuckerman, M. (1991). *Psychobiology of personality*. New York: Cambridge University Press.

PART III

Socialization across the Lifespan

CHAPTER 7

Early Socialization
A Relationship Perspective

DEBORAH LAIBLE and ROSS A. THOMPSON

Early socialization is rarely underestimated but often oversimplified. Traditional formulations emphasize the importance of nurturant, sensitive caregivers, a theme adopted also by contemporary theorists. But traditional views also portray socialization influences as unidirectional and straightforward, with the young child's sense of trust, security, and other characteristics shaped directly by the quality of parental care. Many years ago, Harriet Rheingold (1969) offered a novel portrayal of the "social and socializing infant" that profiled bidirectional socialization influences, recognizing how much young children affect the quality of care they receive. That view has been profoundly influential, and today it is complemented by other perspectives that emerge from efforts to understand the complexity of early socialization. Most prominent among these is a *relational* approach, arguing that close relationships foster the development of unique social capacities because of the behavioral, emotional, and representational contingencies that emerge between two people who know each other well (Collins & Laursen, 1999; Dunn, 1993; Reis, Collins, & Berscheid, 2000). These views are contributing to the emerging field of developmental relational science (Thompson, 2006b) and are the focus of this chapter.

A relationship can be defined as an integrated network of enduring emotional ties, mental representations, and behaviors that connect one person to another over time and across space. What does a relational approach contribute, therefore, to the study of early socialization? First, each relationship is unique because it is created from the mutual contributions of each partner over time. This begins early, as the infant's temperament juxtaposes with the parent's personality and socialization goals to inaugurate a unique partnership. Viewed in this light, therefore, bidirectional influences in relationships must be conceived as the compounding, transactional and mutual influences of relational partners over time. Parents and children respond not only to the partner's current behavior but also to the history of their relationship. The efficacy of parental discipline practices, for example, is affected by the child's temperamental qualities, and this creates outcome expectancies that affect the parent's future disciplinary efforts and, through them, the child's subsequent compliance and moral development (Holden, Thompson, Zambarano, & Marshall, 1997; Kochanska, 1995). Socialization arises from these integrated, bidirectional effects over time because of the opportunities afforded by relationships for transactional influences as development proceeds.

Second, each partner's behavior toward the other is also influenced by mental representations that derive from their shared history and the expectations, relational schemas, affective biases, and other representations they have fostered. This is what is meant by knowing, and being known by, another person to whom one is close, emotionally engaged, and in regular contact. To attachment theorists, these relational representations consist of "internal working models" of the self, the partner, and the relationship that color social expectations and social development from infancy, but mental representations of relationships must be an important facet of socialization in any theoretical view (Dweck, & London, 2004). Relationships thus entail the interaction of mental representations as well as of behavioral contingencies between two people, and this also begins early in life.

Third, relationships encompass influences that are both broad (e.g., mutual responsiveness, warmth, and security) and immediate (e.g., routines and rituals, rewards and sanctions, and modeling). These broad and immediate relational processes are mutually influential. The effects of a parent's emotional references in conversation, for example, interact with the overall security of their relationship to influence the growth of emotion understanding, and similar processes affect early conscience development (Thompson, Laible, & Ontai, 2003). This suggests that early socialization entails dyadic interactions that are meaningful within their broader relational context, and that the impact of specific socialization practices depends on quality of the relationships in which they are embedded.

Fourth, relationships are dynamic and affective. They change over time owing to developmental changes in each partner as well as the growth of the relationship and the influences of other events in each partner's life. Although newer relationships are colored by an individual's prior relationship history, as attachment theorists claim, relationships are also unique because they include different partners. Relationships are also colored by the emotional connection between two people that contributes to the salience of the behavior of relational partners and each person's unique influence over the other. This is why emotional constructs figure prominently in how the quality of early relationships are characterized (e.g., warmth, security, and hostility), and why emotional communication is such an important feature of relational interaction, especially early in life.

Understanding the influences of relationships in socialization involves comprehending how these emotional, mental, and behavioral constituents of relationships unfold developmentally and how social functioning and representations are affected by relational experience. This task is facilitated by developmental researchers who study relational proceses, such as parental scaffolding of children's social and cognitive skills, the influence of parental sensitivity on attachment security, young children's construal of the behavior of relational partners, the importance of the emotional climate of the home for developing self-regulation, children's imitative learning from siblings, parent–child conversations and children's mental representations of the psychological world, and the influences of proactive discipline, negotiation and bargaining, emotional synchrony, and other relational processes on social development. Although relational influences do not exhaust the range of early socialization processes, their consequences are likely to be the most profound, enduring, and ubiquitous because of the regular impact of relational partners on each other. Early relational experiences are especially important, moreover, because of the psychological foundation they create for sociopersonality growth, and a relational perspective to early socialization is best illuminated through exploration of infancy and early childhood when the quality of relationships is developmentally most formative.

Our goal is to outline a relational perspective to early socialization by exploring these broad and immediate relational influences—and their interaction—that are catalysts to social and personality development. We begin by examining research concerning the general quality of early relationships, whether conceptualized in terms of warmth, in terms of security, or in terms of mutual responsiveness. Relational quality has always been important in conceptualizing relational influences because of how it affects each partner's receptiveness to the other, especially in early childhood. In the next section, we examine more immediate relational processes that are important to socialization, distinguishing those that are primarily under the control of the parent (e.g., sensitivity and proactive regulation) from those that are mostly under the control of the child (e.g., interpretations of the partner's behavior and the influence of self-awareness) from those that are more genuinely dyadic in shared regulation (e.g., conversational discourse). Although we focus primarily on parent–child relationships in this chapter, we also consider other significant relationships for young children within this framework. In a concluding section, we consider the implications of this approach for conceptualizing early socialization.

THE QUALITY OF EARLY RELATIONSHIPS

Developmental theorists characterize early relationships in broad, qualitative ways, such as the warmth that is given and received between partners, shared security or trust, mutual positive affect or responsiveness, and other dimensions. They do so because the quality of early relationships defines their affective impact and moderates the influence of many specific relational processes, such as parental discipline practices or shared conversation. Early relationships initiate the child into a system of reciprocity and mutuality that influences children's identification with their relational partners (primarily parents, but also peers and siblings) and their motivation to respond cooperatively and affectionately to them. Children are motivated to attend to parental messages, for example, because of the close emotional attachment they share with them. As a consequence, the general quality of the relationship enhances or diminishes young children's receptivity to the socialization initiatives of others and, in this manner, also affects the responsiveness of others to the child.

In this section, we consider three features of relational quality that have been the focus of early socialization research: warmth, security, and mutual reciprocity. Although these constructs are often measured together in family research, several studies have found that when they are independently assessed, they are empirically distinctive and sometimes nonoverlapping (see Kochanska, 1998; Laible & Thompson, 2000). This may derive from differences in how these constructs are conceptualized and, in turn, measured. Whereas warmth typically involves noncontingent displays of affection, security is believed to derive from parental sensitivity or responsiveness but (especially within attachment theory) is assessed by the child's response to perceived threat or challenge. Mutual reciprocity, by contrast, is a fully dyadic construct typically assessed in nonstressful circumstances. Thus although all three constructs index relational harmony, the quality of the relationship is conceptualized and measured differently, and, consequently, their effects on the child may be different. For these and related reasons, other scholars have also urged distinguishing among these constructs (e.g., Grusec, Goodnow, & Kuczynski, 2000).

Warmth

Warmth has been almost universally recognized as a central influence in early socialization in classic and contemporary formulations. Warmth is most often studied as a characteristic of partners that promotes relational harmony and the young child's developing trust and socioemotional competence, whether those partners are parents, siblings, or child-care providers. Alternatively, warmth is sometimes portrayed as a mediator of the efficacy of other features of parental socialization practices, such as the warmth that is a component of authoritative (or democratic) parenting styles or of inductive discipline (Baumrind & Black, 1967; Hoffman, 1970). More recently, warmth has become increasingly portrayed as a dyadic construct, with the "shared positive affect" of the mother–child dyad found to be an important contributor to early conscience development (Kochanska, 1997). The latter approach underscores the bidirectional quality of warmth and its influence on overall relational quality. Although warmth has been portrayed, over the years, as either a characteristic of specific partners (typically parents) or the dyad, we believe that warmth is more strongly a *relational* construct when it indexes the shared affect of each partner toward the other.

Warmth is influential in early socialization in several ways. First, warm and supportive relationships with caregivers and other partners provide children with a sense that they are loved and respected. As a result, young children are more likely to develop trust in the caregiver's good intentions and, with it, a willingness to share activities, feelings, discoveries, and other features of personal experience (Waters, Kondo-Ikemura, Posada, & Richters, 1991). Second, warm relationships enhance children's motivation to comply and cooperate with relational partners, in part through their identification with them (Grusec et al., 2000; Hoffman, 1970). Taken together, warm relationships expand the opportunities for children to be influenced significantly by relational partners and their receptiveness to their socialization incentives. Finally, the influence of warmth through mood induction is also an important facet of early socialization. High amounts of warmth and positive affect in the context of close relationships heighten children's mood, and children and adults are more likely to be mutually attentive in the context of positive affect (Dix, 1991; Maccoby & Martin, 1983). Moreover, positive mood induction also enhances the compliance of young children with parental requests (Kochanska, 1995; Lay, Waters, & Park, 1989). As a broad index of relational quality, therefore, the warmth of one or both partners is an avenue by which partners become mutually responsive and influential.

Security

According to attachment theorists, a young child's need for secure trust in the protection of caregivers derives from biologically based motives that are deeply rooted in species evolution (Ainsworth, Blehar, Waters, & Wall, 1978; Bowlby, 1969/1982). A caregiver's sensitive responsiveness offers protection and nurturance that enabled human young to survive in the savannah grasslands of human evolution, and a young child's confidence in the adult's solicitude promotes exploration and the competence that it fosters. The confidence to explore provided by a secure attachment has many implications for early socialization because it creates opportunities for individual exploration of the environment and encounters with other people within the secure base afforded by the child's secure attachment. Security in the caregiver–child relationship thus moderates child-environment transactions that influence early experience and socialization.

Attachment research has also shown that a secure attachment significantly colors the parent–child relationship (see Thompson, 2006b, for a review). Young children in secure relationships are more receptive, cooperative, and responsive to the caregiver's socialization efforts, whether these entail enlisting the child's participation in shared activity or requesting compliance or the direct transmission of values (Bretherton, Golby, & Cho, 1997; Kochanska & Thompson, 1997; Thompson, Meyer, & McGinley, 2006). Thus security enhances a young child's willingness to be socialized, and this may be especially apparent for children with particular temperamental profiles. Kochanska (1991, 1995) has reported in several studies, for example, that for young children who are temperamentally relatively fearless, a secure attachment is a central predictor of early conscience development. By contrast, for temperamentally fearful children, attachment security is not directly associated with early conscience (although it remains an important relational resource). Instead, maternal discipline strategies that deemphasize power and are more "gentle" in approach promote the growth of conscience. These findings suggest that there are multiple relational pathways to early moral development, and that the influence of the relational incentives of a secure attachment depends, in part, on characteristics of the child.

Security has other important influences. The social competencies associated with a secure parent–child relationship contribute to more positive social relationships with other partners, such as other adults and peers. Attachment research suggests that security especially facilitates the child's capacities to experience greater closeness and intimacy in close relationships, such as with friends and teachers (Thompson, 2006b). As a result, a secure attachment may offer the child other rich relational contexts in which socialization occurs.

Finally, attachment theory also proposes that based on their history of sensitive parental care, young children create mental representations of relationships, as well as of their attachment figures and themselves, that influence how they experience subsequent relationships (Bretherton & Munholland, 1999; Thompson, 2006b). These "internal working models" constitute interpretive filters by which young children reconstruct their experience of new associations in ways that are consistent with their expectations from past relationships, and thus they color the child's responsiveness to new partners. As a result, children with secure or insecure attachment histories respond to other people in ways that may cause them, for better or worse, to evoke the kinds of responses from others that confirm their expectations for how people would react to them. Insecurely attached children may, for example, so anticipate a new partner's unfriendliness or unreliability that they remain distant and unengaged and, in so doing, evoke the kind of disinterested response from the person they expect. A securely attached child may, by contrast, evoke a much more positive response from the same partner, guided by a prior relationship history to respond more affirmatively and thus contribute to creating a warmer, more intimate relationship with that person.

Internal working models also color children's mental representations in ways that are relevant to socialization outcomes, including their understanding of people (such as their emotions), relationships (e.g., attributional biases, rules, and expectations), and themselves (Thompson et al., 2003). Although direct study of internal working models is difficult (Thompson & Raikes, 2003), research on the associations between attachment security and psychological understanding reveals that secure children show greater emotional understanding (Laible & Thompson, 1998), advances in conscience development (Kochanska, 1991, 1995; Laible & Thompson, 2000), more positive and constructive representations of relationships (Cassidy, Kirsh, Scolton, & Parke, 1996; Laible, 2004a) and more positive conceptions of self (Goodvin, Meyer, Thompson, & Hayes, 2005; see Thompson, 2006b).

Although these benefits of a secure attachment derive not only from a sense of security established early in life but also from the continuing influences of sensitive parental care, they together suggest that security is an important definer of broad relational quality in early socialization. Moreover, these studies indicate that the influence of security arises in the parent–child relationship and extends to other relationships partly through young children's mental representations of themselves and other people.

Mutual Reciprocity

A related but different portrayal of the importance of early relationships has been proposed by several researchers who argue that, at its best, the parent–child relationship introduces young children into a relational system of reciprocity involving the mutual obligations of each partner (Kochanska, 1995, 2002; Maccoby, 1984; Waters et al., 1991). In such a relationship, children who experience positive responsiveness from their caregivers become motivated to respond constructively to parental initiatives, accept parental values, and value the maintenance of emotional harmony with the adult as part of their reciprocal attention to the partner's needs and desires. Young children who are part of a relationship of mutual reciprocity are, in essence, eager and willing to be socialized because they experience an internalized obligation to respond constructively to the parent's initiatives owing to their history of responsive care from the adult. Parpal and Maccoby (1985) found, for example, that preschoolers were significantly more willing to cooperate with their mothers in a clean-up task if they had previously engaged in a session of mutually reciprocal play with them, compared to children who had not. As a consequence, parents can use less coercive or punitive methods to achieve their socialization goals because children more readily cooperate with the parent's goals. More broadly, a parent–child relationship of mutual reciprocity orients young children to the human dimensions of moral conduct (e.g., consequences for another for whom the child cares; see Hoffman, 1970) and provides experience with the kinds of "communal" relationships that children may also share with other partners in the years that follow.

The development of a relationship of mutual reciprocity begins with the parent's responsiveness to the child in the context of their shared positive affect. Research by Kochanska has found that, in addition, children and adults in such relationships exhibit greater empathic responsiveness and mothers use less coercive discipline approaches (Kochanska, 1997; Kochanska, Forman, & Coy, 1999). Once established, there is considerable consistency across situations and over time in individual differences in mutual recproicity between parents and young children (Kochanska & Murray, 2000), and it is related to important socialization outcomes, including conscience development (Kochanska, 1997; Kochanska et al., 1999; Kochanska & Murray, 2000; Laible & Thompson, 2000).

Taken together, research on early relational quality indicates that the general warmth, security, and/or mutual reciprocity of the parent–child relationship affects their specific transactions by enhancing or diminishing the child's receptivity to the caregiver's socialization incentives. At the same time, these relational features have somewhat different consequences, with attachment security influencing children's social skills and mental representations of self and relationships, mutual reciprocity contributing to developing sensitivity to the needs of the partner, and warmth fostering an identification of interests between parent and child (see also Grusec et al., 2000). In a manner analogous to how child temperament colors the impact of parental behavior on the child, the "relational temperament" created by mutual warmth or trust—or its absence—colors the influence of parents and children on each other. Relationship quality moderates the influence of the rewards and sanctions, emotional communication, content and quality of parent–child discourse, child's constructions of parental behavior, and other specific relational processes on young children's developing understanding, values, and character.

RELATIONAL PROCESSES

Within the broad context of relational warmth, security, or mutuality, a variety of immediate, specific practices by the parent or child provide the foundations of early socialization. Some of these practices are, as they are traditionally conceived, primarily under parental control; these include rewards and reinforcement, modeling, sensitive responsiveness, proactive regulation, emotional communication, and establishing family routines and rituals. Other processes are primarily under the control of the child, including how the child construes and interprets the adult's initiatives. Finally, although all relational processes are mutual to some extent, some relational processes are most evidently a matter of dyadic regulation, such as the influence of parent–child conversation on developing sociomoral understanding. Each of these interactional processes can occur with partners to whom a child is not in a close relationship, of course, such as with an occasional babysitter or a temporary child-care provider. But their impact on early socialization has been studied most extensively between relational partners, usually parents and offspring. In doing so, researchers have also begun to examine how the influence of these relational processes is moderated by the broader quality of the relationship they share.

Relational Processes Primarily under Parental Control

Although parents are not the only important socialization agents in early childhood, their influence is primary because of their ubiquitous role in the child's life, the deep emotional attachment of offspring to them, and the adult's behavioral sophistication which enables them to influence child socialization in diverse ways. Indeed, although bidirectional influences in the parent–child relationship are now widely recognized, parents still regulate many relational processes that are central to socialization outcomes.

Reinforcement, Rewards, Incentives—and Punishment

From the days of secondary drive and secondary reinforcement theories to explain infant–parent attachment, the significance of the rewards and reinforcement provided by the parent has long been recognized. Even before verbal praise and more tangible rewards are used to reinforce appropriate child conduct, the adult's warm hug and approving smile are believed to contribute to a toddler's self-esteem and motivaton to please the adult through compliance to behavioral expectations, and maternal warmth makes her affirmation a powerful reinforcer to the baby. Negative reinforcement can also be a powerful influence on child behavior, although, unfortunately, it is often the basis for coercive family processes, as illustrated by Patterson's influential program of research (Patterson & Fisher, 2002). During the preschool years, for example, young children's aggressive conduct is significantly influenced by the extent to which it is effective in ending family conflict when parents withdraw (Snyder & Patterson, 1995).

Parents seek to acccomplish both explicit and implicit socialization goals in their use of rewards and punishments. As noted by Grusec and her colleagues (Grusec & Goodnow, 1994; Grusec et al., 2000), parents' interventions into the lives of children are guided by diverse rather than homogeneous goals, and this begins early in life. Especially in Western industrialized cultures, for example, parents seek to reward self-initiative and assertiveness along with compliance and cooperation, and in specific situations parents may value communication, negotiation, and relational harmony as much as they do compliance (Hastings & Grusec, 1998). Thus a parent who is trying to enlist a young child's cooperation in rushing off to preschool may linger approvingly while the child tries to dress him- or herself, even though it delays their departure. Thus parents provide incentives for the development of many competencies in young children although, in practical terms, this can result in mixed incentives for young children's behavior in specific circumstances.

With increasing age, it becomes more important that children respond to internal incentives rather than merely to external reinforcement of competent conduct, and thus parental use of incentives must be subtle to ensure that children attribute their compliance to internal rather than external motives (Grusec & Redler, 1980). A socialization emphasis on fostering internal incentives proceeds in earnest in middle childhood but begins much earlier. Mothers help to provide a foundation for prosocial motivation, for example, when they provide their young children with emotionally powerful messages concerning the distress of another person and also clarify, when relevant, the child's culpability for that distress (Zahn-Waxler & Robinson, 1995). By focusing on the other person's distress, mothers encourage the child to respond prosocially based on emotional need rather than external rewards for doing so.

In recent years, there has been lively debate about the role of parental punishment, particularly spanking, in early socialization. According to a research review by Gershoff (2002), parental use of physical discipline has few positive effects besides inducing immediate compliance. Beyond this, she concluded, corporal punishment has considerable potential for undermining the parent–child relationship through the anger and humiliation it creates in offspring, fostering later aggression and undermining moral internalization and self-esteem. This literature has led researchers such as Strauss (1994) to argue that spanking should be culturally sanctioned because of its potential to lead to abusive parental conduct as an outlet for parental frustration and anger. By contrast, Baumrind (1996), Larzelere (2000), and Baumrind, Larzelere, and Cowan (2002) argue that prior research has failed to distinguish the effects of punitive, harsh discipline from the mild use of spanking as a normative discipline method and thus has overstated the detriments of spanking. They also argue, consistent with Kochanska's findings earlier reviewed, that child temperament influences the impact of spanking on moral internalization. Baumrind and Larzelere have concluded that spanking can be an appropriate discipline method, especially with young children, when it is used with reasoning, employed flexibly when other methods have proven ineffective, and motivated primarily out of concern for the child. The debate over spanking is important not only because of its practical relevance but also because it exemplifies the challenges of deriving proscriptive recommendations from complex behavioral data on an issue of significant cultural values. In the end, each of these views portrays the effects of spanking as being moderated by broader qualities of the parent–child relationship, predicting that spanking will have significantly different outcomes depending on whether it occurs in the context of an angry parent–child confrontation or reasoned child-centered discipline. They differ, however, in their expectations for which kind of relational context will predominate when spanking is used by parents in everyday circumstances.

Another illustration of how the quality of the parent–child relationship can moderate the effects of parental discipline practices is a study by Kochanska and her colleagues (Kochanska, Aksan, Knaack, & Rhines, 2004). In their longitudinal study, the security of attachment was assessed at 14 months, maternal discipline practices were assessed at 14–45 months, and measures of conscience development were obtained at 56 months. They found that the security of attachment moderated the association between maternal discipline and conscience. For securely attached children, there was a significant positive longitudinal association between measures of maternal gentle discipline/responsiveness and later conscience, but for insecure children, there was no association. Thus the influence of the parent's discipline practices depended, in part, on its meaning within the context of the security of their relationship. In secure relationships, offspring were attentive to maternal discipline practices and responsive to the parent's socialization efforts. Taken together, this literature suggests that the impact of parental practices related to discipline must be regarded not only in the context of bidirectional influences between parent and offspring but also in the context of their broader relational quality.

Modeling

With evidence for neonatal imitation and theoretical views of the relevance of early imitation to emergent understanding of persons (see contributors to Meltzoff & Prinz, 2002), scientific interest in modeling and imitative processes in early socialization has emerged afresh. One reason is the realization that even early imitative activity is cognitively complex, involving sophisticated inferences of the intentional activity of the model and that person's desires and goals (e.g., Carpenter et al., 1998). This means that, consistent with their emerging "theory of mind," young children perceive the behavior of a model with considerable psychological depth (Wellman, 2002). Imitative activity with a responsive partner is also attentionally and emotionally engaging to infants and young children because it enlists contingency perception and contributes to a sense of interactive control (Tarabulsy, Tessier, & Kappas, 1996). Another reason for renewed interest in modeling and imitation is the awareness that individual differences in young children's imitative activity may reflect broader relational influences, such as the child's identification with the other person (Forman & Kochanska, 2001). For these reasons, Meltzoff (2002) has argued that imitation may be central to the development of social and moral understanding.

Forman and his colleagues (Forman & Kochanska, 2001; Forman, Aksan, & Kochanska, 2004) have argued that a young child's willingness to engage in responsive imitation reflects motivational processes in the parent–child relationship that contribute to the efficacy of parental socialization incentives. Emphasizing that imitation entails the young child's active interest in emulating the parent's actions, these researchers argue that the same interest can also underlie the child's positive responsiveness to other aspects of parental socialization. In their research, Forman and Kochanska (2001) found that individual differences in 14-month-olds' willingness to imitate their mothers in a teaching task were longitudinally stable (to 22 months) and predicted children's compliance with the mother in disciplinary control assessments, as well as multiple assessments of conscience nearly 2 years later (Forman et al., 2004). Thus, along with classic views of how the imitation of specific behaviors contributes to behavioral competence in childhood, imitative activity may also reflect a child's broader responsiveness to the parent's socialization incentives from the relationship they share.

Parents are not the only targets of responsive imitation. Young children are also likely to imitate siblings, who are closer in age than are adults and who are also highly attractive models, and there is considerable research indicating that children develop important social and emotional competences from their observations of siblings (Barr & Hayne, 2003; Dunn, 1983; Sawyer et al., 2002). No research has examined how the quality of their relationship affects a child's willingness to imitate a sibling, however, and this remains an important topic for future study.

Sensitive Responsiveness

Sensitive responding involves both contingency and appropriateness: A sensitive partner responds in a manner that is both prompt and suitable to the need (Damast, Tamis-LeMonda, & Bornstein, 1996). Caregiver sensitivity is a central contributor to the development of relational security in infants and young children, but sensitivity also contributes to other important developmental outcomes, including attentional and cognitive skills, early language acquisition, play, and positive emotional expressivity (Bornstein & Tamis-LeMonda, 1997; Damast et al., 1996; Nicely, Tamis-LeMonda, & Grolnick, 1999; Tamis-LeMonda & Bornstein, 2002). For example, mothers who are verbally responsive to the behavior of young offspring facilitate early language acquisition (Tamis-LeMonda & Bornstein, 2002). The context of sensitive responding is important, however. Maternal sensitivity in play and other nondistress situations primarily fosters competence in play and cognitive and language development, whereas sensitivity to the infant's signals of distress is primarily associated with the development of attachment security and other kinds of socioemotional functioning (Bornstein & Tamis-LeMonda, 1997). A recent study by Rodriguez et al. (2005) showed, for example, that maternal unresponsiveness in a high-stress situation predicted toddlers' subsequent problems with self-regulation, but maternal unresponsiveness in a low-stress context did not.

Caregiver sensitivity has similar developmental influences outside the family. The sensitivity of teachers in preschool and child care classrooms predicts the security of children's attachment to their teachers and broader assessments of social competence in the classroom (Howes, 1999; Howes & Galinsky, 1998). Longitudinal research by the NICHD Early Child Care Research Network (2002a, 2002b) has found consistent associations over time between child care quality (a composite of measures including caregiver sensitivity in nondistress situations) and later assessments of social and cognitive competence, even after controlling for family factors.

Why is a caregiver's sensitivity important? One reason is that it contributes to a sense of agency and effectance for infants and young children: Sensitive responding to children's behavior contributes to their perception that their actions make a difference (Bornstein & Tamis-LeMonda, 1997). In stressful circumstances, sensitive responding contributes to the perceived efficacy of distress signals and of the child's capacity to access assistance when needed, together with confidence in the availability of the adult. This contributes to security, of course, but it also fosters the child's sense of control. In nondistress circumstances, sensitive responding affirms the intentionality and goal-directedness of the child's efforts at mastery, whether in the verbal responsiveness of the mother to the toddler's early word usage or in the assistance provided to a young child's efforts to build a tower. In each case, sensitive responding affirms and builds on the child's initiative and contributes to the growth of self-confidence. Moreover, sensitivity is essential to the scaffolding of new conceptual and socioemotional competencies that are created through the shared activity of young children with older people (Rogoff, 1990).

Proactive Regulation

Relationships afford opportunities for partners to have proactive influence: that is, to structure circumstances or experiences to create desired outcomes for the other person. Proactive regulation is an important feature of parent–child relationships. Accident prevention is one example of proactive regulation, especially because accidents are the leading cause of death and disability for young children (Peterson & Stern, 1997). Immunizations, pediatric health care, and nutrition have similarly proactive functions.

Another form of proactive regulation consists of the anticipatory prevention of discipline confrontations. Holden (1983) reported that mothers use a variety of strategies in the supermarket to avoid child misbehavior, such as circumventing aisles with tempting items and distracting the child through talk. Mothers who used such techniques had children who misbehaved less frequently than the children of mothers using only reactive control (i.e., responding only after misbehavior had begun) (see also Holden & West, 1989). Holden has argued that proactive control techniques have several benefits for parent–child relationships. They minimize conflict between partners and, by structuring the environment in such a manner that children behave appropriately, scaffold children's understanding of appropriate conduct.

As children mature, parents use other proactive strategies to shape children's values. For example, they may conceptually "prearm" children against competing values from outside the family by exposing them to these values conflicts and how to resolve them, such as by helping children to understand that other families have different beliefs about watching televised violence than they do (Goodnow, 1997; Padilla-Walker & Thompson, 2005). Parents monitor media exposure and other influences that may compete with family values. Parents also proactively manage children's activities—and the exposures they entail—by regulating permission and access (e.g., through transportation) and often supervising activities while they occur (Bhavnagri & Parke, 1991). Parents' strategies to guide children's values through proactive strategies like these must evolve as children develop from trusting dependents to offspring with independent mobility and ideas, but parental efforts to engage proactively in values socialization begins early.

Parents also engage in proactive regulation of young children's emotional lives (Thompson, 1990, 1994). They do so by structuring everyday routines and demands to remain within the child's developing capacities for emotional self-control, and by assisting offspring in anticipating emotional demands and how to cope with them. Mothers take care to maintain a supportive presence when young children are being introduced to stresses such as new child-care arrangements, for example, and visits to the doctor or dentist may be anticipated by conversations about what will happen and how the child will feel (Fields & Prinz, 1997). Proactive emotion regulation of these kinds is especially important for young children who are more vulnerable to becoming overwhelmed by stress because of their limited understanding of challenging events and their limited capacities for managing their own feelings. Beyond these, of course, parents manage children's emotional experience by keeping the child's stress within manageable levels through their own interventions. Parents who respond promptly to an infant's distress foster the child's developing capacities for emotional self-regulation by keeping the child's arousal within tolerable limits (Thompson, 1990).

In a study examining toddlers' coping with stress in relation to maternal support and the security of mother–child attachment, Nachmias, Gunnar, Mangelsdorf, Parritz, and Buss (1996) found that toddlers who were temperamentally inhibited in insecure attachment relationships showed the strongest physiological stress responses to novel events. Moreover, the behaviors of mothers in insecure attachments were also the least effective in aiding the toddler's coping efforts because they encouraged children to approach unfamiliar objects of which they were wary. These findings suggest, therefore, that toddlers' emotional coping was influenced by the interaction of an index of broad relational quality (i.e., security of attachment) with the specific coping strategies promoted by the mother. Further study of how relational quality affects the salience and influence of the adult's efforts at proactive regulation seems warranted.

Emotional Communication

Emotional communication is a central feature of relational discourse, especially early in life. Emotional communication can be seen in parent–infant face-to-face play, the emotional signals that are conveyed through social referencing, the effects on the child of affectionate or conflicted encounters between other family members, the influence of parental stress or emotional problems, and many other ways. These processes of emotional communication influence important socialization outcomes, including the development of young children's emotional expression and emotion regulation, social expectations, and psychological well-being. Thus although early relational quality can be broadly characterized in terms of warmth and other features, immediate processes of emotional communication are also important to socialization.

The influence of the emotional communication between parent and child begins early in infancy, with the emergence of episodes of face-to-face play at 2 to 3 months of age, and research on these early interactions illustrates the importance of emotional communicative influences. Face-to-face play has no other purpose than mutual enjoyment. Studies of these early interactions indicate that infants respond animatedly to the contingency in the adult's behavior, and from these encounters infants acquire general social expectations that partners will be responsive and interactive, person-specific expectations concerning the adult's interactive style, and understanding of the nature and influence of emotional signals (see Adamson & Frick, 2003, and Thompson, 2006b, for reviews). The importance of the emotional reciprocity of these exchanges is also reflected in studies of the interactions of depressed mothers with their infants. Depressed mothers are less responsive and emotionally more negative and subdued in face-to-face play with their infants compared with typical mothers, and their offspring become less responsive and emotionally animated as early as 2–3 months, even when interacting with another person (e.g., Cohn, Campbell, Matias, & Hopkins, 1990; Field, Healy, Goldstein, & Guthertz, 1990; Field et al., 1988). Furthermore, research by Dawson indicates that the infants of depressed mothers exhibit atypical patterns of frontal brain activity during social interactions with their mothers or other partners. These patterns remain apparent by age 3 if maternal depression persists, at which time young children also begin to show signs of the emergence of behavior problems (Dawson et al., 1999; Dawson et al., 2003).

By the end of the first year, infants are good consumers of the emotional signals they detect in the behavior of those around them, and the affirmative or cautionary messages they receive alter their subsequent behavior. This phenomenon, "social referencing," is especially apparent when infants are uncertain about how to interpret novel situations, and through this mode of emotional communication caregivers influence the young child's interpretation of events as dangerous, amusing, desirable, or forbidden (Bretherton, 1992). Social referencing is especially important in potentially hazardous situations, but it is also a broader means of conveying standards and expectations through emotional cues. The parent's emotional signals of caution or disapproval help toddlers to become aware of prohibited acts, for example, even when they are not necessarily seeking this information, and contribute to self-regulation as toddlers derive a new emotional appraisal of anticipated disapproved behavior (Kochanska & Thompson, 1997).

Vicarious emotional influences also occur within the broader family environment, as young children's emotional expressiveness and understanding are affected by emotional communication among family members (Denham, 1998; Halberstadt, Crisp, & Eaton, 1999; Halberstadt & Eaton, 2002). Not only is early emotional development affected by parents' direct responses to children's emotional expressions (see Eisenberg, Cumberland, & Spinrad, 1998), but it is also significantly influenced by emotional communication between other family members. Research based on the "emotional security hypothesis" of Cummings and Davies (1994) shows, for example, that in addition to the security derived from the parent–child relationship, children also experience security or threats to their emotional well-being based on the harmony of their parents' marital relationship. Parents' negative expressions toward each other provide young children with especially salient lessons in how and whether disturbing feelings such as anger are confronted or resolved, and the extent to which close relationships are preserved or strained by intense emotional exchanges. The emotional impact of parental conflict extends beyond behavioral modeling of aversive conduct to influence children's emotion self-regulation and

representations of relationships (Davies & Forman, 2002). In more extreme circumstances, in families characterized by domestic violence, parental psychopathology, or
heightened stress, young children's exposure to negative emotion is often so arousing that
it interferes with the child's processing of social and emotional information and psychological well-being, and this is one of many reasons why these conditions confer significantly enhanced risks for the development of clinically relevant problems in children (see
Thompson & Calkins, 1996).

In these diverse contexts, therefore, emotional communication is important because
it imbues social interactions with affective valence (and, in so doing, contributes to the
emotional quality of relationships), scaffolds developing understanding of emotional signals and their meaning, cues young children's appraisals of unfamiliar events and anticipated behavior, provides models for children's developing emotionality, creates demands
requiring emotional self-regulatory skills, and contributes to children's experience of
well-being or uncertainty within the family. These influences are particularly important
early in life when young children's social expectations and capacities for emotion management are rapidly developing.

Routines and Rituals

The structure of daily life is important to very young children who are seeking predict-
ability and control to everyday experience, and family routines and rituals provide much
of that organization (Fiese, Hooker, Kotrary, & Schwagler, 1993; Howe, 2002). Routines
involve recurrent patterns of family activity in which some or all family members participate, such as practices associated with meals, bedtime, and morning activity. Rituals are
routines that assume metacognitive meaning for family members because of their symbolic and affective significance, such as birthdays, weddings, and anniversaries (Sameroff
& Fiese, 1992). Family routines and rituals are unique to each family, vary across culture,
and are one important means by which young children acquire culturally appropriate
conduct (Serpell, Sonnenscein, Baker, & Ganapathy, 2002). Children's participation in
these family activities increases during the preschool years, and preschoolers also begin to
negotiate their participation in these family routines as they mature (Fiese et al., 1993).
Family routines and rituals are thus an important avenue for defining the roles and responsibilities of family members, expectations concerning everyday events, and family
identity and values.

Routines and rituals are important influences on early socialization also because of
how they are represented by young children. Research on early memory development
shows that young children bootstrap their recall of unique events on their representations
of familiar recurrent routines, such as how recollections of yesterday's trip to McDonald's
are organized around the internalized "script" for a typical visit to McDonald's (Hudson,
1993; Nelson, 1978). Likewise, children's expectations for future events are also boot-
strapped on their recall of analogous past events (e.g., a mother helps her young child
anticipate going out to a fast-food restaurant by talking about visits to McDonald's)
(Hudson, 2002). Thus everyday routines are a foundation for how young children represent their experiences, and this is one reason why young children become emotionally
committed to routines happening the same way on every occasion (such as bedtime).
Routines also become a socialization avenue for this reason. Parents' behavioral expectations for children are often related to familiar routines, whether they concern appropriate

conduct during meals, admonitions concerning self-care, simple manners, or participation in family activities (Gralinski & Kopp, 1993; Smetana, Kochanska, & Chuang, 2000). Because of young children's sensitivity to normative obligations (Wellman & Miller, in press), these behavioral expectations are likely to become incorporated into their "scripts" for familiar situations even though children have difficulty consistently complying with them (Thompson et al., 2006). In a sense, expectations for *how things are done* (during mealtime, bedtime, etc.) incorporate standards for *how one should act* in these situations.

Taken together, these relational processes—rewards and incentives (and punishment), modeling, sensitive responsiveness, proactive regulation, emotional communication, and routines and rituals—do not exhaust the range of avenues by which, in the context of close relationships, parents and other partners contribute to early socialization. They illustrate, however, that even early in life, socialization is far more than a matter of behavioral control and fostering internalized values. Early socialization also involves developing the relational incentives that enhance the partner's attractiveness as a behavioral model and the child's interest in maintaining relational harmony through cooperative conduct. It entails constructively structuring everyday behavioral and emotional demands to support the child's developing self-regulation and self-control. Early socialization involves fostering social and emotional understanding through nonverbal cues as well as explicit instruction. It also entails contributing to the child's self-awareness as effective, self-controlled, and compliant—what Kochanska (2002) has called the moral self—through cooperative responsiveness. As the studies reviewed in this section indicate, moreover, the influence of these socialization processes is shaped by the broader quality of the parent–child relationship, such that the impact of discipline practices or coping support in stress depends on the broader warmth or security of the parent–child relationship. It is important, in other words, not only who the partner is but the meaning of the partner's behavior in the context of the relationship shared with the child.

Relational Processes Primarily under the Child's Control

Socialization is not entirely under parental control, of course, even early in life. This is clear in the research earlier reviewed that shows how young children are influential through their choices of models and their motivation to responsively imitate them, their capacities for self-management that influence parental proactive regulation efforts, and their negotiated participation in family rituals and representations of the routines of everyday life. Furthermore, research on early socialization highlights the moderating influence of child temperament, by which parental discipline practices have differential impact depending on whether children are temperamentally bold or fearful (see, e.g., Kochanska, 1991, 1995). In this section, we highlight two other relational processes related to early socialization that are also primarily under the control of the child: interpretive constructions of the adult's behavior and self-understanding.

Constructing Social Experience

Socialization theorists now recognize that children are not passive recipients of social knowledge but actively construct understanding from their experiences. Consequently, how children respond to a caregiver's initiatives depends in part on how they perceive the message and meaning of the adult's behavior, which is based on the clarity and relevance of the parent's words, whether the intervention is perceived as appropriate, whether the parent's behavior is experienced as a threat to the child's autonomy or security, and other factors (Grusec & Goodnow, 1994). As children develop more sophisticated conceptual skills for interpreting and appraising parental behavior, their capacity to respond thoughtfully and appropriately expands significantly.

During infancy and early childhood there are remarkable advances in social cognition that influence how young children interpret parental initiatives. Many of these accomplishments are described as advances in developing "theory of mind" by which, beginning in infancy, children interpret people's actions in terms of their inferences of the mental states motivating behavior (see Wellman, 2002). Before the first birthday, for example, infants begin to regard others' actions as intentional and goal-directed, which contributes to the development of social referencing and social expectations for the behavior of parents and other familiar partners (Thompson, 2006b). Social expectations are important to the development of secure relationships (especially when expectations concern the adult's responsiveness when the child is distressed) and affect how infants and young children respond in social interaction, which is shown in studies of face-to-face play with typical and depressed mothers discussed earlier. Perceiving others as intentional partners also influences toddlers' social behavior, especially in their efforts to alter the partner's subjective, intentional orientation through communicative gestures and sounds (such as reaching toward the cookie jar while making imperative grunts and looking at the adult). By the beginning of the third year, young children interpret others' actions further in terms of desires and feelings and thus understand that a parent might be unhappy when his or her intentions or desires are frustrated. By age 5, young children understand the representational nature of mental phenomena and thus that one's thoughts and beliefs can be mistaken. This contributes to young children's dawning awareness of the privacy of mental experience (i.e., one can hide one's feelings and thoughts from others), developing capacities for deception, and growing ability to enlist display rules for emotional expressions in social situations (Thompson, 2006b). Thus young children's developing theories of mind enable them to interpret the reasons for others' behavior within a psychologically more sophisticated context, and this influences their expectations for social partners and their behavior toward them.

Developing conceptions of rules and obligations—or "deontic" reasoning—also advances significantly and enables young children to interpret parental socialization efforts more insightfully. Preschoolers strive to comprehend normative standards for their appearance, language (the meanings of words), social routines ("scripts"), and the integrity of objects (whole, not broken), and with respect to rules of conduct they likewise become attuned to normative obligations (Thompson, 2006b; Wellman & Miller, in press). Three- and 4-year-olds can easily understand and apply prescriptive rules (e.g., "painting is permitted if an apron is worn"), although children of the same ages have more difficulty applying descriptive norms (e.g., "Samantha always wears an apron when painting") (Cummins, 1996; Harris & Nunez, 1996). Preschoolers also understand that an actor's intentions are important in evaluating rule violations, but despite this, they are still prone to asserting inflexibly that rules and obligations cannot be violated. As noted by Piaget (1965) in his similar description of the "moral realism" of young children, this can cause preschoolers to be absolutists with respect to the application of behavioral standards to others, although not always to themselves because of the mental challenges of balancing knowledge of an external standard against awareness of one's own subjective intent in rule-violation situations.

Young children also become proficient at distinguishing between different types of obligations, differentiating moral rules from social conventional obligations (Smetana, 1981, 1985; Smetana & Braeges, 1990). By age 3, children regard moral violations as more serious and less revocable than social conventional violations (e.g., responding negatively to "Would it be OK if there was not a rule about it here?"), reflecting how these domain obligations are conveyed by their mothers (Smetana et al., 2000). This is important not only as a foundation for values socialization, but also because it instills early in young children an appreciation of the greater seriousness of the human costs involved in moral violations.

Taken together, these studies indicate that by age 5, young children are likely to be attuned to the psychological motivations underlying parents' actions, that parents can be mistaken or deceived, the obligatoriness of behavioral standards, and why certain standards of conduct are more obligatory than others. Much more research is needed to understand how these developing facets of theory of mind and domain understanding are applied in the everyday contexts in which socialization occurs, but together they suggest that young children enlist formidable conceptual resources in their interpretation of the parent's message and behavior. There may also be important differences between children in how they interpret parental conduct based on the quality of the parent–child relationship. Attachment theorists argue that from their personal history of care, young children begin to construct mental representations (or "working models") that are enlisted to appraise and forecast the parent's behavior. Thus attributions concerning the caregiver's intentions, motives, and emotional reactions may be biased by the representations derived from past caregiving experiences and how they are interpreted by the child. Young children in secure relationships may develop more positive expectations for the adult's emotional and behavioral dispositions than children in insecure relationships that cause them to perceive the adult's socialization initiatives as more constructive and appropriate. There has been little research directly testing these formulations, but studies in the attachment literature indicate that securely attached young children are more positively responsive to their caregivers and are more advanced on measures of conscience development, emotion understanding, and other psychological processes (see Thompson, 2006b, for a review). Taken together, they suggest that young children's construction of experiences of parent–child interaction are moderated by the broader quality of the parent–child relationship.

Self-Understanding

Infancy and early childhood also witness remarkable advances in the development of self-awareness and self-understanding. These influence how young children are socialized in at least three ways.

First, developing self-understanding contributes to a toddler's awareness of the self as a competent, causal agent whose actions are appraised by others in positive or negative ways. Beginning late in the second year, toddlers begin to develop conceptual self-representations that are manifested in verbal self-referential behavior, assertions of competence and responsibility, self-assertiveness, assertions of ownership, and greater sensitivity to the evaluative standards of others (see Thompson, 2006b; Thompson et al., 2006).

Young children's incentives to cooperate with parents are enhanced by their striving to be perceived as competent, responsible, and "big" and because of how their sense of self has become strongly linked with behaviors that evoke caregiver approval or disapproval (Stipek, Recchia, & McClintic, 1992).

Second, growing capacities for self-control and self-regulation enable preschoolers to develop internalized capacities to comply with parents' expectations. The growth of self-regulation in early childhood is a complex process that entails sophisticated cognitive abilities, including the capacity to understand the self as an independent agent, to remember and spontaneously apply behavioral standards, and to modify behavior and make adjustments according to these remembered guidelines (Kopp, 1987; Kopp & Wyer, 1994). These abilities emerge at the same time that young children are striving to be perceived by parents as cooperative, which is why parental expectations must be within children's capacities to comply.

Third, the development of self-referential emotions in early childhood enhances the affective incentives to comply with parents' socialization initiatives. Late in the second year and early in the third, young children begin to exhibit signs of pride when their behavior elicits praise from adults, and guilt or shame when their behavior violates explicit or internal standards of conduct (Lewis, 2000). Caregivers enlist these feelings in their discipline practices by explicitly linking their response to the standards that the parent has previously conveyed ("You know better than to hit your sister!"), invoking salient attributions of responsibility ("Why did you hit her?"), and often directly inducing the self-referent evaluation and affect ("Bad boy!"). In doing so, they provide a cognitive structure for the child's understanding of the association between prohibited behavior, the relevant standard, the child's responsibility for misbehavior, and the appropriate self-referential emotion.

These remarkable advances in self-understanding in early childhood underscore how much the efficacy of socialization processes depends on the child's developing self-image and capacities for self-control and suggest that variations in the content and affective quality of young children's self-concept may significantly moderate the influence of parental socialization incentives. Appeals to be a "good girl" or to earn the parent's praise may be of little value in a parent–child relationship characterized by hostility or avoidance and suggest that the association between the development of self-understanding and early socialization processes may be influenced by other features of the parent–child relationship, such as their shared warmth or the security of attachment.

Relational Processes under Dyadic Control

Although we have sought to distinguish relational processes that are primarily under the control of either the parent (or another socialization agent) or the child, it is arguable that the studies we have surveyed also illustrate the mutual, dyadic regulation of these socialization processes. After all, these literatures indicate that (1) the influence of many parental initiatives depends on the child's interpretation of the parent's behavior and capacities for self-control; (2) parents' disciplinary strategies are affected by their estimations of their effectiveness based on the child's past responsiveness; (3) childrens' responsive imitation of the parent as a behavioral model depends on the child's motivation to identify with the parent; and (4) processes of negotiation, bargaining, and compromise influence many aspects of parent–child interaction. In addition, because the quality of the parent–

child relationship moderates the influence of parent discipline and other socialization initiatives, dyadic influences are underscored.

Some early socialization processes are, however, more distinctively dyadic in how the
child and parent together create understanding as a result of their mutual interaction. The
contributions of parent–child conversation to early sociomoral understanding is one example. Beginning almost as soon as young children can participate in simple conversations, mothers and their offspring converse about shared experiences, storybooks they
have read, the behavior of others that they observe, pretend play, and even the conflicts
that divide them. Each partner contributes to the content and quality of these early conversations, with mothers and children together shaping the themes, affective tone, and
style of the verbal interactions they share. Equally important, research indicates that the
content, emotional tone, and style of these conversations contribute to early socialization
by influencing developing understanding of emotion, morality, and the self (see Thompson, 2006a, 2006b; Thompson et al., 2003, for recent reviews). Conversations with many
family members, including siblings, are significant catalysts to developing psychological understanding, but mother–child conversations are especially relevant to early socialization.

How mothers and children discuss shared experiences related to compliance and
cooperation, for example, influences early conscience development. In one study, the frequency of mothers' references to emotion when discussing the child's prior behavior at 30
months predicted children's performance on assessments of behavioral internalization
and cooperation at age 3 (Laible, 2004a). Interestingly, the frequency of maternal discussions of rules and the consequences of violating them was unrelated to later conscience in
this study, suggesting the special potency of conversing about the feelings of the child,
mother, or others involved in the child's good and bad behavior (Laible & Thompson,
2000). In another study, 2- to 3-year-old children whose mothers used reasoning and appeals to humanistic concerns in resolving conflict with them were more advanced in measures of moral understanding in kindergarten and first grade (Dunn, Brown, & Maguire,
1995). By contrast, mothers who were conversationally "power assertive" when recounting the child's misbehavior in the recent past—conveying a critical or negative attitude,
feelings of disappointment or anger, or involving reproach or punishment—had preschool
children who obtained lower scores on measures of "moral cognition" assessed via their
story-completion responses to moral dilemmas (Kochanska, Aksan, & Nichols, 2003).
Likewise, mothers who take the initiative to resolve conflict, who employ justifications to
explain their views and do not aggravate the conflict (such as with threats or teasing),
have children with greater moral understanding (Laible & Thompson, 2002).

These findings are important for at least two reasons. First, they indicate that conversations that occur outside the discipline encounter may be important forums for early
moral socialization, perhaps because younger children are more capable of understanding
parental messages when the child's cognitive resources are less consumed by managing
distress or negotiating with parents (Crockenberg & Litman, 1990; Thompson et al.,
2006). Second, they indicate that even in early childhood, conversational prompts that
focus on humanistic concerns (i.e., reasoning about people's feelings) are influential in
fostering the growth of conscience, and that conversations that arouse the child's defen-
siveness are less constructive in doing so. That these conversational influences emerge in
longitudinal analysis suggests, together with the findings of intervention studies and other
research, that these discourse features have a causal influence in stimulating the development of psychological understanding in young children (Thompson, 2006a).

Other aspects of parental conversational discourse may also be important, including how caregivers morally evaluate behavior, their attributions for culpability and causality, and the characteristics they attribute to the child and to others (Thompson et al., 2003). There is evidence, moreover, that how mothers talk about shared experiences is associated with other aspects of developing psychological understanding, including emotion understanding, conceptions of relationships, and young children's self-understanding (Laible & Song, 2006; see Thompson, 2006b, for a review). Miller and her colleagues found in a culturally comparative study, for example, that Anglo American and Chinese or Chinese American mothers emphasized different aspects of their child's character in recounting 2-year-olds' prior misbehavior (Miller, Fung, & Mintz, 1996; Miller, Potts, Fung, Hoogstra, & Mintz, 1990). Anglo American mothers tended to emphasize that misbehavior was the result of the young child's mischievousness or spunk, whereas Chinese or Chinese American mothers empasized the shame inherent in the child's misconduct, consistent with their cultural values. These conversational differences are related to how young children think about themselves in each culture (Wang, 2004).

In addition to conversational content, the style of parent–child discourse also influences young children's sociomoral understanding. In particular, the elaborativeness of the mother's narrative style is an important influence on developing moral and emotion understanding and their representations of their experiences (Thompson et al., 2003). In one study, mothers who were more elaborative when discussing shared events in the recent past—that is, who provided rich background detail and asked open-ended and varied questions—had offspring with more advanced emotional and moral understanding compared with mothers with a less elaborative narrative style (Laible, 2004a, 2004b). By providing children with rich detail about their personal experiences, mothers help children to understand better the causes and consequences of their actions and feelings, as well as the reasons for maternal expectations and requests.

Young children contribute to the content and style of parent–child conversation in many ways: by their willingness or resistance to participate (especially when discussing difficult or sensitive topics), by their topic-switching or introduction of new topics, by disputing the mother's interpretation of events, by their emotional demeanor during conversations, and by their capacities to put into words their emotional or psychological experience. Consider the following example of a reminiscing conversation between a mother and a 4-year-old (from Laible, 2005):

> Mother: So, when we went to Washington, did you have a good time?
>
> Child: Yeah.
>
> Mother: Yeah? Good.
>
> Child: But I really wanted to play with her toys and she did not let me play with them!
>
> Mother: Yeah. Sometimes it's hard to learn to share, isn't it? It makes some people feel bad when you don't share.
>
> Child: Sometimes I don't share.
>
> Mother: Yeah.

In this example, the child's topic-switching transforms the content, focus, and emotional tone of the conversation and, interestingly, leads to the child's acknowledgement of inappropriate behavior.

Other research has found that in conversations with their mothers about recent emotional experiences, 3-year-olds varied not only in their use of emotion words but also in their capacity to spontaneously generate labels for their own emotional states in the absence of a maternal prompt (Raikes & Thompson, 2005; see also Raikes & Thompson, 2006). These two facets of emotion language had different determinants: The security of attachment (assessed a year earlier) predicted emotion labeling but not the child's use of emotion words, while the reverse was true for differences in language ability. Most important, the child's use of emotion words and the child's capacities for emotion labeling each significantly influenced the course of parent–child conversation about emotion.

When conversing about shared experiences, both the adult and the child have their own representations of what occurred, and they may not agree. When they differ, shared conversation becomes a tutorial in divergent mental representations of the same event (Thompson, 2006a). This can happen frequently: One study indicated that mothers and their young children often differed about how the child felt during shared experiences, sometimes when the mother attributed goals or intentions to the child that were inaccurate (Levine, Stein, & Liwag, 1999). This indicates how much conversational content and quality is dyadically constructed.

Researchers have also found that the style of maternal conversation is adapted to young children's temperamental qualities (Laible, 2004b; Lewis, 1999). This is not surprising, given the variety of ways that temperamental features can influence conversational quality through their effects on the young child's interest in conversing about certain topics, prior behavior (that might be the topic of conversation), and behavior during the act of conversation itself. There are, in short, a variety of ways that children influence the course of conversation with adults.

Finally, just as the broader affective quality of the parent–child relationship is an important moderator of the effects of discipline on young children (Kochanska et al., 2004), the same is true of the effects of parent–child conversational discourse. Mothers' references to people's feelings interacts with the shared warmth of the parent–child relationship in its association with conscience development (Laible & Thompson, 2000; Thompson et al., 2003). Thus broader relational quality combines with specific features of parent–child discourse to shape young children's conscience development.

CONCLUSION

A relational approach to early socialization highlights the diversity of relational processes that contribute to important socialization outcomes in the early years. Far more than simply consistently enforcing behavioral standards, parents and other socialization agents contribute to socialized conduct by fostering warm relationships of mutuality that motivate young children to cooperate with the adult's expectations and goals. They contribute to socialization through nonverbal and verbal conversation that shapes young children's representations of normative standards of conduct, as well as their understanding of themselves and their relationships with others. Socialization is advanced through direct instruction and discipline practices, and also through the adult's proactive regulation of events to promote the child's cooperation, creation of routines and rituals within which behavioral standards are integrated, and sensitive responding in everyday circumstances. Even in the early years, young children are active participants in early socialization through their developing conceptual skills by which they interpret the parent's behavior and messages, developing capacities for self-regulation that promote cooperation and compliance, and participation in parent–child conversations that foster understanding of values and self. Beyond these specific relational influences, it is also apparent that early socialization is significantly shaped by the broader quality of the parent–child relationship. The warmth, security, and mutuality of the mother–child relationship moderates the influence of many specific socialization processes because of how the quality of their relationship confers meaning and significance to the adult's socialization initiatives.

These processes influence young children in a wealth of ways: values internalization, a developing "moral self," comprehension of the psychological processes underlying human conduct, conscience development, capacities for self-regulation and self-control, emotion understanding, and a sympathetic orientation to the needs of others are among the socialization outcomes that are fostered by relational influences in the early years. In this respect, the study of early socialization offers a new view of the developing young child. By contrast with traditional theories of moral judgment, for example, it is clear that young children are motivated by far more than punishment and self-interest. Their desire to maintain relationships of warm congeniality with people who matter to them, their developing understanding of people's feelings and needs, and their efforts to perceive themselves as cooperative and mature are also powerful incentives toward socialized conduct. The processes and outcomes of early socialization are highly consistent with the processes and outcomes of socialization at later ages, suggesting that infancy and early childhood establishes a foundation for lifelong socialization.

If this is so, future research could fruitfully be devoted to elucidating the diverse relational influences that shape young children's earliest comprehension of the values, norms, and purposes of socialized conduct in the early years. A relational perspective emphasizes the interaction of broad and immediate relational influences that shape development within the context of the mutual influences of two people who are behaviorally, emotionally, and representationally associated with each other. The research summarized in this chapter suggests that much is known about how these relational processes enlist young children into the human community, and more has yet to be learned.

REFERENCES

Adamson, L., & Frick, J. (2003). The still face: A history of a shared experimental paradigm. *Infancy, 4,* 451–473.

Ainsworth, M. D. S., Blehar, M., Waters, E., & Wall, S. (1978). *Patterns of attachment.* Hillsdale, NJ: Erlbaum.

Barr, R. & Hayne, H. (2003). It's not what you know, it's who you know: Older siblings facilitate imitation during infancy. *International Journal of Early Years Education, 11,* 7–21.

Baumrind, D. (1996). The discipline controversy revisited. *Family Relations, 45,* 405–414.

Baumrind, D., & Black, A. (1967). Socialization practices associated with dimensions of competence in preschool boys and girls. *Child Development, 38,* 291–327.

Baumrind, D., Larzelere, R., & Cowan, P. (2002). Ordinary physical punishment: Is it harmful? Comment on Gershoff. *Psychological Bulletin, 128,* 580–589.

Bhavnagri, N., & Parke, R. (1991). Parents as direct facilitators of children's peer relationships: Effects of age of child and sex of parent. *Journal of Abnormal Child Psychology, 8,* 423–440.

Bornstein, M., & Tamis-LeMonda, C. (1997). Maternal responsiveness and infant mental abilities: Specific predictive relations. *Infant Behavior and Development, 20,* 283–296.

Bowlby, J. (1982). *Attachment and loss: Vol. 1. Attachment* (2nd ed.). New York: Basic Books. (Original work published 1969)

Bretherton, I. (1992). Social referencing, intentional communication, and the interfacing of minds in infancy. In S. Feinman (Ed.), *Social referencing and the social construction of reality in infants* (p. 57–77). New York: Plenum Press.

Bretherton, I., Golby, B., & Cho, E. (1997). Attachment and the transmission of values. In J. Grusec & L. Kuczynski (Eds.), *Parenting and children's internalization of values* (pp. 103–134). New York: Wiley.

Bretherton, I., & Munholland, K. (1999). Internal working models in attachment relationships: A construct revisited. In J. Cassidy & P. Shaver (Eds.), *Handbook of attachment* (pp. 89–111). New York: Guilford Press.

Carpenter, M., Akhtar, N., & Tomasello, M. (1998). Fourteen- to 18-month-old infants differentially imitate intentional and accidental actions. *Infant Behavior and Development, 21*, 315–330.

Cassidy, J., Kirsh, S., Scolton, K., & Parke, R. (1996). Attachment and representations of peer relationships. *Developmental Psychology, 32*, 892–904.

Cohn, J., Campbell, S., Matias, R., & Hopkins, J. (1990). Face-to-face interactions of postpartum depressed and nondepressed mother-infant pairs at 2 months. *Developmental Psychology, 26*, 15–23.

Collins, W. A., & Laursen, B. (1999). *Relationships as developmental contexts. The Minnesota symposia on child psychology* (Vol. 30). Mahwah, NJ: Erlbaum.

Crockenberg, S., & Litman, C. (1990). Autonomy as competence in 2-year-olds: Maternal correlates of child defiance, compliance, and self-assertion. *Developmental Psychology, 26*, 961–971.

Cummings, E., & Davies, P. (1994). *Children and marital conflict.* New York: Guilford Press.

Cummins, D. (1996). Evidence of deontic reasoning in 3- and 4-year-old children. *Memory and Cognition, 24*, 823–829.

Damast, A., Tamis-LeMonda, C., & Bornstein, M. (1996). Mother–child play: Sequential interactions and the relation between maternal beliefs and behaviors. *Child Development, 67*, 1752–1766.

Davies, P. T., & Forman, E. M. (2002). Children's patterns of preserving emotional security in the interparental subsystem. *Child Development, 73*, 1880–1903.

Dawson, G., Ashman, S. B., Panagiotides, H., Hessl, D., Self, J., Yamada, E., et al. (2003). Preschool outcomes of children of depressed mothers: Role of maternal behavior, contextual risk, and children's brain activity. *Child Development, 74*, 1158–1175.

Dawson, G., Frey, K., Panagiotides, H., Yamada, E., Hessl, D., & Osterling, J. (1999). Infants of depressed mothers exhibit atypical frontal electrical brain activity during interactions with mother and with a familiar, nondepressed adult. *Child Development, 70*, 1058–1066.

Denham, S. (1998). *Emotional development in young children.* New York: Guilford Press.

Dix, T. (1991). The affective organization of parenting: Adaptive and maladaptive processes. *Psychological Bulletin, 110*, 3–25.

Dunn, J. (1983). Sibling relationships in early childhood. *Child Development, 54*, 787–811.

Dunn, J. (1993). *Young children's close relationships: Beyond attachment.* Newbury Park, CA: Sage.

Dunn, J., Brown, J. R., & Maguire, M. (1995). The development of children's moral sensibility: Individual differences and emotion understanding. *Developmental Psychology, 31*, 649–659.

Dweck, C. S., & London, B. (2004). The role of mental representation in social development. *Merrill–Palmer Quarterly, 50*, 428–444.

Eisenberg, N.., Cumberland, A., & Spinrad, T. L. (1998). Parental socialization of emotion. *Psychological Inquiry, 9*, 241–273.

Field, T., Healy, B., Goldstein, S., & Guthertz, M. (1990). Behavior-state matching and synchrony in mother–infant interactions of nondepressed versus depressed dyads. *Developmental Psychology, 26*, 7–14.

Field, T., Healy, B., Goldstein, S., Perry, S., Bendell, D., Schanberg, S., et al. (1988). Infants of depressed mothers show "depressed" behavior even with nondepressed adults. *Child Development, 59*, 1569–1579.

Fields, L., & Prinz, R. (1997). Coping and adjustment during childhood and adolescence. *Clinical Psychology Review, 17*, 937–976.

Fiese, B., Hooker, K., Kotrary, L., & Schwagler, J. (1993). Family rituals in the early stages of parenthood. *Journal of Marriage and the Family, 57*, 633–642.

Forman, D., Aksan, N., & Kochanska, G. (2004). Toddlers' responsive imitation predicts preschool-age conscience. *Psychological Science, 15*, 699–704.

Forman, D., & Kochanska, G. (2001). Viewing imitation as child responsiveness: A link between teaching and discipline domains of socialization. *Developmental Psychology, 37*, 198–206.

Gershoff, E. T. (2002). Corporal punishment by parents and associated child behaviors and experiences: A meta-analytic and theoretical review. *Psychological Bulletin, 128*, 539–579.

Goodnow, J.J. (1997). Parenting and the transmission and internalization of values: From social–cultural perspectives to within-family analyses. In J. E. Grusec & L. Kuczynski (Eds.), *Parenting and children's internalization of values* (pp. 333–361). New York: Wiley.

Goodvin, R., Meyer, S., Thompson, R. A., & Hayes, R. (2005). *Self-understanding in early childhood: Associations with attachment security, maternal perceptions of the child, and maternal emotional risk.* Manuscript in preparation, University of Nebraska-Lincoln.

Gralinski, J., & Kopp, C. (1993). Everyday rules for behavior: Mothers' requests to young children. *Developmental Psychology, 29*, 573–584.

Grusec, J., & Goodnow, J. (1994). Impact of parental discipline methods on the child's internalization of values: A reconceptualization of current points of view. *Developmental Psychology, 30*, 4–19.

Grusec, J., Goodnow, J., & Kuczynski, L. (2000). New directions in analyses of parenting contributions to children's internalization of values. *Child Development, 71*, 205–211.

Grusec, J. E., & Redler, E. (1980). Attribution, reinforcement, and altruism: A developmental analysis. *Developmental Psychology, 16*, 525–534.

Halberstadt, A., Crisp, V., & Eaton, K. (1999). Family expressiveness: A retrospective and new directions for research. In P. Philippot, R. Feldman, & E. Coats (Eds.), *The social context of nonverbal behavior* (pp. 109–155). Cambridge, UK: Cambridge University Press.

Halberstadt, A., & Eaton, K. (2002). A meta-analysis of family expressiveness and children's emotion expressiveness and understanding. *Marriage and Family Review, 34*, 35–62.

Harris, P. L., & Nunez, M. (1996). Understanding of permission rules by preschool children. *Child Development, 67*, 1572–1591.

Hastings, P. D., & Grusec, J. (1998). Parenting goals as organizers of responses to parent-child disagreement. *Developmental Psychology, 34*, 465–479.

Hoffman, M. (1970). Moral development. In P. Mussen (Ed.), *Carmichael's handbook of child psychology* (Vol. 2, 3rd ed., pp. 261–359). New York: Wiley.

Holden, G. W. (1983). Avoiding conflict: Mothers as tacticians in the supermarket. *Child Development, 54*, 233–240.

Holden, G. W., Thompson, E. E., Zambarano, R. J., & Marshall, L. A. (1997). Child effects as a source of change in maternal attitudes toward corporal punishment. *Journal of Social and Personal Relationships, 14*, 481–490.

Holden, G. W., & West, M. J. (1989). Proximate regulation by mothers: A demonstration of how differing styles affect young children's behavior. *Child Development, 60*, 64–69.

Howe, G. (2002). Integrating family routines and rituals with other family research paradigms: Comment on special issue. *Journal of Family Psychology, 16*, 437–440.

Howes, C. (1999). Attachment relationships in the context of multiple caregivers. In J. Cassidy & P. Shaver (Eds.), *Handbook of attachment* (pp. 671–687). New York: Guilford Press.

Howes, C., & Galinsky, E. (1998). Child care caregiver sensitivity and attachment. *Social Development, 7*, 25–36.

Hudson, J. (1993). Understanding events: The development of script knowledge. In M. Bennett (Ed.), *The child as psychologist: An introduction to the development of social cognition* (pp. 142–167). New York: Harvester Wheatsheaf.

Hudson, J. A. (2002). "Do you know what we're going to do this summer?": Mothers' talk to young children about future events. *Journal of Cognition and Development, 3*, 49–71.

Kochanska, G. (1991). Socialization and temperament in the development of guilt and conscience. *Child Development, 62*, 1379–1392.

Kochanska, G. (1995). Children's temperament, mother's discipline, and security of attachment: Multiple pathways to emerging internalization. *Child Development, 66*, 597–615.

Kochanska, G. (1997). Mutually responsive orientation between mothers and their young children: Implications for early socialization, *Child Development, 68*, 94–112.

Kochanska, G. (1998). Mother–child relationship, child fearfulness, and emerging attachment: A short-term longitudinal study. *Developmental Psychology, 34*, 480–490.

Kochanska, G. (2002). Committed compliance, moral self, and internalization: A mediated model. *Developmental Psychology, 38*, 339–351.

Kochanska, G., Aksan, N., Knaack, A., & Rhines, H. (2004). Maternal parenting and children's conscience: Early security as a moderator. *Child Development, 75*, 1229–1242.

Kochanska, G., Aksan, N., & Nichols, K. (2003). Maternal power assertion in discipline and moral discourse contexts: Commonalities, differences, and implications for children's moral conduct and cognition. *Developmental Psychology, 39,* 949–963.

Kochanska, G., Forman, D. R., & Coy, K. C. (1999). Implications of the mother–child relationship in infancy for socialization in the second year of life. *Infant Behavior and Development, 22,* 249–265.

Kochanska, G., & Murray, K. T. (2000). Mother–child mutually responsive orientation and conscience development: From toddler to early school age. *Child Development, 71,* 417–431.

Kochanska, G., & Thompson, R. A. (1997). The emergence and development of conscience in toddlerhood and early childhood. In J. E. Grusec & L. Kuczynski (Eds.), *Parenting and children's internalization of values* (pp. 53–77). New York: Wiley.

Kopp, C. B. (1987). The growth of self-regulation: Caregivers and children. In N. Eisenberg (Ed.), *Contemporary topics in developmental psychology* (pp. 34–55). New York: Wiley.

Kopp, C. B., & Wyer, N. (1994). Self-regulation in normal and atypical development. In D. Cicchetti & S. L. Toth (Eds.), *Disorders and dysfunctions of the self* (pp. 31–56). Rochester, NY: University of Rochester Press.

Laible, D. (2004a). Mother–child discourse surrounding a child's past behavior at 30 months: Links to emotional understanding and early conscience development at 36 months. *Merrill–Palmer Quarterly, 50,* 159–180.

Laible, D. (2004b). Mother–child discourse in two contexts: Links with child temperament, attachment security, and socioemotional competence. *Developmental Psychology, 40,* 979–992.

Laible, D. (2005). *Patterns of discourse between mothers and children.* Unpublished manuscript, Southern Methodist University.

Laible, D., & Song, J. (2006). Affect and discourse in mother-child co-constructions: Constructing emotional and relational understanding. *Merrill–Palmer Quarterly, 52,* 44–69.

Laible, D. J., & Thompson, R. A. (1998). Attachment and emotional understanding in preschool children, *Developmental Psychology, 34,* 1038–1045.

Laible, D. J., & Thompson, R. A. (2000). Mother–child discourse, attachment security, shared positive affect, and early conscience development. *Child Development, 71,* 1424–1440.

Laible, D. J., & Thompson, R. A. (2002). Mother–child conflict in the toddler years: Lessons in emotion, morality, and relationships. *Child Development, 73,* 1187–1203.

Larzelere, R. (2000). Child outcomes of nonabusive and customary physical punishment by parents: An updated literature review. *Clinical Child and Family Review, 3,* 199–221.

Lay, K., Waters, E., & Park, K. (1989). Maternal responsiveness and child compliance: The role of mood as a mediator. *Child Development, 60,* 1405–1411.

Levine, L., Stein, N., & Liwag, M. (1999). Remembering children's emotions: Sources of concordant and discordant accounts between parents and children. *Developmental Psychology, 35,* 790–801.

Lewis, K. (1999). Maternal style in reminiscing: Relations to child individual differences. *Cognitive Development, 14,* 381–399.

Lewis, M. (2000). Self-conscious emotions: Embarrassment, pride, shame, and guilt. In M. Lewis & J. M. Haviland-Jones (Eds.), *Handbook of emotions* (pp. 563–573). New York: Guilford Press.

Maccoby, E. E. (1984). Socialization and developmental change. *Child Development, 55,* 317–328.

Maccoby, E., & Martin, J. (1983). Socialization in the context of the family: Parent–child interaction. In P. Mussen (Ed.), *Handbook of child psychology, Vol. IV. Socialization, personality, and social development* (E. Hetherington, Vol. Ed., pp. 1–101). New York: Wiley.

Meltzoff, A. (2002). Elements of a developmental theory of imitation. In A. Meltzoff & W. Prinz (Eds.), *The imitative mind* (pp. 19–41). Cambridge, UK: Cambridge University Press.

Meltzoff, A., & Prinz, W. (Eds.). (2002). *The imitative mind.* Cambridge, UK: Cambridge University Press.

Miller, P., Fung, H., & Mintz, J. (1996). Self-construction through narrative practices: A Chinese and American comparison of early socialization. *Ethos, 24,* 237–280.

Miller, P., Potts, R., Fung, H., Hoogstra, L., & Mintz, J. (1990). Narrative practices and the social construction of self in childhood. *American Ethologist, 17,* 292–311.

Nachmias, M., Gunnar, M., Mangelsdorf, S., Parritz, R. H., & Buss, K. (1996). Behavioral inhibition and stress reactivity: The moderating role of attachment security. *Child Development, 67,* 508–522.

Nelson, K. (Ed.). (1978). *Event knowledge: Structure and function in development.* Hillsdale, NJ: Erlbaum.

Nicely, P., Tamis-LeMonda, C., & Grolnick, W. (1999). Maternal responsiveness to infant affect: Stability and prediction. *Infant Behavior and Development, 22,* 103–117.

NICHD Early Child Care Research Network. (2002a). The interaction of child care and family risk in relation to child development at 24 and 36 months. *Applied Developmental Science, 6,* 144–156.

NICHD Early Child Care Research Network. (2002b). Child-care structure → process → outcome: Direct and indirect effects of child-care quality on young children's development. *Psychological Science, 13,* 199–206.

Padilla-Walker, L. M., & Thompson, R. A. (2005). Combating conflicting messages of values: A closer look at parental strategies. *Social Development, 14,* 305–323.

Parpal, M., & Maccoby, E. (1985). Maternal responsiveness and subsequent child compliance. *Child Development, 56,* 1326–1339.

Patterson, G. R., & Fisher, P. A. (2002). Recent developments in our understanding of parenting: Bidirectional effects, causal models, and the search for parsimony. In M. H. Bornstein (Ed.), *Handbook of parenting, Vol 5. Practical issues in parenting* (pp. 59–88). Mahwah, NJ: Erlbaum.

Peterson, L., & Stern, B. (1997). Family processes and child risk for injury. *Behavior Research and Therapy, 35,* 179–190.

Piaget, J. (1965). *The moral judgment of the child.* New York: Harcourt, Brace.

Raikes, H. A., & Thompson, R. A. (2005). *Children's emotion language in mother–child conversations.* Manuscript in preparation, University of California, Davis.

Raikes, H. A., & Thompson, R. A. (2006). Family emotional climate, attachment security, and young children's emotion understanding in a high-risk sample. *British Journal of Developmental Psychology, 24,* 89–104.

Reis, H. T., Collins, W. A., & Berscheid, E. (2000). Relationships in human behavior and development. *Psychological Bulletin, 126,* 844–872.

Rheingold, H. H. (1969). The social and socializing infant. In D. Goslin (Ed.), *Handbook of socialization theory and research* (pp. 779–790). Chicago: Rand McNally.

Rodriguez, M. L., Ayduk, O., Aber, J. L., Mischel, W., Sethi, A., & Shoda, Y. (2005). A contextual approach to the development of self-regulatory competencies: The role of maternal unresponsivity and toddlers' negative affect in stressful situations. *Social Development, 14,* 136–157.

Rogoff, B. (1990). *Apprenticeship in thinking.* New York: Oxford University Press.

Sameroff, A., & Fiese, B. (1992). Family representations of development. In E. Sigel & A. V. McGillicuddy (Eds.), *Parental belief systems* (pp. 347–369). Hillsdale, NJ: Erlbaum.

Sawyer, K., Denham, S., DeMulder, E., Blair, K., Auerbach-Major, S., & Levitas, J. (2002). The contribution of older siblings' reactions to emotions to preschoolers' emotional and social competence. *Marriage and Family Review, 34,* 183–212.

Serpell, R., Sonnenschein, S., Baker, L., & Ganapathy, H. (2002). The intimate culture of families in the early socialization of literacy. *Journal of Family Psychology, 16,* 391–405.

Smetana, J. G. (1981). Preschool children's conceptions of moral and social rules. *Child Development, 52,* 1333–1336.

Smetana, J. G., (1985). Preschool children's conceptions of transgressions: The effects of varying moral and conventional domain-related attributes. *Developmental Psychology, 21,* 18–29.

Smetana, J. G., & Braeges, J. L. (1990). The development of toddler's moral and conventional judgments. *Merrill–Palmer Quarterly, 36,* 329–346.

Smetana, J. G., Kochanska, G., & Chuang, S. (2000). Mothers' conceptions of everyday rules for young toddlers: A longitudinal investigation. *Merrill–Palmer Quarterly, 46,* 391–416.

Snyder, J., & Patterson, G. (1995). Individual differences in social aggression: A test of a reinforcement model of socialization in the natural environment. *Behavior Therapy, 26,* 371–391.

Stipek, D., Recchia, S., & McClintic, S. (1992). Self-evaluation in young children. *Monographs of the Society for Research in Child Development, 57*(Serial No. 226).

Strauss, M. A. (1994). *Beating the devil out of them: Corporal punishment in American families.* New York: Lexington.

Tamis-LeMonda, C., & Bornstein, M. H. (2002). Maternal responsiveness and early language acquisition. In R. V. Kail & H. W. Reese (Eds.), *Advances in child development and behavior* (Vol. 29, pp. 89–127). San Diego, CA: Academic Press.

Tarabulsy, G., Tessier, R., & Kappas, A. (1996). Contingency detection and the contingent organization of behavior in interactions: Implications for socioemotional development in infancy. *Psychological Bulletin, 120,* 25–41.

Thompson, R. A. (1990). Emotion and self-regulation. In R. A. Thompson (Ed.), *Socioemotional develop-*

ment. Nebraska symposium on motivation (Vol. 36, pp. 383–483). Lincoln: University of Nebraska Press.

Thompson, R. A. (1994). Emotion regulation: A theme in search of definition. In N. Fox (Ed.), *The develop-ment of emotion regulation and dysregulation: Biological and behavioral aspects. Monographs of the Society for Research in Child Development, 59* (Serial no. 240), 25–52.

Thompson, R. A. 2006a). Conversation and developing understanding: Introduction to the special issue. *Merrill–Palmer Quarterly, 52*, 1–16.

Thompson, R. A. (2006b). The development of the person: Social understanding, relationships, self, conscience. In W. Damon & R. M. Lerner (Series Eds.) & N. Eisenberg (Vol. Ed.), *Handbook of child psychology: Vol. 3. Social, emotional, and personality development* (6th ed., pp. 24–98). Hoboken, NJ: Wiley.

Thompson, R. A., & Calkins, S. (1996). The double-edged sword: Emotional regulation for children at risk. *Development and Psychopathology, 8*(1), 163–182.

Thompson, R. A., Laible, D. J., & Ontai, L. L. (2003). Early understanding of emotion, morality, and the self: Developing a working model. In R.V. Kail (Ed.), *Advances in child development and behavior* (Vol. 31, pp. 137–171). San Diego, CA: Academic Press.

Thompson, R. A., Meyer, S., & McGinley, M. (2006). Understanding values in relationship: The develop-ment of conscience. In M. Killen & J. Smetana (Eds.), *Handbook of moral development* (pp. 267–297). Mahwah, NJ: Erlbaum.

Thompson, R. A., & Raikes, H. A. (2003). Toward the next quarter-century: Conceptual and methodologi-cal challenges for attachment theory. *Development and Psychopathology, 15*, 691–718.

Waters, E., Kondo-Ikemura, K., Posada, G., & Richters, J. (1991). Learning to love: Mechanisms and mile-stones. In M. Gunnar & L. Sroufe (Eds.), *Self processes and development. Minnesota symposia on child psychology* (Vol. 23, pp. 217–255). Hillsdale, NJ: Erlbaum.

Wang, Q. (2004). The emergence of cultural self-constructs: Autobiographical memory and self-description in European American and Chinese children. *Developmental Psychology, 40*, 3–15.

Wellman, H. (2002). Understanding the psychological world: Developing a theory of mind. In U. Goswami (Ed.), *Handbook of childhood cognitive development* (pp. 167–187). Oxford, UK: Blackwell.

Wellman, H. M., & Miller, J. G. (in press). Including deontic reasoning as fundamental to theory of mind. *Psychological Review.*

Zahn-Waxler, C., & Robinson, J. (1995). Empathy and guilt: Early origins of feelings of responsibility. In J. Tangney & K. Fischer (Eds.), *Self-conscious emotions* (pp. 143–173). New York: Guilford Press.

CHAPTER 8

Socialization in Emerging Adulthood

*From the Family to the Wider World,
from Socialization to Self-Socialization*

Emerging adulthood is a period of life that has developed in recent decades in industrialized societies, lasting from about age 18 to 25. A number of influences led to the rise of this new period. Economic changes from a manufacturing to an information-based world economy increased the need and desirability of obtaining additional education and training beyond secondary school. A scientific advance, the invention of the birth control pill, made it relatively easy for young people to become sexually active in their late teens without a high risk of pregnancy. Corresponding social changes, specifically, increased acceptance of premarital sexuality and cohabitation, further weakened the traditional belief that marriage must be entered before sexual activity begins. Median ages of entering marriage and parenthood rose into the late 20s.

Thus the period of life lasting from the late teens through (at least) the mid-20s changed in less than a half century from being a period of entering and settling into adult roles of marriage, parenthood, and long-term work to being a period when young people typically focus on their self-development as they gradually lay the foundation for their adult lives. During this time they gradually attain a subjective sense that they have reached adulthood and are ready to take on the full range of adult responsibilities (Arnett, 1998). It has been proposed that, developmentally, emerging adulthood can be characterized as *the age of identity explorations, the age of instability, the self-focused age, the age of feeling in between,* and *the age of possibilities* (Arnett, 2004, 2006a). These features have received empirical support (Reifman, Arnett, & Colwell, 2006). Further empirical investigation may change our understanding of the specific features that characterize this age period developmentally and reveal important variations according to socioeconomic status, ethnic/cultural group, and other characteristics, but this much seems clear: Full adulthood is reached later than in the past, and a new period of life has opened up in recent decades, as reflected in broader participation in higher education and later ages of marriage and parenthood (Arnett, 2004). I proposed the term "emerging adulthood" in order to apply a new term to this new period of life, and to distinguish it from the adolescence that precedes it or the young adulthood that follows it.

The question of the nature of socialization in emerging adulthood presents a variety of intriguing problems and challenges. The focus of most theory and research on socialization has been on the family–that is, on how parents socialize their children (Bornstein, 2002). But most emerging adults leave their parents' household and consequently are much less exposed to parental socialization than they were at younger ages. Even those who remain home or return home tend to be much more autonomous than they were in adolescence, as both parents and emerging adults adjust in response to emerging adults' increasing capabilities (Aquilino, 2006). So, the first challenge for a conception of socialization in emerging adulthood is to assess whether socialization still takes place during this period.

IS THERE SOCIALIZATION IN EMERGING ADULTHOOD?

Because the focus of socialization theory and research as been on childhood and adolescence, there is little to draw on directly for conceptualizing socialization in emerging adulthood. Some previous theoretical ideas have indirect implications. Erikson (1950, 1968), in his psychosocial theory of development across the life course, described early adulthood as a time when the focus of development is on the capacity for forming an intimate partnership. In discussing the challenge of intimacy versus isolation, Erikson implied that socialization was largely over by this time; the challenge is to risk one's identity, newly formed in the course of the socialization experiences of childhood and adolescence, by forming a committed intimate relationship with another person. Erikson also discussed the concept of a "psychosocial moratorium" during this period, which was the idea that some young people delay forming an intimate relationship for some years after adolescence and spend this time exploring various possibilities for their future. Here again, however, there was no suggestion that socialization was a major part of development during these years. The young person experiencing the psychosocial moratorium was depicted as an independent agent, guided by individual choice.

Other theorists have also contributed ideas that have limited application to socialization in emerging adulthood. Keniston (1971) described a period of "youth" between adolescence and young adulthood. However, Keniston (1971) viewed youth as a time of "refusal of socialization" (p. 9) and rejection of what the adult world has to offer to the young. His views were based on the student protesters of the 1960s and have an anachronistic quality by now. Levinson (1978) called ages 17–33 "the novice phase" of development, and argued that the central task of this phase is to move into the adult world and build a stable life structure. He emphasized the primacy of mentors as socialization influences during these years, but no research since then has verified this claim.

Thus the question whether and how socialization takes place in emerging adulthood remains wide open and in need of a fresh conceptualization that would apply to contemporary emerging adults. This question can be addressed by focusing on what socialization entails. According to Grusec (2002), socialization is how "individuals are assisted in the acquisition of skills necessary to function as members of their social group" (p. 143). In this process, elders and novices collaborate, with the elders helping the novices to develop the values, behaviors, and motives necessary to becoming a part of the social community. By this standard, socialization clearly continues through emerging adulthood. In fact, as noted, one of the social changes that has led to the development of emerging adulthood is the increased pervasiveness of post-secondary education and training, where emerging adults acquire from "elders" (i.e., teachers, professors, trainers, employers, and experienced workers) the skills that will enable them to participate in the modern economy. This process involves acquiring not only knowledge and behaviors but also values such as reliability and motives such as the attainment of self-sufficiency (Arnett, 1998).

Grusec (2002) further proposes that socialization involves three specific outcomes: (1) the development of self-regulation of emotion, thinking, and behavior; (2) the acquisition of a culture's standards, attitudes, and values, including a willingness to accept the authority of others; and (3) the development of role-taking skills, strategies for resolving conflicts, and ways of viewing relationships. I have proposed a similar framework of three goals of socialization (Arnett, 1995a), but here I use Grusec's (2002) conceptualization, as it applies especially well to socialization in emerging adulthood. However, I prefer "goals" to "outcomes," because the term implies intentionality and volition. All cultures have a conception of what it means to become an adult (Arnett, 1998), and the adults in a culture typically socialize the young toward gradually developing the beliefs and behavior they believe an adult should have. As part of the socialization process, adults convey to young people whether or not they are making adequate progress toward those goals.

In industrialized cultures, all three of the goals of socialization arguably continue to be developed in emerging adulthood. Self-regulation is by no means attained by the end of adolescence, for most people. With respect to emotional self-regulation, mood fluctuations are greater in adolescence than in childhood or adulthood, and depressed moods are common (Larson & Richards, 1994; Arnett, 1999). Emotional self-regulation improves substantially in the course of emerging adulthood, and consequently overall emotional well-being rises steadily from age 18 to 25 (Schulenberg & Zarrett, 2006). With respect to behavioral self-regulation, emerging adulthood is a period when a variety of types of risk behavior are highest, including substance use, driving while intoxicated, and unprotected sex (Arnett, 2000, 2005; Schulenberg & Zarrett, 2006). However, toward the end of emerging adulthood, in the mid-to-late 20s, frequencies of risk behavior decline substantially, suggesting the attainment of behavioral self-regulation.

With respect to the second goal of socialization, the acquisition of a culture's standards, attitudes, and values, here, too, socialization is incomplete at the end of adolescence and continues into emerging adulthood. Most notably, in Western societies, a central cultural standard is that, in order to attain adult status, young people should learn to become self-sufficient, to accept responsibility for themselves (Arnett, 1998). In numerous studies, across a variety of socioeconomic classes, ethnic groups, and nationalities, accepting responsibility for one's self has been found consistently to be the top criterion for reaching adulthood (Arnett, 1997, 1998, 2001, 2003, 2004; Facio & Micocci, 2003; Nelson, Badger, & Wu, 2004; Mayseless & Scharf, 2003). Furthermore, this criterion is rarely met by the end of adolescence; in these studies, few adolescents believe they have reached adulthood. It is during emerging adulthood that the cultural standard of accepting responsibility for one's self is gradually attained and people move from feeling in between adolescence and adulthood to feeling that they have reached adulthood.

Emerging adulthood may also be a key time for the development of the third goal of socialization, that of learning role-taking skills, strategies for resolving conflicts, and ways of viewing relationships. In their relationships with parents, emerging adults become notably more adept at role-taking, and their relationships with parents improve in part because they are better at taking their parents' perspectives (Aquilino, 2006; Arnett, 2004). Whether parents actually teach (explicitly or implicitly) role-taking skills that promote this change or whether the skills simply develop as a consequence of other social and cognitive changes in emerging adults is uncertain. It also seems likely that emerging adults change in their methods for resolving conflicts and in their ways of viewing relationships. Certainly, in their romantic relationships emerging adults become capable of a greater degree of interpersonal intimacy with a romantic partner than they had as adolescents (Collins & van Dulmen, 2006). However, whether this is due to advances in resolving conflicts and in viewing relationships is an intriguing but heretofore unexamined research question.

Overall, it seems clear that socialization is not complete by the end of adolescence and important developments in socialization take place in emerging adulthood. This leads to a second key problem in conceptualizing socialization in emerging adulthood: If parents play less of a role in the socialization of emerging adults than they do for children or adolescents, what are the sources of socialization in emerging adulthood? Most of this chapter is devoted to this question. First, however, I summarize my socialization theory and offer a few comments on the contexts of socialization.

CULTURAL, HISTORICAL, AND DEVELOPMENTAL CONTEXTS

As a framework for the remainder of the chapter, I use my theory of broad and narrow socialization (Arnett, 1995a, 2004). In this theory, I specify seven levels on which socialization takes place: the cultural belief system, the family, peers (including friends and romantic partners), neighborhood/community, school/work, media, and the legal system. The cultural belief system is the level that underlies all the others. Cultures tending toward broad socialization have cultural beliefs that value individualism, independence, and self-expression. Cultures tending toward narrow socialization have cultural beliefs that prize obedience, duty, and conformity. These beliefs then influence how parents parent, how teachers teach, and so on.

This basic contrast in socialization, between an emphasis on individualism and self-expression on the one hand and conformity and obedience on the other, has been a staple of theory and research on parenting in the United States for decades, using a variety of terminology. Two characteristics distinguish the theory of broad and narrow socialization from other approaches. First, it is a cultural theory, meaning that the focus is on the cultural beliefs that underlie socialization rather than on the parenting practices that reflect cultural beliefs. Second, the theory emphasizes the range of individual differences that cultures allow or encourage—relatively broad in the case of broad socialization, relatively narrow in the case of narrow socialization. In my view, the heart of socialization lies in the boundaries cultures set on the development of individuals. As Scarr (1993) observed, "cultures set a range of opportunities for development; they define the limits of what is desirable, 'normal' individual variation. . . . Cultures define the *range* and *focus* of personal variation that is acceptable and rewarded" (pp. 1335, 1337; emphasis in original). Similarly, Child described socialization as "the whole process by which an individual born with behavioral potentialities of enormously wide range, is led to develop actual behavior which is confined within a much narrower range—the range of what is customary and acceptable for him according to the standards of his group" (quoted in Clausen, 1966, p. 3).

It is important to emphasize that broad and narrow socialization are not two homogeneous categories but two points at either end of a continuum. Most cultures are not either broad or narrow, as pure types, but somewhere along the continuum, relatively broad or relatively narrow. Furthermore, in some cultures socialization is relatively broad on some levels, relatively narrow from others. Still, the various levels are interrelated and tend to reinforce one another, because the cultural belief system underlies and influences all the others. For example, if socialization in the family is narrow, it is likely to be partly because the cultural belief system is narrow. However, because each culture may be evaluated for the extent to which it is broad or narrow on each of the seven levels, the theory makes it possible to accommodate the great diversity in socialization practices of different cultures while also making a useful distinction between different general types of socialization.

The range of acceptable individual differences can vary between cultures, across history, and through the life course. Cultures differ in the degree of restrictiveness they impose, based on their cultural beliefs. Across history, as cultural beliefs change, socialization changes as well. Through the life course, socialization changes as people become more subject to or more exempt from the prohibitions and restrictions of others.

All three of these considerations, culture, history, and life course period, are important for understanding the socialization of emerging adults today. Culturally, emerging adulthood exists mainly in cultures that allow their young people a substantial amount of freedom from their late teens through at least their mid-20s—that is, cultures with relatively broad socialization. Emerging adulthood is a period in which people focus on their self-development as they consider the possible life paths available to them and gradually move toward making the choices that will structure their adult lives (Arnett, 2004). This requires a cultural belief system that values individual development over obligations and duties to others, especially the family. Such individualistic beliefs tend to develop mainly in cultures that are industrialized enough that economic interdependence among kin is not necessary for daily survival (Schlegel & Barry, 1991). Table 8.1 shows median marriage ages in various countries and suggests that emerging adulthood is experienced by the majority in economically developed countries but is not normative in developing countries.

Historically, emerging adulthood developed only in the past half century, as young people began to focus on their self-development in their late teens and early 20s and consequently the median ages of marriage and parenthood rose. There is substantial evidence that socialization in the U.S. majority culture broadened in the second half of the 20th century, when the individualism that has long been part of Western cultural beliefs became substantially more pronounced (Alwin, 1988; Bellah, Madsen, Sullivan, Swidler, & Tipton, 1986).

Within cultures, socialization may vary among subgroups, including periods of the life course. Socialization tends to be notably broader in emerging adulthood than at any other

TABLE 8.1 Median Marriage Age (Females) in Selected Countries

Industrialized countries	Age	Developing countries	Age
United States	25	Nigeria	17
Canada	26	Egypt	19
Japan	27	Indonesia	19
Spain	27	Ghana	19
Germany	28	India	20
France	28	Morocco	20
Holland	29	Brazil	21

age. Children have the boundaries for their behavior set by adults, even in a culture characterized by broad socialization. Adults generally decide what children will do and when they will do it, and adults communicate to children what is acceptable and unacceptable behavior in the culture, sometimes explicitly, sometimes by example. Adolescents, too, are under the authority of their parents. They may have greater autonomy than children (although not necessarily; in cultures that value female virginity before marriage, socialization may become narrower for girls when they reach adolescence; Schlegel & Barry, 1991), but their parents still set the rules and boundaries for their daily lives. Beyond emerging adulthood, once the adult roles of spouse, parent, and long-term worker are entered those roles set standards for behavior that adults are compelled to follow.

Socialization is broadest in emerging adulthood in the sense that this is when people have the most freedom to decide for themselves how to live and what to do and when to do it. Parents no longer have as much power as they did in childhood and adolescence, and obligations to a spouse or long-term partner, children, and long-term employer have not yet been entered. Emerging adulthood is a self-focused age, when social control is at an ebb and people have the greatest freedom to focus on their self-development (Arnett, 2004).

Consequently, emerging adulthood is the most diverse, heterogeneous period of the life course (Arnett, 2006a, 2006b). Nearly all children and adolescents live at home with one or both parents, and the great majority of adults live with a spouse or romantic partner, but emerging adults may live alone, with friends, in a college group setting, with a romantic partner, or with parents, and they change their living arrangements more often than persons at any other age period (Arnett, 2004). Nearly all children and adolescents attend school, and the great majority of adults are employed, but emerging adults have a dizzying range of combinations of school and work, and are also more likely than persons in any other age group to be "disengaged" (i.e., neither working nor in school) (Hamilton & Hamilton, 2006). Thus the consequence of the self-focused freedom conferred by broad socialization in emerging adulthood is that the variance in their living arrangements, school–work combinations, and other areas (to be discussed later) is greater than at any other age period.

THE RISE OF INDIVIDUALIZATION IN THE SOCIALIZATION PROCESS

An important sociological concept that can be applied here is "individualization." According to sociologists and historians of the life course (Beck, 1992; Côté, 2000; Heinz,

2002; Mayer, 2004), the life course has become deinstitutionalized in recent decades. Institutions (such as family and community) have lost their binding power, and individuals have gained more control of and responsibility for the direction of their lives. According to Heinz (2002), there has been "a shift from standardized, institutionalized life course patterns that constitute an age- and gender-bound temporal order of life towards the individualized biography" (p. 43). The result is individualization, meaning that people are no longer as constrained or supported by institutions as they were in the past, and must work out their life course choices for themselves. As Beck (1992) observes, the life course is now a "biography of choice" that requires individuals to weigh alternatives, evaluate outcomes, and repair failures without much help from institutions.

Sociologists rarely frame individualization in developmental terms, instead applying it to the life course in general. Nevertheless, they discuss it especially in relation to life-course transitions that pertain mainly to emerging adulthood, such as transitions related to education, employment, partnership/marriage, and parenthood (Beck, 1992; Heinz, 2002; Mayer, 2004). Applying individualization developmentally to emerging adulthood is useful for emphasizing that socialization is both broader now than in the past and broader in emerging adulthood than in other age periods. As Heinz (2002) notes, due to individualization there has been "a de-standardization of the programmed trajectories, *increasing variations* in the timing and duration of transitions in relation to the family, education, and employment" (p. 49, emphasis added).

Heinz (2002) makes an explicit connection between individualization and socialization with his concept of *self-socialization*. The self-socialization framework has two main principles:

> 1) Individuals construct their own life course by attempting to come to terms with opportunities and constraints concerning transition pathways and life stages. 2) Individuals select pathways, act and appraise the consequences of their actions in terms of their self-identity in reference to social contexts which are embedded in institutions and markets. (p. 58)

Thus individualization requires people to construct their own life course, so that socialization is something that is done by the individual rather than imposed by outside social or institutional forces.

As with individualization, the self-socialization framework is not presented developmentally, but it is easy to see the developmental basis that underlies it and how it pertains especially to emerging adulthood. Children and adolescents have limited freedom to construct their life course and choose their socialization contexts, because many of their choices are either structured by their parents or made by their parents directly. As for adults, once they select their pathways through the choices they make in work and family, the structure of adult life that is set up by those choices tends to perpetuate itself and resists change. It is during emerging adulthood that self-socialization is most pronounced, as people have more freedom to choose their socialization contexts and construct their life course than they did before emerging adulthood or will once they enter the roles and responsibilities of young adulthood.

Let us now return to the question of where and how socialization takes place in emerging adulthood, with a focus on the levels of family, peers/friends, school/work, and media. Family is addressed (even though, as noted, family socialization usually wanes in emerging adulthood) because socialization theory and research have traditionally focused mainly on parenting, and important changes in parental socialization take place in emerging adulthood. Peers/friends, school/work, and media are addressed because these levels of socialization are especially important in emerging adulthood.

FAMILY

If we accept that socialization takes place during emerging adulthood, to what extent do parents continue to be part of the socialization process? And to what extent does parental socialization in childhood and adolescence have effects that endure into emerging adulthood? There is no doubt that the parents' role in socialization diminishes from adolescence to emerging adulthood, as it diminishes from childhood to adolescence. Parents control nearly every aspect of their children's environment from birth through early to middle childhood. Adolescents begin to gain more autonomy from their parents, and consequently they spend a considerable proportion of their time with friends, unmonitored by their parents or other adults (Larson & Richards, 1994). Emerging adults are even more different from adolescents than adolescents are from children with respect to autonomy from parents, because they typically move out of their parents' household. Once they move out, their exposure to socialization from parents becomes voluntary, to a large extent. Indeed, avoiding their parents' efforts to influence their lives on a daily basis is a primary motivation for moving out in emerging adulthood (Arnett, 2004; Dubas & Petersen, 1996). Once they move out, emerging adults are able to control the information their parents have about their lives and let them in on only what they want them to know.

Nevertheless, the influence of parents continues to be evident in emerging adulthood on all three of Grusec's (2002) socialization outcomes. With the respect to self-regulation, parents assist in the development of this quality to the extent that they support their emerging adults' increased capacity for it. This does not mean withdrawing parental support, emotional and financial, once secondary school ends and emerging adulthood begins. On the contrary, it means flexibility in adjusting to emerging adults' needs for autonomy and dependency as the balance of these needs gradually moves more toward autonomy, perhaps in fits and starts, over the course of emerging adulthood (Aquilino, 2006). Most parents of emerging adults do quite well at supporting their emerging adults' development toward greater self-regulation. For example, one study of college students found that 70% of them reported that a parent did or said something that implied that the emerging adult was growing up and gaining in maturity (Bjornsen, 2000). However, some parents express anxiety or reluctance about their emerging adults' growing capacity for autonomy (Bartle-Haring, Brucker, & Hock, 2002).

Moving out promotes the development of self-regulation in emerging adults and also makes it easier for parents to support it. While emerging adults remain home, for most parents the daily presence of their emerging adults in the household proves to be too much of a temptation for attempting to regulate their children's behavior more than most emerging adults believe they need or want. Emotional boundaries, physical privacy, and parental intrusiveness often become critical issues (Arnett, 2004; Aquilino, 2006). Parents' attempts to regulate their emerging adults' daily schedules, eating habits, financial practices, and sexuality become sources of conflict. Emerging adults' progress toward full self-regulation proceeds more smoothly for both parents and emerging adults if they do not live together. For example, Dubas and Petersen (1996) followed a sample of 246 young people from age 13 through 21. At age 21, the emerging adults who had moved at least 1 hour away (by car) from their parents reported the highest levels of emotional closeness to parents and valued their opinions most highly. Emerging adults who remained home had the poorest relations with their parents in these respects, and those who had moved out but remained within an hour's drive were in between the other two groups. This suggests that parents and emerging adults often have different perceptions of the degree of self-regulation the emerging adults can manage. They get along better if they see each other less because the more they are together the more this difference becomes a source of conflict.

The influence of parents is also evident with respect to the second socialization goal, the acquisition of the culture's standards, attitudes, and values. An important standard with respect to emerging adulthood is the expectation that emerging adults will move toward self-sufficiency, an expectation that reflects cultural values of independence and individualism (Arnett, 1998). Parents influence their emerging adults' progress toward this goal by communicating the values of independence and individualism long before their children reach emerging adulthood. By emerging adulthood, both parents and children usually concur that it is best for emerging adults to move toward independence from parents and learn to stand alone.

One area of research that has implications for this issue concerns perceptions of what it means to become an adult (Arnett, 1994, 1997, 1998, 2001, 2003, 2004; Facio & Micocci, 2003; Mayseless & Scharf, 2003; Nelson et al., 2004). Across numerous studies, in a variety of industrialized countries, the consistent finding has been that the top three criteria for adulthood are accepting responsibility for one's self, making independent decisions, and becoming financially independent. All three of these criteria reflect common underlying values of independence and individualism (Arnett, 1998).

Both parents and emerging adults—in fact, persons of all ages—favor those three criteria as the most important criteria for adulthood (Arnett, 2001). Furthermore, all three criteria pertain to emerging adults' independence from parents. Accepting responsibility for one's self means not depending on one's parents to come to the rescue when unpleasant consequences result from one's actions. Making independent decisions means relying on one's own judgment rather than relying on parents for advice. Becoming financially independent means no longer requesting or accepting parents' financial help. By favoring the attainment of these three criteria for adulthood, parents may also communicate the importance of values of independence and individualism. However, studies have yet to be conducted indicating how much parents encourage the attainment of these markers in their emerging adult children, implicitly or explicitly.

Of course, independence and (more generally) individualism are not universal values but cultural values prevalent in industrialized societies, especially Western societies. But even within these societies, some cultural groups have values that depart from the values of the majority culture. With respect to conceptions of what it means to be an adult, an interesting contrast exists between the values of the majority culture in American society and the values of Asian Americans (Arnett, 2003, 2004). Like European Americans, Asian Americans place a high value on the individualistic criteria of accepting responsibility for one's self, making independent decisions, and becoming financially independent. However, a criterion that is highly valued among Asian American emerging adults but almost never mentioned by European Americans is becoming capable of taking care of one's parents. This is a criterion that is clearly derived from the traditional Asian value of *filial piety* (i.e., respecting, obeying, and revering one's parents). (Indeed, emerging adults in China have also been found to place high importance on becoming capable of taking care of one's parents as a criterion of adulthood; Nelson et al., 2004.) Thus, it can be reasonably presumed that Asian American parents (and perhaps others in the cultural community) convey the value of filial piety to their children in the course of childhood socialization, and it is expressed in emerging adulthood in the importance placed on becoming capable of taking care of one's parents.

The third goal of socialization, the development of role-taking skills, strategies for resolving conflicts, and ways of viewing relationships, is strikingly evident in relationships with parents during emerging adulthood. Relationships with parents typically improve greatly in emerging adulthood, compared to adolescence (Aquilino, 2006; Arnett, 2004). Conflict is lower, and warmth and closeness are higher. This is partly because emerging adults typically move out of their parents' household, and it is easier for them to along well when the friction that results from day-to-day living together is avoided. As noted previously, emerging adults get along considerably better with their parents if they move out than if they remain at home (Dubas & Petersen, 1996).

However, there is more to their improved relations than simply seeing each other less, and it is in precisely this area of enhanced role-taking skills and new ways of viewing relationships on the part of emerging adults. Emerging adults are considerably less egocentric than adolescents, and considerably better at role-taking with respect to their parents, which leads them to understand their parents as persons and not merely as parents (Arnett, 2004; Fingerman, 2000). They learn to view their relationships with their parents as more of a relationship among adults rather than strictly in terms of the roles of parents and children.

Whether this change in emerging adults is a consequence of parental socialization is unknown, and it seems unlikely that the direction of effects runs only from parents to children. Emerging adults may even drive the change in the relationship, through their development of new social cognitive skills (Labouvie-Vief, 2006). Parents welcome this change in their children, and parents change, too, becoming less didactic with their children and relating to them more as adults or at least near-adults. Their role as monitor of their children's behavior and enforcer of household rules diminishes, and this results in a more relaxed and amiable relationship with their children. Thus, socialization with respect to relationships between parents and emerging adults appears to be bidirectional, with both changing and both responding to the changes in the other (Arnett, 2004; Fingerman, 2000).

Parental Socialization and Emerging Adults' Psychosocial Development

In addition to research on parental socialization that pertains directly to the three socialization outcomes discussed earlier, there is a considerable amount of research describing the association between relations with parents and psychosocial development in emerging adulthood. This research is mainly in three areas: parenting and emerging adults' psychological well-being, parenting and emerging adults capacity for intimate relations with others, and emerging adults' responses to parental conflict and divorce.

With respect to psychological well-being, research pertaining to emerging adulthood confirms the long-standing finding of socialization research on childhood and adolescence, that the parenting combination of *demandingness* and *responsiveness* that characterizes the authoritative parenting style is consistently related to positive outcomes in children. For example, in a study of college students, Wintre and Yaffe (2000) found that authoritative parenting was related to higher academic achievement and successful adjustment to college life. Similarly, research on attachments to parents in emerging adulthood confirms findings from research on children and adolescents that a secure attachment to parents is related to positive outcomes. For example, a 6-year national longitudinal study in the Netherlands extending through the 20s found that attachments to parents did not diminish over that period and the association between attachment to parents and psychological well-being remained strong and positive (van Wel, Linssen, & Ruud, 2000).

Although authoritative parenting and secure attachment are positively related to favorable psychological outcomes in emerging adulthood as they are in childhood and adolescence, the nature of authoritative parenting and secure attachment change with the age of the children. Authoritative parenting for emerging adults involves a different kind of demandingness than at earlier ages, with broader boundaries and less monitoring; parental responsiveness is likely to be on less than a daily basis, especially once emerging adults move out of their parents' household. Secure attachment, too, is likely to involve less frequent contact with parents in emerging adulthood than at earlier ages, and the "secure base" provided by parents is likely to be more psychological than literal (Allen & Land, 1999). With both authoritative parenting and secure attachment, competent parental socialization includes adapting to the new capacities that children develop in emerging adulthood and fostering their autonomy even as a strong emotional bond to parents is maintained (Aquilino, 2006; Allen, Hauser, O'Connor, & Bell, 2002).

With respect to parental socialization and relations with others in emerging adulthood, research indicates that parental socialization is related to emerging adults' intimate relationships. For example, in one longitudinal study that followed a rural sample from age 12 to 21, authoritative parenting (high in warmth, support, and monitoring) in early adolescence was predictive of behavior toward romantic partners in emerging adulthood that was also warm and supportive (Conger, Cui, Bryant, & Elder, 2000). In another longitudinal study, beginning with a sample ages 13–18 and following up 6 years later at ages 19–25, family cohesion in adolescence predicted self-reported happiness in romantic relationships in emerging adulthood, especially for women (Feldman, Gowen, & Fisher, 1998). These studies appear to indicate that socialization in the family affects the development of interpersonal skills, which are then later carried into emerging adults' romantic relationships (Conger & Conger, 2002).

With respect to the effects of parental divorce, substantial evidence indicates that emerging adults who experienced their parents' divorce during childhood are at risk for depression and other mental health problems in emerging adulthood (Aro & Palosaari, 1992; Zill, Morrison, & Coiro, 1993). One study of a large national sample in Great Britain even showed evidence of a "sleeper effect" of divorce, with its negative influence on mental health becoming more evident in emerging adulthood than it was in childhood (Cherlin, Chase-Lansdale, & McRae, 1998). Furthermore, several studies have found that parental divorce in childhood is negatively related to emerging adults' capacity for intimacy and trust in romantic relationships (Jacquet & Surra, 2001; Summers, Forehand, Armistead, & Tannenbaum, 1998; Toomey & Nelson, 2001).

There is evidence that it is the parental conflict surrounding divorce, and not just divorce per se, that accounts for the relation between parental divorce and negative outcomes in childhood and adolescence as well as emerging adulthood (Sun, 2001). However, studies that control for parental conflict have found that the effects of divorce remain (Amato, 1993). Laumann-Billings and Emery (2000) noted that research on divorce typically focuses on disorders of behavior—how divorce affects functioning in school or work, for example—whereas clinical case studies typically focus on the distress that results from divorce—how divorce feels to those affected by it. In two studies of emerging adults, one with college students and one with a low-income community sample, they found that emerging adults often reported painful feelings, beliefs, and memories concerning the divorce, even if in their behavior they seemed to have recovered from it.

The Question of Parental Influence

Like studies on parental socialization at other ages, studies of parental socialization in emerging adulthood must be examined with respect to questions of interpretation, specifically, the question of the extent to which an association between parental socialization and children's behavior represents the influence of parents on their children or is due instead to other factors. One of the most important considerations is the possibility of passive, evocative, and active genotype–environment processes (Scarr & McCartney, 1983).

Passive genotype–environment processes occur in biological families when parents provide both genes and environment for their children. This seems like a truism at first glance, but it has profound implications for interpreting socialization research. It means that in biological families, when an association is found between parents' behavior and children's outcomes, it is difficult to tell if this association is due to the environment the parents provided or the genes they provided, because they provided both. In socialization research involving emerging adults, including virtually all the studies cited in the previous section, associations between parents' characteristics and emerging adults' characteristics are routinely described in terms of parental "effects" and "influences." However, this interpretation may be questionable, as it ignores the role of passive genotype–environment processes.

Behavioral genetic studies have begun to address this problem in socialization research, mainly using twin studies and adoption studies to unravel the usual confound between genetics and environment that occurs in biological families (see Moffitt & Caspi, Chapter 4, this volume). Few behavioral genetic studies on this topic have included emerging adults, but it could be expected that parental socialization effects would be smaller in emerging adulthood than in childhood or adolescence, due to the fact that emerging adults are less likely to have daily contact with their parents (Aquilino, 2006; Arnett, 2004). However, it is also possible that parental socialization in childhood and adolescence has effects that endure into emerging adulthood.

Evocative genotype–environment processes exist when children's genetically based characteristics evoke responses from parents (and others) so that the children's socialization is due not simply to the effects of parents on children but to the children's effects on the parents. This is part of the broader idea of bidirectional effects (i.e., the idea that socialization is an interactive process in which the direction of effects goes not only from parents to children but from children to parents). There is substantial evidence for this in the literature on socialization in childhood (e.g., Deater-Deckard, Fulker, & Plomin, 1999; Reiss, Neiderhiser, Hetherington, & Plomin, 2000). In emerging adulthood, the child-to-parent effect could be expected to be even stronger, because relationships be-tween emerging adults and their parents becomes closer to a relationship between equals (or at least near-equals) than it is in childhood or adolescence (Arnett, 2004). But re-search on bidirectional effects in emerging adulthood is scarce.

Finally, the concept of active genotype–environment processes means that people pursue environmental niches on the basis of their genetically based characteristics (Rutter & Silberg, 2002). It could be expected that active genotype–environment processes would be more evident in emerging adulthood than at earlier ages, because emerging adults have the freedom to leave the environment provided by their parents and seek out their own niches, to an extent that children and adolescents do not. Here as with the other varieties of genotype–environment processes, few studies have been conducted that involve emerg-ing adults.

There is substantial evidence that parental socialization influences development in childhood and adolescence, especially when parental socialization is at the negative ex-treme and especially in the area of antisocial behavior (Rhee & Waldman, 2002; Scarr, 1991, 1992). However, the extent to which parental socialization is influential in emerg-ing adulthood has yet to be investigated in a way that takes genotype–environment pro-cesses into account.

PEERS AND FRIENDS

What kind of role do peers and friends play in the socialization of emerging adults? Because research on peers and friends in emerging adulthood is very limited, it may be useful to begin by examining the research on peer/friend socialization in adolescence, then consider how it might change from adolescence to emerging adulthood. The abun-dant research on peer/friend socialization in adolescence has led to several conclusions. First, peers and friends are highly important in the lives of adolescents. Adolescents are happiest in the company of friends (Larson & Richards, 1994, 1998), and are closer to friends than to parents in many respects (Youniss & Smollar, 1985). Over the course of adolescence, the amount of time adolescents spend with friends increases while the time they spend with family decreases (Larson, Richards, Moneta, Holmbeck, & Duckett, 1996). Issues of popularity and unpopularity are prominent in secondary schools, and adolescents are acutely aware of how they and others rank (Stone & Brown, 1999). Thus, because of their importance in the lives of adolescents, peers and friends have a great deal of potential power in the socialization process.

Second, like people in other age groups, adolescents tend to choose friends who are similar to themselves in many ways, a process known as *selective association* (Berndt, 1996; Rose, 2002). Consequently, when similarities are found among friends, it is likely that the similarities were there before they became friends and in fact led to their friend-ship rather than that the similarities were produced by "peer pressure" or peer influence. Adolescent friends do influence one another, but those influences are complex. Although the influence of friends in adolescence is often assumed to be negative, toward violations of the socialization outcomes of self-regulation and conforming to authority figures (e.g., toward illicit substance use), in fact adolescent friends tend to reinforce their preexisting similarities (Berndt, 1996; Hamm, 2000). That is, adolescent friends who have a ten-dency for deviance encourage each other toward deviance, whereas adolescent friends who tend to follow the rules reinforce that tendency in each other (Maxwell, 2002).

Third, intimacy in friendships is higher in adolescence than in childhood and rises over the course of adolescence (Berndt, 1996). Prior to adolescence, friendships are based mainly on shared activities, but adolescents rate intimate features such as trust and loyalty as more important to friendship than younger children do, and adolescents are more likely to value their friends as persons who understand them and with whom they can share personal information (Buhrmester & Furman, 1987). Thus, with respect to the third socialization goal, of teaching role-taking skills, strategies for resolving conflicts, and ways of viewing relationship, friends also play an important part.

Unfortunately, research on friendships is as sparse in emerging adulthood as it is abundant in adolescence. Nevertheless, a number of contrasts can be drawn between the socialization role of peers and friends in adolescence and in emerging adulthood, based on what is known. First, peers and friends play a less prominent role in emerging adulthood than they did in adolescence. Emerging adults leave the peer-centered context of secondary school, so they are no longer part of a peer culture on a daily basis and are no longer guaranteed to see their friends at least 5 days a week. Emerging adults who enter a residential college context may also have a wide circle of friends, but this is a minority of emerging adults even at ages 18–22 (National Center for Education Statistics, 2002), and after college the number of friends in emerging adults' social support networks drops sharply (Fischer, Sollie, Sorell, & Green, 1989). Emerging adults also spend more of their time alone than adolescents do; in fact, emerging adults ages 19–29 spend more of their leisure time alone than any group except the elderly (Larson, 1990). Furthermore, emerging adults are more likely than adolescents to be involved with a romantic partner, which typically leads a selective withdrawal from friendships with peripheral friends while close friends are retained (Fischer et al., 1989). Overall, it seems clear that the opportunities for socialization influence by peers and friends decreases from adolescence to emerging adulthood. With peers and friends as with parents, emerging adults' relationships become more volitional, that is, emerging adults have more control over the extent to which they are exposed to the socialization influences of others.

Second, selective association in friendships may be even more pronounced in emerging adulthood than in adolescence. Although adolescents tend to seek out friends who are similar to themselves, parents are able to influence the peer networks their adolescents are likely to experience and the pool of peers from which adolescents are likely to select their friends, through the parents' choices about where to live, where to send their adolescents to school (e.g., public vs. private school), and where (or whether) to attend religious services (Cooper & Ayers-Lopez, 1985). Parental control in all these respects diminishes in emerging adulthood. Furthermore, emerging adults may be less responsive to the influence of their friends than they were as adolescents. Even in the course of adolescence peer influence diminishes, after peaking in early adolescence (Berndt, 1996). In emerging adulthood this decrease is likely to continue, as emerging adults see their friends less often and have more control over when and where they see them. In addition, emerging adults become very intent on learning to make their own decisions as part of becoming an adult (Arnett, 1998, 2003, 2004), which may make them less responsive still to the socialization attempts of their friends.

Third, with respect to intimacy in friendships, evidence indicates that it increases from adolescence to emerging adulthood (Collins & van Dulmen, 2006). Friendships in emerging adulthood tend to be characterized by greater emotional depth and complexity and greater communication about topics of personal importance. Thus, in contrast to the decline in friends' socialization influence that takes place in most respects, with respect to the socialization goal of learning role-taking skills, strategies for resolving conflicts, and ways of viewing relationships, friendships may rise in importance from adolescence to emerging adulthood (although little research has addressed this question directly).

What about romantic relationships as a source of socialization? There is a large literature on romantic relationships in emerging adulthood, mostly from studies of college students (Hatfield & Rapson, 2006). These studies generally focus on relationship quality and sexual issues. Although the results of the studies are rarely framed in terms of socialization effects, they pertain to the third goal of socialization, that of learning role-taking, conflict resolution skills, and ways of viewing relationships. These are all things that emerging adults learn in the course of having romantic relationships (Collins & van Dulmen, 2006). As with friends, the relationship skills learned in romantic relationships occur bidirectionally, between equals, in contrast to the power differential that usually applies when parents are socializing children.

In addition to the research on romantic relationships in emerging adulthood, suggestions regarding romantic relationships as a source of socialization can be found in the literature on the socializing effects of cohabitation and marriage. It has long been established that marriage has a variety of positive effects on physical and mental health (Waite & Gallagher, 2000). Emerging adulthood, the period just prior to marriage for most people, is a low-risk period for physical illness and disease but the highest-risk period of the lifespan for a variety of disorders and injuries caused by behavior, such as substance use and risky sexual behavior (Bachman, Wadsworth, O'Malley, Johnston, & Schulenberg, 1997; Schulenberg & Zarrett, 2006). Marriage has the effect of reducing the behaviors that lead to problems and thereby improving physical and mental health. It is single men who especially engage in high-risk behavior in emerging adulthood, so the change in their behavior once they enter marriage is especially striking (Waite & Gallagher, 2000). Although studies on the effects of marriage rarely frame their findings in terms of socialization, it seems evident that the decline in emerging adults' risky behaviors following marriage reflects increased conformity to their culture's standards, attitudes, and values. It also seems evident that their behavior becomes more well regulated after marriage, although this may be not so much self-regulation as mutual regulation in the marriage relationship.

The socializing effects of marriage presumably result at least in part from having a person around on a daily basis who monitors one's behavior and discourages behavior that reflects a lack of self-regulation or that violates cultural norms. It is surprising, then, that cohabitation appears to have little of the socializing influence of marriage (Waite & Gallagher, 2000). For example, with respect to substance use, the Monitoring the Future surveys have followed a sample from senior of high school through 10 years later (Bachman et al., 1997). Even in high school, the future cohabitors reported higher levels of drinking and marijuana use than those who had married or remained single a decade later. However, in the course of the decade following high school, the cohabitors reported very high and increasing levels of smoking, drinking, and other drug use, whereas those who married during that decade showed declines in all those substance use behaviors following marriage.

What explains these findings? Although emerging adults who cohabit are different in some ways from those who do not, such as being less religious and having higher rates of risk behavior in high school, these differences do not account for the differential effects of cohabitation and marriage. Even when these differences are taken into account statistically, the differential effects remain (Waite & Gallagher, 2000). Instead, there seems to be something about the institution of marriage itself that modifies the behavior of people who enter into it. Despite marked increases in cohabitation and divorce, young people continue to believe in what Waite and Gallagher (2000) call "the power of the vow" (i.e., in marriage as a permanent union that obligates those entering it to modify their behavior so that it is less risky and less violative of cultural norms). Thus, the socializing influence of marriage may be derived mainly from the beliefs that people have about what marriage requires of them.

SCHOOL AND WORK

Once adolescents finish secondary school, the main context of their daily experience becomes college, work, or some combination of the two (Hamilton & Hamilton, 2006). What kind of socialization takes place in these two contexts? Here again, few studies have looked at this question explicitly in terms of socialization issues, but other evidence can be used that has implications for socialization.

Let us examine school first. Although the majority of emerging adults in most industrialized countries are involved in some kind of schooling or occupational training in the first years of emerging adulthood, the nature of the school experience changes considerably from adolescence to emerging adulthood. The secondary school experience of adolescents is highly structured and closely monitored by adults. Adolescents are typically required by law to attend (at least until some time in their late teens, with the upper age varying among countries). They spend 4 to 7 hours a day in the classroom, where teachers record their attendance and monitor their behavior. Although they usually have some discretion in which courses to take, many of their courses are required as part of their general education. Thus, in addition to educating them, teachers and other school personnel are socializing adolescents to acquire cultural standards of doing what is required and conforming to or at least cooperating with the direction of authority figures.

The role of school in socialization broadens considerably in emerging adulthood. Involvement in school at all is discretionary, as there is no longer a legal requirement for attendance. There is a wider variety of schooling options to choose from, including an array of colleges and universities as well as vocational programs. For most of these options, the amount of time spent receiving direct instruction is relatively small, compared to secondary school, and more learning is to be done through assigned work that the students do on their own. Instructors are less likely to monitor whether or not the students come to class. Thus schooling in emerging adulthood requires greater capacities for self-regulation in order to succeed.

Like school, work takes place in both adolescence and emerging adulthood, but the nature of it as a socialization context changes, especially in the United States. Over 80% of U.S. adolescents have held a part-time job by the time they leave high school (Barling & Kelloway, 1999), and by their senior year of high school adolescents who are employed work over 15 hours a week, on average. However, the purpose of these jobs is mainly to obtain money to finance an active leisure life, not to obtain useful occupational training for the future. Most of the jobs U.S. adolescents hold are in restaurant work or retail sales (Loughlin & Barling, 1999) and are unrelated to the work they expect to be doing as adults (Schneider & Stevenson, 1999).

This has important implications for socialization. Because they have no personal investment in the long-term future of their work, adolescents have little reason to cultivate self-regulation on the job or to learn cultural standards of behavior that may be desired by their employers. Thus, although U.S. adolescents say they learn culturally valued qualities on the job such as responsibility, money management, and time management, longitudinal studies have shown that the more they work, the more they tend to engage in deviant behavior such as substance use, fighting, and vandalism (Mortimer, 2003). Also, a majority of working adolescents report some form of "occupational deviance" in the workplace such as stealing from employers or coworkers or giving away items for free or for less than their value (Ruggiero, Greenberger, & Steinberg, 1982). Thus, working in adolescence often undermines rather than promotes the socialization process.

Work in emerging adulthood has a much different nature. The stakes are higher, because most emerging adults are looking for employment not just as a way to provide money for the moment but as a way of building the foundation for the kind of work they will be doing in adulthood. This does not mean they suddenly become more responsible and less deviant in the workplace than they were as adolescents. On the contrary, employers are often reluctant to hire applicants younger than age 25 who have not obtained a college education, regardless of their secondary school achievements, because of the employers' experiences with emerging adults who have been irresponsible and did not prove to be worth the effort and expense involved in training them (Hamilton & Hamilton, 2006; Wilson, 1996). Nevertheless, most people gain in responsibility, future orientation, and planful competence over the course of emerging adulthood (Masten, Obradovic, & Burt, 2006; Roisman, Masten, Coatsworth, & Tellegen, 2004). The workplace rewards these qualities, so emerging adults have a strong incentive to respond to the socialization requirements of the workplace in order to succeed. If they fail to cultivate these qualities, they soon experience the painful consequences of being fired or failing to get the jobs and promotions they would like.

In European countries, there is not such a sharp contrast between work in adolescence and in emerging adulthood as there is in the United States. Work and school are more integrated, as most adolescents receive education and training in secondary school that is directly related to the occupation they plan to have once they leave school. Many adolescents are involved in apprenticeship programs that combine work with schooling that pertains directly to their work (Flammer & Alsaker, 2001). Thus in European countries there is more continuity in workplace socialization from adolescence though emerging adulthood, as self-regulation and cultural standards of responsibility and diligence are required and promoted consistently. However, this system is changing in response to economic changes resulting from globalization and becoming more flexible. The consequences of these changes for socialization in the workplace remain to be seen.

MEDIA

Media have held a substantial and growing place in the socialization environment of industrialized societies in recent decades (Arnett, 1995b; Dubow, Huesmann, & Greenwood, Chapter 16, this volume). For today's emerging adults, the media environment is more diverse and complex than it has ever been before. They are the "new media generation" (Brown, 2006), that is, the first to grow up with the Internet, virtual games, virtual friends (e.g., chat rooms), and make-your-own CDs, in addition to the traditional media of radio, television, recorded music, movies, newspapers, and magazines.

The importance of media in the socialization process can be seen with respect to the three goals of socialization. First, the goal of self-regulation pertains in part to sexuality and aggression, especially in emerging adulthood when risk behavior in these areas tends to be high (Lefkowitz & Gillen, 2006), and a large proportion of media content, especially the content most popular among young people, contains sexual and aggressive themes. Second, the goal of learning cultural standards, attitudes, and values is communicated in the media, through cognitive and social learning processes. Moral situations are depicted, certain behaviors are shown as rewarded and others as punished, some characters are depicted as admirable and others as despicable. Also, values of materialism and consumerism are communicated through the abundant advertising that accompanies most media. Third, the goal of learning knowledge and skills concerning relationships is promoted through media depictions of relationships, including between parents and children, romantic partners, and friends (Ward, Gorvine, & Cytron-Walker, 2002).

However, media also differ in an important way from other socialization sources, especially parents, school, and work (Arnett, 1995b). The goal of these other socializers is for children and young people to become socialized members of their culture, in the sense that they have attained adequate self-regulation; accepted mainstream cultural standards, attitudes, and values; and learned culturally appropriate ways of behaving in relationships. In contrast, the goal of most media is profit, the bigger the better. Thus the goal of the media is not necessarily consistent with and in fact may undermine the goal of the other socializers. Media companies are generally willing to sell content with sexual and aggressive themes even if it undermines self-regulation, which most media researchers believe it does (e.g., Cantor, 2000). Similarly, media content violating mainstream cultural standards, attitudes, and values will be sold if people will buy it, irrespective of whether it undermines that socialization goal. The cultural appropriateness of the ways that relationships are depicted is unlikely to be a major consideration among media makers, and content that is culturally inappropriate will be offered as long as it sells.

What role, then, do media play in the socialization of emerging adults, in particular? A good framework for answering this question is the media practice model (Brown, 2006; Brown, Steele, & Walsh-Childers, 2002; Steele & Brown, 1995). As shown in Figure 8.1, this model portrays media use as a dynamic process between the person and the media environment. The person's Identity (and, more broadly, personality) leads to the Selection of some media products rather than others. Even among those who select the same media products, their Interaction with those products results in differences in how they experience and make sense of them. They also vary in the Application of the media messages (i.e., the extent to which they incorporate or resist the messages). Their acceptance of the messages contributes to the further development of their identity. "Lived Experience" refers to the interconnections between media use and other contexts (e.g., when friends gather to see a movie or listen to music, or when parents and children disagree about the media content the children should consume).

Each of the elements of the model takes a distinctive form in emerging adulthood. Although Identity has traditionally been associated with adolescence, today identity issues are perhaps even more central to development in emerging adulthood (Arnett, 2004; Côté, 2000, 2006). With respect to media and identity development, in one study 70% of Canadian college students reported that they had a "celebrity idol," usually movie stars

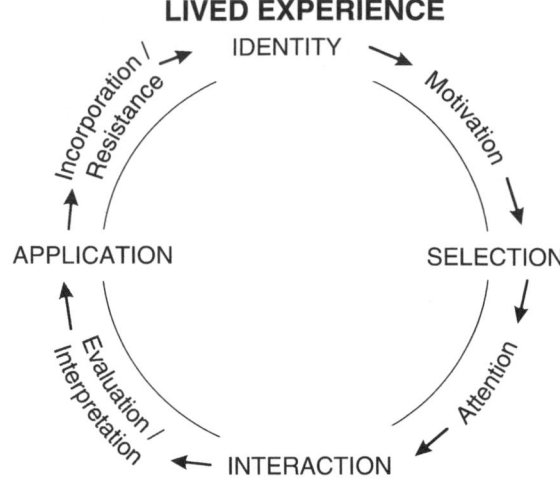

FIGURE 8.1. The media practice model. Copyright 1999 by Jeanne R. Steele, University of St. Thomas. Reprinted by permission.

or musicians (Boon & Lemore, 2001). More than half said their idols had influenced their attitudes and values, indicating the role of media with respect to that socialization goal. More than one-fourth said they had sought to change aspects of their personality to make it more like that of their favorite idol.

With respect to Selection, it is notable that media selection is less constrained in emerging adulthood than in any other age period. Children and adolescents have parents in the household who may disapprove, restrict, or prohibit their selection of certain media products. Beyond emerging adulthood, most adults have a spouse or live-in partner who may express disapproval or criticism of certain media choices. But in emerging adulthood, media choices are virtually unconstrained by any social influences. This may explain why the most avid audience for violent video games and Internet pornography is emerging adult men (Brown, 2006). Here, as in some other respects, socialization is never broader than it is in emerging adulthood.

However, the effects of media on emerging adults may be different than they are for children and adolescents, due to developmental differences in interaction and application. Although very few studies have compared adolescents and emerging adults in their responses to media, research on cognitive development has demonstrated that emerging adults think in ways that are more complex, reflective, and insightful (Labouvie-Vief, 2006), and this may mean that they are more capable than adolescents of stepping back from media content, evaluating it, and consciously resisting it. Even in adolescence, the effects of media are not as strong as they are in childhood (Huesmann, Moise-Titus, Podolski, & Eron, 2003), and it seems likely that the dilution of direct media effects continues into emerging adulthood. In emerging adulthood even more than earlier development, media effects are likely to be subtle and conditional. Nevertheless, media effects on college students have been reported in diverse areas, including aggression, body image, occupational choice, and political ideology (Brown, 2006). But more research is needed on non-college emerging adults and comparing adolescents and emerging adults. More research is also needed on potential positive effects of media use in emerging adulthood (see Dubow et al., Chapter 16, this volume), such as providing information in areas of education and occupation.

CONCLUSION

In industrialized societies, and in the growing middle class of developing countries, adulthood is reached later today than in the past (Arnett, 1998). Economic changes have made it more desirable for young people to obtain education and training past secondary school in order to qualify for jobs in the new information-based world economy. More important, growing individualism has allowed young people greater freedom to decide when to enter adult roles of marriage, parenthood, and long-term work, and given this freedom many of them wait until at least their mid-20s before doing so. As a result, a new period of the life course, emerging adulthood, has developed in between adolescence and young adulthood.

For emerging adults, the socialization goals of self-regulation, developing a set of beliefs and values, and learning roles and relationship skills are still very much in progress, not yet reached. However, the nature of the socialization process changes from adolescence to emerging adulthood. Parents and peers/friends are still involved in socialization for emerging adults, but to less of an extent than they were in adolescence. School remains a socialization context for emerging adults, but in a broader, less restrictive form, and only for *some* emerging adults. Thus institutional frameworks weaken in the socialization process and emerging adults experience individualization, as they are left on their own to make their way to adulthood through self-socialization. This freedom can be exhilarating, but some find it disconcerting and disorienting. Socialization can become so broad that it provides inadequate support and guidance, so that the goals of socialization may remain elusive. But the extent to which emerging adults thrive or struggle under their exceptionally broad socialization is still largely unknown.

The field of emerging adulthood is new, and the study of socialization in emerging adulthood is in a nascent stage. Although quite a bit is known about parental socialization in emerging adulthood, research on socialization with respect to peers/friends, school and work, and the media is sparse. This limits the extent to which a full picture of socialization in emerging adulthood can be drawn, but it presents great opportunities for creative theory and research for scholars seeking to contribute to this growing field.

REFERENCES

Allen, J., Hauser, S., O'Connor, T., & Bell, K. (2002). Prediction of peer-rated adult hostility from autonomy struggles in adolescent-family interactions. *Development and Psychopathology, 14,* 123–137.

Allen, J., & Land, P. (1999). Attachment in adolescence. In J. Cassidy & P. R. Shaver (Eds.), *Handbook of attachment: Theory, research, and clinical applications.* New York: Guilford Press.

Alwin, D. F. (1988). From obedience to autonomy: Changes in desired traits in children, 1928–1978. *Public Opinion Quarterly, 52,* 33–52.

Amato, P. R. (1993). Family structure, family process, and family ideology. *Journal of Marriage & the Family, 55,* 50–54.

Aquilino, W. S. (2006). Family relationships and support systems in emerging adulthood. In J. J. Arnett & J.

L. Tanner (Eds.), *Coming of age in the 21st century: The lives and contexts of emerging adults* (pp. 193–217). Washington, DC: American Psychological Association.

Arnett, J. J. (1995a). Broad and narrow socialization: The family in the context of a cultural theory. *Journal of Marriage and the Family, 57,* 617–628.

Arnett, J. J. (1995b). Adolescents' uses of media for self–socialization. *Journal of Youth and Adolescence, 24,* 519–533.

Arnett, J.J. (1997). Young people's conceptions of the transition to adulthood. *Youth and Society, 29,* 1–23.

Arnett, J. J. (1998). Learning to stand alone: The contemporary American transition to adulthood in cultural and historical context. *Human Development, 41,* 295–315.

Arnett, J. J. (1999). Adolescent storm and stress, reconsidered. *American Psychologist, 54,* 317–326.

Arnett, J. J. (2000). Emerging adulthood: A theory of development from the late teens through the twenties. *American Psychologist, 55,* 469–480.

Arnett, J. J. (2001). Conceptions of the transition to adulthood: Perspectives from adolescence to midlife. *Journal of Adult Development, 8,* 133–143.

Arnett, J. J. (2002). The psychology of globalization. *American Psychologist, 57,* 774–783.

Arnett, J. J. (2003). Conceptions of the transition to adulthood among emerging adults in American ethnic groups. *New Directions in Child and Adolescent Development, 100,* 63–75.

Arnett, J. J. (2004). *Emerging adulthood: The winding road from the late teens through the twenties.* New York: Oxford University Press.

Arnett, J. J. (2005). The developmental context of substance use in emerging adulthood. *Journal of Drug Issues, 35,* 235–253.

Arnett, J. J. (2006a). Emerging adulthood: Understanding the new way of coming of age. In J. J. Arnett & J. L. Tanner (Eds.), *Coming of age in the 21st century: The lives and contexts of emerging adults* (pp. 3–19). Washington, DC: American Psychological Association.

Arnett, J. J. (2006b). The psychology of emerging adulthood: What is known, and what remains to be known? In J. J. Arnett & J. L. Tanner (Eds.), *Coming of age in the 21st century: The lives and contexts of emerging adults* (pp. 303–330). Washington, DC: American Psychological Association.

Aro, H. M., & Palosaari, U. (1992). Parental divorce, adolescence, and the transition to young adulthood: A follow-up study. *American Journal of Orthopsychiatry, 62,* 421–429.

Bachman, J. G., Wadsworth, K. N., O'Malley, P. M., Johnston, L. D., & Schulenberg, J. E. (1997). *Smoking, drinking, and drug use in young adulthood: The impacts of new freedoms and new responsibilities.* Mahwah, NJ: Erlbaum.

Barling, J., & Kelloway, E. K. (1999). *Young workers: Varieties of experience.* Washington, DC: American Psychological Association.

Bartle-Haring, S., Brucker, P., & Hock, E. (2002). The impact of parental separation anxiety on identity development in late adolescence and early adulthood. *Journal of Adolescent Research, 17,* 439–450.

Beck, U. (1992). *Risk society: Toward a new modernity.* London: Sage.

Bellah, R. N., Madsen, R., Sullivan, W. M., Swidler, A., & Tipton, S. M. (1985). *Habits of the heart: Individualism and committment in American life.* New York: Harper & Row.

Berndt, T. J. (1996). Transitions in friendship and friends' influence. In J. A. Graber, J. Brooks-Gunn, & A. C. Petersen (Eds.), *Transitions through adolescence: Interpersonal domains and context.* Mahwah, NJ: Erlbaum.

Bjornsen, C. (2000). The blessing as a rite of passage in adolescence. *Adolescence, 35,* 357–363.

Boon, S. D., & Lemore, C. D. (2001). Admirer-celebrity relationships among young adults: Explaining perceptions of celebrity influence on identity. *Human Communication Research, 27,* 432–465.

Bornstein, M. (Ed.). (2002). *Handbook of parenting.* Mahwah, NJ: Erlbaum.

Brown, J.D. (2006). Emerging adults in a mediated world. In J.J. Arnett & J.L. Tanner (Eds.), *Coming of age in the 21st century: The lives and contexts of emerging adults* (pp. 279–299). Washington, DC: American Psychological Association.

Brown, J. D., Steele, J., & Walsh-Childers, K. (Eds.). (2002). *Sexual teens, sexual media.* Mahwah, NJ: Erlbaum.

Buhrmester, D., & Furman, W. (1987). The development of companionship and intimacy. *Child Development, 58,* 1101–1113.

Cantor, J. (2000). Violence in films and television. In R. Lee (Ed.), *Encyclopedia of international media and communications.* New York: Academic Press.

Cherlin, A. J., Chase-Lansdale, P. L., & McRae, C. (1998). Effects of parental divorce on mental health throughout the life course. *American Sociological Review, 63,* 239–249.

Clausen, J. A. (1966). *Socialization and society.* Boston: Little, Brown.

Collins, W. A., & van Dulmen, M. (2006). Friendships and romance in emerging adulthood: Assessing distinctiveness in close relationships. In J.J. Arnett & J.L. Tanner (Eds.), *Coming of age in the 21st century: The lives and contexts of emerging adults* (pp. 219–234). Washington, DC: American Psychological Association.

Conger, R., & Conger, K. (2002). Resilience in midwestern families: Selected findings from the first decade of a prospective, longitudinal study. *Journal of Marriage and Family, 64,* 361–373.

Conger, R., Cui, M., Bryant, C., & Elder, G. (2000). Competence in early adult romantic relationships: A developmental perspective on family influences. *Journal of Personality and Social Psychology, 79,* 224–237.

Cooper, C. R., & Ayers-Lopez, S. (1985). Family and peer systems in early adolescence: New models of the role of relationships in development. *Journal of Early Adolescence, 5,* 9–22.

Côté, J. (2000). *Arrested adulthood: The changing nature of maturity and identity in the late modern world.* New York: New York University Press.

Côté, J. (2006). Emerging adulthood as an institutionalized moratorium: Risks and benefits to identity formation. In J. J. Arnett & J. L. Tanner (Eds.), *Coming of age in the 21st century: The lives and contexts of emerging adults* (pp. 85–116). Washington, DC: American Psychological Association.

Deater-Deckard, K., Fulker, D. W., & Plomin, R. (1999). A genetic study of the family environment in the transition to early adolescence. *Journal of Child Psychology and Psychiatry, 40,* 769–775.

Dubas, J. S., & Petersen, A. C. (1996). Geographical distance from parents and adjustment during adolescence and young adulthood. *New Directions for Child Development, 71,* 3–19.

Erikson, E. H. (1950). *Childhood and society.* New York: Norton.

Erikson, E. H. (1968). *Identity: Youth and crisis.* New York: Norton.

Facio, A., & Micocci, E. (2003). Emerging adulthood in Argentina. *New Directions in Child and Adolescent Development, 100,* 21–31.

Feldman, S., Gowen, L., & Fisher, L. (1998). Family relationships and gender as predictors of romantic intimacy in young adults: A longitudinal study. *Journal of Research on Adolescence, 8,* 263–286.

Fingerman, K. L. (2000). "We had a nice little chat": Age and generational differences in mothers' and daughters' descriptions of enjoyable visits. *Journal of Gerontology, 55B,* 95–106.

Fischer, J. L., Sollie, D. L., Sorell, G. T., & Green, S. K. (1989). Marital status and career stage influences on social networks of young adults. *Journal of Marriage and the Family, 51,* 521–534.

Flammer, A., & Alsaker, F. D. (2001). Adolescents in school. In L. Goossens & S. Jackson (Eds.), *Handbook of adolescent development: European perspectives.* Hove, UK: Psychology Press.

Grusec, J. (2002). Parental socialization and children's acquisition of values. In M. Bornstein (Ed.), *Handbook of parenting* (pp. 143–168). Mahwah, NJ: Erlbaum.

Hamilton, S. F., & Hamilton, M. A. (2006). School, work, and emerging adulthood. In J. J. Arnett & J. L. Tanner (Eds.), *Coming of age in the 21st century: The lives and contexts of emerging adults* (pp. 257–277). Washington, DC: American Psychological Association.

Hamm, J. V. (2000). Do birds of a feather flock together? The variable bases for African American, Asian American, and European American adolescents' selection of similar friends. *Developmental Psychology, 36,* 209–219.

Hatfield, E., & Rapson, R. L. (2006). *Love and sex: Cross-cultural perspectives.* Boston: Allyn & Bacon.

Heinz, W. R. (2002). Self-socialization and post-traditional society. *Advances in Life Course Research, 7,* 41–64.

Huesmann, L. R., Moise-Titus, J., Podolski, C., & Eron, L. D. (2003). Longidudinal relations between children's exposure to TV violence and their aggressiveness in young adulthood. *Developmental Psychology, 39,* 201–221.

Jacquet, S., & Surra, C. (2001). Parental divorce and premarital couples: Commitment and other relationship characteristics. *Journal of Marriage and the Family, 63,* 627–638.

Keniston, K. (1971). *Youth and dissent: The rise of a new opposition.* New York: Harcourt Brace Jovanovich.

Labouvie-Vief, G. (2006). *Emerging structures of adult thought.* In J. J. Arnett & J. L. Tanner (Eds.), *Coming of age in the 21st century: The lives and contexts of emerging adults* (pp. 59–84). Washington, DC: American Psychological Association.

Larson, R. (1990). The solitary side of life: An examination of the time people spend alone from childhood to old age. *Developmental Review, 10,* 155–183.

Larson, R., & Richards, M. H. (1994). *Divergent realities: The emotional lives of mothers, fathers, and adolescents.* New York: Basic Books.

Larson, R., & Richards, M. H. (1998). Waiting for the weekend: Friday and Saturday nights as the emotional climax of the week. *New Directions for Child and Adolescent Development, 82,* 37–52.

Larson, R. W., Richards, M. H., Moneta, G., Holmbeck, G., & Duckett, E. (1996). Changes in adolescents' daily interactions with their families from ages 10 to 18: Disengagement and transformation. *Developmental Psychology, 32,* 744–754.

Laumann-Billings, L., & Emery, R. E. (2000). Distress among young adults from divorced families. *Journal of Family Psychology, 14,* 671–687.

Lefkowitz, E.S., & Gillen, M.M. (2006). "Sex is just a normal part of life": Sexuality in emerging adulthood. In J.J. Arnett & J.L. Tanner (Eds.), *Coming of age in the 21st century: The lives and contexts of emerging adults* (pp. 235–255). Washington, DC: American Psychological Association.

Levinson, D. J. (1978). *The seasons of a man's life.* New York: Ballantine.

Lewis, M., Feiring, C., & Rosenthal, S. (2000). Attachment over time. *Child Development, 71,* 707–720.

Loughlin, C., & Barling, J. (1999). The nature of youth employment. In J. Barling & E. K. Kelloway (Eds.), *Youth workers: Varieties of experience* (pp. 17–36). Washington, DC: American Psychological Association.

Masten, A. S., Obradovic, J., & Burt, K. B. (2006). Resilience in emerging adulthood. In J. J. Arnett & J. L. Tanner (Eds.), *Coming of age in the 21st century: The lives and contexts of emerging adults* (pp. 173–190). Washington, DC: American Psychological Association.

Maxwell, K. A. (2002). Friends: The role of peer influence across adolescent risk behaviors. *Journal of Youth and Adolescence, 31,* 267–277.

Mayer, K. U. (2004). Whose lives? How history, societies, and institutions define and shape life courses. *Research in Human Development, 1,* 161–187.

Mayseless, O., & Scharf, M. (2003). What does it mean to be an adult? The Israeli experience. *New Directions in Child and Adolescent Development, 100,* 5–20.

Mortimer, J. T. (2003). *Working and growing up in America.* Cambridge, MA: Harvard University Press.

National Center for Education Statistics. (2002). *The condition of education, 2002* [Online]. Washington, DC: U.S. Department of Education. Available: www.nces.gov.

Nelson, L. J., Badger, S., & Wu, B. (2004). The influence of culture in emerging adulthood: Perspectives of Chinese college students. *International Journal of Behavioral Development, 28,* 26–36.

Reifman, A., Arnett, J. J., & Colwell, M. J. (2006). *The IDEA: Inventory of Dimensions of Emerging Adulthood.* Manuscript submitted for publication.

Reiss, D., Neiderhiser, J., Hetherington, E. M., & Plomin, R. (2000). *The relationship code: Deciphering genetic and social influences on adolescent development.* Cambridge, MA: Harvard University Press.

Rhee, S. H., & Waldman, I. D. (2002). Genetic and environmental influences on antisocial behavior: A meta-analysis of twin and adoption studies. *Psychological Bulletin, 128,* 490–529.

Roisman, G. I., Masten, A. S., Coatsworth, J. D., & Tellegen, A. (2004). Salient and emerging developmental tasks in the transition to adulthood. *Child Development, 75,* 1–11.

Rose, R. J. (2002). How do adolescents select their friends? A behavior-genetic perspective. In L. Pulkinnen & A. Caspi (Eds.), *Paths to successful development: Personality in the life course* (pp. 106–125). New York: Cambridge University Press.

Ruggiero, M., Greenberg, E., & Steinberg, L. (1982). Occupational deviance among first-time workers. *Youth and Society, 13,* 423–448.

Rutter, M., & Silberg, J. (2002). Gene–environment interplay in relation to emotional and behavioral disturbance. *Annual Review of Psychology, 53,* 463–490.

Scarr, S. (1991). The construction of the family reality. *Behavioral and Brain Sciences, 14,* 403–404.

Scarr, S. (1992). Developmental theories for the 1990's: Development and individual differences. *Child Development, 63,* 1–19.

Scarr, S. (1993). Biological and cultural diversity: The legacy of Darwin for development. *Child Development, 64,* 1333–1353.

Scarr, S., & McCartney, K. (1983). How people make their own environments. *Child Development, 54,* 424–435.

Schlegel, A., & Barry, H. (1991). *Adolescence: An anthropological inquiry.* New York: Free Press.

Schneider, B., & Stevenson, D. (1999). *The ambitious generation: America's teenagers, motivated but directionless.* New Haven, CT: Yale University Press.

Schulenberg, J. E., & Zarrett, N. R (2006). Mental health in emerging adulthood: Continuity and disconti-nuity in courses, causes, and functions. In J. J. Arnett & J. L. Tanner (Eds.), *Coming of age in the 21st century: The lives and contexts of emerging adults* (pp. 135–172). Washington, DC: American Psycho-logical Association.

Steele, J. R., & Brown, J. D. (1995). Adolescent room culture: Studying media in the context of everyday life. *Journal of Youth and Adolescence 24,* 551–576.

Stone, M. R., & Brown, B. B. (1999). Identity claims and projections: Descriptions of self and crowds in sec-ondary schools. *New Directions for Child and Adolescent Development, 84,* 7–20.

Summers, P., Forehand, R., Armistead, L., & Tannenbaum, L. (1998). Parental divorce during early adoles-cence in Caucasian families: The role of family process variables in predicting the long-term conse-quences for early adult psychosocial adjustment. *Journal of Consulting and Clinical Psychology, 66,* 327–336.

Sun, Y. (2001). Family environment and adolescents' well-being before and after parents' marital disrup-tion: A longitudinal analysis. *Journal of Marriage and the Family, 63,* 697–713.

Toomey, E., & Nelson, E. (2001). Family conflict and young adults' attitudes toward intimacy. *Journal of Divorce and Remarriage, 34,* 49–69.

Vandell, D. L. (2000). Parents, peer groups, and other socializing influences. *Developmental Psychology, 36,* 699–710.

van Wel, F., Linssen, H., & Ruud, A. (2000). The parental bond and the well-being of adolescents and young adults. *Journal of Youth and Adolescence, 29,* 307–318.

Waite, L. J., & Gallagher, M. (2000). *The case for marriage: Why married people are happier, healthier, and better off financially.* New York: Doubleday.

Ward, L. M., Gorvine, B., & Cytron-Walker, A. (2002). Would that really happen? Adolescents' perceptions of sexual relationships according to prime-time television. In J. D. Brown, J. R. Steele, & K. Walsh-Childers (Eds.), *Sexual teens, sexual media: Investigating media's influence on adolescent sexuality* (pp. 95–123). Mahwah, NJ: Erlbaum.

Wilson, W. J. (1996). *When work disappears: The world of the new urban poor.* New York: Knopf.

Wintre, M., & Yaffe, M. (2000). First-year students' adjustment to university life as a function of relation-ships with parents. *Journal of Adolescent Research, 15,* 9–37.

Youniss, J., & Smollar, J. (1985). *Adolescent relations with mothers, fathers, and friends.* Chicago: Univer-sity of Chicago Press.

Zill, N., Morrison, R. D., & Coiro, M. (1993). Long-term effects of parental divorce on parent–child rela-tionships, adjustment, and achievement in young adulthood. *Journal of Family Psychology, 7,* 91–103.

CHAPTER 9

Socialization in Old Age

Karen L. Fingerman and Lindsay Pitzer

People enter old age after years of adulthood when they were young and middle aged. During those earlier years, healthy adults may build strong relationships with family members and friends, take on leadership and mentoring roles, acquire a sense of themselves as autonomous and worthy, and experience a degree of physical comfort within the ranges of their capacities. Old age involves continuity and growth in these areas of prior strength but also ushers in biological and social changes and detriments. Discussion of socialization in old age requires acknowledgment of this accumulated life experience, coupled with recognition of the positive and negative changes that accrue as individuals approach the end of life.

Of course, "old age" is not a unified stage of life. Scholars generally demarcate the start of old age as beginning around age 60 or 65 and lasting until the end of life. Adults often experience good health and active engagement during the early period of old age (young old age, 60–75 years) followed by accumulated health problems and social losses toward the end of life (oldest old age, older than 85 years; P. Baltes, 1997; Smith, Borschelt, Maier, & Jopp, 2002).

Given that old age is a potentially prolonged period of senescence, socialization in old age is complex. It differs from socialization in early life with regard to time perspective, tasks, and influences. Socialization in early life is future oriented. Bugental and Grusec (2006) suggested that socialization involves preparation of the young to manage the tasks of social life in adulthood. Of course, children learn how they are expected to act in the present in school, family, religious settings, and community, but the overarching goals of socialization focus on establishing the child as a functional adult in the long term future. By contrast, the time perspective of socialization in old age is multifaceted. Older adults are concerned not only with the future but with their past and with present adaptation to challenges and gains.

Likewise, tasks of socialization in late life may be distinct from tasks of socialization in early life. In Chapter 1 of this volume, Maccoby suggests that tasks of socialization in early life include imparting "the skills, behavior patterns, values, and motivations needed for competent functioning in the culture in which the child is growing up." In late life, tasks of socialization may be broader and include (1) continuity in prior achievements, self, and relationships; (2) adaptation to changes in health or social partners in the present; and (3) continued growth. These tasks are accomplished in the context of established identity, past life experiences, practiced modes of coping, and cumulative social resources or deprivations. In this chapter, we consider extant literature pertaining to how the social milieu influences the following: (1) improvements in late life (e.g., emotion regulation), (2) declines in late life (e.g., physical health), and (3) attempts at maintenance (e.g., relationships with offspring).

Researchers and theorists have also been interested in the agents who socialize young people and have considered family members, peers, romantic partners, neighborhoods, school or work contexts, the media, and the broader culture in socializing young people (Arnett, 1995a). Similar forces may influence elderly adults, but researchers have rarely considered the impact of different types of socialization forces in old age.

Indeed, research and theory pertaining to socialization in late life are scant. The dearth of systematic data is in stark contrast to the plethora of scholarship pertaining to this topic at earlier stages of life. Gerontological studies do suggest cultural institutions and social partners influence the aging process, but studies are not framed in terms of *socialization*, per se. Thus, in this chapter, we draw on scholarship pertaining to related topics to develop an understanding of socialization in old age. We consider the forces that socialize older adults, tasks of socialization in late life, the mechanisms through which individuals are socialized, and, finally, how research pertaining to socialization in late life might inform an understanding of aging. We draw on a definition of socialization that involves processes through which older individuals internalize experiences from their social world in ways that alter their behavior, beliefs, and emotions. This definition is less specific than more common definitions applied to socialization in early life that involve preparation for future roles. Rather, this definition allows examination of existing literature pertaining to social influences and aging.

AGENTS OF SOCIALIZATION IN LATE LIFE

To start, we consider forces that may influence or socialize older adults through the last decades of life. Socialization in childhood, adolescence, and early adulthood involves different socialization agents who may affect individuals in different ways: parents, siblings, friends, peer groups, the broader neighborhood and school context, the media, and the culture (Arnett, 1995a, Chapter 8, this volume). For example, theorists have suggested that peers and parents shape distinct aspects of adolescents' lives (for a debate, see Harris, 1995, 2000; Maccoby, 2002; Vandell, 2000). It is difficult to differentiate the functions of specific social partners in late life, but close social partners may serve different functions than more peripheral social contacts.

Further, individuals are proactive in shaping their social networks and their development across adulthood (Brandtstadter & Greve, 1994). Children evoke socialization influences in early life as a function of their temperament or developmental stages

(Bugental & Grusec, 2006). In late life, socialization forces reflect not only older adults' predispositions or developmental states but also choices they have made earlier in life, social partners they have selected (or not selected), and their own efforts to influence their development.

In this section, we consider three types of socialization agents in late life: (1) social partners, (2) broader cultural forces, and (3) individual agency. Of course, these influences are not discrete; individuals derive a sense of agency from their social partners and from the broader culture. Nonetheless, the literature is organized to encourage separate discussions of these socialization influences.

Social Partners

Studies consistently find that older adults have small social networks than do younger adults. Yet, this diminishment in size of network does not reflect a lack of *available* social partners (Fingerman & Birditt, 2003). Rather, Carstensen's socioemotional selectivity theory posits that when individuals confront a foreshortened future, they favor emotional goals, but when they experience an open time horizon, they are more likely to seek informational goals (e.g., Carstensen, Isaacowitz, & Charles, 1999; Lang, 2001). Thus, as older adults sense that their future is curtailed (Fingerman & Perlmutter, 1995), they engage in selection processes to maximize investment in the most emotionally meaningful relationships (Carstensen et al., 1999). The process is akin to the cliché of a deathbed wish for more time with friends and family and less time at the office. Older adults spend much of their time and energy with people they have known for years and to whom they feel close.

Shifts in social networks occur with regard to more peripheral friends or acquaintances. Antonucci and colleagues have examined the configuration of social networks in Japan, Germany, France, and the United States. On average, adults of all ages report feeling close or very close to 5 to 10 social partners, but younger adults also include more people to whom they only feel somewhat close in their social networks (Antonucci et al., 2002).

Types of Social Partners

Nonetheless, the configuration of close social partners is highly variable in late life. Some individuals enter old age married with offspring and grandchildren, other individuals are embedded in a circle of friends, and still others are connected to siblings. Systems of compensation and substitution allow older people who lack a given social partner (e.g., a grown child) to derive benefits from a different type of social partner (e.g., a church member; Chatters, Taylor, Lincoln, & Schroepfer, 2002; Connidis & Davies, 1992). Individuals who are married list their spouse as their closest social partner, widowed older adults list a child, and a never married older adult list a close friend. Many older adults also derive benefits from connections to community or church groups as well, particularly in African American communities (Chatters et al., 2002; Krause, 2002).

In early life, individuals care about family and close friends, but friendships and peer groups also exert socialization pressures. In late life, adults rely primarily on their closest social partners for emotional and instrumental support (Antonucci & Akiyama, 1987; Krause, 2001). Studies suggest that older adults turn to close sons and daughters for information about health care (Fingerman, Hay, Kamp-Dush, Cichy, & Hosterman, 2005; Logan & Spitze, 1996). Likewise, research finds that older adults are particularly susceptible to the effects of criticism or support from their spouses when health problems occur in late life (Manne & Zautra, 1989).

Obviously, older adults interact with people who are not psychologically close to them. They talk with health care personnel, live near neighbors, and interact with acquaintances through religious or community gatherings (Fingerman, 2004). Such peripheral social contacts, may treat older adults in ways that diminish their sense of well-being if they rely on stereotypes of elderly people in their interactions. Of course, close social contacts can also exert detrimental effects. Given motivational features of socioemotional selectivity, however, older adults often select social situations where they benefit from their closest social partners.

Duration of Relationships

Older adults' close relationships may be distinct from close relationships involving younger people due to two features: (1) the relationships may have lasted for decades, and (2) the social partners may have infrequent contact. Family members and friends may have known the older adult for half a century or more. The older adults may have little contact with these social partners, however, particularly if they reside far away.

Indeed, when given the choice, older adults seem to prefer relationships of longer duration over relationships that offer greater opportunity for contact. Adams (1985–1986) examined this issue by asking older women about long-term friends who resided at a distance in comparison to newer friends who lived nearby. The women preferred their older friends because they knew them better and felt closer to them. The older women believed these older friends accepted negative qualities in them that they feared their new friends might not accept. As such, older adults may be more receptive to input, advice, or efforts to assist them proffered by long-term social partners. Newly founded relationships may serve functions of companionship or entertainment rather than socialization of values, beliefs, and behaviors, per se.

Furthermore, individuals who have known the older adult for decades may treat them in ways that retain references to younger stages of life. The memory of an elderly friend as a virile, energetic young man may taint interactions even after this man has begun to show physical declines of old age. A friend may treat an older man as though he were still middle-aged. Social partners who only meet this older man after he has begun to show signs of decline may be quicker to offer assistance or treat him in a way that conveys his elderly state (Nussbaum, Hummert, Williams, & Harwood, 1996). The impact of such differential treatment is discussed in greater detail with regard to socialization of dependency in late life.

It is also important to consider theoretical implications of long-lasting relationships on socialization processes. For example, Bronfenbrenner and Morris (1998) described the concept of "proximal processes" through which children develop. Specifically, they asserted that development takes place through reciprocal interaction between individuals and other persons, objects, and symbols in the immediate environment and that repeated interactions must occur over time for these processes to be meaningful. Thus, parents and young children engage in repeated interactions that set a foundation for their relationship as well as for the child's socialization.

However, individuals who have been in relationships for decades may not require repeated interactions to retain strong ties. The prolonged nature of a relationship may permit socialization influences in late life, even in the absence of direct contact. For example, we examined adults' subjective interpretation of the holiday cards they receive in December and January. Participants completed a survey for each card they received, as well as a survey assessing their well-being and adjustment (Fingerman & Griffiths, 1999). Many older adults exchanged holiday greetings with people they had not seen in decades. From the perspective of a younger adult, these liaisons might not truly qualify as *relationships*— they do not provide interaction, emotional connection, or resources. Yet, older adults reported that these relationships meant a great deal to them as connections to their personal past because, for example, they involved a last remaining relative from the participant's youth, a college roommate, or a neighbor from a long-time residence.

Social partners with whom older adults no longer visit or communicate may continue to influence their decisions and beliefs, thus socializing them without direct engagement. Studies have not examined this issue empirically, but in situations in which older adults must apply values or make decisions, it would be worth investigating the extent to which they think about viewpoints of social partners whom they no longer encounter on a daily basis. It is easy to imagine an older adult who even considers social partners who are deceased, "How would my mother handle this situation?" or "What would my late husband have done?" Therefore, the scope of socialization agents in late life may be different than in early life.

In sum, older adults spend most of their time and energy with social partners who are emotionally meaningful and important and whom they have known for decades. Socialization agents in late life tend to have known the older adult for years. In fact, many individuals who affect older adults' behaviors, emotions, and beliefs may themselves have been socialized *by* these older adults (e.g., their son or daughter). They may have infrequent contact with the older adult, but the older adult may still solicit their opinions and input.

Past Influences on Socialization Partners

Early relationship processes on late life may also continue to affect late-life adaptation. Such processes might be considered delayed effects of socialization agents. For example, a vast literature pertaining to attachment theory in adults' romantic relationships presumes that effects of early relationships between parents and infants carry over into an individual's subsequent romantic relationship patterns (e. g., Hazan & Shaver, 1994; Shaver, Belsky, & Brennan, 2000). Further, studies have shown that adults' memories of relationships with parents in childhood shape their relationships with those parents in old age (Carpenter, 2001); the ways in which adults care for their parents in old age are associated with their earlier memories of how the parents treated them.

Yet, empirical evidence for *direct* socialization effects from infancy to old age are scant. Studies have not examined infant attachment patterns and subsequent adaptation in old age longitudinally and, therefore, must rely on retrospective memories of relationships. Thus, it is not always clear whether presumed early effects reflect memories tainted by present circumstances or accurate portraits of the past. Nonetheless, scholars have generated a vast literature pertaining to attachment style influences on later life adaptation (see special issue of *Attachment and Human Development* focusing on late life;

Magai & Consedine, 2004; Magai, Consedine, Gillespie, O'Neal, & Vilker, 2004). Theoretically, this literature suggests social and emotional styles in old age have their roots in much earlier socialization.

In addition to relationships, sociologists who study life-course theory have examined other early life precursors to patterns of adaptation in late life (for reviews see Elder, 1998; Settersten, 2003). The life-course perspective suggests that early experiences influence subsequent adjustment later in life. For example, Elder and Liker (1982) argued that early-life stresses may socialize individuals in ways that permit better adaptation to late-life stressors. The scholars examined 81 mothers from the Berkeley Growth study (born 1890–1910). These women were interviewed in the 1930s and again in 1969–1970 at approximately age 70. The study revealed that women who were initially from a middle-class background but who suffered hardships (i.e., 35% loss of family income) during the Great Depression fared better in late life than women who were either perpetually in lower or upper social strata. Learning to cope with stress (with ample resources before and after the stress) may provide individuals with adaptive resources for old age.

Similarly, Kahana, Kahana, Harel, and Kelly (1997) argued that accumulated stresses may lead to maladaptive reactions to stress in old age. These scholars found that individuals who survived the Holocaust sometimes showed maladaptive reactions to stress in old age. When Holocaust survivors grow ill in late life, they may mistrust the health care system, fear that their illness makes them susceptible to further injury (as during the Holocaust), and otherwise engage in maladaptive behaviors.

In sum, socialization in late life occurs after accumulated experiences. Individuals who have had positive relationships with others and certain types of stressors may be better prepared and more receptive to positive socialization in old age. Alternately, excessive trauma in early life may socialize individuals in ways that render adjustment to late life more difficult.

Culture

The larger culture influences children, young people, and the social agents who interact with them by shaping social relationships, individual values, and behaviors (Arnett, 2001). Children and adolescents acquire cultural ideas from family, peers, and social partners, from larger institutions such as school and work, and through a variety of media including radio, movies, television, and computer venues. Such cultural influences may also influence aspects of the aging process.

Cultures influence the types of socialization partners individuals encounter in late life. Although size of social network tends to diminish with age across cultures (e.g, Antonucci et al., 2002), the configuration of the social network in late life varies across cultures. For example, in the United States, older adults are generally closer to and receive support from their daughters' families, whereas in Asian nations such as China and Japan, the tendency is to align with a son's family and to receive support from a daughter-in-law (Antonucci, Akiyama, & Birditt, 2005).

Support patterns in late life also vary by culture. Within the United States, for example, family exchanges vary across ethnic groups. In a 10-year longitudinal, qualitative investigation of 270 older Filipino, Latino, African American, and Cambodian Americans, Becker, Beyene, Newsom, and Mayen (2003) found ethnic differences in values, living situations, and relationship patterns with younger generations. For example, all but 3 of 48 elderly Cambodian adults resided with their offspring or younger family members and believed this was the norm for older adults. African American adults stated a preference for intergenerational autonomy, as well as for emotionally supportive ties, but they were the most likely to live alone in old age and to state a preference for doing so. Latino older Americans were more likely than other groups to expect their offspring to provide for them financially and to be disappointed when they did not do so. Elderly Filipino Americans made considerable sacrifices to send money home to extended family. Although the literature suggests that overall benefits or detriments in late life reflect the presence or absence of *close* social partners (Antonucci et al., 2002), Becker et al. (2003) suggest that cultures influence the adaptation of older adults in specific ways, such as whether they reside with offspring, whether they provide for others or expect to be provided for, and the values they place on different types of social liaisons. These differences, in turn, set the forum for subsequent decisions and adaptation in advanced old age.

Moreover, cultures vary in their attitudes toward the elderly and aging in general. Individuals within cultures appear to share stereotypes of older people (Hummert, Garstka, Shaner, & Strahm, 1994; Levy, 2003). Research indicates that Asian cultures tend to place greater value on the elderly than American or Western cultures do (Levy & Langer, 1994). Such cultural variability in value for the elderly may affect the ways in which individuals in different cultures experience the aging process (Levy, 1999).

Furthermore, macrolevel cultural influences shape support of older adults who require care. Political systems differ considerably in the structure of their health care systems and long-term care models for older adults, even among Western cultures. For example, the Swedish socialized medical system provides extensive support for older adults to remain in their homes, including remodeling aspects of the physical environment and sending in a night patrol health care aid to assist in taking medication. Thus, older adults in the Swedish system are socialized to value their independence, their autonomy, and their right to grow frail in their own abode. By contrast, few states in the United States support such initiatives, and there is a general emphasis on familial and institutional care (Feinberg, & Newman, 2004). As discussed here, the U.S. approach may increase dependency behaviors among older adults (M. Baltes, 1995).

Thus, cultural differences are evident in the types of support older adults expect from family, in their living situations, in how individuals view the ageing process, and in the larger political and health support systems available to the elderly. Nonetheless, there may be limits in the impact of culture on the aging process.

Possible Limitations in the Influence of Culture on Aging

Although culture is obviously an important socialization force throughout life, culture may have less impact on individuals' aging per se than it does on shaping behaviors and development in early life. The fact that old age differs across cultures does not mean that culture shapes the aging process individuals experience. The differences may arise from earlier experiences that simply persist in old age. There are several reasons why this might be the case: (1) culture may be most efficacious during early stages of life when individuals are seeking information about themselves and the positions they may hold in society, (2) older adults may attempt to sustain themselves relative to traditions rather than incorporating new elements of the culture, (3) cultural media target younger individuals, and (4) as physical declines become paramount, the ability of culture to remediate disabilities may diminish.

Culture, per se, may be most efficacious in shaping behaviors of the young, rather than the elderly (for discussions of culture and socialization of the young, see Rothbaum & Trommsdorff, Chapter 18, this volume; Rogoff et al., Chapter 19, this volume). Previously, we described socioemotional selectivity theory and the processes through which individuals become increasingly invested in emotionally rewarding social partners as their future diminishes. This shift in motivation reflects a move away from seeking social partners who can provide information about the culture to a move toward emotional rewards (Carstensen et al., 1999). By reducing their social networks to close friends and family, older adults may decrease the chances of encountering new information from the culture. Of course, younger relatives engage in behaviors that are culturally acceptable for their time period and may socialize older relatives in doing so. For example, an older adult may grow to accept the idea of cohabitation after a beloved grandchild moves in with a partner. Older adults are not impermeable to the impact of cultural changes, but they may not actively seek out new information concerning cultural expectations.

Indeed, studies have found that older adults transmit culture to younger generations. For example, an early study of grandparents, Neugarten and Weinstein (1964) described the grandparent role of conveying the culture to younger generations. Other studies have also found that older adults communicate traditions embedded within the larger culture to family members (Fingerman, 2001; Wiscott & Kopera-Frye, 2000). In situations in which cultural expectations conflict, older adults tend to retain identification with the culture they knew when they were younger. For example, when families immigrate to the United States, generations may experience tension over the desire to acculturate into ways of life in the United States but to preserve traditions from the prior culture. Older adults tend to serve as the liaison to the prior culture. In the study described by Becker et al. (2003), older adults who had immigrated to the United States in the past decade conveyed family traditions from the former culture as part of their role in the extended family.

In comparison to younger adults, older adults may also encounter less exposure to media that convey cultural messages. Young adults rely on cultural media such as popular music, movies, and Internet blogs to help establish a sense of identity (Arnett, 1995b). The content and advertising in these media tend to target adolescents and young adults rather than older adults (Arnett, 1995b). Thus, when older adults go to the movies or watch television, they are unlikely to see older adults portrayed as models of cultural imperatives. Many of the images of older adults in the mass media are negative or comical (Carrigan & Szmigin, 1999).

This is not to say that older adults avoid contact with cultural media. For example, older adults spend 3.5–6 hours a day on average watching television (National Opinion Research Center, 1997). Further, online research reports indicate that over half of adults ages 55–64 use the Internet (Burstmedia, 2002; iMedia, 2004). Yet, Internet usage is lower in the oldest age groups; fewer than 2% of adults over age 80 use the Internet (iMedia, 2004). Furthermore, studies suggest that older adults use the Internet to send messages to family members rather than to learn about current events, ideas, or entertainment (White et al., 2002). Of course, as current cohorts enter old age, this pattern may change. Nonetheless, socioemotional selectivity theory suggests that regardless of familiarity with computers and the Internet, older adults may be more interested in communicating with relatives than with searching for cultural information when they use the computer.

Finally, P. Baltes (1997) argued that culture loses the ability to impact individuals as biological detriments accumulate in late late life. In early life, social influences may take advantage of plasticity and assist individuals to rebound from physical, cognitive, or social losses. In old-old age, P. Baltes (1997) has suggested that severe deficits and losses accrue and cast a shadow over other features of life. As a result, the efficacy of the social milieu to remediate problems is not as strong as it was at prior stages of life. According to Baltes, biology supersedes cultural interventions in determining quality of life and well-being. At one level, this argument has obvious validity; elderly adults suffering severe dementia, arthritis, and shortness of breath can no longer accomplish daily activities, regardless of their family, social class, or cultural context.

Nonetheless, the social milieu may still serve interpretive functions when elderly adults suffer severe impairments. As mentioned previously, political systems vary considerably in the long-term care policies they initiate and, thus, in the experiences offered to the most debilitated elderly adults. Further, Baltes's discussion pertains to severe disability rather than to cultural differences in aging per se. Recent scholarship suggests that older adults experience many years in good health before experiencing physical disabilities and impairments at the end of life (Freedman, Martin, & Schoeni, 2002). Thus, although the final years of life may involve severe physical or mental impairment that culture cannot ameliorate, these conditions remain relatively rare in comparison to the greater number of older adults who are not severely disabled and who may be susceptible to cultural input.

In sum, with regard to culture and socialization, older adults may be more likely to view themselves as vehicles of traditions within their families and less likely to actively seek new information from media or social partners. Studies have not examined the extent to which older adults adopt attitudes and beliefs embraced by younger family members, but it is likely that such socialization occurs. Finally, cultural institutions that provide health care or other forms of support also influence the aging process.

Individual Agency

Individuals become increasingly responsible for their own socialization in adulthood. Indeed, forces that reside in the social context in early life may come under individual control in later life. Beginning in young adulthood, in Western cultures, individuals are expected to make decisions and guide the course of their own development. For example, Arnett (2001) found that Americans ages 13–55 viewed the onset of adulthood as involving responsibility for one's actions, deciding on one's beliefs and values, establishing an equal relationship with parents, and becoming financially independent. These shifts then persist throughout adulthood, such that individuals attempt to shape their own behavior and adaptations to the aging process.

Furthermore, Schulz and Heckhausen (1999) argue that attempts to control the self increase by late life. The authors distinguish between primary control, behavioral attempts to influence external circumstances, and secondary control, behavioral and cognitive responses to regulate internal responses. Individual histories, personality, and culture influence the nature of secondary control responses. Primary control increases dramatically throughout childhood and adolescence, but as adults traverse old age, they are less able to control external circumstances. During midlife and old age, individuals increasingly cope with losses in primary control by attempting to exert secondary control and to deal with their own emotional reactions.

Efforts to control oneself and one's emotions are evident in situations involving physical limitations. For example, Heckhausen, Wrosch, and Fleeson (2001) examined loss of fertility with menopause. Couples often increased attempts at primary control prior to the transition, such as fertility treatments to become pregnant, but eventually, individuals applied secondary control strategies to cope with their childless state. Social settings can alleviate some consequences of age-associated losses (e.g., one-child-family laws in China makes infertility less difficult for older Chinese couples with no children), but individuals rely on the ability to regulate their emotional reactions to losses as biological imperatives take hold in late life. In other words, functions that might occur in a social setting through mutual behaviors between individuals in early adulthood may occur *within* the individual in old age.

TASKS AND PROCESSES OF SOCIALIZATION IN LATE LIFE

As discussed, forces of socialization in late life include social partners whom individuals have known for years and to whom they feel psychologically close as well as a shift toward internalized control. Older adults also encounter acquaintances, health care professionals, neighbors, and peripheral social partners. They reside within larger cultures that generate values toward family, convey stereotypes of the elderly, and involve political systems that support different forms of long-term care.

It is difficult, however, to delineate the *processes* through which these socialization forces influence older adults. Part of the dilemma involves a lack of clarity with regard to outcomes of socialization in late life. For example, it is possible to examine how expectations about achievement in childhood translate into actual academic or career outcomes in young adulthood (for a discussion, see Eccles, Chapter 26, this volume). Because adults enter old age with a lifetime of prior experience, it is difficult to delineate the specific effects of socialization in old age. Across the lifespan, individuals experience canalization into distinct social milieus based on their personalities, decisions, and earlier experiences. For example, in late life, socioeconomic status reflects accumulated resources, decisions, and socialization forces from decades previously.

As such, rather than attempt to delineate specific tasks of socialization in old age, we consider three types of changes in late life: (1) areas where older adults generally show improvements or benefits (e.g., emotion regulation), (2) events to which older adults must adapt in late life (e.g., widowhood), and (3) declines and problems of late life. Socialization agents may have positive effects—as evidenced by increased survival rates and decreased morbidity among older adults who have strong social ties (Bassuk, Glass, & Berkman, 1999; Berkman, Glass, Brissette, & Seeman, 2000). Likewise, social partners can have negative effects on older adults—as evidenced by findings that younger people who communicate with older adults with condescension harm their self-images (Coupland, Coupland, Giles, & Henwood, 1988). We do not mean to imply that certain socialization forces exert influences that are wholly beneficial or wholly detrimental, nor do we intend to argue that these forces act uniquely in late life. Rather, we examine the ways in which the social milieu may enhance or detract from well-being during the final decades of life.

Our overarching model involves the premise of reciprocal influences through the social input model (Fingerman & Baker, 2006). Older adults bring characteristics to their relationships as a function of their maturational state, their health status, their experiences, and their individual social roles or personality. Social partners respond to these attributes in ways what may enhance or inhibit relationship qualities and well-being. Other models of social relationships have provided information about the social world of late life (e.g., Antonucci & Akiyama, 1987; Carstensen et al., 1999), but these models have not considered reciprocal influences suggestive of socialization processes. We do so here.

Socialization of Positive Gains in Late Life

Certain aspects of cognitive (e.g., knowledge for facts) and socioemotional (e.g., qualities of relationships and decreased experience of negative emotions) functioning may improve in later life. Socialization forces may deter physical and cognitive declines and may contribute to improvements in well-being. Research with regard to these issues stems from two literatures: (1) epidemiological studies examining social relationship effects on mortality and morbidity in late life, and (2) studies examining emotional aspects of relationships in late life.

Relationships and Decreased Morbidity and Mortality in Late Life

A vast literature has shown that good relationships in late life are linked to better well-being (for a review, see Charles & Mavandadi, 2004). The presence of close social partners has been associated with survival in old age. Over 25 years ago, Berkman and Syme (1979) reported that adults ages 30–69 who had poor social networks were at greater risk of mortality than adults who were socially embedded. Subsequent epidemiological studies found that close relationships were associated with better health, better cognitive functioning, and decreased morbidity in old age (Fratiglioni, Wang, Ericsson, Maytan, & Winblad, 2000; Uchino, Cacioppo, & Kiecolt-Glaser, 1996).

Studies have found that perceptions of good relationships prevent cognitive decline and dementia in old age. Fratiglioni et al. (2000) studied 1,203 older people in Stockholm who were assessed as having good cognitive functioning and who did not reside in nursing homes at baseline. They assessed objective (e.g., live alone or with other people) and subjective (e.g., satisfaction) aspects of social networks. Three years later, the older adults participated in a follow-up study, and 176 of them had developed dementia. After controlling for baseline cognitive performance, depression, and vascular diseases, risk of developing dementia was associated with subjective and objective indicators of poor social networks. Individuals who lived alone and who reported no close ties at baseline had nearly double the risk of developing dementia. It is possible that during the 3-year interval between assessments, individuals developed premorbid symptoms that adversely affected their social skills, but risk of dementia was not associated with frequency of contact with social partners. Rather, objective indicators and subjective ratings of satisfaction with relationships 3 years previously appeared to better predict onset of dementia.

In sum, evidence that relationships affect positive adjustment in late life is compelling. Individuals who have had positive relationships throughout life reported fewer physiological risk factors for cardiovascular, neuroendocrine, metabolic, and sympathetic nervous system problems than individuals who had problematic or few relationships (Ryff & Singer, 2005). Indeed, House, Landis, and Umberson (1988) argued that evidence for the impact of social relationships on mortality and morbidity is as strong as evidence for the association between smoking and these outcomes.

MECHANISMS THROUGH WHICH SOCIAL PARTNERS AFFECT WELL-BEING

Berkman et al. (2000) reviewed literature pertaining to social networks and positive health outcomes among adults in their 30s through 60s. These authors suggested social partners might socialize individuals to benefit well-being through (1) increased self-efficacy, (2) decreased risk taking, and (3) better regulation of emotions.

In late life, these mechanisms may be more complex, however. There may be bidirectional effects between good relationships and self-efficacy in old age. For example, in one study, women who experienced greater self-efficacy within a given relationship also reported more satisfaction with support in that relationship (Martini, Grusec, & Bernardini, 2001). Studies have also found that social contacts can hinder self-efficacy among older adults suffering impairments if social partners encourage dependency (M. Baltes, 1995). Nonetheless, the mechanisms by which this occurs may not involve socialization. Individuals who are more self-efficacious may attract better social partners. Indeed, these effects may be enhanced in late life, when individuals narrow their social networks to close partners whom they have known for years. Such findings suggest that social contacts can support self-efficacy in old age, but additional information is needed to understand the mechanisms through which they do so.

Similarly, reciprocal patterns may occur with regard to risk-taking behaviors. Berkman et al. (2000) point out that studies find consistent but small associations with regard to risk taking; individuals with more social ties engage in somewhat fewer risky behaviors (e.g., smoking) and somewhat more risk-minimizing behaviors (e.g., exercising) than individuals with fewer social ties. Yet, it is not clear that these associations indicate that social partners socialize older adults to avoid risk-taking behaviors. Rather, individuals who engage in high risk-taking behaviors may be less attractive to social partners. Furthermore, individuals who engage in risky behaviors may be dead before they reach old age.

A more promising mechanism to explain the positive impact of social ties may involve emotion regulation. Scholars have posited that emotional reactions mediate some of the observed effects of personal relationships on well-being in old age (Charles & Movandadi, 2004; Ryff & Singer, 2005). Indeed, studies reveal that individuals who survive into old age maximize positive emotions and minimize negative emotions in the context of meaningful relationships (Carstensen et al., 1999). In other words, social partners may affect positive outcomes in late life by allowing older adults to experience positive emotions and buffering against negative emotions. Studies do not explain how social partners evoke emotions that benefit health, but we discuss this issue with regard to the social input model in the next section.

OLDER ADULTS AS SOCIALIZATION AGENTS

In addition, social partners may enhance health outcomes by providing older adults with opportunities to remain active and generative (Liang, Krause, & Bennett, 2001; Brown, Consedine, & Magai, 2005). By the time they reach old age, most people are likely to have spent more time serving as "socialization agents" than as objects of socialization. Adults who are parents spend the better part of two or three decades engaged in raising and socializing their children. Regardless of their own parental status, older adults may have assisted younger adults to achieve cultural and social belonging in their families; at work; in community groups; as members of their churches, synagogues, and mosques; and in other contexts. Retaining such roles may contribute to continued sense of self-worth.

Unfortunately, research examining older adults as socialization agents is not well established. Studies have focused on formal programs where older adults serve as mentors in some capacity to youth they have never previously met. Evidence suggests that older adults benefit from these experiences (Herrmann, Sipsas-Herrmann, Stafford, & Herrmann, 2005; Bullock & Osborne, 1999). Unfortunately, these studies suffer from sample selectivity. Older adults who volunteer to participate in intergenerational programs may be distinct from the population of older adults in general. Furthermore, given that older adults prefer to spend time with close friends and family rather than unknown young people, it is not clear whether these findings generalize to real-world daily settings.

Another context associated with socialization might involve older adults' provision of support to familiar partners. The findings are not compelling that providing support helps older adults, however. In a sample of more than 1,000 adults over age 65, Liang et al. (2001) found that providing tangible, informational, and emotional support to others was not significantly associated with well-being (though receiving support was). The study examined social support exchanges, however, rather than mentoring or offering advice. Scholars might examine the extent to which older adults provide advice, mentoring, and socialization of young people in their everyday life and the effects of doing so. Intuitively, it seems that serving as a socialization agent may be more beneficial than others' attempts to socialize the older adult.

Improvements in Relationship Qualities

Qualities of relationships appear to improve in late life. Older adults report less difficulty with their social partners than do younger adults (Akiyama, Antonucci, Takahashi, & Langfahl, 2003; Birditt & Fingerman, 2005; Fingerman & Birditt, 2003). In comparison to younger adults, older adults report better relationships with their: parents and offspring (Fingerman, 1996, 2001; Umberson, 1989), grandchildren (Fingerman, 1998), spouses (Akiyama et al., 2003), friends (Rook, 1984), and siblings (Bedford, 1989).

Explanations for the improved quality of relationships are multifaceted. As mentioned previously, socioemotional selectivity theory suggests that individuals selectively cull their networks to retain those social partners they find emotionally rewarding, while minimizing contact with individuals they find annoying (Carstensen et al., 1999). Furthermore, older adults are better able to regulate their reactions to potentially upsetting situations that do arise, thus minimizing problems in their relationships (Birditt & Fingerman, 2005). Emotion regulation also appears to improve with age, allowing older adults to experience fewer and less intense negative emotions with their social partners (Carstensen, Fung, & Charles, 2003; Birditt & Fingerman, 2003).

The social input model suggests that reciprocal processes in late life result in a diminution of problematic aspects of relationships, improved qualities of relationships, and better emotion regulation within these relationships (Fingerman & Baker, 2006). This model addresses the experiences older adults evoke from their social world by considering the types of social partners older adults have, what they bring to their relationships, and the types of behaviors they evoke from their social partners. Older adults interact with older social partners (i.e., older spouses and older offspring). Given improvements in emotional and behavioral repertoires as individuals grow older, older adults are likely to receive positive social input from these older social partners. From a socialization perspective, this positive social input generates internalized positive emotional gains. In other words, reciprocal processes are involved. Individuals limit their social networks to rewarding social partners, react to these partners in positive ways, and, in turn, receive positive input that reinforces the cycle of warm regard in the relationship.

The few studies that have examined close social partners' reactions to older adults support the social input model. Studies of parent/offspring relationships indicate that older offspring are more solicitous of their parents than are younger offspring (Fingerman, 2000). In a study examining aging mothers and their adult daughters, every daughter described at least one thing about her mother that irritated her when she was interviewed alone. Yet, these middle-aged women did not discuss these problems with their mothers or show their negative feelings to their mothers in audiotaped joint conversations (Lefkowitz & Fingerman, 2003). Rather, middle-aged daughters generally valued their mother and did not wish to hurt her feelings. In a similar vein, Martini, Grusec, and Bernardini (2003) asked middle-aged women and their mothers to report how the daughters initiated help (requested by mother, offered by daughter, imposed by daughter), how comfortable the mothers were with that help, and how comfortable they might be in receiving additional help. These scholars found that middle-aged daughters had a good understanding of when their elderly mothers desired help and how these mothers felt about receiving that help. Yet, daughters underestimated their mothers' comfort with imposed help, again suggesting that middle-aged women are particularly solicitous of their mothers' feelings.

Findings suggest that even less close relatives and friends provide input that enhances older adults' emotional experiences. In the study of holiday greetings described previously, Fingerman and Griffiths (1999) reported that older adults received more sentimental holiday greetings than did younger adults. Social contacts sent cards with pictures of reindeer drinking cappuccino to their young adult friends and family members, and cards with meaningful emotional messages to their grandmother or great uncle. These findings do not imply that friends and family coddle or pamper older adults in well-functioning relationships. Rather, selectivity of relationships and enhanced emotion regulation of late life evoke positive reactions from social partners.

In sum, social partners clearly exert positive benefits throughout life. The importance of close relationships may be particularly evident during periods of life when humans are most vulnerable, at the start and end of the lifespan (Charles & Movandadi, 2004). The mechanisms through which social partners enhance outcomes in late life are unclear. Research supports the social input model; age-associated changes in emotion regulation and the sense that the individual is aging appear to generate positive social input (Fingerman & Baker, 2006). From a socialization perspective, we further argue that this positive input reinforces and enhances older adults' positive emotionality. Thus, reciprocal socialization is present between older adults and social partners.

Socialization and Adaptation to Transitions in Late Life

Socialization effects also may be evident in adaptation in late life. Older adults deal with transitions they can plan, such as retirement, and adverse events such as widowhood, which may be less predictable (and certainly less desirable). Adaptation to such events may involve anticipatory socialization.

Several mechanisms of anticipatory socialization that occur at earlier stages of life may not apply in late life, however. For example, children can draw on their parents' experiences to learn about their possible future. By late life, older people who have experienced the events of old age may have passed away or are in poor health. Furthermore, old age has changed in recent decades, with additional years of life and lower rates of disability (Freedman et al., 2002). These increases in longevity and health render today's older adults distinct, with fewer models for them to follow in preparing for future events of old age.

Furthermore, evidence is mixed regarding the effects of anticipatory socialization in old age. For example, Carr, House, Wortman, Neese, and Kessler (2001) examined anticipation of widowhood in late life. These scholars initially posited that in comparison to widows whose spouses died suddenly, widows who were able to anticipate a spouse's death might fare better due to socialization processes, "Couples who anticipate a death may use the forewarning period to make practical adjustment for the survivor's economic and social adjustment, thus enabling a smoother transition" (p. S238). They used the Changing Lives of Older Couples (CLOC) study involving over 1,000 older couples interviewed in 1987–1988. The researchers then monitored monthly death records and obituaries and interviewed widows at 6 months and 18 months following loss or postloss. The scholars' careful controls of extraneous variables (e.g., caregiving demands during the predeath period) and multiple measures revealed complexities in outcomes. The findings did not support expectations of a smoother transition for widows who anticipated their spouse's death. Rather, older widows whose spouses died suddenly suffered *different* outcomes than widows whose spouses died with forewarning. In comparisons, widows whose spouses died suddenly experienced increased rates of intrusive thoughts 6 months following the loss, but individuals whose spouses died of predictable causes suffered increased anxiety at 6 and 18 months postloss.

Findings such as these suggest that even when adverse events are anticipated and social partners attempt to assist older adults to prepare for future losses, the magnitude of the losses can overwhelm coping resources. In the case of widowhood, spouses, who might best serve as socialization agents to guide them, offer advice, or assist them are no longer available.

Yet, it might be overstating the case to assume that the social milieu cannot provide resources to adults as they anticipate events in late life. The paucity of findings pertaining to socialization influences on adaptation in old age may stem from research foci. Widowhood is an abrupt transition of negative valence. Anticipatory socialization may have more positive effects when transitions are fertile for positive outcomes in late life. For example, individuals who are highly invested in their careers may make a positive transition into retirement when they have the opportunity to experience a partial retirement or anticipatory socialization of their subsequent life roles (Moen, 2001). Adults appear to discuss retirement with their social partners as they near this transition. Ekerdt, Kosloski, and De Viney (2000) examined anticipation of retirement in a nationally representative sample of 4,921 adults ages 51–61. Participants answered three questions: How much have you thought about retirement? How much have you discussed retirement with your partner? and How much have you discussed it with your friends/coworkers? Not surprisingly, individuals who considered themselves near retirement spent time thinking about these events and conferring with social partners about it.

Studies further show that adults respond to marital partners, family members, cultural expectations, and government programs in making a decision to retire (Sczinovacz & Ekerdt, 1995), but the effects of this input on subsequent satisfaction with retirement are unclear. For example, Smith and Moen (1998) examined couples from the Cornell Retirement and Well-being Study and found that spouses influenced one another with regard to retirement decisions. In fact, retired husbands viewed their wives as having more influence on their retirement decision than the wives reported having. By contrast, women often tied their retirement decisions to their husband's retirement decisions. Nonetheless, women were most satisfied with retirement when they felt their husbands had *not* been overly influential in their decision to retire (Smith & Moen, 2004). Such research highlights a distinction between socialization to influence an older adult's decisions versus socialization to assist with decisions the older adult has made. Older adults may favor autonomy with regard to decision making but appreciate assistance with transitions resulting from such decisions.

In sum, studies concerning socialization to assist older adults with transitions and challenges of late life are mixed. In situations in which adversity is severe, such as widowhood, the ability to anticipate and prepare for the event may not affect quality of life. In situations in which positive outcomes are possible, such as the transition to retirement, anticipation and preparation can be effective. Socialization efforts appear to have the most satisfactory outcomes when older adults are preparing for such an event and social partners assist them. In other words, anticipatory socialization can be effective but is not *always* effective in late life.

Socialization of Detriments in Late Life

Finally, socialization forces can induce declines or exacerbate detriments of late life. The processes through which social influences generate negative outcomes in old age range from macrolevel cultural phenomena to microlevel one-on-one social interactions. The detriments scholars have examined range from the psychological (loss of self-esteem) to the physical (loss of functional abilities). We consider these issues next.

Cultural Influences on Detriments

Culturally shared images of the elderly may affect individuals as they age. Theorists suggest that in cultures in which negative stereotypes of the aged abound, older adults may suffer lower self-esteem and lower self-efficacy than in cultures in which the aged are more respected (Levy, 2003). Cultures may socialize older adults into a loss of self-esteem by conveying the message that older adults are unworthy.

Stereotypes of the aged in a given culture may not be purely positive or negative. For example, cultural messages that denigrate aging are obvious across a variety of media in North America. The birthday card industry produces sayings, drawings, and jokes that mock the idea of aging. Advertisers rarely portray older adults in advertisements that attempt to sell everyday products, instead relegating older adults to advertisements pertaining to health care products (Carrigan & Szmigin, 1999). Yet, Chasteen, Schwartz, and Park (2002) found that adults of all ages demonstrated stronger activation for elderly stereotypes than for young adult stereotypes, but those stereotypes tended to be *positive* in valence. In another experiment, older and younger participants responded to scenarios in which a target adult leaves a store without paying for a hat. Participants of all ages were more forgiving of forgetfulness in an older target than in a younger target (Erber, Szuchman, & Prager, 2001). In other words, even in cultures in which negative messages about aging are evident, individuals may simultaneously hold positive feelings about the elderly.

Further, whether older adults incorporate cultural stereotypes of the aged also varies. For example, Levy (1999) examined American, Chinese, and Japanese older adults' views of themselves relative to stereotypes of the aged in these cultures. Levy investigated these groups because Japanese people tend to maintain highly developed and dichotomous views of outer or public self (the omote) and inner or private self (the ura). In comparison to older adults in China and the United States, Japanese elderly adults expressed more negative attitudes toward old people in general but more positive concepts of the self.

The mechanism through which stereotypes might affect older adults is a subject of debate. Given that older adults may be less involved with cultural media than younger adults, it is difficult to explain how media could influence them to internalize negative attributes about aging. Yet, older adults may apply stereotypes of older adults they acquired when they were younger. Levy (2003) argues:

> When individuals reach old age, the aging stereotypes internalized in childhood, and then reinforced for decades, become self-stereotypes. . . . Self-stereotypes may be acquired in two stages. When the individual reaches an age that is formally defined by institutions or informally by other individuals, as old, she or he joins the aged membership group, which constitutes the first stage. . . . [T]he next stage involves identification with others in the same category (i.e., a belief that one is old). (p. 204)

Other theorists debate whether older adults apply stereotypes of the aged to themselves. Older adults often report feeling they are younger than their chronological age and resist being labeled "elderly" (Zebrowitz, 2003). Indeed, even the very elderly may view those who are older than themselves as the *true* old people and believe that other adults their age are worse off than they are (Heckhausen & Brim, 1997).

In sum, as with regard to socialization in childhood, some individuals may be more susceptible to cultural stereotypes of the aged than other individuals. It is likely that some older adults internalize the stereotypes they have formed in early life, whereas other older adults do not. Personality, external pressures, and social partners' reactions to the older adult may help explain these differences. Scholarship suggests that in particular, more distant social partners may reinforce culturally negative views of the elderly and induce dependency in doing so. This may be particularly the case for health care professionals or other individuals who do not know the older adult well.

Socialization When Older Adults Experience Health Problems

Socialization influences may have detrimental effects when older adults begin to experience physical declines in late life. Social partners appear to differentiate between elderly adults in good health and elderly adults with health problems; they generally view their relationships more negatively if the older adult is unwell. For example Fingerman et al. (2005) interviewed adults over age 70 who incurred common health impairments of old age (e.g., vision and hearing loss) and the grown child who knew most about their health.

Parents and offspring were more likely to indicate that their relationship had gotten worse if the parent experienced functional disabilities or serious diseases, regardless of whether or not the adult offspring assisted the parent with tasks of daily living.

Furthermore, adults who have health problems spend a great deal of time with health care professionals. In contrast to the positive experiences older adults may have in relationships that have endured throughout life (e.g., with spouses and grown offspring), older adults may encounter negative interactions with individuals whom they first encounter as an elderly adult. Communication theorists suggest that younger adults in formal situations, such as health care settings, tend to speak to older adults in ways that can be condescending (Coupland et al., 1988); this differential treatment may undermine older adults' sense of autonomy and self-esteem. For example, Ryan, Meredith, Maclean, and Orange (1995) found that medical personnel tended to guess a patient's age based on appearance (white hair) and behaviors (trouble hearing) and roles (retiree), even if their actual age was not known. When these health care personnel perceived a patient as elderly, they engaged in inappropriate communication based on stereotypes. These modifications included slower speech, exaggerated intonation, high pitch, loudness, repetition, simpler vocabulary, and reduced grammatical complexity. The authors argued that older adults who were unsure about their current abilities infer that they are not doing well and reduce self-esteem and efforts at remediation.

The negative effects of socialization agents may be particularly evident as adults begin to experience frailty. Margret Baltes and her colleagues conducted a series of detailed observational studies in which they demonstrated that social influences encourage frail older adults to relinquish autonomy (e.g., M. Baltes, 1988, 1995). Care providers who work in nursing homes encouraged older adults to accept help and to become more dependent over time. The staff rewarded behaviors that involved their assistance, such as pushing a wheelchair to the dining hall, and ignored behaviors that asserted autonomy, such as an older adult's insistence on pushing himself to the dining hall. This approach resulted in increased dependency and loss of competencies among the older adults (M. Baltes & Horgas, 1997). Indeed, M. Baltes referred to this process as a "dependency script" and demonstrated that social partners induced dependent behaviors among older adults in a variety of settings.

In sum, in support of the social input model, social partners may reinforce the detriments or declines that older adults experience. Peope react to older adults who have health problems differently than they react to older adults who are healthy. Of course, social partners can proffer help without undermining older adults (Martini et al., 2001, 2003), but as older adults start to experience physical problems, they may question their own abilities. Coupled with the evidence pertaining to older adults' reactions to stereotypes, evidence further suggests that social input may reinforce existing negative perceptions and, thus, undermine self-efficacy and esteem.

CONCLUSION

At the start of this chapter, we noted the dearth of literature pertaining to socialization in old age. A synthesis of research related to this topic raises as many questions as it answers. Do social partners socialize older adults? If so, what are the mechanisms through which they do so? Does socialization change in form in old age, or is it continuous from socialization in the past? Is socialization effective in old age? This chapter considered these questions.

Do social partners socialize older adults? Research has linked close relationships to better physical and cognitive functioning and to decreased rates of mortality in old age (Berkman & Syme, 1979; Charles & Mavandadi, 2004; Fratiglioni et al., 2000). Yet, the mechanisms through which the social milieu affects older adults are not well specified. It is unclear whether partners socialize older adults in ways that change the older adults or simply proffer support. Social partners may influence physiological mechanisms and health through emotion regulation (Ryff & Singer, 2005). Yet, clearly, additional research is needed to understand these issues.

Does socialization change in form in old age, or is it continuous from socialization in the past? When and how do older adults serve as socialization agents? Many socialization influences in old age stem from continuity with prior stages of life. For example, older adults tend to prefer enduring relationships over newly formed relationships in late life. Events in early life, such as trauma, may affect later life patterns of coping. Nonetheless, research also suggests changes in socialization across adulthood. For example, adults' sense of control changes by late life, such that they exert increased efforts on regulating their own internal reactions rather than the environment (Schulz & Heckhausen, 1999). Further, even within long-lasting relationships, such as ties to offspring, patterns of socialization may shift in late life (Fingerman et al., 2005).

Thus, there is complexity with regard to continuity and discontinuity of socialization in old age. Older adults experience socialization from close social partners in long-lasting ties with established patterns of interactions. Research examining socialization might commence with relationships in early adulthood or midlife to capture the processes that lead to socialization in old age. Given the expense and impracticality of conducting longitudinal research on aging, cross-sectional studies might examine processes thought to arise in old age, such as increased emotion regulation and shifts in control.

Is socialization effective in old age? Socialization agents appear to exert negative, positive, and no influence in different settings. As individuals accrue disabilities in late life, socialization agents can impede autonomous functioning, harm self-esteem, and encourage dependent functioning (M. Baltes, 1995; Nussbaum et al., 1996). The literature suggests mechanisms through which this occurs, including microlevel behavioral interchanges (e.g., ageist communication styles and reinforcement of dependency behaviors) and macrolevel structural constraints (e.g., a Medicaid system that pays for nursing home placement, but not for in-home services that would allow the older adult to remain in place). The literature also suggests contexts in which socialization is ineffective, such as in preparation for widowhood (Carr et al., 2001); older adults who are able to anticipate their spouse's death fare no better on indicators of mental health than older adults who lose a spouse suddenly. The literature is least developed with regard to the positive effects of socialization in old age. Evidence for the social input model suggests that older adults may evoke positive responses from their close social partners (Fingerman & Baker, 2006). Yet, there are few studies specifically examining social partners' perceptions and treatment of old adults. Future research might specifically examine how close social partners respond to older adults and the positive influences they exert.

On the whole, older adults report high well-being and satisfaction with their social world until they begin to experience severe health declines of old age. The social world appears to help compensate for some of the losses and transitions that individuals incur, and individuals in turn develop their own strategies to deal with these challenges after a lifetime of practice. Furthermore, improved emotion regulation and greater investment in relationships appear to pay off in better relationship quality and less negative emotionality in late life (Carstensen et al., 2003). These changes in emotion regulation may set off reciprocal processes whereby individuals evoke, receive, and transmit positive emotions in relationships.

In sum, gerontologists have paid little attention to socialization forces or processes in late life. Extant literature suggests that the social milieu may influence older adults' beliefs, behaviors, and emotions. Future research is needed to specifically examine these issues.

ACKNOWLEDGMENT

This chapter was written with support from Grant No. R01 AG17916 from the National Institute on Aging, "Problems between Parents and Offspring in Adulthood."

REFERENCES

Adams, R. G. (1985–1986). Emotional closeness and physical distance between friends: Implications for elderly women living in age-segregated and age-integrated settings. *International Journal of Aging and Human Development, 22,* 55–76.

Akiyama, H., Antonucci, T., Takahashi, K., & Langfahl, E. S. (2003). Negative interactions in close relationships across the lifespan. *Journal of Gerontology: Psychological Sciences, 58B,* P70–P79.

Antonucci, T. C., & Akiyama, H. (1987). Social networks in adult life and a preliminary examination of the convoy model. *Journals of Gerontology, 42,* 519–527.

Antonucci, T. C., Akiyama, H., & Birditt, K. S. (2005). Intergenerational exchange in the United States and Japan. In M. Silverstein (Ed.), *Intergenerational relations across time and place: Annual review of gerontology and geriatrics* (pp. 224–248). New York: Springer.

Antonucci, T. C., Lansford, J. E., Akiyama, H., Smith, J., Baltes, M. M. Takahashi, K., et al. (2002). Differences between men and women in social relations, resource deficits, and depressive symptomatology during later life in four nations. *Journal of Social Issues, 58,* 767–783.

Arnett, J .J. (1995a). Broad and narrow socialization: The family in the context of a cultural theory. *Journal of Marriage and the Family, 57,* 617–628.

Arnett, J.J. (1995b). Adolescents' uses of media for self-socialization. *Journal of Youth and Adolescence, 24,* 519–553.

Arnett, J. J. (2001). Conceptions of the transition to adulthood: Perspectives from adolescence through midlife. *Journal of Adult Development, 8,* 133–143.

Baltes, M. M. (1988). The etiology and maintenance of dependency in the elderly: Three phases of operant research, *Behavior Therapy, 19,* 301–319.

Baltes, M. M. (1995). Dependency in old age: Gains and losses. *Current Directions in Psychological Science, 4,* 14–19.

Baltes, M. M., & Horgas, A. L. (1997). Long-term care institutions and the maintenance of competence: A dialectic between compensation and overcompensation. In S. L. Willis & K. W. Schaie (Eds.), *Societal mechanisms for maintaining competence in old age. Societal impact on aging.* (pp. 142–181). New York: Springer.

Baltes, P. (1997). On the incomplete architecture of human ontogeny. *American Psychologist, 52,* 366–380.

Bassuk, S. S., Glass, T., & Berkman, L. F. (1999). Social disengagement and incident of cognitive decline in community-dwelling elderly persons. *Annals of Internal Medicine, 131,* 165–173.

Becker, G., Beyene, Y., Newsom, E., & Mayen, N. (2003). Creating continuity through mutual assistance:

Intergenerational reciprocity in four ethnic groups. *Journal of Gerontology: Social Sciences, 58*, S151–S159.

Bedford, V. H. (1989). Understanding the value of siblings in old age: A proposed model. *American Behavioral Scientist, 33*, 33–44.

Berkman, L. F., Glass, T. Brissette, I., & Seeman, T. E. (2000). From social integration to health: Durkheim in the new millennium. *Social Science and Medicine, 51*, 843–857.

Berkman, L. F., & Syme, S. L. (1979). Social networks, host resistance, and mortality: A nine year follow-up study of Alameda County residents. *American Journal of Epidemiology, 109*, 186–204.

Birditt, K. S., & Fingerman, K. L. (2003). Age and gender differences in adults' emotional reactions to interpersonal tensions. *Journal of Gerontology: Psychological Sciences, 58B*, P237–P245.

Birditt, K. S., & Fingerman, K. L. (2005). Do we get better at picking our battles?: Age differences in descriptions of behavioral reactions to interpersonal tensions. *Journals of Gerontology: Psychological Sciences, 60B*, 121–128.

Brandtstadter, J., & Greve, W. (1994). The aging self: Stabilizing and protective processes. *Developmental Review, 14*, 52–80.

Bronfenbrenner, U., & Morris, P (1998). The ecology of developmental processes. In W. Damon & R. Lerner (Eds.). *Handbook of child psychology: Volume 1: Theorectical models of human development* (5th ed., pp. 993–1028). New York: Wiley.

Brown, W. M., Consedine, N. S., & Magai, C. (2005). Altruism relates to health in an ethnically diverse sample of older adults. *Journals of Gerontology: Psychological Sciences and Social Sciences, 60*, P143–P152.

Bugental, D. B., & Grusec, J. E. (2006). Socialization processes. In N. Eisenberg (Vol. Ed.), *Handbook of child psychology: Vol. 3. Social, emotional, and personality development* (pp. 366–428). Hoboken, NJ: Wiley.

Bullock, J. R., & Osborne, S. S. (1999). Seniors', volunteers', and families' perspectives of an intergenerational program in a rural community. *Educational Gerontology, 25*, 237–251.

Burstmedia. (2002). Online insights: Volume 2–9. Retrieved January 14, 2005, from www.burstmedia.com/release/advertisers/online_insights/december_2002.pdf.

Carpenter, B. D. (2001). Attachment bonds between adult daughters and their older mothers: Associations with contemporary caregiving. *Journals of Gerontology: Psychological Sciences*, P257–P266.

Carr, D., House, J. S., Wortman, C. , Nesse, R., & Kessler, R. C. (2001). Psychological adjustment to sudden and anticipated spousal loss among older widows. *Journals of Gerontology: Social Sciences, 56B*, S237–S248.

Carrigan, M., & Szmigin, I. (1999). The representation of older people in advertisements, *Journal of the Market Research Society, 41*, 311–326.

Carstensen, L. L., Fung, H. H., & Charles, S. T. (2003). Socioemotional selectivity theory and the regulation of emotion in the second half of life. *Motivation and Emotion, 27*, 103–123.

Carstensen, L. L., Isaacowitz, D. M., & Charles, S. T. (1999). Taking time seriously: A theory of socioemotional selectivity. *American Psychologist, 54*, 165–181.

Charles, S. T, & Mavandadi, S. (2004). Social support and physical health across the life span: Socioemotional influences. In F. Lang & K. L. Fingerman (Eds.), *Growing together: Personal relationships across the life span* (pp. 240–267). New York: Cambridge University Press.

Chasteen, A. L., Schwarz, N., & Park, D. C. (2002). The activation of aging stereotypes in younger and older adults. *Journal of Gerontology: Psychological Sciences, 57B*, P540–P547.

Chatters, L. M., Taylor, R. J., Lincoln, K. D., & Schroepfer, T. (2002). Patterns of informal support from family and church members among African Americans. *Journal of Black Studies, 33*, 66–85.

Connidis, I. A., & Davies, L. (1992). Confidants and companions: Choices in later life. *Journals of Gerontology: Social Sciences, 47*, S115–S122.

Coupland, N., Coupland, J., Giles, H., & Henwood, K. (1988). Accommodating the elderly: Invoking and extending theory. *Language and Society, 17*, 1–41.

Ekerdt, D. J., Kosloski, K., & De Viney, S. (2000). The normative anticipation of retirement by older workers. *Research on Aging, 22*, 3–22.

Elder, G. H. Jr. (1998). The life course as developmental theory. *Child Development, 69*, 1–12.

Elder, G. H., Jr., & Liker, J. K. (1982). Hard times in women's lives: Historical influences across forty years. *American Journal of Sociology, 88*, 241–269.

Erber, J. T., Szuchman, L. T., & Prager, I. G. (2001). Ain't misbehavin': The effects of age and intentionality on judgments about misconduct. *Psychology and Aging, 16,* 85–95.

Feinberg, L. F., & Newman, S. L. (2004). A study of 10 states since passage of the national family caregiver support program: Policies, perceptions and program development. *The Gerontologist, 44,* 760–769.

Fingerman, K. L. (1996). Sources of tension in the aging mother and adult daughter relationship. *Psychology and Aging, 11,* 591–606.

Fingerman, K. L. (1998). The good, the bad, and the worrisome: Complexities in grandparents' relationships with individual grandchildren. *Family Relations, 47,* 403–414.

Fingerman, K. L. (2000). "We had a nice little chat": Age and generational differences in mothers' and daughters' descriptions of enjoyable visits. *Journals of Gerontology: Series B: Psychological Sciences and Social Sciences, 55B,* 95–106.

Fingerman, K. L. (2001). *Aging mothers and their adult daughters: A study in mixed emotions.* New York: Springer.

Fingerman, K. L. (2004). The consequential stranger: Peripheral ties across the life span. In F. Lang & K. L. Fingerman (Eds.), *Growing together: Personal relationships across the life span* (pp. 183–209). New York: Cambridge University Press.

Fingerman, K. L., & Baker, B. (2006). Socioemotional aspects of aging. In J. Wilmouth & K. Ferraro (Eds.), *Perspectives in gerontology* (3rd ed., pp. 183–202). New York: Springer.

Fingerman, K. L., & Birditt, K. S. (2003). Do age differences in close and problematic family ties reflect the pool of available relatives? *Journal of Gerontology: Psychological Sciences, 58,* P80–P87.

Fingerman, K.L., & Griffiths, P.C. (1999). Season's greetings: Adults' social contacts at the holiday season. *Psychology and Aging, 14,* 192–205.

Fingerman, K. L., Hay, E. L., Kamp-Dush, C. M., Cichy, K., & Hosterman, S. (2005). *Role Revisions: Parents' and offspring's perceptions of change and continuity in later life.* Manuscript under review.

Fingerman, K. L., & Perlmutter M. (1995). Future time perspective across adulthood. *Journal of General Psychology, 122,* 95–112.

Fratiglioni, L., Wang, H. X., Ericsson, K., Maytan, M., & Winblad B. (2000). Influence of social network on occurrence of dementia: A community based longitudinal study. *The Lancet, 355,* 1315–1319.

Freedman, V. A., Martin, L. G., & Schoeni, R. F. (2002). Recent trends in disability and functioning among older adults in the United States. *Journal of the American Medical Association, 288,* 3137–3146.

Harris, J. R. (1995). Where is the child's environment? A group socialization theory of development. *Psychological Review, 102,* 458–489.

Harris, J. R. (2000). Socialization, personality development, and the child's environment: Comment on Vandell (2000). *Developmental Psychology, 36,* 711–723.

Hazan, C., & Shaver, P. (1994). Attachment as an organizational framework for research on close relationships. *Psychological Inquiry, 5,* 1–22.

Heckhausen, J., & Brim, O. G. (1997). Perceived problems for self and others: Self-protection by social downgrading throughout adulthood. *Psychology and Aging, 12,* 610–619.

Heckhausen, J., Wrosch, C., & Fleeson, W. (2001). Developmental regulation before and after a developmental deadline: The sample case of a biological clock for childrearing. *Psychology and Aging, 16,* 400–413.

Herrmann, D. S., Sipsas-Herrmann, A., Stafford, M., & Herrmann, N. C. (2005). Benefits and risks of intergenerational program participation by senior citizens *Educational Gerontology, 31,* 123–138.

House, J. S., Landis, K. R., & Umberson, D. (1988). Social relationships and health. *Science, 241,* 540–544.

Hummert, M. L., Garstka, T. A., Shaner, J. L., & Strahm, S. (1994). Stereotypes of the elderly held by young, middle-aged and older adults. *Journals of Gerontology: Psychological Sciences, 49,* P240–249.

iMedia. (2004). Older adults leading net usage growth. Retrieved January 14, 2005, from www.imediaconnection.com/news/4747.asp.

Kahana, B., Kahana, E., Harel, Z., & Kelly, K. (1997). A framework for understanding the chronic stress of Holocaust survivors. In B.H. Gottlieb (Ed), *Coping with chronic stress. The Plenum series on stress and coping* (pp. 315–342). New York: Plenum Press.

Krause, N. (2001). Social support. In R. H. Binstock (Ed.), *Handbook of aging and the social sciences* (5th ed., pp. 272–294). San Diego: Academic Press.

Krause, N. (2002). Church-based social support and health in old age: Exploring variations by race. *Journal of Gerontology: Social Sciences, 57B,* S332–S347.

Lang, F. R. (2001). Regulation of social relationships in later adulthood. *Journals of Gerontology: Psychological Sciences, 56,* P321–P326.

Lefkowitz, E. S., & Fingerman, K. L. (2003). Positive and negative emotional feelings and behaviors in mother–daughter ties in late life. *Journal of Family Psychology, 17,* 607–617.

Levy, B. R. (1999). The inner self of the Japanese elderly: A defense against negative stereotypes of aging. *International Journal of Aging and Human Development, 48,* 131–144.

Levy, B. R. (2003). Mind matters: Cognitive and physical effects of aging self-stereotypes. *Journals of Gerontology: Psychological Sciences, 58B,* P203–P211.

Levy, B., & Langer, E. (1994). Aging free from negative stereotypes: Successful memory in China and among the American deaf. *Journal of Personality and Social Psychology, 66,* 989–997.

Liang, J., Krause, N. M., & Bennett, J. M. (2001). Social exchange and well-being: Is giving better than receiving? *Psychology and Aging, 16,* 511–523.

Logan, J. R., & Spitze, G. D. (1996). *Family ties: Enduring relations between parents and their grown children.* Philadelphia: Temple University Press.

Maccoby, E. E. (2002). Gender and group process: A developmental perspective. *Current Directions in Psychological Science, 11,* 54–58.

Magai, C., & Consedine, N. S. (2004). Introduction to the special issue: Attachment and aging. *Attachment and Human Development, 6,* 349–351.

Magai, C., Consedine, N. S., Gillespie, M., O'Neal, C., & Vilker, R. (2004). The differential roles of early emotion socialization and adult attachment in adult emotional experience: Testing a mediator hypothesis. *Attachment and Human Development, 6,* 389–417.

Manne, S. L., & Zautra, A. J. (1989). Spouse criticism and support: Their association with coping and psychological adjustment among women with rheumatoid arthritis. *Journal of Personality and Social Psychology, 56,* 608–617.

Martini, T. S., Grusec, J. E., & Bernardini, S. C. (2001). Effects of interpersonal control, perspective taking, and attributions on older mothers' and daughters' satisfaction with their helping relationships. *Journal of Family Psychology, 15,* 688–705.

Martini, T. S., Grusec, J. E., & Bernardini, S. C. (2003). Perceptions of help given to healthy older mothers by adult daughters: Ways of initiating help and types of help given. *International Journal of Aging and Human Development, 57,* 237–257.

Moen, P. (2001). The gendered life course. In R. H. Binstock & L. K. George (Eds.), *The handbook of aging and the social sciences* (5th ed., pp. 179– 196). New York: Academic Press.

National Opinion Research Center. (1997). *General Social Survey.* Chicago: Author.

Neugarten, B. L., & Weinstein, K. K. (1964). The changing American grandparent. *Journal of Marriage and the Family, 26,* 199–204.

Nussbaum, J. F., Hummert, M. L., Williams, A., & Harwood, J. (1996). Communication and older adults. In B. R. Burleson (Ed.), *Communication yearbook* (pp. 1–47). Thousand Oaks, CA: Sage.

Rook, K. S. (1984). The negative side of social interaction: Impact on psychological well-being. *Journal of Personality and Social Psychology, 46,* 1097–1108.

Ryan, E. B., Meredith, S. D., Maclean, M. J., & Orange, J. B. (1995). Changing the way we talk with elders: Promoting health using the communication enhancement model. *International Journal of Aging and Human Development, 41,* 89–107.

Ryff, C. D., & Singer, B. H. (2005). Social environments and the genetics of aging: Advancing knowledge of protective health mechanisms. *Journals of Gerontology, 60B,* 12–23.

Schulz, R., & Heckhausen, J. (1999). Aging, culture, and control: Setting a new research agenda. *Journals of Gerontology: Psychological Sciences and Social Sciences, 54,* P139–P145.

Sczinovacz, M., & Ekerdt, D. J. (1995). Families and retirement. In R. Blieszner & V. H. Bedford (Eds.), *Handbook of aging and the family* (pp. 375–400). Westport, CT: Greenwood Press.

Settersten, R. A. Jr. (2003). Propositions and controversies in life course scholarship. In R. A. Settersten (Ed.), *Invitation to the life course: Toward new understandings of later life* (pp. 15–45). New York: Baywood.

Shaver, P. R., Belsky, J., & Brennan, K. A. (2000). The adult attachment interview and self-reports of romantic attachment: Associations across domains and methods. *Personal Relationships, 7,* 25–43.

Smith, D. B., & Moen, P. (1998). Spousal influence on retirement: His, her, and their perceptions. *Journal of Marriage and the Family, 60,* 734–744.

Smith, D. B., & Moen, P. (2004). Retirement satisfaction for retirees and their spouses: Do gender and the retirement decision-making process matter? *Journal of Family Issues, 25,* 262–285.

Smith, J., Borchelt, M., Maier, H., & Jopp, D. (2002). Health and well-being in the young old and the oldest old. *Journal of Social Issues, 58,* 715–732.

Uchino, B. N., Cacioppo, J. T., & Kiecolt-Glaser, J. K. (1996). The relationship between social support and physiological processes: A review with emphasis on underlying mechanisms and implications for health. *Psychological Bulletin, 119,* 488–531.

Umberson, D. (1989). Relationships with children: Explaining parents' psychological well-being. *Journal of Marriage and the Family, 51,* 999–1012.

Vandell, D. L. (2000). Parents, peer groups, and other socializing influences. *Developmental Psychology, 36,* 699–710.

White, H., McConnell, E., Clipp, E., Branch, L., Sloane, R., Pieper, C., et al. (2002). A randomized controlled trial of the psychosocial impact of providing internet training and access to older adults. *Aging and Mental Health, 6,* 213–221.

Wiscott, R., & Kopera-Frye, K. (2000). Sharing the culture: Adult grandchildren's perceptions of intergenerational relations. *International Journal of Aging and Human Development, 51,* 199–215.

Zebrowitz, L. (2003). Aging stereotypes: Internalization or inoculation: A commentary. *Journals of Gerontology: Psychological Sciences, 58B,* P214–P215.

PART IV

Socialization within the Family

CHAPTER 10

Agency and Bidirectionality in Socialization

Interactions, Transactions, and Relational Dialectics

Leon Kuczynski and C. Melanie Parkin

During much of the previous century socialization was viewed primarily as a mechanism for intergenerational continuity and the reproduction of culture (Corsaro, 1997; Valsiner 1988, Wrong, 1961). Conceptions of how socialization came about tended to be unidirectional and deterministic. Empirical studies attempted to connect static characteristics of parents, conceptualized as causes, to static characteristics of children, conceptualized as outcomes. Major outcomes of socialization such as compliance and the intergenerational transmission of ideas, roles, and values were narrowly conceptualized as the conformity of the younger generation to the norms and regulations of the previous generation.

As the chapters in this handbook attest, contemporary researchers have a much more dynamic conception of the process and outcomes of socialization. The new approaches generally address the actions and interpretive activity of both parents and children and are beginning to consider that innovation and change, not just intergenerational continuity, are to be expected as outcomes of the socialization process. This revitalization of socialization theory can be traced to two important ideas that took hold during the 1960s. The first is that children and, correspondingly, parents, are agents who initiate and resist influence (Rheingold, 1969) and construct new meanings through their interpretation of their social experiences (e.g., Kohlberg, 1969). The second is that socialization is a bidirectional interactive process incorporating the influence of both children and parents (Bell, 1968; Sameroff, 1975a). The purpose of this chapter is to explore how these ideas have played out in contemporary models of socialization in the context of the family. In the first part, we examine current conceptions of parents and children as agents in the context of their relationship. Then we contrast behavioral and dialectical conceptions of bidirectional influence in socialization. Finally, we explore three theories that depict socialization as a dynamic process—social interactional theory, transactional theory, and social relational theory—with respect to their positions concerning human agency and the nature of bidirectional influence. We argue that social relational theory is particularly useful for the analysis of socialization processes between parents and children considered as agents.

PARENTS AND CHILDREN AS AGENTS IN SOCIALIZATION

Contemporary scholars consider human agency to be a multifaceted construct (Bandura, 2001; Cummings & Schermerhorn, 2003; Kuczynski, 2003) that includes cognitive, behavioral, and motivational dimensions. Parents and children have capacities to initiate purposeful behavior and strategically choose methods for influencing each other's behavior. They have the capacity to reflect on their behavior and interpret messages communicated during interaction. They also have the capacity to assert themselves, resist demands that threaten their autonomy (Crockenberg & Littman, 1990; Kuczynski & Kochanska, 1990; Wenar, 1982), block their goals, or contravene their self-constructed understanding of social situations (Kuczynski & Navara, 2005).

Direct personal control over outcomes is not the only way that parents and children exercise agency. Bandura (2001) identified two modes of human agency "proxy agency" and "collective agency" that enable individuals to enlist their network of relationships to extend their effectiveness in achieving their goals. Individuals engage in proxy agency when they get others to act for them. "People also turn to proxy control in areas in which they cannot exert direct influence, when they have not developed the means to do so, when they believe others can do it better, or when they do not want to saddle themselves with the burdensome aspects that direct control entails" (Bandura, 2001, p. 12). The use of proxy agency to augment personal power is an important part of family life. Children go to parents to obtain resources or instrumental aid for themselves. They enlist the support of parents to intercede for them with their siblings, or with teachers and institutions outside the home. They also use their multiple relationships strategically, for instance, approaching their mothers when resources are denied by their fathers. Mothers and fathers exercise proxy agency when they divide up responsibilities for their children's care and socialization. Human agents also increase their power to exert influence through collective agency. When families act collectively as a whole or when subunits of the family form parental or sibling alliances, parents and children may achieve goals that would not be possible if they had acted as individuals.

Contributions of Agency Perspectives

A focus on human agency both contributes to the understanding of the processes of socialization and clarifies the contributions of parents and children to those processes. In their review of the correlational research on parenting styles, Darling and Steinberg (1993) noted that despite consistent evidence that authoritative parents produce competent children, the underlying interactive processes remain obscure. Similarly, children's influence on parents generally has been studied under the rubric of "child effects," an approach that considers global features such as age, gender, physical characteristics, and temperament. Such research is useful in identifying associations between child variables and parental variables but does not illuminate the intervening processes of social interaction and relationship formation that underlie abstract measured variables. The perspective of human agency guides researchers to be curious about what parents and children do in social interactions or how they interpret their experiences.

In addition, considering parents and children equally as agents guides researchers to ask questions about their influence and agency in a parallel manner (Kuczynski, 2003; Valsiner, Branco, & Dantas, 1997). Considering children's perspectives, goals, meaning making, and influence techniques is a corrective strategy for filling in knowledge regarding the neglected children's side of a bidirectional process. For example, research on parental goals has richly described the goal-directed activities of parents during interactions with children. Parents have been found to act on long-term and short-term socialization goals (Kuczynski, 1984), empathic goals, parent-centered goals (Dix & Branca, 2003), and relationship goals (Hastings & Grusec, 1998). In contrast, until recently, the only goals attributed to children concerned short-term goals such as evading parental demands (Patterson, 1982). In a recent study of adolescent conflict, six different goals were identified (Lundell, Grusec, McShane, & Davidson, 2005). These included dyadic concern, a counterpart to parental relationship goals, as well as goals that were self-serving in nature such as goals for emotional support, instrumental help, autonomy, dominance, and conflict avoidance. Younger adolescents reported having instrumental goals more often than older adolescents who reported more goals for emotional support and dominance. An enhanced perspective on children's agency is likely to uncover that as children develop, they will increasingly form and act on a range of short-term and long-term goals that impact on their own socialization and their interactions with parents.

Parental agency has also been discounted by early socialization theories. Although there has been much research on children's internalization, the parent's own internalization processes remain unexplored. A by-product of unidirectional models of socialization is that parents were implicitly considered to be passive conduits of their own socialization experiences in a process of intergenerational transmission (Kuczynski, Marshall, & Schell, 1997; Kuczynski & Navara, 2005). Regarding parents more fully as agents focuses attention on parents' interpretive and constructive activities with regard to their own continuing processes of resocialization and internalization. Parents, like children, are engaged in a lifelong process of socialization and development and, like children, one source for their continuing development is their experiences of interactions within family relationships (Frankel, 1991; Kuczynski et al., 1997; Palkovitz, Marks, Appleby, & Holmes, 2003). Research conducted from the perspective of parental agency would also explore how parents evaluate, reconstruct, and act on or adapt their values in their everyday life and in their childrearing decisions. Parents do not care equally about all values (Grusec, Goodnow, & Kuczynski, 2000). They may not view everything in their own repertoire of socialized behaviors as adaptive for their children's success in society (Kuczynski et al., 1997). Intergenerational change may result from choices that parents make regarding which values they will hold on to and which they allow to be shelved. A challenge for the future is to develop models that consider parents and children interacting simultaneously as agents and adapting to each other's agency during interactions (Kuczynski, Lollis, & Koguchi, 2003).

Bidirectionality and Agency

Kuczynski and colleagues (Kuczynski et al. 2003; Kuczynski, Harach, & Bernardini, 1999) proposed that socialization research could be advanced within a "bilateral framework" that emphasized the role of human agency in bidirectional processes in parent–child interactions. However, not all influence is the result of people's actions as agents. For example, children have a comprehensive but inadvertent influence on parental lives and on the family without exercising agency. Many of the ways that children influence parental lives stem from the mere presence of children in the parents' environment. These include children's impact on parental health, the physical location and social position that parents occupy in society, their daily routines, parental employment (especially that of the mother), disposable income, the quality of marital relations, the parents' interactional and emotional experiences, the parents' participation in the community, the parent's future life plans, and, the parents' feelings of control over their own lives (Ambert, 1992). Children's presence also influences parents' continuing adult development by exposing them to an environment of continuous caregiving and problem solving. The experience of involved parenting is implicated in adult's changes in attitudes and values, increased maturity and responsibility, and identity development (Frankel, 1991; Palkovitz et al., 2003). Although children mediate these processes, their agency is not implicated.

Other areas have been identified in which automaticity and habit rather than intentional action or deliberative construction appears to be the dominant process (Patterson, Reid, & Dishion, 1992). Goodnow (1997) suggests that a great deal of human action is unconsciously channeled by cultural practices. Thus, much of socialization comes about through parents' and children's participation in the everyday routines and practices of their social group where habitual ways of thinking and acting are not subject to questioning or creative thought. Human agency in such situations is constrained unless extraordinary events or therapeutic interventions cause the individual to reflect on and track his or her behaviors and reactions. Clearly, future models of socialization need to incorporate the contribution of both agentic and nonagentic processes in bidirectional influence.

BEHAVIORAL VERSUS DIALECTICAL MODELS OF BIDIRECTIONALITY

There is considerable diversity in the ways in which bidirectional influence is conceptualized in research on socialization (Kuczynski, 2003). However, two general approaches can be distinguished: those that consider bidirectionality in terms of immediate reciprocal exchanges of behaviors producing linear, incremental change and those that consider bidirectionality as a dialectical process in which human agents construct meanings out of each other's behavior and, thereby, produce transformational change.

An early way of conceiving of bidirectional influence in social interactions was in terms of an immediate exchange of behaviors between the parent and child. Sears (1951) conceived of social interactions as an interconnected series of stimulus–response sequences in which each person's behavior was simultaneously a reaction to the other's previous behavior and a stimulus for the partner's subsequent response. These stimulus–response exchanges have been conceived in various ways. Children may reciprocate parents' smiles or irritable responses with smiles or irritable behaviors of their own, a parent may soothe a crying child in the manner of a homeostatic control system (Bell & Harper,

1977), or a parent and child may reciprocally provide contingent negative reinforcement for each other's coercive behavior (Patterson, 1982). Generally speaking, such models consider behavior change to be explained by incremental shaping of behaviors rather than the goal-directed choices, actions, and constructions of parents and children.

In contrast, researchers from cognitive perspectives such as sociocultural theory (Lawrence & Valsiner, 1993), social domain theory (Smetana, 1997), and goal-directed models of parenting (Dix & Branca, 2003; Holden & Hawk, 2003; Grusec, Goodnow, & Kuczynski, 2000) are guided by a dialectical conception of bidirectionality. In this view, bidirectional influence comes about as parents and children interpret each other's behaviors, construct meanings from their experiences of interactions and relationships, and anticipate and accommodate each other's perspectives and goals during interaction. Such models generally conceive of bidirectionality in socialization as a process of mutual adaptation brought about by changing cognitive representations of the interaction or the relationship (Kuczynski et. al., 2003).

Why call these approaches dialectical? First, the processes of mutual interpretation and accommodation of goals based on meanings ascribed to behaviors in interaction clearly cannot be understood by reactive notions of bidirectionality implied by reciprocal exchanges of behavior. Second, even though the term "dialectical" has been used infrequently in socialization research, dialectical concepts are implicit in most current interactional perspectives that conceive of development or change as resulting from interactions between an organism and its environment and that place the organism as an active participant in that process (Salkind, 1985). We suggest, therefore, that a dialectical model of bidirectionality currently provides the best fit for describing interactions between parents and children as human agents.

In the past, dialectical ideas gradually have been co-opted by various theories without attribution. Examples include Piagetian and Vygoskian accounts of cognitive development, attachment theory accounts of working models, and ecological systems theory (Glassman, 2000). However, new accounts of parenting (Holden & Ritchie, 1988, Valsiner et al., 1997), conflict (Valsiner & Cairns, 1992), and social relationships (Baxter & Montgomery 1996; Hinde, 1997) are beginning to explicitly acknowledge their roots in dialectics.

Glassman (2000) suggests that the paradox of the great influence but low recognition of dialectics stems from the philosophical rather than empirical origins of the concept. Glassman traced different stages in the recent evolution of dialectics in the writings of Hegel, Feuerbach, Marx, Lévy-Bruhl, Vygotsky, and Riegel. In this section, we provide an overview of the basic premises of dialectics as a way of encouraging further systematic exploration of dialectics as a conceptual framework for bidirectional processes in theories of socialization.

There are many approaches to dialectics with different theoreticians drawing on or developing different aspects of the concept (see Baxter & Montgomery, 1996, for a review). Common to most conceptions of dialectics are three general principles: *contradiction, the unity of opposites,* and *continuous change* (Altman Vinsel, & Brown, 1981).

Contradiction

The principle of *contradiction* assumes that all phenomena contain opposing elements ("thesis" and "antithesis") as an inherent aspect of their makeup. The tension between these opposing forces produces both cumulative and qualitative change. An important step in a dialectical analysis is the identification of contradictions that are inherent or implicit in the phenomenon under consideration.

The parental role generates many such contradictions on a daily basis. For example, parents must allow exploration yet guard against danger, be responsive yet avoid spoiling the child, seek obedience and respect yet allow autonomy, be involved yet not overinvolved, promote independence yet maintain dependence (Holden & Ritchie, 1988). The parental role itself involves diverse conflicting functions and roles such as authority, caretaker, attachment figure, intimate, and companion that must be kept in balance (Harach & Kuczynski, 2005). Parent–child socialization, considered from the perspective of parents and children interacting as agents, also constantly creates contradictions that feed into the dialectical process. Interactions where parents make demands of their children often pit the parent's needs against the child's needs, the parent's will against the child's will, the parent's understanding of values against the child's understanding, the parent's definitions of a behavior against the child's definitions, and the parent's influence strategies against the child's influence strategies. In addition, parents and children continually come up against a larger ecological context of values and understandings including those of peers, television, Internet, and school that offer up contradictions and opportunities for further change as parents and children adapt to each others' actions and choices.

Unity of Opposites

Unity of opposites implies that individual elements must be understood as interrelated parts of a whole system. "Dialectical psychology takes a fundamental stand in rejecting any contention that a thing or system can be adequately understood without reference to the whole of which it is a part. In particular, it rejects the investigation of individual actions without reference to interpersonal, individual-group and individual-society relations" (Ho, 1998, p. 8). In dialectics, the meaning of a whole system is complex because systems contain both shared and contradictory elements that coexist and continually interact. For example, parents and children may frequently come into conflict because of their needs for autonomy, but they are united by the bonds of their mutual relationship (Kuczynski & Hildebrandt, 1997). The interplay between interdependence coexisting with contradiction produces an ongoing tension between the parent and the child that generates mutual accommodation, adaptation, and negotiation so that independence is achieved within an interdependent relationship context. According to Baxter and Montgomery (1996), "A healthy relationship is not one in which the interplay of opposites has been extinguished or resolved, because these opposing features are inherent in the very fabric of relating. Instead a healthy relationship is one in which the parties manage to satisfy both oppositional demands, that is, relational well-being is marked by the capacity to achieve "both/and" status" (p. 6).

Continuous Change

The interactions between the opposing elements that exist within individuals, between individuals, and between dyadic relationships and other contexts in which they are embedded set the conditions for continuous interaction and continuous change. Holden and Ritchie (1988) suggest that dialectics are suitable for the analysis of parent–child socialization because "the task of parents is, by definition, to rear a rapidly changing organism; change rather than stability is the *modus operandi*. As a result, parental behavior must be adaptive. Parents must modify their behavior in response to their offspring; the process of adaptation is inherent in the task of parenting." (p. 41). Valsiner (1989) describes the dialectical processes as follows: "The relations between X and Y is *contradictory* (a basic assumption of the dialectical perspective) in the sense that the two parts (X and Y) are opposing each other while remaining mutually necessary parts of the system. As a result of the opposition of the subparts of the whole, the whole system 'leaps' to a novel state of being (incorporating a new part Z)" (p. 67). With each new synthesis the very meaning of contradiction shifts and sets the stage for new contradictions and further change.

The dialectical idea of continuous change has a number of advantages for conceptualizing outcomes of socialization over earlier deterministic models of socialization. First, dialectics alerts researchers that the outcomes of socialization processes must be more than the mere transmission of similarity from the older generation to the younger generation. Change and the emergence of novel syntheses in addition to continuity are also to be expected outcomes of socialization and development. Second, contextual dialectics suggest that these syntheses can be positive or negative in direction. A parent's strategies can produce a range of unintended responses beyond compliance or intergenerational transmission, including resistance and children's novel interpretations and syntheses of values from parental and peer cultures. Children's responses may also cause parents to change their own positions. Thus socialization is better understood as producing a range of positive or negative trajectories rather than precisely determined outcomes.

In summary, contemporary socialization theory includes both behavioral and cognitive conceptions of bidirectional causality. Two core models of bidirectionality include the idea of parents and children engaging in reciprocal initiations and reactions and the idea of parents and children as engaging in a dialectical process of adaptation to contradictory meanings represented by each other's actions and their fit with changing contexts. As discussed in the following section these two views of bidirectionality also lie at the core of major theories of socialization in the family and guide the way researchers identify critical processes of socialization and ask new questions about them.

DYNAMIC MODELS OF SOCIALIZATION PROCESSES

In this section we review three different theoretical frameworks for understanding dynamic bidirectional processes of influence in socialization. Social interactional theory is based on a behavioral, reciprocal exchange model of bidirectionality and has a limited view of human agency and social context. In contrast, transactional theory and social relational theory are based on a dialectical conception of bidirectionality and are concerned with parents and children conceptualized as human agents who make sense of and strategically interact with their social and physical contexts. Cutting across these models is a tension between complementary goals of research: that of prediction and control of child outcomes on the one hand, and that of understanding intervening processes on the other. Researchers interested in prediction operate in the theory-testing mode of research (Cook, 2003) and tend toward global, aggregated measures conceptualized as causes and outcomes. Researchers interested in understanding operate in the theory-generating mode of research (Kuczynski & Daly, 2003) and tend toward de-scribing microprocesses of interaction and specify the meanings, attributions, behav-iors, and strategies that underlie the aggregated variables and statistical associations of predictive models. This more descriptive approach to exploring the structure and orga-nization of socialization phenomena has generally utilized inductive and qualitative methodologies such as direct observation and open-ended interviews. Both theory test-ing and theory generation need to be represented within a comprehensive methodology for socialization research.

Social Interactional Theory

Social interactional theory (Patterson 1982, 1997) has its roots in the unidirectional so-cialization traditions of behaviorism and social learning theories of the 1960s but became transformed into a dynamic process model through the efforts of Gerald Patterson and his colleagues at the Oregon Social Learning Center (Patterson, 1982; Patterson et al., 1992). An important theoretical achievement of this group was the recognition of the central role of children's aversive behaviors in shaping antisocial behavior. According to Patterson (1997), "to some extent, the social environment is selected by the child; fur-thermore the child shapes those environments that are selected (i.e. the child is an active agent)" (p. 194).

The theory consists of a micromodel, which explores the dynamics of coercive social interaction and a macromodel, which explores the developmental consequences of coer-cive interactions from early childhood to young adulthood. According to Patterson (1997), both levels of analysis are needed.

> First, knowing that ineffective parental discipline, monitoring, and family problem-solving are related to negative child outcomes does not explain how these practices bring about changes in the child. . . . Second, these macro models cannot satisfactorily explain why the child maintains these behaviors across time and settings. Third, and most important, macro models cannot address the key developmental question: How does the child's behavior change its form? (p. 209)

Patterson believes that the answer lies in a research program that combines the macromodel research methodology focused on structural equation modeling with a microprocess research methodology based on the functional analysis of coercive behaviors during immediate interactions. We argue later that developmental models of socialization also could benefit from a research framework that includes macro- and microlevels of analysis.

In the micromodel of social interactional theory, a reciprocal coercive cycle begins when a parent makes a request to which the child does not comply. The parent and the child may then exchange aversive behaviors such as shouting or whining at a higher level of intensity until the parent or child withdraws and terminates an aversive interaction. According to operant functional analysis of this sequence, the mother's escalation and re-traction of her command would be interpreted as being negatively reinforced by the child's cessation of a coercive response and the child's aversive escalation is negatively re-inforced by mother's retraction of a coercive demand. However, this immediate reward occurs at the expense of future interactions. By responding to the child's current behavior with coercion and then withdrawal, the parent influences the child's future behavior by making aversive strategies and repetitions of the coercive cycle more likely.

The macromodel describes how, as noncompliance becomes more frequent, the coercive processes between parent and child escalate and become consolidated into habitual patterns of interacting as children age. Once the child enters school, the child's habitual use of coercion sends the child on a negative trajectory that cuts the child off from prosocial activities and peers and contributes to poor academic performance, negative self-esteem, and involvement with peers who are similarly unskilled and antisocial. Interactions with deviant peers become the site of new interactions in which the adolescent's coercive behavior is maintained and may escalate further. For example, Dishion, Andrews, and Crosby (1995) found that dyads of deviant peers were more likely to reinforce each other for "rule-breaking talk." Such antisocial behavior in early adolescence may lead to deviant peer associations in later adolescence and hostile talk about women in late adolescence (Capaldi, Dishion, Stoolmiller, & Yoerger, 2001). Therefore, the coercive process macromodel postulates a series of reciprocal behavioral interactions that begin in the home, escalate, and consolidate in adolescent peer groups and set the stage for further negative interactions in romantic relationships and eventual coercive styles of parenting.

Despite invaluable advances in understanding of coercive family processes and negative developmental trajectories of antisocial boys, social interactional theory has important limitations from the perspective of a comprehensive theory of socialization. One limitation of social interactional theory concerns the generalizability of its key findings and hypotheses. Empirically, support for the premises of social interactional theory has been based almost entirely on clinic families with antisocial boys. An important product of this research is a behavioral model of parenting interventions for reducing noncompliant behavior in clinic-referred samples. However, the implications of the model are regularly applied to families with normally developing children who are experiencing moderate levels of noncompliance (Patterson, 1993; Patterson & Forgatch, 1987). Thus, the assumption appears to be that learning what clinic families do wrong might shed light on what normal families do right. Patterson (1982) has argued that external negative contingencies for enforcing parental demands, especially time out, is the key to competent parenting, despite a lack of evidence that nonclinic parents regularly use such a technique.

Research with nonclinic populations, to be reviewed in the section on social relational theory, in contrast, has suggested a competing view that the foundation of children's cooperation lies in processes having to do with constructing and maintaining good parent–child relationships. Thus, the question facing both developmental and behavioral researchers is how to integrate the two bodies of research (Kuczynski & Hildebrandt, 1997). Patterson and Fisher (2002) suggest that relational perspectives could be subsumed under a social interactional perspective if key relational constructs such as "parental responsiveness" were stripped of surplus meaning and were translated to "contingent reinforcement." In contrast, McMahon and Forehand (2003) argued that research on the cognitive and relational processes that has informed the understanding of normal family processes should not be generalized to high-risk clinic-referred populations. The implication of this second position is that the two bodies of research cannot be integrated because there are different processes at work in the two populations with different underlying principles for successful socialization. Proposals also exist for integrating the two bodies of research (Cavell & Strand, 2003; Kuczynski & Hildebrandt, 1997). For example, Kuczynski and Hildebrandt (1997) suggest that definitions of conformity corre-sponding to internally controlled compliance in parent's absence, externally controlled immediate compliance, and mutual accommodation and negotiation within close rela-tionships are all valid but come into play in different childrearing situations. The resolu-tion of this issue awaits future research and debate.

In terms of what the theory attempts to explain, social interaction theory is focused on the development of antisocial behavior and noncooperative orientations to authority and norms of society. Missing is an analysis of socialization more broadly defined as the fostering of values, attitudes, roles, and cultural ideas and practices. Social interactional theory is also at odds with contemporary developmental approaches to socialization in its narrow focus on immediate antecedents and consequences as causes of behavior and a distain for cognitive constructs (Patterson et al., 1992; Patterson & Fisher, 2002). Thus, social interactional theory avoids considering the way parents and children interpret each other's behaviors as well as internal constructs such as "internalization," "goals," "moti-vation," and "relationship." Social interactions are considered to be regulated by auto-matic, reactive processes such that parents and children are not aware of the contingen-cies they provide to one another in the interaction (Chamberlain & Patterson, 1995). Despite acknowledging children's active participation in behavioral sequences, social interactional theory has a limited view of human agency that excludes the significance of parents and children's interpretive capacities. Patterson (1997) states, "The determinants of aggression are not found in the mind of the child but rather in the reactions of the social environment" (p. 194). There is no suggestion of agency in terms of children ac-tively interpreting information from their environment or assessing their relationships or the moral status of their parent's actions or of a motivational agency in terms of children protecting their autonomy. As a result, the social interactional model adopts a reactive model of bidirectional influence and a nominal view of child agency in the socialization process.

Patterson and Fisher (2002) recently suggested that competing behavioral and devel-opmental theories of socialization should be judged using the criterion of parsimony. Spe-cifically, Patterson suggests that social interactional theory's focus on the direct behav-ioral contingencies found in the child's environment adds fewer assumptions than developmental theories of socialization. Internal states and representations are considered by Patterson (1997) to "add a degree of complexity that is unnecessary in accounting for outcomes" (p. 62). Clearly, by not including cognitive variables in the model, social interactional theory is more parsimonious than theories that do consider cognitions. However, this is a view of parsimony that favors a narrow definition of successful social-ization as immediate compliance and a constrained set of concepts for the understanding of the processes of socialization.

For developmental researchers, the goal of understanding socialization processes has promoted a more comprehensive definition of socialization as a phenomenon and the in-clusion of situational contexts and cognitions in descriptions of social interactions in the natural environment. Sameroff and Mackenzie (2003) recently used research on the esca-lation of coercive processes as an illustration of transactional models of development. In doing so, they suggest that qualitative transformation in behavior occurs in the cognitive representations of behaviors and relationships over time. Research to be reviewed in the section on the social relational model has led, for example, to a fine-grain exploration of the form and function of constructs such as compliance and noncompliance (Crockenberg & Litman, 1990; Kochanska & Aksan, 1995; Kuczynski & Kochanska, 1990). The admission of such distinctions may well be parsimonious to the extent that they promote greater understanding of children's skill as agents in disciplinary encounters than simpler definitions of conformity as immediate compliance.

Transactional Model

The transactional model (Sameroff 1975a, 1975b) is the most influential developmental framework for understanding bidirectional causal processes in social development. Transactional models of causality emphasize that social development is a product of continuous interactions between children and their family environments. The bidirectional process as originally envisioned was based on dialectics. Causes cannot be reduced to particular dispositions, cognitions, or behaviors of the parent or the child because these constantly change as parents and children interact over time. Parents and children are engaged in continual transformation as each partner responds to new emerging characteristics of the other. "The child alters his environment and in turn is altered by the changed world he has created" (Sameroff, 1975a, p. 281).

Dialectical processes involving an interaction between contradictory meaning systems were discussed by Sameroff (1975b) as the underlying mechanism of the transactional model. The agency of parents and children is recognized in their attempts to make sense of the contradictions generated by their interactions. Children's transactions with the environment lead to cumulative changes which eventually cause qualitative change in children's interpretation of the environment. "In every developing system, contradictions are generated and it is these contradictions which provide the motivation which lead the organisms to the higher level of organization found in developmental series" (Sameroff, 1975b, p. 74). An important question is whether points of qualitative change are to be found in the behaviors or in the cognitions of parents and children, or in both. Sameroff (1975b) suggests that changes in meaning systems are especially important in transformational processes.

> The contradiction that has occurred consists between a meaning system which sees the child as an object to be manipulated, and one which sees the child as a center of needs and desires existing independently of the needs and desires of his parents. . . . The dialectical model would posit at each stage the contradictions with which the mother is faced in trying to understand her child. (p. 77)

Many of the examples of transaction cited by Sameroff and MacKenzie (2003) such as studies by Bugental and Shennum (1984), Rubin, Nelson, Hastings, and Asendorpf (1999), and Stern and Hildebrandt (1986) focused on changes in mothers' interpretations of their children's behavior or cognitive representations of relationships as the locus of qualitative changes that give rise to changes in behavior.

Research that demonstrates a parent to child and also a separate child to parent direction of influence provides support for the most basic assumption of a transactional model (Cook, 2003). More advanced tests of the transactional model reviewed by Cook (2003) use variations of structural equation modeling to test both directions of influence simultaneously in the same statistical model. Ideally, a complete test of a transactional model requires a longitudinal design, with data for parent and child measured a minimum of 3 points in time. In a review of recent advances in testing transactional models Sameroff and MacKenzie (2003) pointed to another criterion that must be met in a transactional model, a demonstration that bidirectional influences lead to qualitative transformations in the usual behaviors of interactive partners. This dialectical element of transactional models has been neglected such that the bidirectional transactions were viewed in terms of each partner reacting to the stimulus qualities of the other (Valsiner, 1989). "All too often . . . it is used to emphasize a linear environmentalism at the expense of the more complex interplay between dynamic systems" (Sameroff & MacKenzie, 2003, p. 619). Sameroff and MacKenzie also argued that the distinction between mediating variables and moderating variables (Baron & Kenny, 1986) represented a major advance in statistical tests of transactional processes. In their view, mediator analyses are important for identifying linear processes that underlie changes between two points in time. However, moderator analyses, in which differences in the quantity or quality of one partner's response are related to changes in the relation between the other partner's earlier and later behavior, are required to find transactions. Examples of relevant moderator variables indicative of qualitative change include differences in cognitive representations of relationships and, presumably, major transitions such as moves to deviant peer groups that Patterson (1997) refers to as escalations.

Transactional models, particularly when they are used in large-scale longitudinal designs, allow statistical testing of predictions at a macrolevel of analysis. However, these designs can only be considered to be a part of a methodology for understanding dynamic socialization processes. In part, the difficulty lies with the process of developing measures for the purposes of statistical analysis. According to Sameroff and MacKenzie (2003), "Although the transactional model originates from a strongly dialectic, organismic orientation, any operationalization requires a mechanistic measurement model, in which dynamic processes are reduced to static scores that can be entered into statistical analyses" (p. 617). Discrete behaviors and test scores need to be aggregated, a process that can obscure the meaning of the resulting abstract global variable. The interpretations of key processes underlying such variables have been questioned at various times. For example, constructs such as "parental monitoring" and "effective discipline" are not directly measured but are inferred from other measures that are subject to multiple interpretations. In structural equation models, effective discipline is sometimes inferred not from directly observed contingent punishment such as time out but from the absence of coercive interaction. This leaves the possibility that a different process may be implicated, such as sensitive responsivity to children's cues or mutually responsive relationships (Kochanska, 2002; Kuczynski & Hildebrandt, 1997). Similarly, the construct of parental monitoring has been inferred not from direct measures of parental solicitation of information or surveillance but from measures of parental knowledge of the child's whereabouts and activities. Recent reinterpretations of the monitoring construct include not only parental control and surveillance but also adolescents' willingness to disclose information about their thoughts, actions, friends and whereabouts to their parents (Fletcher, Steinberg, & Williams-Wheeler, 2004; Stattin & Kerr, 2000). In other research, measures of authoritarian, authoritative, and permissive parenting styles have been critiqued because they represent not the independent behavior of a parent but a complex amalgam of parent and child behaviors (Lewis, 1981; Shanahan & Sobolewski, 2003). For this reason, transactional models also require research into microprocesses of social interaction as an overall methodology for understanding the dynamic processes involved in socialization.

Social Relational Theory

Social relational theory emphasizes that socialization and the dynamics of parent–child interactions should be understood as occurring in the context of close personal relationships. In earlier socialization research, dimensions of parent–child relationships such as parental acceptance, nurturance, and warmth were considered background variables that enhanced the effectiveness of parental discipline practices. However, during the past two decades, new relational perspectives proposed that parent–child relationships rather than parental discipline strategies are the foundation for successful socialization (Bretherton, Golby, & Cho, 1997; Kuczynski & Hildebrandt 1997; Maccoby & Martin, 1983; Richters & Waters, 1992). In this section we present a new consolidation of social relational theory that integrates three converging streams of theory and empirical research. These are theory on relationships as contexts for interaction, research on the relational origins of parent–child cooperation, and research on parent–child conflict.

Relationships as Contexts

In the relational perspective, human relationships are considered to be the proximal contexts for understanding socialization processes and the dynamics of parent–child interaction. Socialization and social development throughout the lifespan occur within a system of close personal relationships (Laursen & Bukowski, 1997; Maccoby, 1992; Reis, Collins, & Berscheid, 2000). Different relationships, including relationships with parents, siblings, peers, teachers, and other adults (Piniata, 1999), come into salience as contexts for socialization as children develop.

The embeddedness of social interactions in relationships has implications for the study of socialization. In bilateral perspectives, processes having to do with bidirectional influence and the experience of agency and power depend on the relationship context (Kuczynski, 2003). Children's agency and children's effectiveness as agents are enabled by the relationship, and for both parent and child, the competent expression of agency involves accommodating to the mutual constraints of a reciprocal relationship (Kuczynski & Hildebrandt, 1997). The relationship context helps to explain numerous bidirectional phenomena of family life, including parental receptivity to children's influence, mutual cooperation, negotiation, and parent–child conflict. Parents have more opportunities for power than children, but they do not, as agents, always use the power that they have and they are vulnerable to even a young child's influence despite their greater power.

In a recent study, Belgian parents and children between the ages of 11 and 15 were interviewed regarding their understanding of children's agency using Q-sort methodology (De Mol & Buysse, 2004). Parents emphasized children's influence on their own personal development, feelings, and thoughts and the burden on parenting that such influence entails. Children recognized that their effectiveness as agents were derived from their parents' sensitivity and responsiveness to their needs and requests. In other words, both adults and children recognized that agency was constrained and enabled by the context of a reciprocal parent–child relationship.

Kuczynski and Grusec (1997) argue that parents are well placed to constrain and channel children's behavior and internalization processes. Parents' special position in a long-term relationship and society's legitimization of the parents' power and responsibility over early socialization give parents more resources and opportunity to influence the child than any other adults or peers. However, the relationship context also enables children's agency by affording them considerable scope to negotiate the nature of the constraints placed on them (Kuczynski 2003). Qualities of parent–child relationships, such as parents' sense of obligation to their children and their love, ego investment, and long-term goals for their children, place limits on the use of coercive power by parents and thus enable children's capacity for strategic action (Maccoby, 2000). In addition, parents may be willing to tolerate resistance to their requests because they seek to maintain a positive parent–child relationship or wish to foster autonomy, independence, and assertiveness in their children (Hastings & Grusec, 1998).

Hinde's (1979) model of relationships has been used to identify specific dynamics of parent–child interaction that stem from the special context of the parent–child relationship. According to Hinde, as dyads accumulate a history of interactions over time, they form relationships, and the emergent relationships subsequently become contexts for their future interactions. The relationship itself is a cognitive construction that represents more than the sum of interactions that objectively occurred in the history of the relationship. Each partner in the dyad makes sense of the other's behavior through psychological processes such as perception and interpretation. These meanings and expectancies become consolidated in representations of the relationship, which then form the filter through which parent and child behaviors are experienced (Hinde, 1997; Lollis, 2003). Thus, during interactions parents and children not only interpret situational demands but also integrate that information with the emerging relationship.

Children and parents do not act merely on the immediate contingencies found in each other's behavior as suggested by social interactional theories. They are also influenced by the cognitive representations and expectations that they developed from a long history of interactions (Lollis & Kuczynski, 1997; Lollis, 2003; Reis et al., 2000). Parent–child relationships also have a future dimension which shows up when parents act on the basis of long-term rather than immediate goals for children (Lollis, 2003).

Relationship cognitions are readily apparent in "own versus other" research designs that compare a parent or a child's reaction to people who vary in their relationship with the informant. Parents and children use different influence strategies in their own relationships than they do with unfamiliar adults or children and justify their behaviors by referring to knowledge of personality, past behavior, and predictions of future behavioral or cognitive reactions. Mothers feel more responsible and more often use strategies indicative of long-term socialization goals with their own children than with unrelated children (Dawber & Kuczynski, 1999). Children, for their part, are more confident that they can influence their own mothers than unfamiliar women because they were able to draw on knowledge gained from their past experience with their mothers (Hildebrandt & Kuczynski, 1998).

Interdependence is another feature of close relationships that affect social interactions. Interdependence refers to the frequency, duration, and intensity of the impact of each partner's behavior on the other (Kelley et al., 1983). The interdependence of parents and children is a source of both mutual receptivity and mutual vulnerability because each person's behaviors matter to the other. The child depends on the parent for love, security, care, and other resources for physical and psychological needs. Parents also depend on children to have their various needs met. The cross-cultural "Value of Children" studies (Hoffman, 1988; Trommsdorff, Zheng, & Tardif, 2002) document parents' perceptions of the economic, social prestige, and psychological benefits that they receive from children. In traditional and subsistence cultures, children are valued for their contributions to the household economy from an early age and also for the economic security they are expected to provide to aging parents. In industrialized cultures, and increasingly worldwide, the emotional value of children is more important. The emotional value of children, defined as joy, fun, companionship, pride, and the sense of accomplishment that parents gain from having children, suggests that the principal reason that parents have children is for meeting their needs for intimacy and meaning in their own lives.

The concept of the parent–child relationship as a context for socialization raises a host of basic questions about which there is surprisingly little information. Among these are questions about the structure of parent–child relationships, differences between mother–child and father–child relationships, and cultural differences in parent–child relationships.

New research suggests that parent–child relationships cannot be understood as a monolithic relationship of vertical power. Instead, different domains coexist and mutually influence each other within the same relationship (Lollis & Kuczynski, 1997; Russell, Pettit, & Mize, 1998). Bugental and Goodnow (1998) suggested that there are at least three relationship domains—attachment, hierarchical, and reciprocal—that play a role in parent–child relationships. Each of these domains may have different underlying rules governing power and dynamics during social interactions. Depending on the context, the parent may be engaged in interaction roles analogous to authority figure, attachment figure, or playmate and intimate companion (Harach & Kuczynski, 2005). The question therefore emerges how these relationship domains interact in episodes involving the socialization of children. As one example, having an intimate and responsive relationship with a parent may increase the child's receptivity to the parent's requests. However, it is also likely that intimacy may increase the parents' receptivity to children's influence. Moreover the goal of having an intimate relationship with a child sometimes conflicts with the responsibility of socializing and controlling children's behavior (Youniss & Smollar, 1985).

In pursuing questions regarding the structure of parent–child relationships, it may be necessary to distinguish mother–child relationships from father–child relationships as contexts for socialization. Mother–child relationships tend to be more intimate than father–child relationships (Youniss & Smollar, 1985; Harach & Kuczynski, 2005) and this may explain the greater frequency of conflicts in the mother–child relationship (Steinberg, 1987) as well as the more frequent self-disclosure of life events by adolescents to mothers rather than fathers (Smetana, Metzger, Gettman, & Campione-Barr, 2006). In our research (Kuczynski, Lollis, McCullough, Parkin, & Oliphant, 2006) we are studying children as agents of influence in the family as well as how relational representations and other cognitions enter into parents' and children's reasoning about influence interactions. Interviews with mothers, fathers, and children were consistent in indicating that children often strategically choose between the mother or the father as targets of influence attempts, thereby, making use of their knowledge of the separate relationships in meeting their goals. For most issues, such as attempting to change parental attitudes regarding friends, obtaining help with emotional difficulties, or negotiating changes in standing rules, children preferred to approach mothers. Fathers, however, were preferred for one-on-one time outside the home. Children refer to parents' differential expertise, personality, goals, receptivity to influence, availability, and past experiences as reasons for their choices. Other studies document the importance of gender pairings, where parents spend more time with, and are more intimately involved in, the life of a same sex child

(Maccoby, 2003; McHale & Crouter, 2003). Such findings indicate that there may be considerable relationship specificity in children's socialization experiences and also that social interactions may have distinctive dynamics.

It is also important to recognize that there are cross-cultural differences in the structure of parent–child relationships (Kuczynski, 2003; Trommsdorff & Kornadt, 2003). There are variations in the norms for how much power children have in parent–child relationships, norms for intimacy in mother–child versus father–child relationships, and how much of the responsibility for socialization of children rests on parents rather than other relatives or the community. Because parent–child relationships are embedded in culture, culture is important in understanding socialization processes and dynamics of bidirectionality, agency, and power in parent–child interactions.

The Relationship Origins of Cooperation

A second foundation of relational theory is research indicating that socialization and the development of self-regulation may originate from a different source than the parental disciplinary practices that were emphasized in earlier socialization theories. In this view, parenting that contributes to the formation and maintenance of positive relationships provides the early foundation of children's cooperation with parental requests and demands. Stayton, Hogan, and Ainsworth (1971) linked the development of secure attachment relationships with children's compliance with maternal requests. They argued, in line with Bowlby's theory of attachment, that young children are predisposed to cooperate with parental requests because such obedience increases the child's chances of survival in dangerous environments. Empirically, maternal behaviors that facilitate attachment, such as sensitive, accepting, and responsive behavior with regard to the communications of infants, were found to be associated both with children's cooperation with mothers' immediate commands and with self-inhibition of actions that mothers had forbidden in the past. Subsequent research found links between early compliance and secure attachment as assessed using Ainsworth's Strange Situation procedure (Londerville & Main, 1981; Matas, Arend, & Sroufe, 1978).

In a related body of research, Maccoby and Martin (1983) distinguished two processes, "situational compliance," and "receptive compliance," as different motivational bases for children's self-regulation. Receptive or willing compliance (Kochanska & Aksan, 1995) was viewed as growing out of a well-functioning parent–child relationship in which children and parents were engaged in cycles of positive affect, mutual responsivity, and compliance. In contrast, situational compliance stems from power-based parental strategies and is dependent on external controls. Children develop an early disposition for cooperation from experiences of reciprocal cooperation with their parents during the interaction history of their relationship. Over time, children may develop a positive stance toward parental socialization efforts that increases the influence that parents have on their children. Discipline and control strategies subsequently shape children's conformity to the requirements of specific situational contexts (Maccoby & Martin, 1983).

Research suggests that child compliance is more likely to follow responsive interchanges such as play (Gardner, Ward, Burton, & Wilson, 2003; Parpal & Maccoby, 1985). Kochanska and her colleagues found that willing compliance and situational compliance are distinguished by the positive or negative affect that accompanies the behavior and the degree to which the child engages wholeheartedly in the task or needs prompting from the parent. This research has demonstrated that committed compliance and not situational compliance is associated with later measures of internalization and is related to positive responsive parenting rather than power-based techniques (Forman & Kochanska, 2001; Kochanska, 2002).

In the relational perspective children may be motivated to cooperate with parental wishes because they have a stake in the parent–child relationship (Kuczynski & Hildebrandt, 1997). Cavell and Strand (2003) described how a poor parent–child relationship may lead to high levels of noncompliance in clinic populations. Children's unwillingness to adopt parental standards may signal a problem in the relationship that is much larger than parental responses to acts of noncompliance. In normative populations the implication is that children may experience cooperation as intrinsically rewarding (Grolnick, Deci, & Ryan 1997) or as compatible with their own shared goals with the parent. The relational perspective on conformity also broadens the focus on socialization strategies to include parents maintaining their own side of a reciprocally cooperative relationship and strategies for repairing relationships temporarily damaged by excessive parental coercion and control (Harach & Kuczynski, 2005).

Parent–Child Conflict and the Dialectics of Control

A third source for social relational theory is research on parent–child conflict. In early socialization research, parent–child conflict was understood from the perspective of discipline and control. Conflict was equated with children's noncompliance to legitimate authority and, therefore, was viewed as dysfunctional or deviant. The focus of research was on parents' use of discipline strategies that ensured that conflicts ended with children's conformity with their wishes.

An important step toward a relational view of conflict took place when researchers shifted from a view of conflict as deviant opposition to legitimate authority to a view of conflict as an inevitable and mutually tolerated aspect of living in close relationships (Dunn & Munn, 1985; Shantz, 1987). Research from this perspective found outcomes of parent–child conflict to be much more varied than compliance and noncompliance and to include negotiation, compromise, withdrawal from conflict without resolution, mutual standoff (Eisenberg, 1992; Vuchinch, 1987), and relationship repair following interactional missteps by the parent or child (Harach & Kuczynski, 2005).

The relational view of conflict also introduced dialectics as an alternative to a deterministic view of causality in parent–child relationships and socialization. A dialectical conception of process would consider change as an outcome of contradictions in states, needs, knowledge, and goals of parents and children who have unique personalities and perspectives but who nevertheless share a close relationship. In a relational view, conflict is viewed as a necessary condition for change, for better or for worse. "Many different functions—cognition, social cognition, emotions, and social relations—are thought to be formed and/or transformed by conflict. Putting this thesis another way, ontogeny is thought to be impossible without conflict. In this sense, most developmental theories are dialectical ones, with functions ascribed to conflict in ontogeny that are similar to its functions in social and cultural evolution" (Shantz & Hartup, 1992, p. 2).

The dialectical conception of bidirectional influence within social relational theory offers a way of reformulating the outcomes of socialization in a dynamic way. In a dialec-

tical view, internalization and compliance to socialization pressures are not final outcomes of socialization but steps in an ongoing process that set the stage for further
change. Building on Lawrence and Valisiner's (1993) conception of internalization as an
individuals' mental reconstruction of the world, Kuczynski et al. (1997) proposed that internalization is a process by which parents and children construct *personal working models* of the beliefs, attitudes, and values of their family and cultural contexts. The concept
of a working model of internalization suggests that parents' and children's beliefs, values,
skills, attitudes, and motives are continuously under development and reconstruction
throughout life. Because of different life experiences; different transactions with each
other; and their different exposure and susceptibility to ideas of peers, media, or other institutions in their ecological contexts, each member of the family develops somewhat different personal working models as a product of his or her internalization processes
(Kuczynski & Navara, 2005).

Similarly, it is unrealistic to conceive of conformity as an exact match between the
child's response and the parent's command as is implied by standard operational definitions such as compliance in 6 seconds (McMahon & Forehand, 2003). Parental commands and children's responses to them occur in an interdependent relationship context
that supports children's expression of agency. Within close relationships, the goal is less
often to obtain exact compliance than it is to obtain conflict resolution, or some compromise of the original desires of the participants (Miller & Steinberg, 1975). Accommodation and negotiation are proposed as a dialectical replacement for the constructs of compliance and noncompliance. These terms convey the coregulated and nondeterminate
nature of the process and outcomes of many episodes of socialization (Kuczynski &
Hildebrandt, 1997). According to Dix and Branca (2003), "Because they are interdependent, parents and children must adjust to the needs and interests of the other if each is to
succeed in promoting his or her concerns and if the interactions that do so are to be well
coordinated and harmonious" (p. 170). Dix and Branca (2003) discuss various accommodation strategies that parents use to address their children's concerns on the way to
achieving their goals. These included sequencing incompatible goals over time, compro-
mising, replacing a less desirable activity with a somewhat more desirable activity,
reframing, adapting, and convincing through explanation. Such accommodations may be
a lengthy process that involves transformations of the parent's wishes in the short term.
Crockenberg and Litman (1990) found in their sample of preschool children that "obtaining compliance was quite extended; mothers reasoned, persuaded, suggested and
adapted their request to what they thought the child would accept" (p. 970).

Children also play a role in the accommodation process. Socially competent children
display a coregulated but inexact form of conformity and resistance that represents their
expression of agency within the constraints of a close parent–child relationship (Kuczynski
& Hildebrandt, 1997). During the history of their relationship, parents and children
evolve shared understandings of what will pass for compliance in different situations.
Often, what parents accept as compliance, and what children understand to be compliance, is closer to the idea of accommodation than exact, immediate submission. Children
who are inclined to cooperate with a parent's request but under different terms than the
parent had in mind may acknowledge that the parent has been heard, that they will attempt to coordinate their own plans with the parent's wishes, or that they are willing to
negotiate an mutually acceptable course of action. Similarly, the construct of negotiation
implies children's attempts to resist a request within the constraints of an interdependent
relationship.

Fine-grained analyses of children's noncompliant behaviors have found that children's uncooperative responses take a number of forms, including *negotiation, accommodation, unwilling compliance, passive noncompliance, simple refusal,* and *defiance* (Crockenberg & Litman, 1990; Kuczynski & Kochanska, 1990; Lollis, Kuczynski, Navara, & Koguchi, 2003). These can be interpreted from a relational perspective as reflecting variations in children's assertiveness and skill as agents within the bounds of a mutual relationship (Kuczynski & Hildebrandt, 1997). A recent study of control interactions initiated by mothers of children between the ages of 3 and 5 (Lollis et al., 2003) found that only 46% of episodes of control ended with exact compliance (30% freely given by child and 16% forced by the parent). Twenty-six percent of episodes ended in complete failure by the mother to obtain her requests and 22% ended with mother modifying her request in response to children's resistance. This variety of resolutions indicates both the substantial effect of children's agency in outcomes of parent-initiated control episodes and parents' accommodation of children's agency.

The foregoing analysis is limited because it considers only interactions taking place in the parent's presence. What has received little research are the further transformations that may occur over time in the absence of parental surveillance. Parents' capacity to monitor their children's out-of-sight behavior is constrained by children's willingness to disclose relevant information (Kerr & Stattin, 2000). Although a child might comply in the parent's presence, the child might privately reject the parent's message (Grusec & Goodnow, 1994). Even when behaving contrary to a parent's wishes in the parent's absence, children may still choose an accommodative form of resistance to maintain their parents positive regard or to avoid damaging their relationships with their parents. Siblings and peers also play an important role in children's creative interpretation or evasion of evading adult rules and messages (Corsaro, 1997). The implication is that multiple transformations occur between the input of the parent's initial command and the final output of the child's response. The child's conformity is not exact and represents a synthesis of the parents' and children's interpretations and actions.

A question for future research is whether parents take a dialectical perspective in their role as socializing agents. Parents do not always expect exact transmission of messages and exact conformity as outcomes (Grusec et al., 2000), and it is possible that when parents give commands or hold forth on values, they have some expectation that their requests will be compromised or transformed through interpretation. A nondeterministic view of parenting would suggest that parents have a range of goals, from a rigid desire for exact transmission when the child's safety is at risk or strongly held beliefs are at stake to more indulgent attitudes regarding children's interpretations of their demands when less important personal and conventional issues are at stake (Kuczynski & Hildebrandt, 1997). Parents, therefore, may communicate a variety of positions with regard to their acceptance of their child's behaviors ranging from what is ideal to what is acceptable, tolerable, or "out of the question" (Goodnow, 1994). Children, in turn, discover how much stretch their parents' position affords and how much leeway there is for their own creative interpretation (Goodnow, 1997).

Although parents may have bottom lines beyond which they are less likely to accept children's resistance or independent action, such bottom lines can still be tested successfully by a determined child. Children are agents who may or may not accept the parent's ideas despite being compelled behaviorally (Grusec & Goodnow, 1994) and may choose to believe and behave as they see fit out of the parent's sight. Parents who pursue their bottom lines without taking children's agency into account might do so at the cost of their relationship. In addition they may invite deception and noncompliance when supervision is not possible. Even when bottom lines are transgressed, parents and children may choose to agree to disagree (Goodnow, 1994) or not to talk about areas of disagreements so that they can continue to maintain a close relationship.

In summary, social relational theory has much to offer as framework for socialization research. The relational perspective provides a conceptual home to disparate developmental approaches that have an interest in parent and child agency, including their goals, cognitions, and representations of relationships, as critical factors in understanding socialization processes. With regard to the transactional model social relational theory is a complementary conceptual partner at the microlevel of analysis for understanding transformational change. Methodologically, it adds qualitative and observational descriptive methods to unpack key processes that are implicated in qualitative changes uncovered by structural statistical techniques used in transactional models of development. With regard to social interactional theory, the social relational theory guides the researcher to consider the broader temporal context in which processes of social interactions occur. "A relationship-based perspective can be used to understand how parents and children co-adapt to past interactions as well as how they plan to respond to future interactions. There are multiple factors that influence the outcome of a given parent-child interaction, only some of which exist within the finite space and time immediately before, during, and after an interaction takes place" (Cavell & Strand, 2003, p. 407).

CONCLUSION

An implication of dynamic perspectives on socialization is that parents do not have the sort of direct effect on their children predicted in unidirectional models. Parents' influence on children inherently occurs within a causal system that includes the influence and agency of children. Moreover, a dialectical view of causality would suggest that this influence is not deterministic, is mediated by parents' and children's complex interactions as agents, and is moderated by changed interpretive processes and relationships.

An important challenge for future research concerns working out the practical and ethical implications of such a complex perspective for parents. As a beginning, it is important to stress that parents do matter and they do have an influence on their children's socialization and development. This is important because parental beliefs that they cannot influence their children are themselves associated with negative child outcomes (Baumrind, 1993). Bidirectional causality, whether construed as reciprocal exchanges of behavior or mutual dialectics is not a denial of parental influence but a statement that parental influence is complex and not deterministic. Parents play a role in influencing the general trajectory of children's development and may be prepared to accept a considerable range of possibilities as acceptable outcomes.

Even if parents cannot directly determine final outcomes, they are still best placed to have considerable influence on the intervening processes of interaction, the quality of the relationship, and for their role in the positive or negative trajectories on which children are initially launched. Moreover, as stated by advocates of the extreme thesis that parents have little influence over child outcomes (Harris, 1998), parents do matter in that they can make children's experience of socialization and parent–child relationships a happy or unhappy one. This is no small detail from a relational view of socialization!

Regarding parental responsibility, it is important to note that responsibility is a legal and ethical construct, not a causal one. There are many examples of cases in which a person in power is not a direct cause of an outcome but is still held morally responsible. The reverse is particularly true of children, where a child may directly cause even a fatal outcome but would not be held morally responsible for it before a certain legally determined age. Thought needs to be given to establishing a view of responsibility that is appropriate for a bilateral and relational perspective of socialization. Although parental causality is less clear than under a unidirectional model, parents remain responsible for their efforts to adequately care for and support their developing children and for launching them on a positive trajectory toward competence and success in their future lives in society. Thought also is required in conceptualizing the responsibility of children in the complex bilateral processes of socialization. Presumably, very young children would be viewed as influencing parental behavior, but they would not be held responsible for it. However, it is also not consistent with a bilateral view for children to blame parents for all manner of ills that befall them as adults. At some point children must also be held responsible for overcoming negative trajectories through their own actions as agents.

REFERENCES

Altman, I., Vinsel, A., & Bown, B. (1981). Dialectical conceptions in social psychology: An application to social penetration and privacy regulation. *Advances in Experimental Social Psychology 14*, 107–160.

Ambert, A. M. (1992). *The effect of children on parents*. New York: Haworth Press.

Bandura, A. (2001). Social cognitive theory: An agentic perspective. *Annual Review of Psychology, 52*, 1–26.

Baron, R. M., & Kenny, D. A. (1986). The mediator–moderator variable distinction in social psychological research: Conceptual, strategic, and statistical considerations. *Journal of Personality and Social Psychology, 51*, 1173–1182.

Baumrind, D. (1993). The average expectable environment is not good enough: A response to Scarr. *Child Development, 64*, 1299–1317.

Baxter, L. A., & Montgomery, B. M. (1996). *Relating: Dialogues and dialectics*. New York: Guilford Press.

Bell, R. Q. (1968). A reinterpretation of the direction of effects in studies of socialization. *Psychological Review, 75*, 81–95.

Bell, R. Q., & Harper, L. V. (1977). *Child effects on adults*. Hillsdale, NJ: Erlbaum.

Bretherton, I., Golby, B., & Cho, E. (1997). Attachment and the transmission of values. In J. Grusec & L. Kuczynski (Eds.), *Parenting and children's internalization of values: A handbook of contemporary theory* (pp. 103–134). New York: Wiley.

Bugental, D. B., & Goodnow, J. J. (1998). Socialization processes. In N. Eisenberg (Vol. Ed.), *Handbook of child psychology. Vol. 3: Social, emotional, and personality development* (pp. 389–414). New York: Wiley.

Bugental, D. B., & Shennum, W. A. (1984). "Difficult" children as elicitors and targets of adult communication patterns: An attributional–behavioral transactional analysis. *Monographs of the Society for Research in Child Development, 49*.

Capaldi, D. M., Dishion, T. J., Stoolmiller, M., & Yoerger, K. (2001). Aggression toward female partners by at-risk young men: The contribution of male adolescent friendships. *Developmental Psychology, 37*, 61–73.

Cavell, T. A., & Strand, P. S. (2003). Parent-based interventions for aggressive children: Adapting a bilateral lens. In L Kuczynski (Ed.), *Handbook of dynamics in parent–child relationships* (pp. 395–420). Thousand Oaks, CA: Sage.

Chamberlain, P., & Patterson, G. R. (1995). Discipline and child compliance in parenting. In M.H. Bornstein (Ed.), *Handbook of parenting: Vol. 4. Applied and practical parenting* (2nd ed., pp. 205–226). Mahwah NJ: Erlbaum.

Cook, W. L. (2003). Quantitative methods for deductive (theory-testing) research on parent–child dynamics. In L. Kuczynski (Ed.), *Handbook of dynamics in parent–child relationships* (pp. 347–372). Thousand Oaks, CA: Sage.

Corsaro, W. A. (1997). *The sociology of childhood*. Thousand Oaks CA: Pine Forge Press.

Crockenberg, S., & Litman, C. (1990). Autonomy as competence in 2-year-olds: Maternal correlates of child defiance, compliance, and self-assertion. *Developmental Psychology, 26*, 961–971.

Cummings, E. M., & Schermerhorn, A. C. (2003). A developmental perspective on children as agents in the family. In L. Kuczynski (Ed.), *Handbook of dynamics in parent–child relations* (pp. 91–108). Thousand Oaks CA: Sage.

Darling, N., & Steinberg, L. (1993). Parenting style as context: An integrative model. *Psychological Bulletin, 113*(3), 487–497.

Dawber, T., & Kuczynski, L. (1999). The question of owness: Influence of relationship context on parental socialization strategies. *Journal of Social and Personal Relationships, 16*, 475–493.

De Mol, J., & Buysse, A. (2004, July). *The filiating concept: An explorative analysis of children's agency in parent–child relations* Poster presented at the Conference of the International Association for Relationship Research, Madison, WI.

Dishon, T. J., Andrews, D. W., & Crosby, L. (1995). Antisocial boys and their friends in adolescence: Relationship characteristics, quality, and interactional processes. *Child Development, 66*, 139–151.

Dix, T., & Branca, S. H. (2003). Parenting as a goal-regulation process. In L. Kuczynski (Ed.), *Handbook of dynamics in parent–child relations* (pp. 167–188). Thousand Oaks CA: Sage.

Dunn, J. F., & Munn, P. (1985). Becoming a family member: Family conflict and the development of social understanding in the second year. *Child Development. Special Issue: Family Development, 56*(2), 480–492.

Eisenberg, A. R. (1992). Conflicts between mothers and their young children. *Merrill-Palmer Quarterly, 38*, 21–44.

Fletcher, A. C., Steinberg, L., & Williams-Wheeler, M. (2004). Parental influences of adolescent problem behavior: Revisiting Stattin and Kerr. *Child Development, 75*(3), 781–796.

Forman, D., & Kochanska, G. (2001). Viewing imitation as child responsiveness: A link between teaching and discipline domains of socialization. *Developmental Psychology, 37*(2), 198–206.

Frankel, J. (1991) On being reared by your children: State of art as reflected in the literature. *Free Inquiry in Creative Sociology, 19*, 193–200.

Gardner, F., Ward, S., Burton, J., & Wilson, C. (2003). The role of mother–child joint play in the early development of children's conduct problems: A longitudinal observational study. *Social Development, 12*(3), 361–378.

Glassman, M. (2000). Negation through history: dialectics and human development. *New Ideas in Psychology, 18*, 1–22.

Goodnow, J. J. (1994). Acceptable disagreement across generations. *New Directions for Child Development, 66*, 51–63.

Goodnow, J. J. (1997). Parenting and the transmission and internalization of values: From social-cultural perspectives to within-family analyses. In J. E. Grusec & L. Kuczynski (Eds.), *Parenting and children's internalization of values: A handbook of contemporary theory* (pp. 333–361). New York: Wiley.

Grolnick, W. S., Deci, E. L, & Ryan, R. M. (1997). Internationalization within the family: The self-determination theory perspective. In J. E. Grusec, & L. Kuczynski (Eds.), *Parenting and children's internalization of values: A handbook of contemporary theory* (pp. 135–161). New York: Wiley.

Grusec, J. E., & Goodnow, J. J. (1994). Impact of parental discipline methods on the child's internalization of values: A reconceptualization of current points of view. *Developmental Psychology, 30*, 4–19.

Grusec, J. E., Goodnow, J. J., & Kuczynski, L. (2000). New directions in analyses of parenting contributions to children's acquisition of values. *Child Development, 71*, 205–211.

Harach, L., & Kuczynski, L. (2005). Construction and maintenance of parent–child relationships: Bidirectional contributions from the perspective of parents. *Infant and Child Development, 14*, 327–343.

Harris, J. R. (1998). *The nurture assumption*. New York: Simon & Shuster.

Hastings, P. D., & Grusec, J. E. (1998). Parenting goals as organizers of responses to parent–child disagreement. *Developmental Psychology, 34*(3), 465–479.

Hildebrandt, N., & Kuczynski, L. (1998, May). *Children's sense of agency within parent–child and other–child relationships*. Paper presented at the 10th biennial conference on Child Development, University of Waterloo, Waterloo, Ontario.

Hinde, R. A. (1979). *Toward understanding relationships*. London: Academic Press.

Hinde, R. A. (1997). *Relationships: A dialectical perspective*. Hove, UK: Psychology Press.

Ho, D. Y. F. (1998). Interpersonal relationships and relationship dominance: An analysis based on methodological relationalism. *Asian Journal of Social Psychology, 1*, 1–16.

Hoffman, L. W. (1988). Cross-cultural differences in child rearing goals. In R. A. LeVine, P. M. Miller, & M. M. West (Eds.), *Parental behavior in diverse societies* (pp. 99–122). San Francisco: Jossey-Bass.

Holden, G. W., & Hawk, K. H. (2003). Meta-parenting in the journey of child rearing: a cognitive mechanism for change. In L. Kuczynski (Ed.), *Handbook of dynamics in parent–child relations* (pp. 189–210). Thousand Oaks CA: Sage.

Holden, G. W., & Ritchie, K. L. (1988). Child rearing and the dialectics of parental intelligence. In J. Valsiner (Ed.), *Child development within culturally structured environments. Parental cognition and adult–child interaction, Vol. 1: Parental cognition and adult–child interaction* (pp. 30–59). Norwood, NJ: Ablex.

Kelley, H. H., Berscheid, E., Christensen, A., Harvey, J. H., Huston, T. L., Levinger, G., et al. (1983). *Close relationships*. New York: Freeman.

Kerr, M., & Stattin, H. (2000). What parents know, how they know it, and several forms of adolescent adjustment: Further support for a reinterpretation of monitoring. *Developmental Psychology, 36*, 366–380.

Kochanska, G. (2002). Committed compliance, moral self and internalization: A mediational model. *Developmental Psychology, 38*(3), 339–351.

Kochanska, G., & Aksan, N. (1995). Mother–child mutually positive affect, the quality of child compliance to requests and prohibitions, and maternal control as correlates of early internalization. *Child Development, 66*(1), 236–254.

Kohlberg, L. (1969). Stage and sequence: The cognitive-developmental approach to socialization. In D. A. Goslin (Ed.), *Handbook of socialization: Theory and research* (pp. 347–480). Chicago: Rand McNally.

Kuczynski, L. (1984). Socialization goals and mother–child interaction: Strategies for long-term and short-term compliance. *Developmental Psychology, 20*, 1061–1073.

Kuczynski, L. (2003). Beyond bidirectionality: bilateral conceptual frameworks for understanding dynamics in parent–child relations (pp. 1–24). In L. Kuczynski (Ed.), *Handbook of dynamics in parent–child relations*. Thousand Oaks CA: Sage.

Kuczynski, L., & Daly, K. (2003). Qualitative methods for inductive (theory generating) research: Psychological and sociological approaches. In L. Kuczynski (Ed.), *Handbook of dynamics in parent–child relationships* (pp. 372–393). Thousand Oaks, CA: Sage.

Kuczynski, L., & Grusec, J. E. (1997). Future directions for a theory of parental socialization. In J. E. Grusec & L. Kuczynski (Eds.), *Parenting and the internalization of values: A handbook of contemporary theory* (pp. 398–413). New York: Wiley.

Kuczynski, L., Harach, L., & Bernardini, S. C. (1999). Psychology's child meets sociology's child: Agency, power and influence in parent–child relations. In C. Shehan (Ed.), *Through the eyes of the child: Revisioning children as active agents of family life* (pp. 21–52). Stamford, CT: JAI Press.

Kuczynski, L., & Hildebrandt, N. (1997). Models of conformity and resistance in socialization theory. In J. E. Grusec & L. Kuczynski (Eds.), *Parenting and the internalization of values: A handbook of contemporary theory* (pp. 227–256). New York: Wiley.

Kuczynski, L., & Kochanska, G. (1990). The development of children's noncompliance strategies from toddlerhood to age 5. *Developmental Psychology, 26*, 398–408.

Kuczynski, L., Lollis, S., & Koguchi, T. (2003). Reconstructing common sense: Metaphors of bidirectionality in parent–child relations. In L. Kuczynski (Ed.), *Handbook of dynamics in parent–child relations* (pp. 421–438). Thousand Oaks, CA: Sage.

Kuczynski, L., Lollis, S., McCullough, L., Parkin, C. M., & Oliphant, A. (2006, March). *Children's influence on parents from the perspective of mothers, fathers, and children*. Poster presented at the Biennial Meeting of Society for Research on Adolescence, San Francisco, CA.

Kuczynski, L., Marshall, S., & Schell, K. (1997). Value socialization in a bidirectional context. In J. E. Grusec & L. Kuczynski (Eds.), *Parenting and the internalization of values: A handbook of contemporary theory* (pp. 23–50). New York: Wiley.

Kuczynski, L., & Navara, G. (2005). Sources of change in theories of socialization and internalization. In M. Killen & J. Smetana (Eds.), *Handbook of moral development* (pp. 299–327). Mahwah, NJ: Erlbaum.

Laursen, B., & Bukowski, W. A. (1997). A developmental guide to the organization of close relationships. *International Journal of Behavioral Development, 21*, 747–770.

Lawrence, J. A., & Valsiner, J. (1993). Conceptual roots of internalization: From transmission to transformation. *Human Development, 36*(3), 150–167.

Lewis, C. C. (1981). The effects of parental firm control: A reinterpretation of findings. *Psychological Bulletin, 90*(3), 547–563.

Lollis, S. (2003). Conceptualizing the influence of the past and the future in present parent–child relationships. In L. Kuczynski (Ed.), *Handbook of dynamics in parent–child relationships* (pp. 67–89). Thousand Oaks, CA: Sage.

Lollis, S., & Kuczynski, L. (1997). Beyond one hand clapping: Seeing bidirectionality in parent–child relations. *Journal of Social and Personal Relationships, 14,* 441–461.

Lollis, S., Kuczynski, L., Navara, J., & Koguchi, Y. (2003). *Children's agency within compliance and noncompliance.* Poster presented at the biennial meeting of the Society for Research in Child Development, Tampa FL.

Londerville, S., & Main, M. (1981). Security of attachment, compliance and maternal training methods in the second year of life. *Developmental Psychology, 17,* 289–299.

Lundell, L., Grusec J. E., McShane, K., & Davidson, M. (2005). *Adolescent goals in conflict with their mothers.* Unpublished manuscript, University of Toronto.

Maccoby, E. E. (1992). The role of parents in the socialization of children: An historical overview. *Developmental Psychology, 28,* 1006–1017.

Maccoby, E. E. (2000). The uniqueness of the parent–child relationship. In W. A. Collins & B. Laursen. *Relationships as developmental contexts* (pp. 157–175). Mahwah, NJ: Erlbaum.

Maccoby, E. E., & Martin, J. A. (1983). Socialization in the context of the family: Parent–child interaction. In P. H. Mussen (Ed.) & E. M. Hetherington (Vol. Ed.), *Handbook of child psychology: Vol. 4. Socialization, personality, and social development* (4th ed., pp. 1–101). New York: Wiley.

Matas, L., Arend, R., & Sroufe, L. (1978). Continuity of adaptation in the second year: The relationship between quality of attachment and later competence. *Child Development, 49,* 547–556.

McMahon, R. J., & Forehand, R. L. (2003). *Helping the noncompliant child: Family-based treatment for oppositional behavior* (2nd ed.). New York: Guilford Press.

McHale, S. M., & Crouter, A. C. (2003). How do children exert an impact on family life? In A. C. Crouter & A. Booth (Eds.). *Children's influence on family dynamics: The neglected side of family relationships* (pp. 207–220). Mahwah, NJ: Erlbaum.

Miller, G., & Steinberg, M. (1975). *Between people: A new analysis of interpersonal communication.* Chicago: Science Research Associates.

Palkovitz, R., Marks, L. D., Appleby, D. W., & Holmes, E. K. (2003). Processes and products of intergenerational relationships. In L. Kuczynski (Ed.) *Handbook of dynamics in parent–child relations* (pp. 307–324) Thousand Oaks, CA: Sage.

Parpal, M., & Maccoby, E. E. (1985). Material responsiveness and subsequent child compliance. *Child Development, 56,* 1326–1334.

Patterson, G. R. (1982). *Coercive family process.* Eugene, OR: Castalia.

Patterson, G. R. (1993). Orderly change in a stable world: The antisocial trait as a chimera. *Journal of Consulting and Clinical Psychology, 61,* 911–919.

Patterson, G. R. (1997). Performance models for parenting: A social interactional perspective. In J. E. Grusec & L. Kuczynski (Eds.), *Parenting and the internalization of values: A handbook of contemporary theory* (pp. 193–226). New York: Wiley.

Patterson, G. R., & Fisher, P. A. (2002). Recent developments in our understanding of parenting: Bidirectional effects, causal models, and the search for parsimony. In M.H. Bornstein (Ed.), *Handbook of parenting. Vol. 5: Practical issues in parenting* (3rd ed., pp. 59–88). Mahwah NJ: Erlbaum.

Patterson, G. R., & Forgatch, M. (1987). *Parents and adolescents: Living together.* Eugene, OR: Castalia Press.

Patterson, G., Reid, J., & Dishion, T. (1992). *Antisocial boys: Vol. 4. A social interactional approach.* Eugene, OR: Castalia.

Piniata, R. C. (1999). *Enhancing relationships between children and teachers.* Washington, DC: American Psychological Association.

Reis, H. T., Collins, W. A., & Berscheid, E. (2000). The relationship context of human behavior and development. *Psychological Bulletin, 126,* 844–872.

Rheingold, H. L. (1969). The social and socializing infant. In D. A. Goslin (Ed.), *Handbook of socialization theory and research.* Chicago: Rand McNally.

Richters, J. E., & Waters, E. (1992). Attachment and socialization: The positive side of social influence. In M. Lewis & S. Feinman (Eds.), *Social influences and behavior* (pp. 185–214). New York: Plenum Press.

Rubin, K. H., Nelson, L. J., Hastings, P., & Asendorpf, J. (1999). The transaction between parents' perceptions of their children's shyness and their parenting styles. *International Journal of Behavioral Development, 23,* 937–957.

Russell, A., Petit, G., & Mize, J. (1998). Horizontal qualities in parent–child relationships: Parallels with and possible consequences for children's peer relationships. *Developmental Review, 18,* 313–352.

Salkind, N. (1985). *Theories of human development* (2nd. ed.). New York: Wiley.

Sameroff, A. (1975a). Transactional models of early social relations. *Human Development, 18,* 65–79.

Sameroff, A. (1975b). Early influences on development: Fact or fancy? *Merrill-Palmer Quarterly, 21,* 267–293.

Sameroff, A. J., & MacKenzie, M. J. (2003). Research strategies for capturing transactional models of development: The limits of the possible. *Development and Psychopathology. 15*(3), 613–640.

Sears, R. R. (1951). A theoretical framework for personality and social behavior. *American Psychologist, 6,* 476–482.

Shanahan, L., & Sobolewski, J. M. (2003). Child effects as family process. In A.C. Crouter & A. Booth (Eds.), *Children's influence on family dynamics: The neglected side of family relationships* (pp. 237–252). Mahwah, NJ: Erlbaum.

Shantz, C. U. (1987). Conflicts between children. *Child Development, 58*(2), 283–305.

Shantz, C. U., & Hartup, W. W. (1992). *Conflict in child and adolescent development.* Cambridge, MA: Cambridge University Press.

Smetana, J. (1997). Parenting and the development of social knowledge reconceptualized: A social domain analysis. In J. E. Grusec, & L. Kuczynski (Eds.), *Parenting and the internalization of values: A handbook of contemporary theory* (pp. 162–192). New York: Wiley.

Smetana, J. G., Metzger, A., Gettman, D. C., & Campione-Barr, N. (2006). Disclosure and secrecy in adolescent–parent relationships. *Child Development, 77,* 201–217.

Stattin, H., & Kerr, M. (2000). Parental monitoring: A reinterpretation. *Child Development, 71,* 4, 1072–1085.

Stayton, D., Hogan, R., & Ainsworth, M. D. S. (1971). Infant obedience and maternal behaviour: The origins of socialization reconsidered. *Child Development, 42,* 1057–1069.

Steinberg, L. (1987). Impact of puberty on family relations: Effects of pubertal status and pubertal timing. *Developmental Psychology, 23,* 451–460.

Stern, M., & Hildebrandt, K. A. (1986). Prematurity stereotyping: Effects on mother–infant interaction. *Child Development, 57,* 308–315.

Trommsdorff, G., & Kornadt, H. (2003). Parent–child relations in cross-cultural perspective. In L. Kuczynski (Ed.), *Handbook of dynamics in parent–child relations* (pp. 271–306). Thousand Oaks, CA: Sage.

Trommsdorff, G., Zheng, G., & Tardif, T. (2002). Value of children and intergenerational relations in cultural context. In P. Boski, F. J. R. van de Vijver, & A. M. Chodynicka (Eds.), *New directions in cross-cultural psychology* (pp. 581–601). Warsaw: Polish Psychological Association.

Valsiner, J. (1988). Ontogeny of co-construction of culture within socially organized settings. In J. Valsiner (Ed.), *Child development within culturally structured environments* (Vol. 2, pp. 283–297). Norwood, NJ: Ablex.

Valsiner, J. (1989). *Human development and culture.* Lexington, MA: Heath.

Valsiner, J., Branco, A. U., & Dantas, C. M. (1997). Co-construction of human development: Heterogeneity within parental belief orientations. In J.E. Grusec & L. Kuczynski (Eds.), *Parenting and the internalisation of values: A handbook of contemporary theory* (pp. 283–304). New York: Wiley.

Valsiner, J., & Cairns, R. (1992). Theoretical perspectives on conflict and development. In C. U. Shantz & W. W. Hartup (Eds.), *Conflict in child and adolescent development* (pp. 15–35). New York: Cambridge University Press.

Vuchinich, S. (1987). Starting and stopping spontaneous family conflicts. *Journal of Marriage in the Family, 49,* 591–601.

Wenar, C. (1982). On negativism. *Human Development, 25,* 1–23.

Wrong, D. H. (1961). The oversocialized conception of man in modern sociology. *American Sociological Review, 26,* 183–193.

Youniss, J., & Smollar, J. (1985). *Adolescent relations with mothers, fathers, and friends.* Chicago: The University of Chicago Press.

CHAPTER 11

Socialization in the Family
The Roles of Parents

JOAN E. GRUSEC and MAAYAN DAVIDOV

Parents, siblings, teachers, peers, and the media all function as agents of socialization for children. We would argue, however, that parents are the most important in their impact. In this chapter we explore research relevant to the role that parents play in socialization. A complete understanding of this role depends on knowledge of how the human species has evolved to parent and to be parented, of behavior genetics, of the neurological and hormonal processes that operate during the socialization process, and of the cultural context. Each of these is the primary focus of other chapters in this book. In this chapter we focus on the emotional, cognitive, and behavioral processes associated with socialization and their antecedents in parenting actions. We also focus on parenting in a Western industrialized context in which the bulk of research has been conducted, referring the reader to other chapters in this handbook for reviews of parenting in other cultural contexts. However, we draw on findings from these other cultural contexts when they appear relevant. Maccoby (Chapter 1, this volume) has provided a historical survey of parenting research that provides the background for what follows.

Socialization involves the acceptance of values, standards, and customs of society as well as the ability to function in an adaptive way in the larger social context. These values, standards, and customs are not simply transmitted from one generation to the other but, to some extent at least, constructed by each generation. Thus parents are not so much purveyors of information as helpers in setting the stage for their children to become well-functioning members of the social group. Also, an important (but not the only) goal of socialization is that values and standards be internalized in the sense that members of the group behave in accord with them willingly, rather than out of fear of external consequences or hope of reward. In this chapter we briefly comment on parents as primary agents of socialization as well as on issues having to do with direction of effect in parent–child interactions. We then move to a discussion of socialization as situation- or domain-specific, expanding on this idea as a way of presenting what is known about the function of parents in the socialization process. Space limitations mean that our treatment of socialization in the family is far from comprehensive. We say nothing, for example, about the importance of the relationship between parents and how that interacts with socialization goals and outcomes (but see Maccoby, Chapter 1, this volume, for a discussion of some of the relevant literature).

THE PRIMACY OF PARENTS

Few contemporary researchers would argue with the proposition that parents are primary in socialization (Collins, Maccoby, Steinberg, Hetherington, & Bornstein, 2000). First, parents and children are part of a biosocial system that functions to protect offspring and to ensure that they are able to deal with the demands of social life. Thus they are both biologically prepared to be attracted to and remain in close proximity to each other (see Beaulieu & Bugental, Chapter 3, this volume, and Bugental & Grusec, 2006, for a review of the relevant literature). Second, the strong human need for interrelatedness plays a substantial role in the socialization process, and opportunities for such interrelatedness abound in the parent–child relationship as parents protect, nurture, and express affection and warmth to their offspring. Moreover, the bonds of relatedness between parent and child can never be formally severed, unlike those between peers, teachers, and other biologically unrelated individuals. Next, in most societies, parents are formally assigned the role of primary agents of socialization. Fourth, practical reasons facilitate parents' motivation to socialize their children, given that they must live in close proximity to these children and that the lives of all are more comfortable when there is some agreement about the nature of appropriate behavior. Finally, parents are in a position in which they can control resources available to their children as well as manage their environments to ensure that they are either protected from or forewarned about undesirable influences.

DIRECTION OF EFFECT IN SOCIALIZATION

Whereas there may be excellent reasons for arguing that parents are central in socialization, there are challenges to demonstrating empirically the extent to which their actions affect their children's outcomes. Thus researchers have long acknowledged that children also influence parents during the course of socialization and are currently making considerable strides in untangling the complexities of family interactions (Kuczynski, 2003). Behavior geneticists have argued that children affect their own outcomes by triggering particular responses (e.g., harshness) from their parents or by actively seeking out particular environments (e.g., Scarr & McCartney, 1983). Patterson (e.g., 1980) has documented how children can lead to maternal loss of control through negative reinforcement, for example, by ceasing to whine when their mothers stop making aversive demands. Moreover, the mothers' repeated inability to gain compliance leads to feelings of incompetence that further interfere with attempts to control their children's actions. Others have described the parent–child interaction as transactional (e.g., Sameroff, 1975), with one member of the dyad changing the actions of the other which, in turn, alter the actions of the first member. Thus there is a constant process of reciprocal interchange that leads to constant transformation of interactions. What this all indicates is that children are highly involved in their own socialization process.

The nature of reciprocal interactions can be untangled in a number of ways in order to allow greater confidence in inferences that parents cause the behavior of their children. More and more researchers are utilizing longitudinal approaches: By controlling for levels of variables of interest at earlier points in time, they can suggest with considerably more conviction that parents are indeed making a difference. Behavior genetics studies allow for a separation of genetic and environmental contributions to outcomes of interest. Animal analogue studies, parenting intervention studies, and "experiments of nature," such as studies of Romanian orphans raised under conditions of deprivation and then adopted (e.g., Chisholm, 1998; Rutter & O'Connor, 2004), also contribute to an increasing understanding of direction of influence.

SOCIALIZATION AS SITUATION-SPECIFIC

Traditionally, analyses of socialization focused not only on the role of parenting styles and parenting strategies such as discipline and modeling (see Maccoby, Chapter 1, this volume), but they also assumed that there are general socialization processes that operate across all settings. Increasingly, however, it has become evident that socialization involves different processes in different social contexts. Indeed, it has long been evident that organisms are prepared to learn certain responses such as food aversion and fear of animals more easily than others (see Seligman, 1970). Bell and Ainsworth (1972) found that, contrary to the principles of reinforcement theory (which appeared to apply in many aspects of a child's development), maternal responding to infant cries in the first few months of life led to decreased crying toward the end of the first year. Distinctions have also been made between the child's need for protection and need for warmth, with the argument that these two needs are biologically separate systems (MacDonald, 1992). Youniss, McLellan, and Strouse (1994) noted that peer relationships were governed by the principle of cooperation among equals as opposed to the asymmetrical power relationship that exists between parents and children. And Turiel and his colleagues (Turiel, 1998) have demonstrated that even very young children differentiate among moral (harm to others), social conventional (customs), prudential (harm to self), and personal issues, judging moral ones as obligatory and unalterable but seeing social conventional ones as able to be changed by agreement or consensus.

Distinctions of context also appear in the actions of parents with respect to the goals that are activated in different socialization situations. Dix (1992) notes that parents on different occasions espouse personal goals relevant to obtaining obedience, empathic goals oriented to satisfaction of their children's emotional needs and socialization goals relevant to the acquisition of values. Similarly, Hastings and Grusec (1998) found that parents, in response to their children's misbehaviors, report a variety of goals including achieving obedience, teaching values, and maintaining harmony. In each case they employ different strategies ranging from power assertion (for obedience) through reasoning (for value acquisition) to negotiation and acceptance (for harmony).

Finally, social domain theorists (e.g., Fiske, 1992; Bugental, 2000) talk about domains of social life where there are different tasks to be solved and where different rules or algorithms operate. Four domains relevant to socialization include safety and protection of the young, interaction in social settings involving authority, sharing of benefits in the ingroup, and exchange relationships (Beaulieu & Bugental, Chapter 3, this volume; Bugental & Goodnow, 1998; Bugental, 2000; Bugental & Grusec, 2006). In each of these domains, it has been argued, different mechanisms underlying socialization are operating and different practices are needed to achieve the desired goal of the domain.

In this chapter we suggest that a useful way of organizing knowledge about socialization processes is around behavioral systems that are activated in different situations during the course of socialization. Each system reflects different states in the child and each requires different kinds of interventions in order to satisfy the current needs of the child. In the course of appropriate parenting, different skills relevant to the socialization process are acquired. The four systems, which map onto Bugental's (2000) domains of social life, have to do with the child's need for protection and security, the child's developing sense of autonomy that can be threatened when parents attempt to impose control on or direct the child's actions, the child's need to identify with or be part of a social group, and the child's proclivity to reciprocate the behavior of others. We suggest that different mechanisms of socialization operate and different child outcomes are addressed in each of these four behavior systems. In essence, there are different routes to socialization and somewhat different outcomes at the end of each route, with each requiring different parenting practices.

The protection system, most extensively studied by attachment theorists, entails the evolved need of children to seek protection and safety from their parents by maintaining proximity to them. It is here that they learn to trust adults as responsible and well-intentioned caregivers and to regulate negative affect associated with distress that could potentially interfere with positive social behavior. Parents, in turn, need to be sensitively responsive to the child's distress and manage it in a way that promotes positive socialization outcomes. The control domain has been the primary focus of most socialization researchers as they studied parenting styles and discipline. In the control domain children learn through discussion, explanation, and the experience of consequences for their actions what is deemed socially appropriate and what is not. Parents, in turn, need to impose control in a way that is not coercive and that does not threaten the child's autonomy. The third system—group identification—includes the adoption of observed behavior as well as the practice of routines and rituals: Children are eager to acquire and act in accordance with the rules, standards, and actions of the group with which they identify. Parents, in turn, serve as models of socially acceptable behavior as well as managing their children's environment so that they are protected from exposure to unacceptable ways of acting. The fourth system, that of mutual reciprocity, is particularly in evidence as children reciprocate the actions of others. Thus parents, to take advantage of this tendency, need to be responsive to the wishes of their children, cooperate with their desires, and engage in harmonious, positive exchanges. To some degree all these systems operate both within and outside the family, although parents play an important role in all of them. In the remainder of this chapter we elaborate on this analysis of socialization domains.

SOCIALIZATION IN THE CONTEXT OF PROTECTIVE CAREGIVING

Humans at birth are far from able to care for themselves and so they have evolved to seek protection and nurturing from adults during infancy and childhood and to provide protection and nurturing for their offspring during adulthood. Seeking the proximity of the caregiver in the face of threats to well-being is organized by the child's attachment behavioral system, whereas parental behavior aimed at ensuring the safety and well-being of the young is organized by the parent's caregiving system (Bowlby, 1969/1982; Cassidy, 1999; George & Solomon, 1999). These two behavioral systems are complementary and have likely evolved in parallel. Thus, when either the attachment or caregiving system is activated, proximity between child and caregiver is increased and protection is thereby enhanced (Cassidy, 1999; George & Solomon, 1999). The systems are activated by internal or external cues indicating that the child is in real or potential danger. The actions taken by the parent to protect the child from harm will vary depending (among other things) on the situation and the age of the child. With infants, protection includes such behaviors as retrieving, maintaining proximity, calling, signaling the child to follow, holding, soothing and comforting (with soothing and comforting important because they enable the parent to ascertain that the child is no longer in danger; Cassidy, 1999). Children whose mothers are sensitively responsive to their distress cues become securely attached and able to be easily soothed when they are upset. Those whose mothers are rejecting or inconsistent become insecurely attached, either appearing to minimize their signaling of distress or being difficult to soothe (Ainsworth, Blehar, Waters, & Wall, 1978).

This analysis of parent–child relationships focuses on protective caregiving specifically, whereas much work in the area of attachment has assessed positive parenting more generally (Goldberg, Grusec, & Jenkins, 1999). Yet both theory and accumulating empirical evidence suggest that different aspects of the parent–child relationship require different abilities and skills from parents and lead to different outcomes. Thus many parents who are responsive in the protection domain may not be equally responsive in other contexts and situations, and vice versa (Cassidy, 1999; Goldberg et al., 1999). Moreover, there are numerous examples that protection-related and unrelated aspects of parental behavior have separate linkages to child outcomes. Thus maternal soothing and comforting at 3 months predict attachment security whereas exchanges of positive affect or interactions centering on physical objects do not (Del Carmen, Pederson, Huffman, & Bryan, 1993). Roberts and Strayer (1987) report that parents' responsiveness to their preschoolers' distress was correlated with children's overall competence at school, even after statistically controlling for parental warmth. Similarly, Davidov and Grusec (2006) found that parental responsiveness to distress, but not parental warmth, predicted children's capacity to self-regulate their negative emotions and to respond with empathy and prosocial behavior to another's distress. Contrarily, maternal warmth, but not responsiveness to distress, was a significant predictor of children's competent regulation of positive affect and of boys' peer acceptance. Finally, Rodriguez et al. (2005) demonstrated that 2-year-old children whose mothers were responsive during an emotionally demanding task were better able to regulate their own behavior in a resistance-to-temptation task 3 years later, whereas maternal responsiveness when the task was not emotionally demanding had no impact on subsequent self-regulation.

It is thus clear that protective caregiving does not encompass all aspects of positive, responsive parenting. Rather, protection denotes parenting behavior aimed at ensuring the safety and well-being of the child (e.g., Goldberg et al., 1999; Cassidy, 1999). It comes into play in situations involving real or potential threat, such as when the child is hurt, ill, in physical danger, or emotionally upset. Sensitive protective caregiving involves the provision of help and emotional support in times of need in a manner suitable to the particular needs of the child, as well as the provision of a safe environment for the child. Finally, it does not involve overly protective or overly restrictive practices, which can interfere with the development of competent self-regulatory abilities.

Sensitively protective parenting can facilitate positive socialization outcomes in several ways, including self-regulation of negative emotion, facilitation of empathic responding, and fostering of trust in the parent. We now discuss each of these ways.

Effective Regulation of Negative Emotions

Protective caregiving facilitates children's ability to self-regulate their negative emotions and to cope in an adaptive, flexible manner, expressing negative emotion in an appropriate, controlled, and modulated way (Cassidy, 1994). Infants whose parents are consistent in alleviating distress and discomfort expect their signals to be effective at recruiting parental assistance. Thus they come to perceive negative events as less threatening, and thus these events are less likely to trigger a physiological stress response. In contrast, when parents repeatedly fail to protect, infants experience high levels of stress, which can adversely affect the development and subsequent functioning of neurobiological systems responsible for the regulation of stress and negative emotion (Gunnar, 2000). Early exposure to stressors results in chronic hyperresponsiveness of these systems, which means that relatively mild events come to trigger intense physiological stress reactions. Protective parents also model competent coping behavior in response to stress, as well as coach their children in and scaffold their acquisition of effective coping strategies (Gottman, Katz, & Hooven, 1996; Thompson, 1994). They can also help their children gain control and understanding of negative emotions by allowing an outlet for the child's negative affect in a supportive context (Fabes, Leonard, Kupanoff, & Martin, 2001; Roberts & Strayer, 1987). Although encouraging the restraint of negative expressions can be appropriate in some situations (Roberts, 1999), devaluing the child's negative emotions and attempting to suppress them altogether have been linked to poor regulation of negative affect (Fabes et al., 2001; Gottman et al., 1996).

Children's successful self-regulatory capacities promote positive socialization outcomes in two important ways. First, they increase children's ability to attend to parental teaching about appropriate behavior because children are less likely to be overly aroused in the discipline situations where much of this teaching occurs. Second, self-regulatory abilities enable children to manifest socialization values in action. Thus, well-regulated children can inhibit negative emotions that fuel antisocial action or undermine prosocial action. Accordingly, Eisenberg et al. (1999) found that the children of mothers who had responded punitively or with distress to their negative emotions subsequently displayed more aggressive and disruptive behavior with peers and adults; moreover, this relation was partially mediated by the children's poorer self-regulation. Similarly, Gottman et al. (1996) found that parents who had a coaching meta-emotional philosophy, that is, accepted their 5-year-olds' negative emotions and tried to help their children understand and manage them, had children who could regulate their physiological arousal more effectively as indicated by measures of vagal tone. This regulation, in turn, predicted their

ability to self-regulate their emotions 3 years later, which further predicted their competent, nonaggressive behavior with peers (teacher report). Davidov and Grusec (2006)
have also provided evidence that effective self-regulation of negative affect partially mediates the linkage between parental responsiveness to distress and children's prosocial responding to another's distress.

Empathy

Parents' sensitive responding to child distress can also facilitate children's empathic capacity (e.g., Davidov & Grusec, 2006; Eisenberg & Fabes, 1998). Empathy and sympathy are other-oriented emotional responses to the distress or need state of another and are
important motivators of prosocial action. Parents who respond with sensitivity to their
children's distress model empathy and compassion, which children are likely to emulate
later when interacting with others. Responsive reactions to children's negative emotions
also facilitate their ability to accurately read others' emotions (Fabes, Poulin, Eisenberg,
& Madden-Derdich, 2002) which can promote empathy. Finally, as noted previously,
sensitive caregiving can promote empathic responding by fostering a balanced style of
negative affect regulation. Such a regulatory style facilitates empathy because it enables
individuals to identify with the emotion experienced by another but without becoming
overly aroused and distressed as a result (Eisenberg, Wentzel, & Harris, 1998; van
IJzendoorn, 1997). Absence or suppression of any negative sympathetic feeling in response to another's misfortune marks lack of concern for others, while overarousal produces personal distress, a self-focused response (e.g., disturbance, anxiety) that distracts
from prosocial behavior.

Deficits in empathic capacity not only may reduce prosocial responding but also may
make antisocial behavior more likely. Individuals who cannot reflect on and identify with
other persons' feelings and mental states will not experience guilt or discomfort as a consequence of hurting others (Fonagy, Target, Steele, & Steele, 1997). Indeed, Bowlby's first
empirical paper, which focused on the etiology of juvenile delinquency, drew linkages between early experiences of lack of a consistent, supportive caregiver and the development
of an "affectionless" personality and delinquent behavior (Bowlby, 1944).

Trust in the Parent

A final process linking protection to positive socialization outcomes involves trust in the
parent to act fairly and in the best interests of the child. Thus, children whose parents are
typically available and supportive in times of need should be more likely to perceive parental prescriptions and prohibitions as manifestations of caring and goodwill than as
malevolent and coercive (Grusec & Goodnow, 1994; Bretherton, Golby, & Cho, 1997).
As a result they would be more likely to comply and cooperate with their parents (and
subsequently with others with whom they establish a secure relationship), and to accept
parental values as appropriate and just (see also Richters & Waters, 1991).

Stayton, Hogan, and Ainsworth (1973) have argued that the tendency to cooperate
with the parent develops in concert with the formation of the attachment bond, as both
would have been essential for survival during human evolution. In fact, the results of research looking at links between attachment and compliance have been mixed. Stayton et
al. (1973) found that mothers who provided sensitive cargiving to their infants (a dimen-

sion shown to be predictive of a secure attachment in the same sample; Ainsworth et al., 1978) had infants who, when observed in their homes, were more likely to comply with maternal verbal commands as well as inhibit a previously forbidden behavior. Similarly, Londerville and Main (1981) found that secure toddlers, when observed in free play in a laboratory room containing potential safety hazards (e.g., an electric fan), were more compliant with maternal directives, less likely to actively disobey their mothers, more cooperative with strangers, and more likely to self-inhibit previously prohibited behavior. Securely attached toddlers were found to comply more with maternal suggestions during a challenging problem-solving task but not when asked to clean up toys in the laboratory (Matas, Arend, & Sroufe, 1978). Nor did van der Mark, Bakermans-Kranenburg, and van IJzendoorn (2002) find much evidence that securely attached toddlers were more compliant when asked to clean up toys or to refrain from touching attractive toys at home and in the laboratory.

These seemingly inconsistent findings raise the possibility that the linkage between protective caregiving and compliance might depend on the area in which compliance is being sought. Thus, protective caregiving (and the secure attachment it engenders) may facilitate compliance in some situations but not in others. Perhaps protection and attachment security are primarily important for compliance in the area of safety, in which conformity to parental commands is indeed important for ensuring the child's health and well-being. For adolescents, the impact of parental responsiveness to distress might be particularly great with respect to health-threatening activities such as alcohol and drug use and unsafe sexual activity. Protection is also important for the ability to openly seek help when in need and is thus likely linked to the ability to accept and cooperate with such help once it is offered. In contrast, protection might not play a role in more benign situations, such as when a child is asked to clean up, for which other behavioral systems (discussed below) might be more central. These possible domain distinctions, however, await direct empirical examination. Also deserving of attention are children's feelings of trust in the parent and their perceptions of parental intentions and fairness, to examine whether such cognitions mediate between sensitive protection and children's willingness to cooperate and accept parental values in these domains (Grusec & Goodnow, 1994).

SOCIALIZATION IN THE CONTEXT OF PARENTAL CONTROL AND CHILD AUTONOMY

In the domain of protection parents serve as "stronger and wiser" guardians who provide support, help, and reassurance in times of need. But the superior strength and resources of parents compared to children has additional implications. Thus, the hierarchical aspect of the parent–child relationship means that parents are not only providers of protection but are also enforcers of rules. We now turn to discuss socialization processes involved in the discipline encounter, as parents attempt to direct their children's behavior in the face of children's resistance and desire for autonomy.

The exertion of parental control can take many forms including persuasion, reasoning, and punishment or power assertion. These tactics are also applied in the context of different styles, either in a warm and supportive way or in a harsh and rejecting way. When control involves the clarifying of limits and the keeping of order it is positive in its outcomes (e.g., Baumrind, 1971). When it involves rigidity, inflexibility, and insensitivity to the needs of the child it is negative in its outcomes (e.g., Deci & Ryan, 1985; Rothbaum & Weisz, 1994). Another way of framing the issue has to do with the extent to which control threatens the autonomy of the child with, for example, reasoning conceived of as less threatening to autonomy than more power-assertive interventions (Hoffman, 1970a). As we noted at the beginning of this chapter, children need to feel that their behavior is self-generated and that they are not impelled by external forces over which they have no power (although we note that too much autonomy is problematic because it leads to indecisiveness and dissatisfaction; see Schwartz, 2000). A desire for reasonable amounts of autonomy is a feature of human behavior that many have suggested is not limited to a Western cultural context but is universal. Indeed, there is physiological evidence that supports the assertion of universality. Thus long-term occupation of a subordinate role has been shown in primates to have high costs with its accompanying detrimental levels of cardiovascular strain and activation of the hypothalamic–pituitary–adrenocortical (HPA) system (Abbott et al., 2003). Also, it has been demonstrated that even in so-called collectivist societies, with their emphasis on group harmony and interconnectedness, autonomy is still valued (Killen & Wainryb, 2000; Ryan & Deci, 2000). At a different level of analysis, actual or perceived lower socioeconomic status (SES) predicts poorer health and, particularly, higher rates of stress-related diseases, with the SES/health gradient steeper the greater the degree of income inequality (e.g., Sapolsky, 2004): This observation provides another demonstration of the impact of perceptions of low power and restricted autonomy on human functioning.

The partitioning of control into forms that are positive and negative in outcome has led to two avenues of investigation. One has to do with the variety of kinds of control and the other with the fact that different children perceive what is objectively the same kind and amount of control as differentially threatening to their sense of autonomy. We discuss research related to each of these aspects of control in turn.

Varieties of Control

Psychological versus Behavioral Control

Baumrind's (e.g., 1971) distinction between authoritative and authoritarian parenting styles, involving sensitive and rigid control, respectively, has guided socialization research for many years. More recently, control has been divided into the two categories of behavioral and psychological control (Barber, 1996; Steinberg, 1990). Behavioral control involves reasonable setting of rules for children's behavior and their reasonable (non autonomy-threatening) enforcement, as well as monitoring of children's activities. Low levels of behavioral control are associated with externalizing problems that include drug use, truancy, and antisocial behavior (Barber & Harmon, 2002; Crouter & Head, 2002). High levels of behavioral control, if they involve feelings of being controlled, however, also appear to predict maladjustment (Kerr & Stattin, 2000). Psychological control involves attempts to direct children by influencing their emotional state. It includes the use of guilt-inducing strategies, withdrawal of love, and parental intrusiveness. Parents who are highly psychologically controlling are manipulative and insensitive to the emotional needs of their children, undermining their sense of self-esteem and self-identity. High levels of psychological control are associated with internalizing problems, including anxiety, depression, loneliness, low academic achievement, low self-esteem, low self-reliance, and self-derogation (Barber & Harmon, 2002). Behavioral and psychological control, then, are qualitatively different and have different consequences for child development.

Self-Determination Theory and Autonomy Support

Another, related perspective on control comes from self-determination theory (e.g., Deci & Ryan, 1985; Grolnick, Deci, & Ryan, 1997). Proponents of the theory suggest that although children have a natural tendency to engage in many intrinsically rewarding prosocial behaviors, there are other prosocial behaviors that are not intrinsically rewarding and so conditions must be in place to encourage their internalization. These behaviors need to be fully internalized (coherent, that is, fully integrated or assimilated with all aspects of the self), a condition that is facilitated by autonomy support (gentle control, provision of appropriate choice), as well as by structure (setting clear expectations), and interpersonal involvement (being warm and caring, demonstrating interest in the child). Autonomy support facilitates the perception that behavior is self-generated rather than externally imposed. Structure is required so that children know what it is they are supposed to do, and interpersonal involvement and relatedness so that children are willing to accept the structure. Self-determination theorists have provided considerable empirical evidence that these three conditions do in fact facilitate children's autonomous self-regulation (Grolnick, 2003).

Similar analyses of autonomy support are seen in the work of investigators such as Pomerantz (e.g., Pomerantz & Eaton, 2001) who refer to intrusive support, with examples being parents checking their children's homework when they are not requested to do so (monitoring) and helping with their homework when such assistance is not requested (helping). Intrusive support has both positive and negative qualities. Thus it communicates caring but it also undermines autonomy. In fact, at least in the area of academic achievement, such intrusive support appears to have more negative consequences for children who are less successful academically, presumably because they are more sensitive to the inference of incompetence that such intrusive parenting offers (Ng, Kenney-Benson, & Pomerantz, 2004). This last observation underlines the fact that the impact of control is not a uniform one and that control interacts with a great many features of the situation. We turn now to some of these features.

Moderators of Control

Current analyses of the socialization process and, particularly, the role of parental control, increasingly point to the importance of interactions. Examinations of the main effects of particular discipline strategies and approaches have produced a limited set of consistent findings because, as has become more and more evident, different characteristics of children and of situations alter the outcomes of different forms of discipline (Collins et al., 2000; Grusec, Goodnow, & Kuczynksi, 2000; Grusec & Goodnow, 1994). A main focus of the work has been on interactions between parenting strategies and features of child temperament. There are also a variety of other attributes of children and of the context that interact with features of parenting. We discuss some representative examples of such interactions, without intending to be at all exhaustive in our treatment.

Temperament

There is considerable evidence that temperament is a moderator of reactions to control, and Bates and Pettit (Chapter 6, this volume) have reviewed this research literature. They suggest that children with fearful temperaments internalize values better when gentle rather than harsh control is used, whereas those with fearless temperaments respond better when their relationship with the mother is warm. Children who are high in negative emotionality are more affected by the quality of parenting they receive than are those who are less irritable, with highly directive parenting reducing behavioral inhibition in irritable children and harsh parenting increasing the risk of externalizing problems in these same children. As well, children who are low in self-regulatory ability are less likely to exhibit externalizing behaviors when their mothers are controlling.

Age

There are developmental differences in reactions to control or what is perceived as threatening to one's sense of autonomy. Young children are more likely to accept strong forms of parental intervention and direction as fair and appropriate than are older children, and the range of issues that children and adolescents consider to be under their own personal jurisdiction rather than that of their parents' increases with age (Siegal & Cowen, 1984; Smetana, 1988). Indeed, links between harsh parenting and externalizing behavior are greater for older children than for preschoolers (Rothbaum & Weisz, 1994), presumably because older children are more likely to see such parenting as infringing on their sense of autonomy. This increase in association with age may also reflect a qualitative change in children's underlying motivations to engage in externalizing conduct. Thus, instrumental and autonomy-seeking motives, which parents are less likely to react to negatively and are more capable of deterring, are central at a younger age (at least in nonclinical samples), whereas externalizing behavior in older children appears to have an underlay of hostility that is further exacerbated by increasingly interwoven mutual negative expectations (Rothbaum & Weisz, 1994). Childrearing strategies also change in the role they play with age, with contingent responding to child misbehavior being a more important factor in the minimization of antisocial behavior early in childhood and monitoring and guidance more important during adolescence (Patterson, Crosby & Vuchinich, 1992; Pettit, 1997). This change may result from the fact that the use of external contingencies to manage behavior works better with younger children because they see it as less threatening of autonomy than do older children and it is therefore less undermining of intrinsic motivation. For older children, parents may have to turn to more subtle interventions in order to achieve the same outcomes. Age differences also arise in the ability to understand complex rationales (Grusec & Goodnow, 1994) and to deal with messages whose content and method of delivery are at odds, for example, approval expressed in a neutral tone of voice (Bugental, Kaswan, & Love, 1970; Morton & Trehub, 2001).

Sex

There is considerable evidence that boys react more negatively to control than girls, at least when the outcome variable is externalizing behavior. Thus, a meta-analysis and review by Rothbaum and Weisz (1994) suggests that maternal caregiving is more strongly linked to externalizing behavior in preadolescent boys as compared to girls. Similarly, boys are more likely than girls to be involved in coercive cycles of escalating negative behavior with their mothers (McFadyen-Ketchum, Bates, Dodge, & Pettit, 1996; Patterson, 1982). These findings could reflect boys' predisposition to react more negatively, or at least in a more antisocial manner, to harsh parenting, as well as mothers' different relationship dynamics with boys and girls. In another demonstration of sex differences in response to control, Awong, Grusec, and Sorenson (2005) assessed externalizing problems in 12-year-old children as a function of maternal control (operationalized as demands for family deference and parental respect) at the time of their children's birth. They found high levels of this particular form of control to be predictive of high levels of externalizing problems for boys but not for girls. In addition, boys are more likely to resist parental intervention as their testosterone levels increase and they become more aggressive (Panksepp, 1993). However, it should be noted that high levels of testosterone predict aggressive and destructive behavior when the parent–child relationship is poor but not when it is good (Booth, Johnson, Granger, Crouter, & McHale, 2003). There is some suggestion in the literature that girls are more likely than boys to respond to control with internalizing problems, but the evidence is mixed (e.g., Awong et al., 2005; Compton, Snyder, Schrepferman, Bank, & Shortt, 2003; Crockenberg & Lourie, 1996).

Nature of the Misdeed

There is abundant evidence that parents respond differentially to different kinds of misdeeds (Grusec & Goodnow, 1994). Moreover, any given response is effective for certain misdeeds but less so for others. In other words, the effectiveness of a chosen intervention is influenced by its suitability to the nature of the particular misdeed. This process is likely mediated, at least in part, by children's perceptions of the fairness of the parental control strategy given the type of social rule that has been violated (e.g., moral standard, social convention, failure to act prosocially, and personal issue) (Smetana, 1997). Differential usage of discipline techniques has been linked to positive child outcomes. Thus, Hoffman (1970b) found that reliance on different forms of discipline as a function of the nature of the misdeed was particularly great in mothers of children with a strong moral orientation. Moreover, authoritative mothers, who are more likely to produce good outcomes in their children, make appropriate distinctions among moral misdeeds (physical and psychological damage to others), social conventional misdeeds (rules governing appropriate social interactions), and personal issues, whereas authoritarian mothers moralize social conventional acts and treat personal issues as though they were conventional and appropriately subject to parental intervention (Smetana, 1995). Similarly, Trickett and Kuczynski (1986) found that physically abusive mothers employed primarily power assertive strategies in contrast to nonabusive mothers who were governed in their interventions by the nature of their child's misdeed.

Affective Context

Parenting interventions assume different meanings for children as a function of the affective context in which they occur. If control signifies, means, or represents love or concern, then children's sense of autonomy is less threatened, and they would be more likely to accept and internalize parental direction, perhaps to please a warm and caring parent or because psychological reactance has not been aroused. But when control signifies rejection and hostility, its outcomes may be detrimental. For example, although power-assertive and controlling parenting, when used in association with nurturance and warmth, is often linked to positive outcomes for African American children (e.g., Brody & Flor, 1998), it is a negative predictor for these same children when it is operationalized as observed rejection, criticism, and failure to say good-bye or to greet children in a day-care setting (Kilgore, Snyder, & Lentz, 2000). As another example, control in the form of parental demands for respect has a positive impact on self-esteem, but not when it is used in a context of anger (Awong et al., 2005).

Additional evidence for the importance of the affective context emerges from studies that have compared so-called authoritarian parenting in different cultural contexts. Rudy and Grusec (2001, 2006), for example, have demonstrated that authoritarian parenting is associated with lack of warmth, feelings of inefficacy, negative cognitions about the child, and anger in Anglo Canadian parents, linkages not evident in Middle Eastern Canadian parents. Moreover, they found that children's self-esteem was more strongly predicted by these negative emotions and cognitions than it was by parental control or authoritarianism. They suggest that it is association with negative cognition and affect that accounts for the deleterious impact of authoritarian parenting in Western cultural contexts. In non-Western cultural contexts the same parenting style has fewer harmful outcomes and does not occur in this same negative context (e.g., Lindahl & Malik, 1999; Leung, Lau, & Lam, 1998) or is even positively associated with warmth and acceptance (Rohner & Pettengill, 1985; Stewart et al., 1998). In these same cultures, however, when authoritarian parenting is operationalized as domineering or overprotective behavior, it has negative effects (Herz & Gullone, 1999; Stewart et al., 1998), just as it does in a Western cultural context.

Implications of Moderation Effects on Control for Socialization

The existence of so many variables that moderate the impact of parental control suggests that the traditional focus on specific parenting strategies and on the control process itself cannot provide a comprehensive understanding of parenting. Indeed, Grusec and Goodnow (1994) were led to argue, on the basis of the evidence, that internalization of values should not be seen as arising from the use of specific strategies. Instead, it would be better seen as a function of children's accurate perception of the parental message and acceptance of that message, with the latter determined by such variables as appropriateness of the strategy (e.g., fairness), the child's motivation (e.g., to please a warm parent), and the child's feeling that the message was self-generated and not threatening to autonomy. Accordingly, Grusec et al. (2000) argued that effective parenting in the control domain is at least in part a reflection of the ability of parents to know how their children will react to different forms of intervention, that is, to accurately identify the meaning of the intervention to their child or the impact of the intervention on the child's sense of autonomy. Good parenting involves problem solving and flexibility in the sense of the parent being able and willing to modify interventions so that they are suited to the current situation (including features of the child, of the behavior under consideration, and of the context). Parents who are knowledgeable about their children's perceptions and reactions can tailor their interventions accordingly and thus promote positive socialization outcomes. For example, they can accurately assess if their children understand what they are supposed to do, if their children feel they are being treated fairly or noncoercively, whether a particular strategy is seen as a manifestation of caring behavior or of hostility, or if a power assertive intervention is seen as an indication of the importance of the issue to the parent rather than as an angry outburst.

In accord with this analysis, Hastings and Grusec (1998) found that parents who were accurate in perceiving their adolescents' thoughts and feelings during conflict felt greater satisfaction with the outcomes of conflict (in the case of mothers) and had fewer conflicts (in the case of fathers). Similarly, Lundell, Grusec, McShane, and Davidov (2005) found that mothers who took the perspective of their adolescents were likely to have less intense conflicts with them, and that the link between perspective-taking and reduced conflict intensity was through a reduction in the adolescents' desire to retaliate against the mother or alter her behavior. Thus they reasoned that mothers who can take their child's point of view into account are able to manage the situation in a way that reduces the probability of escalation. As well, Davidov and Grusec (in press) found that mothers who were more knowledgeable about their children's reactions to different discipline strategies were more likely to have children who complied, after initial resistance, to a request to tidy a playroom. Moreover, they found that mothers' responsive reactions to their children's protests mediated between maternal accuracy and children's ultimate compliance.

This analysis of effective childrearing assumes that parents are motivated as well as able to put their knowledge into effect. Given these conditions, however, one can ask about the best way to acquire knowledge. Inquiries about thoughts and emotions, done in a noncoercive and accepting way, would be one good approach. Modeling and reciprocation of such sharing by appropriate discussion of the parents' own feelings and thoughts with the child is yet another. Setting the conditions for a positive and warm relationship or a trusting relationship, which facilitate the child's sharing of information about thoughts, feelings, and reactions, is another approach. Parents can also observe their children closely in order to assess their reactions to events. Good relationships also make it easier for both parent and child to spend time with each other, another essential ingredient of knowledge gathering.

SOCIALIZATION IN THE CONTEXT OF GROUP IDENTIFICATION

Close attention to and explicit direction of behavior is an important feature of socialization. But much socialization occurs that is less explicit in nature and that is less often the result of the imposition of specific rules of conduct. Thus we move to the domain of observational learning and the practice of cultural routines. In this domain, socialization occurs as children watch others and match their actions. Many of these actions involve routinized or ritualized ways of doing things, and they often easily become part of the child's behavioral repertoire. Moreover, parents manage their children's daily lives so that they are exposed to models of desirable behavior and protected from models of undesirable behavior. Finally, unlike interactions in the control domain, those involving observation and imitation of others do not involve conflict between agent of socialization and child.

One source of the human tendency to observe and imitate has been located in the desire for group affiliation or belongingness. Preference for the ingroup has long been recognized to be a primary feature of human thinking, carrying with it feelings such as pride, loyalty, and perceived superiority (Allport, 1954). Evolutionary theorists have proposed that ingroups arise because humans have moved beyond isolated individuals or pairs of individuals to rely on the wider social group as a source of assistance and resources. Such mutual cooperation requires a degree of trust that is depersonalized (i.e., goes beyond kin) but must not be indiscriminate and so is limited to the boundaries of an identified set of individuals (Brewer & Gardner, 1996). Symbols and behaviors that differentiate the ingroup from the outgroup become important as a way of decreasing the chance that ingroup benefits will be inadvertently extended to members of the outgroup as well as ensuring that ingroup members receive the benefits that are their due. The ingroup, then, becomes a place where one can expect to be treated well and liked. Brewer (1999) suggests that as ingroups increase in size and become more depersonalized, the rules and customs of the group are seen as better, rather than just different, from those of the outgroup. Although, as noted, the ingroup consists of more than just kin, it does include them. Moreover, it is with kin, in the family context, that children have their first exposure to the group's way of doing things. Thus we suggest that a powerful force for socialization in the family is the predisposition to emulate the actions of parents, as well as other members of the ingroup.

The evolutionary perspective suggests that young children are biologically predisposed to adopt the customs, rules, and standards of the group. Kagan (1982) has argued that children have a natural interest in standards and that they become upset when they see an adult normative standard violated. As well, they become distressed when they are unable to model the actions of an adult because it is too difficult to do so. From an early age children are aware of "proper" ways of doing things (Dunn & Munn, 1985; Smetana, 1997) and engage in compulsive-like ritualistic and repetitive behavior (Evans et al., 1997). They value family routines and react negatively to their omission. This interest in abiding by rules and conventions and engaging in ritualized actions fits with the notion of a predisposition to avoid exclusion from the group. It reflects the importance of cultural practices, routines, and rituals (i.e., everyday ways of doing things).

Learning Novel Responses through Observation

Although cultural practices as such have not taken center stage in analyses of socialization, their study was a major part of the analysis of socialization made by imitation theorists. Bandura and Walters (1963), in their sociobehavioristic approach, suggested that researchers to that point had relied too heavily on a narrow range of learning principles that had been derived from the study of animals, and that greater emphasis needed to be placed on the social nature of human functioning, particularly in the case of the acquisition of novel responses. They suggested that observational learning was the primary means by which novel responses were acquired. Moreover, they maintained that observational learning was the primary or most important, as well as most efficient, form of learning for human beings. Their thesis was supported by a great many demonstrations of the role of observational learning in the acquisition of a wide variety of behaviors including aggression and self-regulation (see Bandura, 1977, for a review). These studies demonstrated that models can teach novel responses and that this learning is not affected by knowledge that rewards for imitation will be forthcoming. The probability of performance of observed actions can be increased if models are rewarded for their actions, although the evidence with respect to punitive consequences decreasing the frequency of modeling over baseline is somewhat more equivocal (Hoffman, 1970a). Nevertheless, the basic conclusion is that people cannot be kept from learning what they have seen. This conclusion is buttressed by the recent discovery of "mirror neurons" in primates, in which the same neural firings occur when individuals are observing an action executed by another individual as when they carry out the action themselves (Gallese, Ferrari, Kohler, & Fogassi, 2002).

Learning through Participation

Anthropologists have addressed the role of observational learning in the acquisition of societal norms, particularly in settings in which formal instruction of children by adults is less the norm. Lave and Wenger (1991), for example, used the phrase "legitimate peripheral participation" to describe the way in which younger members of the cultural group observe older ones performing activities that are valued by the group. Rogoff, Paradise, Arauz, Correa-Chavez, and Angelillo (2003) and Rogoff et al. (Chapter 19, this volume) describe "learning through community intent participation," that is, learning through keen observation and listening in anticipation of engaging in a specific endeavor. This is a form of learning that occurs more frequently in cultural communities that are particularly inclined to involve children in adult activities as opposed to communities that segregate children in formal school settings. Nevertheless, learning through intent participation does occur in these latter communities too, as parents and children interact during the course of accomplishing everyday tasks together. Rheingold (1982), for example, describes the desire of young children to help with work around the house, even though they are not proficient at it and are even discouraged by their mothers. Young children also "play house," an indication of their motivation to engage in closely observed adult activity.

Routines and Rituals

Routines include a multitude of social expectations such as gender-based activities, work around the house, modes of dressing, what can be done in public and what is to be done in private, and where to eat and sleep. They can also include structured play. An important feature of practices and routines in the group identification domain is that they are habit-driven, develop a momentum of their own, and are frequently not questioned and therefore do not offer a basis for conflict (Bugental & Goodnow, 1998; Goodnow, Miller, & Kessel, 1995). Indeed, once they are questioned, the interaction moves into the arena of conflict and autonomy-preservation that forms the control domain. Routines and practices mark individuals as members of the group and they allow learning about principles of behavior in action beyond discussion and persuasion. The importance of one particular kind of routine, the ritual (described by one young child as "doing the same old thing—only it's still fun"), has been underlined by researchers who link family rituals and routines to well-being. Thus Eaker and Walters (2002) report that more psychosocially mature adolescents feel more closely connected to family rituals. Dubas and Gerris (2002), in a longitudinal study of Dutch families, found that the time fathers spent with their young adolescents in activities such as eating together, watching television, and sharing activities and places visited was a predictor of reduced conflict. Finally, Grusec, Goodnow, and Cohen (1997) have demonstrated how routinely performed work around the house, when it is done for the benefit of other family members, is linked with greater spontaneous prosocial behavior.

The importance of observational learning and routines and cultural practices as involving unquestioned action is echoed in self-determination theory's proposal that humans have a natural motivational propensity to internalize or take over cultural values, attitudes, and behaviors and that when agents of socialization force children to engage in socially acceptable action they inhibit or stifle this natural desire to be like the group, thereby undermining intrinsic motivation (Deci & Ryan, 1985). Self-determination theorists argue that the maintenance of intrinsic motivation is dependent on the satisfaction of three basic psychological needs—autonomy, competence, and relatedness. Thus the introduction of external incentives, threats, demandingness, and surveillance—events that undermine autonomy—are likely to shift the child from an internal to an external locus of causality and to move the interaction to the control domain. And intrinsically motivated behavior is maintained by the child's need to feel competent as well as being part of a social group.

Managing the Child's Environment

Parents can take advantage of their children's desire to be like others by exposing them to favorable role models, limiting their access to negative ones, and managing their activities to encourage emulation of prosocial behavior and the acquisition of socially acceptable routines and rituals. They also need to know where their children are and to what they are being exposed. A major source of this knowledge is children's spontaneous volunteering or willing disclosure of information to their parents (Kerr & Stattin, 2000). Presumably such spontaneous volunteering of information is more likely to occur in the context of a warm, loving, and accepting parent–child relationship. Although Kerr and Stattin argue for the primacy of spontaneous disclosure as a source of parents' knowledge of their children, Waizenhoffer, Buchanan, and Jackson-Newsom (2004) have found that parental participation in the activities of children and their questioning of knowledgeable adults about their children is also predictive of their knowledge.

SOCIALIZATION IN THE CONTEXT OF MUTUAL RECIPROCITY

In the area of routines, observational learning, and intent to participate, parents and other agents of socialization set the conditions for socialization. As well, they might encourage children to pay attention and learn through observation. But they do not specifically demand action as in the control domain or need to be sensitively responsive as in the protection domain. We turn to a final context in which parents' responsive behavior again becomes important in yet another way, that involving mutual reciprocity.

Humans appear to have an inborn tendency to reciprocate the actions of others (Trevarthen, Kokkinski, & Flamenghi, 1999), an evolutionarily adaptive response given the survival and reproductive benefits that arise from assisting others. They are also alleged to be endowed with a "cheater mechanism" that makes them sensitive to times when they provide benefits to others but do not receive benefits in return (Cosmides & Tooby, 1992). This tendency to reciprocate what others have done forms the basis for a final domain of socialization. By willingly cooperating with their children's reasonable requests and bids for attention and reciprocating their positive expressions, parents can induce children into a system of mutual reciprocity. In such a relationship parents and children are each attuned and responsive to the needs of the other and share common goals, in contrast to the conflict of goals that exists when parents actively attempt to alter undesirable behavior. Children's responsiveness in the context of mutual reciprocity therefore reflects a genuine willingness and interest in compliance that is not externally forced. Play interactions provide an important context for engaging in social reciprocity, as they allow child and parent equal influence in determining the course of the interaction. The sharing of pleasure and joy, during play and other rewarding activities, can also facilitate the establishment of mutual interests and goals and thus contribute to a mutually responsive stance. In the reciprocity domain, in contrast to the protection and control domains, parents and children operate as equal-status partners and their interactions are marked by symmetry (e.g., Bugental, 2000).

The importance of a mutually responsive orientation during socialization was first demonstrated by Parpal and Maccoby (1985), who showed that when mothers acceded to the reasonable demands of their children, their children were subsequently more responsive to their mothers' demands. Considerable evidence has since accumulated for the significance of parental compliance and mutual reciprocity in socialization. For example, Kochanska and her colleagues (e.g., Kochanska & Aksan, 1995; Kochanska & Murray, 2000) have found that parent–child relationships that are mutually compliant, harmonious, and positive during the preschool and toddler years not only predict cooperative action but also are precursors of conscience in later childhood as indexed by internalized conduct and guilt following perceived wrongdoing. Gardner, Ward, Burton, and Wilson (2003) observed that children whose mothers had engaged with them in joint cooperative play at the age of 3 years were less likely to have conduct problems at 4 years of age (controlling for level of conduct problems at 3 years). They suggest that one reason for this association may be that joint play allows children to experience parental responsiveness and therefore to be more likely to comply with parental wishes in the future. Mutual reciprocity appears to be important beyond early childhood. Thus Criss, Shaw, and Ingoldsby (2003) found that mother–son interactions during a discussion that were reciprocal, responsive, interconnected, and engaged were predictive of the boys' lower antisocial behavior after controlling for earlier levels of antisocial behavior. Criss et al. argue that in these engaged or synchronous interactions boys engage in mutual exchange with their parents and that this facilitates the development of prosocial behavior. In all these cases, then, another significant element of socialization is manifested. Finally, the importance of parental willing responsiveness to children's requests, as specific to the context of mutual reciprocity, is seen in the finding that maternal willing compliance predicted children's immediate compliance with a maternal request to clean up a playroom, but not children's compliance once they had protested and thereby moved the interaction into the control domain (Davidov & Grusec, in press).

CONCLUSION

In this chapter we have argued that socialization happens in a variety of domains or settings. These domains or settings can be identified by a focus on different motives experienced by children and different actions required by agents of socialization in response to those different motives. Children need to be protected, want to feel autonomous, want to be like other members of the group, and reciprocate the behavior of others. Socialization goes on in all these contexts. In the course of parent–child interactions different domains become activated and deactivated, depending on features of the situation as well as the characteristics, goals, and needs of both parent and child. In the domain of protection, parents who respond sensitively to their children's distress socialize them by helping them to regulate negative emotions that otherwise interfere with socially appropriate behavior. These parents also model empathy and compassion, and foster trust in their children that parental demands (especially, perhaps, in the area of safety) are reasonable and fair. In the control domain parents need to impose their greater power in a nonthreatening way such that their children come to accept and internalize the norms and standards that parents wish to impart. The challenge for the parent is to direct the child's behavior by using the minimal amount of force needed, so as not to undermine the child's sense of autonomy. The use of too little power will not cause a change in behavior, while too much power will generate resentment and feelings of external coercion and thus undermine the internalization of the desired value. Because various characteristics of the child, parent, and context influence children's subjective experience of parental control attempts, parents are more likely to achieve this delicate balance if they can accurately perceive their children's point of view and thus tailor their interventions accordingly. In the group affiliation domain parents set up conditions that lead to the automatic and (more or less) unquestioning adoption of standards. The incorporation of routines and structure in daily activities is effective in the group affiliation domain because it encourages children to expect that life is predictable and involves the seemingly universally accepted (and therefore unquestioned) repetition of events. When societal standards and socially approved actions are folded over into routinized daily actions (e.g., helping others at prescribed times and in prescribed places) the performance of those actions is made more likely to occur. And in the domain of mutual responsiveness parents promote a sense that socialization is not about conflict and conflict resolution but, rather, about people sharing goals and accommodating each other's needs. By cooperating willingly with children's reasonable influence attempts and engaging in mutually rewarding positive exchanges, parents can foster a cooperative stance in their children. In the context of such mutual reciprocity, cooperation occurs without the elicitation of antagonism and perceived threats to autonomy that are all too likely when the goals of the self and the other appear to be in conflict.

This analysis suggests that what works effectively in one domain may be counterproductive when another domain is activated. Attention and comfort for a child who is crying because of distress will have a different impact than attention and comfort for a child who is crying in order to avoid an unpleasant task. Compliance with the request of a child who wants to play will have a different impact than compliance with the request of a child who wants to stay up too late. Discussion, reasoning, and praise used in connection with household work will work well in the control domain but will undermine the helpfulness of a child who sees such work as a badge of membership in the group. Belief that virtue should be its own reward and that reinforcement should not be given for positive action because it undermines intrinsic motivation will be problematic if the child views that positive action as part of a reciprocal exchange. At the same time, however, some parental behaviors can promote positive outcomes in more than one domain. Monitoring of a child's activities can aid both in effectively correcting that child's behavior through discipline and managing that child's environment: In the former case the control domain is activated whereas in the latter it is the group identification domain. Similarly, parental expression of warmth and affection can make children more likely to go along with the demands of their parents in the control domain and can also foster the formation of shared goals and reciprocal positive exchanges in the mutual reciprocity domain. Finally, children's characteristics can, of course, influence the nature of parent–child interactions in the various domains. A particular child attribute might have differential effects as a function of the interaction domain. For example, a child's strong need for autonomy might cause friction in the control domain yet facilitate the establishment of mutual reciprocity. The symmetry of power, parental openness to child's influence, and the pursuit of mutual goals characteristic of the latter domain should be particularly pleasing to children with a strong need to determine their own actions.

In summary, then, we suggest that features of willing or well-socialized behavior differ. They may involve trust that a caregiver makes demands that are in the interest of the child, a feeling that prosocial behavior has been autonomously generated, a desire to be like others, or a feeling of shared goals and enjoyment of exchange. We do not mean to imply, however, that the nature of parent–child interaction is a fragmented one. Whereas it is helpful to outline different roles played by parents in different domains of socialization, in the end these roles are embodied in the same persons and the same overall relationship. The implication is that parental responsivity or competence in one domain may well compensate for insensitivity or incompetence in another domain, and difficulties in one domain may well exacerbate problems in other domains. We know relatively little about these complex processes and their implications. It is clear, however, that they provide important directions for future research on socialization in the family.

REFERENCES

Abbott. D. H., Keverne, E. B., Bercovitch, F. B., Sjively, C. A., Mendoza, S. P., Saltzman, W., et al. (2003). Are subordinates always stressed?: A comparative analysis of rank differences in cortisol levels among primates. *Hormones and Behavior, 43*, 67–82.

Ainsworth, M. D., Blehar, M., Waters, E., & Wall, S. (1978). *Patterns of attachment: A psychological study of the strange situation*. Hillsdale, NJ: Erlbaum.

Allport, G. (1954). *The nature of prejudice*. Reading, MA: Addison-Wesley.

Awong, T., Grusec, J. E., & Sorenson, A. (2005). *Authority-based control and anger as determinants of children's socio-emotional development*. Unpublished manuscript, University of Toronto.

Bandura, A. (1977). *Social learning theory*. Englewood Cliffs, NJ: Prentice-Hall.

Bandura, A., & Walters, R. H. (1963). *Social learning theory and personality development*. New York: Holt, Rinehart, & Winston.

Barber, B. K. (1996). Parental psychological control: Revisiting a neglected construct. *Child Development, 67*, 3296–3319.

Barber, B. K., & Harmon, E. L. (2002). Violating the self: Parental psychological control of children and adolescents. In B.K. Barber (Ed.), *Intrusive parenting: How psychological control affects children and adolescents* (pp. 15–52). Washington, DC: American Psychological Association.

Baumrind, D. (1971). Current patterns of parental authority. *Developmental Psychology, 4*, 1–103.

Bell, S. M., & Ainsworth, M. D. (1972). Infant crying and maternal responsiveness. *Child Development, 43*, 1171–1190.

Booth, A., Johnson, D. R., Granger, D. A., Crouter, A. C., & McHale, S. (2003). Testosterone and child and adolescent adjustment: The moderating role of parent-child relationships. *Developmental Psychology, 39,* 85–98.

Bowlby J. (1944). Forty-four juvenile thieves: Their characters and home life. *International Journal of Psycho-Analysis, 25,* 19–52, 107–127.

Bowlby, J. (1982). *Attachment and loss: Vol. 1. Attachment.* New York: Basic Books. (Original work published 1969)

Bretherton, I., Golby, B., & Cho, E. (1997). Attachment and the transmission of values. In J. E. Grusec & L. Kuczynski Eds.), *Parenting and children's internalization of values* (pp. 103–134). New York: Wiley.

Brewer, M. B. (1999). The psychology of prejudice: Ingroup love and outgroup hate? *Journal of Social Issues, 55,* 429–444.

Brewer, M. B., & Gardner, W. (1996). Who is this "WE"? Levels of collective identity and self representations. *Journal of Personality and Social Psychology, 71,* 83–93.

Brody, G. H., & Flor, D. L. (1998). Maternal resources, parenting practices, and child competence in rural, single-parent African American families. *Child Development, 69,* 803–816.

Bugental, D. B. (2000). Acquisition of the algorithms of social life: A domain-based approach. *Psychological Bulletin, 26,* 187–209.

Bugental, D. B., & Goodnow, J. J. (1998). Socialization processes. In N. Eisenberg (Vol. Ed.), *Handbook of child psychology: Vol. 3. Social, emotional, and personality development* (pp. 389–462). New York: Wiley.

Bugental, D. B., & Grusec, J. E. (2006). Socialization processes. In N. Eisenberg (Vol Ed.), *Handbook of child psychology: Vol. 3. Social, emotional, and personality development* (pp. 366–428). New York: Wiley.

Bugental, D. B., Kaswan, J. W., & Love, L. R. (1970) Perception of contradictory meanings conveyed by verbal and nonverbal channels. *Journal of Personality and Social Psychology, 16,* 647–655.

Cassidy, J. (1994). Emotion regulation: Influences of attachment relationships. *Monographs of the Society for Research in Child Development, 59,* 228–249.

Cassidy, J. (1999). The nature of the child's ties. In J. Cassidy & P. Shaver (Eds.), *The handbook of attachment* (pp. 3–20). New York: Guilford Press.

Chisholm, K. (1998). A three-year follow-up of attachment and indiscriminate friendliness in children adopted from Romanian orphanages. *Child Development, 69,* 1092–1106.

Collins, W. A., Maccoby, E. E., Steinberg, L., Hetherington, E. M., & Bornstein, M. H. (2000). Contemporary research on parenting: The case for nature and nurture. *American Psychologist, 55,* 218–232.

Compton, K., Snyder, J., Schrepferman, L., Bank, L., & Shortt, J. W. (2003). The contribution of parents and siblings to antisocial and depressive behavior in adolescents: A double jeopardy coercion model. *Development and Psychopathology, 15,* 163–182.

Cosmides, L., & Tooby, J. (1992). Cognitive adaptations for social exchange. In J. H. Barkow, L. Cosmides, & J. Tooby (Eds.), *The adapted mind: Evolutionary psychology and the generation of culture* (pp. 163–228). London: Oxford University Press.

Criss, M.M., Shaw, D.S., & Ingoldsby, E.M. (2003). Mother–son positive synchrony in middle childhood: Relation to antisocial behavior. *Social Development, 12,* 379–400.

Crockenberg, S., & Lourie, A. (1996). Parents' conflict strategies with children and children's conflict strategies with peers. *Merrill-Palmer Quarterly, 42,* 495–518.

Crouter, A. C., & Head, M. R. (2002). Parental monitoring and knowledge of children. In M. H. Bornstein (Ed.), *Handbook of parenting: Vol. 3: Being and becoming a parent* (2nd ed., pp. 461–483). Mahwah, NJ: Erlbaum.

Davidov, M., & Grusec, J. E. (2006). Untangling the links of parental responsiveness to distress and warmth to child outcomes. *Child Development, 77,* 44–58.

Davidov, M., & Grusec, J. E. (in press). Multiple pathways to compliance: Mothers' willingness to cooperate and knowledge of their children's reactions to discipline. *Journal of Family Psychology.*

Deci, E. L., & Ryan, R. M. (1985). *Intrinsic motivation and self-determination in human behavior.* New York: Plenum Press.

Del Carmen, R., Pederson, F. A., Huffman, L. C., & Bryan, Y. E. (1993). Dyadic distress management predicts subsequent security of attachment. *Infant Behavior and Development, 16,* 131–147.

Dix, T. (1992). Parenting on behalf of the child: Empathic goals in the regulation of responsive parenting. In I. E. Sigel, A. V. McGillicuddy-DeLisi, & J. J. Goodnow (Eds.), *Parental belief systems: the psychological consequences for children* (2nd ed., pp. 319–346). Hillsdale, NJ: Erlbaum.

Dubas, J. S., & Gerris, J. R. M. (2002). Longitudinal changes in the time parents spend in activities with their adolescent children as a function of child age, pubertal status and gender. *Journal of Family Psychology, 16*, 415–462.

Dunn, J., & Munn., P. (1985). Becoming a family member: Family conflict and the development of understanding. *Child Development, 56*, 480–492.

Eaker, D. G., & Walters, L. H. (2002). Adolescent satisfaction in family rituals and psychosocial development: A developmental systems theory perspective. *Journal of Family Psychology, 16*, 406–414.

Eisenberg, N., & Fabes, R. A. (1998). Prosocial development. In W. Damon (Series Ed.) & N. Eisenberg (Vol. Ed.), *Handbook of child psychology, Vol. 3: Social, emotional, and personality development* (5th ed., pp. 701–778). New York: Wiley.

Eisenberg, N., Fabes, R. A., Shepard, S. A., Guthrie, I. K., Murphy, B. C., & Reiser, M. (1999). Parental reactions to children's negative emotions: Longitudinal relations to quality of children's social functioning. *Child Development, 70*, 513–534.

Eisenberg, N., Wentzel, M., & Harris, J. D. (1998). The role of emotionality and regulation in empathy-related responding. *School Psychology Review, 27*, 506–521.

Evans, D. W., Leckman, J. F., Carter, A., Reznick, J. S., Henshaw, C., King, R. A., et al. (1997). Ritual, habit, and perfectionism: The prevalence and development of compulsive-like behavior in normal young children. *Child Development, 68*, 58–68.

Fabes, R. A., Leonard, S. A., Kupanoff, K., & Martin, C. L. (2001). Parental coping with children's negative emotions: Relations with children's emotional and social responding. *Child Development, 72*, 907–920.

Fabes, R. A., Poulin, R. E., Eisenberg, N., & Madden-Derdich, D. A. (2002). The Coping with Children's Negative Emotions Scale (CCNES): Psychometric properties and relations with children's emotional competence. *Marriage and Family Review, 34*, 285–310.

Fiske, A. P. (1992). The four elementary forms of sociality: Framework for a unified theory of social relations. *Psychological Review, 99*, 689–723.

Fonagy, P., Target, M., Steele, M., & Steele, H. (1997). The development of violence and crime as it relates to security of attachment. In J. D. Osofsky (Ed.), *Children in a violent society* (pp. 150–177). New York: Guilford Press.

Gallese, V., Ferrari, P., Kohler, E., & Fogassi, L. (2002). The eyes, the hand, and the mind: Behavioral and neurophysiological aspects of social cognition. In M. Bekoff, C. Allen, & G. M. Burghardt (Eds.), *The cognitive animal* (pp. 451–461). London: MIT Press.

Gardner, F., Ward, S., Burton, J., & Wilson, C. (2003). The role of mother–child joint play in the early development of children's conduct problems: A longitudinal observational study. *Social Development, 12*, 361–378.

George, C., & Solomon, J. (1999). Attachment and caregiving: The caregiving behavioral system. In J. Cassidy & P. Shaver (Eds.), *Handbook of attachment: Theory, research, and clinical applications* (pp. 649–670). New York: Guilford Press.

Goldberg, S., Grusec, J. E., & Jenkins, J. (1999). Confidence in protection: Arguments for a narrow definition of attachment. *Journal of Family Psychology, 13*, 475–483.

Goodnow, J. J., Miller, P. J., & Kessel, F. (Eds.). (1995). *Cultural practices as contexts for development.* San Francisco: Jossey-Bass.

Gottman, J. M., Katz, L. F., & Hooven, C. (1996). Parental meta-emotion philosophy and the emotional life of families: Theoretical models and preliminary data. *Journal of Family Psychology, 10*, 243–268.

Grolnick W. (2003). *The psychology of parental control: How well-meant parenting backfires.* Mahwah, NJ: Erlbaum.

Grolnick, W. S., Deci, E. L., & Ryan, R. M. (1997). Internalization within the family: The self-determination theory perspective. In J.E. Grusec & L. Kuczynski (Eds.), *Parenting and children's internalization of values: A handbook of contemporary theory* (pp. 135–161). New York: Wiley.

Grusec, J. E., & Goodnow, J. J. (1994). The impact of parental discipline methods on the child's internalization of values: A reconceptualization of current points of view. *Developmental Psychology, 30*, 4–19.

Grusec, J. E., Goodnow, J. J., & Cohen, L. (1997) Household work and the development of children's concern for others. *Developmental Psychology, 32*, 999–1007.

Grusec, J. E., Goodnow, J. J., & Kuczynski, L. (2000). New directions in analyses of parenting contributions to children's acquisition of values. *Child Development, 71*, 205–211.

Gunnar, M. R. (2000). Early adversity and the development of stress reactivity and regulation. In C. A. Nelson (Ed.) *The effects of early adversity on neurobehavioral development. The Minnesota Symposia on Child Development*, (Vol. 31, pp. 163–200). London: Erlbaum.

Hastings, P. D., & Grusec, J. E. (1998). Parenting goals as organizers of responses to parent–child disagreement. *Developmental Psychology, 34*, 465–479.

Herz, L., & Gullone, E. (1999). The relationship between self-esteem and parenting style: A cross-cultural comparison of Australian and Vietnamese Australian adolescents. *Journal of Cross-Cultural Psychology, 30*, 742–761.

Hoffman, M. L. (1970a). Conscience, personality, and socialization techniques. *Human Development, 13*, 90–126.

Hoffman, M. L. (1970b). Moral development. In P.H. Mussen (Ed.), *Carmichael's manual of child psychology* (Vol. 2, pp. 261–360). New York: Wiley.

Kagan, J. (1982). The emergence of self. *Journal of Child Psychology and Psychiatry, 23*, 363–381.

Kerr, M., & Stattin, H. (2000). What parents know, how they know it, and several forms of adolescent adjustment: Further support for a reinterpretation of monitoring. *Developmental Psychology, 36*, 366–380.

Kilgore, K., Snyder, J., & Lentz, C. (2000). The contribution of parental discipline, parental monitoring, and school risk to early-onset conduct problems in African American boys and girls. *Developmental Psychology, 36*, 835–845.

Killen, J., & Wainryb, C. (2000). Independence and interdependence in diverse cultural contexts. In S. Harkness, C. Raeff, & C. M. Super (Eds.), *Variability in the social construction of the child* (pp. 5–21). San Francisco: Jossey-Bass.

Kochanska, G., & Aksan, N. (1995). Mother–child mutually positive affect, the quality of child compliance to requests and prohibitions, and maternal control as correlates of early internalization. *Child Development, 66*, 236–254.

Kochanska, G., & Murray, K. T. (2000). Mother–child mutually responsive orientation and conscience development: From toddler to early school age. *Child Development, 71*, 417–431.

Kuczynski, L. (2003). Beyond bidirectionality: Bilateral conceptual frameworks for understanding dynamics in parent–child relations. In L. Kuczynski (Ed.), *Handbook of dynamics in parent–child relationships* (pp. 3–24). Thousand Oaks, CA: Sage.

Lave, J., & Wenger, E. (1991). *Situated learning: Legitimate peripheral participation*. Cambridge, UK: Cambridge University Press.

Leung, K., Lau, S., & Lam, W. L. (1998). Parenting styles and achievement: A cross-cultural study. *Merrill-Palmer Quarterly, 44*, 157–172.

Lindahl, K. M., & Malik, N. M. (1999). Marital conflict, family processes, and boys' externalizing behavior in Hispanic American and European American families. *Journal of Clinical and Child Psychology, 28*, 12–24.

Londerville, S., & Main, M. (1981). Security of attachment, compliance, and maternal training methods in the second year of life. *Developmental Psychology, 17*, 289–299.

Lundell, L., Grusec, J. E., McShane, K., & Davidov, M. (2005). *Mother–adolescent conflict: Adolescent goals, maternal perspective-taking, and conflict intensity*. Unpublished manuscript, University of Toronto.

MacDonald, K. (1992). Warmth as a developmental construct: An evolutionary analysis. *Child Development, 63*, 753–773.

Matas, L., Arend, R., & Sroufe, L. A. (1978). Continuity of adaptation in the second year: The relationship between quality of attachment and later competence. *Child Development, 49*, 547–556.

McFadyen-Ketchum, S. A., Bates, J. E., Dodge, K. A., & Pettit, G. S. (1996). Patterns of change in early childhood aggressive-disruptive behavior: Gender differences in predictions from early coercive and affectionate mother–child interactions. *Child Development, 67*, 2417–2433.

Morton, J. B., & Trehub, S. E. (2001). Children's understanding of emotion in speech. *Child Development, 72*, 834–843.

Ng, F. F., Kenney-Benson, G. A., & Pomerantz, E. M. (2004). Children's achievement moderates the effects of mothers' use of control and autonomy support, *Child Development, 75*, 764–780.

Panksepp, J. (1993). Rough and tumble play: A fundamental brain process. In K. McDonald (Ed.), *Parent–child play: Descriptions and implications* (pp. 147–184). Albany: State University of New York Press.

Parpal, M., & Maccoby, E. E. (1985). Maternal responsiveness and subsequent child compliance. *Child Development, 56*, 1326–1334.

Patterson, G. R. (1980). Mothers: The unacknowledged victims. *Monographs of the Society for Research in Child Development, 45.*

Patterson, G.R. (1982). *Coercive family process.* Eugene, OR: Castalia Press.

Patterson, G. R., Crosby, L., & Vuchinich, S. (1992). Predicting risk for early police arrest. *Journal of Quantitative Criminology, 8,* 335–355.

Pettit, G. S. (1997). The developmental course of violence and aggression: Mechanisms of family and peer influence. *Psychiatric Clinics of North America, 20,* 283–299.

Pomerantz, E.M., & Eaton, M.M. (2001). Maternal intrusive support in the academic context: Transactional socialization processes. *Developmental Psychology, 37,* 174–186.

Rheingold, H. L. (1982). Little children's participation in the work of adults, a nascent prosocial behavior. *Child Development, 53,* 114–125.

Richters, J. E., & Waters, E. (1991). Attachment and socialization: The positive side of social influence. In M. Lewis & S. Feinman (Eds.), *Social influences and socialization in infancy* (pp. 185–213). New York: Plenum Press.

Roberts, W. L. (1999). The socializaton of emotional expression: Relations with prosocial behavior and competence in five samples. *Canadian Journal of Behavioural Science, 31,* 72–85.

Roberts, W., & Strayer, J. (1987). Parents' responses to the emotional distress of their children: Relations with children's competence. *Developmental Psychology, 23,* 415–422.

Rodriguez, M. L., Avduk, O., Aber, J. L., Mischel, W., Sethi, A., & Shoda, Y. (2005). A contextual approach to the development of self-regulatory competencies: The role of maternal unresponsivity and toddlers' negative affect in stressful situation. *Social Development, 14,* 136–157.

Rogoff, B., Paradise, R., Arauz, R. M., Correa-Chavez, M., & Angelillo C. (2003). Firsthand learning through intent participation. *Annual Review of Psychology, 54,* 175–203.

Rohner, R. P., & Pettengill, S. M. (1985). Perceived parental acceptance-rejection and parental control among Korena adolescent. *Child Development, 56,* 524–528.

Rothbaum, F., & Weisz, J. R. (1994). Parental caregiving and child externalizing behavior in nonclinical samples: A meta-analysis. *Psychological Bulletin, 116,* 55–74.

Rudy, D., & Grusec, J. E. (2001). Correlates of authoritarian parenting in individualist and collectivist cultures and implications for understanding the transmission of values. *Journal of Cross-Cultural Psychology, 32,* 202–212.

Rudy, D., & Grusec, J. E. (2006). Authoritarian parenting in individualist and collectivist groups: Associations with maternal emotion and cognition and children's self-esteem. *Journal of Family Psychology, 20,* 68–78.

Rutter, M., & O'Connor, T. G. (2004). Are there biological programming effects for psychological development? Findings from a study of Romanian adoptees. *Developmental Psychology, 40,* 81–94.

Ryan, R. M., & Deci, E. L. (2000). Self-determination theory and the facilitation of intrinsic motivation, social development, and well-being. *American Psychologist, 55,* 68–78.

Sameroff, A. (1975). Transactional models of early social relations. *Human Development, 18,* 65–79.

Sapolsky, R. M. (2004). Social status and health in humans and other animals. *Annual Review of Anthropology, 33,* 393–418.

Scarr, S., & McCartney, K. (1983). How people make their own environment: A theory of genotype–environment effects. *Child Development, 54,* 424–435.

Schwartz, B. (2000). Self-determination: The tyranny of freedom. *American Psychologist, 55,* 79–88.

Seligman, M. E. (1970). On the generality of the laws of learning. *Psychological Review, 77,* 406–418.

Siegal, M., & Cowen, J. (1984). Appraisals of intervention: The mother's versus the culprit's behavior as determinants of children's evaluations of discipline techniques. *Child Development, 55,* 1760–1766.

Smetana, J. (1988). Adolescents' and parents' conceptions of parental authority. *Child Development, 59,* 321–335.

Smetana, J. (1995). Parenting styles and conceptions of parental authority during adolescence. *Child Development, 66,* 299–316.

Smetana, J. (1997). Parenting and the development of social knowledge reconceptualized: A social domain analysis. In J. E. Grusec & L. Kuczynski (Eds.), *Parenting and the internalization of values: A handbook of contemporary theory* (pp. 162–192). New York: Wiley.

Stayton, D., Hogan, R., & Ainsworth, M. D. S. (1973). Infant obedience and maternal behavior: The origins of socialization reconsidered. *Child Development, 42,* 1057–1070.

Steinberg, L. (1990). Autonomy, conflict, and harmony in the family relationship. In S.S. Feldman & G.R.

Elliott, (Eds.), *At the threshold: The developing adolescent* (pp. 255–276). Cambridge, MA: Harvard University Press.

Stewart, S. M., Rao, N., Bond, M. H., McBride-Chang, C., Fielding, R., & Kennard, B. D. (1998). Chinese dimensions of parenting: Broadening Western predictors and outcomes. *International Journal of Psychology, 33*, 345–358.

Thompson, R. A. (1994). Emotion regulation: A theme in search of a definition. In N. A. Fox (Ed.), The development of emotion regulation: Biological and behavioral considerations. *Monographs of the Society for Research in Child Development, 59*, 25–52.

Trevarthen, C., Kokkinski, T., & Flamenghi, G. A., Jr. (1999). In J. Nadel & G. Butterworth (Eds.). *Imitation in infancy Cambridge studies in cognitive perceptual development* (pp. 127–185). New York: Cambridge University Press.

Trickett, P., & Kuczynski, L. (1986). Children's misbehavior and parental discipline in abusive and nonabusive families. *Developmental Psychology, 22*, 115–123.

Turiel, C. (1998). Notes from the underground: Culture, conflict, and subversion In J. Langer & M. Killen (Eds.). *Piaget, evolution, and development. The Jean Piaget symposium series* (pp. 271–296). Mahwah, NJ: Erlbaum.

Van der Mark, I. L., Bakermans-Kranenburg, M. J., & van IJzendoorn, M. H. (2002). The role of parenting, attachment, and temperamental fearfulness in the prediction of compliance in toddler girls. *British Journal of Developmental Psychology, 20*, 361–378.

van IJzendoorn, M., H. (1997). Attachment, emergent morality, and aggression: Toward a developmental socioemotional model of antisocial behavior. *International Journal of Behavioral Development 21*, 703–727.

Waizenhoffer, R. N., Buchanan, C. M., & Jackson-Newsom, J. (2004). Mothers' and fathers' knowledge of adolescents' daily activities: Its sources and its links with adolescent adjustment. *Journal of Family Psychology, 18*, 348–360.

Youniss, J., McLellan, J. A., & Strouse, D. (1994). "We're popular, but we're not snobs": Adolescents describe their crowds. In R. Montemayor, G. R. Adams, & T. P. Gullotta (Eds.), *Personal relationships during adolescence. Advances in adolescent development: An annual book series* (Vol. 6, pp. 101–122). Thousand Oaks, CA: Sage.

CHAPTER 12

Siblings and Socialization

JUDY DUNN

The great majority of individuals grow up with siblings (around 80% in the United States and in Europe). For many people, their relationships with their sisters and brothers are the longest lasting in their lives—longer than their relationships with parents, partners, or children. All over the world, siblings figure importantly in legends, history, and literature; yet the scientific study of the nature and influence of sibling relationships is relatively recent. From early in the 20th century clinicians and family theorists have argued that siblings can influence individual adjustment and play a key role in family relationships (see Adler, 1928; Freud, 1916/1961, 1938). Ethnographic studies of siblings have shown how widespread and significant sibling caregiving can be (Zukow-Goldring, 2002). Yet systematic study of siblings was relatively rare until the 1970s and 1980s—an important exception being the classic research on siblings carried out by Koch in the 1950s and 1960s (see Koch, 1954, 1960). Over the last two decades the picture has changed markedly, and research interest in siblings has grown notably, focusing particularly on childhood and adolescence (Brody, 1998; Hetherington, Reiss, & Plomin, 1994). Siblings in adulthood remain relatively unstudied (for review, see Cicirelli, 1996).

To consider sibling influences on socialization, we focus first on the nature of relationships between siblings, and on individual differences in those relationships, as well as associations with other family relationships. Second, the evidence that these relationships influence individual socialization is considered with a focus on two domains, children's adjustment and the development of social understanding; third, we discuss comparisons of the influence of siblings and peers on socialization. Finally, we consider how research on siblings has challenged our understanding of family socialization more broadly considered—the issue of why siblings growing up within the same family differ from one another in personality and adjustment. Note that the relationship between twins and triplets is beyond the scope of this chapter; however, we do discuss the issue of nonshared environments, to which behavior geneticists have drawn attention.

SIBLING RELATIONSHIPS AS CONTEXTS FOR SOCIALIZATION

Two characteristics of sibling relationships in childhood and adolescence stand out from systematic research—characteristics that make the potential of the relationship for influence on socialization very high. The first is the emotional quality of the relationship; between siblings, both intense positive and negative feelings are frequently and uninhibitedly expressed from infancy through adolescence. Observational naturalistic studies documented, for instance, that during the toddler and preschool period intense negative emotions were expressed in around 20% of sibling interactions, and intense positive emotions were also frequent (Dunn, Creps, & Brown, 1996). For many young siblings, the relationship is one in which mixed feelings are evident—both positive and negative feelings freely expressed.

The second feature of sibling relationships that heightens their potential for influence on socialization is the familiarity and intimacy of the relationship. From the preschool years through middle childhood siblings spend more time together and in interaction with each other than they do with parents or peers (McHale & Crouter, 1996). They know each other very well, and this intimacy means that they can provide effective support or that they can tease and undermine each other—as they do with great effectiveness from the second year onward (Dunn, 1988a)—or both! Either way, the impact on each child's attitude toward conforming to the social rules of the family is likely to be high.

While the intimacy and emotional intensity of siblings' relationships make their potential for influence on socialization high, a third characteristic of siblings' relationships that mitigates against generalising about sibling influence is the great range of individual differences between siblings that research has documented in observational, interview, and experimental studies. Some siblings describe their affection and interest in their siblings vividly in interviews and show cooperation, insight, and empathy in most of their interactions. Others describe their feelings of irritation, hostility, and dislike and show this hostility and aggression in their interactions with their siblings. Others show and describe their *ambivalent* feelings (for siblings' perceptions of their relationship, see, e.g., McGuire, Manke, Eftekhari, & Dunn, 2000). In assessing the developmental influence of the relationship on patterns of socialization it is clearly crucial to take into account the quality of the sibling relationship and the factors that lead to these notable individual differences.

Individual Differences in Sibling Relationships

Early studies of sibling relationship differences focused chiefly on birth order, gender, and age gap (e.g., Ernst & Angst, 1983; Sutton-Smith & Rosenberg, 1970). It was supposed that these "family constellation" factors affected children's personalities, intelligence, or motivation and thus their relationships with one another. In the last decades, research has broadened to include not only the temperament or personality of the siblings themselves but also the influence of other relationships within the family and of a range of social adversities and risks faced by the family (e.g., Brody, 1998; Brody, Stoneman, & McCoy, 1994; Furman & Lanthier, 1996).

Birth Order, Gender, and Age Gap

There is some evidence that during the early years of childhood the quality of the relationship between siblings who are first- and second-born children is more influenced by the affection, interest, or hostility of the firstborn than by the feelings of the secondborn (see also Tucker, Updegraff, McHale, & Crouter, 1999, for evidence on firstborns' influence on secondborns' empathy, in adolescence). Longitudinal research shows that the reaction of first-born children (their affection and interest, or hostility) to a new sibling is linked over time to the quality of both siblings' behavior toward each other (Dunn & Kendrick, 1982). This would suggest that the socialization influence of the firstborn on the later born was more striking than vice versa. However, the significance of the contribution of second-born siblings to the relationship quality increases during the preschool years (Dunn, 1988b).

Patterns of normative change in the quality of siblings' relationships depend on siblings' birth order, with declines in emotional intimacy toward a sibling during the transition to adolescence being less characteristic of younger siblings than older: Younger siblings tend to place greater value on the support they receive from older siblings than vice versa (Buhrmester, 1992). Research into the associations between sibling and friend relationships has highlighted differences between first-born and second-born adolescents (Updegraff, McHale, & Crouter, 2002). In a study that took the "insider's perspective" by focusing on young adolescents' own reports of their sibling and friendship relationships, Updegraff et al. (2002) predicted that there would be stronger connections between the quality of sibling and peer relationships for secondborns than firstborns, in terms of both dimensions of intimacy and control in the relationships. Support was found for the birth-order effects: secondborns' reports of sibling intimacy were modestly associated with greater friendship intimacy, but this pattern was not found for first-born adolescents. Effects were qualified by sex and by gender constellation. The authors conclude that these results support the notion that adolescents will be most likely to learn from high-status models (McHale, Updegraff, Helms-Erikson, & Crouter, 2001; Tucker et al., 1999). The associations between the two relationships in this research were stronger for sibling and friendship *control*, for both first- and secondborn. Adolescents who reported high levels of controlling behavior with their siblings also reported high levels of control in their friendships. Patterns of longitudinal change in control also were similar in the two relationships. The researchers emphasize that the relationship connections may be more salient when the comparison involves same-sex sibling and friendship dyads but point out that it will be important in the future to consider the possibility that the extent to which siblings model behavior in accordance with masculine or feminine roles (e.g., how expressive or traditionally feminine they are) may be more important than sibling sex in the moderation of cross-relationship linkages.

Birth order is also highlighted in the evidence that older antisocial siblings can have deleterious effects on their younger siblings (Slomkowski, Rende, Conger, Simons, & Conger, 2001; these are discussed later).

Findings on how the quality of the relationship is related to gender and age gap vary with the age and developmental stage of the siblings. In early childhood, the evidence on gender is inconsistent; some studies report that same-sex pairs get along better than different-sex pairs (Dunn, 1983). During middle childhood, research indicates that gender becomes more significant, with boys becoming less likely to describe intimacy and warmth in their sibling relationships (Dunn, Slomkowski, & Beardsall, 1994). It appears that the socialization influences of the wider world outside the family impact increasingly on siblings' relationships within the family in the teenage years. In older adulthood, relationships with sisters become increasingly important (Cicirelli, 1996). This is generally attributed to women's traditional role as nurturers.

Temperament and Personality

Sibling influence on socialization will be linked to the quality of their relationship, and associations between the temperamental or personality characteristics of siblings and the quality of their relationship have been described in preschoolers, in early and middle childhood, and in adolescence (e.g., Brody, Stoneman, & Burke, 1987; Furman & Lanthier, 1996; Munn & Dunn, 1989; Stocker, Dunn, & Plomin, 1989). But the results vary in the different studies; these tend to be based on different populations; they vary in the ages of the children studied and the methods used. It is noted by Furman and Lanthier (1996), however, that a general pattern is evident across studies: Temperamental characteristics are more systematically related to conflict in the sibling relationship than to affection and warmth. This may be because while conflict between siblings is easy to measure—it shows up in a variety of settings and methods—the positive features of the relationship are less evident. In terms of socialization processes, warmth in the relationship may be particularly important in the extent of influence a sibling exerts on another child.

The frequency of conflict and affection in siblings was found to be importantly linked to the *match* between siblings' temperaments, in studies in early and middle childhood (Brody, 1996; Munn & Dunn, 1989). Siblings who were more similar in temperament had more positive relationships—a finding that fits with the evidence on both adult and childhood friends that similarity makes for friendship: "like me" attracts (Hartup, 1996; Hinde, 1979). While inconsistency marks the findings on gender and age gap, and also on temperament, the evidence on connections between sibling relationships and other family relationships is much clearer; these are discussed next.

Associations with Other Family Relationships

A number of general developmental points have been established concerning links between sibling relationships and other relationships within the family. The first concerns parent–child relationships. Attachment research has shown that children who were secure in their attachments to their parents developed more positive sibling relationships than those who were insecure (Teti & Ablard, 1989; Volling & Belsky, 1992). And studies that investigate a broad range of dimensions of parent–child relationships consistently report that positive, prosocial sibling relationships are associated with warm positive parent–child relationships (for review, see Brody, 1998). Punitive, negative, and overcontrolled parent–child relations are associated with aggressive, hostile sibling relations. The evidence for these associations is correlational, and this means we cannot make inferences about the direction of causal influence or the family processes that are implicated. It could be that parental influence explains the associations, but it could also be that children's personal characteristics contribute to the quality of their relationships with both their parents and their siblings—that difficult children, for instance, elicit negative behavior from both parents and siblings. It could also be that siblings who are very aggressive and hostile are so difficult to live with that this hostility contributes in turn to the difficulties in their relationships with their parents. It seems likely that all these family processes may be implicated in the links between relationships.

The second point, established in several research programs, is that the quality of the relationship between parents is associated with differences in the sibling relationship, with more positive marital/spousal relationships linked to more positive sibling relations (Brody, Stoneman, McCoy, & Forehand, 1992; Dunn, Deater-Deckard, Pickering, Beveridge, & ALSPAC Study Team, 1999; Erel, Margolin, & John, 1998; MacKinnon, 1989; Stocker, Ahmed, & Stall, 1997). Both direct pathways from marital to sibling relationships, and indirect pathways via the parent–child relationship are implicated (Dunn et al., 1999). Interestingly, the pattern of associations between marital and sibling relationships differs in stepfamilies: conflict between mother and stepfather showed no relation to conflict between siblings in a study in the United Kingdom, in contrast to the pattern found in families with two biological parents (Dunn et al., 1999; see also Hetherington & Clingempeel, 1992). Siblings' responses to marital conflict, we now know, differ even within the same family, and these differences are linked to their adjustment (Jenkins, Dunn, Rasbash, O'Connor, & Simpson, 2005). Differences in siblings' feelings of self-blame for marital conflict were found to be correlated with differences in their depressed mood and conduct problems (Parke & Buriel, 1998).

The third point also concerns parent–child and sibling relationships. There is some clinical evidence that in families in which parent–child relationships are extremely distant or uninvolved, the siblings can develop intensely supportive relationships with each other (Bank & Kahn, 1982; Boer & Dunn, 1990). This kind of "compensatory" pattern of family relationships may be more likely to be found in families facing extremes of stress and adversity than those within the normal range.

The fourth point is one that has received a great deal of recent research attention. This is that differential parent–child relationships within a family are associated with more conflicted hostile sibling relationships. If parents show more affection, attention, and warmth or less discipline, control, or pressure for socialization in their relationship with one sibling than with another, the siblings are likely to get along less well than the siblings in families in which parents and siblings do not describe such differential treatment (Brody, 1998; Feinberg & Hetherington, 2001; Reiss, Neiderhiser, Hetherington, & Plomin, 2000; Stocker, 1993; Stocker et al., 1989; Volling & Belsky, 1992).

Such differential patterns of treatment of siblings by parents are more evident when families are facing stress, for example those with disabled or sick children, those in which parent have recently separated, or stepfamilies (Bank, Patterson, & Reid, 1996). Differential parent–child relationships are associated with difficulties or distress in the parents' own relationship, and in turn with higher levels of sibling conflict both concurrently and longitudinally over time (Brody, Stoneman, & McCoy, 1992; Brody et al., 1994; Hetherington, Henderson, & Reiss, 1999; McHale & Crouter, 1996). The evidence here again is correlational, and the direction of causal influence is not clear. One process that is seen as important here is children's interpretation of their parents' differential behavior. If children interpret such behavior as evidence that their parents are less concerned about them than their sibling, or that they are less worthy of love than their siblings, the sibling relationship is likely to be less positive (Kowal & Kramer, 1997). Note, however, that children may perceive preferential treatment of one sibling as fair, and in these cases, lower levels of internalizing behavior problems and greater self-esteem have been reported than in families in which the children do not perceive such differential treatment as unfair (Kowal, Kramer, Krull, & Crick, 2002). These processes of monitoring the relations between other family members and reflecting on them are likely to begin very early. Developmental studies have shown that children from a surprisingly early age monitor and respond to the interactions between their siblings and parents (Dunn & Munn, 1985). The frequency of control and conflict between parents and older siblings was found to contribute independent variance to children's social understanding (Dunn, Brown, Slomkowski, Tesla, & Youngblade, 1991), again indicating that the potential effects of one family relationship (between parent and sibling A) on the socialization of sibling B should be taken into account. And the developmental significance of perceived differential treatment for sibling relationships continues into adulthood: A recent study of adult siblings found that the relationships between adult siblings diminished in positivity with increasing favoritism or disfavoritism (Boll, Ferring, & Fillipp, 2003); sibling relationships were less positive in families in which one sibling was favored more than the other.

The final point on links between parent–child and sibling relationships is that the quality of the relationship that develops between young siblings is linked to the *changes* in the relationship between parent and firstborn that accompany the birth of a sibling. Both intensive, observational research (Dunn & Kendrick, 1982; Stewart, Mobley, Van Tuyl, & Salvador, 1987; Stewart, 1990) and large-scale surveys (Baydar, Greek, & Brooks-Gunn, 1997; Baydar, Hyle, & Brooks-Gunn, 1997) report that the birth of a sibling is accompanied by a decline in positive mother–child interactions, an increase in controlling negative interactions, and an increase in behavioral problems in the child who has been "displaced" by a new sibling. There are new socialization pressures on children when a new baby is born, and these may be reflected in increased conflict between parent and child. The large-scale studies show that these changes in family relationships with the birth of a sibling are accompanied by a decline in material resources for the family, and this decline may in itself have sequelae for the children's adjustment and relationships. The general point to be emphasized by such findings is that such *indirect* links between parent–child and sibling relationships (via social or economic adversities or family stress) are implicated as influences on the quality of the siblings' relationships over time, as well as on children's socialization.

Developmental Changes in Sibling Relationships

Before considering sibling relationships as influences on children's socialization, it is important to recognize that there may be significant changes in the nature of the relationship as the siblings grow up that affect the ways in which the siblings influence one another. Longitudinal research has shown that as their powers of social understanding and communication develop in the preschool years, the younger siblings within sibling dyads take an increasingly active role in the relationship. They begin to initiate more games, they cooperate and participate in joint play more effectively (Dunn et al., 1996), and use their powers of understanding to get their own way more effectively in sibling conflict (Tesla & Dunn, 1992). Both their presence and their increasingly powerful actions may be considered influences on older siblings' socialization. Most of the studies of middle childhood and adolescence are cross-sectional, and these have mapped the normative changes in sibling relationships over these years—showing changes in the balance of power between siblings, as the relationship becomes more egalitarian (Buhrmester, 1992; Buhrmester & Furman, 1990; Vandell, Minnett, & Santrock, 1987). It is not clear how far this change in power relations reflects an increase in the ability of the younger sibling to influence the older, and to be autonomous, or a decrease in the caregiving role of the older sibling, or indeed a decrease in dominance that both children attempt to exert on each other. In adolescence, there tends to be a decrease in the warmth and positivity that siblings express about each other (paralleling the changes in child–parent relationships over this period, as adolescents become more involved with peers outside the family).

To answer the question of how far there is continuity in the marked individual differences in sibling relationships in early childhood, as children grow up, and especially to delineate sibling influence over time, longitudinal research is key. With some notable exceptions, such as the research of Brody and his colleagues (e.g., Brody, Stoneman, & McCoy, 1992; Brody, Stoneman, McCoy, & Forehand, 1992; Brody et al., 1994), middle-childhood sibling research has been chiefly cross-sectional. However, in two particular domains we have evidence from which to assess siblings' influence on each other from the early childhood years through adolescence, namely, the children's adjustment and their social understanding, considered next.

SIBLING RELATIONSHIPS AS INFLUENCES ON SOCIALIZATION

Children's Adjustment

Associations between the quality of sibling relationships and children's adjustment have been repeatedly demonstrated, with both concurrent links and associations over time documented. Concurrent associations between sibling conflict and poor adjustment (in terms of internalizing and externalizing behavior) have been demonstrated in 5-year-olds and elementary-school-age children (e.g., Garcia, Shaw, Winslow, & Yaggi, 2000; Stocker, 1994; Stormshak, Bellanti, Bierman, & Conduct Problems Prevention Research Group, 1996), and adolescence (Kim, Hetherington, & Reiss, 1999). The direction of effects in such cross-sectional research is not clear; however, in seminal studies in the 1980s, Patterson and his colleagues in Oregon showed through detailed observations of children in their families that siblings reinforced each other's aggressive behavior by fighting back, escalating conflict (Patterson, 1986). The evidence for direct socialization by siblings was clear. These patterns of coercive behavior were found both in community samples, and in clinical samples of children with conduct disorders. Snyder and Patterson (1995) made the important point that growing up in families in which children were thus "trained" to be coercive and aggressive had the doubly handicapping effect of not only reinforcing aggressive behavior but failing to provide training in prosocial behavior.

In a longitudinal study following children from middle childhood to adolescence, Stocker and her colleagues found that conflict between 7- and 10-year-olds accounted for unique variance in the children's anxiety, depression, and delinquent behavior 2 years later, beyond the variance explained by mothers' hostility, fathers' hostility, and marital conflict at the earlier time point (Stocker, Burwell, & Briggs, 2002). Such patterns begin early in siblings' lives: An observational study found that conflict between 5-year-old and preschool-age siblings was associated with internalizing problems both concurrently and 7 years later (Dunn, Slomkowski, Beardsall, & Rende, 1994), beyond the variance accounted for by mothers' current mood. Such longitudinal patterns may extend beyond adolescence: Interactions with siblings during adolescence have been reported to predict the quality of couples' interactions in young adulthood (Conger, Cui, Bryant, & Elder, 2000).

Socialization Processes Implicated: Direct and Indirect

What are the mechanisms and socialization processes implicated in these associations between sibling relationships and later adjustment outcome? Several possible explanations can be given. First, learning theorists would argue that children learn hostile behavior in conflict with their siblings that then generalizes to other relationship contexts. According to this model, sibling aggressive behavior has a direct shaping effect on a child's own conduct. The research of Patterson and colleagues supports such a view. Second, it can be plausibly argued that growing up with a sibling who continually behaves in a negative way toward one and makes disparaging, diminishing comments lowers children's self-esteem and increases their feelings of depression and anxiety, and increases the likelihood that they will develop a negative attributional style—which in itself is a risk factor for later depression and anxiety (Seligman & Nolen-Hoeksma, 1987). Third, as we saw above, Snyder and Patterson (1995) argued plausibly that children growing up with an aggressive hostile sibling may be deprived of the social contexts in which their prosocial empathetic skills are developed. That is, they may have difficulties in developing powers of social understanding and of emotion regulation—and these limitations in themselves may contribute both to internalizing and to externalizing problems—and may further contribute to the hostility in the sibling relationship.

It is also possible that a third "common causal factor" underlies both the sibling conflict and the child's adjustment problems. An obvious candidate here is the relationship between parent and child, which as we saw previously is implicated in patterns of family relationships and adjustment (see Caspi & Elder, 1988). Similarly, marital conflict or distress can lead to both adjustment problems in children and problems in the sibling relationship. To disentangle these pathways of influence, research like that of Stocker and her colleagues (Stocker et al., 2002) is needed; these authors, as noted earlier, showed that sibling conflict was associated with increases in children's adjustment problems over time even when earlier parent–child hostility and marital conflict were controlled. Moreover, sibling adjustment at Time 1 did not predict significant increases in sibling conflict at Time 2; in contrast, sibling conflict at the first time point predicted increases in internalizing and externalizing problems at Time 2 (i.e., across the developmental transition from elementary to middle school). This study focused on the older sibling in each dyad. However, there is a substantial body of research now showing that *younger* siblings are influenced by their older siblings in the domain of adjustment (in some cases more than vice versa) (see, e.g., Dunn, Slomkowski, Beardsall, & Rende, 1994; Hetherington et al., 1999).

One possible process of sibling influence that has received serious attention—and some empirical support—is the notion of sibling deidentification. This was originally described by Adler (see Ansbacher & Ansbacher, 1956) as a psychological process by which siblings diverge in their development, finding different domains of interest by which they create separate and independent identities (see Schachter, Shore, Feldman-Rotman, Marquis, & Campbell, 1976). According to these theorists, deidentification will be most pronounced for siblings who are more similar in age or sex. Support for the idea of deidentification in the adjustment domain was reported by Feinberg and Hetherington (2000), in a study of adolescents: Siblings who were farther apart in age were more similar in adjustment than those who were close in age. Some evidence indicates that processes of deidentification become more pronounced as individuals reach adolescence (McHale et al., 2001).

While there is then evidence for sibling socialization effects that are independent of parent–child associations, it is also possible (indeed likely) that there are also interactive effects involving both parent–child and sibling relationships in the development of adjustment problems. Thus, Garcia et al. (2000) demonstrated, with a low-income sample of 5-year-old boys, that the interaction between sibling conflict and rejecting parent–child relationships predicted aggressive behavior problems over time. An increase in aggression was found for children who had both high scores on sibling conflict, and also rejecting parent–child relationships. Deidentification processes were also linked to parent–child relationships over time (Feinberg, McHale, Crouter, & Cumsille, 2003).

In addition to these lines of evidence for direct socializing influence of siblings upon one another's adjustment, there are also several sources of evidence suggesting that siblings affect each other's adjustment through less direct processes. A particularly powerful process is the impact of *differential* parent–child relationships within the family, as outlined previously. Thus several studies have shown that the sibling who is perceived or observed to be the least favored shows more adjustment problems than the favored sibling (Conger & Conger, 1994; Reiss et al., 2000). Differential paternal treatment has been included in some studies and also contributes to adjustment outcome (e.g., Brody, Stoneman, & McCoy, 1992; Stocker, 1995; Volling & Elins, 1998). Volling and Elins found, for instance, that preschoolers showed more symptoms of both internalizing and externalizing when both mothers and fathers disciplined them more than their siblings. Differential parental treatment has also been studied in a cross-ethnic framework. Thus one study compared European American and Asian American families with late adolescents, and while in general the findings showed that perceptions of differential treatment predicted up to 13% of the variance in achievement and self-perceptions—a significant amount of variance beyond that predicted by absolute levels of affection and control, several findings were moderated by ethnicity and gender (Barrett Singer & Weinstein, 2000). It is now clear that different cultural and ethnic groups can hold very different attitudes to differential treatment. The research of Mosier and Rogoff (2003) into Guatemalan and U.S. middle-class families with toddlers and preschoolers showed that the Mayan toddlers were accorded a privileged position by both their mothers and their older siblings— and were allowed access to objects that their older siblings also wanted. In contrast, the U.S. toddlers were expected to follow the same rules for sharing as their older siblings. This pattern, the authors argue, fits a cultural model that prioritizes both responsibility and respect for others' freedom of choice.

A further source of evidence on indirect effects concerns the research on the family disruption caused by the birth of a second child, already referred to earlier. Home observations (Dunn & Kendrick, 1982; Stewart et al., 1987) and large-scale surveys (Baydar, Greek, & Brooks-Gunn, 1997; Baydar, Hyle, & Brooks-Gunn, 1997) have documented the disturbance in bodily functions, withdrawal, aggression, and anxiety that follows the birth of a sibling, correlated with changes in the older siblings' changed relationship with the parent. A variety of processes may be implicated here (see Dunn, 1988b); these differ in nature ranging from general emotional disturbance as a mediating link, through a series of processes of increasing specificity and cognitive complexity, such as children's monitoring of differential maternal behavior toward self and sibling to processes involving maternal "attributional style" and communication about others. Even with children who are only preschoolers, it seems, maternal discourse about sibling differences can be linked to differences in children's outcome. It has been argued that individual differences in children and the developmental stage of the child will influence which of these processes is developmentally significant (Dunn, 1988b).

Another indirect process of influence involves peer groups. Evidence has accumulated that antisocial older siblings can affect their younger siblings' antisocial development in part through their involvement with deviant friends (e.g., Slomkowski et al., 2001). Younger siblings are vulnerable not only to the influences of their older siblings but also to the influences of the older siblings' friends (Rowe, Linver, & Rodgers, 1996).

Socialization and Sources of Support

While much of the sibling research on adjustment has focused on the impact of hostility and negative interactions between siblings, there is also evidence that siblings can be an important source of support for children who are faced with stressful experiences. There are reports, for instance, that children growing up in disharmonious homes have fewer adjustment problems if they have a good sibling relationship (Jenkins & Smith, 1990; Jenkins, 1992). It seems that both offering comfort to a sibling and receiving support from a sibling are linked to benefits for children. It should be noted that other studies of family transitions report that siblings are relatively infrequently the source of confiding support (Dunn & Deater-Deckard, 2001). However, children faced with other negative life events, such as paternal unemployment or grandparental death, do report becoming more close and intimate following stressful life events (Dunn, Slomkowski, Beardsall, & Rende, 1994). Whether siblings function in this way to support each other depends crucially on the nature of their relationship—the extent to which they are affectionate and interested in each other. This issue of individual differences is crucial to the second domain of socialization influence we consider, the influence of siblings on the development of social understanding.

The Development of Social Understanding

Sibling research has importantly changed our understanding of the development of children's "discovery of the mind" (Astington, 1993). The growth of children's understanding of other people's emotions, thoughts, and beliefs and their understanding of the links between such inner states and people's actions are topics that have dominated cognitive developmental psychology over the last two decades. It is a domain of development that is clearly implicated in children's socialization. In standard experimental settings designed to assess this ability to "mind read," young preschool children show limited understanding of the connections between what someone thinks and their actions; it is not until 4 years of age that children can reliably succeed in these standard assessments (Wellman, Cross, & Watson, 2001). However, in the context of their interactions with their siblings—

interactions of intense emotions and familiarity—much younger children show powers of anticipating the other's intentions, manipulating the other's emotions. Their ability to deceive, to tease, to manage conflict by anticipating the other's perspective, to share an imaginative world in joint pretend, and to engage in conversations about why people behave the way they do, referring to mental states and feelings as causes and consequences of action, all reflect a growing understanding of connections between inner states and behavior, and all are seen in the interactions between siblings from rising 2 years old to 4 years. Such observations of siblings have provided a new perspective on a central feature of sociocognitive development (Dunn, 2002). The message of the sibling research is not only that these developments begin considerably earlier than suspected but that it is the emotional context and familiarity of the sibling relationship that can play an important part in the growth of understanding.

And the sibling research has been important in highlighting the development of *individual differences* in children's understanding of others, and sibling experiences are importantly linked to the development of such individual differences. Children who have engaged in frequent talk about mental states—with family members (Brown, Donelan-McCall, & Dunn, 1996) or friends (Hughes & Dunn, 1998) are particularly successful on assessments of understanding feelings and mental states (Dunn, 1999). And such conversations are particularly likely to take place in the context of joint pretend play with a sibling or a close friend, when both children have to plan narratives together about how the protagonists in the pretend play behave, and why. Children who have frequently engaged in shared pretend with an older sibling are likely to perform particularly successfully on the standard assessments of understanding of mind (Howe, Petrakos, & Rinaldi, 1998). Some studies find that children with older siblings in general perform better on such assessments than those without older siblings (Perner, Ruffman, & Leekam, 1994); other research indicates that it is family interaction with familiar kin, rather than siblings per se, that is linked to this growth of understanding (Lewis, Freeman, Kyriakidou, Maridaki-Kassotaki, & Berridge, 1996). However, the connection with shared pretend is well established, and this is particularly likely to occur between siblings *who like each other* and have a friendly relationship (Dunn & Dale, 1984), or between close friends (Dunn & Cutting, 1999; Hughes & Dunn, 1998).

This research is chiefly correlational, so again we have to be cautious about inferring causal contributions from sibling interaction to growing understanding. Children who are precocious at understanding feelings and at mind-reading are likely to be rewarding play companions; their abilities may contribute to the growth of shared imaginative experiences with sibling or friend, and these in themselves may contribute to further growth in understanding other people' inner states (Howe et al., 1998). However, although the issue of direction of effects remains a difficult one, what we have learned from studying siblings is that certain social processes within the family are potentially of great significance in the development of such a central feature of human cognitive ability.

Siblings and Peers

How do the relationships that children develop with their siblings within the family relate to the kinds of relationship they form with peers outside the family? If they do, this has to be taken seriously as a "socialization" process, albeit an indirect one, as there is now a wealth of evidence that children's experiences with peers have an important role in their social development (see Bukowski, Brendgen & Vitaro, Chapter 14, this volume).

We might well expect that there are systematic links between the quality of sibling and peer relationships, on the grounds of attachment theory, in terms of social learning theory (which would predict that what is learned within the sibling relationship will generalize to interactions with familiar peers), or because of the evidence that individual characteristics elicit similar responses from different others (Caspi & Elder, 1988). The processes underlying such links differ in these different theoretical frameworks, but each would predict positive connections between sibling and peer relationships.

There are, however, counterarguments, which focus on the clear differences between sibling and peer relationships and suggest that simple positive links should not be expected between them. Friendships involve commitment, trust, and support, and many siblings do not feel this way about each other. Friendships do not involve sharing parental love and attention, or resentment about preferential treatment by parents. Children select their friends but do not choose their siblings.

Given these differences it is perhaps not surprising that evidence for positive associations between sibling and peer relationships is not consistent. Some research on young children reports that the ways in which children behave during disputes is related to their behavior in conflict with peers (Slomkowski & Dunn, 1992), and correlations between aggression with peers and with siblings have been described (Vandell et al., 1987). Other studies of young children report no such links across the relationships (Abramovitch, Corter, Pepler, & Stanhope, 1986). As for the positive dimensions of the relationships, Slomkowski and Dunn (1992) found that individual differences in connected communication were correlated across the relationships. Findings on middle childhood and early adolescence are inconsistent: Links between the two relationships in controlling and positive behavior were reported by (Stocker & Mantz-Simmons, 2006), but the study also noted that children who were especially cooperative with their siblings described lower levels of companionship with their friends. Other evidence that supports this suggestion of "compensatory" patterns across the two relationships has been reported (Mendelson, Aboud, & Lanthier, 1994; Stocker & Dunn, 1990). For instance, in a study of young adolescents, East and Rook (1992) found that the individuals who were isolated from their peers described their sibling relationships as more supportive. And sometimes even within the same study, evidence for both positive associations and negative links is found (e.g., Updegraff & Obeidallah, 1999; Volling, Youngblade, & Belsky, 1997).

Given the mixed findings found for associations across these two important relationships, the conclusion of Parke and Buriel (1998), reviewing the field, remains appropriate: "the challenge for future work is to discover the contexts under which strong, weak, or compensatory connections might be expected between (sibling and peer) relationship systems" (p. 485).

Siblings and Family Influence

The study of siblings has raised an important general issue for developmental psychologists, which concerns the ways in which family experiences affect individual development and influence socialization. Siblings who grow up in the same family nevertheless differ notably in personality and adjustment from one another. These differences, which have now been documented in a wide range of studies (Conger & Conger, 1994; Dunn &

Plomin, 1990; Hetherington et al., 1994; Reiss et al., 2000), do present a major challenge to those who study family influence on socialization. The various features of family life that have been investigated as important influences on children's and adolescents' development—such as parental education and occupation, marital relationship and parents' mental health, social adversities faced by the family, and neighborhood effects—are all apparently shared by siblings within the same family. Why then do the siblings grow up to be so different from one another?

A range of answers to this question have been explored, including the notion that experiences within the family differ very much for siblings, and that it is these "within-family" or "nonshared" experiences that are key to the development of individual differences. To clarify this issue, we need to study the experiences that are specific to each sibling, rather than compare children growing up in different families—the "between-family" differences that have been the chief focus of research. The key message from this research is not that family influences are not important but that families are experienced very differently by the siblings who are members of these families (Hetherington et al., 1994).

This new perspective on family processes is being systematically studied, through a focus on differential parent–child relationships as described earlier, differential experiences within the sibling relationship itself (Dunn & Plomin, 1990), and analytic approaches such as multilevel modeling, which enable the researcher to separate out the variance in outcome that is attributable to *shared* family influence (affecting all the siblings within the family) and *nonshared* family influence, which affects specific children within the family and not others. Examples of such research include studies of the development of adjustment problems in siblings (O'Connor, Dunn, Jenkins, Pickering, & Rasbash, 2001), studies of the impact of marital conflict on siblings (Jenkins et al., 2005), and studies of parenting (O'Connor, Dunn, Jenkins, & Rasbash, 2006). It is clear that individual differences in sibling temperament, adjustment, and intelligence play a key part in eliciting different responses from other family members and from those outside the family, and in their response to shared stresses such as conflict between their parents. But fully to understand how families affect individual development, it is also clear that we need to include more than one in child in each family.

Cross-Cultural Perspectives

We also need to broaden the range of communities that are studied. Research on siblings in minority communities is still relatively sparse, as are cross-cultural and non-Western studies. These lacunae are surprising given that we know from ethnographic studies that siblings play a key role as caregivers for very young children in many cultures (Weisner, 1989; Zukow, 1989; Zukow-Goldring, 2002). Weisner considers that experiences with siblings in many non-Western communities play an important role in socialization for parenthood. Siblings can, anthropological research tells us, be central in adults' lives in many such communities (see e.g., Nuckolls, 1993). Many of the issues discussed in this chapter would be illuminated by systematic cross-cultural comparisons, as the example of the privileged treatment of toddlers in a Mayan community, discussed earlier in the chapter, demonstrated. In this study, Mosier and Rogoff (2003) argued convincingly that the pattern they observed in Guatemala in which older siblings showed voluntary responsibility and the toddlers were privileged "reflects early socialization in this model of individual freedom of choice in support of responsibility to the group" (p. 1056).

A second example is the evidence for the significance of siblings' teaching skills which was highlighted in a study of Mayan children (Maynard, 2002). The Zinocantec older siblings were videotaped in caregiving interactions with their 2-year-old brothers and sisters. In the context of play, older siblings taught their younger siblings how to do everyday tasks such as washing and cooking. Ethnographic observations and discourse analyses were used to show that children's teaching skills increased over the course of middle childhood, and by 8 years old children were highly skilled in using talk combined with demonstrations, to guide their siblings, and thus helped their younger siblings to increase their participation in culturally important tasks. This example illustrates a general point made by Zukow-Goldring (2002) in her review of sibling caregiving—that in agrarian societies sibling caregivers do more than attend to immediate biological needs of their younger siblings: "Siblings are 'culture brokers,' introducing their sisters and brothers to ways of acting and knowing through unique styles of interaction" (p. 278).

We remain largely ignorant about the extent or significance of ethnic differences in sibling relationships, either in childhood or adulthood. A study in the United States compared adult sibling relationships in African American, Hispanic, non-Hispanic whites, and Asian American adults and concluded that the similarities across these groups in support and contact far outweighed the differences (Riedmann & White, 1996). Would the same be true for childhood and adolescence?

SUMMARY: SOCIALIZATION AND SIBLINGS

The study of siblings has provided a powerful new perspective on both normative and individual differences in development and socialization. Research on the growth of social understanding, on social competence, on the links between emotional and cognitive development, on family influence on adjustment and socialization, or on peer relations has been illuminated by a focus on siblings. Recent research on siblings has given us the opportunity to learn more about not only their relationships and their direct socialization influences but about key issues in developmental psychology. The relationships of step- and half-siblings and individual differences in their development is a growing area of research; not only is this an important practical area, with the increasing numbers of families that include step-relationships (Hetherington et al., 1999) but comparison of full, half, and stepsiblings gives a useful approach to the study of the role of genetics in the development of individual differences (Deater-Deckard, Dunn, O'Connor, & Golding, 2002). In the clinical literature there is growing interest in siblings (Boer & Dunn, 1990), as in the example of studies of children's response to illness, disability, or injury in their siblings (Stallard, Mastroyannopoulou, Lewis, & Lenton, 1997); of siblings as donors in bone marrow transplant surgery (Lwin, 2006); and of traumatic experiences of siblings (Newman, Black, & Harris-Hendriks, 1997).

There are nevertheless some striking gaps in what we know about siblings and socialization. Although there is a welcome increase in studies of siblings in adolescence, there is still little longitudinal research into adulthood, or studies with an intergenerational perspective, despite the evidence for the importance of siblings in adulthood (Cicirelli, 1996). The issue of how long term the significance of early experiences with siblings may be remains unclear. There is the notable gap in cross-cultural studies of siblings. However, sibling research is clarifying both normative developmental questions and key issues in socialization theory; the gaps in what is known provide opportunities for further research that is likely to be both illuminating in terms of developmental theory and important in terms of practical issues, and of our understanding of family processes and socialization.

REFERENCES

Abramovitch, R., Corter, C., Pepler, D. J., & Stanhope, L. (1986). Sibling and peer interaction: A final follow-up and a comparison. *Child Development, 57,* 217–229.

Adler, A. (1928). Characteristics of the first, second and third child. *Children, 3.*

Ansbacher, H. L., & Ansbacher, R. R. (1956). *The individual psychology of Alfred Adler.* New York: Basic Books.

Astington, J. W. (1993). *The child's discovery of the mind.* Cambridge, MA: Harvard University Press.

Bank, L., Patterson, G. R., & Reid, J. B. (1996). Negative sibling interactions as predictors of later adjustment problems in adolescent and young adult males. In G. H. Brody (Ed.), *Sibling relationships: Their causes and consequences* (pp. 197–229). Norwood, NJ: Ablex.

Bank, S., & Kahn, M. D. (1982). *The sibling bond.* New York: Basic Books.

Barrett Singer, A. T., & Weinstein, R. S. (2000). Differential parental treatment predicts achievement and self-perceptions in two cultural contexts. *Journal of Family Psychology, 14,* 491–509.

Baydar, N., Greek, A., & Brooks-Gunn, J. (1997). A longitudinal study of the effects of the birth of a sibling during the first 6 years of life. *Journal of Marriage and the Family, 59,* 939–956.

Baydar, N., Hyle, P., & Brooks-Gunn, J. (1997). A longitudinal study of the effects of the birth of a sibling during preschool and early grade school years. *Journal of Marriage and the Family, 59,* 957–965.

Boer, F., & Dunn, J. (1990). *Children's sibling relationships: Developmental and clinical issues.* Hillsdale, NJ: Erlbaum.

Boll, T., Ferring, D., & Fillipp, S. (2003). Perceived parental differential treatment in middle adulthood: Curvilinear relations with individuals' experienced relationship quality to sibling and parents. *Journal of Family Psychology, 17,* 472–487.

Brody, G. H. (1996). *Sibling relationships: Their causes and consequences.* Norwood, NJ: Ablex.

Brody, G. H. (1998). Sibling relationship quality: Its causes and consequences. *Annual Review of Psychology, 49,* 1–24.

Brody, G., Stoneman, Z., & Burke, M. (1987). Child temperaments, maternal differential behavior, and sibling relationships. *Developmental Psychology, 23,* 354–362.

Brody, G., Stoneman, Z., & McCoy, J. (1992). Associations of maternal and paternal direct and differential behavior with sibling relationships: Contemporaneous and longitudinal analyses. *Child Development, 63,* 82–92.

Brody, G. H., Stoneman, Z., & McCoy, J. K. (1994). Forecasting sibling relationships in early adolescence from child temperaments and family processes in middle childhood. *Child Development, 65,* 771–784.

Brody, G., Stoneman, Z., McCoy, J. K., & Forehand, R. (1992). Contemporaneous and longitudinal associations of sibling conflict with family relationship assessments and family discussions about sibling problems. *Child Development, 63,* 391–400.

Brown, J. R., Donelan-McCall, N., & Dunn, J. (1996). Why talk about mental states? The significance of children's conversations with friends, siblings, and mothers. *Child Development, 67,* 836–849.

Buhrmester, D. (1992). The developmental course of sibling and peer relationships. In F. Boer & J. Dunn (Eds.), *Children's sibling relationships: Developmental and clinical issues* (pp. 19–40). Hillsdale, NJ: Erlbaum.

Buhrmester, D., & Furman, W. (1990). Perceptions of sibling relationships during middle childhood and adolescence. *Child Development, 61,* 1387–1398.

Caspi, A., & Elder, G. H., Jr. (1988). Emergent family patterns: The intergenerational construction of problem behaviour and relationships. In R. Hinde & J. Stevenson-Hinde (Eds.), *Relationships within families: Mutual influences* (pp. 218–240). Oxford, UK: Clarendon.

Cicirelli, V. (1996). Sibling relationships in middle and old age. In G. Brody (Ed.), *Sibling relationships: Their causes and consequences* (pp. 47–73). Norwood, NJ: Ablex.

Conger, K., & Conger, R. (1994). Differential parenting and change in sibling differences in delinquency. *Journal of Family Psychology, 8*, 287–302.

Conger, R. D., Cui, M. M., Bryant, C. M., & Elder, G. H., Jr. (2000). Competence in early adult relationships: A developmental perspective on family influences. *Journal of Personality and Social Psychology, 79*, 224–237.

Deater-Deckard, K., Dunn, J., O'Connor, T. G., & Golding, J. (2002). Sibling relationships and social-emotional adjustment in different family contexts. *Social Development, 11*, 571–590.

Dunn, J. (1983). Sibling relationships in early childhood. *Child Development, 54*, 787–811.

Dunn, J. (1988a). *The beginnings of social understanding* (1st ed.). Cambridge, MA: Harvard University Press.

Dunn, J. (1988b). Connections between relationships: Implications of research on mothers and siblings. In R. A. Hinde & J. Stevenson-Hinde (Eds.), *Relations between relationships* (pp. 168–180). Oxford, UK: Oxford University Press.

Dunn, J. (1999). Mindreading and social relationships. In M. Bennett (Ed.), *Developmental Psychology: Achievements and prospects* (pp. 55–71). Philadelphia, PA: Psychology Press.

Dunn, J. (2002). Mindreading, emotion understanding, and relationships. In R. Silbereisen & W. W. Hartup (Eds.), *Growing points in developmental science: An introduction* (pp. 167–176). Oxford, UK: Psychology Press.

Dunn, J., Brown, J., Slomkowski, C., Tesla, C., & Youngblade, L. (1991). Young children's understanding of other people's feelings and beliefs: Individual differences and their antecedents. *Child Development, 62*, 1352–1366.

Dunn, J., Creps, C., & Brown, J. (1996). Children's family relationships between two and five: Developmental changes and individual differences. *Social Development, 5*, 230–250.

Dunn, J., & Cutting, A. (1999). Understanding others, and individual differences in friendship interactions in young children. *Social Development, 8*, 201–219.

Dunn, J., & Dale, N. (1984). I a Daddy: 2-year-olds' collaboration in joint pretend with sibling and with mother. In I. Bretherton (Ed.), *Symbolic play: The development of social understanding* (pp. 131–158). San Diego, CA: Academic Press.

Dunn, J., & Deater-Deckard, K. (2001). *Children's views of their changing families.* York, UK: York Publishing Services/Joseph Rowntree Foundation.

Dunn, J., Deater-Deckard, K., Pickering, K., Beveridge, M., & ALSPAC Study Team. (1999). Siblings, parents and partners: Family relationships within a longitudinal community study. *Journal of Child Psychology and Psychiatry, 40*, 1025–1037.

Dunn, J., & Kendrick, C. (1982). *Siblings: Love, envy and understanding.* London: Grant McIntyre.

Dunn, J., & Munn, P. (1985). Becoming a family member: Family conflict and the development of social understanding in the second year. *Child Development, 56*, 764–774.

Dunn, J., & Plomin, R. (1990). *Separate lives: Why siblings are so different* (1st ed.). New York: Basic Books.

Dunn, J., Slomkowski, C., & Beardsall, L. (1994). Sibling relationships from the preschool period through middle childhood and early adolescence. *Developmental Psychology, 30*, 315–324.

Dunn, J., Slomkowski, C., Beardsall, L., & Rende, R. (1994). Adjustment in middle childhood and early adolescence: Links with earlier and contemporary sibling relationships. *Journal of Child Psychology and Psychiatry and Allied Disciplines, 35*, 491–504.

East, P. L., & Rook, K. S. (1992). Compensatory patterns of support among children's peer relationships: A test using school friends, nonschool friends, and siblings. *Developmental Psychology, 28*, 163–172.

Erel, O., Margolin, G., & John, R. S. (1998). Observed sibling interaction: Links with the marital and the mother–child relationship. *Developmental Psychology, 34*, 288–298.

Ernst, C., & Angst, J. (1983). *Birth order: Its influence on personality.* Berlin and New York: Springer-Verlag.

Feinberg, M., & Hetherington, E. M. (2000). Sibling differentiation in adolescence: Implications for behaviour genetic theory. *Child Development, 71*, 1611–1628.

Feinberg, M., & Hetherington, E. M. (2001). Differential parenting as a within-family variable. *Journal of Family Psychology, 15*, 22–37.

Feinberg, M. E., McHale, S. M., Crouter, A. C., & Cumsille, P. (2003). Sibling differentiation: Sibling and parent relationship trajectories in adolescence. *Child Development, 74*, 1261–1274.

Freud, S. (1938). *An outline of psychoanalysis.* London: Hogarth Press.

Freud, S. (1961). *Introductory lectures on psycho-analysis*. In J. Strachey (Ed. and Trans.), *Standard edition of the complete psychological works of Sigmund Freud Vols. 15–16*. London: Hogarth Press. (Original work published 1916)

Furman, W., & Lanthier, R. P. (1996). Personality and sibling relationships. In G. H. Brody (Ed.), *Sibling relationships: Their causes and consequences* (pp. 127–146). Norwood, NJ: Ablex.

Garcia, M. M., Shaw, D. S., Winslow, E. B., & Yaggi, K. E. (2000). Destructive sibling conflict and the development of conduct problems in young boys. *Developmental Psychology, 36*, 44–53.

Hartup, W. W. (1996). The company they keep: Friendships and their developmental significance. *Child Development, 67*, 1–13.

Hetherington, E. M., & Clingempeel, W. G. (1992). Coping with marital transitions: A family systems approach. *Monographs of the Society for Research in Child Development, 57*, 2–3.

Hetherington, E. M., Henderson, S., & Reiss, D. (1999). Adolescent siblings in stepfamilies: Family functioning and adolescent adjustment. *Monographs of the Society for Research in Child Development, 64*, 1–222.

Hetherington, E. M., Reiss, D., & Plomin, R. (1994). *Separate social worlds of siblings: The impact of nonshared environment on development*. Hillsdale, NJ: Erlbaum.

Hinde, R. A. (1979). *Towards understanding relationships*. London: Academic Press.

Howe, N., Petrakos, H., & Rinaldi, C. (1998). "All the sheeps are dead. He murdered them": Sibling pretense, negotiation, internal state language and relationship quality. *Child Development, 69*, 182–191.

Hughes, C., & Dunn, J. (1998). Understanding mind and emotion: Longitudinal associations with mental-state talk between young friends. *Developmental Psychology, 34*, 1026–1037.

Jenkins, J. M. (1992). Sibling relationships in disharmonious homes: Potential difficulties and protective effects. In F. Boer & J. Dunn (Eds.), *Children's sibling relationships: Developmental and clinical issues*. Hillsdale, NJ: Lawrence Erlbaum Associates.

Jenkins, J. M., Dunn, J., Rasbash, J., O'Connor, T. G., & Simpson, A. (2005). The mutual influence of marital conflict and children's behavior problems: shared and non-shared family risks. *Child Development, 76*, 24–39.

Jenkins, J., & Smith, M. (1990). Factors protecting children living in disharmonious homes: Maternal reports. *Journal of the American Academy of Child and Adolescent Psychiatry, 29*, 60–69.

Kim, J. E., Hetherington, E. M., & Reiss, D. (1999). Associations among family relationships, antisocial peers, and adolescents' externalizing behaviors: Gender and family type differences. *Child Development, 70*, 1209–1230.

Koch, H. L. (1954). The relation of "primary mental abilities" in five- and six-year-olds to sex of child and characteristics of his sibling. *Child Development, 15*, 209–223.

Koch, H. (1960). The relation of certain formal attributes of siblings to attitudes held toward each other and toward their parents. *Monographs of the Society for Research in Child Development, 25*, 1–124.

Kowal, A., & Kramer, L. (1997). Children's understanding of parental differential treatment. *Child Development, 68*, 113–126.

Kowal, A., Kramer, L., Krull, J. L., & Crick, N. R. (2002). Children's perceptions of the fairness of parental preferential treatment and their socioemotional well-being. *Journal of Family Psychology, 16*, 297–306.

Lewis, C., Freeman, N. H., Kyriakidou, C., Maridaki-Kassotaki, K., & Berridge, D. M. (1996). Social influences on false belief access: Specific sibling influences or general apprenticeship? *Child Development, 67*, 2930–2947.

Lwin, R. (2006). *Sibling relationships and bone marrow transplant*. Unpublished manuscript, University of London, London.

MacKinnon, C. (1989). An observational investigation of sibling interactions in married and divorced families. *Developmental Psychology, 25*, 36–44.

Maynard, A. E. (2002). Cultural teaching: The development of teaching skills in Maya sibling interactions. *Child Development, 73*, 969–982.

McGuire, S., Manke, B., Eftekhari, A., & Dunn, J. (2000). Children's perceptions of sibling conflict during middle childhood: Issues and sibling (Dis)similarity. *Social Development, 9*, 173–190.

McHale, S. M., & Crouter, A. C. (1996). The family context of children's sibling relationships. In G. Brody (Ed.), *Sibling relationships: Their causes and consequences* (pp. 173–195). Norwood, NJ: Ablex.

McHale, S. M., Updegraff, K. A., Helms-Erikson, H., & Crouter, A. C. (2001). Sibling influences on gender development in middle childhood and early adolescence: A longitudinal study. *Developmental Psychology, 37*, 115–125.

Mendelson, M., Aboud, F., & Lanthier, R. (1994). Kindergartners' relationships with siblings, peers and friends. *Merrill-Palmer Quarterly, 40*, 416–427.

Mosier, C. E., & Rogoff, B. (2003). Privileged treatment of toddlers: Cultural aspects of individual choice and responsibility. *Developmental Psychology, 39*, 1047–1060.

Munn, P., & Dunn, J. (1989). Temperament and the developing relationship between siblings. *International Journal of Behavioral Development, 12*, 433–451.

Newman, M., Black, D., & Harris-Hendriks, J. (1997). Victims of disaster, war, violence or homicide: Psychological effects on siblings. *Child Psychology and Psychiatry Review, 2*, 140–149.

Nuckolls, C. (1993). *Siblings in South Asia*. New York: Guilford Press.

O'Connor, T., Dunn, J., Jenkins, J., Pickering, K., & Rasbash, J. (2001). Family settings and children's adjustment: Differential adjustment within and across families. *British Journal of Psychiatry, 179*, 110–115.

O'Connor, T. G., Dunn, J., Jenkins, J., & Rasbash, J. (2006). Predictors of between-family and within-family variation in parent–child relationships. *Journal of Child Psychology and Psychiatry, 47*, 498–510.

Parke, R. D., & Buriel, R. (1998). Socialization in the family: Ethnic and ecological perspectives. In W. Damon (Ed.), *Handbook of child psychology: Vol 3. Social, emotional and personality development* (pp. 463–552). New York: Wiley.

Patterson, G. R. (1986). The contribution of siblings to training for fighting: A microsocial analysis. In D. Olweus, J. Block, & M. Radke-Yarrow (Eds.), *Development of antisocial and prosocial behavior* (pp. 235–261). New York: Academic Press.

Perner, J., Ruffman, T., & Leekam, S. R. (1994). Theory of mind is contagious: You catch it from your sibs. *Child Development, 65*, 1228–1238.

Reiss, D., Neiderhiser, J. M., Hetherington, E. M., & Plomin, R. (2000). *The relationship code: Deciphering genetic and social influences on adolescent development*. Cambridge, MA: Harvard University Press.

Riedmann, A., & White, L. (1996). Adult sibling relationships: Racial and ethnic comparisons. In G. Brody (Ed.), *Sibling relationships: Their causes and consequences* (pp. 105–126). Norwood, NJ: Ablex.

Rowe, D. C., Linver, M., & Rodgers, J. L. (1996). Delinquency and IQ: Using siblings to find source of variation. In G. H. Brody (Ed.), *Sibling relationships: Their causes and consequences* (pp. 147–171). Norwood, NJ: Ablex.

Schachter, F. F., Shore, E., Feldman-Rotman, S., Marquis, R. E., & Campbell, S. (1976). Sibling deidentification. *Developmental Psychology, 12*, 418–427.

Seligman, M. E. P., & Nolen-Hoeksma, S. (1987). Explanatory style and depression. In D. Magnusson & A. Oehman (Eds.), *Psychopathology: An interactional perspective* (pp. 125–139). San Diego, CA: Academic Press.

Slomkowski, C. L., & Dunn, J. (1992). Arguments and relationships within the family: Differences in young children's disputes with mother and sibling. *Developmental Psychology, 28*, 919–924.

Slomkowski, C., Rende, R., Conger, K., Simons, R., & Conger, R. (2001). Sisters, brothers, and delinquency: Evaluating social influence during early and middle adolescence. *Child Development, 72*, 271–283.

Snyder, J., & Patterson, G. (1995). Individual differences in social aggression: A test of a reinforcement model of socialization in the natural environment. *Behavior Therapy, 26*, 371–391.

Stallard, P., Mastroyannopoulou, K., Lewis, M., & Lenton, S. (1997). The siblings of children with life-threatening conditions. *Child Psychology and Psychiatry Review, 2*, 26–33.

Stewart, R. B. (1990). *The second child*. Newbury Park, CA: Sage.

Stewart, R., Mobley, L., Van Tuyl, S., & Salvador, M. (1987). The firstborn's adjustment to the birth of a sibling. *Child Development, 58*, 341–355.

Stocker, C. (1993). Siblings' adjustment in middle childhood: Links with mother–child relationships. *Journal of Applied Developmental Psychology, 14*, 485–499.

Stocker, C. M. (1994). Children's perceptions of their relationships with siblings, friends and mothers: Compensatory processes and links with adjustment. *Journal of Child Psychology and Psychiatry, 35*, 1447–1459.

Stocker, C. M. (1995). Differences in mothers' and fathers' relationships with siblings: Links with behavioral problems. *Development and Psychopathology, 7*, 499–513.

Stocker, C., Ahmed, K., & Stall, M. (1997). Marital satisfaction and maternal emotional expressiveness: Links with children's sibling relationships. *Social Development, 6*, 373–385.

Stocker, C. M., Burwell, R. A., & Briggs, M. L. (2002). Sibling conflict in middle childhood predicts children's adjustment in early adolescence. *Journal of Family Psychology, 16,* 50–57.

Stocker, C., & Dunn, J. (1990). Sibling relationships in childhood: Links with friendships and peer relationships. *British Journal of Developmental Psychology, 8,* 227–244.

Stocker, C., Dunn, J., & Plomin, R. (1989). Sibling relationships: Links with child temperament, maternal behavior, and family structure. *Child Development, 60,* 715–727.

Stocker, C., & Mantz-Simmons, L. (2006). *Children's friendships and peer status: Links with family relationships, temperament and social skills.* Unpublished manuscript, University of Denver.

Stormshak, E. A., Bellanti, C., Bierman, K. L., & Conduct Problems Prevention Research Group. (1996). The quality of sibling relationships and the development of social competence and behavioural control in aggressive children. *Developmental Psychology, 32,* 79–89.

Sutton-Smith, B., & Rosenberg, B. (1970). *The sibling.* New York: Holt, Rinehart & Winston.

Tesla, C., & Dunn, J. (1992). Getting along or getting your own way: The development of young children's use of argument in conflicts with mother and sibling. *Social Development, 1,* 107–121.

Teti, D. M., & Ablard, K. E. (1989). Security of attachment and infant–sibling relationships: A laboratory study. *Child Development, 60,* 1519–1528.

Tucker, C. J., Updegraff, K. A., McHale, S. M., & Crouter, A. C. (1999). Older siblings as socializers of younger siblings' empathy. *Journal of Early Adolescence, 19,* 176–198.

Updegraff, K. A., McHale, S. M., & Crouter, A. C. (2002). Adolescents' sibling relationship and friendship experiences: Developmental patterns and relationship linkages. *Social Development, 11,* 182–204.

Updegraff, K. A., & Obeidallah, D. A. (1999). Young adolescents' patterns of involvement with siblings and friends. *Social Development, 8,* 53–69.

Vandell, D. L., Minnett, A. M., & Santrock, J. W. (1987). Age differences in sibling relationships during middle childhood. *Journal of Applied Developmental Psychology, 8,* 247–257.

Volling, B. L., & Belsky, J. (1992). The contribution of mother–child and father–child relationships to the quality of sibling interaction: A longitudinal study. *Child Development, 63,* 1209–1222.

Volling, B. L., & Elins, J. L. (1998). Family relationships and children's emotional adjustment as correlates of maternal and paternal differential treatment: A replication with toddler and preschool siblings. *Child Development, 69,* 1640–1656.

Volling, B. L., Youngblade, L. M., & Belsky, J. (1997). Young children's social relationships: an examination of the linkages between siblings, friends, and peers. *American Journal of Orthopsychiatry, 67,* 102–111.

Weisner, T. S. (1989). Comparing sibling relationships across cultures. In P. Zukow (Ed.), *Sibling interaction across cultures: Theoretical and methodological issues* (pp. 11–25). New York: Springer-Verlag.

Wellman, H. M., Cross, D., & Watson, J. (2001). Meta-analysis of theory of mind development: The truth about false belief. *Child Development, 72,* 655–684.

Zukow, P. (1989). *Sibling interaction across cultures.* New York: Springer-Verlag.

Zukow-Goldring, P. (2002). Sibling caregiving. In M.H. Bornstein (Ed.), *Handbook of parenting* (Vol. 3, pp. 253–286). Mahwah, NJ: Erlbaum.

CHAPTER 13

Socialization in the Context of Family Diversity

CHARLOTTE J. PATTERSON and PAUL D. HASTINGS

The diversity of family structures in the Western world is arguably greater today than at any other point in history. Infants are being born into an array of different family types, some of which were not even recognized as existing as recently as 50 years ago. Babies conceived via reproductive technology may be biologically related to one, two, or none of the adults who intend to rear them. Adoption and remarriage add to the diversity of biologically related and unrelated parent–child relationships. Children today are being reared not only by married, mother–father couples, but also by unmarried heterosexual couples, and by divorced or never-married single heterosexual men and women. Single lesbian women and single gay men, unmarried lesbian couples and unmarried gay couples, and, in a growing number of jurisdictions, married lesbian couples and married gay couples, are also rearing children in an ever-growing number of nonheterosexual families. Substantial numbers of children are not even being reared by parents at all but live instead with grandparents. What does all this mean for the socialization of infants and children?

This question has not always been of such central interest to scholars of human development. For many years, most researchers assumed that they knew the conditions that were most favorable for child development. Those conditions were normally considered to be provided most reliably by families that included two heterosexual parents, one male and one female, who were married to one another and who were biologically related to the child or children whom they were rearing. While fathers in such families were expected to be employed full time outside the home, mothers were expected to stay at home, where they were responsible for child care and household upkeep but did not earn money. Even though the existence of such so-called traditional families has not characterized much of human history, and even though many if not most families today—even in Western countries—do not fit this pattern, it has nevertheless been widely adopted as the norm against which other family rearing environments should be measured (Lamb, 1999a).

Questions about the degree to which children's development might vary as a function of family constellation have been seen as rooted in Freudian psychoanalytic theory (Hay & Nash, 2002). Although he presumed that children identify with their same-sex parents, Freud emphasized that children's relationships with both biological parents were important (e.g., Freud, 1938). Thus, children not raised in homes with both their biological mother and their biological father were seen as being at greater risk for psychosocial problems and, in particular, of not following normative gender role development. Freud's theory should be considered within the historical and sociocultural context of the era in which he lived, when it was more unusual for children to be raised by nonbiologically related parents. However, contemporary theoretical perspectives also call attention to ways in which socialization processes and outcomes might be expected to vary across family structures.

For example, family systems theory regards parent–child relationships as embedded within the larger family unit, which functions as a dynamic whole (Cox & Paley, 1997). Within a two-parent family, a parent is also a partner and therefore has a spousal relationship as well as a childrearing relationship. The absence of a spousal relationship in a single-parent home would provide a different family system context for the parent–child relationship, because each relationship within a family influences the functioning of each individual. Family structure might also be associated with variations in extrafamilial relationships and experiences. From an ecological perspective (Bronfenbrenner, 1989), children and parents living in different family structures might be expected to have access to different economic, social, and community resources, and to experience the broader sociocultural milieu in different ways. Researchers versed in these and other theories, therefore, may have cause to examine differences between "traditional" and other family structures and question whether they have import for socialization.

Some elements of the "traditional" family that were deemed critical in years past have received extensive study. For instance, based on the traditionally expected division of labor involving fathers as "breadwinners" and mothers as "homemakers," some scholars wondered whether children might suffer if fathers served as primary caregivers, while mothers worked outside the home. Research has, however, dispelled that concern (Parke, 2002; Russell, 1999). Others argued that, in families in which both parents were employed, the experience of child care outside the home might be damaging to infants and children. Over time, the powerful secular movement of mothers into the labor force, together with results of extensive research, has largely transformed discussions about whether mothers should pursue employment outside the home into discussions about how best to manage child care when both parents are at work (Clarke-Stewart & Allhusen, 2002; Honig, 2002; Lamb, 1999b). Thus, many of the concerns posed by an earlier generation of researchers studying family diversity have been addressed.

Some of the other critical elements that "traditional" family environments have been expected to exemplify still remain controversial. Two married, heterosexual adults raising children to whom they are both biologically related has been seen as the normative, and ideal, family context for socialization. Currently, these assumptions are all under active discussion. Many children in Western countries grow up in families that differ from this norm. In the Western world today, diversity of family structure is a growing reality (Lamb, 1999a). Even those children whose families correspond to the normative picture are likely to attend school with youngsters from other kinds of families.

In this chapter, the impact of family diversity on human development is considered, with particular focus on processes of socialization. This topic has most often been studied in research focused on family structure. For example, traditions of research have grown up around the study of single-parent families, stepfamilies, and dual-career two-parent families (Hetherington & Stanley-Hagan, 1999; Weinraub, Horvath, & Gringlas, 2002). Results of this research have, however, consistently revealed that family resources, processes, and relationships are more important predictors of successful socialization than are assessments of family structure. As our following examination of the literature reveals, when family processes and relationships are supportive, and when family resources are sufficient to meet children's needs, successful socialization of young children generally ensues, even when structural characteristics of the family may not conform to culturally approved norms.

This chapter begins by considering some key aspects of family environments, interactions, and relationships. In light of these considerations, different nontraditional family structures and the evidence about their impact on human development are reviewed. Although many forms of diversity in family structure occur, space does not permit exploration of them all. In this chapter, nontraditional families—including one-parent families, umarried heterosexual-parent families, families formed using reproductive technology, families with lesbian and gay parents, and grandparent-headed families—are discussed. In the final section, we summarize the overall findings and consider their possible implications.

FAMILY RESOURCES, INTERACTIONS, AND RELATIONSHIPS

It is one thing to assess the possible impact of family structure on children's development. Should there indeed be differences in children's behavior, characteristics, or abilities across family types, it is also important to identify *why* such differences exist. Differences in developmental outcomes that are observed across family types might be attributable to other factors that are confounded with family type. Families that share a given structure may also share similar socioeconomic conditions, for example, or similar ideas about family roles. Indeed, there is abundant evidence that single-parent families, on average, have lower mean annual incomes than two-parent families (see Conger & Dogan, Chapter 17, this volume). Identifying the variables and processes that contribute to similarities and differences in children's development across family structures is important for efforts to promote the well-being and positive development of all children.

Within and across different family types, there are fundamental resources, interactions, and relationships that are likely to be needed in order to support positive socialization. First, it is clear that families need access to sufficient financial resources and to the satisfactory nutrition, adequate shelter, and health care that such financial resources make possible. Second, the qualities of parent–child interactions and relationships are important issues in any family. Third, the emotional climate and stability of families are important elements of environments they provide for the socialization of infants, children, and adolescents. In addition, the social embeddedness of the family and the availability of social support for parents facilitates appropriate socialization. In the sections that follow, we briefly outline the contributions of each of these resources to socialization.

Access to Resources

For socialization to proceed in positive directions, the basic needs of infants and children must be met. These include sufficient nutrition, adequate shelter, protection from dangers, and access to opportunities for socialization. In most parts of the Western world, basic needs such as food and shelter are generally purchased using a family's economic resources. Inasmuch as family financial resources play a central role in providing for the needs of infants, children, and adolescents, wealth and poverty are central issues for research on socialization. When families are impoverished, the difficulties in socialization of infants and children are multiple.

Infants and children from low-income families are less likely than those from more affluent families to receive adequate nutrition and appropriate health care (Brooks-Gunn & Duncan, 1997a, 1997b). Low birthweights, poor childhood health, stunted growth, and poor nutrition (Alaimo, Olson, Frongillo, & Breifel, 2001; Brooks-Gunn & Duncan, 1997a, 1997b) are all more common in impoverished than in affluent families.

Similarly, low-income families are less likely than others to have adequate housing (Bradley, 2002). They have greater exposure to toxins like lead-based paint (Nordin et al., 1998) and to environmental harms such as exposure to air pollution, experience of community or family violence, and direct victimization by physical abuse or neglect (Bolger & Patterson, 2003; Bradley, 2002). Research has consistently shown that parents with low incomes and less access to resources show poorer socialization practices and less authoritative parenting styles, compared to more financially well off parents (Magnuson & Duncan, 2002). Across racial groups (Bradley, Corwyn, McAdoo, & Garcia Coll, 2001; Brody, Flor, & Gibson, 1999), and for both mothers and fathers (Burbach, Fox, & Nicholson, 2004), parents with fewer economic resources have been found to be less confident in their parenting, less warm and engaged with their children, and more verbally and physically punitive than parents with greater financial resources.

Children from impoverished families are less likely than those from more affluent homes to have access to enriching opportunities (Bradley et al., 2001). They are less likely to live in homes that contain many books, less likely to have access to music or to works of art, and less likely to visit libraries and museums (Bradley, 2002). They are less likely to have the opportunity to take music or dance lessons, to participate in clubs, or to play on sports teams (Fields, Smith, Bass, & Lugalia, 2001).

Children in socioeconomically disadvantaged families also fare less well than their more advantaged counterparts, showing more of a variety of adjustment difficulties and problematic behaviors (Offord, Boyle, & Jones, 1987). The effects of socioeconomic stress on children are likely to be at least partially mediated by effects on parents (Hoff, Laursen, & Tardif, 2002; Ross, Roberts, & Scott, 1998). One study showed that socioeconomic status (SES) was positively correlated with better parenting practices in divorced mothers; in turn, better parenting practices predicted children's adaptive and prosocial behavior at school (DeGarmo, Forgatch, & Martinez, 1999). Job loss, income loss, and persistent economic hardship undermine parents' ability to respond in nurturant ways to their children. Overall, family economic circumstances are a major determinant of socialization outcomes for infants and children (Bradley, 2002; Brooks-Gunn & Duncan, 1997b; Conger & Dogan, Chapter 17, this volume).

Quality of Parenting

The consensus of many years of research on infant and child socialization clearly reveals the importance of quality of parenting. Attachment theory emphasizes the influence of sensitive and responsive parenting on the qualities of parent–infant, parent–child, and parent–adolescent relationships (Cassidy & Shaver, 1999). Baumrind (1967, 1971, 1973) and others have emphasized the importance of a parenting style that combines high parental warmth, communication, and control (Parke & Buriel, 1998). Others have suggested the importance of parental ability to monitor child and adolescent activities (Patterson & Fisher, 2002). In all these ways and more, children whose parents exemplify more favorable parenting strategies are more likely to develop well (as discussed in several chapters in this volume). Should these aspects of parenting be found to vary across family types, socialization might be expected to confer relative advantages or disadvantages to children living in different family structures.

Family Climate and Stability

Over and above the qualities of parenting by individual parents, the larger family climate is also an important factor in the socialization of infants, children, and adolescents. The role of marital relations—whether harmonious or conflictual—is one factor here; children exposed to a great deal of conflict between their parents are less likely to show positive developmental outcomes (Cummings & Davies, 1994). In addition, the extent to which families are characterized by mutuality, support, and emotional harmony is an important influence on socialization (McHale et al., 2002).

Another factor that appears to be important to socialization efforts is the stability of children's environments (Adam, 2004). Those who have greater numbers of separations from primary caregivers or greater numbers of residential moves are more likely to have problems in adjustment (Adam & Chase-Lansdale, 2002). Multiple residential moves are often associated with school transfers, and these are important stressors for children and adolescents. Residential moves may often be associated with family disruptions, such as separation or divorce of parents, and so they may be markers for other stresses. In all, children and adolescents whose families provide stable environments seem to be at an advantage over those in less stable homes (Wood, Halfon, Scarlata, Newacheck, & Nessim, 1993).

Social Networks

Positive social relationships outside the family are another element of supportive environments for children. The other family members, adult friends, and community members with whom parents have regular contact may support parental socialization efforts (Cochran & Niego, 2002). Support can be *emotional*, bolstering a parent's confidence and providing an outlet for stress, *informational*, giving useful advice about childrearing, or *instrumental*, offering practical assistance (Crockenberg, 1988). Other adults can also act as additional socialization agents for children, through their involvement in child care, provision of social or material resources to children, or status as models of healthy adult social functioning (Cochran & Brassard, 1979).

Supportive social networks benefit both parents and children. Parents with greater social support are less stressed, are more authoritative, and have warmer interactions with their children (Cochran & Niego, 2002). Children of parents who maintain more frequent and satisfying contacts with their social networks themselves have more friends and are more socially competent (Homel, Burns, & Goodnow, 1987; Krantz, Webb, & Andrews, 1984; Markiewicz, Doyle, & Brendgen, 2001). Access to supportive adults through parents' social networks has also been found to protect children from the adverse effects of risk factors as economic hardship (Stanton-Salazar & Spina, 2003; Zimmerman, Bingenheimer, & Notaro, 2002).

Summary

Overall, then, children's access to physical resources, high-quality parenting, favorable family climate, reasonable stability, and supportive extrafamilial social networks are important resources for socialization. These resources are not necessarily independent factors. Many vary with family income, so that children growing up in poverty receive less of everything. On the other hand, not all children or adolescents from affluent families are well adjusted, and important resources (e.g., parental attention) may be in short supply for some children from wealthy homes (Luthar & Latendresse, 2005). What may matter most for socialization of positive development is access to sufficient physical, psychological and social resources to offset whatever ill effects are incurred through deficiencies in some resources or occurrences of other risk factors.

DIVERSE FAMILY STRUCTURES AND THE SOCIALIZATION OF CHILDREN

We now consider research on socialization in various nontraditional families from the standpoint of the family resources and processes outlined previously. We begin by examining never-married one-parent families, then explore research on unmarried two-parent heterosexual parent families, families formed using assisted reproductive technologies, lesbian and gay parented families, and custodial grandparent families. In each case, we assess research findings to determine how the family structure in question fares in terms of the resources and processes outlined earlier, as well as in terms of socialization outcomes.

Never-Married, Mother-Headed, One-Parent Families

Single-parent families are a sizable and diverse group in the United States today (Weinraub et al., 2002). In addition to those who become single parents after divorce, many single parents have never been married. More than a third of births in the United States were to unmarried women in 2003—more than 1 million babies (Martin, Kochanek, Strobino, Guyer, & MacDornan, 2005). Some never-married mothers are single professional women who decided to have children in their 30s, but the largest number are unmarried adolescent mothers (Martin et al., 2005). These figures vary widely across countries, though. For example, approximately 25% of live births in Canada in 2003 were to unmarried mothers, and less than 20% of these were to teenage mothers (Statistics Canada, 2005). Internationally, it is likely that differences in sex education, access to methods of contraception and terminating pregnancy ("morning-after" pill; abortion), and attitudes about premarital sex all impact the relative proportions of single adolescent and adult women who give birth. Regardless of such percentages, though, the experiences of children born to single adolescent mothers compared to single adult mothers can be extremely different.

Young single mothers face many challenges. Coming, as they most often do, from backgrounds that are educationally and economically disadvantaged, these young mothers face tasks of establishing personal identities, preparing for adulthood, and becoming parents all at the same time (Weinraub et al., 2002). This pattern is especially common among African American adolescents; as we discuss later, these young women often establish residence with their own mothers, who may help in the rearing of children (Smith & Drew, 2002). Because these families often have limited economic resources, they are likely to have access only to less desirable housing, in neighborhoods that may be characterized by violence and other environmental hazards. Parents facing economic hardship also have been found to be more likely than others to act in punitive ways with their children (Hanson, McLanahan, & Thomson, 1997). Given the multiple disadvantages of these families, it is not surprising that their children often experience many problems (McLanahan & Sandefur, 1994; Weinraub et al., 2002).

The fastest growing group of unmarried mothers are employed, college-educated women in their 30s who have become parents without the benefit of marriage (Bachu, 1998). Due to greater educational and employment opportunities for women, to declining stigma associated with single parenthood, and to delayed childbearing, single parenthood has increased dramatically among women in managerial and professional occupations (Weinraub et al., 2002). Research on this group is still somewhat limited, but available results paint a very different picture for children than the one just presented for younger single mothers.

In one study of children reared by older unmarried mothers versus same-age married couples, Weinraub and her colleagues reported that the women had middle-class incomes and were able to provide food, shelter, and many other opportunities for their children. Weinraub and colleagues reported that when levels of stress were relatively low, 8- to 13-year-olds from single and matched two-parent families were equally well adjusted (Gringlas & Weinraub, 1995). When families had experienced many stressful life events, however, children of single parents showed more behavior problems than did those from low-stress one-parent or from two-parent homes (Weinraub et al., 2002). Thus, under difficult circumstances, children of single mothers—even single mothers with many resources—were more vulnerable. Most of the time, however, when life went smoothly, children of older unmarried mothers were well adjusted.

Social support may help single mothers meet the challenges of parenting. Single mothers with young children showed more optimal parenting when they felt that they had more social support (Weinraub & Wolf, 1983, 1987). However, they also felt that they received less social support than mothers in two-parent families. A program designed to strengthen the social networks of low-income mothers with preschool-age children showed that as European American single mothers built larger and closer networks of nonkin friends, the mothers felt greater confidence in their parenting and were more active in preparing their children for school (Cochran, 1991). African American single mothers with strong social connections with relatives and nonkin adults were more engaged with their children. Overall, these studies indicate that social support is associated with better quality parenting at least as strongly for single parents as it is for other family types (Cochran & Niego, 2002; Weinraub et al., 2002).

Resource issues are thus crucial to the parenting issues of single-mother families. For families with few economic resources and little social support, many difficulties arise. For single mothers whose economic resources allow them to provide for children's needs and to offer stimulating opportunities as well, outcomes may be very different. Even in these affluent families, however, and even in the best of times, there is only one parent to talk over problems or help with homework. In stressful circumstances, parental resources may be overwhelmed sooner than in cases in which two parents are involved; and, when this happens, children of single parents are likely to have adjustment problems. Although the research findings are still somewhat limited, the most important explanatory factors appear to be available resources and the qualities of family interactions, rather than the nature of the family structure itself (Hanson et al., 1997; McLanahan & Sandefur, 1994).

Single-Father Families

Although there are far fewer single fathers than single mothers, and fewer studies of single-father families, the number of single-father families is growing (Weinraub et al., 2002). Higher rates of adoption by single men and custody awards to men following divorce and family dissolution are contributing to this social change. Some studies suggest that the socialization by single fathers and single mothers is similar. For example, they have both been found to be more permissive than mothers and fathers in two-parent families (Dornbusch & Gray, 1998).

Compared to single mothers, single fathers have more economic resources, feel more confident, have more authority over their children, and are more positively engaged with children (Hilton & Devall, 1998). Some studies find no difference in the well-being of elementary school age children living in single-father, single-mother, and two-parent families (Hilton, Desrochers, & Devall, 2001; Schnayer & Orr, 1989). However, one study found that daughters of single fathers showed more adjustment difficulties than girls in other family types, including decreased sociability and increased neediness, whereas sons of single fathers did not differ in social competence from their peers (Santrock, Warshak, & Elliott, 1982), suggesting the possibility of gender differences in children's responses to being raised by single fathers.

Like single-mother families, single-father families tend to have fewer economic resources than two-parent families (Meyer & Garasky, 1993). Single fathers who obtained custody after divorce receive more offers of informational and instrumental support from their social networks than newly divorced single mothers (Weinraub et al., 2002), although they may not use the support that is offered. Overall, the limited amount of research available suggests that many of the socialization processes and experiences affecting single-mother families also pertain to single-father families, although clearly more work in this area is needed.

Unmarried Heterosexual Two-Parent Families

Increasing numbers of cohabiting heterosexual couples are choosing to conceive, bear, and rear children within the context of unmarried two-parent families (Cancian & Reed, 2001; Ermisch, 2001). Until recently, little empirical attention had been devoted to child development or parenting practices in this family structure. Even now, there have been only a few studies.

A number of factors associated with problematic socialization have been found to characterize unmarried two-parent families more often than married families. Cohabitating parents, on average, have fewer economic resources than do married couples (McLanahan & Teitler, 1999). Satisfaction with the couple relationship tends to be lower (Nock, 1995), and the stability of unmarried relationships is also lower. Thus, it is not surprising that cohabiting couples separate earlier and more often than do married couples (DeMaris & Rao, 1992; Lillard, Brien, & Waite, 1995). Having a child is associated with greater stability of unmarried couples' relationship (Wu, 1995), especially if the child is conceived within the relationship (Manning, 2004), although this may mean that more committed cohabiting couples are more likely to choose parenthood.

A few recent studies indicate that, compared to married heterosexual two-parent families, children and parents in unmarried heterosexual two-parent families are more likely to manifest difficulties. Examining data from the NICHD Study of Early Child Care, Aronson and Huston (2004) found that infants and mothers in cohabiting relationships were more similar to their counterparts in single-mother families than to those in married two-parent families. Cohabiting mothers were less attentive and positive toward their infants and provided less structured and stimulating home environments than did married mothers. Infants of cohabiting mothers were less positive and less securely attached. Mothers in unmarried families were younger and less educated than mothers in married families, and unmarried families had fewer economic resources. These contextual factors did not account for differences in parenting or infant measures, however. The quality of the partner relationship did, however, mediate the relation of family structure with parenting: The less optimal parenting of unmarried mothers was attributable to lower intimacy, support, and satisfaction they felt with their partner.

Studies with older children and adolescents have shown that compared to children of married heterosexual parents, children of unmarried but cohabiting heterosexual parents experience more academic problems, achieve lower grades, and have more behavioral problems (Brown, 2004; Duniform & Kowaleski-Jones, 2002; Thompson, Hanson, & McLanahan, 1994). Although unmarried parents of children and youth tend to use less optimal socialization practices than married parents, researchers have not found that the differences in warmth, control, and punishment across family structures account for the differences in children's well-being (Duniform & Kowaleski-Jones, 2002; Thompson et al., 1994). Thus, the associations between children's functioning and living in unmarried two-parent families may be explained by other variables and processes, such as access to resources, quality of parent relationship, and social networks.

It is important to note that most of the research on socialization in unmarried two-parent families has been conducted in the United States, where attitudes about unmarried cohabitation are generally negative. Associations between cohabitation and development may be very different in nations and cultures in which childrearing by unmarried couples is more common and accepted. For example, heterosexual couples in Quebec, Canada, are now more likely to cohabitate than marry, and for over a decade there have been more children born to unmarried heterosexual couples than married heterosexual couples (Institut de la Statistic Québec, 2005). It would be informative to pursue cross-cultural research on variations in the relations between parental marriage versus cohabitation and children's development, depending on the relative prevalence of these two family types within societies.

Families Formed Using Reproductive Technologies

With the advent of *alternative reproductive technologies* (ARTs), many new options are available to couples and other adults who would otherwise experience infertility. Since the birth of Louise Brown, the first "test-tube baby," in 1978, many new choices have emerged (Golombok, MacCallum, & Goodman, 2001). *Donor insemination* (DI) involves the insemination of a woman with sperm from a male donor. The donor may be the husband, may be another man known to the woman, or may remain anonymous. *In vitro fertilization* (IVF) involves the fertilization of egg by sperm in the laboratory, with the resulting embryo transferred to the mother's womb for gestation. *Egg donation* (ED) involves the removal of fertile eggs from the body of a female donor (who may be known or may be anonymous), and fertilization via IVF, with the resulting embryo transferred to the womb of a gestational mother. These techniques are sometimes combined with *surrogacy,* in which a woman (called a surrogate) carries to term a baby that she agrees to give up at birth to be raised by others. Thus, ARTs make possible the birth of children who are genetically linked to both mothers and fathers, to mothers but not fathers, to fathers but not mothers, or to neither parent. Considerable controversy has surrounded medical, legal, and ethical questions about these new practices, but here we focus on issues related to parenting and the development of children who have been conceived using the new reproductive technologies (Golombok & MacCallum, 2003).

How might the children conceived via ART be expected to fare? The expenses involved in pursuing ART can be high, and those who become parents in this way are likely to have economic resources. These people were highly motivated to become parents and were willing to undergo arduous medical procedures in order to do so. Given that they have undergone diagnosis and treatment for infertility, these people are also likely to be older than other parents of same-age children. All these are factors that might make for favorable predictions about the parenting circumstances and skills of those who have formed families using ART.

On the other hand, additional factors seem to suggest that children conceived via ART might have difficulties (Golombok, 2002). For instance, the lack of a genetic link between the child and at least one of the parents might be seen as a cause for concern, especially if it is thought to be related to reduced interest in parenting by the parent who is not biologically linked with the child. Consistent with this idea, Dunn, Davies, O'Connor, and Sturgess (2000) reported that in natural conception heterosexual-parent families, stepparents were less affectionate toward and less supportive of stepchildren than of biological children. If the lack of genetic links between some ART parents and their children results in less warmth and less supportive parenting, this might result in negative outcomes for children conceived via ART.

Research addressing these issues has been extensive in recent years, and normal patterns of socialization among children conceived using ART have been reported (Golombok, 2002). For instance, the European Study of Assisted Reproduction Families (Golombok, Cook, Bish, & Murray, 1995; Golombok et al., 1996) examined the quality of parenting as well as outcomes for children among IVF and DI heterosexual parent families, as well as among heterosexual natural conception families, when their children were between 4 and 8 years of age. This original group of families was recruited in the United Kingdom, but observations from more families were later added to the study from Spain, Italy, and the Netherlands (Golombok et al., 1995; Golombok et al., 1996); because the results revealed no national differences, only the overall results are described here. Measures of the quality of parenting included assessments of maternal warmth, emotional involvement in parenting, and qualities of mother–child and father–child interaction. In addition, parents completed assessments of marital adjustment, parenting stress, anxiety and depression. Assessments of child development included social competence as well as behavior problems.

Results revealed positive patterns of parenting as well as favorable outcomes for children (Golombok et al., 1995; Golombok et al., 1996). Child adjustment, parenting, and marital quality among IVF and DI mothers was similar in most respects to that among mothers who had conceived naturally. Mothers who had used ART reported greater warmth toward and higher emotional involvement with their children than did those who had conceived naturally, and they also reported less parenting stress. ART fathers were reported to interact more with their children than did natural conception fathers. Children were found to have few cognitive or behavior problems and to be functioning well. The qualities of ART children's attachment relationships with parents were no different than those of naturally conceived children. No differences between DI and IVF families were reported. Similar findings come from a study in Taiwan, which found that teachers described IVF mothers as more affectionate than natural conception mothers with their children but otherwise similar (Hahn & DiPietro, 2001). Related studies have also given few if any reasons for concern; most differences between ART and other families favor positive development among the ART offspring (Golombok & MacCallum, 2003).

The authors also conducted a follow-up of these families when the children were 12 years of age (Golombok et al., 2001; Golombok, MacCallum, Goodman, & Rutter, 2002), when possible problems with children's self-esteem and sense of positive identity might be expected to emerge. Golombok et al. (2001; Golombok et al., 2002) reported that both ART parents and their youngsters showed good adjustment. Parents who had conceived children via ART were similar to those who had conceived naturally on measures of psychological adjustment, parenting, and marital relations. Children conceived via ART had scholastic records, peer relations, and emotional development that were not significantly different from those of other children (Golombok et al., 2002). Overall, the data suggested that socialization of children conceived via DI and IVF was proceeding in a typical fashion (Golombok & MacCallum, 2003).

Somewhat less information is available about the development of children conceived using ED, though available data are similar to those just reviewed for children conceived using other forms of ART. Both in early studies (e.g., Raoul-Duval, Bertrand-Servais, Letur-Konirsch, & Frydman, 1994) and in more recent ones (Golombok, Murray, Brinsden, & Abdalla, 1999), results of assessments of parenting were similar to those for natural conception families, except that ED mothers reported less parenting stress. The self-esteem and behavioral adjustment of young children in ED families was similar to that in natural conception families (Golombok et al., 1999).

A pair of recent studies of infants and toddlers conceived via ED, as compared with those who were naturally conceived, confirmed the earlier finding of positive parenting profiles in ED and DI families (Golombok, Lycett, et al., 2004; Golombok, Jadva, Lycett, Murray, & MacCallum, 2005). Mothers who had used ART to conceive infants showed greater emotional involvement with them than did mothers who had conceived naturally but did not differ on personal or marital adjustment (Golombok, Lycett, et al., 2004). When children were 2 years of age, follow-up assessments revealed that there were still no differences in parents' personal or marital adjustment as a function of mode of conception. Mothers who had conceived using ART described feeling greater pleasure in their children and saw their children as more vulnerable than did those who had conceived naturally. No developmental differences among the children were noted (Golombok et al., 2005). A similar study of children up to 8 years of age who had been conceived via ED (Golombok et al., 1999) found that adjustment was also similar to that among naturally conceived children.

Little is yet known about the development during childhood of children born through surrogacy (Golombok & MacCallum, 2003). One study (Golombok, Murray, Jadva, MacCallum, & Lycett, 2004) has compared surrogacy, ED, and natural conception families through the first year of the infant's life. Results showed more favorable psychological adjustment and better adjustment to parenthood among surrogacy than among natural conception families (Golombok, Murray, et al., 2004). No differences in infant temperament were observed, but qualities of parent–infant relationships were more favorable among ART than among natural conception parents. Overall, the little evidence that is available suggests that children of surrogacy are developing in typical ways (Golombok, 2002; Golombok, Murray, et al., 2004).

Successful outcomes among offspring conceived via ART suggest that, at least among the families that have been studied, the desire and ability to parent are not related to biological linkages. The greater resources of the older, financially secure ART parents, as well as their greater than average desire for parenthood, appear to have been important elements in their ability to parent as well as to create harmonious family environments. Thus, it would appear that the financial and psychological resources of these parents have been important elements in their success (Golombok, 2002; Golombok & MacCallum, 2003).

Lesbian- and Gay-Parented Families

Whether through the use of ART, through adoption, or by means of earlier heterosexual marriages, many lesbian women and gay men have become parents (Patterson, 2000, 2002, 2005). For instance, of the same-sex couples who identified themselves on the most recent U.S. Census, 33% of women and 22% of men reported that they were rearing at least one child in their home (Simmons & O'Connell, 2003). Children growing up in gay and lesbian parented homes may live with one parent or two, and they may or may not be biologically linked to the adults who are their parents. These children are genetically related to both parents only in rare cases (e.g., in ART conceptions, when one partner is a genetic parent, and the egg or sperm donor is a biological relative of the other parent). Although laws have changed recently in some countries and states, in much of the Western world, same-sex partners still do not have access to the legal institution of marriage, so most children growing up in lesbian and gay parented households live with unmarried—

and many with never-married—parents (Patterson, in press; Patterson, Fulcher, & Wainright, 2002). In addition, of course, children with same-sex parents do not have the male and female parents prescribed by cultural norms. Thus, lesbian and gay-parented families differ from cultural expectations in a number of ways.

What is the impact on children of growing up with lesbian or gay parents? More than two decades of research on children's self-esteem, academic achievement, behavior, and emotional development has revealed that, for the most part, children with lesbian or gay parents develop in much the same ways that other children do (Hastings et al., 2005; Patterson, 2000, 2002, 2005; Perrin & the Committee on Psychosocial Aspects of Child and Family Health, 2002; Stacey & Biblarz, 2001). For instance, in a recent study conducted in England, Golombok et al. (2003) compared psychological development among 7-year-old children with lesbian mothers to that among same-age children with heterosexual parents from the same communities. Only two differences in parenting emerged as a function of sexual orientation. Lesbian mothers were more likely to report engaging in imaginative play with their children and less likely to report "smacking" (i.e., using corporal punishment with) their children—both differences that might be seen as favoring children in the lesbian mother families. On measures of self-concept, peer relations, conduct, and gender development, however, no significant differences emerged between children with lesbian and heterosexual parents (Golombok et al., 2003).

Particularly notable was Golombok et al.'s (2003) finding of no differences in gender development. Golombok et al. (2003) employed an activities inventory that had been designed specifically to identify variations in children's gendered behavior and characteristics (e.g., interest in playing with jewelry), that had been extensively validated against behavioral observations, and that had good reliability (Golombok & Rust, 1993). Especially given the strengths of this instrument, the fact that gender development scores of children with lesbian and heterosexual parents did not differ was of particular interest. The results are, however, consistent with those from a substantial body of research on children of lesbian mothers (Patterson, 1992, 2000, 2005; Perrin & the Committee on Psychosocial Aspects of Child and Family Health, 2002).

The Golombok et al. (2003) study included single lesbian, coupled lesbian, single heterosexual, and coupled heterosexual parent families in a fully crossed design. Thus, the study allowed not only comparisons focused on parental sexual orientation but also comparisons based on number of parents in the home. These latter comparisons provided an instructive contrast to those based on sexual orientation. Regardless of sexual orientation, single mothers reported significantly more dysfunctional interactions with their children, more severe disputes with them, less enjoyment of motherhood, lower overall quality of parenting, and greater parenting stress than did mothers with partners. Parenting stress was a significant predictor of children's behavioral and socioemotional problems, such that greater stress was associated with more problems. Single mothers did not see their children as experiencing more problems than other children, but teachers identified children of single parents as having more emotional and conduct problems than those growing up in homes with two parents (Golombok et al., 2003). Thus, while parental sexual orientation was unrelated to children's outcomes, increased parenting stress and lower-quality parenting in single-parent families were related to difficulties in children's socioemotional development.

Other studies with older children and adolescents have reported similar results (e.g., Gartrell, Deck, Rodas, Peyser, & Banks, 2005; Gershon, Tschann, & Jemerin, 1999;

Huggins, 1989; O'Connor, 1993; Tasker & Golombok, 1997; Wainright, Russell, & Patterson, 2004; for a review, see Hastings et al., 2005). For example, in their longitudinal study of children born to lesbian mothers, Gartrell et al. (2005) interviewed children and their mothers when the children were 10 years of age. Standardized scores for children's social competence and behavior problems on a maternal interview measure were compared to those for the norming group of same-age schoolchildren in the United States. Results showed that both social competence and conduct of children with lesbian mothers were comparable to that of the children in the norming sample. Although a substantial minority of the children acknowledged having experienced antigay incidents (e.g., other children expressing dislike for nonheterosexual people or activities), most reported speaking up in response to them (Gartrell et al., 2005).

Children's and youths' concerns about, or actual experiences of, discrimination due to the sexual orientation of their gay and lesbian parents is not an uncommon finding (Crosbie-Burnett & Helmbrecht, 1993; Gartrell et al., 2000; Javaid, 1993; Ray & Gregory, 2001; van Dam, 2004). Adolescents with gay and lesbian parents may feel more concern than younger children do about negative peer reactions to their family structure. There appears, however, to be little if any impact of discrimination on the overall well-being of the children and youths of gay and lesbian parents.

A study by Wainright et al. (2004) explored personal, social, and academic development among adolescents (12 to 18 years of age) living with same-sex and opposite-sex parents. The two samples were matched on demographic characteristics and drawn from a national sample (the National Longitudinal Study of Adolescent Health). Adolescents living with same-sex parents were at least as well adjusted as their peers living with opposite-sex parents on psychological well-being (e.g., depression, anxiety, and self-esteem), school outcomes (e.g., grades, trouble in school, and connectedness at school), and family and relationship processes (e.g., perceived care from adults and peers, perceived parental warmth, feelings of neighborhood integration, and perceived autonomy). Among both adolescents living with same-sex and adolescents living with opposite-sex parents, the best predictors of overall adjustment were parent reports of warm, close relationships with their teenage offspring. Thus, not only were adolescents with same-sex parents well adjusted, but familial predictors of adolescent adjustment remained the same, regardless of family structure.

Another finding of interest from the Wainright et al. (2004) study was that there were no differences in adolescents' reports of romantic attractions and behaviors as a function of family structure. Few adolescents reported same-sex attractions, so only opposite-sex romantic relationships were examined. When asked whether they had been involved in a romantic relationship within the past 18 months, 68% of adolescents with same-sex parents and 59% of adolescents with opposite-sex parents reported that they had; the difference was not statistically significant. Results also revealed that equal proportions of adolescents with same- and opposite-sex parents reported having ever engaged in sexual intercourse (34% of each group). Thus, romantic and sexual development of adolescents in the two groups appeared to be comparable.

Tasker and Golombok (1997) interviewed the offspring of divorced lesbian and divorced heterosexual mothers when they were young adults. They found no differences in anxiety or depression, employment histories, age at first intercourse, numbers of sexual relationships, current relationship status, or happiness in current romantic relationship (if any). The young adults with lesbian mothers were no more likely than those with hetero-

sexual mothers to describe themselves as attracted to same-sex romantic or sexual partners. If they were attracted to same-sex partners, the offspring of lesbian mothers were
more likely to say that they would consider acting on their attraction, or that they already
done so. In the end, however, the young adult offspring of lesbian mothers were not more
likely than those of heterosexual mothers to describe themselves as lesbian, gay, or bisexual (Tasker & Golombok, 1997).

This last result is consistent with a substantial body of research showing that the
great majority of children with lesbian and gay parents themselves grow up to be heterosexual (Patterson, 1992, 2000, 2005; Patterson & Chan, 1999; Perrin & the Committee
on Psychosocial Aspects of Child and Family Health, 2002). Thus, for better or worse,
parental sexual orientation seems to have little impact on sexual development. The similarities between children raised by heterosexual parents and children raised by gay and
lesbian parents are striking and may be seen as being at odds with some predictions based
on risk models of developmental psychopathology. Children of gay and lesbian parents
may experience some discrimination and are also at increased risk of living in conditions
of economic hardship. Gay men earn less than heterosexual men with the same education, experience, and occupation who live in the same region (Badgett, 1995), although
differences between lesbian and heterosexual women are less dramatic. Lesbian and gay
couples who become parents after coming out have generally been relatively affluent, but
divorced lesbian and gay parents may have fewer economic resources (Patterson, 2000;
van Dam, 2004). The economic disadvantages of lesbian and gay couples (e.g., lack of access to health insurance through partner's job) might be expected to result in disadvantages for families.

However, gay and lesbian parents also appear to be, on average, effective socialization agents. A number of studies have noted no differences in the socialization attitudes
and behaviors of heterosexual parents compared to gay and lesbian parents (Bos, van
Balen, & van den Boom, 2004; Wainright et al., 2004). When researchers have noted differences, these have generally favored gay and lesbian parents. Compared to heterosexual
parents, lesbian parents in two-parent households are able to identify more potential
child-care problems and generate more solutions to those problems (Flaks, Ficher,
Masterpacqua, & Joseph, 1995), and they report more positive relationships with their
children (Brewaeys, Ponjeart, Van Hall, & Golombok, 1997). Lesbian mothers and gay
fathers are less likely than heterosexual parents to report the use of physical punishment
(Golombok et al., 2003; Johnson & O'Connor, 2001). Gay fathers put more emphasis
than heterosexual fathers on the importance of tradition and security in their decision to
have children, and they are more likely to report using an authoritative parenting style
with their children (Bigner & Jacobsen, 1989a, 1989b).

Family relationships and social support networks also play a role in the positive development of children of gay and lesbian parents. Studies have found that lesbian couples
report sharing household tasks and parenting duties more equally than heterosexual couples, and they report high satisfaction with the quality of their spousal relationships (Bos
et al., 2004; Brewaeys et al., 1997; Patterson, 2002). Similar to the research on single-
mother versus two-parent families, gay fathers who share their home with another supportive adult, including a partner, roommate, or parent, report fewer difficulties with
parenting than single gay fathers (Barrett & Tasker, 2001). Support from social networks
appears to be an important part of the lives of gay and lesbian parents. Younger lesbian
mothers were more likely to use informal social support, such as talking to friends, than

were older lesbian mothers, which could protect the young mothers and their children from some of the risks associated with early parenthood (Bos et al., 2004). Children of lesbian mothers may also benefit from their mothers' social networks. Children who had more frequent contacts with their grandparents or with their lesbian mothers' friends reported less anxiety and greater well-being, compared to children who were less involved in their mothers' social networks (Patterson, Hurt, & Mason, 1998). Thus, as has been observed in families with heterosexual parents, well-functioning family systems and supportive social networks contribute to the adjustment and effective socialization of gay and lesbian parents and to their children's overall positive development despite the presence of social and economic risks.

Favorable development among offspring of lesbian mothers and gay fathers suggests that the desire and ability to parent effectively are not related to parental sexual orientation. Because becoming parents often requires significant efforts on their part, lesbian and gay parents as a group may have greater than average desire for parenthood. Lesbians and gay men are less likely to become parents unintentionally than are heterosexual women and men, and thus it is possible that lesbian and gay parents are more of a self-selected group of individuals with better-than-average potential for appropriate socialization of children. Many lesbian and gay parents who choose to become parents through ART or adoption are able to draw on considerable personal, financial, or social resources, which serve to support their ability to exhibit favorable patterns of parenting. Regardless of parental sexual orientation, single parents typically have fewer resources, feel more stressed by parenting, describe more problematic interactions with their children, and have children who are described by teachers as showing more emotional and behavioral problems at school (Golombok et al., 2003). Overall, these findings suggest that while two parents may often be better than one, access to resources and to social support appear to be more important determinants of socialization outcomes than is parental sexual orientation.

Custodial Grandparent Families

Almost 10% of American children live in a household in which a grandparent is present, and a wide range of experiences is represented in this group (Smith & Drew, 2002). In some families, a grandparent needing help lives with parents and children in the parents' household; in this case, parents are generally offering assistance to a grandparent. In other families, parent and child live in the grandparent's home; in this case, a young or unemployed parent (usually, a mother) and child accept help from a grandparent (usually, a grandmother). Finally, due to issues such as parental death, drug addiction, or incarceration, grandparents may be the sole custodial guardians of their grandchildren.

These diverse types of homes are likely to provide very different environments for children (Smith & Drew, 2002). As an example, custodial grandparents in the United States are more likely than any other grandparents to be living below the official poverty line, to have no health insurance, and to be receiving public assistance (Fields, 2003). Younger African American grandmothers who have not graduated from high school are most likely to take custodial roles with grandchildren. Considering the lack of economic power of these women, the fact that they experience financial problems when required to care for grandchildren cannot be viewed as surprising (Minkler & Fuller-Thompson, 2000). Custodial grandparents are also more likely than other grandparents to feel depressed and to report poor health (Minkler & Fuller-Thompson, 1999, 2001; Minkler, Fuller-Thompson, & Driver, 1997). Grandparents raising grandchildren with special needs are particularly likely to feel distressed (Emick & Hayslip, 1999), probably because the task of caring for such children can easily overwhelm the resources of any family. Although parenting by grandparents has not been studied directly, it seems likely that it may suffer from the kinds of problems that affect other single adults in parenting roles, especially those with few financial or other resources. Thus, even though they share genetic links with the grandparents who rear them, children living in these households face many challenges and are likely to experience many problems of adjustment (Smith & Drew, 2002).

SUMMARY AND CONCLUSIONS

Although cultural norms in the Western world describe only a narrow range of family structures as optimal for childrearing, substantial numbers of children are in fact growing up in other kinds of families. The norms prescribe that children should be reared by heterosexual, married couples who are their genetic parents. In reality, however, many children are being reared by never-married couples, by lesbian and gay couples, by parents to whom they are not genetically linked, by single parents, or by their grandparents (Lamb, 1999a).

What are the socialization outcomes for childrearing in these varied family environments? To address this question, we reviewed research on socialization in families that differ from the cultural norm in one or more ways. In this section, we consider each assumption of the cultural norm in turn and examine the evidence regarding its significance. First, however, the issue of economic resources is discussed as it relates to family structure and to socialization processes.

One finding that emerges clearly from the research literature is that children growing up in economically impoverished families are at greater risk of encountering problems in development. These range from poor nutrition and housing to inadequate access to health care to coercive parenting and family instability. Family economic circumstances are related to children's health, behavior, and educational opportunities, and those whose families have fewer economic resources are likely to suffer on all these counts (Brooks-Gunn & Duncan, 1997a, 1997b).

Economic resources are, of course, unevenly distributed across family structures. Because of long-standing patterns of discrimination (e.g., on gender or racial grounds), some family types generally have fewer resources than others. Thus it can be difficult to avoid attribution of the problems associated with economic issues to various family structures. There have been well-known efforts to separate economic from family structure issues (e.g., McLanahan & Sandefur, 1994), and these have served to underline the importance of economic resources. Overall, though, economic inequalities are not always acknowledged fully in research on family structure.

Of all the cultural prescriptions for the "traditional" family, the one that receives the most powerful support from the available research literature is that children are better off when they have two parents rather than only one. First, two parents together generally have access to greater economic resources than either one alone. They may also have more extensive social support networks together than either one alone, and they may provide important support and encouragement for one another. It is clear that some single parents—especially those with considerable economic resources—arrange family life in ways that support positive socialization, but this is more difficult for a lone parent than for two parents working closely together. Other things being equal, two parents are usually better than one.

Does it benefit children if their parents are married? Looking first at heterosexual couples who have access to civil marriage, the evidence suggests that children of married parents show better adjustment. Even though there is an association between marriage and children's adjustment, the reasons or mechanisms for this link are far from clear. Does marriage favor children because of the differences between parents who do or do not marry? Because of the economic and social benefits that flow from marriage? Because of the added family stability that comes with marriage? Or are the benefits of marriage for children due to some combination of these and other factors? We know that those who choose to marry differ in some ways from those who do not (see Arnett, Chapter 8, this volume), and we know that many economic, social, and health benefits are associated with marriage (General Accounting Office, 1997; Horwitz, White, & Howell-White, 1996; Horwitz & White, 1998; Schoenborn, 2004). How important each of these elements may be for children's socialization, however, is not yet known.

For same-sex couples rearing children, the issues regarding marriage have been, and in many jurisdictions continue to be, different. Until recently, no same-sex couples had access to the institution of civil marriage. Thus, the selection factors that apply to married versus unmarried heterosexual couples might not be similarly evident in lesbian or gay couples. As same-sex couples begin to gain access to civil marriage (e.g., in Canada, Massachusetts, and some countries in the European Union), the situation in this regard is in flux. It seems likely that the economic and social rewards of marriage will benefit same-sex couples, just as they have benefited opposite-sex couples. For example, both parents would share legal decision-making capacities for their children, and in the event of the death of one parent, inheritance and custody for the second parent would not be issues. Further, to the degree that civil marriage might encourage family stability, it should be expected to benefit children in same-sex parent families.

Although some of the prescriptions of cultural norms have received support from the research on nontraditional families, others clearly have not. First, it is clear from research on ART that genetic links between parents and children are not necessary for favorable socialization outcomes to occur. Studies of families whose children were conceived via DI, ED, IVF, and surrogacy show that positive parenting and favorable child outcomes can occur in the absence of genetic links between parents and children. Although difficulties in socialization may yet be uncovered, results of research to date are not consistent with the idea that genetic linkages are necessary for favorable parenting and socialization.

Similarly, the research findings to date do not support the view that parental sexual orientation is an important factor in the socialization of children. Other things being equal, the offspring of lesbian and gay parents appear to develop in ways that are very similar to the development of those with heterosexual parents. Although many such children acknowledge encounters with antigay sentiments, these do not seem, on average, to have an appreciable impact on their overall development at home or at school. In all, the childrearing behaviors, parenting style, and family management practices of a parent are much more important than parental sexual orientation for children's psychosocial development.

Finally, we come to the issue of gender in parenting and socialization. Our reading of the socialization literature does not support the traditional view that children need both male and female parents in order to develop in positive ways. It may well be true that two parents are often better than one, but that is not relevant to the issues of gender in parenting. When families are headed by heterosexual parents, number and gender of parents are confounded because parents of each gender are required if there are to be two parents. In gay- and lesbian-headed families, in contrast, number and gender of parents are not confounded. As of this writing, data on children reared by gay couples are still sparse, so arguments in this area cannot be advanced with great confidence. In general, however, the successful socialization of children by lesbian couples suggests that parental gender, like parental sexual orientation, may not be as important for socialization as cultural norms might suggest.

Overall, then, the theoretical yield of research on nontraditional families has already been substantial and holds promise of further contributions. While the results of research uphold the importance of some prescriptions, others receive little or no support. The research has revealed fairly robust support for the importance of having two parents and tentative support for the importance of the two parents being married. Traditional expectations about the importance of genetic linkages, parental sexual orientation, and parental gender have not, however, borne up under close scrutiny. Thus, research on nontraditional families has been valuable in evaluating the significance of widely held views about factors that are most important in socialization.

REFERENCES

Adam, E. K. (2004). Beyond quality: Parental and residential stability and children's adjustment. *Current Directions in Psychological Science, 13*, 210–213.

Adam, E. K., & Chase-Lansdale, P. L. (2002). Home sweet home(s): Parental separations, residential moves, and adjustment problems in low-income adolescent girls. *Developmental Psychology, 38*, 792–805.

Alaimo, K., Olson, C. M., Frongello, E. A., Jr., & Breifel, R. R. (2001). Food insufficiency, family income, and health in U. S. preschool and school-aged children. *American Journal of Public Health, 91*, 781–786.

Aronson, S. R., & Huston, A. C. (2004). The mother–infant relationship in single, cohabiting, and married families: A case for marriage? *Journal of Family Psychology, 18*, 5–18.

Bachu, A. (1998). *Trends in marital status of U. S. women at first birth* (Population Division Working Paper No. 20). Washington, DC: U.S. Government Printing Office.

Badgett, M. V. (1995). The wage effects of sexual orientation discrimination. *Industrial and Labor Relations Review, 48*, 726–739.

Barrett, H., & Tasker, F. (2001). Growing up with a gay parent: Views of 101 gay fathers on their sons' and daughters' experiences. *Education and Child Psychology, 18*, 62–77.

Baumrind, D. (1967). Childcare practices anteceding three patterns of preschool behavior. *Genetic Psychology Mongraphs, 75*, 43–88.

Baumrind, D. (1971). Current patterns of parental authority. *Developmental Psychology Monographs, 4* (1, Pt. 2).

Baumrind, D. (1973). The development of instrumental competence through socialization. *Minnesota Symposium on Child Psychology, 7*, 3–46.

Bigner, J. J., & Jacobsen, R. B. (1989a). Parenting behaviors of homosexual and heterosexual fathers. In F.W. Bozett (Ed.). *Homosexuality and the family.* (pp. 173–186). New York: Haworth Press.

Bigner, J. J., & Jacobsen, R. B. (1989b). The value of children to gay and heterosexual fathers. In F. W. Bozett (Ed.). *Homosexuality and the family* (pp. 163–172). New York: Haworth Press.

Bolger, K. E., & Patterson, C. J. (2003). Sequelae of child maltreatment: Vulnerability and resilience. In S. S.

Luthar (Ed.), *Resilience and vulnerability: Adaptation in the context of childhood adversities* (pp.156–181). New York: Cambridge University Press.

Bos, H. M. W., van Balen, F., van den Boom, D., C. (2004). Experiences of parenthood, couple relationship, social support, and child-rearing goals of lesbian mothers families. *Journal of Child Psychology and Psychiatry, 45,* 755–764.

Bradley, R. H. (2002). In M. H. Bornstein (Ed.), *Handbook of parenting: Vol. 2. Biology and ecology of parenting* (pp. 281–314). Mahwah, NJ: Erlbaum.

Bradley, R. H., Corwyn, R. F., McAdoo, H. P., & Garcia Coll, C. (2001). The home environments of children in the United States, Part I: Variations by age, ethnicity, and poverty status. *Child Development, 72,* 1844–1867.

Brewaeys, A., Ponjeart, I., Van Hall, E. V., & Golombok, S. (1997). Donor insemination: Child development and family functioning in lesbian mother families. *Human Reproduction, 12,* 1349–1359.

Brody, G. H., Flor, D. L., & Gibson, N. M. (1999). Linking maternal efficacy beliefs, developmental goals, parenting practices, and child competence in rural single-parent African American families. *Child Development, 70,* 1197–1208.

Bronfenbrenner, U. (1989). Ecological systems theory. *Annals of Child Development, 6,* 187–250.

Brooks-Gunn, J., & Duncan, G. J. (1997a). The effects of poverty on children. *Future of children, 7,* 58–69.

Brooks-Gunn, J., & Duncan, G. J. (Eds.). (1997b). *Consequences of growing up poor.* New York: Russell Sage.

Brown, S. L. (2004). Family structure and child well-being: The significance of parental cohabitation. *Journal of Marriage and Family, 66,* 351–367.

Burbach, A. D., Fox, R. A., & Nicholson, B.C. (2004). Challenging behaviors in young children: The father's role. *Journal of Genetic Psychology, 165,* 169–183.

Cancian, M., & Reed, D. (2001). Changes in family structure: Implications for poverty and related policy. In S. Danziger & R. Haveman (Eds.), *Understanding poverty in America: Progress and problems* (pp. 69–97). New York: Harvard University Press.

Cassidy, J., & Shaver, P. R. (Eds.). (1999). *Handbook of attachment: Theory, research, and clinical applications.* New York: Guilford Press.

Clarke-Stewart, K. A., & Allhusen, V. D. (2002). Nonparental caregiving. In M. H. Bornstein (Ed.), *Handbook of parenting: Vol. 3. Being and becoming a parent* (pp. 215–252). Mahwah, NJ: Erlbaum.

Cochran, M. (1991). Personal social networks as a focus of support. In D. Unger & D. Powell (Eds.), *Families as nurturing systems* (pp. 45–68). New York: Haworth Press.

Cochran, M., & Brassard, J. (1979). Child development and personal social networks. *Child Development, 50,* 609–615.

Cochran, M., & Niego, S. (2002). Parenting and social networks. In M.H. Bornstein (Ed.), *Handbook of parenting: Vol. 4. Social conditions and applied parenting* (2nd ed., pp. 123–148). Mahwah, NJ: Erlbaum.

Cox, M. J., & Paley, B. (1997). Families as systems. *Annual Review of Psychology, 48,* 243–267.

Crockenberg, S. (1988). Social support and parenting. In W. Fitzgerald, B. Lester, & M. Yogman (Eds.), *Research on support for parents and infants in the postnatal period* (pp. 67–92). New York: Ablex.

Crosbie-Burnett, M., & Helmbrecht, L. (1993). A descriptive empirical study of gay male stepfamilies. *Family Relations, 42,* 256–262.

Cummings, E. M., & Davies, P. (1994). *Children and marital conflict: The impact of family dispute and resolution.* New York: Guilford Press.

DeGarmo, D. S., Forgatch, M. S., & Martinez, C. R. (1999). Parenting of divorced mothers as a link between social status and boys academic outcomes: Unpacking the effects of socioeconomic status. *Child Development, 70,* 1231–1245.

DeMaris, A., & Rao, V. (1992). Premarital cohabitation and subsequent marital stability in the United States: A reassessment. *Journal of Marriage and the Family, 54,* 178–190.

Dornbusch, S. M., & Gray, K. D. (1988). Single-parent families: Perspectives on marriage and the family. In M.H. Strober & Dornbusch, S. M. (Eds), *Feminism, children, and the new families* (pp. 274–296). New York: Guilford Press.

Duniform, R., & Kowaleski-Jones, L. (2002). Who's in the house? Race differences in cohabitation, single parenthood, and child development. *Child Development, 73(4),* 1249–1264.

Dunn, J., Davies, L. C., O'Connor, T. G., & Sturgess, W. (2000). Parents' and partners' life course and family experiences: Links with parent–child relationships in different family settings. *Journal of Child Psychology and Psychiatry, 41,* 955–968.

Emick, M. A., & Hayslip, B. (1999). Custodial grandparenting: Stresses, coping skills, and relationships with grandchildren. *International Journal of Aging and Human Development, 48*, 35–61.

Ermisch, J. (2001). Cohabitation and childbearing outside of marriage in Britain. In B. Wolfe & L. L. Wu (Eds.), *Out of wedlock: Causes and consequences of nonmarital fertility,* (pp. 109–139). New York: Russell Sage.

Fields, J. M., Smith, K., Bass, L. E., & Lugalia, T. (2001). *A child's day: Home, school and play (selected indicators of child well-being)* (Current Population Reports P70–68). Washington, DC: U.S. Census Bureau.

Flaks, D. K., Ficher, I., Masterpasqua, F., & Joseph, G. (1995). Lesbians choosing motherhood: A comparative study of lesbian and heterosexual parents and their children. *Developmental Psychology, 31*, 105–114.

Freud, S. (1938). *An outline of psychoanalysis* (J. Strachey, Trans). London: Hogarth Press.

Gartrell, N., Banks., A., Reeds. N., Hamilton, J., Rodas, C., & Deck, A. (2000). The national lesbian family study: 3. Interviews with mothers of five-year-olds. *American Journal of Orthopsychiatry, 70*, 542–548.

Gartrell, N., Deck, A., Rodas, C., Peyser, H., & Banks, A. (2005). The National Lesbian Family Study: 4. Interviews with the 10-year-old children. *American Journal of Orthopsychiatry, 75*, 518–524.

General Accounting Office. (1997). *Tables of laws in the United States Code involving marital status, by category* [On line]. Available: www.gao.gov/archive/1997/og97016.pdf.

Gershon, T. D., Tschann, J. M., & Jemerin, J. M. (1999). Stigmatization, self-esteem, and coping among the adolescent children of lesbian mothers. *Journal of Adolescent Health, 24*, 437–445.

Golombok, S. (2002). Parenting and contemporary reproductive technologies. In M. H. Bornstein (Ed.), *Handbook of parenting: Vol. 3. Being and becoming a parent* (pp. 339–360). Mahwah, NJ: Erlbaum.

Golombok, S., Brewaeys, A., Cook, R., Giavazzi, M. T., Guerra, D., Mantovanni, A., et al. (1996). The European study of assisted reproduction families. *Human Reproduction, 11*, 2324–2331.

Golombok, S., Cook, R., Bish, A., & Murray, C. (1995). Families created by the new reproductive technologies: Quality of parenting and social and emotional development of the children. *Child Development, 66*, 285–298.

Golombok, S., Jadva, V., Lycett, E., Murray, C., & MacCallum, F. (2005). Families created by gamete donation: Follow-up at age 2. *Human Reproduction, 20*, 286–293.

Golombok, S., Lycett, E., MacCallum, F., Jadva, V., Murray, C., Rust, J., et al. (2004). Parenting infants conceived by gamete donation. *Journal of Family Psychology, 18*, 443–452.

Golombok, S., & MacCallum, F. (2003). Outcomes for parents and children following non-traditional conception: What do clinicians need to know? *Journal of Child Psychology and Psychiatry, 44*, 303–315.

Golombok, S., MacCallum, F., & Goodman, E. (2001). The "test-tube" generation: Parent–child relationships and the psychological well-being of *in vitro* fertilization children at adolescence. *Child Development, 72*, 599–608.

Golombok, S., MacCallum, F., Goodman, E., & Rutter, M. (2002). Families with children conceived by donor insemination: A follow-up at age twelve. *Child Development, 73*, 952–968.

Golombok, S., Murray, C., Brinsden, P., & Abdalla, H. (1999). Social versus biological parenting: Family functioning and the socioemotional development of children conceived by egg or sperm donation. *Journal of Child Psychology and Psychiatry, 40*, 519–527.

Golombok, S., Murray, C., Jadva, V., MacCallum, F., & Lycett, E. (2004). Families created through surrogacy arrangements: Parent–child relationships in the first year of life. *Developmental Psychology, 40*, 400–411.

Golombok, S., Perry, B., Burston, A., Murray, C., Mooney-Somers, J., Stevens, M., et al. (2003). Children with lesbian parents: A community study. *Developmental Psychology, 39*, 20–33.

Golombok, S., & Rust, J. (1993). The Pre-School Activities Inventory: A standardized assessment of gender role in children. *Psychological Assessment, 5*, 131–136.

Gringlas, M., & Weinraub, M. (1995). The more things change: Single parenting revisited. *Journal of Family Issues, 16*, 29–52.

Hahn, C., & DiPietro, J. A. (2001). In vitro fertilization and the family: Quality of parenting, family functioning, and child psychosocial adjustment. *Developmental Psychology, 37*, 37–48.

Hanson, T. L., McLanahan, S., & Thomson, E. (1997). Economic resources, parental practices, and children's well-being. In G. J. Duncan & J. Brooks-Gunn (Eds.), *Consequences of growing up poor* (pp. 190–238). New York: Russell Sage.

Hastings, P. D., Vyncke, J., Sullivan, C., McShane, K. E., Benibgui, M., & Utendale, W. (2005). *Children's development of social competence across family types*. Ottawa, Ontario, Canada: Department of Justice, Canada: Family, Children and Youth Section.

Hay, D. F., & Nash, A. (2002). Social development in different family arrangements. In P. K. Smith & C. H. Hart (Eds.), *Blackwell handbook of childhood social development* (pp. 238–261). Oxford, UK: Blackwell.

Hetherington, E. M., & Stanley-Hagan, M. M. (1999). Stepfamilies. In M. E. Lamb (Ed.), *Parenting and child development in "nontraditional" families* (pp. 137–159). Mahwah, NJ: Erlbaum.

Hilton, J. M., Desrochers, S., & Devall, E. L. (2001). Comparison of role demands, relationships, and child functioning in single-mother, single-father, and intact families. *Journal of Divorce and Remarriage, 35*(1/2), 29–56.

Hilton, J. M., & Devall, E. L. (1998). Comparison of parenting and children's behavior in single-mother, single-father, and intact families. *Journal of Divorce and Remarriage, 29*, 23–54.

Hoff, E., Laursen, B., & Tardif, T. (2002). Socioeconomic status and parenting. In M. H. Bornstein (Ed.), *Handbook of parenting: Vol. 4. Social conditions and applied parenting* (pp. 231–251). Mahwah, NJ: Erlbaum.

Homel, R., Burns, A., & Goodnow, J. (1987). Parental social networks and child development. *Journal of Social and Personal Relationships, 4*, 159–177.

Honig, A. S. (2002). Choosing childcare for young children. In M. H. Bornstein (Ed.), *Handbook of parenting: Vol. 5. Practical issues in parenting* (pp. 375–405). Mahwah, NJ: Erlbaum.

Horwitz, A. V., & White, H. R. (1998). The relationship of cohabitation and mental health: A study of a young adult cohort. *Journal of Marriage and the Family, 60*, 505–514.

Horwitz, A. V., White, H. R., & Howell-White, S. (1996). Becoming married and mental health: A longitudinal study of a cohort of young adults. *Journal of Marriage and the Family, 58*, 895–907.

Huggins, S. L. (1989). A comparative study of self-esteem of adolescent children of divorced lesbian mothers and divorced heterosexual mothers. In F. W. Bozett (Ed.), *Homosexuality and the family* (pp. 123–135). New York: Harrington Park Press.

Institut de la Statistic Québec (2005). *Conjugal life of the parents*. Gouvernement du Québec, Canada: Québec, QC: Available: www.stat.gouv.qc.ca/donstat/societe/demographie/naisn_deces/naissance/410.htm.

Javaid, G. A. (1993). The children of homosexual and heterosexual single mothers. *Child Psychiatry and Human Development, 23*, 235–249.

Johnson, S. M., & O'Connor, E. (2001). *Lesbian and gay parents: The national gay and lesbian family study* (APA Workshop 2). San Francisco: American Psychiatric Association Press.

Krantz, M., Webb, S. D., & Andrews, D. (1984). The relationship between child and parental social competence. *The Journal of Psychology, 188*, 51–56.

Lamb, M. E. (Ed.). (1999a). *Parenting and child development in "nontraditional" families*. Mahwah, NJ: Erlbaum.

Lamb, M. E. (1999b). Parental behavior, family processes, and child development in nontraditional and traditionally understudied families. In M. E. Lamb (Ed.), *Parenting and child development in "nontraditional" families* (pp. 1–14). Mahwah, NJ: Erlbaum.

Lillard, L. A., Brien, M. J., & Waite, L. J. (1995). Premarital cohabitation and subsequent marital dissolution: A matter of self-selection? *Demography, 32*, 437–457.

Luthar, S. S., & Latendresse, S. J. (2005). Children of the affluent: Challenges to well-being. *Current Directions in Psychological Science, 14*, 49–53.

Magnuson, K. A., & Duncan, G. J. (2002). Parents in poverty. In M. H. Bornstein (Ed), *Handbook of parenting: Vol. 4. Social conditions and applied parenting* (2nd ed., pp. 95–121). Mahwah, NJ: Erlbaum.

Manning, W. D. (2004). Children and the stability of cohabiting couples. *Journal of Marriage and Family, 66*, 674–689.

Markiewicz, D., Doyle, A. B., & Brendgen, M. (2001). The quality of adolescents' friendships: Associations with mothers' interpersonal relationships, attachment to parents and friends, and prosocial behaviours. *Journal of Adolescence, 24*, 429–445.

Martin, J., Kochanek, K. D., Strobino, D. M., Guyer, B., & MacDornan, M. F. (2005). Annual summary of vital statistics—2003. *Pediatrics, 115*, 619–634.

McHale, J., Khazan, I., Erera, P., Rotman, T., De Courcey, W., & McConnell, M. (2002). Coparenting in diverse family systems. In M. H. Bornstein (Ed.), *Handbook of parenting: Vol. 3. Being and becoming a parent* (pp. 75–107). Mahwah, NJ: Erlbaum.

McLanahan, S., & Sandefur, G. (1994). *Growing up with a single parent: What hurts, what helps?* Cambridge, MA: Harvard University Press.

McLanahan, S., & Teitler, J. (1999). The consequences of father absence. In M. E. Lamb (Ed.), *Parenting and child development in "nontraditional" families* (pp. 83–102). Mahwah, NJ: Erlbaum.

Meyer, D. R., & Garasky, S. (1993). Custodial fathers: Myths, realities and child support policies. *Journal of Marriage and the Family, 55,* 73–89.

Minkler, M., & Fuller-Thompson, E. (1999). The health of grandparents raising grandchildren: Results of a national study. *American Journal of Public Health, 89,* 1384–1389.

Minkler, M., & Fuller-Thompson, E. (2000). Second time around parenting: Factors predictive of grandparents becoming caregivers for their grandchildren. *International Journal of Aging and Human Development, 50,* 185–200.

Minkler, M., & Fuller-Thompson, E. (2001). Physical and mental health status of American grandparents providing extensive child care to their grandchildren. *Journal of the American Medical Women's Association, 56,* 199–205.

Minkler, M., Fuller-Thompson, E., & Driver, D. (1997). Depression in grandparents raising grandchildren: Results of a national longitudinal study. *Archives of Family Medicine, 6,* 445–452.

Nock, S. L. (1995). A comparison of marriages and cohabiting relationships. *Journal of Family Issues, 16*(1), 53–76.

Nordin, J., Rolnick, S., Ehlinger, E., Nelson, A., Arneson, T., Cherney-Stafford, L., et al. (1998). Lead levels in high-risk and low-risk young children in the Minneapolis–St. Paul metropolitan area. *Pediatrics, 101,* 72–76.

O'Connor, A. (1993). Voices from the heart: The developmental impact of a mother's lesbianism on her adolescent children. *Smith College Studies in Social Work, 63,* 281–299.

Offord, D. R., Boyle, M. H., & Jones, B. R. (1987). Psychiatric disorder and poor school performance among welfare children in Ontario. *Canadian Journal of Psychiatry, 32,* 518–525.

Parke, R. D. (2002). Fathers and families. In M. H. Bornstein (Ed.), *Handbook of parenting: Vol. 3. Being and becoming a parent* (pp. 27–73). Mahwah, NJ: Erlbaum.

Parke, R. D., & Buriel, R. (1998). Socialization in the family: Ethnic and ecological perspectives. In N. Eisenberg (Vol. Ed.) & W. Damon (Series Ed.), *Handbook of child psychology: Vol. 3. Social, emotional, and personality development,* (pp. 463–552). New York: Wiley.

Patterson, C. J. (1992). Children of lesbian and gay parents. *Child Development, 63,* 1025–1042.

Patterson, C. J. (2000). Family relationships of lesbians and gay men. *Journal of Marriage and the Family, 62,* 1052–1069.

Patterson, C. J. (2002). Lesbian and gay parenthood. In M. H. Bornstein (Ed.), *Handbook of parenting: Vol. 3. Being and becoming a parent.* (2nd ed., pp. 317–338). Hillsdale, NJ: Erlbaum.

Patterson, C. J. (2005). *Lesbian and gay parents and their children: Summary of research findings.* Washington, DC: American Psychological Association.

Patterson, C. J. (in press). Lesbian and gay family issues in the context of changing legal and social policy environments. In R. M. Perez, K. A. DeBord, & K. J. Bieschke (Eds.), *Handbook of counseling and psychotherapy with lesbian, gay and bisexual clients.* Washington, DC: American Psychological Association.

Patterson, C. J., & Chan, R. W. (1999). Families headed by lesbian and gay parents. In M. E. Lamb (Ed.), *Parenting and child development in "nontraditional" families* (pp. 191–219). Mahwah, NJ: Erlbaum.

Patterson, C. J., Fulcher, M., & Wainright, J. (2002). Children of lesbian and gay parents: Research, law, and policy. In B. L. Bottoms, M. B. Kovera, & B. D. McAuliff (Eds.), *Children, social science and the law* (pp, 176–199). New York: Cambridge University Press.

Patterson, C., Hurt, S., & Mason, C. (1998). Families of the lesbian baby-boom: Children's contact with grandparents and other adults. *American journal of Orthopsychiatry, 68,* 390–399.

Patterson, G. R., & Fisher, P. A. (2002). Recent developments in our understanding of parenting: Bidirectional effects, causal models, and the search for parsimony. In M. H. Bornstein (Ed.), *Handbook of parenting: Vol. 5. Practical issues in parenting* (pp. 59–88). Mahwah, NJ: Erlbaum.

Perrin, E. C., & the Committee on Psychosocial Aspects of Child and Family Health. (2002). Technical Report: Coparent or second-parent adoption by same-sex parents. *Pediatrics, 109,* 341–344.

Raoul-Duvan, A., Bertrand-Servais, M., Letur-Konirsch, H., & Frydman, R. (1994). Psychological follow-up of children born after in-vitro fertilization. *Human Reproduction, 9,* 1097–1101.

Ray, V., & Gregory, R. (2001) School experiences of the children of lesbian and gay parents. *Family Matters, 59,* 28–34.

Ross, D. P., Roberts, P. A., & Scott, K. (1998). Mediating factors in child development outcomes: Children in lone-parent families. *Applied Research Branch Strategic Policy, Human Resources Development Canada.* Hull, QC.

Russell, G. (1999). Primary caregiving fathers. In M. E. Lamb (Ed.), *Parenting and child development in "nontraditional" families* (pp. 57–81). Mahwah, NJ: Erlbaum.

Santrock, J. W., Warshak, R. A., & Elliott, G. L. (1982). Social development and parent–child interaction in father custody and stepmother families. In M. L. Lamb (Ed.), *Nontraditional families* (pp. 289–314). Hillsdale, NJ: Erlbaum.

Schnayer, R., & Orr, R. (1989). A comparison of children living in single-mother and single-father families. *Journal of Divorce, 12,* 171–184.

Schoenborn, C. A. (2004, December 15). *Marital status and health: United States, 1999–2002.* (Advance Data from Vital and Health Statistics, No. 351). Washington, DC: National Center for Health Statistics.

Simmons, T., & O'Connell, M. (2003). *Married-couple and unmarried-partner households: 2000.* Washington, DC: U.S. Bureau of the Census.

Smith, P. K., & Drew, L. M. (2002). Grandparenthood. In M. H. Bornstein (Ed.), *Handbook of parenting: Vol. 3. Being and becoming a parent* (pp. 141–172). Mahwah, NJ: Erlbaum.

Stacey, J., & Biblarz, T. J. (2001). (How) does the sexual orientation of parents matter? *American Sociological Review, 66,* 159–183.

Stanton-Salazar, R. D., & Spina, S. U. (2003). Informal mentors and role models in the lives of urban Mexican-origin adolescents. *Anthropology and Education Quarterly, 34,* 231–254.

Statistics Canada. (2005). *Births 2003.* (Catalogue No. 84F0210XIE). Ottawa, Ontario: Author.

Tasker, F. L., & Golombok, S. (1997). *Growing up in a lesbian family: Effects on child development.* New York: Guilford Press.

Thompson, E., Hanson, T., & McLanahan, S. (1994). Family structure and child well-being: Economic resources vs. parental behaviors. *Social Forces, 73,* 221–242.

van Dam, M. A. (2004). Mothers in two types of lesbian families: Stigma experiences, supports and burdens. *Journal of Family Nursing, 10,* 450–494.

Wainright, J. L., Russell, S. T., & Patterson, C. J. (2004). Psychosocial adjustment, school outcomes, and romantic relationships of adolescents with same-sex parents. *Child Development, 75,* 1886–1898.

Weinraub, M., Horvath, D. L., & Gringlas, M. B. (2002). Single parenthood. In M. H. Bornstein (Ed.), *Handbook of parenting: Vol. 3. Being and becoming a parent* (pp. 109–140). Mahwah, NJ: Erlbaum.

Weinraub, M., & Wolf, B. M. (1983). Effects of stress and social supports on mother–child interactions in single- and two-parent families. *Child Development, 54,* 1297–1311.

Weinraub, M., & Wolf, B. M. (1987). Stressful life events, social supports, and parent–child interactions: Similarities and differences in single-parent and two-parent families. In C. Boukydis (Ed), *Research on support for parents and infants in the postnatal period* (pp. 114–135). Westport, CT: Ablex.

Wood, D., Halfon, N., Scarlata, D., Newacheck, P., & Nessim, S. (1993). Impact of family relocation on children's growth, development, school function, and behavior. *Journal of the American Medical Association, 270,* 1334–1338.

Wu, Z. (1995). The stability of cohabitation relationships: The role of children. *Journal of Marriage and the Family, 57,* 231–236.

Zimmerman, M. A., Bingenheimer, J. B., & Notaro, P. C. (2002). Natural mentors and adolescent resiliency: A study with urban youth. *American Journal of Community Psychology, 30,* 221–243.

PART V

Socialization outside the Family

CHAPTER 14

Peers and Socialization
Effects on Externalizing and Internalizing Problems

WILLIAM M. BUKOWSKI, MARA BRENDGEN, and FRANK VITARO

Consider the following three examples, one from empirical research, one from popular culture, and one from personal history.

1. In an empirical study of coping and well-being during the school-age years, boys and girls were asked to identify the experience that was most likely to cause them to be "stressed." By far, the modal response was being rejected by one's peers.
2. In *Castaway*, a favorite film of critics and the mass audience, the character played by Tom Hanks finds himself washed up on a desert island following a plane crash. He has hardly anything useful, just a few random items including a volley ball. When he decides to transform the ball into a companion he needed to choose which category of relationship he would assign it to. Instead of choosing spouse, mother, or father, he chooses to refer to it as "friend."
3. At a reception following her wedding, a student of the first author (W. B.) recounted an experience she had had a few days before she was called to the Torah as a *bat mitzvah*. During a meeting with her rabbi, she was asked to identify the two parts of her life that were most important to her. Wanting to impress the rabbi, she immediately replied "God and the Torah." "No!" the wise rabbi exclaimed. "The two parts of your life that are most important to you are your family and your friends." And so it is.

For many children and adolescents, peers are a nearly daily source of many forms of experience. Children find in their peers opportunities for companionship, help, amuse-

---

Each of the three authors contributed equally to this chapter; the authorship order is arbitrary.

ment, intimacy, novelty, instruction, and, alas, challenge, conflict, victimization and rejection. Children who spend 7 or 8 hours each week day in the peer-rich environment of day
care or a school probably spend more time with their peers than with their parents except
on weekends. And when students are at home at night, they often, maybe too often according to some parents, stay in touch with their friends via a range of terrestrial and
wireless communication systems.

Certainly, time spent together cannot be used as an index of whether or how much
children and adolescents influence each other's development. One can, however, turn to a
well-established database to find evidence that peers contribute to children's and adolescents' development in many ways (Rubin, Bukowski, & Parker, 2006). The purpose of
this chapter is to review and comment on the theory and the empirical database related to
the premise that experiences with peers constitute an important socialization domain for
children and adolescents. According to this premise, peers serve an important function in
children's lives and in their socialization beyond companionship. We show that there is
increasing evidence that experiences with peers affect the emotions that children and adolescents experience, how they think about themselves, and how they behave. We show
also that some basic hypotheses about peer relations require more empirical scrutiny than
they have received already.

There have been several large reviews of the literature on peer relations. These reviews written by Hartup (1970, 1983) and others (e.g., Rubin, Bukowski & Parker,
1998, Rubin et al., 2006; Parker & Asher, 1987) have covered a broad set of domains in
which peers appear to influence socialization. These domains include prosocial behavior,
school performance, affect, aggression, the self-concept, and other areas of development.
In this chapter our review is restricted to two broad forms of behavior that have accounted for the lion's share of research on peer relations during the past 25 years, specifically, externalizing problems and internalizing problems.

ORGANIZING THE FEATURES OF PEER RELATIONS

The study of peer relations is not a new domain of developmental psychology. Experiences with peers and their significance for development has been studied for at least a
century (see Rubin et al., 2006). Influenced by ethology and by social psychologists interested in the social mechanisms underlying learning, the study of peers was initially
steeped in observational traditions that emphasized the influence that children had on
each other. In parallel to this interest in influence, there was a concern with the antecedents and consequences of how much a child was liked and disliked by peers. During the
past 25 years the study of peers has grown larger, especially as investigators have recognized the extent to which measures of functioning with peers are related to subsequent
measures of well-being and adjustment.

The term "peer relations" does not refer to one form of experience but instead to
many. These experiences can be organized according to a multilevel model in which
aspects of peer relations can occur at the level of the individual, the dyad, or the group
(Rubin et al., 1998, 2006). This organizational scheme, based largely on the work of
Hinde, claims that phenomena from one level of experience are conceptually and
experientially *interdependent* with phenomena at other levels such that individual,

dyadic, and group variables influence and constrain each other. According to this model the level of the individual refers to the characteristics that children bring with them to their experiences with peers.

Interactions, a form of experience that occurs at the level of the dyad, are believed to be influenced by these individual characteristics, as well as by features of the social situation, such as the partner's characteristics, overtures, and responses. Interactions, in turn, form the basis of relationships. Relationships may take many forms and have properties that are not relevant to interactions. At the same time, the nature of a relationship is defined partly by the characteristics of its members and its constituent interactions, and over the long-term, the kinds of relationships individuals form depend on their history of interactions in earlier relationships. Finally, individual relationships are embedded within *groups*, or networks of relationships with more or less clearly defined boundaries (e.g., cliques, teams, and school classes). Groups are defined by the types and diversity of interactions that are characteristic of the participants in those relationships. Groups are not the same as a mere aggregate of relationships; through emergent properties such as norms or shared cultural conventions, groups help define the type and range of relationships and interactions that are likely or permissible. Further, groups have properties and processes, such as hierarchical organization and cohesiveness that are not relevant to description of children's experiences at lower levels of social complexity.

The interdependency of the phenomena that comprise the peer system places two clear conceptual and methodological demands on persons who study peer relations. First, a central goal of research on peer relations should be the understanding of how the peer system is structured. Following from ideas taken from systems theory (Sameroff, 1983), researchers should show a concern with understanding how the various elements that comprise the peer system are associated with each other. This kind of understanding is a prerequisite for the second goal. Specifically, persons who study peer relations need to comprehend how experiences in the peer system function together as a system as well as to consider how individual experiences affect outcomes and how these effects are moderated by other parts of the system.

THEORY

Dyadic Models

Theoretical models about the contribution of peer relations to socialization emphasize different levels of social complexity. If any level of complexity has been emphasized to the exclusion of others it is probably the level of the dyad. The oldest arguments about the effects of peer relations can be found in psychoanalytic models, especially the writing of Peter Blos. Blos (1967) claimed that the impact of peers would be seen during the adolescent process of individuation wherein adolescents restructure their childhood relationships with their parents and strive to achieve qualitatively different relationships with peers. Blos claimed that at this time of restructuring their relationships with parents, adolescents come to experience turmoil and anxiety accompanied by feelings of despair, worthlessness, discouragement, and vulnerability. According to Blos, adolescents' capacities to cope with these feelings and experiences rest with their ability to establish qualitatively distinct forms of supportive relationships with peers. In the process of separating from parents and prior to achieving a state of personal autonomy, adolescents turn to peers for "stimulation, belongingness, loyalty, devotion, empathy, and resonance" in an effort to regulate their emotions (Blos, 1967, p. 177).

The belief that peer relationships would be most important during adolescence is also seen in the writings of Sullivan (1953). Sullivan proposed that as children enter early adolescence they begin to develop "chumships" or close, intimate mutual relationships with same-sex peers. As a relationship between "co-equals," chumships differ from the hierarchical relationships that children experienced with their parents and from the play-based interactions of childhood. Accordingly, Sullivan argued that this close relationship was a child's first true interpersonal experience of reciprocity and exchange. He proposed that it was within chumships that children had their first opportunities to experience a sense of self-validation. This validation would result from the internalization of the positive regard and care that their chums provided to them. Sullivan went so far as to propose that the positive experiences of having a "chum" in adolescence would be so powerful as to enable adolescents to overcome trauma that may have resulted from prior family experiences. Conversely, Sullivan believed that the experience of being isolated from the group, during the juvenile period, would lead a child to have concerns about his or her own competencies and his or her acceptability as a desirable peer. Consequently, Sullivan suggested that children who are unable to establish a position within the peer group would develop feelings of inferiority that could contribute to a sense of psychological distress. One posited outcome of the lack of supportive chumships was the development of loneliness, or "the exceedingly unpleasant and driving experience connected with the inadequate discharge of the need for human intimacy" (Sullivan, 1953, p. 290).

To some extent the role of the dyad is apparent in the work of Piaget. Piaget claimed that in contrast to relationships with parents, peer relationships were balanced, were egalitarian, and fell along a more or less horizontal plane of dominance and power assertion. Thus, it was in the peer context that children could experience opportunities to examine conflicting ideas and explanations, to negotiate and discuss multiple perspectives, to decide to compromise with, or to reject, the notions held by peers. In these ways, interactions with peers were an ideal context for the development of social constructs such as those related to moral judgment. The influence of Piaget is seen in the work of coconstructivist thinkers such as Azmitia (Azmitia, Lippman, & Ittel, 1999). These writers introduce the notion that the quality of the relationship between the peers who are interacting with each other may contribute to cognitive and social–cognitive growth and development. Given that friends are more sensitive to each others' needs, and more supportive of each others' thoughts and well-being than nonfriends, it may be that children are more likely to talk openly and challenge each others' thoughts and deeds in the company of friends than nonfriends. Accordingly, these relationships are likely to have unique effects on a child's thoughts and behaviors.

Peers play a role in the theory of Vygotsky also. Whereas Piaget emphasized the effects of conflict between peers, Vygotsky proposed that it was *cooperation* and the discussion of ideas that would promote change. According to Vygotsky, the cooperative coconstruction of social events led to the formation of social constructs. Researchers such as Rogoff (1997) have argued that the child's peers can play the role of coconstructivist and that the pairing of a less mature child with a more competent "expert" peer may facilitate a child's development.

Group Approaches

Theories about the specific processes by which peer groups have their effects have been rare. Nevertheless, at least one well-known theory, social learning theory, has specified specific means by which peers influence each other. Although social learning theory may be more specific in the mechanisms it emphasizes, it takes a more general approach to peer relations than is seen in theories that emphasize the dyad in the sense that it does not refer specifically to one level of complexity to the exclusion of others. The traditional learning theory perspective has been that children are agents of behavior control and behavior change for each other. Peers punish or ignore nonnormative social behavior and reward or reinforce positively those behaviors considered culturally appropriate and competent. Thus, to the extent that children behave in a socially appropriate manner, they develop positive relationships with their peers; to the extent that children behave in a socially incompetent or nonnormative manner, peer rejection may result. According to this view, peer relations are believed to constitute developmental contexts which function as miniature cultures, each with its own norms, expectations, opportunities, and practices. Due to participation in a particular context, one's behavior will change in response to the context's demand characteristics The emphasis on the role of modeling and the reinforcement of norms show how the social behaviors of children are quickly and effectively organized, reorganized, and redirected. Observational learning promotes adaptation to new circumstances and new relationships (Cairns, 1979). As Cairns noted, however, once learned, social behaviors are subject to maintenance and change; thus, it is argued that the demonstration of a socially learned behavior will be maintained or inhibited by its actual or expected consequences.

One theory that explicitly emphasizes experience at the level of group and deemphasizes experiences with friends is the socialization model of Judith Harris (1995). Harris claimed that (1) the effects of parenting on development were, at best, small; (2) the effects of genes on development were strong; and (3) the effect of peer relationships, and especially the peer group, was strong also. Harris's claims about the effects of the peer system were, in part, predicated on the view that young people are driven by an atavistic desire to be part of a group. According to Harris, an important repercussion of these tribal motivations is that young people, in an effort to be part of a group, will change their behavior in response to group norms and expectations. Thus, it was proposed that once children find themselves outside the home, they take on the norms prevalent in the groups within which they spend their time, especially those of other children. Drawing from social psychological perspectives on the significance of group norms (a motivation to "fit in"), ingroup biases and outgroup hostilities, and social cognitive views of group processes, it was argued that children's identities develop primarily from their experiences within the peer group. Although some persons have seen value in some aspects of Harris's point of view, this enthusiasm has been far from universal (see Collins, Maccoby, Steinberg, Hetherington, & Bornstein, 2000).

In summary, theories about peer relations have emphasized different levels of analysis. Whereas Sullivan and others have emphasized the dyad, theorists such as Harris have directed attention to experiences in groups per se. Regardless of which aspect of peer relations a theory emphasizes, however, each is aimed at trying to explain some feature of development. In the next two sections we review what is known about peer relations and two broad domains of outcome, specifically, externalizing and internalizing behaviors. In this review we expand on the theoretical issues that have been raised in this section as well as refer to the large empirical data base regarding peers and socialization.

PEERS AND EXTERNALIZING BEHAVIORS

This section covers the links between difficulties in peer interactions and children's/ adolescents' externalizing problems. For practical purposes, externalizing problems are limited to aggressive/antisocial/delinquent behaviors, although substance use and school difficulties are occasionally included to illustrate the negative effects of peer difficulties. The section is divided into two parts. The first part focuses on peer rejection whereas the second part covers affiliation with peers and friends from either the mainstream or deviant groups. Within each part, variables and processes that contribute to peer rejection or to affiliation with mainstream or deviant peers are examined first, followed by discussion of the consequences of peer rejection or affiliation with mainstream or deviant peers. Finally, the factors that might moderate or mediate the impact of peer rejection or the influence of mainstream or deviant peers are also explored. Throughout this section, as throughout the chapter, a developmental perspective is adopted. In consequence, longitudinal studies were preferred over cross-sectional studies whenever possible because of their potential to help disentangle the directionality of the links between peer rejection/ affiliation with deviant peers, on one hand, and externalizing problems, on the other hand, and because of their potential to control for confounding factors. Similarly, studies that collected data directly from the peer group (for rejection) or from friends or clique members (for friends' and cliques' characteristics) were preferred over studies that used teachers to assess children's rejection by their peers or studies in which the participants themselves were the only informants to report on their friends' externalizing behaviors.

Variables and Processes Contributing to Peer Rejection

More than 20 years ago, researchers (e.g., Coie & Kupersmidt, 1983) assembled unacquainted children and assessed their emerging peer status. Verbal and physical aggression was shown to precede the emergence of peer rejection, which suggested that aggressive behaviors could be considered a proximal determinant of peer rejection (see Coie, 1990). Studies that distinguished stable from transient peer rejection and studies that established trajectories of peer acceptance during childhood also concluded that externalizing problems (especially aggression and low prosociality) predicted stable (vs. transient) peer rejection (Vitaro, Tremblay, Gagnon, & Boivin, 1992) or chronic low peer acceptance (Brendgen, Markiewicz, Doyle, & Bukowski, 2001). However, Dodge, Coie, Pettit, and Price (1990) found that this conclusion may depend on the children's age and the types of aggressive behavior considered. In their study, angry reactive aggression and instrumental (i.e., proactive object-oriented) aggression, but not rough play, were associated with peer rejection for both grade 1 and grade 3 children. However, bullying (i.e., proactive person-oriented aggression) was positively related to peer rejection in grade 3 children but negatively related in grade 1 children. In other words, in grade 1, the children who manifested the most bullying were the least rejected by their peers, as if bullying was an accepted means to achieve dominance in the peer group at that young age. The link between aggressiveness and rejection may also depend on the base rate of aggressive behaviors in the peer group and on the social norms about the acceptability of aggression. Hence, a positive relationship between aggressive behaviors and peer popularity can be found in groups in which the norms toward the use of aggression are positive (Chang, 2004). In sum, in most but not all conditions, externalizing problems lead to peer rejection, which, in turn, leads to an increase in externalizing problems, as discussed next.

Consequences of Peer Rejection for Externalizing Problems

There is substantial evidence suggesting that peer rejection is associated with later aggressive/ antisocial/delinquent behaviors as well as other psychopathological problems (see Deater-Deckard, 2001, for a review). However, theorists and researchers continue to disagree on the precise role of peer rejection in the developmental sequence of these problems. Three theoretical models have been proposed to account for the possible role of peer rejection (i.e., low peer acceptance) with respect to later externalizing outcomes. According to the *incidental model*, low peer acceptance is a by-product of children's behavior problems, which serve as the true determinants of later adjustment problems. That is, rejection by peers is seen as an indicator of children's behavior problems but does not contribute on its own to later development: Both peer rejection and later adjustment problems are believed to stem from the same underlying personal difficulty. (This is also called the "common cause" model or the "behavior-continuity" model for this reason; Caspi, Elder, & Bem, 1987.) Controlling for concurrent or antecedent problems should eliminate the links between peer rejection and externalizing adjustment problems. Conversely, according to the *causal model*, peer rejection independently and uniquely contributes to the development of externalizing problems above and beyond children's behavioral dispositions. One version of this model actually views peer rejection as a possible mediator of the link between children's earlier behavior problems and later adjustment problems. Another version views peer rejection as a unique experience that might contribute on its own to later externalizing problems, above and beyond the behavior problems that predicted it in the first place. The causal model could be expanded into a bidirectional causal model whereby externalizing problems predict peer rejection and peer rejection, in turn, predicts increases in externalizing problems. Finally, the *interactional* or *moderator model* (Bierman & Wargo, 1995) suggests that peer rejection exacerbates the link between children's externalizing problems and later adjustment problems. According to this view, peer rejection plays a moderator role although it may not have a main effect in explaining later externalizing problems.

Empirical evidence supports each of the three theoretical models. In support of the incidental model, there is evidence that the link between peer rejection and later social adjustment problems may be accounted for by underlying behavior problems (Woodward & Fergusson, 1999; Hartup, 1983; Parker & Asher, 1987). For example, in Woodward and Fergusson's (1999) study, peer rejection failed to predict criminal offending and substance use in adolescence after controlling for family risk factors and other characteristics of the child, such as cognitive ability.

In support of the causal model, there are studies showing that peer rejection uniquely predicts later adjustment problems even after controlling for concurrent externalizing problems, particularly when accumulative peer rejection (i.e., rejection by peers for more than 1 year) is considered (Brendgen, Vitaro, & Bukowski, 2000; Deater-Deckard,

Dodge, Bates, & Pettit, 1998; Ladd & Troop-Gordon, 2003). For example, Ladd and Troop-Gordon (2003) showed that the number of years children were rejected by their peers during the first 3 years of primary school predicted later externalizing problems (i.e., teacher-rated aggression and delinquency), above and beyond previous aggressive behaviors (which predicted chronic rejection), concurrent peer victimization, and involvement in mutual friendships. Moreover, as argued by Nelson and Dishion (2004), peer rejection during childhood may predict later delinquent-criminal problems at periods during which these problems are declining in most individuals, such as young adulthood. This may help reconcile these results with results from Fergusson and colleagues showing little contribution of peer rejection during childhood to conduct problems assessed by mid-adolescence when these problems tend to peak because some of the delinquents in their study were delinquent only during adolescence. The predictive power of peer rejection with respect to early adulthood outcomes, however, may not be independent from the presence or the absence of friendships. For example, Bagwell, Newcomb, and Bukowski (1998) showed that externalizing problems (i.e., trouble with the law) during early adulthood was predicted only by a combination of peer rejection and absence of mutual friends over 2 consecutive years.

In line with the interactional (or moderator) model, many studies have found that the link between personal dispositions (i.e., aggression) and later externalizing problems was exacerbated for individuals who were also rejected by their peers (Bierman & Wargo, 1995). For example, Dodge et al. (2003) found that peer rejection in kindergarten interacted with early aggression in predicting later aggression. Specifically, children who were initially aggressive and who were also rejected by their peers were most likely to show an increase in their aggressive behavior, compared to rejected classmates who were not initially aggressive. This effect was particularly true for children who were high on reactive but not on proactive aggression and for girls. However, there are also studies that did not find support for peer rejection as a moderator of the link between childhood aggression and later externalizing problems (Miller-Johnson, Coie, Maumary-Gremaud, Bierman, & Conduct Problems Prevention Group, 2002; Woodward & Fergusson, 1999). For example, Miller-Johnson et al. (2002) showed that peer rejection in grade 1 predicted conduct problems 4 years later independently of children's initial levels of aggression and hyperactivity–inattention.

With respect to potential moderators of the link between early peer rejection and subsequent antisocial behavior, some researchers have concluded that the link appears to be stronger and more consistent across studies for boys than for girls (McDougall, Hymel, Vaillancourt, & Mercer, 2001). As noted by Deater-Deckard (2001) this conclusion may very well be an artifact of the number of studies including only males and of the use of measures that apply more to males than to females. The picture may change as girls are more frequently included in studies of externalizing problems.

Some investigators have noted that the link between low peer acceptance and later adjustment problems may depend on children's age, children's awareness of their rejected status, the importance children place on peer acceptance, local norms for aggressive–antisocial behavior, and ethnicity (McDougall et al., 2001). Finally, there is evidence pointing to the fact that recency of peer rejection may be as important as chronicity. For example, De Rosier, Cillessen, Coie, and Dodge (1994) reported that children rejected over several years had more externalizing (and internalizing) problems than children rejected over 1 year only, even after controlling for early behavior problems. However, children who had been rejected in the recent past also experienced more negative outcomes than other children even if they had not been chronically rejected.

Mediating Links between Peer Rejection and Later Externalizing Problems

Despite suggestions by Parker and Asher (1987), few researchers have examined the process through which peer rejection contributes to the development of externalizing problems or related problems such as substance use or dropping out of school. Also, little attention has been directed to the mechanisms though which peer rejection serves as a catalyst for childhood aggression to lead to heterotypical outcomes. As suggested by Hay, Payne, and Chadwick (2004), peer rejection may increase children's later tendencies to be aggressive because they may become more actively victimized by their peers and, in consequence, develop social–cognitive biases or negative retaliatory emotions against peers. This may be especially true for reactively aggressive children (i.e., those who are aggressive in response to provocation), who are prone to peer rejection in the first place and who as a result lack supportive friendships as a possible buffer or compensation with respect to rejection by the peer group (Dodge et al., 2003; Poulin & Boivin, 2000). In other words, it is likely that peer rejection may exacerbate emotion regulation problems and can distort social–cognitive processes related to aggression that may be implicated in the etiology of rejection in the first place. However, this process may be limited to older children and adolescents as negative beliefs toward peers do not seem to mediate the link between peer rejection and increases in externalizing problems in young children (Ladd & Troop-Gordon, 2003).

Peer rejection may also alter self-perceptions and self-capabilities for achieving positive outcomes (McDougall et al., 2001), although, once more, empirical evidence does not seem to support this suggestion with young children (Ladd & Troop-Gordon, 2003). It also certainly reduces rejected children's opportunities to interact with and learn normative values from conventional peers. Moreover, peer rejection can also decrease school motivation and increase school difficulties, which in turn, may exacerbate or trigger externalizing behaviors (Hymel Comfort, Schonert-Reichl, & McDougall, 1996). As proposed by Furman and Robbins (1985), a unique function of peer acceptance is to provide a sense of inclusion and a source of motivation to participate in activities involving peers. The absence of such feelings may very well drive rejected children away from their normative but rejecting peers and the contexts in which they interact with them, including the school. Alternatively, rejected children may be motivated to affiliate with similarly rejected, and possibly aggressive, peers.

Variables and Processes Leading to Affiliation with Deviant Peers

A basic premise of the argument that experiences with peers influence how children behave and develop is that the characteristics of one's peers matters. As a result, knowing how children become associated with one type of peer rather than another is of great importance to understanding socialization processes among peers. Although generally rejected by conventional peers, many aggressive/antisocial children and adolescents have friends, and most of them participate in cliques (Cairns, Cairns, Neckerman, Gest, & Gariépy, 1988; Pellegrini, Bartini, & Brooks, 1999). Dyadic friendships refer to mutual relationships between two children based on affection, reciprocity, and intimacy. In contrast, peer cliques are cohesive groups of children or adolescents who spend time together. Peer clique participation can be assessed in terms of centrality or degree of association in the group. By extension, gangs are defined as cliques involved in deviant–antisocial behaviors.

On average, aggressive–antisocial adolescents' friends and clique members are more aggressive–antisocial than are the friends of nonaggressive–nonantisocial adolescents (Cairns et al., 1988). Some researchers showed that homophily (i.e., the tendency for children and adolescents to affiliate with peers who are similar to themselves) with respect to antisocial behaviors and attitudes is already present in youth even before they actually become friends or clique members (Lahey, Gordon, Loeber, Stouthamer-Loeber, & Farrington, 1999). This seems to be true for preschool children as well as for older children and adolescents, although only a few studies have examined whether homophily with respect to aggression/antisociality exists among young children (Snyder, Horsch, & Childs, 1997).

Dishion, Patterson, and Griesler (1994) proposed the confluence model to account for the coming together of antisocial children and deviant friends. According to this model, the confluence process between deviant children and deviant peers begins by mid-childhood and accelerates thereafter to reach a peak by early adolescence. Some support for the confluence model comes from a study by Vitaro, Brendgen, and Wanner (2005), who found four groups with distinct affiliation profiles with delinquent friends from age 10–13 years: an early affiliative group that already had delinquent friends by age 10, a late affiliative group that started to affiliate with deviant friends by age 12 (i.e., after transition to high school), a desistor group that affiliated with deviant friends early on and desisted by age 12, and, finally, a large group of children who never affiliated with delinquent friends. Interestingly, the proportion of boys was higher in the early affiliative group but not in the late affiliative group. Although these results support the confluence process for at least one group of the children they also reveal more complex patterns of affiliation than is suggested by this model. On the other hand, the existence of a linkage between children's and friends' aggressive/antisocial dispositions already by early childhood poses a challenge to the confluence model with respect to its initiation stage. In sum, similarity in behavioral style seems to serve as the basis for attraction among children and adolescents (Rose, Swenson, & Carlson, 2004). There is evidence also for the converse of homophily: Children tended to be disliked by classmates who were dissimilar to them in behavioral style especially among boys (Nangle, Erdley, Zeff, Stanchfield, & Gold, 2004). Not surprisingly, dissimilarity also seems to play a role in the dissolution of friendships (i.e., deselection) between aggressive children (Poulin & Boivin, 2000).

Rejection by conventional peers has also been found to predict children's association with deviant friends after controlling for children's antisocial behavior and school problems in some studies (Dishion, Patterson, Stoolmiller, & Skinner, 1991; Quinton, Pickles, Maughan, & Rutter, 1993), although other studies have found no such link (Fergusson, Woodward, & Horwood, 1999). The age at which affiliation with deviant peers is measured can partly explain these contradictory results, as illustrated by the work of Dishion and collaborators. These investigators found that peer rejection predicted involvement with deviant peers by early adolescence, in addition to antisocial behavior and academic difficulties (Dishion et al., 1991). However, using the same participants and the same measures, peer rejection did not uniquely predict deviant peer involvement by age 15 anymore (Dishion, Capaldi, Spracklen, & Li, 1995). In consequence, the widely endorsed pathway according to which peer rejection (that follows aggressive behaviors) leads to later delinquent–aggressive behaviors because it fosters affiliation with other aggressive-rejected peers may depend on the time the measures are collected and is yet to be supported empirically (Cairns & Cairns, 1994; Hay et al., 2004; Quinton et al., 1993).

Two theoretical models have been proposed to integrate the available empirical evidence about the process variables leading to affiliation with deviant peers; one model was proposed by Kaplan (Kaplan, Johnson, & Bailey, 1986) and the other by Patterson and colleagues (e.g., Patterson, DeBaryshe, & Ramsey, 1989; Patterson, Reid, & Dishion, 1992). The Kaplan model suggests that poor relationships with valued social agents such as the family or the peer group might lead to feelings of self-rejection and a decrease in children's self-esteem. Because individuals are believed to minimize negative self-views and to maximize positive self-perceptions, they might be less and less motivated to conform to the usually conventional and nondelinquent norms and expectations put forth by the family and normative peers. Instead, in an effort to find alternative sources that will enhance self-esteem, individuals might be increasingly likely to adopt delinquent attitudes and behaviors and to affiliate with other nonnormative, antisocial peers who are similar to themselves and are therefore likely to reinforce the individuals' own antisocial behavior. Thus, a decrease in self-esteem might mediate the relation between the lack of a close affective relationship with parents and youth's subsequent affiliation with delinquent friends. Specifically, the lack of a close relationship with parents might leave youth with low self-esteem, which, in turn, might motivate them to seek the company of delinquent friends for compensatory support.

According to the model proposed by Patterson, Dishion, and colleagues (e.g., Dishion, French & Patterson, 1995; Patterson et al., 1992), it is not so much a poor parent–child relationship but rather poor parenting behavior that is at the root of children's affiliation with antisocial friends. Specifically, maladaptive parenting behavior such as a lack of monitoring or overly harsh punishment, perhaps in reaction to a difficult temperament of the child, is believed to promote aggressive–antisocial behavior in the child. Over time, the child will transfer this aggressive–antisocial disposition from the home to other social environments, such as the school, which then will lead to rejection by the more conventional and better adjusted peers. As in the Kaplan model, the rejected child will eventually try to avoid the environments (i.e., school and home) and people (i.e., conventional peers and adults) that serve as punishment agents and seek social settings and social agents (i.e., deviant friends) that are more supportive of his or her aggressive–antisocial characteristics. As such, although the two theoretical models describe slightly different antecedent pathways, both emphasize two final processes that lead to affiliation with deviant friends, namely, (1) selection based on peer rejection and as a consequence of limited access to conventional peers as friends, and (2) selection based on similarity in attitudes and behaviors (i.e., homophily).

Consequences of Affiliating with Aggressive–Antisocial Peers

Whatever the reason for selecting deviant friends in the first place, there is substantial empirical evidence supporting the negative influence of deviant peers. Several researchers have shown that association with deviant peers at the dyadic level (i.e., one a one-to-one basis) is related to more externalizing problems (Kim, Hetherington, & Reiss, 1999; Simons, Chao, Conger, & Elder, 2001). Other researchers have found that deviant peer associations mediate the links between low self-esteem or rejection by conventional peers and rates of change in problem behaviors (Hymel et al., 1996). Studies examining the influence of deviant friends at the clique level reveal similar results. For example, Keenan, Loeber, Zhang, and Stouthamer-Loeber (1995) found that exposure to deviant peers resulted in subsequent engagement in delinquent behavior for previously nondelinquent male adolescents. Finally, Battin, Hill, Abbott, Catalano, and Hawkins (1998) found that belonging to a deviant clique (i.e., a gang) predicted self-reported and officially recorded delinquency beyond the effects of having delinquent friends and prior delinquency. Similarly, Lacourse, Nagin, Tremblay, Vitaro, and Claes (2003), using a longitudinal person-centered approach, found that being involved in a delinquent group at any specific time during adolescence was associated with an increase in violent behaviors, and that leaving these groups resulted in a decrease in violent behaviors.

Context effects appear to be important also. Most studies examine the effect of deviant peers (friends or clique members) at school and often in the classroom. This is a reasonable strategy because classroom-based studies and school-based studies capture most of the friendships and clique memberships during childhood and early adolescence, respectively (Ennett & Bauman, 1994). However, there is also growing evidence that peers outside school may be important, especially for unpopular children/adolescents who tend to have more friends outside school than well-accepted classmates (George & Hartmann, 1996). For example, Kiesner, Poulin, and Nicotra (2003) showed that being involved in an after-school peer network was concurrently related to externalizing problems (i.e., in-school behavior problems and out-of-school delinquency) above and beyond being involved in an in-school peer network. However, the peers who are part of a child's in-school and the child's out-of-school cliques (i.e., the conjoint peers) seem to be the most influential over a 1-year interval on physical aggression and violence in and outside school (Kerr, Stattin, & Kiesner, 2004). Stattin and collaborators also showed that associations with deviant peers outside the school seem to play important roles not well captured in school-based studies. Specifically, these investigators reported that attending unstructured and unsupervised youth recreation centers in the neighborhood is related to an increase in antisocial behavior, above and beyond personal and sociofamily characteristics (Mahoney & Stattin, 2000). The effects for girls are especially striking. Other researchers also report that unsupervised wandering and deviant peer association predict both onset and frequency of official court records of arrests for early adolescent boys (Stoolmiller, 1994). Particularly for early developing girls, the most influential peers seem to be older boys from outside the school system, especially for those who also manifest behavior problems (Stattin & Magnusson, 1990).

Many of the previous results are in line with the *peer influence model* which views deviant friends as a causal necessity for the development of delinquency. Concordant with social learning principles, behaviors, but also attitudes favorable to aggression can be learned from association with deviant friends (Brendgen, Bowen, Rondeau, & Vitaro, 1999). According to this model, affiliation with deviant friends may mediate the link between aggression and peer rejection on one hand and the emergence or the increases in externalizing problems on the other hand. It can also mediate the link between family dysfunction and antisocial behavior in adolescence (Kim et al., 1999). Finally, affiliation with deviant peers can have a unique additive effect above and beyond other factors. As suggested by findings from Fergusson, Swain-Campbell, and Horwood (2002), the weight of the contribution of deviant peers to criminal activity and substance use may depend on when it is assessed (i.e., during adolescence vs. during early adulthood).

Variables That Moderate the Link between Affiliation with Deviant Peers and Increases in Externalizing Problems

Several studies suggest that a number of factors may mitigate the influence of deviant peers/deviant cliques. For example, some studies have found that children's and adolescents' behavioral or social–cognitive characteristics may exacerbate friends' influence. Thus, Vitaro, Brendgen, and Tremblay (2002) found that young adolescents' disruptiveness profile or attitudes toward deviancy moderated the link between friends' delinquency and increases in participants' delinquent behaviors. Prinstein, Boergers, and Spirito (2001) also found that participants' depressive feelings increased the link between the number of deviant friends and physical violence.

Other researchers have examined the moderating role that factors originating in the family might play with respect to the possible influence of deviant peers. For example, in some studies, attachment to parents weakened the link between exposure to deviant friends and participants' delinquent behaviors (Mason, Cauce, Gozales, & Hiraga, 1994; Vitaro, Brendgen, & Tremblay, 2000). However, Keenan et al. (1995), who used a composite score of supervision, discipline, and affectionate relationships, found no interaction between family variables and association with deviant peers in predicting severe delinquency. Similarly, Vitaro et al. (2000) found no interaction between parental supervision and exposure to deviant friends in predicting later delinquency, but they found that parental supervision had a positive main effect that compensated for the presence of deviant friends. As suggested by Vitaro et al. (2000), it is possible that positive relationships with parents may protect against negative influence of deviant friends whereas disciplinary practices (i.e., monitoring and supervision) may be important with respect to affiliation with deviant friends or deviant clique members

Proximal Processes That Might Help Explain the Influence of Deviant Friends on Externalizing Behaviors

Examining the processes that might help explain the influence of deviant peers assumes that deviant peers actually exert some influence through some form of socialization mechanisms and that this influence is not spurious (i.e., attributable to a third factor). In other words, it assumes that the peer influence or the social interactional models are at least partly true. Work by Dishion and colleagues on rule-breaking talk during dyadic interactions involving deviant adolescents indicates that positive verbal reinforcement by peers for deviant behaviors becomes increasingly important in shaping social behavior (Dishion, French, et al., 1995). This process, labeled "deviancy training," has received substantial empirical support. Specifically, these investigators showed that peers' reinforcement (through laughter or positive nonverbal feedback) of rule-breaking talk during videotaped group discussions devoted to teaching problem-solving strategies to problem youths resulted in an increase in youngsters' subsequent delinquent behavior and substance use, even after controlling for prior levels of these. In another study, antisocial boys elicited fewer positive reactions from their friends following normative talk than normal boys with their friends (Dishion et al., 1994). In a follow-up study, it has been shown that the association between exposure to deviant peers by age 10 and growth in arrests, substance use, and sexual intercourse from ages 10 to 18 was mediated by deviancy training at age 14 (Patterson, Dishion, & Yoerger, 2000). Interestingly, the participants with more externalizing problems who received positive feedback from less deviant peers were the most affected by the deviancy training process. Partly, similar processes may be operating during bullying episodes when peers are involved (which is the case for the majority of episodes).

Negative reinforcement in coercive peer interactions may also shape children's and adolescents' behaviors in the same way it shapes undesirable behavior during child–adult coercive interchanges. For example, Snyder and Brown (1983) found that the use of verbal aggression was followed by termination of a conflict episode for aggressive children, whereas a positive verbal interchange or the absence of a response terminated the conflict episode for nonaggressive children. In other words, aggressive children were negatively reinforced for using coercive behaviors with their peers whereas nonaggressive children were reinforced for using nonaversive strategies.

Although some researchers have not found differences between aggressive or delinquent children and their friends with respect to friendship quality or social competence (Grotpeter & Crick, 1996), antisocial children and adolescents (mainly boys) have also been found to be more bossy with their friends and more frequently involved in coercive exchanges than conventional children and adolescents (Windle, 1994). Increased levels of conflict and training in negative conflictual style in these friendships may lead to aggressive episodes between aggressive friends and may provide a further explanation of how aggressive children's friendships may predict increases in children's and adolescents' aggressive behaviors. In line with this notion, Berndt and Keefe (1996) found that early adolescents who have negative interactions with friends report more disruptive behaviors at the end of the school year even after controlling for initial levels of disruptiveness. Similarly, Kupersmidt, Burchinal, and Patterson (1995) showed that conflict with a best friend predicted delinquency beyond what is already predicted by peer rejection and best friend's aggressiveness. Finally, perceived quality of their friendship among antisocial–delinquent children was found to positively predict their delinquent behavior, in addition to their actual behavior problems (Heaven, Caputi, Trivellion, & Swinton, 2000). Consequently, it is possible that the negative features of children's friendships with their deviant friends directly influence these children's problematic behavioral profiles through coercion training. Negative features of friendship and attitudes toward the use of aggression as a mean to resolve conflicts between "friends" may also serve to establish norms with respect to the use of aggression in interpersonal relationships.

Finally, there is evidence showing that pressure to conform to norm-breaking behaviors may also serve as a mechanism to account for deviant friends' or clique members' influence. For example, Bagwell and Coie (2004) reported that 10-year-old aggressive boys and their friends provided more enticement for rule violations in situations that provided opportunities for rule-breaking behavior and that required conflict management than nonaggressive boys and their friends. Aggressive boys and their friends also engaged in more rule-breaking behavior than did nonaggressive boys and their friends. These data suggest that pressure to conform to norm-breaking behaviors may also serve as a mechanism for deviant peer influence.

In summary, we have presented several models and perspectives regarding the effect of peer experiences on externalizing problems. Different models have been developed to organize the complex associations between rejection, the association with aggressive peers, and children's aggressive behaviors. These models differ according to the causal power that is ascribed to the experience of having aggressive friends. Currently, one cannot claim that one model or perspective clearly provides the most compelling explanation of whether and how peers influence a child's aggressive behaviour. Nevertheless, there is sufficient evidence to conclude that peers can socialize each other to behave in aggressive ways.

PEER RELATIONS AND INTERNALIZING TENDENCIES

The study of peer relations and internalizing problems typically has targeted three aspects of the peer system: (1) peer status, which refers to acceptance vs. rejection by the peer group; (2) peer victimization experiences; and (3) dyadic friendships (see Rubin et al., 1998, for a review). Although these three types of peer relationships are interrelated to some degree, they are conceptually distinct and represent distinct social experiences and they are uniquely associated with developmental outcomes including different forms of internalizing behavior (e.g., Ladd & Troop-Gordon, 2003). The most frequently studied types of internalizing problems in relation to peer difficulties are anxious–withdrawn behavior, depression, and loneliness feelings. Although other variables related to internalizing behaviors, such as self-esteem or general and specific self-perceptions, have also been examined in relation to peer relations, we limit our review to the former three because they either are relevant for clinical diagnoses of psychopathology (in the case of anxiety and depression) or directly refer to children's internal appraisal of their social inclusion in the peer world (in the case of loneliness). Although they do not necessarily assess exactly the same constructs, findings from studies that use different forms of assessment (e.g., categorical vs. continuous measures) and different assessors (e.g., self-reports vs. peer assessments) are considered here because they not only offer complementary views but also lead to similar conclusions. It should also be mentioned that research findings sometimes vary depending on the data source. Thus, links between peer difficulties and internalizing problems are considerably stronger when peer relations are evaluated based on youths' self-reports than when peers or teachers judge the extent of children's peer difficulties (e.g., Brendgen, Vitaro, Turgeon, Poulin, & Wanner, 2004). Although one cannot always rule out the possibility that this association may be the result of shared method variance, the few studies employing multitrait, multimethod assessments support the existence of a link between peer difficulties and internalizing problems (e.g., Nolan, Flynn, & Garber, 2003).

Links between Peer Difficulties and Internalizing Problems

Many cross-sectional studies reveal that peer rejection is significantly related to the presence of internalizing problems. Thus, anxiety has been found to be concurrently related to peer status in elementary school children and adolescents. Similar findings have been reported for the concurrent link between peer status and loneliness and between peer status and depression (Cole & Carpentieri, 1990; Vosk, Forehand, Parker, & Rickard, 1982). Not surprisingly, the concurrent links between peer-related problems at the group level and internalizing behavior are even stronger for harassment by the peer group, a particularly strong indicator of peer rejection (see Hawker & Boulton, 2000, for a review).

In addition to peer-related problems at the group level, difficulties in dyadic friendship relations have also been linked to internalizing problems. Thus, the absence of mutual friends, as indicated by a lack of reciprocal friendship nominations, is significantly correlated with concurrent feelings of loneliness and depression (Brendgen et al., 2000; Bukowski, Hoza, & Boivin, 1993; Parker & Asher, 1993; Windle, 1994). More of a good thing is not necessarily better, however, as children with at least one mutual friend are not worse off than those with more than one mutual friend in terms of their internalizing problems (Asher & Paquette, 2003). Apart from the mere presence of a mutual friend, the quality of the friendship relation is also linked to children's internalizing behavior. For example, Parker and Asher (1993) found that each of six assessed aspects of friendship quality (i.e., validation and caring, conflict, companionship, help and guidance, intimate exchange, and conflict resolution) was significantly related to elementary school-age children's perceived loneliness.

Studies consistently show that peer rejection and—even to a stronger degree—verbal, physical, or indirect victimization by peers lead to increases in children's feelings of loneliness as well as their symptoms of anxiety and depression (Boivin, Hymel, & Bukowski, 1995a; Paul & Cillessen, 2003; Hodges & Perry, 1999; Kiesner, 2002; Panak & Garber, 1992). Similarly, friendlessness as well as a low friendship quality have been found to predict subsequent internalizing problems (e.g., Vernberg, Abwender, Ewell, & Beery, 1992). Some findings suggest that the predictive links between peer-related difficulties and internalizing problems are especially strong for girls (e.g., Oldenburg & Kerns, 1997), which might indicate a relatively greater orientation toward and dependence on social relationships in females than in males.

Not surprisingly, the nefarious effects of peer relationship difficulties on children's internalizing problems increase with the duration of a child's exposure to such difficulties (Goldbaum, Craig, Pepler, & Connolly, 2003). These findings are in line with chronic stress models stating that the likelihood of child maladjustment is directly related to the chronicity of relational stress (e.g., Dohrenwend & Dohrenwend, 1981). A recent study by Ladd and Troop-Gordon (2003) showed that the negative effects of chronic peer difficulties on internalizing problems not only pertain to consistent rejection or harassment by peers but also to a chronic lack of close dyadic friendships. Specifically, chronic exposure to either form of peer difficulties (i.e., peer rejection, peer victimization, or lack of close friendships) over the course of the first 3 years of elementary school uniquely predicted anxious–depressed behavior and loneliness in grade 4, even when children's relationship status in fourth grade was taken into account. These results suggest that children suffering from prolonged exposure to problematic peer relations may be at risk of later internalizing problems even after these problems have waned. In line with this notion, Kochenderfer-Ladd and Wardrop (2001) found that victimized children's feelings of loneliness do not necessarily decrease even when they are no longer harassed by their peers. Indeed, evidence suggests that experiences of victimization by peers have detrimental effects on individuals' emotional well-being well into adulthood. For example, Olweus (1992, 1993) found that boys who had been chronically victimized in grades 6–9 still showed elevated levels of depression at age 23 and were also at increased risk of being harassed by colleagues at the workplace or at school.

Similarly, negative long-term effects have been found for individuals without friends. Thus, a longitudinal study following a Finnish community cohort showed that having no close friends at age 16 predicted depression at age 22 even when controlling for previous levels of depressed mood (Pelkonen, Marttunen, & Aro, 2003). One explanation for this predictive risk status may lie in the fact that peer difficulties tend to be rather stable over time for many affected children (Brendgen, Vitaro, Bukowski, Doyle, & Markiewicz, 2001). Such accumulated negative peer experiences can significantly alter children's beliefs about themselves and about their peers, which in turn foster consistent anxiety and depression and feelings of loneliness. This notion is supported by the finding that children's negative beliefs about themselves as social agents in conjunction with concerns about how they are treated by their peers appear to partially mediate the link between chronic peer difficulties and children's subsequent internalizing problems (Ladd & Troop-Gordon, 2003). This mediating role of children's beliefs about themselves or others in the link between peer difficulties and internalizing outcomes, especially in girls, has also been demonstrated in other studies (e.g., Grills & Ollendick, 2002).

It should be noted that although difficult peer relations at both the group and the dyadic level play a unique predictive role in the development and maintenance of internalizing problems, they are not completely independent from each other. Indeed, recent studies show that especially peer rejection (i.e., being disliked by peers) may contribute to further peer difficulties, which then in turn fosters internalizing problems. For example, Boivin and colleagues (e.g., Boivin & Hymel, 1997; Boivin, Hymel, & Bukowski, 1995a, 1995b; Boivin, Hymel, & Hodges, 2001) have provided empirical support for a sequential model in which anxious–withdrawn behavior increases the likelihood of peer rejection, which in turn increases the risk of being victimized (i.e., harassed and treated badly) by the peer group. Peer victimization then leads to increases in both loneliness and depression. Further evidence that different forms of peer difficulties might be sequentially linked and feed into each other is provided by another recent study linking peer rejection, friendship experiences, and internalizing outcomes in elementary school-age children (Nangle, Erdley, Newman, Mason, & Carpenter, 2003). Specifically, these researchers showed that popularity (which can be considered a negative index of peer rejection) exerted no direct impact on internalizing outcomes. Instead, low popularity was related to children's lack of involvement in dyadic friendships, which, in turn, affected depression through its strong association with loneliness. Together, these findings suggest that peer rejection might be important for setting the stage for the development of other forms of peer difficulties such as peer victimization or a lack of dyadic friendship experiences, which may then more directly influence feelings of loneliness and depression.

Factors That Moderate the Association between Peer Difficulties and Internalizing Problems

Despite substantial empirical support for the link between peer relation difficulties and internalizing problems, effect sizes are often moderate at best, especially in longitudinal studies. Further investigations reveal that these weak associations can be explained by the presence of several moderating factors, which qualify the link between peer difficulties and internalizing problems.

One crucial factor that has been found to moderate the link between children's peer difficulties and the extent of their subsequent internalizing problems are the children's personal characteristics. For example, although the experience of being intensely disliked by their peers is common to all rejected children, there is substantial heterogeneity among these children with respect to their behavioral characteristics. Half of them are highly aggressive whereas the rest are more characterized by withdrawn behavior (Cillessen, van

IJzendoorn, Van Lieshout, & Hartup, 1992). Only withdrawn-rejected children report more concurrent loneliness and depression than nonrejected children, whereas aggressive-rejected children—as long as they are not also withdrawn—do not differ from nonrejected children in this respect (Parkhurst, & Asher, 1992; Hymel, Bowker, & Woody, 1993). Moreover, a recent longitudinal study spanning 5 years from kindergarten through fourth grade (Gazelle & Ladd, 2003) showed that children high in both anxiety and excluded in kindergarten through grade 2 had the most elevated depressive symptom trajectories over the course of elementary school. In contrast, children who were high in either anxiety or peer exclusion but not both exhibited only moderate levels of depressed symptoms during that time period.

Several explanations have been suggested for the differences in internalizing problems between aggressive–rejected and withdrawn–rejected children. One possibility may be that the former are simply less aware of their disadvantaged social status among peers than the latter. Indeed, aggressive–rejected children considerably underestimate their rejection by peers, whereas withdrawn–rejected children are relatively accurate in evaluating their social status (Cillessen et al., 1992; Zakriski & Coie, 1996). Evidence suggests that children's perceived acceptance or rejection among peers is more strongly related to internalizing problems than actual acceptance or rejection (Panak & Garber, 1992). The lack of awareness of their troubled status may thus help explain why, in contrast to withdrawn–rejected children, aggressive–rejected children do not necessarily suffer internalizing problems. Another possible explanation for the difference between aggressive–rejected and withdrawn–rejected children in regard to internalizing outcomes may be that their everyday social experiences with peers differ considerably, although both groups are intensely disliked. Evidence suggests that aggressive–rejected children are less excluded by their peers and suffer less active and passive peer disregard than nonaggressive–rejected children (Boivin & Poulin, 1993). In contrast, as mentioned previously, withdrawn–rejected children are often characterized by insecure, nonassertive, and submissive behavior, which increases the risk of victimization by peers.

Children's friendship experiences appear to moderate the link between peer difficulties at the group level and internalizing problems. In regard to differences between children with friends and those without, several studies have shown that unpopular and rejected children who have at least one mutual friend (as defined by reciprocal friendship nominations) do not differ from their more accepted peers in terms of their reported levels of loneliness and depression (Parker & Asher, 1993). It appears that friends not only protect children against the negative emotional effects of being rejected and excluded from the peer group but also protect them against peer victimization and its negative consequences (Hodges, Boivin, Vitaro, & Bukowski, 1999; Hodges, Malone, & Perry, 1997). For example, a study of fourth and fifth graders by Hodges et al. (1999) revealed that having a reciprocal best friend significantly reduced the likelihood of being victimized over a 1-year period especially among children who were most at risk for victimization. The characteristics of the friend appear to matter also. For children with a best friend, the degree to which this friend came to the rescue during attacks moderated the link between internalizing problems as a risk factor of victimization, on the one hand, and actual victimization experiences, on the other hand. Specifically, as long as their friend was able to provide some protection, even anxious–withdrawn children were not at risk for victimization from their peers. The buffering effect of friends against the negative consequences of peer victimization might also be explained by the fact that friendships—at least those of a high quality—provide important social benefits such as companionship, emotional support, intimacy, and self-validation (Buhrmester & Furman, 1987; Bukowski et al., 1993), which may alleviate the stress associated with repeated attacks from peers.

Internalizing Problems as a Predictor of Experiences with Peers

Relatively few studies have examined the predictive effect of depression or loneliness on subsequent peer rejection and conclusive empirical evidence for such a link is still lacking (e.g., Brendgen, Vitaro, Turgeon, Poulin, 2002; Nolan et al., 2003; Little & Garber, 1995). Nevertheless, studies on the predictive effect of anxious–withdrawn behavior on peer rejection and peer victimization provide support for the notion that internalizing problems may have a negative impact on children's relations with their peers. This effect, however, seems to depend on children's age. Indeed, several studies found no link between withdrawn behavior and subsequent peer status in kindergarten children (e.g., Ladd & Burgess, 1999). However, withdrawn behavior becomes increasingly associated with peer difficulties, especially victimization by peers, over the course of middle childhood (e.g., Boivin et al., 2001). These findings indicate that internalizing behavior may not necessarily be a critical factor in determining subsequent peer status in young children but it gradually becomes more nonnormative and thus more salient for peer relations over the course of middle childhood (Younger, Gentile, & Burgess, 1993).

Most important, however, anxiety and peer relations appear to be involved in a cycle of experiences that influence subsequent functioning. As has been shown by Rubin and Krasnor (1986), anxious–withdrawn children tend to blame themselves for social failures. Rubin, Burgess, and Coplan (2002) argue that the combination of peer rebuff experiences and internal attributions for failing to achieve social goals creates a feedback loop whereby an anxious–withdrawn child attributes social failure to his or her own characteristics, which causes the child to become even more socially wary. Persistent or increasing anxiety then contributes to further social failure, which reinforces the child's beliefs about his or her social incompetence. In some cases, anxious children's social wariness translates into severely maladaptive behavior, which may become so extreme that they risk becoming easy targets of harassment from peers. Thus, anxious–withdrawn children, especially those who are also rejected, are often characterized by high levels of insecurity and nonassertive and submissive behavior, which can increase the risk of victimization by peers (Goldbaum et al., 2003; Hodges & Perry, 1996; Schwartz, Dodge, & Coie, 1993).

The question arises whether this vicious cycle of anxiety-laden emotions and cognitions, maladaptive behavior, and peer relation difficulties also extends to difficulties in children's dyadic friendships. In regard to the number of friends at least, there is little evidence that internalizing problems seriously hamper children's success in developing or maintaining friendship relations. Thus, withdrawn children—as long as they are not also aggressive—are as likely to have a mutual best friend as other children (Ladd & Burgess, 1999). Similarly, depression in a sample of fourth to sixth graders did not predict change in the number of reciprocal friends over a 6-month period (Brendgen et al., 2004). In contrast, internalizing problems do seem to have a negative impact on the quality of children's friendship relations, at least according to the children's own point of view. Thus, prospective analyses in a sample of early adolescents showed that social anxiety impaired the development of self-reported companionship and intimacy in newly formed friendships over the course of a school year (Vernberg et al., 1992). Similarly, depressed children in the Brendgen, Vitaro, Tremblay, and Wanner (2002) study reported a significant decrease in friendship quality. Notably, however, no such decrease in friendship quality could be detected from the depressed children's friends' perspective and no difference was found between depressed children and their nondepressed counterparts in regard to friendship stability. As such, it is still unclear whether the negative effect of internalizing problems really extends to children's dyadic friendship relations or whether internalizing problems merely foster children's negatively biased perceptions of their friendship relations.

CONCLUSION AND EMERGING ISSUES

On the basis of the preceding review it can be concluded that both a child's peer group and his or her dyadic friendships constitute fundamental domains of social experience. As a consequence, a lack of positive experiences in either of these domains suggests significant disadvantages for the child's social development and adjustment. Moreover, the experience of being rejected by one's peers seems to be especially problematic, as it increases the risk of further peer difficulties such as peer victimization and friendlessness. However, being rejected and even being harassed by peers does not necessarily imply being without friends; instead, the negative correlates of peer rejection and peer victimization might be alleviated by having at least one satisfying friendship. Despite the plethora of research supporting the link between peer difficulties and internalizing problems, however, many questions remain.

One issue that has garnered recent interest refers to children's way of coping with peer difficulties, which may have a profound impact on the development of subsequent internalizing problems (e.g., Bowker, Bukowski, Hymel, & Sippola, 2000; Kochenderfer-Ladd & Skinner, 2002; Sandstrom, 2004). Coping refers to individual-specific appraisal and response patterns in light of stressful situations or events (Lazarus & Folkman, 1984). Recent evidence suggests not only that many children experiencing peer difficulties use less effective coping strategies than their less troubled counterparts but that these maladaptive coping styles may exacerbate children's risk of developing internalizing problems. Thus, a recent study by Sandstrom (2004) examining children's coping strategies in regard to experiences of peer exclusion and peer harassment revealed four distinct coping strategies, which were highly consistent across different situations: (1) *active coping*, such as seeking advice from others; (2) *aggressive coping*, such as seeking revenge; (3) *denial coping*, such as ignoring the event; and (4) *ruminative coping*, such as consistent thinking about the event. Although less accepted children significantly differed from their more accepted counterparts only with respect to the frequent use of aggressive coping strategies, there was also a tendency for less accepted children to use ruminative coping more frequently. Moreover, ruminative coping was related to higher levels of concurrent internalizing problems. Even outright denial, however, may not always be successful in curbing the negative effects of peer difficulties, as shown in another study by Kochenderfer-Ladd & Skinner (2002). Examining the role of coping strategies as potential moderators of the link between peer victimization and children's internalizing problems, they found that denial or cognitive distancing from the problem was related to higher rates of anxious–depressed symptoms in victimized boys, although no such moderating effect was found for girls. Together, these results further underline the complexity of the link between peer difficulties and internalizing problems and show that children's own behavioral or cognitive characteristics need to be considered an important moderator, along with potential sex-related differences in this context.

Another promising new avenue of research might be to examine other types of peer experiences in the school and their link to the development of internalizing problems. For example, a retrospective study by Prinstein and LaGreca (2002) revealed that adolescents' affiliation with reputation-based peer crowds such as Populars, Jocks, Brains, Burnouts, Nonconformists, and Average crowds is significantly related to internalizing distress. Specifically, children who classified themselves as Populars/Jocks had experienced significant declines in internalizing distress between childhood and adolescence, whereas Brains exhibited some increases in internalizing distress. Although it is not yet clear whether membership in one of these reputation-based peer crowds affects internalizing behavior, this question certainly merits further investigation. In a related vein, it might be fruitful to further explore peer relations that children establish out of the school context, especially in regard to dyadic friendship relations. The limited evidence that we have already shows that out-of-school friends appear to affect externalizing behaviors; their impact on internalizing problems needs to be examined. In the vast majority of studies, friendship nominations are limited to the classroom or the grade, which limits interpretability of findings. Although elementary school children especially choose most of their friendship relations within the school context (Kupersmidt et al., 1995), some children who are considered friendless may well have friends outside the school context. These out-of-school friends may protect them at least to some extent against the negative effects of peer rejection and friendlessness in the school context even though they might not be able to protect against peer harassment that happens in the school. Some indication for the importance of out-of-school peer relations comes from a study by Kiesner, Poulin, and Nicotra (2003), who examined the in-school and after-school peer relations of early adolescents in Italy. These researchers found that both in-school and after-school peer network inclusion—a measure of friendship involvement—contributed to explaining variance in depressive symptoms, even after controlling for the effect of peer rejection in the classroom on depression. Again, a lack of longitudinal data in this context makes it difficult to establish directionality of effects between out-of-school peer relations and internalizing problems, but further research promises to shed more light on this important issue.

SUMMARY

The study of peer relationships has been an area of interest to developmental psychologists for more than a century. The study of peer relations has been especially intense during the past 25 year as researchers have developed and tested several models of peer influence. In contrast with the study of other socialization domains, the study of the effects of peers poses several unique challenges. Insofar as peers are not "assigned" to a child, in the way that parents are, either through biology or through adoption, the peer domain is fluid and dynamic in ways that the family system cannot be. Research on the socializing effects of peer experiences has emphasized how much a child is liked and disliked, the characteristics of the peers the child associates with, and the features of their interactions and relationships. As the discussion in this chapter shows, these factors affect development via several pathways and processes that involve both mediation and moderation. Moreover, the current data show that different aspects of experiences with peers can affect internalizing and externalizing problems. Whereas the characteristics of the friend appear to affect externalizing behavior, the properties of a child's relationship with peers, especially friends, appears to affect internalizing tendencies. Currently, the results of the studies we have discussed do not always provide clear support for one model of peer influence over another. Nevertheless, there is no doubt that children's behavior, thoughts, and emotions are highly associated with and likely influenced by their experiences with peers. These effects derive from a set of processes rather than from just one mechanism. Ongoing longitudinal studies under way around the world will shed further light on the importance of the various facets of the peer system.

ACKNOWLEDGMENTS

Work on this project was supported by grants to each of the authors from the Social Sciences and Humanities Research Council of Canada and the *Le Fonds québécois de la recherche sur la société et la culture*.

REFERENCES

Asher, S. R., & Paquette, J. A. (2003). Loneliness and peer relations in childhood. *Current Directions in Psychological Science, 12*(3), 75–78.

Azmitia, M., Lippman, D. N., & Ittel, A. (1999). On the relation of personal experience to early adolescents' reasoning about best friendship deterioration. *Social Development, 8*(2), 275–291.

Bagwell, C. L., & Coie, J. D. (2004). The best friendships of aggressive boys: Relationship quality, conflict management, and rule-breaking behavior. *Journal of Experimental Child Psychology, 88*(1), 5–24.

Bagwell, C. L., Newcomb, A. F., & Bukowski, W. M. (1998). Preadolescent friendship and peer rejection as predictors of adult adjustment. *Child Development, 69*(1), 140–153.

Battin, S. R., Hill, K. G., Abbott, R. D., Catalano, R. F., & Hawkins, J. D. (1998). The contribution of gang membership to delinquency beyond delinquent friends. *Criminology, 36*, 93–115.

Berndt, T. J., & Keefe, K. (1996). Friends' influence on school adjustment: A motivational analysis. In J. Juvonen & K. R. Wentzel (Eds.), *Social motivation: Understanding children's school adjustment* (pp. 248–278). New York: Cambridge University Press.

Bierman, K. L., & Wargo, J. B. (1995). Predicting the longitudinal course associated with aggressive-rejected, aggressive (nonrejected), and rejected (nonaggressive) status. *Development and Psychopathology, 7*(4), 669–682.

Blos, P. (1967). *The second individuation process of adolescence. Psychoanalytic study of the child* (Vol. 22). New York: International Universities Press.

Boivin, M., & Hymel, S. (1997). Peer experiences and social self-perceptions: A sequential model. *Developmental Psychology, 33*(1), 135–145.

Boivin, M., Hymel, S., & Bukowski, W. M. (1995a). The roles of social withdrawal, peer rejection, and victimization by peers in predicting loneliness and depressed mood in childhood. *Development and Psychopathology, 7*, 765–785.

Boivin, M., Hymel, S., & Bukowski, W.M. (1995b). Victimization and loneliness as mediators between peer experiences and depression. *Development and Psychopathology, 7*, 765–786.

Boivin, M., Hymel, S., & Hodges, E. V. E. (2001). Toward a process view of peer rejection and harassment. In J. Juvonen & S. Graham (Eds.), *Peer harassment in school: The plight of the vulnerable and victimized* (pp. 265–289). New York: Guilford Press.

Boivin, M., & Poulin, F. (1993). Les camarades de jeu des garçons agressifs. les choix de camarades de jeu et la qualit de l 'insertion sociale des garçons agressifs. *Enfance, 47*(3), 261–278.

Bowker, A., Bukowski, W. M., Hymel, S., & Sippola, L. K. (2000). Coping with daily hassles in the peer group during early adolescence: Variations as a function of peer experience. *Journal of Research on Adolescence, 10*(2), 211–243.

Brendgen, M., Bowen, F., Rondeau, N., & Vitaro, F. (1999). Effects of friends' characteristics on children's social cognitions. *Social Development, 8*(1), 41–51.

Brendgen, M., Markiewicz, D., Doyle, A. B., & Bukowski, W. M. (2001). The relations between friendship quality, ranked-friendship preference, and adolescents' behavior with their friends. *Merrill–Palmer Quarterly, 47*(3), 395–415.

Brendgen, M., Vitaro, F., & Bukowski, W. M. (2000). Stability and variability of adolescents' affiliation with delinquent friends: Predictors and consequences. *Social Development, 9*(2), 205–225.

Brendgen, M., Vitaro, F., Bukowski, W. M., Doyle, A. B., & Markiewicz, D. (2001). Developmental profiles of peer social preference over the course of elementary school: Associations with trajectories of externalizing and internalizing behavior. *Developmental Psychology, 37*(3), 308–320.

Brendgen, M., Vitaro, F., Doyle, A. B., Markiewicz, D., & Bukowski, W. M. (2002). Same-sex peer relations and romantic relationships during early adolescence: Interactive links to emotional, behavioral, and academic adjustment. *Merrill–Palmer Quarterly, 48*(1), 77–103.

Brendgen, M., Vitaro, F., Tremblay, R. E., & Wanner, B. (2002). Parent and peer effects on delinquency-related violence and dating violence: A test of two mediational models. *Social Development, 11*(2), 225–244.

Brendgen, M., Vitaro, F., Turgeon, L., & Poulin, F. (2002). Assessing aggressive and depressed children's social relations with classmates and friends: A matter of perspective. *Journal of Abnormal Child Psychology, 30*(6), 609–624.

Brendgen, M., Vitaro, F., Turgeon, L., Poulin, F., & Wanner, B. (2004). Is there a dark side of positive illusions?: Overestimation of social competence and subsequent adjustment in aggressive and nonaggressive children. *Journal of Abnormal Child Psychology, 32*, 305–320.

Buhrmester, D., & Furman, W. (1987). The development of companionship and intimacy. *Child Development, 58*(4), 1101–1113.

Bukowski, W. M., Hoza, B., & Boivin, M. (1993). Popularity, friendship, and emotional adjustment during early adolescence. In B. Laursen (Ed.), *Close friendships in adolescence* (pp. 23–37). San Francisco: Jossey-Bass.

Cairns, R. B. (1979). *Social development: The origins and plasticity of interchanges.* New York: Freeman.

Cairns, R. B., & Cairns, B. D. (1994). *Lifelines and risks: Pathways of youth in our time.* New York: Cambridge University Press.

Cairns, R. B., Cairns, B. D., Neckerman, H. J., Gest, S. D., & Gariépy, J. (1988). Social networks and aggressive behavior: Peer support or peer rejection? *Developmental Psychology, 24*(6), 815–823.

Caspi, A., Elder, G. H., & Bem, D. J. (1987). Moving against the world: Life-course patterns of explosive children. *Developmental Psychology, 23*(2), 308–313.

Chang, L. (2004). The role of classrooms in contextualizing the relations of children's social behaviors to peer acceptance. *Developmental Psychology, 40*, 691–702.

Cillessen, A. H., Van IJzendoorn, H. W., Van Lieshout, C. F., & Hartup, W. W. (1992). Heterogeneity among peer-rejected boys: Subtypes and stabilities. *Child Development, 63*(4), 893–905.

Coie, J. D. (1990). Towards a theory of peer rejection. In S. R. Asher & J. D. Coie (Eds.), *Peer rejection in childhood* (pp. 365–401). Cambridge, MA: Cambridge University Press.

Coie, J. D., & Kupersmidt, J. B. (1983). A behavioral analysis of emerging social status in boys' groups. *Child Development, 54*(6), 1400–1416.

Cole, D. A., & Carpentieri, S. (1990). Social status and the comorbidity of child depression and conduct disorder. *Journal of Consulting and Clinical Psychology, 58*(6), 748–757.

Collins, W. A., Maccoby, E. E., Steinberg, L., Hetherington, E. M., & Bornstein, M. H. (2000). Contemporary research on parenting: The case for nature and nurture. *American Psychologist, 55*(2), 218–232.

Deater-Deckard, K. (2001). Annotation: Recent research examining the role of peer relations in the development of psychopathology. *Journal of Child Psychology and Psychiatry, 42*, 565–579.

Deater-Deckard, K., Dodge, K. A., Bates, J. E., & Pettit, G. S. (1998). Multiple risk factors in the development of externalizing behavior problems: Group and individual differences. *Development and Psychopathology, 10*(3), 469–493.

DeRosier, M. E., Cillessen, A. H. N., Coie, J. D., & Dodge, K. A. (1994). Group social context and children's aggressive behavior. *Child Development, 65*(4), 1068–1079.

Dishion, T. J., Capaldi, D., Spracklen, K. M., & Li, F. (1995). Peer ecology of male adolescent drug use. *Development and Psychopathology, 7*(4), 803–824.

Dishion, T. J., French, D. C., & Patterson, G. R. (1995). The development and ecology of antisocial behavior. In D. Cicchetti, & D. J. Cohen (Eds.), *Developmental psychopathology: Vol. 2. Risk, disorder, and adaptation* (pp. 421–471). New York: Wiley.

Dishion, T. J., Patterson, G. R., & Griesler, P. C. (1994). Peer adaptations in the development of antisocial behavior: A confluence model. In L. R. Huesmann (Ed.), *Aggressive behavior: Current perspectives* (pp. 61–95). New York: Plenum Press.

Dishion, T. J., Patterson, G. R., Stoolmiller, M., & Skinner, M. L. (1991). Family, school, and behavioral antecedents to early adolescent involvement with antisocial peers. *Developmental Psychology, 27*(1), 172–180.

Dodge, K. A., Coie, J. D., Pettit, G. S., & Price, J. M. (1990). Peer status and aggression in boys' groups: Developmental and contextual analyses. *Child Development, 61*(5), 1289–1309.

Dodge, K. A., Lansford, J. E., Burks, V. S., Bates, J. E., Pettit, G. S., & Fontaine, R., et al. (2003). Peer rejection and social information-processing factors in the development of aggressive behavior problems in children. *Child Development, 74*(2), 374–393.

Dohrenwend, B. P., & Dohrenwend, B. S. (1981). Socioenvironmental factors, stress, and psychopathology. *American Journal of Community Psychology, 9*(2), 128–164.

Ennett, S. T., & Bauman, K. E. (1994). The contribution of influence and selection to adolescent peer group homogeneity: The case of adolescent cigarette smoking. *Journal of Personality and Social Psychology, 67*(4), 653–663.

Fergusson, D. M., Swain-Campbell, N. R., & Horwood, L. J. (2002). Deviant peer affiliations, crime and substance use: A fixed effects regression analysis. *Journal of Abnormal Child Psychology, 30*(4), 419–430.

Fergusson, D. M., Woodward, L. J., & Horwood, L. J. (1999). Childhood peer relationship problems and young people's involvement with deviant peers in adolescence. *Journal of Abnormal Child Psychology, 27*(5), 357–369.

Furman, W., & Robbins, P. (1985). What's the point?: Issues in the selection of treatment objectives. In B. H. Schneider, K. H. Rubin, & J. E. Ledingham (Eds.), *Children's peer relations: Issues in assessment and intervention* (pp. 41–54). New York: Springer.

Gazelle, H., & Ladd, G. W. (2003). Anxious solitude and peer exclusion: A diathesis–stress model of internalizing trajectories in childhood. *Child Development, 74*(1), 257–278.

George, T. P., & Hartmann, D. P. (1996). Friendship networks of unpopular, average, and popular children. *Child Development, 67*(5), 2301–2316.

Goldbaum, S., Craig, W. M., Pepler, D., & Connolly, J. (2003). Developmental trajectories of victimization: Identifying risk and protective factors. *Journal of Applied School Psychology, 19*(2), 139–156.

Grills, A. E., & Ollendick, T. H. (2002). Peer victimization, global self-worth, and anxiety in middle school children. *Journal of Clinical Child and Adolescent Psychology, 31*(1), 59–68.

Grotpeter, J. K., & Crick, N. R. (1996). Relational aggression, overt aggression, and friendship. *Child Development, 67*(5), 2328–2338.

Harris, J. R. (1995). Where is the child's environment?: A group socialization theory of development. *Psychological Review, 102,* 458–489.

Hartup, W. W. (1970). Peer interaction and social organization. In P. H. Mussen (Ed.), *Carmichael's manual of child psychology* (Vol. 2, pp. 361–456). New York: Wiley.

Hartup, W. W. (1983). Peer relations. In P. H. Mussen (Ed.), *Handbook of child psychology: Vol. 4. Socialization, personality, and social development* (pp. 103–196). New York: Wiley.

Hawker, D. S. J., & Boulton, M. J. (2000). Twenty years' research on peer victimization and psychosocial maladjustment: A meta-analytic review of cross-sectional studies. *Journal of Child Psychology and Psychiatry, 41*(4), 441–455.

Hay, D. F., Payne, A., & Chadwick, A. (2004). Peer relations in childhood. *Journal of Child Psychology and Psychiatry, 45*(1), 84–108.

Heaven, P. C. L., Caputi, P., Trivellion-Scott, D., & Swinton, T. (2000). Personality and group influences on self-reported delinquent behaviour. *Personality and Individual Differences, 28*(6), 1143–1158.

Hodges, E. V. E., Boivin, M., Vitaro, F., & Bukowski, W. M. (1999). The power of friendship: Protection against an escalating cycle of peer victimization. *Developmental Psychology, 35*(1), 94–101.

Hodges, E. V. E., Malone, M. J., & Perry, D. G. (1997). Individual risk and social risk as interacting determinants of victimization in the peer group. *Developmental Psychology, 33*(6), 1032–1039.

Hodges, E., & Perry, D. (1996). Victims of peer abuse: An overview. *Reclaiming Children and Youth: Journal of Emotional and Behavioral Problems, 5*, 23–28.

Hodges, E. V. E., & Perry, D. G. (1999). Personal and interpersonal antecedents and consequences of victimization by peers. *Journal of Personality and Social Psychology, 76*(4), 677–685.

Hymel, S., Bowker, A., & Woody, E. (1993). Aggressive versus withdrawn unpopular children: Variations in peer and self-perceptions in multiple domains. *Child Development, 64*(3), 879–896.

Hymel, S., Comfort, C., Schonert-Reichl, K., & McDougall, P. (1996). Academic failure and school dropout: The influence of peers. In J. Juvonen, & K. R. Wentzel (Eds.), *Social motivation: Understanding children's school adjustment.* (pp. 313–345). Cambridge, UK: Cambridge University Press.

Kaplan, H. B., Johnson, R. J., & Bailey, C. A. (1986). Self-rejection and the explanation of deviance: Refinement and elaboration of a latent structure. *Social Psychology Quarterly, 49*(2), 110–128.

Keenan, K., Loeber, R., Zhang, Q., & Stouthamer-Loeber, M. (1995). The influence of deviant peers on the development of boys' disruptive and delinquent behavior: A temporal analysis. *Development and Psychopathology, 7*(4), 715–726.

Kerr, M., Stattin, H., & Kiesner, J. (2004, February). *Peers and problem behavior: Have we missed something?* Presented at Hot Topics in Developmental Research: Peer Relations in Adolescence Conference. Nijmegen, The Netherlands.

Kiesner, J. (2002). Depressive symptoms in early adolescence: Their relations with classroom problem behavior and peer status. *Journal of Research on Adolescence, 12*(4), 463–478.

Kiesner, J., Poulin, F., & Nicotra, E. (2003). Peer relations across contexts: Individual-network homophily and network inclusion in and after school. *Child Development, 74*(5), 1328–1343.

Kim, J. E., Hetherington, E. M., & Reiss, D. (1999). Associations among family relationships, antisocial peers, and adolescents' externalizing behaviors: Gender and family type differences. *Child Development, 70*(5), 1209–1230.

Kochenderfer-Ladd, B., & Skinner, K. (2002). Children's coping strategies: Moderators of the effects of peer victimization? *Developmental Psychology, 38*(2), 267–278.

Kochenderfer-Ladd, B., & Wardrop, J. L. (2001). Chronicity and instability of children's peer victimization experiences as predictors of loneliness and social satisfaction trajectories. *Child Development, 72*(1), 134–151.

Kupersmidt, J. B., Burchinal, M., & Patterson, C. J. (1995). Developmental patterns of childhood peer relations as predictors of externalizing behavior problems. *Development and Psychopathology, 7*(4), 825–843.

Lacourse, E., Nagin, D., Tremblay, R. E., Vitaro, F., & Claes, M. (2003). Developmental trajectories of boys' delinquent group membership and facilitation of violent behaviors during adolescence. *Development and Psychopathology, 15*(1), 183–197.

Ladd, G. W., & Burgess, K. B. (1999). Charting the relationship trajectories of aggressive, withdrawn, and aggressive/withdrawn children during early grade school. *Child Development, 70*(4), 910–929.

Ladd, G. W., & Troop-Gordon, W. (2003). The role of chronic peer difficulties in the development of children's psychological adjustment problems. *Child Development, 74*(5), 1344–1367.

Lahey, B. B., Gordon, R. A., Loeber, R., Stouthamer-Loeber, M., & Farrington, D. P. (1999). Boys who join gangs: A prospective study of predictors of first gang entry. *Journal of Abnormal Child Psychology, 27*(4), 261–276.

Lazarus, R., & Folkman, S. (1984). *Stress, appraisal, and coping.* New York: Springer.

Little, S. A., & Garber, J. (1995). Aggression, depression, and stressful life events predicting peer rejection in children. *Development and Psychopathology, 7*(4), 845–856.

Mahoney, J. L., & Stattin, H. (2000). Leisure activities and adolescent antisocial behavior: The role of structure and social context. *Journal of Adolescence, 23*(2), 113–127.

Mason, C. A., Cauce, A. M., Gonzales, N., & Hiraga, Y. (1994). An ecological model of externalizing behaviors in african-american adolescents: No family is an island. *Journal of Research on Adolescence, 4*(4), 639–655.

McDougall, P., Hymel, S., Vaillancourt, T., & Mercer, L. (2001). The consequences of childhood peer rejection. In M. R. Leary (Ed.), *Interpersonal rejection* (pp. 213–247). Oxford University Press.

Miller-Johnson, S., Coie, J.D., Maumary-Gremaud, A., Bierman, K., & Conduct Problems Prevention Research Group. (2002). Peer rejection and aggression and early starter models of conduct disorder. *Journal of Abnormal Child Psychology, 30*, 217–230.

Nangle, D. W., Erdley, C. A., Newman, J. E., Mason, C. A., & Carpenter, E. M. (2003). Popularity, friendship quantity, and friendship quality: Interactive influences on children's loneliness and depression. *Journal of Clinical Child and Adolescent Psychology, 32*(4), 546–555.

Nangle, D. W., Erdley, C. A., Zeff, K. R., Stanchfield, L. L., & Gold, J. A. (2004). Opposites do not attract: Social status and behavioral-style concordances and discordances among children and the peers who like or dislike them. *Journal of Abnormal Child Psychology, 32*(4), 425–434.

Nelson, S. E., & Dishion, T. J. (2004). From boys to men: Predicting adult adaptation from middle childhood sociometric status. *Development and Psychopathology, 16*(2), 441–459.

Nolan, S. A., Flynn, C., & Garber, J. (2003). Prospective relations between rejection and depression in young adolescents. *Journal of Personality and Social Psychology, 85*(4), 745–755.

Oldenburg, C. M., & Kerns, K. A. (1997). Associations between peer relationships and depressive symptoms: Testing moderator effects of gender and age. *Journal of Early Adolescence, 17*(3), 319–337.

Olweus, D. (1992). Bullying among schoolchildren: Intervention and prevention. In R. D. Peters, R. J. McMahon & V. L. Quinsey (Eds.), *Aggression and violence throughout the life span* (pp. 100–125). London: Sage.

Olweus, D. (1993). Bully/victim problems among schoolchildren: Long-term consequences and an effective intervention program. In S. Hodgins (Ed.), *Mental disorder and crime* (pp. 317–349). Thousand Oaks: Sage.

Panak, W. F., & Garber, J. (1992). Role of aggression, rejection, and attributions in the prediction of depression in children. *Development and Psychopathology, 4*(1), 145–165.

Parker, J. G., & Asher, S. R. (1987). Peer relations and later personal adjustment: Are low-accepted children at risk? *Psychological Bulletin, 102*(3), 357–389.

Parker, J. G., & Asher, S. R. (1993). Friendship and friendship quality in middle childhood: Links with peer group acceptance and feelings of loneliness and social dissatisfaction. *Developmental Psychology, 29*(4), 611–621.

Parkhurst, J. T., & Asher, S. R. (1992). Peer rejection in middle school: Subgroup differences in behavior, loneliness, and interpersonal concerns. *Developmental Psychology, 28*(2), 231–241.

Patterson, G. R., DeBaryshe, B. D., & Ramsey, E. (1989). A developmental perspective on antisocial behavior. *American Psychologist, 44*(2), 329–335.

Patterson, G. R., Dishion, T. J., & Yoerger, K. (2000). Adolescent growth in new forms of problem behavior: Macro- and micro-peer dynamics. *Prevention Science, 1*(1), 3–13.

Patterson, G. R., Reid, J. B., & Dishion, T. J. (1992). *Antisocial boys: Vol. 4. A social interactional approach*. Eugene, OR: Castalia.

Paul, J. J., & Cillessen, A. H. N. (2003). Dynamics of peer victimization in early adolescence: Results from a four-year longitudinal study. *Journal of Applied School Psychology, 19*(2), 25–43.

Pelkonen, M., Marttunen, M., & Aro, H. (2003). Risk for depression: A 6-year follow-up of finnish adolescents. *Journal of Affective Disorders, 77*(1), 41–51.

Pellegrini, A. D., Bartini, M., & Brooks, F. (1999). School bullies, victims, and aggressive victims: Factors relating to group affiliation and victimization in early adolescence. *Journal of Educational Psychology, 91*(2), 216–224.

Poulin, F., & Boivin, M. (2000). The role of proactive and reactive aggression in the formation and development of boys' friendships. *Developmental Psychology, 36*(2), 233–240.

Prinstein, M. J., Boergers, J., & Spirito, A. (2001). Adolescents' and their friends' health-risk behavior: Factors that alter or add to peer influence. *Journal of Pediatric Psychology, 26*(5), 287–298.

Prinstein, M. J., & La Greca, A. M. (2002). Peer crowd affiliation and internalizing distress in childhood and adolescence: A longitudinal follow-back study. *Journal of Research on Adolescence, 12*(3), 325–351.

Quinton, D., Pickles, A., Maughan, B., & Rutter, M. (1993). Partners, peers, and pathways: Assortative pairing and continuities in conduct disorder. *Development and Psychopathology, 5*(4), 763–783.

Rogoff, B. (1997). Evaluating development in the process of participation: Theory, methods and practice building on each other. In E. Amsel, & K. A. Renninger (Eds.), *Change and development: Issues of theory, method, and application* (pp. 265–285). Mahwah, NJ: Erlbaum.

Rose, A. J., Swenson, L. P., & Carlson, W. (2004). Friendships of aggressive youth: Considering the influences of being disliked and of being perceived as popular. *Journal of Experimental Child Psychology, 88*(1), 25–45.

Rubin, K.H., Bukowski, W.M., & Parker, J.G. (1998). Peer interactions, relationships and groups. In W. Damon (Series Ed.) & N. Eisenberg (Vol. Ed.), *The handbook of child psychology* (5th ed., pp. 619–700). New York: Wiley.

Rubin, K.H., Bukowski, W.M., & Parker, J.G. (2006). Peer interactions, relationships and groups. In N. Eisenberg (Vol. Ed.), *The handbook of child psychology* (6th ed., pp. 571–645). New York: Wiley.

Rubin, K. H., Burgess, K. B., & Coplan, R. J. (2002). Social withdrawal and shyness. In P. K. Smith, & C. H. Hart (Eds.), *Blackwell handbook of childhood social development* (pp. 330–352). London: Blackwell.

Rubin, K. H., & Krasnor, L. R. (1986). Social-cognitive and social behavioral perspectives on problem solving. *Minnesota Symposia on Child Psychology, 18,* 1–68.

Sameroff, A. J. (1983). Developmental systems: Contexts and evolution. In P. H. Mussen (Ed.), *Handbook of child psychology: Vol. 1. History, theory, and methods* (pp. 237–294). New York: Wiley.

Sandstrom, M. J. (2004). Pitfalls of the peer world: How children cope with common rejection experiences. *Journal of Abnormal Child Psychology, 32*(1), 67–81.

Schwartz, D., Dodge, K. A., & Coie, J. D. (1993). The emergence of chronic peer vicitimization in boys' play groups. *Child Development, 64*(6), 1755–1772.

Simons, R. L., Chao, W., Conger, R. D., & Elder, G. H. (2001). Quality of parenting as mediator of the effect of childhood defiance on adolescent friendship choices and delinquency: A growth curve analysis. *Journal of Marriage and the Family, 63*(1), 63–79.

Snyder, J., & Brown, K. (1983). Oppositional behavior and noncompliance in preschool children: Environmental correlates and skills deficits. *Behavioral Assessment, 5*(4), 333–348.

Snyder, J., Horsch, E., & Childs, J. (1997). Peer relationships of young children: Affiliative choices and the shaping of aggressive behavior. *Journal of Clinical Child Psychology, 26*(2), 145–156.

Stattin, H., & Magnusson, D. (1990). *Pubertal maturation in female development.* Mahwah, NJ: Erlbaum.

Stoolmiller, M. (1994). Antisocial behavior, delinquent peer association, and unsupervised wandering for boys: Growth and change from childhood to early adolescence. *Multivariate Behavioral Research, 29*(3), 263–288.

Sullivan, H. S. (1953). *The interpersonal theory of psychiatry.* New York: Norton.

Vernberg, E. M., Abwender, D. A., Ewell, K. K., & Beery, S. H. (1992). Social anxiety and peer relationships in early adolescence: A prospective analysis. *Journal of Clinical Child Psychology, 21*(2), 189–196.

Vitaro, F., Brendgen, M., & Tremblay, R. E. (2000). Influence of deviant friends on delinquency: Searching for moderator variables. *Journal of Abnormal Child Psychology, 28*(4), 313–325.

Vitaro, F., Brendgen, M., & Tremblay, R. E. (2002). Reactively and proactively aggressive children: Antecedent and subsequent characteristics. *Journal of Child Psychology and Psychiatry, 43*(4), 495–506.

Vitaro, F., Brendgen, M., & Wanner, B. (2005). Patterns of affiliation with delinquent friends during late childhood and early adolescence: Correlates and consequences. *Social Development, 14*(1), 82–108.

Vitaro, F., Tremblay, R. E., Gagnon, C., & Boivin, M. (1992). Peer rejection from kindergarten to grade 2: Outcomes, correlates, and prediction. *Merrill-Palmer Quarterly, 38*(3), 382–400.

Vosk, B., Forehand, R., Parker, J. B., & Rickard, K. (1982). A multimethod comparison of popular and unpopular children. *Developmental Psychology, 18*(4), 571–575.

Windle, M. (1994). A study of friendship characteristics and problem behaviors among middle adolescents. *Child Development, 65*(6), 1764–1777.

Woodward, L. J., & Fergusson, D. M. (1999). Early conduct problems and later risk of teenage pregnancy in girls. *Development and Psychopathology, 11*(1), 127–141.

Younger, A., Gentile, C., & Burgess, K. (1993). Children's perceptions of social withdrawal: Changes across age. In K. H. Rubin, & J. B. Asendorpf (Eds.), *Social withdrawal, inhibition, and shyness in childhood* (pp. 215–235). Mahwah, NJ: Erlbaum.

Zakriski, A. L., & Coie, J. D. (1996). A comparison of aggressive–rejected and nonaggressive–rejected children's interpretations of self-directed and other-directed rejection. *Child Development, 67*(3), 1048–1070.

CHAPTER 15

Socialization in School Settings

Kathryn R. Wentzel and Lisa Looney

Most American children over the age of 6 spend a minimum of 108 days each year in formal educational settings. Many younger children also spend significant portions of their lives in day care or preschool settings. Although the objectives of schooling are primarily academic in nature, preschools as well as later school settings also represent social worlds of major importance and significance to children. In many respects, schools provide social experiences that are highly similar to and overlap with those provided by families, the broader community, and the peer group. However, children are required to use specific skills on a routine basis if they are to be successful at school. For instance, schoolchildren spend significant amounts of time in large groups, engaged in activities that require the coordination of personal goals and abilities with those of others. The abilities to engage in prosocial interactions, regulate behavior to complement that of others, and delay personal gratification are essential for this task. In addition, children's relationships with teachers are less personal and intimate than their relationships with parents. Therefore, children at school must be more independent and self-reliant and more dependent on other children for social support than would be required in most family settings. Finally, evaluations of children's academic and behavioral competencies are ongoing, necessitating goal-directed, planful, and self-monitoring skills in response to feedback.

In essence, the value systems of schools focus on a relatively small set of characteristics and abilities central to children's future roles as citizens and workers, including those related to being socially responsible and responsive to group goals, and to behaving in prosocial, cooperative ways with peers. While accomplishing these socially integrative tasks, children also are expected to assert themselves academically by competing successfully with others or by developing mastery in specific areas of interest. If these outcomes reflect the primary objectives of educators and nonfamilial caregivers, how might their achievement be accomplished? Rarely have scholars attempted to align school-based objectives with specific socialization processes to identify what might promote the development and achievement of such outcomes. The goal of this chapter, therefore, is to describe what is known about the process of socialization within school contexts and to offer suggestions for future theory development and research in this area.

In this chapter, socialization is defined with reference to contextual affordances, that is, supports and opportunities (e.g., staff and setting characteristics such as teacher:child ratios and class size, the nature and quality of relationships with teachers and peers) that facilitate the development of children's school-based competencies. We consider schools to be complex systems that can provide students with multiple affordances, as a function of the school itself as well as through social interactions and interpersonal relationships that are embedded in the educational process. Based on a competence perspective, our discussion of outcomes of socialization in schools is focused primarily on social outcomes rather than academic achievements (see Eccles, Chapter 26, this volume). Toward this end, we begin with a consideration of how to define competence within the social context of schools. We then review the literature on the processes of socialization, including those associated with structural characteristics of schools as well as more proximal social and interpersonal processes that might support competence development. We consider children's experiences in preschool and child care as well as in K–12 schools. Finally, we end with a discussion of remaining issues and challenges to the field.

DEFINING SOCIAL COMPETENCE AT SCHOOL

In the social developmental literature, social competence has been described from a variety of perspectives ranging from the development of individual skills, such as effective behavioral repertoires, social problem-solving skills, positive beliefs about the self, and achievement of social goals, to more general adaptation within a particular setting as reflected in social approval and acceptance. In addition, central to many definitions of social competence is the notion that contextual affordances and constraints contribute to and mold the development of these outcomes in ways that enable them to support the social good (Bronfenbrenner, 1989). In other words, social contexts are believed to play an integral role in competence development by providing opportunities for the development of intrapersonal outcomes (e.g., the achievement of social goals to make friends), but also in defining the appropriate parameters of social accomplishments such that individual skills and attributes can contribute to the social cohesion and smooth functioning of the group (e.g., establishing friendship groups that are socially inclusive rather than exclusive). In this chapter, therefore, social competence at school is defined as a balance between students' achievement of positive outcomes for themselves and adherence to school-specific expectations for behavior.

Support for this definition can be found in the work of Bronfenbrenner (1989), who argues that competence can only be understood in terms of context-specific effectiveness, being a product of personal attributes such as goals, values, self-regulatory skills, and cognitive abilities, and of ways in which these attributes contribute to meeting situational requirements and demands. Bronfenbrenner further suggests that competence is facilitated by contextual supports that provide opportunities for the growth and development of these personal attributes as well as for learning what is expected by the social group. Ford (1992) expands on this notion of person–environment fit by specifying dimensions of competence that reflect personal as well as context-specific criteria: the achievement of personal goals and those that result in positive developmental outcomes for the individual, and the achievement of goals that are situationally relevant, using appropriate means to achieve these goals.

The application of this definition to the realm of schooling results in a multifaceted description of children who are socially competent. First, competent students achieve goals that are personally valued as well as those that are sanctioned by others. Second, the goals they pursue result in social integration as well as in positive developmental outcomes for the student. Socially integrative outcomes are those that promote the smooth functioning of social groups at school (e.g., cooperative behavior) and are reflected in levels of social approval and social acceptance. Student-related outcomes reflect healthy development of the self (e.g., perceived competence and feelings of self-determination) and feelings of emotional well-being (Bronfenbrenner, 1989; Ford, 1992). Therefore, social competence is achieved to the extent that students accomplish goals that result in personal satisfaction and psychological well-being as well as social approval and acceptance. Achieving these positive personal and social outcomes is accomplished not just by one student's efforts but often as the result of compromise or conflict resolution with classmates and teachers.

A consideration of self-enhancing as well as socially integrative outcomes as dual components of social competence is important because the achievement of personal goals and social acceptance are not always compatible. For example, gaining teacher and peer approval might be a personal goal. In this case, a student would be competent if his or her social approval goal is met. A competent student might also view demonstrations of personally valued behavior (e.g., sharing) and social acceptance as multiple and interrelated goals and might use goal coordination skills to achieve both (e.g., sharing in acceptable ways). However, a student might have goals to engage in behavior without concerns about social approval. For this student, social competence would be achieved only if personal goals and social expectations happen to be similar, with social incompetence being a negative consequence if they are incompatible. For example, a child who achieves personal goals by engaging in potentially harmful acts such as bullying or breaking classroom rules would not be considered to be socially competent if others disapprove of such behaviors. Alternatively, a student might try to gain social approval for ulterior motives such as to enhance feelings of self-worth or to decrease anxiety associated with fear of punishment or social retribution. This student would not be socially competent if maladaptive outcomes for the self such as social anxieties or fears remain despite social approval from others.

Finally, an ecological perspective reminds us that the ability to be socially competent at school is contingent upon opportunities and affordances that allow students to achieve a balance between socially integrative and self-assertive outcomes. In this chapter we review work on several aspects of school contexts that have the potential to provide such supports: structural characteristics, social interactions with teachers and classmates, and interpersonal relationships with teachers and classmates. First, however, we describe the goals that teachers, peers, and students themselves value within school contexts. This section is followed by a discussion of processes by which school contexts might support the achievement of these goals.

GOALS FOR STUDENTS AT SCHOOL

The notion that schools provide children with unique socialization experiences has been acknowledged since the beginning of public schooling in the United States. Indeed, public schools were initially developed with an explicit function of educating children to become healthy, moral, and economically productive citizens. Since then, social behavior in the form of moral character, conformity to social rules and norms, cooperation, and positive styles of social interaction has been promoted consistently as a goal for students to achieve (see Wentzel, 1991c, for a review). Given these overarching social goals for education, are there specific goals that are valued more than others in school settings? Do teachers and peers have goals for students concerning what they value and believe should be accomplished within the classroom? In the following sections, research on teachers', peers', and students' goals for themselves is reviewed.

Teachers' Goals for Students

Researchers rarely have asked teachers about their specific goals for students. In preschool and child-care settings, researchers typically identify desirable outcomes of care, often with an implicit assumption that such arrangements might in fact be detrimental to children's social development in comparison to parental care (e.g., Belsky, 2001). As a result, the focus of empirical investigations has been on outcomes that reflect developmentally appropriate milestones for young children, such as secure attachments to mothers and cooperative interactions with peers (Shonkoff & Phillips, 2000), rather than on specific outcomes that teachers would like children to achieve. In contrast, K–12 teachers have been asked what they think well-adjusted and successful students are like. Elementary school teachers (typically first through fifth grades) report preferences for students who are cooperative, conforming, cautious, and responsible rather than independent, assertive, argumentative or disruptive (e.g., Brophy & Good, 1974). Similarly, in the middle school grades (sixth through eighth graders ranging in age from 11 to 14) teachers describe their "ideal" students as sharing, helpful, and responsive to rules, as persistent, and intrinsically interested, and as earning high grades (Wentzel, 2003).

Researchers also have documented social values and expectations that teachers communicate to their students, including appropriate ways to respond to requests, appropriate contexts for different types of behavior, and expectations for impulse control, mature problem solving, and involvement in class activities (e.g., Shultz & Florio, 1979; Trenholm & Rose, 1981). Teachers also communicate expectations for students' interactions with each other. Preschool teachers tend to focus on the development of prosocial behavior by modeling and encouraging prosocial interactions, discouraging social exclusion, and creating cooperative activities (e.g., Doescher & Sugawara, 1989; Hagens, 1997). Elementary and secondary teachers focus on establishing norms for sharing, working well with others, and adherence to rules concerning aggression, manners, stealing, and loyalty (Hargreaves, Hester, & Mellor, 1975; Sieber, 1979).

Students' Goals for Each Other

The classroom goals that students would like each other to achieve are not well documented. However, it is reasonable to assume that students also communicate to each other expectations concerning valued forms of behavior. For instance, approximately 70% of adolescents from three predominantly middle-class middle schools reported that their peers expected them to be cooperative and helpful in class either sometimes or always, and approximately 80% reported similar levels of peer expectations for academic learning (Wentzel, Looney, & Battle, 2006). Moreover, these perceptions did not appear to differ as a function of middle school grade level. Therefore, at least in some schools, peers actively promote the pursuit of positive social and academic outcomes.

Insights concerning peer expectations and values also can be gleaned from research on social characteristics and outcomes related to peer approval and acceptance at school. Researchers typically have defined children's involvement in peer relationships in three ways: degree of peer acceptance or rejection by the larger peer group, peer group membership, and dyadic friendships. Correlates of each of these types of relationships, however, are similar with respect to school-related outcomes. For example, socially accepted students tend to be highly cooperative, helpful, sociable, and self-assertive, whereas socially rejected students are less compliant, less self-assured, and less sociable, and more aggressive, disruptive, and withdrawn than many of their classmates (Rubin, Bukowski, & Parker, 1998). Similarly, children with friends at school tend to be more sociable, cooperative, prosocial, and emotionally supportive when compared to their classmates without friends (Newcomb & Bagwell, 1995; Wentzel, Barry, & Caldwell, 2004).

Of additional interest are findings that being socially accepted and enjoying popular sociometric status is related to successful academic performance and rejected status and rejection to academic difficulties. Results are most consistent with respect to classroom grades (e.g., Buhs & Ladd, 2001; Wentzel, 1991a), although peer acceptance has been related positively to standardized test scores (Austin & Draper, 1984) as well as to IQ (Wentzel, 1991a). These findings are robust for elementary school-age children as well as adolescents, and longitudinal studies document the stability of relations between peer acceptance and academic accomplishments over time (e.g., Ladd & Burgess, 2001; Wentzel & Caldwell, 1997). Other indices of social acceptance such as the ability to establish close friendships also have been related positively to grades and test scores in elementary school and middle school (Berndt & Keefe, 1995; Wentzel et al., 2004).

Students' Goals for Themselves

Research on students' social goals also has not been frequent (see Eccles, Chapter 26, this volume for work on students' achievement-related goals). However, students consistently express interest in forming positive relationships with their classmates (Allen, 1986; Wentzel, 1989, 1991b). Although children are interested in and even emotionally attached to their peers at all ages, establishing rewarding relationships with peers becomes increasingly important for students in middle school and high school. One reason for this growing interest in peers is that many young adolescents enter new middle school structures that necessitate interacting with larger numbers of peers on a daily basis. In contrast to elementary school classrooms, the relative uncertainty and ambiguity of having multiple teachers and different sets of classmates for each class, new instructional styles, and more complex class schedules often result in middle school students turning to each other for information, social support, and ways to cope.

Establishing positive relationships with teachers is also of concern to most students. However, clear developmental trends are evident. Whereas elementary school-age children often describe teachers as being important sources of support (Reid, Landesman, Treder, & Jaccard, 1989), adolescents rarely mention relationships with teachers as having importance in their lives (Lempers & Clark-Lempers, 1992). Finally, when given a list of possible social and academic goals to pursue at school, high school students indicate frequent attempts to achieve a range of social goals, with having fun, making friends, being dependable and responsible, and being helpful ranking as the most frequently pursued goals (Wentzel, 1989).

Summary

Although teachers' and students' goals for education have not been studied extensively, it is clear that a core set of competencies are valued by teachers as well as students. In addition to academic accomplishments, positive forms of behavior that are reflected in compliance to classroom rules and norms and that demonstrate cooperation and caring for classmates also are related to social approval and acceptance by others. Students themselves also mention trying to achieve these same outcomes although they also mention more personal goals such as to have fun. Given these multiple goals, how might a consensus among the various constituents (i.e., teachers, classmates, and individual students) concerning which goals should be pursued at school be achieved? It is clear that schools can play a powerful role in defining socially valued outcomes for students to achieve and that teachers and students actively promote these outcomes in their day-to-day interactions with each other. In the following section, we discuss processes by which schools as well as teachers and students might influence individuals to pursue these outcomes.

PROCESSES OF SOCIALIZATION WITHIN SCHOOL SETTINGS

Although children try to achieve multiple goals for many reasons, the question of what leads them to willingly engage in the pursuit of goals that are valued by others lies at the heart of research on socialization (e.g., Grusec & Goodnow, 1994). If schools promote the adoption and pursuit of socially valued goals, how then does this influence occur? Models of socialization at school are not well developed. However, models of family socialization suggest at least three general mechanisms whereby social resources and experiences might influence competent functioning. First, the structure and general features of social contexts afford opportunities and resources that can directly support or hinder competence development. Second, ongoing social interactions teach children about themselves and what they need to do to become accepted and competent members of their social worlds. Within the context of these interactions, children develop a set of values and standards for behavior and goals they strive to achieve (Grusec & Goodnow, 1994). Third, the qualities of children's social relationships are likely to have motivational significance. When their interpersonal relationships are responsive and nurturant, children are more likely to adopt and internalize the expectations and goals that are valued by others than if their relationships are harsh and critical (Grusec & Goodnow, 1994; Ryan, 1993).

When considered with respect to educational settings, these mechanisms reflect the nested quality of children's experiences at school. Structural features of schools, such as school and class size, teacher:student ratios, and funding, can influence the amount and quality of resources and opportunities available to students. Social interactions and dyadic relationships with teachers and peers describe the more proximal contexts that can influence student adjustment. In the following sections, we review research on each of these mechanisms.

Structural Characteristics of Schooling

Processes of social influence are rarely discussed with regard to structural features of schools. However, numerous studies have documented significant differences in student outcomes as a function of the structural features of the schools they attend, at the pre-school level as well as in elementary and secondary school settings.

Preschool and Child Care

Out-of-family care of preschool children takes place in a diversity of arrangements and settings. However, there is general agreement that structural aspects of quality care are reflected in specific characteristics of staff and settings (e.g., Brooks-Gunn, Fuligni, & Berlin, 2003; Fitzgerald, Mann, Cabrera, & Wong, 2003). Staff characteristics include staff:child ratios, amount and type of staff education and training, years of experience, turnover, and wages. Setting features include type and availability of developmentally appropriate curricular materials, cleanliness, safety, and group size. Researchers also have examined the amount of time children spend in child-care settings in relation to child outcomes.

In general, research has documented significant relations of staff characteristics to a range of social and cognitive outcomes in children across a variety of child-care settings (see Lamb, 1998; Shonkoff & Phillips, 2000, for reviews). Few studies have examined these features while taking into account other important predictors of child outcomes such as family characteristics or the quality of caregiver–child relationships (Fitzgerald et al., 2003). However, results of the National Institute of Child Health and Human Development (NICHD) Early Child Care Study in which a range of child care, home and family (structural, quality, and parent characteristics), and child characteristics have been assessed (see Brooks-Gunn et al., 2003) are beginning to shed light on the combined impact of these multiple factors on child outcomes over time.

A sampling of these findings indicates that child-care factors by themselves do not predict young children's adjustment (as indexed by attachment classifications) unless mothers' characteristics also are taken into account; time spent in child care is related to young children's increased risk for insecure attachment at 12 and 36 months only if maternal sensitivity also is low (NICHD, 1997, 2001). The more time young children spend in nonmaternal care also predicts externalizing problems and conflict with adults at 54 months and in kindergarten, but not in first grade (NICHD, 2003a, 2003b). In general, these findings are robust, even when quality of caregiver–child interactions, type of setting (e.g., center and home-based), instability of child-care arrangements, and maternal sensitivity, level of education, and depression are taken into account. However, levels of problem behavior (e.g., disobedience and aggression) exhibited by children who spend the most time in child care are not at clinical levels and the effect sizes are relatively small. In addition, significant effects often differ depending on who is rating child behavior (mothers or caregivers), making it difficult to draw definitive conclusions (see, e.g., NICHD, 2003a).

More systematic intervention studies have documented the effects of preschool programs such as Head Start on young children. These studies have documented that in the short term, participation in high-quality preschool programs can have significant, positive effects on cognitive and school readiness outcomes (e.g., Love et al., 2003), especially for children living in poverty (e.g., Farran, 2000). These programs also appear to have short-term and long-term effects on social outcomes such as aggression. These latter effects have been found, however, only when interventions also focus on changing parent behavior (Schweinhart, Barne, Weikart, Barnett, & Epstein, 1993). Therefore, the direct effects of participation in preschool programs on young children's social behavior independent of parental influence have not yet been established. Conclusions concerning preschool effects also must be tempered given that researchers typically cannot randomly assign children to control and intervention groups; comparison groups that are comparable with respect to subject and program characteristics are rare.

Formal Schooling

In contrast to research on day care and preschool settings, research on structural effects of elementary and secondary schooling has been guided by specific goals for enhancing the academic and social skills that form the basis of public education policy. For example, policy-driven work in the 1960s (e.g., Coleman et al., 1966) led to conclusions that physical features and administrative structures of schools such as school size, funding, space, class size, teacher:child ratio, and curricular resources explained minimal variance in student outcomes relative to nonschool variables such as family and demographic factors. Subsequent research has confirmed these findings in that the strength of school effects relative to nonschool factors is typically small, except when comparing schools at the two extremes of quality continua (Scheerens & Bosker, 1997). However, other research has documented the positive effects of small school size on academic outcomes and staying in school, even when teacher characteristics and teacher–student relationships are taken into account (Lee & Burkam, 2003; Lee & Loeb, 2000).

School climate, as defined by students' sense of school community and school belonging, also has been related positively (albeit modestly) to social behavioral (Anderman, 2002; Battistich, Solomon, Kim, Watson, & Schaps, 1995; Brand, Felner, Shim, Seitsinger, & Dumas, 2003) and academic (Anderman, 2002) outcomes, with effects often being moderated by students' sex, race (e.g., Kuperminc, Leadbetter, Emmons, & Blatt, 1997), school size (Anderman, 2002) and poverty levels of the schools' community (Battistich et al., 1995). To illustrate, beliefs that their schools are cohesive, responsive, and caring communities predicts young adolescents' decreased drug use and delinquency, even when accounting for within-school differences and the poverty level of the schools' communities (Battistich & Hom, 1997). Similarly, significant negative relations of school climate to young adolescents' externalizing behavior have been documented, even when controlling for race, socioeconomic status, stress levels, and self-concept, with the greatest effects of positive climate shown for African American and single-parent students (Kuperminc et al., 1997). Intervention studies designed to enhance the quality of school climate also have demonstrated that when students begin to experience a greater sense of school community they also display more positive social skills (e.g., Watson, Solomon, Battistich, Schaps, & Solomon, 1989).

The effects of school structures on student outcomes also can be gleaned from school transition studies in which students move from one school level to another, each level being marked by somewhat unique characteristics. Research on transitions of preschool children entering into kindergarten and then into elementary school is rare. However, in contrast to elementary schools, middle schools tend to be larger, require students to interact with larger numbers of peers on a daily basis, and to adjust to new instructional styles (Brophy & Evertson, 1978; Eccles & Midgley, 1989). The transition into high school is associated with similar changes, as the focus on academic accomplishments becomes even more demanding, peer groups are once again disrupted, and the school environment becomes even more impersonal. Predictable changes associated with transitions to middle school are student perceptions that teachers are less caring (Feldlaufer, Midgley, & Eccles, 1988; Midgley, Feldlaufer, & Eccles, 1989) and that they become more focused on students earning high grades, promoting competition between students, and maintaining control (Harter, 1996) than in elementary school. The transition to high school is associated with predictable declines in academic performance, attendance, participation in extracurricular activities (e.g., Alspaugh, 1998; Felner, Aber, Primavera, & Cauce, 1985), and in a perceived loss of teacher and school social support (e.g., Seidman, Allen, Aber, Mitchell, & Feinman, 1994) for many adolescents. Students who do not display these declines often report higher levels of self-esteem and perceived support from teachers and peers than those who do not.

In summary, a number of features that characterize school settings at the preschool and K–12 level appear to be related to children's overall social and academic adjustment to school. For the most part, however, the effects are small, especially when family characteristics are taken into account. Moreover, specific processes that might explain these relations are rarely examined. However, several researchers have demonstrated that classroom-level processes can explain associations between school-level features and student outcomes (e.g., Finn, Pannozzo, & Achilles, 2003). These processes entail teacher and peer communications of goals and expectations for specific behavioral outcomes and creation of interpersonal contexts that motivate students to achieve them (Grusec & Goodnow, 1994).

Social Interactions: Transmitting Values and Providing Help, Advice, and Instruction

How might students learn what is valued by their teachers and peers? Here we review research on ways in which teachers and peers communicate specific values concerning what it means to be competent, and on interactions with teachers and peers that provide help, advice, and instruction with respect to socially valued outcomes.

Social Interactions with Teachers

In the classroom, teachers play the central pedagogical function of transmitting knowledge and training students in academic subject areas. However, during the course of instruction, teachers also promote the development of behavioral competencies by way of classroom management practices (see Doyle, 1986), and by structuring learning environments in ways that make social goals more salient to students (Cohen, 1986; Solomon, Schaps, Watson, & Battistich, 1992). For example, cooperative learning activities can be designed to promote the pursuit of social goals to cooperate and help each other, to be responsible to the group, and to achieve common objectives (Cohen, 1986; Solomon et al., 1992). Indeed, students report stronger levels of social satisfaction when given the opportunity to learn within cooperative learning settings (Slavin, Hurley, & Chamberlain, 2003). Direct instruction of social skills also has been related to decreases in students' aggressive and victimizing behavior toward each other (e.g., Aber, Brown, & Jones, 2003).

Teachers also can convey expectations about ability and performance differentially to students. In this regard, researchers have documented that many teachers hold negative stereotypes of minority and low-achieving students, expecting less competent behavior and lower levels of academic performance from them than from other students (Weinstein, 2002). Of particular importance is that teachers' false expectations can become self-fulfilling prophecies, with student performance changing to conform to teacher expectations (Weinstein, 2002). Although the effects of these expectations tend to be fairly weak (e.g., Jussim, 1991), self-fulfilling prophecies tend to have stronger effects on African American students, students from low socioeconomic backgrounds, and low achievers (Smith, Jussim, & Eccles, 1999). Moreover, teachers who communicate high expectations can bring about positive changes in performance: Teachers' overestimations of ability seem to have a somewhat stronger effect in raising levels of achievement than teachers' underestimations have on lowering achievement, especially for low-performing students (Madon, Jussim, & Eccles, 1997).

Social Interactions with Peers

Interactions with peers also can lead directly to resources and information that help students to be socially competent. Even in preschool settings, peers can create beneficial (as well as risky) contexts for the development of self-regulatory skills (Fabes, Hanish, & Martin, 2003). At older ages, peers provide information and advice, modeled behavior, or specific experiences that facilitate learning social expectations for behavior (Sieber, 1979). Students frequently clarify and interpret their teacher's instructions concerning what they should be doing and how they should do it and provide mutual assistance in the form of volunteering substantive information and answering questions (Cooper, Akers-Lopez, & Marquis, 1982). Classmates also provide each other with important information about themselves; information concerning social self-efficacy and skills can be gleaned by observing social competencies and skills demonstrated by peers (Bandura, 1986; Price & Dodge, 1989).

Other evidence suggests that peer expectations have the potential to provide the most proximal input concerning whether doing something might be important or fun. For instance, middle school students who perceive relatively high expectations for prosocial behavior from their peers also pursue goals to behave prosocially for internalized reasons, or because they think it is important; in contrast, perceived expectations from teachers are associated with prosocial goal pursuit in order to stay out of trouble or to gain social approval (Wentzel, Filisitti, & Looney, 2006). Therefore, peers who communicate a sense of importance or enjoyment with regard to specific types of behavior are likely to lead others to form similar attitudes (Bandura, 1986). This is especially true if students are friends; strong emotional bonds associated with friendships tend to increase the likelihood that friends will imitate each other's behavior (Berndt & Perry, 1986). This latter point highlights the quality of students' interpersonal relationships as an additional, potential influence on their social and academic functioning. This aspect of socialization in school settings is discussed next.

Interpersonal Relationships: Providing Responsive and Emotionally Supportive Contexts

Systems concepts, such as attachment and models of person–environment fit (Eccles & Midgley, 1989; Pianta, Hamre, & Stuhlman, 2003) are used most often to discuss the motivational effects of children's interpersonal relationships at school, especially those with teachers. Similar to parent–child relationships, interpersonal relationships at school are believed to provide children with responsive and nurturing environments that promote personal growth as well as adaptive social functioning. In particular, feelings of relatedness and belongingness at school are expected to contribute directly to positive feelings of self-worth and self-esteem (Pianta et al., 2003). In turn, levels of emotional well-being are believed to contribute to social as well as academic competence (e.g., Harter, 1996).

Perspectives on children's interpersonal relationships at school tend to differ according to the age of the child. Using a developmental systems approach, Pianta and his colleagues (e.g., Pianta et al., 2003) argue for the centrality of teacher–student attachments in the lives of preschool and elementary students. They describe qualities of the teacher–child relationship in terms of three features: closeness (e.g., warmth and open communication), conflict, and dependency. Research on middle childhood and adolescence has focused more often on specific qualities of teacher–student interactions. These qualities correspond closely to parenting styles reflecting consistent enforcement of rules, expectations for self-reliance and self-control, solicitation of children's opinions and feelings, and expressions of warmth and approval (see Wentzel, 2002). In general, these qualities of teacher–student attachments and interactions reflect broad-level relationship provisions of responsiveness (e.g., safety, structure, and autonomy–support) and warmth (e.g., emotional and social support).

Although these aspects of teacher–student relationships have been the focus of most research in this area, relationships with peers also appear to play an important role in creating responsive and emotionally supportive contexts at school. Next we describe research on provisions of responsiveness and warmth from teachers and peers.

Responsive and Warm Relationships with Teachers

During the preschool years, changes in the quality of child–teacher attachments as children move to new child-care settings are related to changes in various aspects of their social functioning (Howes & Hamilton, 1993). Secure attachments to teachers appear to have some positive compensatory effects on the prosocial behavior of preschool children who are insecurely attached to their mothers (Mitchell-Copeland, Denham, & DeMulder, 1997). Findings from the NICHD Early Child Care Study have demonstrated that close relationships with teachers (as perceived by teachers) are related positively to children's social behavior concurrently in kindergarten and 2 years later, with stronger effects for children with less-well-educated mothers (Peisner-Feinberg et al., 2001). However, in observational studies of quality of caregiver–child relationships, emotionally supportive interactions with caregivers are not related significantly to child outcomes when family and child characteristics (e.g., child sex and maternal sensitivity) are taken into account (NICHD, 2003b, 2003c).

Over time, preschool children who enjoy emotionally secure relationships with their teachers also are more likely to demonstrate prosocial, gregarious, and complex play and less likely to show hostile aggression and withdrawn behavior toward their peers (e.g., Howes & Hamilton, 1993). Young children's reports of caring teachers also have been related to positive attitudes about school (Valeski & Stipek, 2001). Following children from kindergarten through eighth grade, Hamre and Pianta (2001) found that kindergartners' relationships with teachers marked by conflict and dependency predicted not only lower grades and standardized test scores but fewer positive work habits and increased numbers of disciplinary infractions through eighth grade, especially for boys (Hamre & Pianta, 2001). Similarly, Birch and Ladd (1998) found teacher–child closeness to be associated positively with children's academic performance, school liking, and self-directedness, whereas relationships marked by conflict and dependency were associated with less than positive outcomes, including declines in children's prosocial behavior over time.

In the elementary school years, student reports of close and supportive teacher–student relationships predict low levels of aggression, especially for African American and Hispanic students (Meehan, Hughes, & Cavell, 2003). This latter finding is especially important in that African American students at this age tend to enjoy less positive relationships with teachers than do white children (e.g., Hamre & Pianta, 2001; Meehan et al., 2003). In late elementary school, students' reports of negative relationships with teachers also are related to externalizing behavior problems, anxiety, and depression (Murray & Greenberg, 2000) and positive relationships to identification with teachers' values and positive social self-concept (Davis, 2001).

In older students, much research has documented significant, positive relations between teacher provisions of structure, guidance, and autonomy and various aspects of academic motivation, engagement, and performance outcomes (e.g., Skinner & Belmont, 1993; Wentzel 2002). Studies relating responsive teaching to social outcomes have been far less frequent. However, Wentzel (2002) documented significant relations of perceived high expectations and low levels of criticism on the part of teachers to students' pursuit of goals to be prosocial and socially responsible. Schoolwide interventions in which teachers are taught to provide students with clear expectations for behavior, developmentally appropriate autonomy, and warmth and support result in increased levels of students' sense of community and displays of socially competent behavior (Watson et al., 1989).

Adolescents' perceptions that teachers are emotionally supportive and caring have been related most often to positive motivational outcomes, including the pursuit of goals to learn and to behave prosocially and responsibly; academic interest; educational aspirations and values; and positive self-concept (e.g., Harter, 1996; Roeser, Midgley, & Urdan, 1996; Wentzel, 1994, 1997). Having supportive relationships with teachers also appears to predict in part, whether students at this age drop out of school (Rumberger, 1995). In a study of perceived support from teachers, parents, and peers (Wentzel, 1998), perceived support from teachers was unique in its relation to students' interest in class and pursuit of goals to adhere to classroom rules and norms.

Responsive and Warm Relationships with Peers

Researchers have not adapted parenting models to the study of peer relationships (cf. Wentzel, 2004). However, it is reasonable to assume that when peers create responsive and emotionally supportive interpersonal contexts, students will benefit in positive ways. In young children, high levels of peer acceptance and positive friendships have been linked to academic and socioemotional adjustment in school, including positive affect, academic and social engagement, and positive attitudes toward school (e.g., Buhs & Ladd, 2001; Ladd, Kochenderfer, & Coleman, 1996). Older students (in middle childhood and adolescence) who are accepted by their peers and who have established friendships with classmates are more likely to enjoy a relatively safe school environment and less likely to be the targets of peer-directed violence and harassment than their peers who do not have friends (Hodges, Bovin, Vitaro, & Bukowski, 1999). In contrast, children who are rejected by their peers tend to be bullied and victimized more frequently than others (Olweus, 1993). Even among young children, rejected children are treated more negatively by their peers than are their more socially accepted classmates (Buhs & Ladd, 2001).

During adolescence, students also report that their peer groups and crowds provide them with a sense of emotional security and a sense of belonging (Brown, Eicher, & Petrie, 1986). In contrast, adolescents without friends or who are socially rejected are often lonely, emotionally distressed, and depressed and suffer from poor self-concepts (Guay, Boivin, & Hodges, 1999; Wentzel & Caldwell, 1997). Perceived social and emotional support from peers has been associated positively with prosocial outcomes such as helping, sharing, and cooperating and negatively to antisocial forms of behavior (e.g., Wentzel, 1994). Perceived support from peers also has been related to pursuit of academic goals and interests; in contrast, students who perceive little peer support tend to be at risk for academic problems (see Wentzel, 2003).

Summary

The extant literature supports the notion that structural features, social interactions with teachers and peers, and the provisions of responsiveness and warmth have the potential to provide tangible resources, opportunities, and experiences that support competence development at school. In this regard, children's experiences at school, whether in preschool or K–12 settings, appear to support the pursuit and achievement of goals that are espoused by teachers and peers, as well as the development of positive outcomes for students themselves. In the following section, we offer remaining questions and challenges for continued work in this area.

CONCLUSIONS AND FUTURE DIRECTIONS

In this chapter, we have described social competence at school as the achievement of personal goals that include healthy developmental outcomes, such as emotional well-being, in balance with the achievement of socially valued goals, such as displays of prosocial forms of behavior. Further, we have argued that the socialization of these competencies within school settings can be understood as a function of the amount and quality of structural-level resources of schools as well as interpersonal contacts with teachers and peers that support students' efforts to achieve personal as well as socially valued goals. Social interactions are likely to teach students what they are expected to accomplish and how to achieve it. In turn, the transmission of values and knowledge is more likely to occur if students enjoy supportive and caring relationships at school. In conclusion, we would like to raise several general issues that require additional consideration and empirical investigation if the field is to make progress in understanding the socialization functions of schools. These issues concern the nature of social competence at school and how it is socialized, the unique role of schools in promoting the development of competent outcomes, and the need for more sophisticated research methods and designs that can test theoretical models relevant for school settings.

Social Competence at School

Although we are beginning to understand the basic social outcomes that most teachers and students value at school, we know little about how and why students come to learn about and to adopt these goals as their own. For instance, it is clear that teachers communicate their expectations and goals to students on a daily basis. However, less is known about factors that predispose students to accept or reject these communications. The family socialization literature suggests that parental messages are more likely to be perceived accurately by children if they are clear and consistent, are framed in ways that are relevant and meaningful to the child, require decoding and processing by the child, and are perceived by the child to be of clear importance to the parent and as being conveyed with positive intentions (Grusec & Goodnow, 1994). Adapting this work to the realm of the classroom might provide important insights into effective forms of teacher and peer communication that lead to the adoption of socially valued goals.

Similarly, a greater focus on understanding student characteristics that facilitate their acceptance of teachers' communications is needed. Factors such as students' beliefs regarding the fairness, relevance, and developmental appropriateness of teachers' goals and expectations (e.g., Smetana & Bitz, 1996) and aspects of social–cognitive processing, such as selective attention, attributions, and social biases and stereotypes (Price & Dodge, 1989) are likely to influence students' interpretations and acceptance of social communications. Other individual characteristics such as attachment security and family functioning (e.g., Fuligni, Eccles, Barber, & Clements, 2001), racial identity (Graham, Taylor, & Hudley, 1998), and the extent that students are oriented toward gaining social approval also are likely to influence the degree to which they are influenced by teacher and peer expectations.

Consideration of student characteristics also must take into account age-related capabilities. For example, primary developmental tasks of young children under age 6 involve basic self-regulatory skills (managing physiological arousal, emotions, and attention), executive functions such as the ability to monitor and plan behavior, language and communication skills, and peer interaction skills (Shonkoff & Phillips, 2000). As they make their way through school, children are challenged with school transitions requiring skills related to social integration, flexible coping, and adaptation to new environments. In part, these successful adaptations require the development of positive self-perceptions of autonomy, competence, and personal identity (Grolnick, Kurowski, & Gurland, 1999).

In general, mastery of these developmental tasks as they relate to children's understanding and adoption of socially valued goals and objectives of teachers and peers needs to be incorporated into models of school success. A developmental focus also is necessary for understanding the demands of teachers on students of different ages. A few researchers (e.g., Brophy & Good, 1974; Eccles & Midgley, 1989) have observed that teachers treat students differently and focus on different tasks and goals depending on the age of their students. For example, teachers of early elementary (i.e., first grade) and junior high school students tend to spend more of their time on issues related to social conduct than do teachers at other grade levels. However, little else is known about these differences. Therefore, a critical look at the normative requirements for competent classroom functioning also is necessary for knowledge of school socialization processes to advance.

An additional issue concerns what it is that develops or is changed on the part of students as a result of exposure to supportive teacher and peer contexts. In part, responsive and warm relationships are likely to promote a sense of emotional well-being and corresponding desires to contribute to the smooth functioning of classroom activities. Continued research that focuses on additional psychological mediators might be particularly fruitful in determining specific ways in which students' social interactions and interpersonal relationships at school ultimately influence their social competence at school. For example, an additional area for consideration is the influence of social relationships on self-regulatory processes that promote goal pursuit, such as positive beliefs about ability, personal values, and attributions for success and failure (see Wentzel, 2004). The role of these intrapersonal processes in mediating relations between aspects of socialization and competent functioning has not been studied extensively. The differential impact of teachers and peers in contributing to these outcomes also deserves further study (see e.g., Wentzel, 1997).

Schools as Unique Socializing Contexts

One of the enduring issues with respect to school-related influence concerns the possibility that school experiences mainly afford the practice, refinement, and reinforcement of skills and values learned at home. If so, continuity across home and school settings might explain children's competence at school more so than experiences unique to schools. This notion is supported by findings that family socialization models are useful for describing socialization processes at school (Wentzel, 2002). In addition, family factors are typically strong predictors of school outcomes (e.g., Rumberger, 1995) and often completely explain variance predicted by school variables when they are taken into account (e.g., Jimerson, Egeland, Sroufe, & Carlson, 2000). Research that examines core socialization processes that are common across multiple settings and domains of functioning is a natural extension of this work. An additional question, however, concerns the extent to which exposure to socialization processes at school might influence children for whom experiences at home and at school are not highly similar. It is likely that school effects might be most noticeable for these children, with degrees of home-school continuity moderating the effects of schooling on child outcomes.

Another intriguing issue concerns the role of peers in the school socialization process. As noted at the beginning of this chapter, a fairly unique aspect of schooling is the requirement that students learn to cooperate and get along with each other. Although this implies that socializing children to function well in formalized peer groups might be a central function of schools, the development of cooperative, prosocial behavior is often attributed to interactions with peers rather than with adults (Younnis, 1994). Few researchers have documented ways in which teachers and school settings might influence the development and quality of peer interactions independently of the influence that students exert on each other. However, teachers' verbal and nonverbal behavior toward certain children has been related to how these children are treated by their peers (Harper & McCluskey, 2003; White & Kistner, 1992). Therefore, it is reasonable to assume that the development of positive forms of behavior might be due in large part to systematic regulation of peer interactions in formal school settings. We suggest that this is an important area of inquiry for developmental as well as educational psychologists to pursue.

Theory, Methods, and Designs

Most of our conclusions concerning socialization in school settings are based on findings from nonexperimental correlational studies. These correlational strategies have resulted in a wealth of data that can serve as a strong foundation for further theory building and research. Descriptive designs also are useful for developing profiles of behavior that characterize competent students. However, more extensive research that can identify variations in these characterizations across classrooms and schools requires in-depth conversations with and extensive observations of students and teachers as they carry out their day-to-day lives at school. In addition, correlational designs typically have focused on a limited number of variables at one point in time. As a result, it is rare that process-oriented variables such as teacher–student interactions are included in studies of structural effects, or familial and nonschool predictors in studies of classroom processes. It also is likely that schools can have effects on children by way of their positive impact on the economic (Sederberg, 1987) and political (Reynolds, 1995) life of communities; school-to-work and service learning programs are good examples of school-based resources that have the potential to provide positive benefits to communities and families. The notion that community and family effects might mediate the impact of schools on children is intriguing but rarely studied in systematic fashion. Therefore, a necessary next step is the development of conceptual models that consider ways in which children and the various social systems in which they develop, including home, peer groups, communities, and schools, interact to support the development of school-related competence.

In addition, correlational research cannot advance understanding of causal influence or direction of effects. Indeed, is it that responsive and supportive teachers and peers have the potential to influence the development of competencies and skills they value, or is it that competent students influence teachers and peers to interact with them in specific ways? Although the answer is likely that both are true, identifying ways in which teachers and peers actively promote the development of social competencies at school requires systematic longitudinal and experimental research. Large-scale longitudinal studies have begun to document school-based predictors of young children's competence over time (e.g., NICHD Child Care Study). Others have begun to document correlates of change related to qualities of older students' relationships with teacher and peer relationships (e.g., Hamre & Pianta, 2001; Ladd & Burgess, 2001; Wentzel & Caldwell, 1997).

Experimental studies designed to examine processes that support social competence development in schools are rare (cf. Solomon et al., 1992). Unfortunately, most school reform efforts focus on improving achievement test scores and other academic outcomes (e.g., No Child Left Behind Act of 2001), without consideration of the social and psychological consequences of these efforts. However, given the strong interrelations among qualities of relationships with teachers and peers, forms of classroom behavior and academic outcomes (see Wentzel, 2003), it seems essential that reform initiatives involving experimentation in schools and evaluation of student progress incorporate assessments of outcomes across multiple social and academic domains.

Our current understanding of school socialization also is based primarily on studies of white middle-class children. Therefore, more diverse samples with respect to race and socioeconomic status also are needed in this area of research. For instance, in response to findings reported by the NICHD Child Care Study, researchers have argued that when child-care variables are assessed in more diverse samples that include a broader range of socioeconomic status (SES) and ethnicity, different results are obtained (e.g., Sagi, Koren-Karie, Gini, Ziv, & Joels, 2002). Researchers of older children also have found that race moderates relations between dropping out of school and features of schools and families, such that the SES of families and schools predicts dropping out for white and Hispanic adolescents but not for African American students (Rumberger, 1995). Some studies also have demonstrated differential teacher treatment of students as a function of student gender, race, (Irvine, 1986), and behavioral styles (Chang, 2003), with these differences sometimes attributed in part, to teachers' own race and gender (Saft & Pianta, 2001).

Although it is likely that the underlying psychological processes that contribute to school adjustment are similar for all students regardless of race, ethnicity, gender, or other contextual and demographic variables, the degree to which these latter factors interact with psychological processes to influence adjustment outcomes is not known. Achieving a better understanding of such interactions deserves our full attention. To illustrate, goal coordination skills, such as planning, monitoring, and regulation of behavior, that support the achievement of multiple objectives might be more important for the adjustment of children from minority backgrounds than for children who come from families and communities whose goals and expectations are similar to those of the educational establishment (e.g., Fordham & Ogbu, 1986). Peer relationship skills might be especially important for adjustment in schools in which peer cultures are particularly strong or in which collaborative and cooperative learning is emphasized. Similarly, beliefs about how to characterize a competent student are likely to vary as a function of race, gender, neighborhood, or family background. The fact that many results concerning child outcomes and schooling differ as a function of who provides the assessments of behavior (e.g., parents, teachers, or students themselves) attests to this possibility (e.g., NICHD, 2003a; Toro et al., 1985). Expanding our database to include the voices of underrepresented populations both as research participants and as researchers can only enrich our understanding of how and why children make successful adaptations to school.

In conclusion, we have argued that being a competent student requires children to achieve positive developmental outcomes and personal goals while meeting social objectives that are imposed externally by teachers and peers. Identifying the precise socialization experiences that lead to a healthy balance between personal growth and social integration remains a significant challenge to the field. However, we have gained some initial insights into students' experiences within school settings as they relate to social approval and acceptance as well as the development of personal competencies and interests. Socialization of these outcomes within school settings can be understood in part, as a function of the amount and quality of structural-level resources of schools as well as interpersonal contacts with teachers and peers. Ideally, these insights can serve as a foundation for continued research on the social antecedents of children's competent functioning at school.

REFERENCES

Aber, J. L., Brown, J. L., & Jones, S. M. (2003). Developmental trajectories toward violence in middle childhood: Course, demographic differences, and response to school-based intervention. *Developmental Psychology, 39*, 324–348.

Allen, J. D. (1986). Classroom management: Students' perspectives, goals, and strategies. *American Educational Research Journal, 23*, 437–459.

Alspaugh, D. (1998). Achievement loss associated with the transition to middle school and high school. *Journal of Educational Research, 92*, 20–25.

Anderman, E. M. (2002). School effects on psychological outcomes during adolescence. *Journal of Educational Psychology, 94*, 795–809.

Austin, A. B., & Draper, D. C. (1984). The relationship among peer acceptance, social impact, and academic achievement in middle school. *American Educational Research Journal, 21*, 597–604.

Bandura, A. (1986). *Social foundations of thought and action: A social cognitive theory.* Englewood Cliffs, NJ: Prentice-Hall.

Battistich, V., & Hom, A. (1997). The relationship between students' sense of their school as a community and their involvement in problem behaviors. *American Journal of Public Health, 87*, 1997–2001.

Battistich, V., Solomon, D., Kim, D., Watson, M., & Schaps, E. (1995). Schools as communities, poverty levels of student populations, and students' attitudes, motives, and performance: A multilevel analysis. *American Educational Research Journal, 32*, 627–658.

Belsky, J. (2001). Emanuel Miller lecture: Developmental risks (still) associated with early child care. *Journal of Child Psychology and Psychiatry and Allied Disciplines, 42*, 845–859.

Berndt, T. J., & Keefe, K. (1995). Friends' influence on adolescents' adjustment to school. *Child Development, 66*, 1312–1329.

Berndt, T. J., & Perry, T. B. (1986). Children's perceptions of friendships as supportive relationships. *Developmental Psychology, 22*, 640–648.

Birch, S. H., & Ladd, G. W. (1998). Children's interpersonal behaviors and the teacher–child relationship. *Developmental Psychology, 34*, 934–946.

Brand, S., Felner, R., Shim, M., Seitsinger, A., & Dumas, T. (2003). Middle school improvement and reform: Development and validation of a school-level assessment of climate, cultural pluralism, and school safety. *Journal of Educational Psychology, 95*, 570–588.

Bronfenbrenner, U. (1989). Ecological systems theory. In R. Vasta (Ed.), *Annals of child development* (Vol. 6, pp.187–250). Greenwich, CT: JAI Press.

Brooks-Gunn, J., Fuligni, A. S., & Berlin, L. J. (2003). *Early childhood development in the 21st century.* New York: Teachers College Press.

Brophy, J. E., & Evertson, C. M. (1978). Context variables in teaching. *Educational Psychologist, 12*, 310–316.

Brophy, J. E., & Good, T. L. (1974). *Teacher–student relationships: Causes and consequences.* New York: Holt, Rinehart & Winston.

Brown, B. B., Eicher, S. A., & Petrie, S. (1986). The importance of peer group ("crowd') affiliation in adolescence. *Journal of Adolescence, 9*, 73–96.

Buhs, E. S., & Ladd, G. W. (2001). Peer rejection as an antecedent of young children's school adjustment: An examination of mediating processes. *Developmental Psychology, 37*, 550–560.

Chang, L. (2003). Variable effects of children's aggression, social withdrawal, and prosocial leadership as functions of teacher beliefs and behaviors. *Child Development, 74*, 535–548.

Cohen, E. G. (1986). *Designing group work: Strategies for the heterogeneous classroom.* New York: Teachers College Press.

Coleman, J. S., Campbell, E. Q., Hobson, C. J., McPartland, J., Mood, A. M., Weinfeld, F. D., et al. (1966). *Equality of educational opportunity.* Washington, DC: U.S. Government Printing Office.

Cooper, C. R., Ayers-Lopez, S., & Marquis, A. (1982). Children's discourse during peer learning in experimental and naturalistic situations. *Discourse Processes, 5*, 177–191.

Davis, H. A. (2001). The quality and impact of relationships between elementary school students and teachers. *Contemporary Educational Psychology, 26*, 431–453.

Doescher, S. M., & Sugawara, A. I. (1989). Encouraging prosocial behavior in young children. *Childhood Education, 65*, 213–216.

Doyle, W. (1986). Classroom organization and management. In M. C. Witrock (Ed.), *Handbook of research on teaching* (pp. 392–431). New York: Macmillan.

Eccles, J. S., & Midgley, C. (1989). Stage-environment fit: Developmentally appropriate classrooms for young adolescents. In C. Ames & R. Ames (Eds.), *Research on motivation in education* (Vol. 3, pp. 139–186). New York: Academic Press.

Fabes, R. A., Hanish, L. D., & Martin, C. (2003). Children at play: The role of peers in understanding the effects of child care. *Child Development, 74*, 969–1226.

Farran, D. (2000). Another decade of intervention for children who are low income or disabled: What do we know now? In J. P. Shonkoff & S. J. Meisels (Eds.), *Handbook of early childhood intervention* (2nd ed., pp. 510–548). New York: Cambridge University Press.

Feldlaufer, H., Midgley, C., & Eccles, J. S. (1988). Student, teacher, and observer perceptions of the classroom before and after the transition to junior high school. *Journal of Early Adolescence, 8*, 133–156.

Felner, R. D., Aber, M. S., Primavera, J., & Cauce, A. M. (1985). Adaptation and vulnerability in high-risk adolescents: An examination of environmental mediators. *American Journal of Community Psychology, 13*, 365–379.

Finn, J. D., Pannozzo, G. M., & Achilles, C. M. (2003). The "why's" of class size: Student behavior in small classes. *Review of Educational Research, 73*, 321–368.

Fitzgerald, H., Mann, T., Cabrera, N., & Wong, M. (2003). Diversity in caregiving contexts. In R. Lerner, A. Easterbrooks, & J. Mistry (Ed.), *Handbook of psychology, Vol. Six: Developmental psychology* (pp. 135–167). Mahwah, NJ: Erlbaum.

Ford, M. E. (1992). *Motivating humans: Goals, emotions, and personal agency beliefs.* Newbury Park, CA: Sage.

Fordham, S., & Ogbu, J. U. (1986). Black students' school success; Coping with "the burden of 'acting white.'" *The Urban Review, 18*, 176–206.

Fuligni, A. J., Eccles, J. S., Barber, B. L., & Clements, P. (2001). Early adolescent peer orientation and adjustment during high school. *Developmental Psychology, 37*, 28–36.

Graham, S., Taylor, A., & Hudley, C. (1998). Exploring achievement values among ethnic minority early adolescents. *Journal of Educational Psychology, 90*, 606–620.

Grolnick, W. S., Kurowski, C. O., & Gurland, S. T. (1999). Family processes and the development of children's self-regulation. *Educational Psychologist, 34*, 3–14.

Grusec, J. E., & Goodnow, J. J. (1994). Impact of parental discipline methods on the child's internalization of values: A reconceptualization of current points of view. *Developmental Psychology, 30*, 4–19.

Guay, F., Boivin, M., & Hodges, E. V. E. (1999). Predicting change in academic achievement: A model of peer experiences and self-system processes. *Journal of Educational Psychology, 91*, 105–115.

Hagens, H. E. (1997). Strategies for encouraging peer interactions in infant/toddler programs. *Early Childhood Education Journal, 25*, 147–149.

Hamre, B. K., & Pianta, R. C. (2001). Early teacher-child relationships and the trajectory of children's school outcomes through eighth grade. *Child Development, 72*, 625–628.

Hargreaves, D. H., Hester, S. K., & Mellor, F. J. (1975). *Deviance in classrooms.* London: Routledge & Kegan Paul.

Harper, L. V., & McCluskey, K. S. (2003). Teacher–child and child–child interactions in inclusive preschool settings: Do adults inhibit peer interactions? *Early Childhood Research Quarterly, 18*, 163–184.

Harter, S. (1996). Teacher and classmate influences on scholastic motivation, self-esteem, and level of voice in adolescents. In J. Juvonen & K. Wentzel (Eds.), *Social motivation: Understanding children's school adjustment* (pp. 11–42). New York: Cambridge University Press.

Hodges, E. V., Boivin, M., Vitaro, F., & Bukowski, W. M. (1999). The power of friendship: Protection against an escalating cycle of peer victimization. *Developmental Psychology, 35*, 94–101.

Howes, C., & Hamilton, C.E. (1993). The changing experience of child care: Changes in teachers and in teacher–child relationships and children's social competence with peers. *Early Childhood Research Quarterly, 8*, 15–32.

Irvine, J. J. (1986). Teacher–student interactions: Effects of student race, sex, and grade level. *Journal of Educational Psychology, 78*, 14–21.

Jimerson, S., Egeland, B., Sroufe, L. A., & Carlson, B. (2000). A prospective longitudinal study of high school dropouts: Examining multiple predictors across development. *Journal of School Psychology, 38*, 525–549.

Jussim, L. (1991). Social perception and social reality: A reflection–construction model. *Psychological Review, 98*, 9–34.

Kuperminc, G. P., Leadbetter, B. J., Emmons, C., & Blatt, S. J. (1997). Perceived school climate and difficulties in the social adjustment of middle school students. *Applied Developmental Psychology, 1*, 76–88.

Ladd, G. W., & Burgess, K. B. (2001). Do relational risks and protective factors moderate the linkages between childhood aggression and early psychological and school adjustment? *Child Development, 72*, 1579–1601.

Ladd, G. W., Kochenderfer, B. J., & Coleman, C. C. (1996). Friendship quality as a predictor of young children's early school adjustment. *Child Development, 67*, 1103–1118.

Lamb, M. E. (1998). Nonparental child care: Context, quality, correlates. In W. Damon, I. E. Sigel, & K. A. Renninger (Eds.), *Handbook of child psychology, Vol. 4: Child psychology in practice* (pp. 73–134). New York: Wiley.

Lee, V. E., & Burkam, D. T. (2003). Dropping out of high school: The role of school organization and structure. *American Educational Research Journal, 40*, 353–393.

Lee, V. E., & Loeb, S. (2000). School size in Chicago elementary schools: Effects on teachers' attitudes and students' achievement. *American Educational Research Journal, 37*, 3–31.

Lempers, J. D., & Lempers-Clark, D. S. (1992). Young, middle, and late adolescents' comparisons of the functional importance of five significant relationships. *Journal of Youth and Adolescence, 21*, 53–96.

Love, J. M., Harrison, L., Sagi-Schwartz, A., van IJzendoorn, M. H., Ross, C., Ungerer, J. A., et al. (2003). Child care quality matters: How conclusions may vary with context. *Child Development, 74*, 1021–1033.

Madon, S., Jussim, L., & Eccles, J. (1997). In search of self-fulfilling prophecy. *Journal of Personality and Social Psychology, 72*, 791–809.

Meehan, B. T., Hughes, J. N., & Cavell, T. A. (2003). Teacher–student relationships as compensatory resources for aggressive children. *Child Development, 74*, 1145–1157.

Midgley, C., Feldlaufer, H., & Eccles, J. (1989). Student/teacher relations and attitudes toward mathematics before and after the transition to junior high school. *Child Development, 60*, 981–992.

Mitchell-Copeland, J., Denham, S. A., DeMulder, E. K. (1997). Q-Sort assessment of child–teacher attachment relationships and social competence in the preschool. *Early Education and Development, 8*, 27–40.

Murray, C., & Greenberg, M.T. (2000). Children's relationships with teachers and bonds with school: An investigation of patterns and correlates in middle childhood. *Journal of School Psychology, 38*, 423–445.

Newcomb, A. F., & Bagwell, C. L. (1995). Children's friendship relations: A meta-analytic review. *Psychological Bulletin, 117*, 306–347.

NICHD Early Child Care Research Network. (1997). The effects of infant child care on infant-mother attachment security: Results of the NICHD study of early child care. *Child Development, 68*, 860–879.

NICHD Early Child Care Research Network. (2001). Child-care and family predictors of preschool attachment and stability from infancy. *Developmental Psychology, 37*, 847–862.

NICHD Early Child Care Research Network. (2003a). Does amount of time spent in child care predict socioemotional adjustment during the transition to kindergarten? *Child Development, 74*, 976–1005.

NICHD Early Child Care Research Network. (2003b). Social functioning in first grade: Associations with earlier home and child care predictors and with current classroom experiences. *Child Development, 74*, 1639–1662.

NICHD Early Child Care Research Network. (2003c). Does quality of child care affect child outcomes at age 4½? *Developmental Psychology, 39*, 451–469.

Olweus, D. (1993). Victimization by peers: Antecedents and long-term outcomes. In K. Rubin & J. B. Asendorf (Eds.), *Social withdrawal, inhibition, and shyness in childhood* (pp. 315–341). Chicago: University of Chicago Press.

Peisner-Feinberg, E.S., Burchinal, M.R., Clifford, R.M., Culkin, M.L., Howes, C., Kagan, S.L., et al. (2001). The relation of preschool child-care quality to children's cognitive and social development trajectories through second grade. *Child Development, 72*, 1534–1553.

Pianta, R. C., Hamre, B., & Stuhlman, M. (2003). Relationships between teachers and children. In W.

Reynolds & G. Miller (Eds.), *Handbook of psychology: Vol. 7. Educational psychology* (pp. 199–234). New York: Wiley.

Price, J. M., & Dodge, K. A. (1989). Peers' contributions to children's social maladjustment: Description and intervention. In T. J. Berndt & G. W. Ladd (Eds.), *Peer relationships in child development* (pp. 341–370). New York: Wiley.

Reid, M., Landesman, S., Treder, R., & Jaccard, J. (1989). "My family and friends": Six-to twelve-year-old children's perceptions of social support. *Child Development, 60,* 896–910.

Reynolds, D. R. (1995). Rural education: Decentering the consolidation debate. In E. N. Castle (Ed.), *The changing American countryside: Rural people and places* (pp. 451–480). Lawrence: University Press of Kansas.

Roeser, R. W., Midgley, C., & Urdan, T. C. (1996). Perceptions of the school psychological environment and early adolescents' psychological and behavioral functioning in school: The mediating role of goals and belonging. *Journal of Educational Psychology, 88,* 408–422.

Rubin, K. H., Bukowski, W., & Parker, J. G. (1998). Peer interactions, relationships, and groups. In W. Damon (Series Ed.) & N. Eisenberg (Vol. Ed.), *Handbook of child psychology: Vol. 3. Social, emotional, and personality development* (5th ed., pp. 619–700). New York; Wiley.

Rumberger, R. W. (1995). Dropping out of middle school: A multilevel analysis of students and schools. *American Educational Research Journal, 32,* 583–625.

Ryan, R. M. (1993). Agency and organization: Intrinsic motivation, autonomy, and the self in psychological development. In J. Jacobs (Ed.), *Nebraska symposium on motivation* (Vol. 40, pp. 1–56). Lincoln: University of Nebraska Press.

Saft, E. W., & Pianta, R. C. (2001). Teachers' perceptions of their relationships with students: Effects of child age, gender, and ethnicity of teachers and children. *School Psychology Quarterly, 16,* 125–141.

Sagi, A., Koren-Karie, N., Gini, M., Ziv, Y., & Joels, T. (2002). Shedding further light on the effects of various types and quality of early child care on infant–mother attachment relationship: The Haifa study of early child care. *Child Development, 73,* 1166–1186.

Scheerens, J., & Bosker, R. J. (1997). *The foundations of educational effectiveness.* Oxford, UK: Elsevier.

Schweinhart., L. J., Barne, H. V., Weikart, D. P., Barnett, W. S., & Epstein, A. S. (1993). *Significant benefits: The High/Scope Perry Preschool Study through age 27.* Ypsilanti, MI: High/Scope Press.

Sederberg, C. H. (1987). Economic role of school districts in rural communities. *Research in Rural Education, 4,* 125–130.

Seidman, E., Allen, L., Aber, J. L., Mitchell, C., & Feinman, J. (1994). The impact of school transitions in early adolescence on the self-esteem and perceived social context of poor urban youth. *Child Development, 65,* 507–522.

Shultz, J., & Florio, S. (1979). Stop and freeze: The negotiation of social and physical space in a kindergarten/first grade classroom. *Anthropology and Education Quarterly, 10,* 166–181.

Shonkoff, J. P., & Phillips, D. A. (2000). *From neurons to neighborhoods: The science of early childhood development.* Washington, DC: National Academy Press.

Sieber, R. T. (1979). Classmates as workmates: Informal peer activity in the elementary school. *Anthropology and Education Quarterly, 10,* 207–235.

Skinner, E. A., & Belmont, M. J. (1993). Motivation in the classroom: Reciprocal effects of teacher behavior and student engagement across the school year. *Journal of Educational Psychology, 85,* 571– 581.

Slavin, R. E., Hurley, E. A., & Chamberlain, A. (2003). Cooperative learning and achievement: Theory and research. In W. Reynolds & G. Miller (Eds.), *Handbook of psychology: Vol. 7. Educational Psychology* (pp. 177–198). New York: Wiley.

Smetana, J., & Bitz, B. (1996). Adolescents' conceptions of teachers' authority and their relations to rule violations in school. *Child Development, 67,* 1153–1172.

Smith, A. E., Jussim., & Eccles, J. (1999). Do self-fulfilling prophecies accumulate, dissipate, or remain stable over time? *Journal of Personality and Social Psychology, 77,* 548–565.

Solomon, D., Schaps, E., Watson, M., & Battistich, V. (1992). Creating caring school and classroom communities for all students. In R. Villa, J. Thousand, W. Stainback, & S. Stainback (Eds.), *Restructuring for caring and effective education: An administrative guide to creating heterogeneous schools* (pp. 41–60). Baltimore: Brookes.

Toro, P. A., Cowen, E. L., Gesten, E. L., Weissberg, R. P., Rapkin, B. D., & Davidson, E. (1985). Social environmental predictors of children's adjustment in elementary school classrooms. *American Journal of Community Psychology, 13,* 353–363.

Trenholm, S., & Rose, T. (1981). The compliant communicator: Teacher perceptions of appropriate class-room behavior. *The Western Journal of Speech Communication, 45*, 13–26.

Valeski, T. N., & Stipek, D. J. (2001). Young children's feelings about school. *Child Development, 72*, 1198–1213.

Watson, M., Solomon, D., Battistich, V., Schaps, E., & Solomon, J. (1989). The child development project: Combining traditional and developmental approaches to values education. In L. Nucci (Ed.), *Moral development and character education: A dialogue* (pp. 51–92). Berkeley, CA: McCutchan.

Weinstein, R. S. (2002). *Reaching higher: The power of expectations in schooling.* Cambridge, MA: Harvard University Press.

Wentzel, K. R. (1989). Adolescent classroom goals, standards for performance, and academic achievement: An interactionist perspective. *Journal of Educational Psychology, 81*, 131–142.

Wentzel, K. R. (1991a). Relations between social competence and academic achievement in early adolescence. *Child Development, 62*, 1066–1078.

Wentzel, K. R. (1991b). Social and academic goals at school: Achievement motivation in context. In M. Maehr and P. Pintrich (Eds.), *Advances in motivation and achievement* (Vol. 7, pp. 185–212). Greenwich, CT: JAI Press.

Wentzel, K. R. (1991c). Social competence at school: Relations between social responsibility and academic achievement. *Review of Educational Research, 61*, 1–24.

Wentzel, K. R. (1994). Relations of social goal pursuit to social acceptance, classroom behavior, and perceived social support. *Journal of Educational Psychology, 86*, 173–182.

Wentzel, K. R. (1997). Student motivation in middle school: The role of perceived pedagogical caring. *Journal of Educational Psychology, 89*, 411–419.

Wentzel, K. R. (1998). Social support and adjustment in middle school: The role of parents, teachers, and peers. *Journal of Educational Psychology, 90*, 202–209.

Wentzel, K. R. (2002). Are effective teachers like good parents? Interpersonal predictors of school adjustment in early adolescence. *Child Development, 73*, 287–301.

Wentzel, K. R. (2003). School adjustment. In W. Reynolds & G. Miller (Eds.), *Handbook of psychology: Vol. 7. Educational psychology* (pp. 235–258). New York: Wiley.

Wentzel, K. R. (2004). Understanding classroom competence: The role of social-motivational and self-processes. In R. Kail (Ed.), *Advances in child development and behavior, Vol. 32* (pp. 214–242). San Diego, CA: Academic Press.

Wentzel, K. R., Barry, C., & Caldwell, K. (2004). Friendships in middle school: Influences on motivation and school adjustment. *Journal of Educational Psychology, 96*, 195–203.

Wentzel, K. R., & Caldwell, K. (1997). Friendships, peer acceptance, and group membership: Relations to academic achievement in middle school. *Child Development, 68*, 1198–1209.

Wentzel, K. R., Filisetti, L., & Looney, L. (2006). *Predictors of prosocial behavior in young adolescents: Self-processes and contextual factors.* Unpublished manuscript, University of Maryland, College Park.

Wentzel, K. R., Looney, L., & Battle, A., (2006). *Teacher and peer contributions to classroom climate in middle school and high school.* Unpublished manuscript, University of Maryland, College Park.

White, K. J., & Kistner, J. (1992). The influence of teacher feedback on young children's peer preferences and perceptions. *Developmental Psychology, 28*, 933–940.

Youniss, J. (1994). Children's friendship and peer culture: Implications for theories of networks and support. In F. Nestmann & K. Hurrelmann (Eds.), *Social networks and social support in childhood and adolescence* (pp. 75–88). Berlin, Germany: Degrader.

CHAPTER 16

Media and Youth Socialization

Underlying Processes and Moderators of Effects

ERIC F. DUBOW, L. ROWELL HUESMANN, and DARA GREENWOOD

Consider this quote: "By the time most Americans are eighteen years old, they will have spent 15,000 hours in front of a television set, about 4,000 hours more than they have spent in school, and far more than they have spent talking with their teachers, their friends, or even their parents" (Minnow & LaMay, 1995, p. 5). Today's youth are exposed to a "media-saturated environment" (Roberts, Foehr, Rideout, & Brodie, 1999), which has long been a concern of parents, educators, policymakers, professional groups, and researchers, and there is much empirical evidence of meaningful effects of media exposure on youth (see, e.g., Anderson et al., 2003; Singer & Singer, 2001).

Concern with the effects of communicated words and images on youth is not new; it has been around as long as humans have been able to write and draw. Scientists were not needed to convince Greeks that audience members are influenced by the plays they saw, or to convince European kings that the populace is influenced by what they read, or to convince the 19th-century British middle class that children tend to imitate what they see others doing. However, with every step that society has taken toward greater "mass" communication, with each introduction of a new medium (e.g., photography, radio, movies, television, video games, and the world wide web), the concerns have increased. Increases in research have accompanied increases in concerns, and the outcomes of even the very early research tended to validate society's concerns. In the 1930s, studies by Peterson and Thurstone (1933) showed that movie viewers' attitudes about ethnic groups were altered by what they saw. By the 1940s, Lazersfeld had established an "Office of Radio Research" at Columbia University that investigated the effects of radio, ranging from the influence of daytime serials on women to the influence of political advertisements on voting (Lowery & DeFleur, 1995). However, the real explosion of research occurred in the latter half of the 20th century as television became a primary element in every child's life. As we argue in this chapter, this accumulating research, taken together, indicates that the mass media is in fact a key socializing influence in almost every child's life.

To make this point, we first present recent statistics describing the prevalence of children's exposure to television, video games, and the computer, paying particular attention to age, gender, and socioeconomic differences. Next, we examine theoretical explanations describing the underlying processes by which media exposure influences youth. Because this research generally shows that some youth are more affected by media exposure than other youth, we examine factors that moderate the effects of media exposure on youth. Finally, we present a section on selected examples of media effects; here, we highlight selected empirical research on the degree to which media exposure is associated with specific outcomes for youth at three developmental levels (preschool age, middle childhood, adolescence). Specifically, we examine the socializing impact of educational programming on preschoolers, the effect of violent content on children, and the impact of sexual content on adolescents.

CHILDREN'S EXPOSURE TO MEDIA

The data describing children's exposure to different types of media reported in this section come from three recent national large-scale surveys in the United States. The Kaiser Family Foundation reported on two studies: (1) the *Generation M: Media in the Lives of 8–18 Year-Olds* survey (Roberts, Foehr, & Rideout, 2005), a school-based survey administered to 2,032 students in grades 3–12, supplemented by media diaries from 694 of these students; and (2) *The Kids & Media @ the New Millennium* survey (Roberts et al., 1999), based on samples of 2,065 children in 3rd through 12th grades surveyed in their schools, 1,090 children ages 2–7 interviewed in their homes, and 621 children for whom media use diaries were completed by parents or the children themselves. The third data set is *The Media in the Home* survey (Woodard, 2000), supported by the Annenberg Public Policy Center, which was based on telephone interviews of 1,235 parents of children ages 2–17 and 416 children ages 8–16.

Television

Roberts et al. (2005) found that 51% of youth reported that the television is on "most of the time" in their homes; 63% said the television is on during meals. Children watch 184 minutes per day of television (Roberts et al., 2005). Woodard (2000) reported that boys watched more TV than girls, but Roberts et al. (2005) found no gender difference, and whereas Woodard (2000) found that children from higher-income homes watched less TV than children from lower-income homes, Roberts et al. (2005) found no income-level differences.

There are strong age-related viewing trends (Comstock & Paik, 1991) with viewing hours peaking at age 11–13 and declining slightly thereafter. Twelve-year-olds average about 28 hours per week of viewing, and 25% of 12-year-olds watch 40 or more hours per week. Of course, this is more time than they spend in school. On a typical day, 59% of infants (ages 0–2 years) and 73% of 0- to 6 year-olds watch TV (Kaiser Family Foundation, 2003a). Forty-three percent of 4- to 6-year-olds and 68% of children age 8 and older have a TV in their bedroom (Roberts et al., 2005). Younger children (ages 2–7) overwhelmingly watched entertainment and educational programs, 8–13-year-olds preferred entertainment and comedy programs, and 14–18-year-olds preferred comedy, drama, and sports programs (Roberts et al., 1999).

Parental viewing behavior also seems to influence how much children watch. Woodard (2000) found that children's frequency of TV viewing was related to their parents' frequency of TV viewing. Woodard also reviewed data that raise the concern that parents might be using television as a babysitter. Specifically, a higher percentage of children living in single-parent households had a television in their bedrooms compared to children in homes with multiple adult caretakers. Roberts et al. (1999) also reported that TV use was higher among children in single-parent homes. Even in dual-parent homes, parental coviewing with the child is relatively low. On average, 2- to 7-year-olds watch TV *without* a parent present more than 80% of the time, and for teenagers that number increases to 98% (Kaiser Family Foundation, 2003b, p. 2). Correspondingly, coviewing with peers increases as the child gets older.

One other recent trend in television programming has become very important for the issue of how television socializes children. With the introduction of cable television in the 1970s and the explosion of multiple networks and stations that followed in the 1980s and 1990s, TV programming became much more diverse. Specialized channels targeting children or subsets of adults emerged, and niche programming became more frequent. Programs could be successful that were aimed at smaller proportions of the general audience and that would offend or "turn off" the majority of viewers. The consequences are that youth are now exposed to a greater variety of material than ever before on TV, some of which is specifically targeted at them (e.g., Nickelodeon, and MTV), and some of which was never intended for viewing by children.

Video Games

Video game units are now present in 83% of homes with children (Roberts et al., 2005). Children spent 49 minutes per day playing video games (Roberts et al., 2005). Each day, 52% of children ages 8–18 years play a video game. The surveys found that boys played video games far more frequently than girls. In the most recent survey, video game playing was unrelated to family income level. Regarding age trends, video game use declined from an average of 65 minutes per day for 8–10-year-olds to 33 minutes per day for 15–18-year-olds (Roberts et al., 2005). Action, adventure, and sports games were the most popular choices, with role-play games increasing in interest for the 14–18-year-olds (Roberts et al., 1999).

Computers and Online Access

Roberts et al. (2005) found that 86% of homes with children ages 8–18 have a computer, 74% have Internet access, and the average time spent on the computer for recreational purposes (not school related) was 62 minutes. Neither Roberts et al. (2005) nor Woodard (2000) found gender differences in amount of time spent on the computer. All three surveys found that computer ownership was related to family income level: Roberts et al. (2005) found that 78% of families in the "less than $35,000/year" income range versus 93% of families in the "over $50,000" range reported owning a computer. Nevertheless,

Roberts et al. did not find significant family-income-level differences in total recreational computer use per day. Regarding age trends, Woodard (2000) and Roberts et al. (1999) reported that young children (below age 8) used the computer less frequently than did older children. Woodard found that Internet use was 8 minutes per day for preschoolers, 15 minutes per day for school-age children (ages 6–11), and 46 minutes per day for teens. More recently, Roberts et al. (2005) reported that total recreational computer use increased from 37 minutes per day for 8–10-year-olds, to 62 minutes per day for 11–14-year-olds, to 82 minutes per day for 15–18-year-olds. In addition, use of the computer for instant messaging increased with age from an average of 3 minutes per day for 8–10-year-olds, to 18 minutes per day for 11–14-year-olds, to 27 minutes per day for 15–18-year-olds. Woodard (2000) reported that children ages 8–13 years preferred entertainment and gaming websites, whereas 14–18-year-olds preferred entertainment and sports websites.

The "Media Budget" and Parents' Views

Roberts et al. (1999; Roberts et al., 2005) calculated a "media budget" that represents the portion of time youth were exposed to each media type. Through age 14, Roberts et al. (2005) reported that the largest proportion of time was spent with television. In fact, television accounts for more than half the leisure time of 6–11-year-old children (Comstock & Paik, 1991). For the 2–7-year-olds, the second largest portion was spent with print media (18% of their time). But by age 11, Roberts et al. (2005) found that the second largest portion of youth's media time was spent with audio media (radio, tapes, and CDs). For the 14–18-year-olds, audio media occupied the largest proportion of youth's media budget (30%, compared to 28% for television). Interestingly, Roberts et al. (2005) found that across these age groups, less than 13% of children's media budget was allocated to video games and less than 16% also was allocated to the computer.

Many have investigated what activities diminish when children devote more and more time to the mass media (Comstock & Paik, 1991). The overarching principle to describe what happens has been called the replacement of "functionally similar" activities. As children watch more television, their reading time, study time, and library time, for example, all decrease, while there is little change in their time spent in sports or socializing (Comstock & Paik, 1991). In other words, the mass media substitutes for what might be called functionally similar activities. However, more recently, Roberts et al. (2005) reported that heavy users of any one medium (i.e., TV, print media, computer, and video games) tend to be heavy users of the other media and that one should exercise caution in assuming "that time spent with media is synonymous with time taken from other activities." Rather, it is important to examine the specific "medium (or media) under consideration, the 'other' activity under consideration, and the individual youth" (p. 50). For example, whereas heavy TV users reported spending more time with their parents compared to light TV users, they also reported spending less time on their homework.

Surveys also show that a large portion of parents are concerned about their children's exposure to media. Woodard (2000) reported that over 70% of parents were at least "somewhat" concerned with their children's exposure to TV, the Internet, and music, and 53% were concerned with video games. Almost half of all parents believe that "viewing violence and sex on TV contributes a lot to children adopting violent behavior or becoming involved in sexual situations before they are ready" (Kaiser Family Foundation, 2001). A survey by Common Sense Media (2003) found that 80–90% of American parents believe that today's media contribute to children "becoming too materialistic, using more coarse and vulgar language, engaging in sexual activity at younger ages, experiencing a loss of innocence too early, and behaving in violent or anti-social ways." Still, most parents recognize the media can have a positive effect on children (Kaiser Family Foundation, 2003b). They are most conflicted about Internet use. For example, most parents recognize the educational value of the Internet for their children (Corporation for Public Broadcasting, 2003) but worry that online time will displace more important activities and expose them to negative content (Lenhart, Rainie & Lewis, 2001).

THE MASS MEDIA AS A SOCIALIZING INFLUENCE

Given the sheer amount of time from infancy to adolescence that youth devote to media consumption, given the lack of parental awareness and control over that media exposure, and given the reduction in time that some children might spend on other socializing activities, one has to be concerned with the role of the mass media in socializing children. The very act of engaging with the mass media either alone or with peers provides learning opportunities that socialize children, and what children observe through the mass media's window on the world alters their beliefs, attitudes, and behaviors, as we demonstrate later in this chapter in our review of studies of media effects. Some (e.g., Huesmann, 1995) have characterized the time since the introduction of television in the 1950s as a period in which the mass media steadily gained influence in socializing children while parents and more traditional socializing organizations (e.g., schools, churches) steadily lost influence. Because much of the content of the mass media to which children are exposed contains stereotyped, unrealistic, and/or antisocial models of social behavior (Kilbourne, 1999; Mastro & Greenberg, 2000; Yokota & Thompson, 2000), it is only natural that social scientists have focused more on understanding the negative influences of the mass media in socializing children. Yet, the mass media also provides opportunities for positive socialization. As becomes clear below, the powerful psychological processes that account for the influence of the mass media in socializing children do not distinguish between the positive and negative, though some content may be more likely than others to invoke certain processes. For example, sexual scenes and scenes of blood and gore may be more innately arousing than prosocial scenes. However, one can produce scenes that innately stimulate positive emotions or sad emotions that are just as intense. Whether the mass media teaches prosocial or antisocial behavior more easily certainly depends on how the behavior is presented, but the same learning processes are involved in both cases.

UNDERLYING PROCESSES BY WHICH MEDIA EXPOSURE AFFECTS YOUTH OUTCOMES

Huesmann and his colleagues (Anderson et al., 2003; Bushman & Huesmann, 2001; Huesmann, 1988, 1998, 2005; Huesmann, Moise-Titus, Podolski, & Eron, 2003; Huesmann & Taylor, 2006) have described a set of psychological processes that they believe explain most of the effects that exposure to the mass media has on youth. It is important to realize that these processes (described in detail later) apply to observations of behavior in real life (e.g., at home, in school, and in the neighborhood) as well as in the media. The social–cognitive psychological processes of observational learning, priming, desensitization, and so on, always have been defined as processes that occur when behavior is observed anywhere, not just in the mass media (Bandura, 1986; Huesmann, 1998). Furthermore, empirical examples of all these processes working in the real world are readily available (Fiske, 2004; Guerra, Huesmann, & Spindler, 2003; Wolpe, 1958). In addition, although the theoretical explanations were developed initially to account for the effects of exposure to media violence, the processes also are applicable to understanding the ways in which exposure to positive media content can affect behavior (Mares & Woodard, 2001). These processes generally fall under the rubric of social–cognitive information-processing models, which focus on the ways in which people perceive, interpret, learn, and come to behave in their interactions with their social world.

One of the most important distinctions that Huesmann (Huesmann et al., 2003) makes is to divide these information processes into those that account for short-term effects of media exposure and those that account for long-term effects. In this chapter, we are more concerned with the long-term effects that account for the socializing influence of the mass media, but they can only be understood in the context of the short-term processes. Short-term processes are those through which exposure to the mass media stimulates immediate changes in behaviors, emotions, or cognitions, but the changes are very transient.

Short-Term Effects

Huesmann (1988, 1998; Huesmann et al., 2003) proposes that most short-term effects of exposure to television, films, video games, or Internet web pages are a consequence of three processes: (1) priming of already existing cognitions or scripts for behavior; (2) immediate mimicking (imitation) of observed behaviors; or (3) changes in emotional arousal and the misattribution of that arousal (excitation transfer).

Priming

Neuroscientists and cognitive psychologists posit that the human mind acts as an associative network in which ideas are partially activated, or primed, by stimuli with which they are associated (Fiske & Taylor, 1984). The activation produced by an observed stimulus spreads in the network and moves even remotely related concepts more toward a threshold of influence. Thus, an encounter with an event or object can prime related concepts, ideas, and emotions in a person's memory, even without the person being aware of it (Bargh & Pietromonaco, 1982). For example, the mere presence of a weapon in a person's visual field can increase aggressive thoughts or behavior (Berkowitz & LePage, 1967). Alternatively, exposure to a scene of helping behavior can stimulate related prosocial thoughts and supportive feelings. The external stimulus can be inherently linked to a cognition; for example, the sight of a gun is inherently linked to the concept of aggression, or the external stimulus can be something inherently neutral like a particular ethnic group (e.g., African American) that has become linked in the past to certain beliefs or behaviors (e.g., welfare) (Valentino, Traugott, & Hutchings, 2002). The primed concepts make thoughts, emotions, and behaviors linked to them more easily activated.

Repeated exposure to specific media content, therefore, has the potential to bias individuals toward thinking, feeling, or behaving in ways relevant to that content. For example, priming men to view women as sexual objects via exposure to sexually objectify-ing commercials not only increases the speed with which men recognize sexist words, illustrating construct activation, but also increases the likelihood that the men will behave in a sexist manner during subsequent interactions with a female (Rudman & Borgida, 1995). In a related vein, priming women who excel at math and for whom math achieve-ment is central to self-worth with gender-stereotyped commercials predicted decreased performance on a subsequent math exam (Davies, Spencer, Quinn, & Gehardstein, 2002). Importantly, this decrease was mediated by the extent to which gender stereotypes were made cognitively accessible, as measured by increased speed of recognizing words relevant to the female stereotype.

Imitation

Immediate mimicry of specific behaviors can be viewed as a special case of the more gen-eral long-term process of observational learning (Huesmann, 2005). Human and primate young have an innate tendency to imitate whomever they observe (Butterworth, 1999; Meltzoff & Moore, 2000; Wyrwicka, 1996). Neuroscientists (e.g., Rizzolati, Fadiga, Gallese, & Fogassi, 1996) have discovered so-called mirror neurons in primates that seem to promote such processing. Although theorists argue over whether immediate mimicry is "true" imitation (see Hurley & Chater, 2004), no one doubts that it happens automati-cally in human youth. Consequently, observation of specific facial expressions or social behaviors increases the likelihood of children immediately displaying those expressions or behaviors (Bandura, Ross, & Ross, 1963; Meltzoff & Moore, 2000). In fact, many stud-ies have shown that most young children frequently mimic the behaviors of those charac-ters they observe in the media (e.g., Paik & Comstock, 1994).

Arousal and Excitation Transfer

Media portrayals are often high-action sequences that can be very arousing for youth, as measured by increased heart rate, skin conductance of electricity, and other physiological indices of arousal. To the extent that mass media presentations arouse the observer, cer-tain behaviors may become more likely in the short run for two possible reasons—general arousal (Berkowitz, 1993; Geen & O'Neal, 1969) and excitation transfer (Bryant & Zillmann, 1979; Zillmann, Bryant, & Cominsky, 1981).

First, high arousal generated by exposure to rapid action sequences and loud music makes any dominant response tendency more likely to be carried out. The increased gen-eral arousal stimulated by a media presentation may simply reach such a peak that per-formance on complex tasks declines, inhibition of inappropriate responses is diminished, and dominant learned responses tend to be displayed in response to an immediately en-countered social situation (e.g., direct instrumental aggression in response to a highly arousing social conflict situation). Second, when a child has been generally aroused by a media stimulus, the specific emotion (e.g., anger) generated by a subsequent real-world event (e.g., an insult) may be "felt" as more severe than it is because some of the emo-tional response stimulated by a preceding media presentation is misattributed as due to the provocation (Bryant & Zillmann, 1979; Zillmann et al., 1981). This process differs from priming in that the causal stimulus is not specifically linked to anger in any way, but simply increases general arousal.

Long-Term Effects

Although short-term effects have important influences on children's day-to-day behaviors, emotions, and thinking, they do not result in lasting changes in children's cognitions, behaviors, or the links between emotions and cognitions and behaviors. The more lasting changes that could be called "mass media socialization" occur when new cognitions or behavioral scripts are firmly encoded as a consequence of exposure to the mass media or new links between emotions and these cognitions and behaviors are acquired. Three long-term processes seem to be most important for socialization of the child: (1) observational learning of behavioral scripts, world schemas, and normative beliefs; (2) activation and desensitization of emotional processes; and (3) didactic learning processes.

The Observational Learning Process

By "observational learning" we mean the process of encoding lasting behavioral scripts and cognitions simply as a consequence of observing others. Whereas short-term mimicry requires only one exposure to an observed behavior, long-term observational learning usually requires repeated exposures. The more the child's attention is riveted on the observed behavior, the fewer repetitions are needed. However, numerous other factors besides attention affect the extent of the learning. Current conceptions of this process have grown out of the convergence of Bandura's (1986) social learning theory with more recent theories of social information processing (Dodge, 1985; Huesmann, 1988, 1998). The more the child identifies with the observed people (e.g., responds that he or she acts like or does the things a certain character does; Huesmann & Eron, 1986), the more the child is likely to encode the behavioral scripts the people are using, adopt the schemas about the world that the people seem to hold, or acquire the beliefs that the observed behaviors seem to imply (Huesmann, 1988, 1998, 2005). The more the observed scripts for behavior are rewarded and portrayed as appropriate, the more firmly the scripts will be encoded, and the more likely it is that more general beliefs about such behaviors will be extracted and encoded (Bandura, 1986; Huesmann, 1998).

As children grow older, they learn progressively more complex, generalized scripts for behavior through repeated observations of family members, peers, others in the community, and characters portrayed in the mass media. The scripts become more complex, abstract, and automatic as children's social–cognitive schemas about the world around them become more elaborated and as children mentally rehearse the scripts (Huesmann, 1988, 1998). For example, extensive observation of violence biases children's world schemas toward attributing hostility to others' actions (Dodge, 1985; Gerbner, Gross, Morgan, & Signorielli, 1994), which in turn increases the likelihood of children behaving aggressively themselves (e.g., Dodge, Pettit, & Bates, 1995). Through repeated observation of real-life models and models portrayed in the media, as well as by reflecting on the consequences of their own behaviors in social situations, children develop normative beliefs about what social behaviors are appropriate. During middle childhood, these beliefs become crystallized and begin to act as filters to evaluate scripts that are accessed in a given situation (Guerra et al., 2003; Guerra, Huesmann, Tolan, Van Acker, & Eron, 1995; Huesmann & Guerra, 1997; Huesmann, Moise, & Podolski, 1995).

This observational learning interacts with conditioning by family and peers to build behavioral scripts and social cognitions that are highly resistant to change. The reinforcements that a child receives from imitating a positive or negative behavior strongly influence the likelihood of that behavior persisting (Bandura, 1986; Berkowitz, 1993). One of the powerful aspects of the interactive nature of video games as a socializing tool is that the act of playing the game not only provides for observation of behaviors that can be acquired but also provides for the reinforcement of the behaviors that "win" the game (Gentile & Anderson, 2003). Similarly, if the world schemas and normative beliefs that a child acquires through observing others (again, in real life and in the media) lead to valuable outcomes for the child, they will become more firmly encoded and more resistant to change (Huesmann & Guerra, 1997).

Long-term socialization effects of the mass media also are increased by the way the mass media and especially interactive video games affect emotions. Through classical conditioning, fear or anger can become linked with specific stimuli after only a few exposures (Cantor, 2002; Harrison & Cantor, 1999). These emotions influence behavior in social settings away from the media source through stimulus generalization. A child may then react with inappropriate fear or anger in a novel situation similar to one that the child has observed in the media.

Activation and Desensitization of Emotional Processes

Repeated exposure to emotionally arousing media or video games can lead to habituation of certain natural emotional reactions. This process is often called "desensitization," and it has been used to explain a reduction in distress-related physiological reactivity to media portrayals of violence (Carnagey, Anderson, & Bushman, in press). Indeed, violent scenes do become less arousing over time (Cline, Croft, & Courrier, 1973), and brief exposure to media violence can reduce physiological reactions to real-world violence (Carnagey et al., in press).

If we apply this concept more broadly to children's media exposure, behaviors observed by the child viewer that might seem unusual at first might begin to seem more normative after repeated presentations. For example, most humans seem to have an innate negative emotional response to observing blood and violence, as evidenced by increased heart rates, perspiration, and self-reports of discomfort that often accompany such exposure. However, with repeated exposure, this negative emotional response habituates, and the child becomes "desensitized." The child can then think about and plan proactive aggressive acts without experiencing negative affect. For example, Moise-Titus (1999) and Kirwil and Huesmann (2003) have shown that more aggressive college students show less negative emotional reactions to observing violence than do less aggressive students. Although it is difficult to know if the individual differences in those studies stemmed from dispositional differences or habituation, Drabman and Thomas (1974a, 1974b) have shown that young children become less emotionally aroused by violent scenes and more tolerant of aggression after just one exposure.

Didactic Learning Processes

Most persuasion theorists distinguish between influences on viewers' attitudes and beliefs that operate through "peripheral" processing and influences that require "central" processing (see Petty & Priester, 1994). These concepts are usually applied to persuasive communications, but they represent a more general theoretical proposition that attitudes and beliefs can be changed by what the child observes through relatively "automatic" cognitive processes of which the child may be unaware or through more "controlled and effortful" cognitive processes including thoughtful elaboration of observed information. The social–cognitive theory of observational learning allows that scripts, world schemas, and normative beliefs about behaviors can be acquired from observations without viewer awareness. Similarly, emotional desensitization does not require conscious awareness. Consequently, much of the media socialization process can happen outside the child's awareness. For example, the ethnicity and gender of characters, the behaviors they accept as normative, the emotions they display in response to events—all these influence the child viewer's cognitions, and the child may not be aware of the influence of these elements.

Nevertheless, research has shown that properly crafted didactic material and persuasive arguments that engender "central, effortful" processing can produce enduring well-integrated cognitions (Chaiken, Lieberman, & Eagly, 1989), as illustrated by carefully scripted depictions about social relations such as those found on *Sesame Street* and *Mr. Rogers' Neighborhood*. Further, cognitive changes in middle childhood make children more active processors of media information, applying the schemas they have acquired and becoming more interested in the abstract, conceptual meanings of the material presented (Huston & Wright, 1997). Children during this developmental period become more receptive to the counterstereotypical (or stereotypical) messages and nuanced perceptions provided by both content directed at children and content directed at adults. Counterstereotypical messages received from the media during middle childhood and early adolescence (e.g., about alternative lifestyles) are probably particularly likely to be processed effortfully resulting in more lasting effects.

MODERATORS OF MEDIA SOCIALIZATION FOR CHILDREN AND ADOLESCENTS

The previous section reviewed the basic psychological processes by which media exposure influences children's attitudes, behaviors, and emotions. However, as illustrated by the media effects studies we review later in this chapter, we know that youth are not equally affected by even the same media portrayal (e.g., a specific violent scene in a movie, a music video with sexual content). Thus, a crucial question is, "Why are there individual differences in the ways in which exposure to a specific type of media content affects the development of youths' attitudes, behaviors, and emotions?" Researchers have identified many variables that act as moderators of the effects of media exposure. In this review, we present an organizational framework for understanding media effects on cognitions, behaviors, and emotions, based on our interpretation of the current body of research (see Figure 16.1). This framework includes the theoretical processes believed to underlie media effects, as well as five categories of moderators hypothesized to affect the degree to which media content will influence outcomes: the user's motivations for viewing, the user's characteristics, attributes of the media content, the viewing context, and cultural factors. In the next section, we review studies that provide empirical support for some of these moderators.

The User's Motivations

According to the uses and gratifications theory of media effects (Katz, Blumler & Gurevitch, 1974; Rubin, 1986), children engage with the mass media for multiple rea-

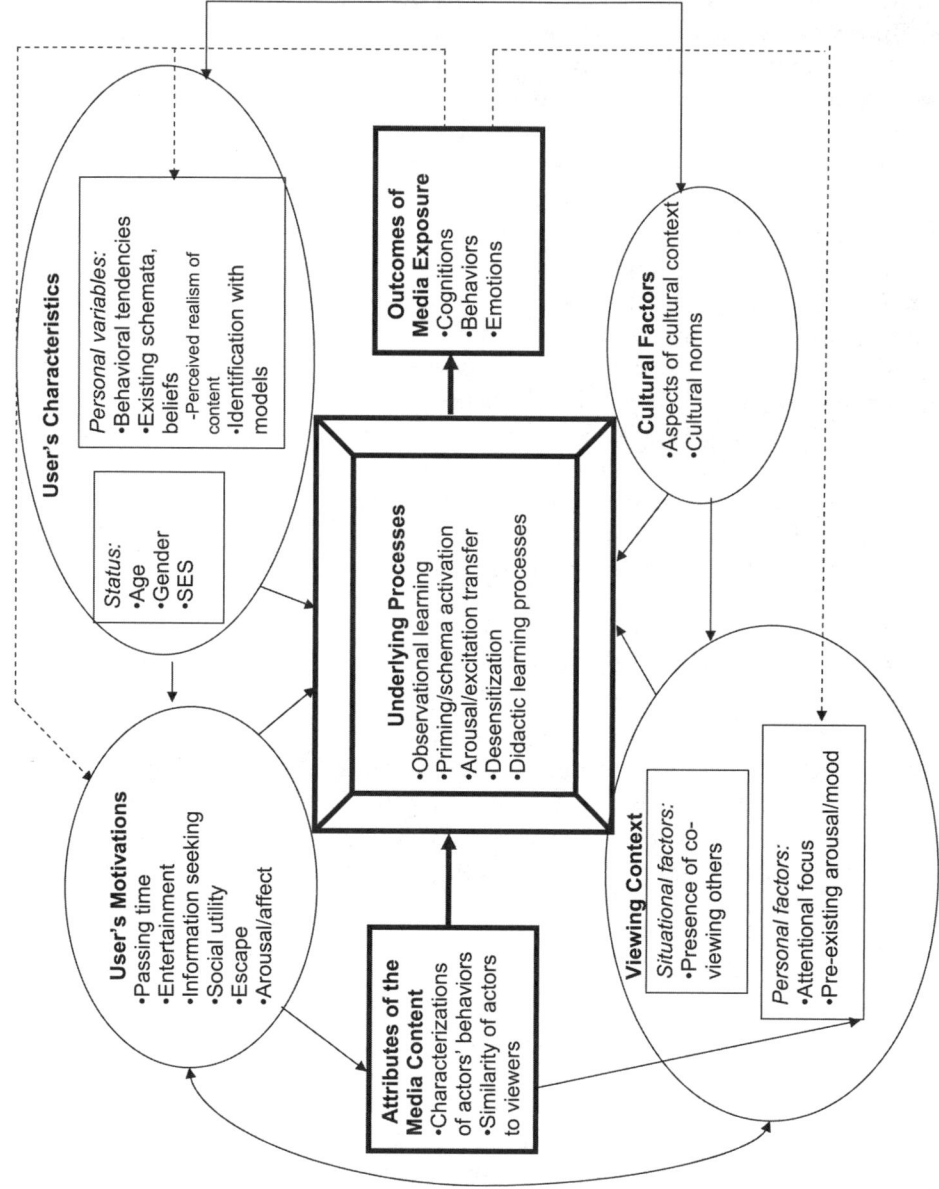

FIGURE 16.1. Organizational framework for understanding media effects on cognitions, behaviors, and emotions.

414

sons: simply to pass the time, to be entertained, to seek specific information, for social utility purposes (e.g., social comparison, to fit in with the peer group, to support identity formation), to escape boredom or aversive activities, and to achieve a certain level of arousal/mood state (Comstock & Scharrer, 2001; Roberts & Christenson, 2001; Valkenburg & Cantor, 2000). Of course, uses of and gratifications derived from media consumption are not static but evolve in step with developmental interests and needs. In any case, to the extent that an adolescent chooses a particular genre of media for the purposes of identity formation (see Larson, 1995), we can expect that the content can contribute significantly to the development of attitudes, emotions, and behaviors differently than if the genre were selected for another reason. For example, another adolescent might use the same media for entertainment purposes and not encode the content in a way that connects him or her to identity constructs, so we would not expect a similar effect of the media for that adolescent. As another example of the role of users' motivations, adolescent females, who are socialized to conflate social identity and feelings of self-worth with physical appearance concerns, may be motivated to selectively consume and idealize images of female beauty in media programs and magazines. Although research generally finds an association between exposure to idealized images and increased body image concerns (Harrison & Cantor, 1997; Stice & Shaw, 1994), individual differences motivating selective exposure moderate the degree of media impact. For example, Thomsen, McCoy, and Gustafson (2002) found that selective consumption of women's magazines for the purposes of feeling motivated to lose weight was associated more strongly with disordered eating and body image concerns than was sheer frequency of reading.

The User's Characteristics

Age

Paik and Comstock (1994), in a meta-analysis of the effects of TV/movie viewing on aggression, found that the strongest effects were on children less than 5 years old. The conclusion that even very young children are influenced strongly by what they observe around them and in the mass media is supported by the research described earlier showing that imitation is an innate process that operates from infancy on (Meltzoff & Moore, 2000).

Existing Behavioral Tendencies

Individuals who already have tendencies toward behaving a particular way are more likely to be influenced in that direction by relevant mass media exposures. For example, multiple studies show that aggressive individuals are more likely than less aggressive individuals to show short-term effects of viewing media violence and playing violent video games on subsequent aggressive outcomes (see Anderson et al., 2003; Josephson, 1987), although viewing violent TV programs has been shown to increase later aggression among children initially displaying even low levels of aggression as well (Eron, Huesmann, Lefkowitz, & Walder, 1972; Huesmann et al., 2003). More aggressive youth already have developed more aggressive scripts for dealing with conflict situations, and when they are exposed to violent content, these scripts are easily primed. In addition, new aggressive scripts can more easily be encoded if they are consistent with existing scripts, schemas, and beliefs.

Schemas and Beliefs

Children's existing schemas and beliefs about aggression and violence moderate the effects of media violence. Huesmann and colleagues (Huesmann & Eron, 1986; Huesmann et al., 2003) have shown that school-age children who believed that the violent programs they watched were realistic portrayals of life scored higher on measures of physical and verbal aggression 1 year and 15 years later compared to youth who perceived the programs as less realistic and who were less identified with aggressive protagonists. A compelling illustration of the importance of perceiving the media portrayal as realistic is a case study by Coleman (2002); in response to an ongoing dialogue with a young African American male, convicted of being party to a copycat murder after watching *Menace II Society*, Coleman notes, "[he] saw ghetto-centric media (in mythic proportions) and real life conflate to create a series of acceptable courses of action for him to choose from in a given situation" (p. 265).

Identification with Characters

Theoretically, individual differences in intensity of character identification should be one of the most important determinants of the media impact of idealized images. According to social–cognitive observational learning theory, children should learn most from characters with whom they identify. Indeed, the empirical evidence seems to support this prediction. In a classic study by Vidmar and Rokeach (1974), viewers high and low in prejudice alike reported finding *All in the Family* enjoyable and humorous. However, whereas high-prejudice viewers identified with the bigoted views of the main character, Archie Bunker, low-prejudice viewers dismissed Archie's prejudicial attitude and instead identified with the egalitarian struggle of the liberal son-in-law. Of course the attitudes acquired and reinforced from watching the shows would then differ for the two types of viewers.

The importance of identification has been illustrated even more clearly in the research on how exposure to certain media can increase eating disorders in young women. The degree to which young women identify with and idealize female icons increases the power of such role models. For example, Harrison (1997) found that women's "interpersonal attraction" (e.g., liking, wanting to be like, and feeling similar) to a favorite female character was associated with increased eating disorder symptomatology after controlling for mere exposure to shows featuring thin characters. Young women's levels of relational anxiety also may motivate more intense engagement with idealized images. Greenwood and Pietromonaco (2004) found that women with anxious ambivalent attachment styles (women who rely on others for emotional regulation and validation of self-worth) were most likely to identify with, idealize, and feel close to favorite female characters. Appearance idealization in particular was associated with increased body anxiety. Although young women who already are concerned with body image may be more prone to identify with and idealize ultrathin characters, this research highlights the relevance of understanding the interpersonal processes that may link these two phenomena. Further, it is likely that the recent "downward spiral" model—applied to the interaction between existing aggressive tendencies and increased aggression following selective exposure to media violence (Slater, Henry, & Swaim, 2003)—also is relevant to the complex relation between body anxiety and selective exposure to idealized images. Specifically, emotional engagement with idealized media icons may reflect, reinforce, and exacerbate existing body concerns.

Research on media violence also has provided strong evidence of the importance of identification to the observational learning process. Identification with the aggressive character moderates the effect of violence viewing on aggression. Huesmann and colleagues (Huesmann & Eron, 1986; Huesmann et al., 2003) found that both over the course of a year and over the course of 15 years, those boys who viewed violence and identified more with the aggressive character behaved more aggressively than the boys who viewed violence but did not identify as much. For females, identification with aggressive characters also predicted increased subsequent aggression, but the interaction was not as strong.

Attributes of the Media Content

Characteristics of the media content moderate effects on outcomes. For example, children's attentional focus during media exposure plays a role in learning effects, and format and content can compel or repel children's attention. Rapid character movements, colorful characters, changes in sound, and frequent changes in camera angles attract attention (Comstock & Paik, 1991). Bickham, Wright, and Huston (2001) suggested that by "layering" bits of novel, slightly more complicated material into content that is familiar to the child, not only is the child's attention maintained, but the complex material becomes more familiar, enhancing learning effects.

The extent to which a child identifies with a character as discussed earlier depends on how the character is portrayed. According to observational learning theory, the likelihood that a child will acquire a certain modeled behavior is increased by the model's perceived attractiveness, power, charisma, and similarity to the viewer (e.g., similar age, gender, and race) (Huesmann, 1998; Huesmann et al., 2003). Advertisers have long used such models to promote products such as tobacco and alcohol among targeted populations, and studies have shown that adolescents' increased exposure to such ads are associated with adolescents' positive beliefs about the product as well as more positive perceptions of users (Atkin & Block, 1983; Atkin, Neuendorf, & McDermott, 1983). However, an equally important implication is that most children are more likely to be influenced in their behavior by powerful, attractive, charismatic heroes in dramas than by villains or undesirables. Scenes in crime dramas, westerns, and science fiction in which heroes use violence will teach more violence to the child viewer than scenes in which characters with whom they cannot identify use violence.

Another important moderating attribute of the content of a media presentation is whether the behaviors being observed in the scene are portrayed as justified and are rewarded. Both characteristics have been shown to increase the likelihood of behaviors being learned (Anderson et al., 2003; Bandura, 1986; Bandura et al., 1963). For example, Berkowitz and his colleagues (Berkowitz & Geen, 1967; Berkowitz & Powers, 1979) showed that to the degree to which violence was portrayed as justified, research participants were more likely to exhibit aggression in a laboratory setting in response to a prior provocation. Consequently, one should expect, for example, the greatest socialization toward acceptance of aggression to occur when a child is exposed to a movie with a physically attractive, charismatic hero who uses violence for justified reasons, to achieve desirable goals, and who is rewarded extensively for what was done.

The Viewing Context

The social context of media use is another viewing factor that moderates its effects. Parents can perform important coviewing functions. Coviewing parents can discuss the media content with their children by commenting critically about the realism of the portrayals and the potential consequences of protagonists' behaviors if enacted in the real world. These parent behaviors can reduce the potentially negative impact of violent media content (Anderson et al., 2003; Nathanson, 1999; Singer & Singer, 1986).

Siblings and peers are more likely than parents to be the coviewing others. Roberts et al. (1999) reported that one-third to one-half of children coviewed with siblings or peers. As an example of potential effects of coviewing with siblings, Wilson and Weiss (1993) found that preschool-age children who coviewed a frightening television program with their older siblings became less emotionally aroused than preschoolers watching the program alone; the older siblings provided emotional and physical comfort to their younger siblings. Regarding coviewing with peers, Huntemann and Morgan (2001) suggested that youths' media preferences reflected a "badge of identity that young people use to define themselves, both to themselves and to others" (p. 313). The authors argued that coviewing with peers can strengthen group identity, in both positive and negative ways. Huesmann and Taylor (2006) similarly suggested that video games often are played as part of a peer network, which is especially concerning given findings that both boys and girls across grade levels prefer violent video games (see Funk, 2002) and that playing violent video games influences aggressive behavior, thoughts, and emotions (Bushman & Anderson, 2001). Coviewing with peers also may function to reinforce traditional gender role socialization. Research suggests that opposite-sex coviewing of horror films, for example, may provide a context for boys to rehearse stereotypically masculine displays of stoicism, whereas the same context may socialize girls to exhibit stereotypically feminine displays of fear and dependence (Zillmann & Weaver, 1996).

Cultural Factors

The impact that media exposure has on a given individual is often relevant to his or her surrounding social–cultural context. The socializing influence of media may increase when the television content is resonant with everyday lived experience (Gerbner et al., 1994). For example, research has shown that television exposure was related to both general and personal perceptions of crime risk only for those individuals who had direct experience with crime in their own lives (Shrum & Bischak, 2001). Media images seemed to magnify their perceptions of real-life experience. On the other hand, the effects of exposure to media violence on aggression toward peers were lessened for children raised in kibbutz environments that emphasized prosociality (Huesmann & Eron, 1986).

Another interesting study illustrating the impact of cultural context on media influence comes from research on television consumption and body image disturbance among women in Fiji (Becker, Burwell, Herzog, Hamburg, & Gilman, 2002). Prior to the introduction of Western media programs, Fijian women seemed buffered against subscribing to a thin ideal of female beauty; "going thin" frequently was used in the pejorative, suggesting declining health or well-being. However, 3 years after television viewing became more normative among Fijian residents and programs such as *Melrose Place* made their way into homes, young women reported increased disordered eating symptoms and weight concerns. Although this increased symptomatology might reflect the impact of TV viewing becoming more normative in Fijian society, the authors raised the possibility that media effects on body image were actually exacerbated by the changing climate of Fijian social and economic life. The glamorous career women depicted on television may have represented attractive social models for Fijian women, who were increasingly entering the work force and imagining a different life from older generations. The authors also raised the possibility that peer culture moderated this impact, as the women described the extent to which new ideals for female roles and attractiveness influenced their peers, which further affected their own perceptions. Of course, in this study it is not easy to isolate the effects of multiple variables (e.g., changing cultural norms, media effects, and peer effects), or the directions of relations among those variables. Nevertheless, the study illustrates an interesting interplay among cultural norms, media portrayals, and individual adjustment.

SELECTED EMPIRICAL STUDIES OF MEDIA EFFECTS

Two recent volumes (Singer & Singer, 2001; Strasburger & Wilson, 2002) reviewed the wide range of research on media effects on children and adolescents, including effects on cognitive and academic skills, prosocial and aggressive behaviors, fears and anxieties, sexual attitudes and behaviors, gender role images, identity development, body image concerns, and substance use. In this section, our intent is not to provide an exhaustive review of those findings. Rather, for each of three developmental levels (preschoolers, elementary school-age children, adolescents), we review media effects on selected outcomes, and within those studies, we highlight findings for moderator effects.

Media Socialization and Preschoolers: A Focus on the Educational and Social Impact of Children's Programming

In 1968, the Children's Television Workshop (CTW) created *Sesame Street* with a major goal of fostering the educational progress of preschool children, especially those from low-income families (Palmer & Fisch, 2001). From its outset, CTW paired TV producers with educators and researchers to assess whether *Sesame Street* was effective in enhancing children's preacademic (language, reading, math) and social–affective skills. And, indeed, research has shown that those preschoolers who viewed *Sesame Street* most frequently gained the most in literacy and number skills, and in the following year, their teachers judged them to be more proficient in school readiness skills, quantitative skills, positive attitudes toward school, and peer relations (Mielke, 2001). In a nationally representative telephone survey in which data were collected from parents of 10,888 preschool through first-grade children, Zill (2001) found that the effects of more frequent *Sesame Street* viewing on parent-reported preacademic skills (e.g., letter recognition, counting to 20 or more, and telling connected stories when pretending to read) were stronger for lower-income viewers than for middle-income viewers. Although this cross-sectional study could not provide strong evidence about changes induced by viewing *Sesame Street*, it is possible that *Sesame Street* provided resources for learning for children from lower-income homes that already might be available to children from higher-income homes. Perhaps more impressive are results of short-term (Wright, Huston, Scantlin, & Kotler, 2001) and long-term (Anderson, Huston, Schmitt, Linebarger, & Wright, 2001) longitudinal studies of the educational value of *Sesame Street*. Regarding long-term effects, Anderson et al. (2001) reported on the results of "The Recontact Study," which followed up 570 preschoolers in two cities (Topeka, Kansas, and Springfield, Massachusetts) when they were adolescents (average ages at follow-up were 16.6 years for the Topeka youth, 18.2 years for the Springfield youth). For both boys and girls, more frequent viewing of *Sesame Street* at age 5 predicted higher high school math and science grades and a composite score reflecting leisure reading. For boys, viewing *Sesame Street* also predicted higher high school English grades. These results held even after controlling for background variables (i.e., parents' education level and birth order).

In addition to underscoring the educational impact of specific programming targeting children, research also suggests that exposure to certain programs influences children's social attitudes and behaviors. Interestingly, however, this research generally indicates that prosocial content is most effective and lasting when program exposure is combined with and reinforced by additional interactive interventions (Mares & Woodard, 2001). For example, viewing a series of prosocial episodes of the program *Freestyle* was associated with decreases in fourth to sixth graders' gender stereotypes; however, the positive attitudinal impact of viewing was most pronounced when episodes were followed by teacher-facilitated classroom discussion (Johnston & Ettema, 1982). Similarly, Singer and Singer (1998) found that repeated viewing of episodes of *Barney* had a positive impact on preschool children's knowledge about polite social behavior, and that these results were notably stronger when combined with a postviewing lesson compared to viewing alone, or lesson alone.

Media Socialization in Middle Childhood: A Focus on the Effects of Violent Content on Aggression

Children's exposure to violent media is probably the most widely studied media socialization effect, dating back to the 1954 Kefauver hearings, and followed by other high-profile investigations (e.g., National Institute of Mental Health, 1982; Steinfeld, 1972; Eron, Gentry, & Schlegel, 1994; Joint Statement of Congress, 2000; Anderson et al., 2003), most of which concluded that media violence is a cause of aggressive behavior, particularly among children. It is impossible in this chapter to review adequately the large number of empirical studies that led to these conclusions; thus we focus here on a few meta-analytic reviews and one longitudinal study that illustrates the socialization effect. Extensive recent reviews exist that cover the material in much greater depth (e.g., Anderson et al., 2003).

The theory that explains how exposure to media violence would socialize children into behaving more aggressively has been described earlier. The longer-term socializing effects are best explained as due to the child's acquisition through observational learning of social cognitions (e.g., world schemas, normative beliefs, and scripts) that promote aggression and from desensitization of the child's negative emotional reactions to violence through repeated exposures to violence. Once acquired, such cognitions and lack of reactivity may persist throughout life and increase the risk of aggression throughout life.

In 1994, Paik and Comstock conducted the most comprehensive meta-analysis to date about the relation between TV viewing and aggressive or antisocial behavior. They analyzed 217 key studies conducted from 1957 to 1990. The studies included laboratory and field experiments, surveys, and time series designs. They found that the average effect size for experiments was $r = .40$ and for field studies was $r = .19$. These effect sizes, while moderate to small in absolute terms, were highly significant. The effect sizes were significant for college-age students ($r = .39$), preschoolers ($r = .49$), 6- to 11-year-olds ($r = .32$), and 12- to 17-year-olds ($r = .23$). The overall effect sizes were also somewhat stronger for males ($r = .37$) than for females ($r = .26$). The Paik and Comstock review did not include many studies of video games, but in 2001 Anderson and Bushman published a meta-analysis of the effects of violent video games. They found 35 research reports through 2000. The results showed highly significant relations for aggressive behavior ($r = .19$), aggressive cognitions ($r = .27$), and aggressive affect ($r = .17$), which were similar across ages (children below age 19 vs. adults), gender, and study design (experimental vs. nonexperimental). These same authors (Bushman & Anderson, 2001; Anderson & Bushman, 2002) also conducted a new meta-analysis of the effects of violent media content for 280 studies conducted up to the year 2000 across multiple media types (television, movies, video games, comic books, and music). They found effect sizes very comparable to those reported earlier by Paik and Comstock (1994). Effect sizes across study designs (laboratory and field experiments, cross-sectional and longitudinal studies) ranged from $r = .17$ to $r = .23$.

Researchers of effects of violent media content on aggressive behavior generally have reached a consensus that "media violence increases the likelihood of aggressive and violent behavior in both immediate and long-term contexts" (Anderson et al., 2003, p. 1). This conclusion has emerged from the combination of the laboratory studies in which causation has been unambiguously demonstrated, the cross-sectional field studies in which correlations have been found in many different "real-world" settings, and the longitudinal studies in which it has been found that children who are exposed to more violence grow up to be more aggressive independently of any of the third variables that have been examined as potential explanations (existing aggression, low IQ, low socioeconomic status, poor parenting, etc.). A number of scholars (e.g., Abelson, 1985; Anderson et al., 2003; Rosenthal, 1986) also have noted that although correlations around .20 may seem to explain only small proportions of variance, it is the wrong statistic with which to evaluate the social significance of a public health threat. Effect sizes of $r = .20$ are very socially meaningful because a very large population is exposed to the risk factor, the effects are likely to accumulate with repeated exposure, and no other explanatory factors have much larger effect sizes. A number of writers have disputed the importance of media violence in socializing children into aggression (e.g., Fowles, 1999; Freedman, 2002; Rhodes, 2000), and numerous scholarly rejoinders to their critiques have been written (Huesmann, Eron, Berkowitz, & Chaffee, 1992; Huesmann & Moise, 1996; Huesmann & Taylor, 2006).

Let us now turn to one specific study that illustrates the long-term socializing effect of habitual exposure to media violence in childhood. This recent longitudinal study demonstrates empirically that repeated exposure to TV violence in childhood has lasting effects; it also illustrates the influence of moderator variables (Huesmann et al., 2003; Huesmann & Eron, 1986). The study began in the late 1970s when 748 children in two cohorts (6-year-olds, 8-year-olds) were assessed each year for 3 consecutive years. Children reported on their TV violence viewing and peers reported on the children's aggressive behavior using a classroom-based peer-nomination procedure. It was found that those boys and girls who regularly watched more TV violence in the first 2 years were significantly more aggressive in the third year than children who were equally aggressive initially but did not watch the violence. However, for boys the effect was strongest when the boy not only watched the violence but strongly identified with the character (usually a "hero") who was being aggressive.

Huesmann et al. (2003) reinterviewed the U.S. children 15 years later when they were in their early 20s. They then found that for both men and women childhood TV violence viewing measured 15 years earlier now predicted how aggressive they were as adults. This was true for predicting physical, verbal, and indirect aggression, even when the researchers controlled for childhood aggression, socioeconomic status, and academic achievement. (Alternatively, childhood aggressiveness was not related to adult TV violence viewing.) For example, compared to males who were low childhood TV violence viewers, males who were high childhood TV violence viewers were more likely to report having "pushed, grabbed, or shoved" their spouses (42% vs. 22%). Compared to females who were low childhood TV violence viewers, females who were high childhood TV violence viewers were more likely to report "shoving, punching, beating, or choking" someone who had made them angry (17% vs. 4%). The extent to which this effect is a product of "socialization into cognitions approving" of aggression was indicated by the fact that for both males and females normative beliefs approving of aggression was found to be a significant "mediator" of the 15-year effect (Huesmann et al., 1995).

Media Socialization and Adolescents: The Effect of Sexual Content on Attitudes and Behaviors

Perhaps the only other type of content that rivals the amount of violent content in the mass media is sexual content. Researchers have found that young people are likely to encounter up to 14,000 sexual images or messages on television per year (Harris & Associates, 1988, as cited in Strasburger & Wilson, 2002). It is important to note that sexual and violent content are not always separable; sexually explicit content is frequently confounded with violent content in the media (Malamuth & Spinner, 1980; Yang & Linz, 1990), a combination that has been cause for concern among researchers and parents alike. Another concern about the potential socializing influence of sexual media content is the way in which certain genres of media, such as music videos, depict women as passive sexual objects relative to men (Jhally, 1995). Researchers also have noted an asymmetry between the high frequency of sexual innuendo and behavior occurring on prime-time television programs (Kunkel, Cope, & Colvin, 1996) and the relatively low frequency of discussion surrounding abstinence, contraception, or the health risks of sexual activities (Cope-Farrar & Kunkel, 2002, as cited in Strasburger & Wilson, 2002). Although the sexual media landscape looks bleak, there are some media programs that raise public awareness of sexual health issues from rape to AIDS and contraception use (Agha, 2003; Folb, 2000).

Correlational investigations frequently find an association between exposure to sexual content and sexual attitudes and behaviors (e.g., Brown & Newcomer, 1991; Strouse, Buerkel-Rothfuss, & Long, 1995). However, this body of research also indicates that viewing habits and sexual behaviors are often moderated by gender, family environment, and/or viewing context. For example, Strouse et al. (1995) found that the associations between exposure to sexual content (e.g., in music videos) and increased sexual behavior and sexually permissive attitudes were stronger for adolescent girls than boys. These effects were most pronounced for girls who reported unhappiness and dissatisfaction with their family environments. Further, research on exposure to sexually explicit media and onset of sexual intercourse is complicated by questions of causal direction. Although researchers have found increased likelihood of having engaged in intercourse to be associated with increased exposure to sexual content in the media (Brown & Newcomer, 1991), the authors note that it is unclear whether this suggests a selection effect (i.e., those who are already interested in sexual activity choose to consume sexually relevant media) or a socializing impact (i.e., increased sexual behavior is motivated by media depictions).

Experimental manipulations of sexually oriented media content appear to have at least short-term effects on adolescents' attitudes and behaviors that outweigh individual differences in motive and engagement. Greeson and Williams (1986) found that adolescents (7th and 10th graders) exposed to only 10 minutes of music videos were more likely to report acceptance of premarital sex than those who were not exposed. Much work also has been devoted to understanding the effects of violent sexual content on viewers' attitudes and behaviors (e.g., Donnerstein & Berkowitz, 1981; Linz, Donnerstein, & Penrod, 1984; Malamuth, 1984). That research has found evidence of a desensitization effect as a result of viewing violence; specifically, men who watched sexually explicit and violent films over a period of 5 days perceived less violence on the final day of viewing (suggesting that they had habituated to the violence) and evaluated a hypothetical rape victim more harshly than men who were not exposed to such content (Linz et al., 1984). Other research has found that the way a female character responds to sexual violence may play a critical role in men's subsequent perceptions (Donnerstein & Berkowitz, 1981). Viewing scenes in which a woman is portrayed as responding positively to sexual violence (what has been termed "rape myth sexual violence"; Harris, 1999, p. 226) relate to increased aggressiveness toward females but not males.

Not all portrayals of sexual behavior in the media are negative in impact. To the extent that sexual content in the media may stimulate open communication between parents and children, it may prove to be a highly useful medium. For example, although the former hit TV show *Sex and the City* (now in syndication) has sparked much controversy over its explicit focus on sexual activities and issues, it also has won awards for "accurate and honest representation of sexuality" (Hepola, 2003). In particular, the show has been lauded for its candid dialogue regarding abortion, an issue that is frequently avoided in many other programs, in which a strategically timed miscarriage might preclude the debate over termination considerations (Strasburger, 1995). Media programs also may disseminate valuable information about sexually transmitted diseases, such as AIDS, and increase public awareness. For example, increased exposure to contraception advertisements (e.g., condoms) in Kenya was associated with increased perceptions of self-efficacy in the domain of contraception and decreased discomfort in buying condoms (Agha, 2003). Moreover, fictional programming also may be useful in educating adolescent viewers about sexual awareness; a plot line in the popular teen program *Felicity* focused on date rape and included a rape crisis number at the end of the episode, and calls to the hotline increased significantly after the episode aired (Folb, 2000).

In general, the research evidence linking media exposure to sexual attitudes and behaviors in young adults is fairly persuasive. Correlational and experimental studies find that increased exposure to sexual content is associated with media-perpetuated attitudes about sex. Integrating the findings from one-shot exposures and habitual viewing patterns, it seems plausible that chronic exposure to sexual-themed media might cultivate and perpetuate media-congruent attitudes. More research is needed to clarify the specific interactions among exposure, involvement, and personal experience on viewers' sexual schemas.

SUMMARY AND CONCLUSIONS

In this chapter, we first reviewed the frequency with which youth are engaging in media consumption. Next, we examined the underlying psychological processes by which exposure to media content exerts its effects. We stressed that it is necessary to distinguish between processes accounting for short-term effects (e.g., priming and excitation transfer and simple imitation) and processes accounting for long-term effects (e.g., observational learning and desensitization of emotional processes), as well as the relation between the two (e.g., chronically primed images and messages may become more easily accessible over time). In addition, we reviewed factors that act as moderators of the effects of media exposure on youth (e.g., characteristics of the user and characteristics of the viewing context). Finally, we illustrated how these processes and moderators were relevant to understanding the effects of educational content on preschoolers, the effects of violent content on children, and the effects of sexual content on adolescents. As some of the studies illustrate, by understanding the processes and moderators accounting for media effects, researchers can develop interventions that can weaken potential negative effects and strengthen the potentially positive effects of media content (e.g., promoting active adult coviewing and postpresentation discussions).

A media socialization model that stresses ongoing interactions among content, moderators, processes, and outcomes also may prove highly useful for asking and answering questions about the impact of the latest interactive media (e.g., instant messaging, web-based games, and chat rooms). Researchers are just beginning to scratch the surface of how Internet use may influence the social development of children and adolescents (Wartella, Caplovitz, & Lee, 2004), and to date, "the empirical research on children and interactive media has yet to match the myriad of questions posed about its effects" (Wartella et al., 2004, p. 3). However, early investigations into this particular domain of media already highlight the utility of considering multiple moderators such as the user's age, gender, and motivation that may interact with medium-specific features to predict facilitation or inhibition of educational and social development (Lenhart et al., 2001). Ongoing research must keep pace with the emerging trends in media technology that command the interest and attention of young consumers.

REFERENCES

Abelson, R. P. (1985). A variance explanation paradox: When a little is a lot. *Psychological Bulletin, 97,* 129–133.

Agha, S. (2003). The impact of a mass media campaign on personal risk perception, perceived self-efficacy and on other behavioural predictors. *AIDS Care, 15,* 749–762.

Anderson, C. A., Berkowitz, L., Donnerstein, E., Huesmann, L. R., Johnson, J., Linz, D., et al. (2003). The influence of media violence on youth. *Psychological Science in the Public Interest, 4*(3), 81–110.

Anderson, C. A., & Bushman, B. J. (2001). Effects of violent video games on aggressive behavior, aggressive cognition, aggressive affect, physiological arousal, and prosocial behavior: A meta-analytic review of the scientific literature. *Psychological Science, 12,* 353–359.

Anderson, C. A., & Bushman, B. J. (2002, June/July). Media violence and the American public revisited. *American Psychologist,* pp. 448–450.

Anderson, D. A., Huston, A. C., Schmitt, K. L., Linebarger, D. L., & Wright, J. C. (2001). Early childhood television viewing and adolescent behavior. *Monographs of the Society for Research in Child Development, 66*(1).

Atkin, C. K., & Block, M. (1983). Effectiveness of celebrity endorsers. *Journal of Advertising Research, 23,* 57–61.

Atkin, C. K., Neuendorf, K., & McDemott, S. (1983). The role of alcohol advertising in excessive and hazardous drinking. *Journal of Drug Education, 13,* 313–325.

Bandura, A. (1986). *Social foundations of thought and action: A social cognitive theory.* Upper Saddle River, NJ: Prentice-Hall.

Bandura, A., Ross, D., & Ross, S. A. (1963). Imitation of film-mediated aggressive models. *Journal of Abnormal and Social Psychology, 66,* 3–11.

Bargh, J. A., & Pietromonaco, P. (1982). Automatic information processing and social perception: The influence of trait information presented outside of conscious awareness on impression formation. *Journal of Personality and Social Psychology, 43,* 437–449.

Becker, A. E., Burwell, R. A., Herzog, D. B., Hamburg, P., & Gilman, S. E. (2002). Eating behaviors and attitudes following prolonged exposure to television among ethnic Fijian adolescent girls. *British Journal of Psychiatry, 180,* 509–514.

Berkowitz, L. (1993). *Aggression: Its causes, consequences, and control.* Boston: McGraw-Hill.

Berkowitz, L., & Geen, R. G. (1967). Stimulus qualities of the target of aggression: A further study. *Journal of Personality and Social Psychology, 5,* 364–368.

Berkowitz, L., & LePage, A. (1967). Weapons as aggression-eliciting stimuli. *Journal of Personality and Social Psychology, 7*(2), 202–207.

Berkowitz, L., & Powers, P. C. (1979). Effects of timing and justification of witnessed aggression on the observers' punitiveness. *Journal of Research in Personality, 13,* 71–80.

Bickham, D. S., Wright, J. C., & Huston, A. C. (2001). Attention, comprehension, and the educational influences of television. In D. G. Singer & J. L. Singer (Eds.), *Handbook of children and the media* (pp. 101–119). Thousand Oaks, CA: Sage.

Brown, J. D., & Newcomer, S. F. (1991). Television viewing and adolescents' sexual behavior. *Journal of Homosexuality, 21,* 77–91.

Bryant, J., & Zillmann, D. (1979). Effect of intensification of annoyance through unrelated residual excitation on substantially delayed hostile behavior. *Journal of Experimental Social Psychology, 15*(5), 470–480.

Bushman, B. J., & Anderson, C. A. (2001). Media violence and the American public: Scientific facts versus media misinformation. *American Psychologist, 56,* 477–489.

Bushman, B. J., & Huesmann, L. R. (2001). Effects of televised violence on aggression. In D. Singer & J. Singer (Eds.), *Handbook of children and the media* (pp. 223–254). Thousand Oaks, CA: Sage.

Butterworth, G. (1999). Neonatal imitation: Existence, mechanisms and motives. In J. Nadel & G. Butterworth, (Eds.), *Imitation in infancy* (pp. 63–88). New York: Cambridge University Press.

Cantor, J. (2002). Fright reactions to mass media. In J. Bryant & D. Zillmann (Eds.), *Media effects: Advances in theory and research* (2nd ed., pp. 287–306). Mahwah, NJ: Erlbaum.

Carnagey, N. L., Anderson, C. A., & Bushman, B. J. (in press). The effect of video game violence on physiological desensitization to real life violence. *Journal of Experimental Social Psychology.*

Chaiken, S., Lieberman, A., & Eagly, A. H. (1989). Heuristic and systematic processing within and beyond the persuasion context. In J. Uleman & J. Bargh (Eds.), *Unintended thought* (pp. 212–252). New York: Guilford Press.

Cline, V. B., Croft, R. G., & Courrier, S. (1973). Desensitization of children to television violence. *Journal of Personality & Social Psychology, 27*(3), 360–365.

Coleman, R. R. (2002). The Menace II Society copycat murder case and thug life: A reception study with a convicted criminal. In R. R. Coleman (Ed.). *Say it loud: African American audiences, media, and identity* (pp. 249–284). New York: Routledge.

Common Sense Media (2003). *The 2003 Common Sense Media poll of American parents* [Online]. Available: www.commonsensemedia.org.

Comstock, G. A., & Paik, H. (1991). *Television and the American child*. San Diego, CA: Academic Press.

Comstock, G., & Scharrer, E. (2001). The use of television and other film-related media. In D. G. Singer & J. L. Singer (Eds.), *Handbook of children and the media* (pp. 47–72). Thousand Oaks, CA: Sage.

Cope-Farrar, K. M., & Kunkel, D. (2002). Sexual messages in teens' favorite prime-time TV programs. In J. D. Brown, J. R. Steele, & K. Walsh-Childers (Eds.), *Sexual teens, sexual media* (pp. 59–78). Hillsdale, NJ: Erlbaum.

Corporation for Public Broadcasting (2003). *Connected to the future: A report on children's internet use* [Online]. Washington, DC. Available: www.cpb.ord.

Davies, P. G., Spencer, S. J., Quinn, D. M. & Gerhardstein, R. (2002). Consuming images: How television commercials that elicit stereotype threat can restrain women academically and professionally. *Personality and Social Psychology Bulletin, 28*, 1615–1628.

Dodge, K. A. (1985). Attributional bias in aggressive children. In P. C. Kendall (Ed.), *Advances in cognitive-behavioral research and therapy* (Vol. 4, pp. 73–110). San Diego, CA: Academic Press.

Dodge, K. A., Pettit, G. S., & Bates, J. E. (1995). Social information-processing patterns partially mediate the effect of early physical abuse on later conduct problems. *Journal of Abnormal Psychology, 104*(4), 632–643.

Donnerstein, E., & Berkowitz, L. (1981). Victim reactions in aggressive erotic films as a factor in violence against women. *Journal of Personality and Social Psychology, 41*, 710–724.

Drabman, R. S., & Thomas, M. H. (1974a). Does media violence increase children's toleration of real-life aggression? *Developmental Psychology, 10*, 418–421.

Drabman, R. S., & Thomas, M. H. (1974b). Exposure to filmed violence and children's tolerance of real life aggression. *Personality and Social Psychology Bulletin, 1*(1), 198–199.

Eron, L. D., Gentry, J. H., & Schlegel, P. (Eds.). (1994). *Reason to hope: A psychological perspective on violence and youth*. Washington, DC: American Psychological Association.

Eron, L. D., Huesmann, L. R., Lefkowitz, M. M., & Walder, L. O. (1972). Does television violence cause aggression? *American Psychologist, 27*(4), 253–263.

Fiske, S. T. (2004). *Social beings*. New York: Wiley.

Fiske, S. T., & Taylor, S. E. (1984). *Social cognition*. Reading, MA: Addison-Wesley.

Folb, K. L. (2000). "Don't touch that dial!" TV as a—what? positive influence. *SIECUS Report, 28*, 16–18.

Fowles, J. (1999). *The case for television violence*. Thousand Oaks, CA: Sage.

Freedman, J. (2002). *Media violence and its effect on aggression*. Toronto, Ontario, Canada: University of Toronto Press.

Funk, J. B. (2002). Electronic games. In V. C. Strasburger & B. J. Wilson (Eds.), *Children, adolescents, and the media* (pp. 117–144). Thousand Oaks, CA: Sage.

Geen, R. G., & O'Neal, E. C. (1969). Activation of cue-elicited aggression by general arousal. *Journal of Personality & Social Psychology, 11*(3), 289–292.

Gentile, D. A., & Anderson, C. A. (2003). Violent video games: The newest media violence hazard. In D. Gentile (Ed.), *Media violence and children* (pp. 131–152). Westport, CT: Praeger.

Gerbner, G., Gross, L., Morgan, M., & Signorielli, N. (1994). Growing up with television: The cultivation perspective. In J. Bryant & D. Zillmann (Eds.), *Media effects* (pp. 17–41). Hillsdale, NJ: Erlbaum.

Greenwood, D. N., & Pietromonaco, P. R. (2004). The interplay among attachment orientation, idealized media images of women, and body dissatisfaction: A social psychological analysis (pp. 291–308). In L. J. Shrum (Ed.) *The psychology of entertainment media: Blurring the lines between entertainment and persuasion*. Mahwah, NJ: Erlbaum.

Greeson, L. E., & Williams, R. A. (1986). Social implications of music videos for youth: An analysis of the contents and effects of MTV. *Youth and Society, 18*, 177–189.

Guerra, N. G., Huesmann, L. R., & Spindler, A. (2003). Community violence exposure, social cognition, and aggression among urban elementary school children. *Child Development, 74*(5), 1561–1576.

Guerra, N. G., Huesmann, L. R., Tolan, P. H., Van Acker, R., & Eron, L. (1995). Stressful events and individual beliefs as correlates of economic disadvantage and aggression among urban children. *Journal of Consulting and Clinical Psychology, 63*(4), 518–528.

Harris, R. J. (1999). *A cognitive psychology of mass communication* (2nd ed., pp. 14–30). Mahwah, NJ: Erlbaum.

Harrison, K. (1997). Does interpersonal attraction to thin media personalities promote eating disorders? *Journal of Broadcasting and Electronic Media, 41*, 478–500.

Harrison, K., & Cantor, J. (1997). The relationship between media consumption and eating disorders. *Journal of Communication, 47*, 40–67.

Harrison, K., & Cantor, J. (1999). Tales from the screen: Enduring fright reactions to scary media. *Media Psychology, 1*(2), 97–116.

Hepola, S. (2003, June 22). Her favorite class: "Sex" education. *New York Times*, AR 1, AR 29.

Huesmann, L. R. (1988). An information processing model for the development of aggression. *Aggressive Behavior, 14*(1), 13–24.

Huesmann, L. R. (1995). *Screen violence and real violence: Understanding the link* [Brochure]. Auckland, NZ: Media Aware.

Huesmann, L. R. (1998). The role of social information processing and cognitive schema in the acquisition and maintenance of habitual aggressive behavior. In R. G. Geen & E. Donnerstein (Eds.), *Human aggression: Theories, research, and implications for social policy* (pp. 73–109). San Diego, CA: Academic Press.

Huesmann, L. R. (2005). Imitation and the effects of observing media violence on behavior. In S. Hurley & N. Chater (Eds.), *Perspectives on imitation: From neuroscience to social science: Vol. 2. Imitation, human development, and culture* (pp. 257–266). Cambridge, MA: MIT Press.

Huesmann, L. R., & Eron, L. D. (Eds.). (1986). *Television and the aggressive child: A cross national perspective*. Hillsdale, NJ: Erlbaum.

Huesmann, L. R., Eron, L. D., Berkowitz, L., & Chaffee, S. (1992). The effects of television violence on aggression: A reply to a skeptic. In P. Suedfeld & P. E. Tetlock (Eds.), *Psychology and social policy* (pp. 191–200). New York: Hemisphere.

Huesmann, L. R., & Guerra, N. (1997). Children's normative beliefs about aggression and aggressive behavior. *Journal of Personality and Social Psychology, 72*(2), 408–419.

Huesmann, L. R., & Moise, J. (1996). Media violence: A demonstrated public health threat to children. *Harvard Mental Health Letter, 12*(12), 5–7.

Huesmann, L. R., Moise, J. & Podolski, C. L. (1995, May). *Fantasy and normative beliefs as mediators of the relation between media violence and aggression*. Paper presented at the annual meeting of the Midwest Psychological Association, Chicago.

Huesmann, L. R., Moise-Titus, J., Podolski, C., & Eron, L. (2003). Longitudinal relations between children's exposure to TV violence and their aggressive and violent behavior in young adulthood: 1977–1992. *Developmental Psychology, 39*(2), 201–221.

Huesmann, L. R., & Taylor, L. D. (2006). Developmental contexts in middle childhood: Bridges to adolescence and adulthood. In A. C. Huston & M. N. Ripke (Eds.), *Middle childhood: Contexts of development* (pp. 303-326). Cambridge, UK: Cambridge University Press.

Huntemann, N., & Morgan, M. (2001). Mass media and identity development. In D. G. Singer & J. L. Singer (Eds.), *Handbook of children and the media* (pp. 309–322). Thousand Oaks, CA: Sage.

Hurley, S., & Chater, N. (2004). *Perspectives on imitation: From cognitive neuroscience to social science*. Cambridge, MA: MIT Press.

Huston, A. C., & Wright, J. C. (1997). Mass media and children's development. In W. Damon (Series Ed.), I. Sigel, & A. Renniger (Volume Eds.), *Handbook of child psychology: Vol. 4. Child psychology in practice* (5th ed., pp. 999–1058). New York: Wiley.

Jhally, S. (1995). *Dreamworlds II*. [Video] Northampton, MA: Media Education Foundation.

Johnston, J., & Ettema, J. (1982). *Positive images: Breaking stereotypes with children's television*. Beverly Hills, CA: Sage.

Joint Statement of Congress. (2000). *Joint statement on the impact of entertainment violence on children*. Retrieved December 2, 2003, from http://www.apa.org/advocacy/release/jstmtevc.htm.

Josephson, W. L. (1987). Television violence and children's aggression: Testing the priming, social script, and disinhibition predictions. *Journal of Personality and Social Psychology, 53*(5), 882–890.

Kaiser Family Foundation. (2001). *Parents and the V-chip* [Online]. Menlo Park, CA. Available: www.kff.org.

Kaiser Family Foundation. (2003a). *Zeros to six: Electronic media in the lives of infants, toddlers, and preschoolers* (Publication #3378). Menlo Park, CA: Author.

Kaiser Family Foundation. (2003b). *Key facts: Parents and the media* (Publication #3353). Menlo Park, CA: Author.

Katz, E., Blumler, J. G., & Gurevitch, M. (1974). Utilization of mass communication by the individual. In J. G. Blumler & E. Katz (Eds.), *The uses of mass communications: Current perspectives on gratifications research* (pp. 19–32). Beverly Hills, CA: Sage.

Kilbourne, J. (1999). *Deadly persuasion: Why women and girls must fight the addictive power of advertising*. New York: Free Press.

Kirwil, L., & Huesmann, L. R. (2003, May). *The relation between aggressiveness and emotional reactions to observed violence*. Paper presented at the annual meeting of the Midwestern Psychological Association, Chicago.

Kunkel, D., Cope, K. M., & Colvin, C. (1996). *Sexual messages on family hour television: Content and context*. Menlo Park, CA: Henry J. Kaiser Family Foundation.

Larson, R. (1995). Secrets in the bedroom: Adolescents' private use of media. *Journal of Youth and Adolescence, 24*, 535–550.

Lenhart, A., Rainie, L., & Lewis, O. (2001). *Teenage life online: The rise of the instant-message generation and the internet's impact on friendships and family relationships*. Washington, DC: Pew Foundation. Available: www.pewinternet.org.

Linz, D., Donnerstein, E., & Penrod, S. (1984). The effects of multiple exposures to filmed violence against women. *Journal of Communication, 34*, 130–147.

Lowery, S. A., & DeFleur, M. L. (1995). *Milestones in mass communication research: Media effects* (3rd ed.). White Plains, NY: Longman.

Malamuth, N. M. (1984). Aggression against women: Cultural and individual causes. In N. M. Malamuth & E. Donnerstein (Eds.), *Pornography and sexual aggression* (pp. 19–52). Olrando, FL: Academic Press.

Malamuth, N., & Spinner, B. (1980). A longitudinal content analysis of sexual violence in the best selling erotica magazines. *Journal of Sex Research, 16*, 226–237.

Mares, M., & Woodard, E. H. (2001). Prosocial effects on children's social interactions. In D. G. Singer & J. L. Singer (Eds.), *Handbook of children and the media* (pp. 183–205). Thousand Oaks, CA: Sage.

Mastro, D., & Greenberg, B. S. (2000). The portrayal of racial minorities on prime-time television. *Journal of Broadcasting and Electronic Media, 44*, 690–703.

Meltzoff, A. N., & Moore, M. K. (2000). Imitation of facial and manual gestures by human neonates: Resolving the debate about early imitation. In D. Muir & A. Slater (Eds.), *Infant development: The essential readings* (pp. 167–181). Malden, MA: Blackwell.

Mielke, K. W. (2001). A review of research on the educational and social impact of *Sesame Street*. In S. M. Fisch & R. T. Truglio (Eds.), *"G" is for growing: Thirty years of research on children and Sesame Street* (pp. 83–94). Mahwah, NJ: Erlbaum.

Minnow, N. M., & LaMay, C. L. (1995). *Abandoned in the wasteland: Children, television, and the first amendment*. New York: Hill & Wang.

Moise-Titus, J. (1999). *The role of negative emotions in the media violence–aggression relation*. Unpublished dissertation, University of Michigan.

Nathanson, A. I. (1999). Identifying and explaining the relationship between parental mediation and children's aggression. *Communication Research, 26*, 124–143.

National Institute of Mental Health. (1982). *Television and behavior: Ten years of scientific progress and implication for the eighties: Vol. 1. Summary report* (DHHS Publication No. ADM 82–1195). Washington, DC: U.S. Government Printing Office.

Paik, H., & Comstock, G. (1994). The effects of television violence on antisocial behavior: A meta-analysis. *Communication Research, 21*(4), 516–546.

Palmer, E. L., & Fisch, S. M. (2001). The beginnings of *Sesame Street* research. In S. M. Fisch & R. T. Truglio (Eds.), *"G" is for growing: Thirty years of research on children and Sesame Street* (pp. 3–23). Mahwah, NJ: Erlbaum.

Peterson, R. C., & Thurstone, L. L. (1933). *Motion pictures and the social attitudes of children*. New York: Macmillan.

Petty, R. E., & Priester, J. R. (1994). Mass media attitude change: Implications of the elaboration likelihood model of persuasion. In J. Bryant & D. Zillmann (Ed.), *Media effects: Advances in theory and research* (pp. 91–122). Hillsdale, NJ: Erlbaum.

Rhodes, R. (2000). Hollow claims about fantasy violence. *New York Times*, §4, p. 19.

Rizzolati, G., Fadiga, L., Gallese, V., & Fogassi, L. (1996). Premotor cortex and the recognition of motor actions. *Cognitive Brain Research, 3*, 131–141.

Roberts, D. F., & Christenson, P. G. (2001). Popular music in childhood and adolescence. In D. G. Singer & J. L. Singer (Eds.), *Handbook of children and the media* (pp. 395–413). Thousand Oaks, CA: Sage.

Roberts, D. F., Foehr, U. G., & Rideout, V. J. (2005). *Generation M: Media in the lives of 8–18 year-olds.* Menlo Park, CA: Henry J. Kaiser Family Foundation.

Roberts, D. F., Foehr, U. G., Rideout, V. J., & Brodie, M. (1999). *Kids & media @ the new millenium: A comprehensive national analysis of children's media use.* Menlo Park, CA: Henry J. Kaiser Family Foundation.

Rosenthal, R. (1986). Media violence, antisocial behavior, and the social consequences of small effects. *Journal of Social Issues, 42,* 141–154.

Rubin, A. M. (1986). Uses, gratifications, and media effects research. In J. Bryant & D. Zillmann (Eds.), *Perspectives on media effects* (pp. 281–301). Hillsdale, NJ: Erlbaum.

Rudman, L. A., & Borgida, E (1995). The afterglow of construct accessibility: The behavioral consequences of priming men to view women as sexual objects. *Journal of Experimental Social Psychology, 31,* 493–517.

Shrum, L. J., & Bischak, V. D. (2001). Mainstreaming, resonance and impersonal impact: Testing moderators of the cultivation effect for estimates of crime risk. *Human Communication Research, 27,* 187–215.

Singer, J. L., & Singer, D. G. (1986). Family experiences and television viewing as predictors of children's imagination, restlessness, and aggression. *Journal of Social Issues, 42,* 107–124.

Singer, J. L., & Singer, D. G. (1998). *Barney & Friends* as entertainment and education. In J. K. Asamen & G. Berry (Eds.), *Research paradigms, television, and social behavior* (pp. 305–367). Thousand Oaks, CA: Sage.

Singer, D. G., & Singer, J. L. (Eds.). (2001). *Handbook of children and the media.* Thousand Oaks, CA: Sage.

Slater, M. K., Henry, K. L., & Swaim, R. C. (2003). Violent media content and aggressiveness in adolescents: A downward spiral model. *Communication Research, 30,* 713–736.

Steinfeld, J. (1972). *Statement in hearings before Subcommittee on Communications of Committee on Commerce* (U.S. Senate, Serial No. 92–52, pp. 25–27). Washington, DC: U.S. Government Printing Office.

Stice, E., & Shaw, H. (1994). Adverse effects of the media portrayed thin-ideal on women and linkages to bulimic symptomatolgy. *Journal of Social and Clinical Psychology, 13,* 288–308.

Strasburger, V. C. (1995). *Adolescents and the media: Medical and psychological impact.* Thousand Oaks, CA: Sage.

Strasburger, V. C., & Wilson, B. J. (Eds.). (2002). *Children, adolescents, and the media.* Thousand Oaks, CA: Sage.

Strouse, J. S., Buerkel-Rothfuss, N., & Long, E. C. (1995). Gender and family as moderators of the relationship between music video exposure and adolescent sexual permissiveness. *Adolescence, 30,* 505–521.

Thomsen, S. R., McCoy, J. K., & Gustafson, R. L. (2002). Motivations for reading beauty and fashion magazines and anorexic risk in college age women. *Media Psychology, 4,* 113–135.

Valentino, N. A., Traugott, M., & Hutchings, V. (2002). Group cues and ideological constraint: A replication of political advertising effects studies in the lab and in the field. *Political Communication, 19,* 29–48.

Valkenburg, P. M., & Cantor, J. (2000). Children's likes and dislikes of entertainment programs. In D. Zillmann & P. Vorderer (Eds.), *Media entertainment: The psychology of its appeal* (pp. 135–152). Mahwah, NJ: Erlbaum.

Vidmar, N., & Rokeach, M. (1974). Archie Bunker's bigotry: A study in selective perception and exposure. *Journal of Communication, 24,* 36–47.

Wartella, E., Caplovitz, A. G., & Lee, J. H. (2004). From Baby Einstein to Leapfrog, from Doom to the Sims, from Instant Messaging to internet chat rooms: Public interest in the role of interactive media in children's lives. *Social Policy Report, XVIII.*

Wilson, B. J., & Weiss, A. J. (1993). The effects of sibling coviewing on preschoolers' reactions to a suspenseful movie scene. *Communication Research, 20,* 214–248.

Wolpe, J. (1958). *Psychotherapy by reciprocal inhibition.* Stanford, CA: Stanford University Press.

Woodard, E. H. (2000). *Media in the Home 2000: The fifth annual survey of parents and children* (Survey Series No. 7). Philadelphia: Annenberg Public Policy Center of the University of Pennsylvania.

Wright, J. C., Huston, A. C., Scantlin, R., & Kotler, J. (2001). The Early Window Project: *Sesame Street* prepares children for school. In S. M. Fisch & R. T. Truglio (Eds.), *"G" is for growing: Thirty years of research on children and Sesame Street* (pp. 97–114). Mahwah, NJ: Erlbaum.

Wyrwicka, W. (1996). *Imitation in human and animal behavior.* New Brunswick, NJ: Transaction.

Yang, N., & Linz, D. (1990). Movie ratings and the content of adult videos: The sex–violence ratio. *Journal of Communication, 40,* 28–32.

Yokota, F., & Thompson, K. M. (2000). Violence in G-rated animated films. *Journal of the American Medical Association, 283,* 2716–2720.

Zill, N. (2001). Does *Sesame Street* enhance school readiness?: Evidence from a national survey of children. In S. M. Fisch & R. T. Truglio (Eds.), *"G" is for growing: Thirty years of research on children and Sesame Street* (pp. 115–130). Mahwah, NJ: Erlbaum.

Zillmann, D., Bryant, J., & Comisky, P. W. (1981). Excitation and hedonic valence in the effect of erotica on motivated inter-male aggression. *European Journal of Social Psychology, 11*(3), 233–252.

Zillmann, D., & Weaver, J. B. (1996). Gender-socialization theory of reactions to horror. In J. B. Weaver & R. Tamborini (Eds.), *Horror films: Current research on audience preferences and reactions* (pp. 81–101). Mahwah, NJ: Erlbaum.

PART VI

Class and Cultural Perspectives on Socialization

CHAPTER 17

Social Class and Socialization in Families

RAND D. CONGER and SHANNON J. DOGAN

Current concerns about the influence of social class or socioeconomic status (SES) on processes of socialization and human development arise from a long history of research in this area, dating back to the middle of the last century (e.g., Davis & Havighurst, 1946; Sears, Maccoby, & Levin, 1957). Economic changes in the United States and other industrialized and developing countries during the last two decades (e.g., increasing income inequality) have enhanced this ongoing interest in how social position and economic resources affect families and the development of children (e.g., Conger & Conger, 2002; Duncan & Brooks-Gunn, 1997; Keating & Hertzman, 1999; Prior, Sanson, Smart, & Oberklaid, 1999; Schoon et al., 2002). Indeed, research by developmental scholars joins with a broader initiative within the field of social epidemiology that focuses on *health disparities* or the general trend for more socially and economically disadvantaged people to suffer above-average rates of physical, emotional, and behavioral problems (Berkman & Kawachi, 2000; Oakes & Rossi, 2003).

Consistent with this broader concern for social position and health in general, recent reviews provide significant evidence that important indicators of SES are positively related both to effective socialization strategies by parents (Parke, 2004) and to the physical, intellectual, social, and emotional health of children and adolescents (Bradley & Corwyn, 2002). Indeed, a host of research now suggests a link between various dimensions of SES and physical health, social–emotional well-being, and cognitive functioning for both children and adults (e.g., Berkman & Kawachi, 2000; Bradley & Corwyn, 2002; McLeod & Shanahan, 1996). With respect to the development of children and adolescents, recent findings demonstrate a clear connection between poverty and mental health (e.g., Ackerman, Brown, & Izard, 2004; Dearing, McCartney, & Taylor, 2001; McLeod

433

& Shanahan, 1996), SES and cognitive development (e.g., Ackerman et al., 2004; Dearing et al., 2001; Hoff, 2003; Hughes et al., 2005; Mezzacappa, 2004), and social class position and physical well-being (e.g., Evans & English, 2002; McLoyd, 1998).

This chapter provides a selective review of recent research and theory related to the role of social class or SES in the socialization and development of children. We focus primarily on advances in the field during the past 5–10 years because there has been tremendous growth in both empirical and theoretical work during this period (e.g., Bornstein & Bradley, 2003; Bradley & Corwyn, 2002; Conger & Conger, 2002). Moreover, increasingly sophisticated research designs and statistical strategies have shed important new light on how social disadvantage affects the behaviors of parents and the development of their offspring.

We focus particular attention on the avenues through which SES is hypothesized to influence the childrearing practices that parents and other caregivers in the family employ in efforts to socialize their children. That is, the central concern of the chapter is how social position affects parent behaviors that contribute to whether or not children become well-adjusted members of the broader community in terms of their personal attributes and relationships with others. There are two reasons for this emphasis in this review. First, identifying the family pathways through which SES plays a role in children's lives holds promise for the development of effective community programs that might help overcome the potentially adverse consequences of socioeconomic disadvantage.

Second, although social position also affects socialization within other relevant contexts, such as peer relationships and the school environment (Ensminger & Fothergill, 2003; Leventhal & Brooks-Gunn, 2003), the most significant progress on understanding the relationship between SES and child development has been made in terms of family socialization goals and practices. For example, recent reviews of the research show that lower- compared to middle-SES parents are more likely to demand compliance from their children, more likely to use physical punishment, and less likely to reason with their children about the consequences of their behavior (e.g., Hoff, Laursen, & Tardif, 2002; Hoffman, 2003). Most important, the more authoritarian style of lower-SES parents has been linked to less competent social and emotional development for children. With regard to cognitive functioning, middle- compared to lower-SES parents are more likely to use richer vocabularies and to engage in cognitively stimulating activities with their children. Thus, current evidence suggests that SES is related both to important socialization practices in families and to the health and well-being of children. As demonstrated in the remainder of this chapter, different theoretical perspectives interpret these sets of empirical relationships in different ways.

ORGANIZATION OF THE CHAPTER

The following sections of the chapter are organized to address several major issues. The first section considers definitions of social class or SES, how these definitions have been translated into measures used in empirical studies, and how the construct is best conceptualized. We next consider some of the primary theoretical frameworks that attempt to explain the relationships among social class, socialization, and child development. Some of these models propose that social position influences parental behavior and, in turn, child development. This perspective represents an instance of the *social causation argu-*

ment, which predicts that social conditions lead to variations in health and well-being. Other models propose that the relationship between SES and parenting is an artifact that is explained by individual differences in the personal characteristics of parents that affect both their SES and relationships with their children. This view represents the *social selection perspective*, which proposes that the traits and dispositions of individuals influence both their social circumstances and their future emotions and behaviors (McLeod & Kaiser, 2004). The social selection hypothesis has been offered as a serious challenge to the presumption that social disadvantage has a causal influence on families and children, and we consider these theoretical arguments in this review.

Following consideration of each model of SES and socialization, we discuss a wide range of empirical work that addresses important predictions from these theoretical perspectives. This rapidly developing literature involves diverse research strategies, from cross-sectional survey research to randomized experiments. Taken together, these research efforts have significantly advanced understanding of the relationship between social status and socialization. As will become clear, however, the association between individual development and SES represents a dynamic process which is far more complex than the static notion of an individual's response to social constraint that many earlier theories envisioned. With this idea in mind, the next to last section of this review proposes an integrated perspective on the interconnections among SES, socialization strategies, and human development. The chapter concludes with a discussion of promising future directions for research on the relationships among social class, socialization, and child and adolescent development.

WHAT IS SOCIAL CLASS?

Social class as a construct relates to various dimensions of social position, including prestige, power, and economic well-being (Hoff et al., 2002; Liu et al., 2004; Oakes & Rossi, 2003). Measures of social class can be objective or subjective, and there is no consensus as to how the construct should be assessed (Liu et al., 2004). Earlier research often used categorical variables such as "working class" as markers of social position, whereas more recent research tends to employ continuous measures of the construct (Duncan & Magnuson, 2003; Hoff et al., 2002). Despite the ambiguity surrounding the meaning and measurement of social class, for several reasons important progress has been made in recent work relating social position to family processes and child development.

To begin with, there appears to be an emerging consensus in the developmental literature that social class and SES are equivalent constructs (e.g., Ensminger & Fothergill, 2003; Hoffman, 2003), although some researchers suggest caution in this regard (Hoff et al., 2002). This consensus creates the opportunity for greater comparability across studies concerned with social status and family socialization practices. Second, most investigators agree that there are three quantitative indicators of social class or SES that provide reasonably good coverage of the domains of interest: income, education, and occupational status (Bradley & Corwyn, 2002; Ensminger & Fothergill, 2003). Despite the fact that these indicators of social position are positively correlated (Ensminger & Fothergill, 2003), there also is general agreement that they should not be combined into simple composite scores, such as the Hollingshead Four Factor Index which combines measures of education and occupation (Hollingshead, 1975). Duncan and Magnuson (2003), for example, note that one indicator of SES is inadequate and that these three measures should be used separately in data analyses. They suggest that each of these markers of social status demonstrates different levels of stability across time and also differentially predicts family processes and child adjustment. Only by including each of them as a separate variable in data analyses can the investigator understand their unique and combined contributions to the relationship between SES and socialization.

Perhaps most fundamental to contemporary understanding of social class in developmental research, though, is the view that education, occupation, and income represent separate yet related personal, social, and economic resources that have important implications for the health and well-being of both parents and children. These resources can be thought of as "capital" that differentiates persons, households, and neighborhoods (Bradley & Corwyn, 2002; Hoff et al., 2002; Oakes & Rossi, 2003). As an illustration, Oakes and Rossi (2003) draw on Coleman (1990) to propose that SES should be defined in terms of material or financial capital (economic resources), human capital (knowledge and skills), and social capital (connections to and the status and power of individuals in one's social network). Income and other forms of wealth obviously relate to material or financial capital and education to human capital. Although the connection is not as straightforward for occupational status, it can be considered a marker of social capital inasmuch as people in higher-status occupations are more likely to associate with others who have higher than average occupational status, advanced skills, and economic resources (Bradley & Corwyn, 2003; Oakes & Rossi, 2003).

Conceptualizing social class or SES in terms of important economic, personal, and social resources provides several advantages in terms of theory building and theory testing. For example, human capital in the form of advanced education may influence a parent's approach to socialization in terms of the priority he or she places on academic achievement and the assistance he or she can provide to foster success in school. On the other hand, material capital can be used to finance enriching educational experiences, adequate housing and nutrition, and residential location in a neighborhood that supports the well-being of children. Equally important, social capital in the form of occupational status may both increase the parent's capacity to serve as a mentor for success in work and help the parent connect the child to important social resources in the community. Interestingly, most of the recent theoretical work relating SES to socialization and child development has focused on income and economic hardship, as will become evident in the next section of this chapter. Also important, however, is consideration of how economic models might be extended to include parents' educational attainment and occupational status.

SOCIAL CAUSATION PERSPECTIVES ON SOCIAL CLASS AND SOCIALIZATION

As noted earlier, some theories argue that social class affects the socialization strategies of parents and, in that fashion, influences the development of children. These models are consistent with the *social causation perspective*. In this section we describe two major approaches consistent with this view of SES effects and evaluate empirical evidence related to these perspectives. The first theoretical paradigm, the family stress model (FSM) of economic hardship, proposes that financial difficulties have an adverse effect on parents' emotions, behaviors, and relationships which, in turn, negatively influence their parenting or socialization strategies (Conger & Conger, 2002). The second perspective, what we call the extended investment model (EIM), takes a very different approach to SES effects. Whereas the FSM emphasizes the stress-inducing properties of low SES, the EIM focuses on the ways in which the resources conveyed by higher social status increase the tendency and ability of parents to promote the talents and well-being of their children.

The EIM builds on the notion that higher compared to lower SES parents are likely to have greater financial (e.g., income), social (e.g., occupational status), and human (e.g., education) capital. Earlier theory and empirical evidence suggest that these types of resources are associated with more successful development of children. For example, economists propose that financial resources increase the investments parents make in their children's development, thus promoting a wide range of academic and social competencies that accrue to the benefit of the child (Bradley & Corwyn, 2002; Mayer, 1997). Sociologists have argued that greater occupational status affects parents' values and priorities in a fashion that positively influences their childrearing strategies (Kohn, 1959, 1969). Finally, parental education is considered to be one of the most important and influential markers of SES in terms of socialization practices and child adjustment (Bradley & Corwyn, 2002). The following review combines these insights to propose the EIM and to evaluate evidence that may support it.

The Family Stress Model of Economic Hardship

The Theory

The FSM builds on a tradition of research dating back to the Great Depression years of the 1930s. A series of studies at that time provided evidence that severe hardship could undermine family functioning and socialization practices in a fashion that negatively affected the lives of both parents and children (e.g., Angell, 1936; Cavan & Ranck, 1938; Komarovsky, 1940). Elder's research extended this earlier work in a series of reports demonstrating the response of depression-era parents to economic loss (Elder, 1974; Elder & Caspi, 1988). These themes have been carried forward in contemporary investigations that both support and modify many of the conclusions reached in these earlier studies (Leventhal & Brooks-Gunn, 2003; McLoyd, 1998). Mayer (1997) calls the conceptual ideas emanating from this line of research the "good parent theory," which proposes that poverty or low income has a negative impact on parents' psychological well-being. These psychological disruptions, in turn, are expected to reduce effective socialization practices.

Consistent with this line of research, Conger and his colleagues coined the term "family stress model," which was developed in their efforts to understand how financial problems influenced the lives of Iowa families going through a severe downturn in the agricultural economy during the 1980s (Conger & Conger, 2002; Conger & Elder, 1994; Conger et al., 2002). As shown in Figure 17.1, the FSM proposes that economic hardship leads to economic pressure in the family. Markers of hardship include low income, high debts relative to assets, work instability, and negative financial events (i.e., increasing economic demands and/or declining material resources). These indicators of hardship are consistent with the concept of economic or material capital, which includes the notion of accumulated wealth as well as current income. These hardship conditions are expected to affect family functioning and individual adjustment primarily through the economic pressures they generate. The FSM proposes that economic pressures include (1) unmet mate-

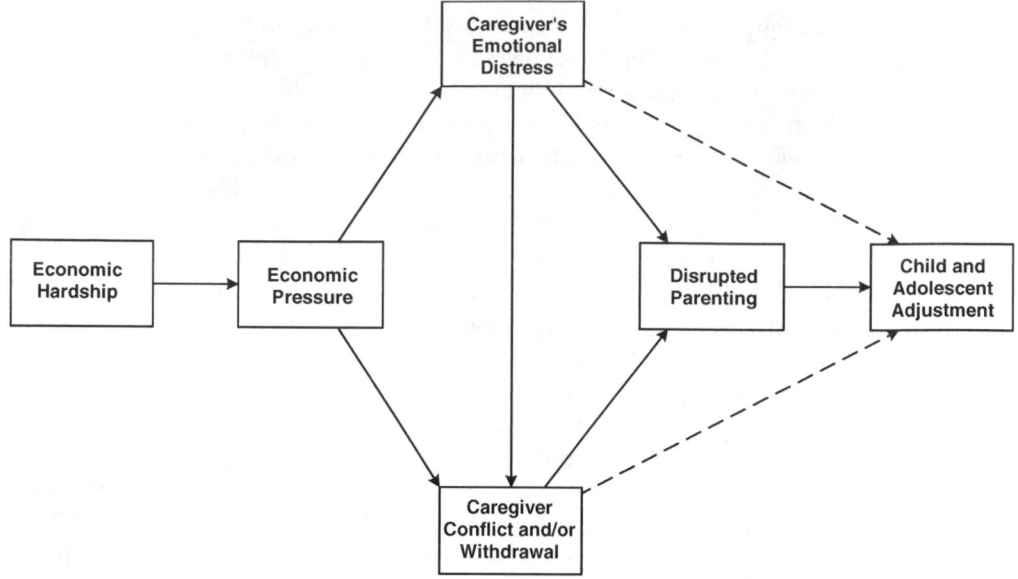

FIGURE 17.1. The family stress model of economic hardship.

rial needs involving necessities such as adequate food and clothing, (2) the inability to pay bills or make ends meet, and (3) having to cut back on even necessary expenses (e.g., health insurance and medical care). Conger and his colleagues argue that experiencing these kinds of pressures or strains gives psychological meaning to living with economic hardship (Conger & Conger, 2002; Conger et al., 1992, 1993; Conger & Elder, 1994; Conger, Ge, Elder, Lorenz, & Simons, 1994; Conger et al., 2002).

In addition, the model predicts that when economic pressure is high, parents and other caregivers (e.g., members of the extended family) living with children are at increased risk for becoming emotionally distressed as indicated by feelings of depression, anxiety, anger, and alienation. These markers of emotional problems are broadly conceived and may also be reflected in related problems such as substance use or antisocial behavior, as suggested by earlier research (Conger, 1995). According to the model, emotional distress and economic pressure both predict increased conflict and reduced warmth and support in the relations between caregivers (Conger & Conger, 2002; Conger et al., 2002). The FSM also proposes that caregivers' emotional distress and relationship problems will be directly related to disruptions in parenting (e.g., being harsh and inconsistent, relatively uninvolved, and low in nurturance and affection). The dashed lines from distress and relationship problems to child development indicate that there may be some direct effect from these constructs to child adjustment; however, the primary hypothesis is that disrupted parenting will mediate or explain the influence of parental distress and conflicts on child development.

According to the model, then, when families experience economic hardship, children are at risk for suffering both decrements in positive adjustment (e.g., cognitive ability, social competence, school success, and attachment to parents) and increases in internalizing (e.g., symptoms of depression and anxiety) and externalizing (e.g., aggressive and antisocial behavior) problems. The model also proposes, however, that these economic effects on children will only be indirect through their impact on the lives of parents and other family caregivers. For single-parent families, caregiver conflicts with one another may be omitted from the model or conflicts with an ex-spouse or current romantic partner might be substituted, as economic problems are expected to affect these relationships as well (Conger et al., 2002). Although elaborations of the FSM include factors that promote resilience or exacerbate vulnerability to these mediating pathways, the model in Figure 17.1 provides the basic tenets of this theoretical framework (Conger & Conger, 2002; Conger et al., 2002).

Empirical Findings Related to the Family Stress Model

An important characteristic of the FSM is that it focuses on only one domain of SES or social class (i.e., the economic dimension of family life). Despite the fact that the financial fortunes of families have been shown to be relatively unstable, with a significant proportion of households entering or leaving poverty in any given year, low income has been associated with significant developmental difficulties for children, especially when poverty is severe or persistent (Dearing et al., 2001; Duncan & Magnuson, 2003; Magnuson & Duncan, 2002; McLoyd, 1998). Thus, the FSM's focus on economic hardship has merit in terms of identified relationships with child and adolescent development. An important feature of the FSM, however, is that it proposes that economic conditions involve much more than just the level of family income. It places financial life within the context of the economic demands that families face as well as the resources available for meeting those demands. It also considers wealth, in the form of assets and debts. As noted earlier, the concept of financial or material capital involves more than just income; it also encompasses all forms of accumulated wealth (Oakes & Rossi, 2003). Thus, the FSM specifically incorporates the notion of wealth in the conception of family economic circumstances.

Because several studies of families and children have now evaluated significant portions of the FSM using the same labels for constructs as described in Figure 17.1, this review focuses on the findings from these six investigations. These studies represent a rich array of ethnic or national groups, geographic locations, family structures, children's ages, and research designs. Following a brief description of each study, findings from these investigations are summarized in relation to the FSM (Figure 17.1). The first study in this group is the *Iowa Youth and Families Project* (IYFP), which involved 451 rural Iowa families and was initiated in 1989. Two initial reports from this study evaluated the FSM, first for 205 seventh-grade boys (Conger et al., 1992) and then for 220 seventh-grade girls (Conger et al., 1993). These rural, European American families included mothers, fathers, and the seventh-grade children.

The second investigation, the *Family and Community Health Study* (FACHS), replicated and extended the original Iowa research in several important ways. First, it involved 422 two-caregiver African American families living in Iowa and Georgia who were raising the focal child, a fifth grader at study initiation. Second, these families primarily came from urban rather than rural areas, although these were not large urban centers of the type that have been the focus of most research with African American parents and children. Eligible families were randomly recruited from schools and neighborhoods in Iowa and Georgia in a manner that generated a true community sample with a wide range of SES characteristics. Third, the caregiver relationship took several different forms including the married, biological parents of the focal child (39%) or stepparents (33%), or children living with some other form of caregiver arrangement such as mothers and grandmothers (28%). These important variations in caregiver relationships made it possible to determine whether the processes described by the FSM would apply only to married, biological parents or to a broader array of possible caregiving arrangements. The results indicated that different forms of caregiver relationships demonstrate the same types of responses to economic hardships and pressures (Conger et al., 2002).

The third study, the *New Hope Project* (Mistry, Vandewater, Huston, & McLoyd, 2002), focused on a poor urban sample of primarily ethnic minority (57% African American, 28% Hispanic) families headed by a single parent (83%). Children ranged in age from 5 to 12 years for the 419 families in the study. This experimental study was designed to determine whether financial assistance and job training efforts would improve the life conditions of poor families. Mistry and her colleagues examined how economic pressures influenced parenting behaviors and child outcomes using program evaluation data from the larger investigation. Because almost all of these families involved only a single parent, information was not collected on caregiver conflicts. The fourth study related to the FSM involved findings from the *Panel Study of Income Dynamics*, a nationally representative investigation of families and their economic experiences (Yeung, Linver, & Brooks-Gunn, 2002). This research addressed the family stress process for younger children, ages 3–5 years. The sample for the study is quite diverse in terms of ethnicity, place of residence, SES, and family structure. Yeung and her colleagues examined predictions from the FSM for 753 preschool children, a relatively neglected age group in previous tests of the model. The results in the report considered here were based on information about the children and their mothers. The relationship between caregivers was not examined in these analyses. Also important, all models were estimated controlling for mother's education and cognitive ability.

In the fifth study considered here, the *Finnish Replication Study*, Solantaus, Leinonen, and Punamäki (2004) attempted a major replication of the original Iowa findings based on an investigation of 527 two-parent families in Finland. Not only did they include all of the major constructs in the model in their assessment package, they also predicted to child externalizing and internalizing symptoms at time 2 controlling for the same problems at time 1, approximately 4 years earlier. Thus, they predicted rank-order change in child adjustment. In addition, all the families included both a mother and a father along with a focal child between 12 and 13 years of age, characteristics consistent with the original Iowa research. There were approximately the same number of boys and girls in the sample. The replication study took place during a period of economic crisis in Finland, similar to the agricultural depression experienced by the Iowa families. To our knowledge, this study represents the only attempted replication of the complete FSM outside the United States. Finally, the sixth study related to the FSM was the *Riverside Economic Stress Project*. This replication study involved European American ($N = 111$) and Mexican American ($N = 167$) families of fifth graders and was conducted in urban areas of Southern California (Parke et al., 2004). Significant and theoretically meaningful differences were found for the two ethnic groups.

With regard to the connection between economic hardship and economic pressure (see Figure 17.1), the degree of association across these six studies ranged from .20 to .88, with a median standardized path coefficient of .68, a robust association. The findings with regard to this predicted association also underscore the importance of the FSM emphasis on a broad array of measures for economic hardship, including indicators of income, income loss, financial resources, and economic demands. That is, all the studies that included multiple measures of economic hardship produced much higher associations with economic pressure (median coefficient = .70) than those that only used a measure of family income (studies 3 and 4, median coefficient = .20). These findings highlight the importance of the idea that economic status or capital as a dimension of social class requires a richer assessment than a measure of income alone. That is, an adequate evaluation of economic standing requires measures of other material resources and demands in addition to income (Bradley & Corwyn, 2002; Oakes & Rossi, 2003). Also consistent with the model, for all six studies the link between economic hardship and other endogenous variables was indirect through economic pressure.

The next step in the FSM involves the path from economic pressure to the emotional distress of parents and other caregivers. Across the six studies this predicted relationship was always statistically significant and the median association between these two constructs was respectable (standardized path coefficient = .42). Given the fact that many of the studies used different indicators for economic pressure and emotional distress, this degree of replication is quite remarkable. Also consistent with the FSM, each of the model tests found that emotional distress was directly related to caregiver conflict after economic pressure was taken into account (median path coefficient = .33). Inconsistent with the model as illustrated in Figure 17.1 was the hypothesis that economic pressure would directly predict caregiver conflict net of emotional distress. This expected association was never statistically significant. It appears that the FSM should be modified so that economic pressure predicts caregiver conflict only indirectly through its association with emotional distress. In this set of findings, emotional distress is clearly the parental response that connects economic problems to conflicts between caregivers.

For five out of the six studies, emotional distress also predicted disrupted parenting in at least some instances, consistent with the model. It is not clear why this hypothesized relationship occurred in some cases but not in others, and the variability in the connection between the two constructs is an important issue for future research. In most instances emotional distress did not directly predict child and adolescent adjustment once disrupted parenting was taken into account, a finding that is consistent with the dashed line in Figure 17.1 suggesting that this relationship may or may not occur. For three of the four studies that included a measure of caregiver conflict, this measure was associated with disrupted parenting (median path coefficient = .45). The major exception to this finding was the Parke et al. (2004) study in Southern California. Future research is needed to clarify whether the null finding in the Riverside study was an anomaly of that investigation or an indication that this expected pathway does not hold under certain types of social, economic, or cultural conditions.

For almost all of the studies, caregiver conflict was not directly related to child and adolescent adjustment, consistent with the dashed line in Figure 17.1 suggesting that this link may or may not be significant. However, there was one intriguing exception to this pattern of results. For the Mexican American families in the Parke et al. (2004) study, caregiver conflict demonstrated a substantial direct path with child and adolescent adjustment problems (standardized path coefficient = .53). It may be that this result represents something unique about this study. This view is contradicted, though, by the fact that caregiver conflict did not directly predict child and adolescent adjustment for the European American families in the study. We believe this unique finding may result from the high value Mexican American parents and children place on the family unit. Because threats to the family itself engendered by interparental conflict may be especially distressing for Mexican American children, caregiver conflict may directly affect the emotional and behavioral problems of these children independently of styles of parenting (Parke et al., 2004). This possibility needs to be investigated in future research.

Finally, all six studies provided some support for the hypothesis that disrupted parenting is significantly associated with child and adolescent adjustment, consistent with the FSM. Each of the first four studies included a measure of child or adolescent positive adjustment, and eight of the nine estimated path coefficients were statistically significant (median path coefficient = −.31). All six studies included measures of poor child or adolescent adjustment, and 17 of the 21 estimated relationships were statistically significant (median path coefficient = .44). These results provide substantial evidence that the socialization or childrearing strategies of caregivers provide the most proximal mechanism through which the economic fortunes of the family affect the development of children and adolescents, consistent with the FSM.

In addition to the original tests of the FSM using data from the IYFP that were just discussed (Conger et al., 1992, 1993), subsequent findings from this longitudinal study have shown that the model predicts adolescent adjustment in the future and that family conflicts resulting from economic pressure can include children as well as parents (Conger, Conger, Matthews, & Elder, 1999; Conger et al., 1994). Other research from the Iowa project has shown that economic pressure predicts change in the emotional distress of parents over time (Conger, Rueter, & Elder, 1999). These follow-up, longitudinal studies increase confidence in the causal ordering of the variables proposed in the model (Figure 17.1). Especially important, the evidence from the reviewed studies shows that the model applies to (1) different racial and ethnic groups, (2) families in at least one other nation (see Robila & Krishnakumar, 2005, for additional evidence of cross-national replication), (3) urban and rural children and families, and (4) families with different structural arrangements (e.g., both single- and two-parent families). Taken together, these studies suggest that the FSM provides a reasonably good heuristic model for helping to understand how the economic or financial capital aspects of low social class influence family members, socialization processes, and the positive or problematic adjustment of children and adolescents.

In this review of findings related to the FSM, we have chosen to focus on studies that included (1) the same labeling for constructs as in the theory and (2) all or almost all of the central constructs in the model. For example, all the investigations discussed thus far in relation to the FSM included the key construct of economic pressure. Many studies in this literature use a related but somewhat different variable, economic stress or strain, to serve a similar role as economic pressure within an explanatory framework (e.g., Mistry, Biesanz, Taylor, Burchinal, & Cox, 2004). Other studies omit this aspect of the model altogether (e.g., Brody, Murry, Kim, & Brown, 2002; Linver, Brooks-Gunn, & Kohen, 2002). Despite these small variations in conceptualization, most of this related research also provides substantial support for the FSM. Also noteworthy is the fact that these related studies extend across racial and ethnic groups and involve other nations in addition to the United States (e.g., Borge, Rutter, Cote, & Tremblay, 2004; Dodge, Pettit, & Bates, 1994; Prior et al., 1999; Zevalkink & Riksen-Walraven, 2001). And, in an interesting extension of the model, Sobolewski and Amato (2005) found that the economic stress processes proposed in the FSM influence the psychological well-being of a child grown to adulthood. That is, these findings indicated that these economic stress processes during childhood and adolescence have a continuing influence on psychological functioning after a child becomes an adult.

Especially exciting are recent experimental or quasi-experimental studies that also report results consistent with the FSM. For instance, Costello, Compton, Keeler, and Angold (2003) found that the opening of a casino in an American Indian community moved a number of families out of poverty. Children in these families demonstrated a significant drop in psychiatric disorders as their economic situations improved. Children in families that remained poor did not show evidence of a reduction in adjustment problems. Moreover, the investigators reported that an increase in effective parenting behaviors accounted for the connection between improved family finances and child well-being. These findings are quite consistent with predictions from the FSM, and it is likely that the increases in income reduced economic pressures and emotional distress for parents leading, in turn, to improved parenting and child adjustment. Other experimental research on income supplementation for poor families or on moving poor families to more economically advantaged neighborhoods has produced some evidence that these programs can have a positive influence on parents' well-being and on developmental outcomes for children and adolescents. Although these findings remain preliminary, there is a growing body of evidence suggesting that improvements in family income may have beneficial effects consistent with predictions from the FSM (Gennetian & Miller, 2002; Leventhal & Brooks-Gunn, 2003).

The Extended Investment Model

The Theory

In terms of financial capital, the EIM draws on the investment model from the field of economics, which proposes that families with greater economic resources are able to make significant investments in the development of their children whereas more disadvantaged families must invest in more immediate family needs (Becker & Thomes, 1986; Bradley & Corwyn, 2002; Corcoran & Adams, 1997; Duncan & Magnuson, 2003; Haveman & Wolfe, 1994; Linver, et al., 2002; Mayer, 1997). These investments involve several different dimensions of family support, including (1) learning materials available in the home, (2) parent stimulation of learning both directly and through support of advanced or specialized tutoring or training, (3) the family's standard of living (adequate food, housing, clothing, medical care, etc.), and (4) residing in a location that fosters a child's competent development. For example, wealthier parents are expected to reside in areas that promote a child's association with conventional friends, access to good schools, and involvement in a neighborhood or community environment that provides resources for the developing child such as parks and child-related activities. Notice also that the investment model assumes certain socialization goals and practices. That is, the theory predicts that economic well-being will be positively related to childrearing activities expected to foster the academic and social success of a child.

Basically, this economic model proposes that financially well-to-do families can provide a variety of resources that increase human capital for the developing child. The model reflects its economic heritage in this regard. That is, the theory proposes that families, just like businesses, invest in the products or services they provide. Presumably, businesses with greater resources can make greater capital investments and, thus, maintain a competitive edge in the world of commerce. Similarly, families with greater resources can invest them in a fashion that will produce a more competent and successful child. Children in more well-to-do families are more likely to have the nourishment, medical care, environmental safety and support, and educational and social opportunities they require to succeed in life. And, although the theory primarily is concerned with income and wealth, we propose that it can be extended to include family differences in education and occupation as well.

Figure 17.2 provides an illustration of our EIM of SES effects on children and families. The traditional model links family economic resources to investments in children which, in turn, are expected to increase the likelihood that youth will become competent and successful adults. We extend the basic model by proposing that the educational achievements and occupational positions of parents and other caregivers will be similarly related to investments in children. For example, parents with greater education would be expected to place a priority on activities, goods, and services that foster academic and social competence, a prediction consistent with the idea that the human capital of parents will tend to promote the development of human capital in their children. With regard to occupational position, the extended model proposes that parents with more prestigious and higher-paying work roles will tend to invest in their children in at least two important ways. First, they should provide social capital by increasing access to employment and other career-related activities. Second, they should provide human capital by guiding their children toward activities that will promote their eventual career success.

Especially important, Kohn's (1963, 1969, 1995) model of the linkages among occupational status, socialization practices, and child development is consistent with the EIM perspective. Kohn proposed perhaps the best known theory regarding the connection be-

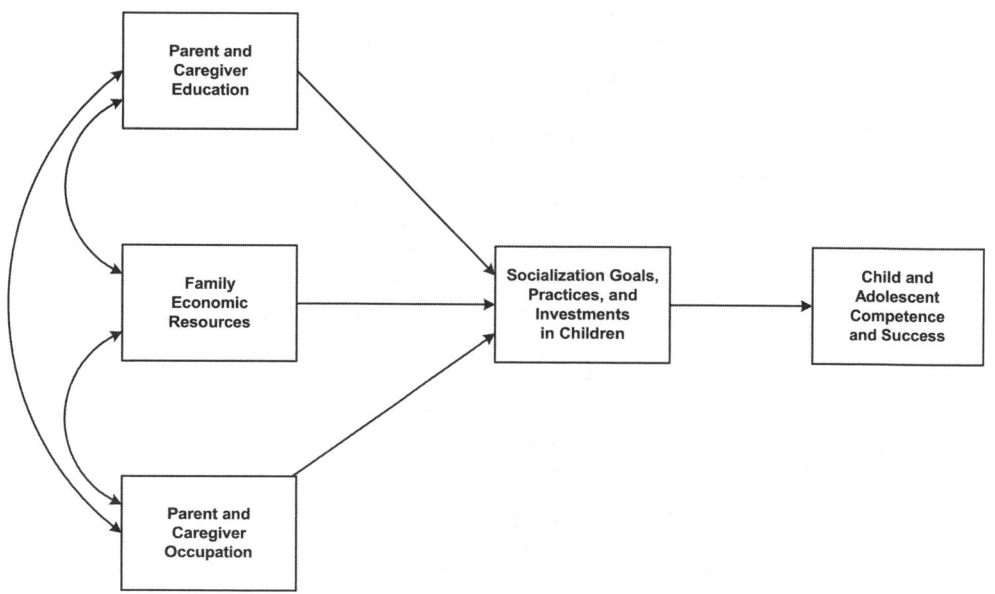

FIGURE 17.2. The extended investment model.

tween occupational status and patterns of socialization in families. He argued that occupational prestige or status was related to parental goals, values, and childrearing practices. According to Kohn, parents in middle-class compared to working-class occupations operate in a more complex and autonomous work environment. The demands of their positions are more likely to focus on interpersonal relations, ideas, and symbols. Moreover, they tend to operate independently in the accomplishment of their occupational responsibilities. In contrast, the jobs of working-class parents tend to involve the manipulation of things such as tools and machines. In addition, parents in the working-class experience greater direct supervision and are less likely to operate independently in their jobs.

Based on these observations, the theory suggests that success in middle-class occupations requires independence, self-direction, the ability to work effectively with abstract ideas, and the capacity to supervise or direct the work of other people. In contrast, success in working-class occupations requires the ability to conform to the rules of the workplace, to be responsive to direct supervision, and to effectively perform standardized and repetitive tasks. Kohn also reasoned that the personalities and life orientations of middle- and working-class parents would differ, and that these differences would affect their goals and priorities for their children.

Specifically, he proposed that middle-class parents would value self-direction in their children. When it came to discipline, they would be more likely to consider the intent of a child's actions and to use reasoning and withdrawal of rewards rather than physical punishment. Given their job demands, he proposed that working-class parents would be more likely to value conformity and obedience in their children. As a result, their approach to discipline would emphasize what the child has done rather than their reasons for their behavior, and they would be more likely to use physical punishment as a disciplinary response. Some researchers have extended Kohn's ideas to other dimensions of occupational influences (Parcel & Menaghan, 1994), but the basic structure of the theory is the same today as when it was originally proposed.

These observations suggest that Kohn's model clearly fits within the broader set of propositions included in the EIM. For example, Kohn suggests that parents in more prestigious occupations will tend to invest more time and energy in their children by reasoning with them, encouraging their independence and talents, and taking time to consider their perspectives on their behaviors and activities. This approach to socialization places greater time demands on the parent than simply responding to noncompliance with harsh or physical punishment. It also creates a richer learning environment in terms of the development of social and academic competence, consistent with the EIM. That is, Kohn's perspective proposes that higher compared to lower SES parents will engage in a broad range of time intensive activities that have the goal of teaching their children the social and academic skills they will need to succeed in life. This view is consistent with the original economic model upon which the EIM is based. To summarize, the EIM proposes that economic, educational, and occupational resources in the family of origin will tend to promote investments in children that are linked to increasing competence during childhood and adolescence and eventual success during the adult years.

Empirical Findings Related to the Extended Investment Model

Unlike the extensive literature on the FSM and variations of the FSM, there is only a limited amount of recent research on the parameters included in the proposed EIM (Figure

17.2). In part, this paucity of findings results from the fact that these demographic measures typically are treated as control variables in developmental research, rather than as phenomena of theoretical interest in their own right (Hoff et al., 2002; Hoffman, 2003). For that reason it is not possible to enumerate a range of findings involving specific theoretical constructs from a number of theoretical tests of the model as we did for the FSM. Instead, we organize this review of recent empirical findings considering in turn each of the exogenous constructs in the model involving income, education, and occupational status. Because the basic investment model proposed by economists is the core of the conceptual framework, we begin by considering studies focusing on family income.

In terms of *family income*, the emphasis in research on the investment model has been on the means by which parents and other caregivers foster the academic, economic, and social success of children. For this reason, cognitive and academic performance has been an especially important focus in this line of research. The family stress perspective, on the other hand, has tended to focus on social and emotional adjustment problems of children and adolescents, consistent with the greater mental health orientation of the approach. As we saw with research on the FSM, however, some work in this area also addresses competent development and it is also the case that the investment model has sometimes been used to predict behavioral and emotional problems.

A number of studies have confirmed the most basic propositions of the investment model; that is, that family income during childhood and adolescence is positively related to academic, financial, and occupational success during the adult years (Bradley & Corwyn, 2002; Corcoran & Adams, 1997; Mayer, 1997; Teachman, Paasch, Day, & Carver, 1997) and that family income affects the types of investments parents make in the lives of their children (Bradley & Corwyn, 2002; Mayer, 1997). The central aim of research on the model is to determine whether these investments explain the connections between income and developmental outcomes. With regard to the proposed association between income and investments, a seminal study by Bradley, Corwyn, McAdoo, and García Coll (2001) demonstrated the pervasiveness of this association.

Bradley and his colleagues used data from several waves of the National Longitudinal Survey of Youth to evaluate differences in parental investments and parental behavior, as measured by the Home Observation for Measurement of the Environment (HOME) scale (Bradley & Caldwell, 1980), for several thousand children ranging in age from infancy to early adolescence. For three major ethnic groups (European American, African American, and Hispanic American) the study indicated consistent differences on these dimensions between poor (families below the official poverty guidelines) and nonpoor families. For example, compared to poor families, parents in families with incomes above the official poverty guidelines were more likely to engage their children in conversation, learning activities, and discussions of events in their daily lives. Children in more financially secure families also had greater access to books, magazines, toys, and games that stimulate learning, cultural events and activities outside the home, and special lessons that encourage particular talents in music, sports, and so on.

Parents in the nonpoor families were also more likely to demonstrate affection and respect for their children and less likely to use physical punishment or restraint. Moreover, the physical environments in which more advantaged children lived tended to be safer, cleaner, roomier, and less dark and cluttered. This finding underscores the material disadvantage of poor children, which also extends to nutrition, medical care, clothing, and other basic necessities (e.g., Mayer, 1997). Finally, the poor children in the study were less likely to spend time with or even know their fathers, a reduction in the social capital available to them. Taken together, the results of this study of a large-scale, nationally representative, multiethnic sample of families demonstrate a clear link between family income and the investments that are made in the human capital of children. Especially important, these investments extend beyond tutoring and material goods to include parental affection and respect as well.

Other research has shown that family income and the investments in children it predicts appear to have a beneficial influence on long-term developmental success. For example, children from more economically advantaged compared to poorer families accrue more years of education; are less likely to experience adverse, life-altering events such as a teenage pregnancy; and are more likely to have an adequate income as an adult (Corcoran & Adams, 1997; Mayer, 1997). A significant limitation in most of this earlier research, however, is that the full mediating process proposed by the investment model has not been evaluated. Linver et al. (2002) provided perhaps the best evidence for the set of empirical relationships proposed by the model.

In their paper, Linver and her associates used information from several hundred families participating in the Infant Health and Development Program, a large-scale, multiethnic study of children from birth to 5 years of age at the time of their analysis. A particularly important feature of this study is that it examines economic influences at an early age, influences which likely set the stage for later child success or failure. Consistent with the investment model, the association between family income and child cognitive development at ages 3 and 5 years (standardized intelligence test scores, $b = .70$ without control variables and .52 with control variables) was significantly reduced ($b = .36$) when the investment mediator was introduced into the analyses. A test of indirect effects also supported the conclusion that the influence of family income on cognitive development was partially due to parental investments. The measure of parental investment was derived from the HOME, as in the Bradley et al. (2001) study just discussed, and included items related to parental behaviors expected to stimulate cognitive development such as language stimulation, teaching colors and numbers, providing books and other learning materials, and exposing the child to learning experiences outside the home. The investigators also found that the measure of parental investment completely mediated the association between income and child behavior problems at 3 and 5 years of age. Thus, the basic investment model in this study partially explained not only child competence but also child maladjustment.

A particularly important feature of the Linver et al. (2002) study is that the investigators controlled for the influence of parent education and intelligence in the analyses, as well as other social–demographic characteristics. These controls reduced the likelihood that the results could be attributed simply to the educational attainment and intelligence of the parent, which might indicate a direct genetic effect on the child's cognitive abilities. Thus, this report provides substantial support for the basic investment model. In a similar set of analyses using data from the Panel Study of Income Dynamics, Yeung et al. (2002) also controlled for parent personal and demographic characteristics in a test of the investment model. Even with these controls, they found evidence that family income had an influence on child outcomes at least in part through parental investments in the competent development of children. These findings provide suggestive evidence regarding the utility of the EIM using income as the exogenous variable. The connections between income and parental investment and between parental investment and child competence appear to be fairly well established (Bradley & Corwyn, 2002; Mayer, 1997). Required now are additional tests regarding the proposition that parental investments of various types actually account for the basic relationship between income and successful child development.

Returning to Figure 17.2, the EIM proposes that parent *education* will have a similar influence on parental investments as income, and that these investments, in turn, will have a similar relationship with competent development. It seems reasonable to predict an association between parental education and investments. Presumably a better educated parent will acquire more knowledge about child and adolescent development, will have a greater understanding of strategies for encouraging academic and social competence, and will generally be more skillful and effective in teaching children to negotiate the many environments to which they must adapt (Bornstein, Hahn, Suwalsky, & Haynes, 2003). Despite the reasonableness of this hypothesized mediating process, there are no specific empirical tests of this proposition cast in terms of the EIM. However, there is some evidence consistent with these ideas.

To begin with, several studies demonstrate that parental education predicts competent child development even when a number of other variables are controlled, such as family income and occupational status, parent's cognitive ability and emotional well-being, and family structure (Dearing et al., 2001; Duncan & Magnuson, 2003; Han, 2005; Kohen, Brooks-Gunn, Leventhal, & Hertzman, 2002). Moreover, recent research is consistent with a long history of empirical findings that relate parent education to socialization practices and priorities (Hoff et al., 2002). For example, Huston and Aronson (2005) investigated the influence of several demographic characteristics in a sample of 1,053 families from the NICHD Study of Early Child Care. They found that maternal education was positively correlated with maternal sensitivity toward the focal child at 36 months ($r = .50$) and also with parental investments involving a more enriched and positive home environment as assessed by the HOME ($r = .52$). These positive relationships still existed after controlling for a variety of other maternal, child, and family characteristics. Moreover, this study also replicated earlier findings regarding the association between education and competent child development including cognitive ability, social competence, and low rates of problem behavior. Similarly, Tamis-LeMonda, Shannon, Cabrera, and Lamb (2004) found that maternal and paternal education were positively associated with sensitivity, positive regard, and cognitive stimulation of a young child and also with the child's cognitive development.

In addition to this more general evidence for the plausibility of education as an important part of the investment process, two recent studies provide credible tests of a mediating pathway. These findings are consistent with predictions from the EIM even though neither investigation referred specifically to an investment model in describing their theoretical approaches. In an intensive study of 33 families in which both parents had a college education and 30 families in which neither parent had gone beyond the receipt of a high school diploma, Hoff (2003) examined the pathways through which these educational differences affected the vocabulary development of 2-year-old children. The findings showed that more highly educated parents create a richer, more complex language environment for their children. This environment includes a greater variety of words, more verbal interaction, and more frequent response by the mother to topics addressed by the child. These dimensions of speech are very consistent with phenomena addressed by the HOME in terms of identifying a more stimulating learning environment. Thus, they can be thought of as parental investments in the cognitive development of the child. Hoff also predicted and found that parental education was positively associated with the diversity of children's vocabulary in terms of the number of different types of words they emitted in interactions with their mothers. Especially important for the investment hypothesis, the richness of maternal speech completely mediated the association between parent education and child productive vocabulary. Thus, Hoff's findings are quite consistent with the education component of the EIM.

In the second study that investigated education, parental investments, and child developmental outcomes, Bradley and Corwyn (2003) used data from the National Longitudinal Survey of Youth to evaluate the impact of SES on development from early childhood through early adolescence. Among a number of analyses, the investigators examined the degree to which the learning stimulation provided by parents mediated the relationship between parent education and a child's cognitive and behavioral development. The HOME was used to evaluate the learning environment in terms of (1) interactions between parent and child that fostered learning, (2) the provision of material goods like books and magazines, and (3) support for lessons and tutoring in various skills. At each of three age levels, ranging from 3 to 6 to 10 to 15 years, Bradley and Corwyn found that education was positively related to a child's vocabulary, reading, and mathematical skills and negatively related to behavioral problems. Moreover, for each age level and each developmental outcome they discovered that the association between education and child development was reduced in magnitude once learning stimulation was added to the prediction equation. From these findings, they concluded that the parent's stimulation of learning mediated the relationship between education and child competence, a conclusion that is consistent with the EIM.

The final exogenous variable in the EIM involves parent or caregiver *occupational status*. The two most common measures of occupational standing are the Hollingshead Index (HI) and the Socioeconomic Index of Occupations (SEI; Bornstein et al., 2003). The HI uses a combination of occupation and education to create an occupational score as a marker of SES (Hollingshead, 1975), and the SEI uses the educational and income levels associated with a specific occupation to estimate an occupational prestige score (Duncan, 1961). Thus, the usual way to estimate an occupational effect is to create a composite score based on some combination of the exogenous variables in the EIM. Moreover, as noted earlier, Kohn's (1995) theory of occupational effects on socialization has been the primary framework for considering the influence of occupation on parenting practices. In much of his early research, Kohn (1959) used the HI as his measure of social class. The question for the moment concerns the degree to which findings related to occupational status fit the EIM as proposed in Figure 17.2.

In addition to presenting evidence that learning stimulation (as measured by the HOME) mediated the relationship between parents' educational attainment and child competence, Bradley and Corwyn (2003) also reported a similar mediating process for occupation, as assessed by the SEI. The investigators concluded that parenting behaviors related to an enriched learning environment for children ranging in age from 3 to 15 years and of mixed ethnic backgrounds helped to account for the relationship between occupational status and a child's cognitive and behavioral competence. These findings are consistent with the EIM. In another study, Gottfried, Gottfried, Bathurst, Guerin, and Parramore (2003) followed a cohort of 130 1-year-old children and their parents for almost two decades. They reported results separately for the constituent measures of education and occupation contained within the HI. Thus, they were able to look specifically at the relationship between occupational status, ranging from laborer to business executive or professional, socialization practices, and child developmental outcomes. Across the almost two decades of the study, they found that father's occupational status reliably predicted an enriched cultural, intellectual, and learning environment for children, as measured by the HOME and by the Family Environment Scale (correlations from .27 to .52). Mother's occupation also predicted these markers of parental investment, but not as frequently or at the same level as father's occupation.

The investigators also found that father's occupation predicted children's cognitive ability, academic achievement, and socioemotional well-being, but in most instances the mother's occupational status did not. The lack of mother influence may reflect the fact that these were generally traditional two-parent families in which fathers were most likely to be the primary breadwinners. Unfortunately, the authors did not directly examine the mediating role of parental investments in explaining the association between occupation and child outcomes; however, the pattern of reported correlations suggests that a mediating process is likely.

Although these two studies found significant evidence for occupational effects consistent with the EIM, neither of them controlled for education in the estimates of occupational influences. This is an important problem inasmuch as many investigators have concluded that education tends to be the more important predictor of both socialization practices and child development (Bornstein et al., 2003; Hoff et al., 2002; Hoffman, 2003).

In addition, there are many qualities of lower- and higher-status occupations that may play an important role in child development. For example, Kohn proposed that occupational differences primarily affect children through parental values. He hypothesized and found evidence to support the idea that the demands of parents' occupations should influence the degree to which they place a higher priority on obedience and conformity versus independence and self-direction, and these values should determine their parenting practices (Kohn, 1995).

There are many other differences between less and more prestigious occupations that might influence parents and children. For example, less prestigious occupations are (1) less stable, (2) less likely to have important benefits related to health care or paid vacations, (3) more likely to involve hourly rather than salaried compensation, and (4) more likely to involve difficult or even dangerous physical labor within a somewhat toxic working environment. In a recent article, Kalil and Ziol-Guest (2005) reported that parental work characteristics such as these had an adverse influence on the academic attainment of adolescents. These dimensions of work also need to be considered in future tests of the EIM.

Taken together, the studies reviewed in relation to the social causation perspective provide a great deal of suggestive evidence consistent with the idea that several markers of social class involving income, education, and occupation are significantly related to child and adolescent development. In addition, these dimensions of SES appear to have their effects on children primarily through specific mediating processes involving socialization practices. Thus, the empirical evidence reviewed here provides some support for both the FSM and the EIM and the social causation perspective in general. Despite these supportive findings, however, other researchers have proposed that these results are likely spurious, the result of social selection (e.g., Mayer, 1997). Moreover, many investigators have noted the difficulties in drawing firm causal inferences from the types of primarily nonexperimental studies that have addressed these issues (Bornstein et al., 2003; Bradley

& Corwyn, 2002; Duncan & Magnuson, 2003; Hoff et al., 2002). With these ideas in mind, the next section of this review considers evidence for social selection as an alternative explanation for the links among social class, socialization, and life-course development.

SOCIAL SELECTION, SOCIAL CLASS, AND SOCIALIZATION

The Social Selection Perspective

As noted earlier, the connections among social class, childrearing practices, and child development may be interpreted as a process of social selection rather than social causation. This view draws heavily from both economic arguments about how parents influence the lives of their children and from suggestions by behavioral geneticists (e.g., Becker, 1981; Lerner, 2003; Rowe & Rodgers, 1997). For example, Mayer (1997) notes that parents pass on a range of endowments to their children that not only include the kinds of economic investments discussed earlier but also genes, behavioral dispositions, values, and priorities in life. The basic argument is that certain parental characteristics help to account both for their economic success and for the adjustment of their children. Corcoran and Adams (1997) have called this the "non-economic parental resources" perspective. Indeed, based on the findings from her analyses of income differentials between families, Mayer (1997) notes that "parental income is not as important to children's outcomes as many social scientists have thought. This is because the parental characteristics that employers value and are willing to pay for, such as skills, diligence, honesty, good health, and reliability, also improve children's life chances, independent of their effect on parents' income. Children of parents with these attributes do well even when their parents do not have much income" (pp. 2–3).

Figure 17.3 provides an illustration of the central propositions of this noneconomic parental resources or social selection argument. The theoretical model hypothesizes that individual characteristics of parents based on genes, personality dispositions, and physical traits will predict their degree of achievement in terms of family income, occupational status, and educational attainment—the major indicators of social class or SES. Moreover, once these individual differences among caregivers are taken into account, the theory proposes that there will be no direct relationship between SES and either socialization strategies or child adjustment. Rather, any associations between social status and child development will be spurious, a result of their common dependence on the personal qualities of parents.

Although it is not essential to the argument, we propose that individual differences among parents that affect their SES should also influence the way they socialize their children. For example, parents who are skilled, diligent, honest, in good health, and reliable should be better informed and more responsible in raising their children than caregivers without these positive attributes. Consistent with the model in Figure 17.3, they should engage in more effective parenting practices and, as a result, their children should be better adjusted and more competent as they move from childhood to adulthood.

Empirical Findings Related to the Social Selection Perspective

Almost no research has directly addressed this counterproposal to the social causation argument; however, some interesting new findings are beginning to shed light on the issue.

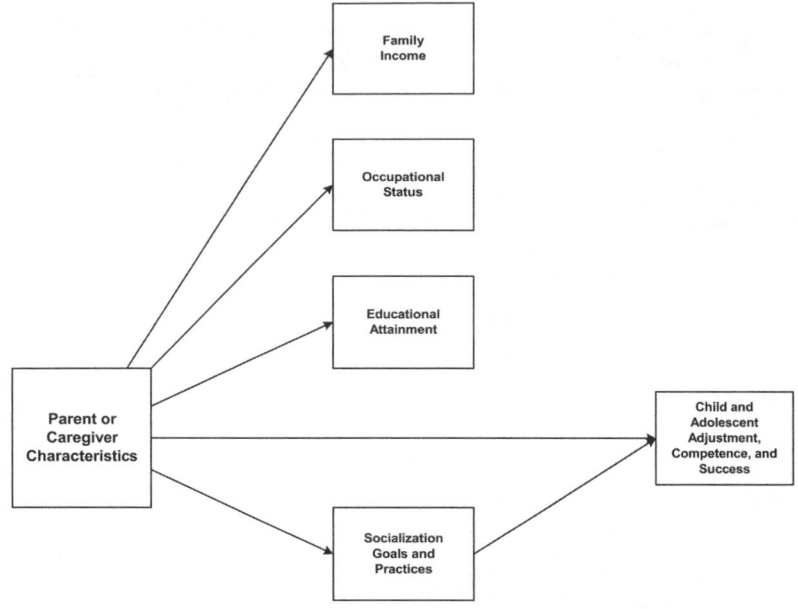

FIGURE 17.3. The noneconomic parental resources or social selection model.

For example, two recent investigations found evidence that characteristics of family members may affect SES. In a study of preschool children, Hyde, Else-Quest, Goldsmith, and Biesanz (2004) discovered that a young child with a difficult temperament exacerbates feelings of parental incompetence and depressed affect for mothers. These maternal characteristics, in turn, reduced the quality and rewardingness of the mother's work life. Over time, one might expect that these types of family processes could actually decrease the mother's success in work and the family's overall SES. With regard to the FSM, Conger and Conger (2002) showed that parents who were high in mastery actually reduced their economic pressure over time, suggesting that this parental trait likely led to extra efforts to deal with economic problems. Presumably, this orientation to dealing with financial difficulties should help to maintain or improve family SES.

Perhaps even more relevant to the question of selection effects is a series of studies showing that the traits and dispositions of children and adolescents predict to their SES as an adult. For instance, McLeod and Kaiser (2004) found that internalizing and externalizing problems occurring as early as 6 years of age predict lower adult educational attainment. In a separate study, Kokko and Pulkkinen (2000) showed that aggressive behavior at 8 years of age was related to long-term unemployment during the adult years. In their investigation, Feinstein and Bynner (2004) discovered that poor cognitive performance during early and middle childhood predicted lower educational attainment, lower income, and less work success during the adult years. Presumably these earlier behavioral, emotional, and cognitive problems reduced the competence of these children in social and academic pursuits, thus jeopardizing their eventual success as adults. Consistent with this hypothesis, Schoon et al. (2002) showed that low SES in a child's family of origin predicted lower academic achievement and continuing life stress across the years of childhood and adolescence. Lower academic competence and higher life stress, in turn, were associated with lower SES when the child became an adult. These results suggest a recip-rocal process in which low SES in the family of origin is associated with low SES in the next generation of adults as a result of diminished academic performance and greater life stress. These studies provide suggestive evidence regarding the plausibility of the selection argument.

Even more difficult to address is the argument that at least part of the presumed in-fluence of SES on child development is a function of shared genes. One recent study, how-ever, used a twin design to evaluate children's resilience to low SES and found that resil-ience was in part genetic and in part a function of environmental influences such as parental warmth and stimulating activities (Kim-Cohen, Moffitt, Caspi, & Taylor, 2004). Moreover, a study cited by Duncan and Magnuson (2003) found that children adopted between 4 and 6 years of age demonstrated greater IQ gains in higher compared to lower SES adoptive families (Duyme, Dumaret, & Tomkiewicz, 1999). This research is espe-cially important inasmuch as adopted children and their adoptive parents share no genes in common; thus, the association between SES and child cognitive development in this study cannot be explained as a genetic effect.

Preliminary evidence, then, suggests that genes may play a role in the connection be-tween SES and child development, but they do not seem to explain away the basic linkage between the two. From the present review it appears that an integrated perspective on SES, socialization, and child development that addresses issues of both social causation and social selection would provide the best fit with available empirical evidence.

AN INTEGRATED PERSPECTIVE ON SOCIAL CLASS AND SOCIALIZATION

Based on the earlier sections of this review, Figure 17.4 illustrates an integrated perspec-tive on social class, socialization, and child development. The model systematically inter-relates and extends predictions from the two social causation perspectives considered here, the EIM and FSM, and the social selection argument. All the dashed lines in Figure 17.4 represent predictions from the social selection perspective; the solid lines represent predictions from a social causation view.

To address the social selection approach, this general model begins with the charac-teristics of future parents during childhood and adolescence (Figure 17.4, Box 1). The se-lection framework proposes that these characteristics should predict adult experiences in the areas of socioeconomic circumstances (Box 2), the stresses and strains associated with low SES (Box 3), and abilities–investments as a parent (Box 4). The path from Box 1 to Box 5 also proposes a direct association between the earlier characteristics of the parent and developmental outcomes for children in the next (G2) generation. This direct path-way could occur biologically (e.g., through genes or intrauterine environment) or could reflect continuities in G1 characteristics that are observed and emulated by the G2 child. According to the selection argument, earlier G1 cognitive abilities, social competence, persistence, planfulness, and ambition will be positively related to later SES, negatively related to economic pressure and its associated social and emotional problems, positively related to adequate parenting and parental investments, and positively related to compe-tent child (G2) development.

The social causation aspects of the integrated model propose that the exogenous SES variables, primarily from the EIM (Box 2), should predict the various dimensions of the

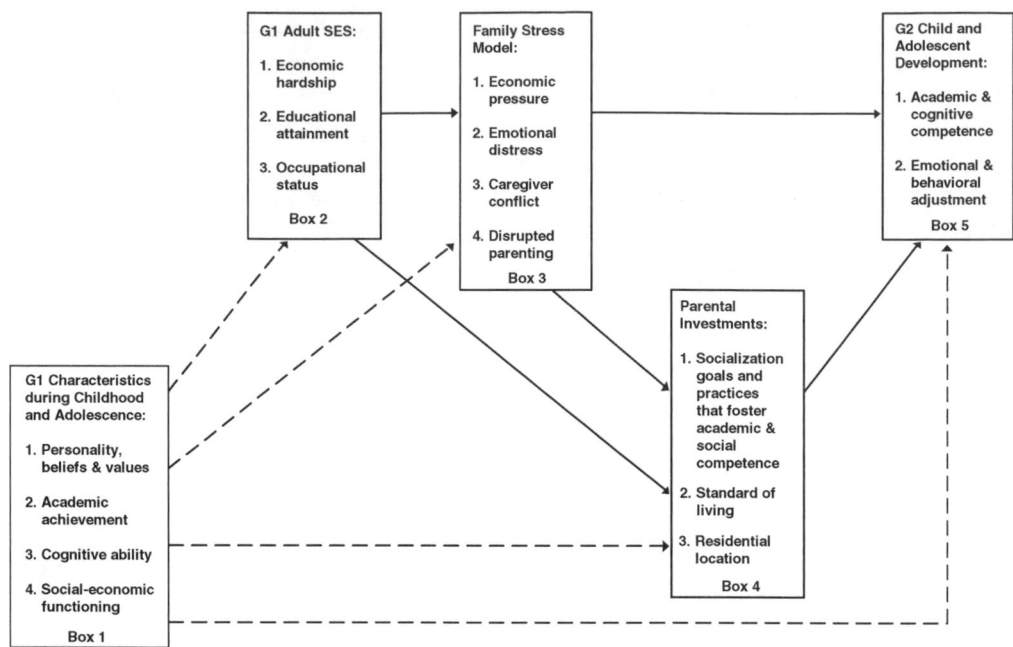

FIGURE 17.4. The integrated perspective on social class, socialization, and child development. Solid arrows represent predictions consistent with the social causation perspective. Dashed arrows represent predictions consistent with the social selection perspective or genetic effects.

FSM (Box 3). Consistent with the results of this review, the integrated model of hypothesized SES influences proposes a broad evaluation of economic circumstances, educational accomplishments, and occupational status (also see Duncan & Magnuson, 2003). Notice that economic hardship is included in Box 2, inasmuch as the hardship variable includes a much broader range of economic conditions than income alone (e.g., debts and assets), an important element in the predictive ability of the studies related to the FSM. Thus, the integrated model includes elements of two major approaches to understanding SES effects on socialization and child development: the FSM and the EIM. Especially important, the integrated perspective proposes that the indicators of both SES (Box 2) and family stress processes (Box 3) will affect parental investments (Box 4) and, in turn, the development of children (Box 5). This model also proposes that SES will have an indirect influence on investments and child development through family stress processes, an important issue to be addressed in future research. That is, the integrated model specifically merges two of the primary approaches to understanding the social influence of SES on parents and children, a step that has not been taken in previous theory or research.

The most important aspect of the integrated model, however, is that it incorporates the competing hypotheses from both the social selection and social causation perspectives. The social selection aspects of the model suggest that the personal characteristics of the eventual G1 parents will account for their adult SES, stresses and strains proposed to be associated with low SES, effective parenting behaviors, and, directly or indirectly through parental investments, the competent development of the second generation child. If all these hypotheses were supported, they would run contrary to the social causation argument that SES, family stress processes, and parental investments represent a causal network that operates independent of, or in conjunction with, earlier G1 characteristics. On the other hand, if the social causation pathways in the model are supported net of the social selection predictions, such findings would provide strong support for a social causation perspective.

It must be noted that tests of the integrated model require very special types of studies conducted over long periods of time. Data must be collected during childhood or adolescence on future parents and this G1 generation must be followed far enough into adulthood to evaluate the competing theoretical processes proposed in Figure 17.4. Fortunately, an increasing number of such studies are now available that can be used for the types of analyses required to test the integrated perspective (e.g., Capaldi, Conger, Hops, & Thornberry, 2003). Although the demands and costs of such research are quite high, without such long-term investigations it will be impossible to disentangle the degree to which the relationships among SES, socialization practices, and child development represent processes of social selection, social causation, or a combination of the two. The present review of the most recent research and theory suggests that both social selection and social causation will likely play a role in a reciprocal process that reaches across generations.

CONCLUDING COMMENTS AND FUTURE DIRECTIONS

This chapter began with a discussion of SES differences in socialization practices and developmental outcomes for children. This discussion was placed within the context of a larger concern for health disparities in general. Consistent with the health disparities argument, research findings show that lower SES children are at risk not only for higher than average rates of physical illness and reduced life expectancies but also for truncated life opportunities and behavioral or emotional problems. Various theoretical perspectives were reviewed that propose to account for these SES differences, and empirical findings were frequently consistent with predictions from these theories, including perspectives that link SES to children's lives through socialization practices. The final conclusion from this review, however, is that additional research will be required to more adequately evaluate these and other approaches to understanding the relationships among SES, socialization, and child development. We proposed an integrated model as a heuristic guide for future research. The following brief comments explore future research needs in a bit more detail.

First, we believe it will be especially important for investigators who now have long-term data on children or adolescents grown to adulthood to begin to evaluate aspects of the integrated perspective illustrated in Figure 17.4. Although most studies will not have all the variables required to test the full model, many ongoing studies can test many of the connections of interest. This type of prospective, longitudinal research will begin to shed new light on the various predictions from theoretical models based on either a social causation or a social selection perspective. It will also be important to evaluate both the integrated and other more limited conceptual models across different ethnic and national groups and types of families. For example, the Parke et al. (2004) study showed that certain aspects of the FSM might operate differently for Mexican American compared to European American families. And the findings from Mistry et al. (2002) and Yeung et al.

(2002) indicated that emotional distress relates directly to disrupted parenting for single-parent families, while other research showed that emotional distress usually relates indirectly to disrupted parenting through caregiver conflict when two caregivers are raising a child. Also worth noting is the inclusion in the model of neighborhood or community effects under the rubric of parental investments. We have addressed this issue only tangentially in this chapter, but it remains an important issue for future investigations.

Another important direction for future research concerns experiments and quasi-experiments related to the theoretical frameworks we have discussed. As noted earlier, some income supplementation or residential relocation programs have shown promising effects in terms of family processes and child outcomes (Leventhal & Brooks-Gunn, 2003). These effects appear to be relatively limited, however, and we suspect for good reasons. Income supplementation as provided by governmental programs is unlikely to fundamentally alter a family's socioeconomic standing. For the most part, planned interventions are unable to provide sufficient material resources to create real change for families. On the other hand, naturally occurring experiments in which family incomes rise substantially as a result of new economic opportunities in a geographic area can trace the effects of truly significant changes in income. Costello et al. (2003) demonstrated the robustness of such effects and their research serves as a model for future inquiries of this type. Also important, however, will be interventions that address other aspects of the models discussed in this chapter, such as mental health services relevant to family stress processes or supplemental learning programs consistent with the EIM. These types of experimental tests through randomized preventive interventions are important for increasing confidence in the causal significance of predictions from the various theoretical frameworks reviewed here.

The primary message of this chapter is that SES-related health disparities are quite real for both adults and children (Berkman & Kawachi, 2000; Repetti, Taylor, & Seeman, 2002). The evidence reviewed here suggests that the mechanisms accounting for the associations among SES, socialization, and child and adolescent development may be complex and even bidirectional. What is fundamentally important, however, is the need to improve understanding of these processes so that appropriate steps can be taken to help improve the lives of families, parents, and children.

ACKNOWLEDGMENTS

Grants from the National Institute of Child Health and Human Development (HD047573, HD051746), the National Institute of Mental Health (MH51361), and the National Institute on Drug Abuse (DA017902, HD047573) supported work on this chapter.

REFERENCES

Ackerman, B. P., Brown, E. D., & Izard, C. E. (2004). The relations between persistent poverty and contextual risk and children's behavior in elementary school. *Developmental Psychology, 40*, 367–377.

Angell, R. C. (1936). The *family encounters the depression*. New York: Charles Scribner's Sons.

Becker, G. S. (1981). *A treatise on the family*. Cambridge, MA: Harvard University Press.

Becker, G. S., & Thomes, N. (1986). Human capital and the rise and fall of families. *Journal of Labor Economics, 4*, S1–S139.

Berkman, L. F., & Kawachi, I. (Eds.). (2000). *Social epidemiology*. New York: Oxford University Press.

Borge, A. I. H., Rutter, M., Cote, S., & Tremblay, R. E. (2004). Early childcare and physical aggression: Differentiating social selection and social causation. *Journal of Child Psychology and Psychiatry, 45*, 367–376.

Bornstein, M. H., & Bradley, R. H. (Eds.). (2003). *Socioeconomic status, parenting, and child development*. Mahwah, NJ: Erlbaum.

Bornstein, M. H., Hahn, C.-S., Suwalsky, J. T. D, & Haynes, O. M. (2003). Socioeconomic status, parenting, and child development: The Hollingshead Four-Factor Index of Social Status and The Socioeconomic Index of Occupations. In M. H. Bornstein & R. H. Bradley (Eds.), *Socioeconomic status, parenting, and child development* (pp. 29–82). Mahwah, NJ: Erlbaum.

Bradley, R. H., & Caldwell, B. M. (1980). The relation of the home environment, cognitive competence, and IQ among males and females. *Child Development, 51*, 1140–1148.

Bradley, R. H., & Corwyn, R. F. (2002). Socioeconomic status and child development. *Annual Review of Psychology, 53*, 371–399.

Bradley, R. H., & Corwyn, R. F. (2003). Age and ethnic variations in family process mediators of SES. In M. H. Bornstein & R. H. Bradley (Eds.), *Socioeconomic status, parenting, and child development* (pp. 161–188). Mahwah, NJ: Erlbaum.

Bradley, R. H., Corwyn, R. F., McAdoo, H. P., & García Coll, C. (2001). The home environments of children in the United States: Part I. Variations by age, ethnicity, and poverty status. *Child Development, 72*, 1844–1867.

Brody, G. H., Murry, V., Kim, S., & Brown, A. C. (2002). Longitudinal pathways to competence and psychological adjustment among African American children living in rural single-parent households. *Child Development, 73*, 1505–1516.

Capaldi, D. M., Conger, R. D., Hops, H., & Thornberry, T. P. (2003). Introduction to special section on three-generation studies. *Journal of Abnormal Child Psychology, 31*, 123–125.

Cavan, R. S., & Ranck, K. H. (1938). *The family and the depression: A study of one hundred Chicago families*. Chicago: University of Chicago Press.

Coleman, J. S. (1990). *The foundations of social theory*. Cambridge, MA: Belknap.

Conger, R. D. (1995). Unemployment. In D. Levinson (Ed.), *Encyclopedia of marriage and the family* (pp. 731–735). New York: Macmillan.

Conger, R. D., & Conger, K. J. (2002). Resilience in midwestern families: Selected findings from the first decade of a prospective, longitudinal study. *Journal of Marriage and Family, 64*, 361–373.

Conger, R. D., Conger, K. J., Elder, G. H., Jr., Lorenz, F. O., Simons, R. L., & Whitbeck, L. B. (1992). A family process model of economic hardship and adjustment of early adolescent boys. *Child Development, 63*, 526–541.

Conger, R. D., Conger, K. J., Elder, G. H., Jr., Lorenz, F. O., Simons, R. L., & Whitbeck, L. B. (1993). Family economic stress and adjustment of early adolescent girls. *Developmental Psychology, 29*, 206–219.

Conger, R. D., Conger, K. J., Matthews, L. S., & Elder, G. H., Jr. (1999). Pathways of economic influence on adolescent adjustment. *American Journal of Community Psychology, 27*, 519–540.

Conger, R. D., & Elder, G. H., Jr. (Eds.). (1994). *Families in troubled times: Adapting to change in rural America*. Hawthorne, NY: Aldine de Gruyter.

Conger, R. D., Ge, X., Elder, G. H., Jr., Lorenz, F. O., & Simons, R. L. (1994). Economic stress, coercive family process, and developmental problems of adolescents. *Child Development, 65*, 541–561.

Conger, R. D., Rueter, M. A., & Elder, G. H., Jr. (1999). Couple resilience to economic pressure. *Journal of Personality and Social Psychology, 76*, 54–71.

Conger, R. D., Wallace, L. E., Sun, Y., Simons, R. L., McLoyd, V. C., & Brody, G. (2002). Economic pressure in African American families: A replication and extension of the family stress model. *Developmental Psychology, 38*, 179–193.

Corcoran, M., & Adams, T. (1997). Race, sex, and the intergenerational transmission of poverty. In G. J. Duncan & J. Brooks-Gunn (Eds.), *Consequences of growing up poor* (pp. 461–517). New York: Russell Sage.

Costello, E. J., Compton, S. N., Keeler, G., & Angold, A. (2003). Relationships between poverty and psychopathology: A natural experiment. *Journal of the American Medical Association, 290*, 2023–2029.

Davis, A., & Havighurst, R. J. (1946). Social class and color differences in child-rearing. *American Sociological Review, 11*, 698–710.

Dearing, E., McCartney, K., & Taylor, B. A. (2001). Change in family income-to-needs matters more for children with less. *Child Development, 72,* 1779–1793.

Dodge, K. A., Pettit, G. S., & Bates, J. E. (1994). Socialization mediators of the relation between socioeconomic status and child conduct problems. *Child Development, 65,* 649–665.

Duncan, G. J., & Brooks-Gunn, J. (1997). Income effects across the life span: Integration and interpretation. In G. J. Duncan & J. Brooks-Gunn (Eds.), *Consequences of growing up poor* (pp. 596–610). New York: Russell Sage.

Duncan, G. J., & Magnuson, K. A. (2003). Off with Hollingshead: Socioeconomic resources, parenting, and child development. In M. H. Bornstein & R. H. Bradley (Eds.), *Socioeconomic status, parenting, and child development* (pp. 83–106). Mahwah, NJ: Erlbaum.

Duncan, O. D. (1961). A socioeconomic index for all occupations. In A. L. Reiss, Jr., O. D., Duncan, P. K. Hatt, & C. C. North (Eds.), *Occupations and social status.* New York: Free Press.

Duyme, M., Dumaret, A.-C., & Tomkiewicz, T. C. (1999). How can we boost IQs of "dull children"?: A late adoption study. *Proceedings of the National Academy of Sciences, 96,* 8790–8794.

Elder, G. H., Jr. (1974). *Children of the Great Depression: Social change in life experience.* Chicago: University of Chicago Press.

Elder, G. H., Jr., & Caspi, A. (1988). Economic stress in lives: Developmental perspectives. *Journal of Social Issues, 44,* 25–45.

Ensminger, M. E., & Fothergill, K. (2003). A decade of measuring SES: What it tells us and where to go from here. In M. H. Bornstein & R. H. Bradley (Eds.), *Socioeconomic status, parenting, and child development* (pp. 13–27). Mahwah, NJ: Erlbaum.

Evans, G. W., & English, K. (2002). The environment of poverty: Multiple stressor exposure, psychophysiological stress, and socioemotional adjustment. *Child Development, 73,* 1238–1248.

Feinstein, L., & Bynner, J. (2004). The importance of cognitive development in middle childhood for adulthood socioeconomic status, mental health, and problem behavior. *Child Development, 75,* 1329–1339.

Gennetian, L. A., & Miller, C. (2002). Children and welfare reform: A view from an experimental welfare program in Minnesota. *Child Development, 73,* 601–620.

Gottfried, A. W., Gottfried, A. E., Bathurst, K., Guerin, D. W., & Parramore, M. M. (2003). Socioeconomic status in children's development and family environment: Infancy through adolescence. In M. H. Bornstein & R. H. Bradley (Eds.), *Socioeconomic status, parenting, and child development* (pp. 189–207). Mahwah, NJ: Erlbaum.

Han, W.-J. (2005). Maternal nonstandard work schedules and child cognitive outcomes. *Child Development, 76,* 137–154.

Haveman, R. H., & Wolfe, B. S. (1994). *Succeeding generations: On the effects of investments in children.* New York: Sage.

Hoff, E. (2003). The specificity of environmental influence: Socioeconomic status affects early vocabulary development via maternal speech. *Child Development, 74,* 1368–1378.

Hoff, E., Laursen, B., & Tardif, T. (2002). Socioeconomic status and parenting. In M. H. Bornstein (Ed.), *Handbook of parenting: Vol 2. Biology and ecology of parenting* (2nd ed., pp. 231–252). Mahwah, NJ: Erlbaum.

Hoffman, L. W. (2003). Methodological issues in the studies of SES, parenting, and child development. In M. H. Bornstein & R. H. Bradley (Eds.), *Socioeconomic status, parenting, and child development* (pp. 125–143). Mahwah, NJ: Erlbaum.

Hollingshead, A. B. (1975). *Four-factor index of social status.* Unpublished manuscript, Yale University, New Haven, CT.

Hughes, C., Jaffee, S. R., Happé, F., Taylor, A., Caspi, A., & Moffitt, T. E. (2005). Origins of individual differences in theory of mind: From nature to nurture? *Child Development, 76,* 356–370.

Huston, A. C., & Aronson, S. R. (2005). Mothers' time with infant and time in employment as predictors of mother–child relationships and children's early development. *Child Development, 76,* 467–482.

Hyde, J. S., Else-Quest, N. M., Goldsmith, H. H., & Biesanz, J. C. (2004). Children's temperament and behavior problems predict their employed mothers' work functioning. *Child Development, 75,* 580–594.

Kalil, A., & Ziol-Guest, K. M. (2005). Single mothers' employment dynamics and adolescent well-being. *Child Development, 76,* 196–211.

Keating, D. P., & Hertzman, C. (Eds.). (1999). *Developmental health and the wealth of nations.* New York: Guilford Press.

Kim-Cohen, J., Moffitt, T. E., Caspi, A., & Taylor, A. (2004). Genetic and environmental processes in young children's resilience and vulnerability to socioeconomic deprivation. *Child Development, 75,* 651–668.

Kohen, D. E., Brooks-Gunn, J., Leventhal, T., & Hertzman, C. (2002). Neighborhood income and physical and social disorder in Canada: Associations with young children's competencies. *Child Development, 73,* 1844–1860.

Kohn, M. L. (1959). Social class and parental values. *American Journal of Sociology, 64,* 337–351.

Kohn, M. L. (1963). Social class and parent–child relationships: An interpretation. *American Journal of Sociology, 68,* 471–480.

Kohn, M. L. (1969). *Class and conformity: A study in values.* Oxford, UK: Dorsey.

Kohn, M. L. (1995). Social structure and personality through time and space. In P. Moen, G. H. Elder, Jr., & K. Lüscher (Eds.), *Examining lives in context: Perspectives on the ecology of human development* (pp. 141–168). Washington, DC: American Psychological Association Press.

Kokko, K., & Pulkkinen, L. (2000). Aggression in childhood and long-term unemployment in adulthood: A cycle of maladaptation and some protective factors. *Developmental Psychology, 36,* 463–472.

Komarovsky, M. (1940). *The unemployed man and his family: The effect of unemployment upon the status of the man in fifty-nine families.* New York: Dryden Press.

Lerner, R. M. (2003). What are SES effects effects of? A developmental systems perspective. In M. H. Bornstein & R. H. Bradley (Eds.), *Socioeconomic status, parenting, and child development* (pp. 231–255). Mahwah, NJ: Erlbaum.

Leventhal, T., & Brooks-Gunn, J. (2003). Moving on up: Neighborhood effects on children and families. In M. H. Bornstein & R. H. Bradley (Eds.), *Socioeconomic status, parenting, and child development* (pp. 209–230). Mahwah, NJ: Erlbaum.

Linver, M. R., Brooks-Gunn, J., & Kohen, D. (2002). Family processes as pathways from income to young children's development. *Developmental Psychology, 38,* 719–734.

Liu, W. M., Ali, S. R., Soleck, G., Hopps, J., Dunston, K., & Pickett, T., Jr. (2004). Using social class in counseling psychology research. *Journal of Counseling Psychology, 51,* 3–18.

Magnuson, K. A., & Duncan, G. J. (2002). Parents in poverty. In M. H. Bornstein (Ed.), *Handbook of parenting: Vol 4. Social conditions and applied parenting* (2nd ed., pp. 95–121). Mahwah, NJ: Erlbaum.

Mayer, S. (1997). *What money can't buy: Family income and children's life chances.* Cambridge, MA: Harvard University Press.

McLeod, J. D., & Kaiser, K. (2004). Childhood emotional and behavioral problems and educational attainment. *American Sociological Review, 69,* 636–658.

McLeod, J. D., & Shanahan, M. J. (1996). Trajectories of poverty and children's mental health. *Journal of Health and Social Behavior, 37,* 207–220.

McLoyd, V. C. (1998). Socioeconomic disadvantage and child development. *American Psychologist, 53,* 185–204.

Mezzacappa, E. (2004). Alerting, orienting, and executive attention: Developmental properties and sociodemographic correlates in an epidemiological sample of young, urban children. *Child Development, 75,* 1373–1386.

Mistry, R. S., Biesanz, J. C., Taylor, L. C., Burchinal, M., & Cox, M. J. (2004). Family income and its relation to preschool children's adjustment for families in the NICHD Study of Early Child Care. *Developmental Psychology, 40,* 727–745.

Mistry, R. S., Vandewater, E. A., Huston, A. C., & McLoyd, V. C. (2002). Economic well-being and children's social adjustment: The role of family process in an ethnically diverse low-income sample. *Child Development, 73,* 935 951.

Oakes, J. M., & Rossi, P. H. (2003). The measurement of SES in health research: Current practice and steps toward a new approach. *Social Science and Medicine, 56,* 769–784.

Parcel, T. L., & Menaghan, E. G. (1994). *Parents' jobs and children's lives.* Hawthorne, NY: Aldine de Gruyter.

Parke, R. D. (2004). Development in the family. *Annual Review of Psychology, 55,* 365–399.

Parke, R. D., Coltrane, S., Duffy, S., Buriel, R., Dennis, J., Powers, J., et al. (2004). Economic stress, parenting, and child adjustment in Mexican American and European American families. *Child Development, 75,* 1632–1656.

Prior, M. Sanson, A., Smart, D., & Oberklaid, F. (1999). Psychological disorders and their correlates in an

Australian community sample of preadolescent children. *Journal of Child Psychology and Psychiatry*, *40*, 563–580.

Repetti, R. L., Taylor, S. E., & Seeman, T. E. (2002). Risky families: Family social environments and the mental and physical health of offspring. *Psychological Bulletin*, *128*, 330–366.

Robila, M., & Krishnakumar, A. (2005). Effects of economic pressure on marital conflict in Romania. *Journal of Family Psychology*, *19*, 246–251.

Rowe, D. C., & Rodgers, J. L. (1997). Poverty and behavior: Are environmental measures nature and nurture? *Developmental Review*, *17*, 358–375.

Schoon, I., Bynner, J., Joshi, H., Parsons, S., Wiggins, R. D., & Sacker, A. (2002). The influence of context, timing, and duration of risk experiences for the passage from childhood to midadulthood. *Child Development*, *73*, 1486–1504.

Sears, R. R., Maccoby, E. E., & Levin, H. (1957). *Patterns of child rearing*. Oxford, UK: Peterson.

Sobolewski, J. M., & Amato, P. R. (2005). Economic hardship in the family of origin and children's psychological well-being in adulthood. *Journal of Marriage and Family*, *67*, 141–156.

Solantaus, T., Leinonen, J., & Punamäki, R. L. (2004). Children's mental health in times of economic recession: Replication and extension of the family economic stress model in Finland. *Developmental Psychology*, *40*, 412–429.

Tamis-LeMonda, C. S., Shannon, J. D., Cabrera, N. J., & Lamb, M. E. (2004). Fathers and mothers at play with their 2- and 3-year-olds: Contributions to language and cognitive development. *Child Development*, *75*, 1806–1820.

Teachman, J. D., Paasch, K. M., Day, R. D., & Carver, K. P. (1997). Poverty during adolescence and subsequent educational attainment. In G. J. Duncan & J. Brooks-Gunn (Eds.), *Consequences of growing up poor* (pp. 382–418). New York: Russell Sage.

Yeung, W. J., Linver, M. R., & Brooks-Gunn, J. (2002). How money matters for young children's development: Parental investment and family processes. *Child Development*, *73*, 1861–1879.

Zevalkink, J., & Riksen-Walraven, J. M. (2001). Parenting in Indonesia: Inter- and intracultural differences in mothers' interactions with their young children. *International Journal of Behavioral Development*, *25*, 167–175.

CHAPTER 18

Do Roots and Wings Complement or Oppose One Another?

The Socialization of Relatedness and Autonomy in Cultural Context

Fred Rothbaum and Gisela Trommsdorff

For centuries in Western civilization, politicians, economists, psychologists and laypeople alike have assumed that the desirability of individual choice was inherent in humankind. From Mill to Locke, from Rousseau to Jefferson, choice has been hailed as an inalienable human right–an essential human need. . . . Might our theories of motivation require modification among people whose fundamental values are fate, duty, and the pursuit of interdependence [versus life, liberty and the pursuit of happiness].
—Iyengar and Lepper (1999, p. 364)

This chapter examines cultural similarities and differences in the development of autonomy and relatedness. We are interested in whether *autonomy and relatedness are positively or negatively correlated, and whether they have similar or different socialization antecedents.*

Conflicting findings regarding the association between autonomy and relatedness reflect, in part, profound cultural differences in the valuing of autonomy. Western theories highly value autonomy, as suggested in the opening quote, and Western research points to a close association between autonomy and relatedness. Cultural studies, which indicate that autonomy is less valued in non-Western cultures, point to an inverse association between autonomy and relatedness across cultures. It is not unusual for within-culture findings to be opposite than between-culture findings,[1] but it is important to understand the difference (Kagitcibasi, 1997; Smith & Schwartz, 1997). At the end of our review we suggest a synthesis of Western and cross-cultural findings.

Borrowing from Grusec (2002) we define *socialization* as "the way in which individuals are assisted in the acquisition of skills necessary to function in their social group" (p. 143). *Autonomy* refers to a constellation of phenomena, centering on personal choice, self agency, and psychological independence (e.g., in decision making), and it is closely associated with both intrinsic motivation and an emphasis on individual rights (Bridges, 2003; Ryan & Deci, 2000; Smetana, 2002; Smith & Schwartz, 1997). We do not define autonomy in terms of separation because doing so would ensure a negative association between autonomy and relatedness. *Relatedness* is also defined broadly. It encompasses love, attachment, intimacy, caring, support, loyalty, mutual obligations, and belongingness.

Our distinction between Western and non-Western cultures is, at best, imprecise. By "Western" we are referring primarily to English-speaking (United States, Canada, Australia, and New Zealand) and Western- and Northern-European communities. The authors of the major theories of development, the participants in most empirical studies, and the audience for these theories and studies overwhelming reside in these communities. "Non-Western" refers to the rest of the world—the overwhelming majority of the world's cultures and the vast majority of the world's population, including but not limited to Asian, African, Middle Eastern, Southern and Eastern European, and Hispanic/Latino communities. We do not believe that there is homogeneity within either of these groups (particularly the latter), nor within individual countries, but our point is that prevailing theories and evidence apply much better to the former group.

While we focus on generalizations regarding cultural differences, we are mindful of the complexity of each culture—in terms of practices, contexts, development, and the meaning of relatedness and autonomy. The Amish practice of *rumspringa* (runningaround) provides an excellent example of this complexity. At age 16, children in this collectivistic, close-knit, and sheltered community are free to sample the outside world and all its vices. This poignant experience of Amish autonomy occurs within a larger context of obligations, expectations, and constraints of personal choice; it occurs in particular settings (with peers in situations outside the home) and involves a particular life choice (deciding whether to dedicate the rest of one's life to Jesus). Similarly, Miller (2003) notes how notions of choice and agency are infused with notions of duty in many collectivistic cultures. The experience of autonomy and relatedness in each culture reviewed in this chapter is colored by a unique pattern of practices, contexts, and beliefs.

The chapter is divided into five sections. First, we provide an overview of the theories from which we borrow most heavily. Second, we review Western theories and research that highlight the close association between relatedness and autonomy on an "individual level" (i.e., individuals high in relatedness are high in autonomy). Third, we review research from different cultures that point to an inverse association between relatedness and autonomy on a "cultural level" (i.e., Western cultures are higher in autonomy and lower in relatedness than non-Western cultures). Fourth, we review research on socialization practices in different cultures that help explain this inverse association. Fifth, we distinguish between two notions of relatedness—general trust (a faith in new relationships) and assurance (a guarantee that relationships are stable). This distinction helps resolve conflicting individual-level and cultural-level findings. To foreshadow our conclusion, general trust, prevalent in the West, complements autonomy, whereas assurance, prevalent in many other cultures, conflicts with autonomy.

THEORETICAL STARTING POINTS

This chapter is based on (1) socioecological theories, which provide richly textured descriptions of the myriad levels of culture and of child development; and (2) theories concerned with individualism–collectivism and related constructs, which identify fundamental distinctions between cultural groups and provide robust evidence pertaining to these distinctions.

Socioecological Theories

We borrow heavily from socioecological theories of culture, particularly as they have been elaborated by Bruner (1996), LeVine et al. (1994), Rogoff (2003), Harkness and Super (1995), Valsiner (2001), and, before them, Whiting and Whiting (1975). Of particular interest are these investigators' emphases on the meaning of behavior, developmental processes, children's role in their socialization, and the nested settings in which behavior is embedded. The settings include tangible artifacts, such as infant slings or playpens, local arrangements such as extended family courtyards or nuclear family dwellings, and economic, political and religious institutions. Socioecological theory is concerned with continuity as well as change.

   In contrast to Western theories of socialization and cultural transmission theories, both of which have historically emphasized parents' direct role in the socialization process, socioecological theorists maintain that the influences of parents, siblings, other kin, ingroup members, the immediate context and larger values and meanings, as well as children's own influence, are difficult to disentangle from one another. Parents do not exert their influence in a vacuum but, rather, in the context of other socialization influences (Bronfenbrenner, 1986; Lerner, 1991).

Individualism–Collectivism and Related Dimensions

We rely heavily on theory and research on individualism–collectivism and related dimensions such as independence–interdependence. In individualistic societies ties between individuals are usually loose; people are expected to look after themselves and their immediate families only. In collectivistic societies people are usually integrated into cohesive ingroups which, throughout people's lives, protect them in exchange for unquestioning loyalty (Triandis, 1995). An independent self is one which is more separate, decontextualized, autonomous, unique, self-expressive, and self-maximizing. An interdependent self is more connected to others, contextualized, dependent, conformist, self-controlled, and group maximizing.

   These dimensions have generated a great deal of evidence pertaining to the constructs of relatedness (which underlies collectivism and the interdependent self) and autonomy (which underlies individualism and the independent self). The convergence in findings involving these dimensions is remarkable given that the investigators championing them (e.g., Hofstede, 1980; Kitayama & Markus, 2000; Smith & Schwartz, 1997; Triandis, 1995) differ in their theoretical backgrounds, methods employed, and cultures studied.

   Despite criticisms that these dimensions treat cultures as internally consistent and externally distinctive (Kagitcibasi, 1997, Smetana, 2002), the investigators cited previously do *not* ignore the complexity of cultures. Like them, we view the overarching dimensions as encompassing loosely connected elements rather than as coherent unitary constructs (cf. Smith & Schwartz, 1997), and we do not view the dimensions as bipolar (Tafarodi, Lang, & Smith, 1999).

All societies have elements of individualism and collectivism.[2] Within culture, individualism and collectivism are more or less emphasized by different individuals/subgroups (Kagitcibasi; 1997; Killen & Wainryb, 2000; Triandis, 1995), with respect to different behaviors (Oyserman, Coon, & Kemmelmeier, 2002), at different time periods (Kwak, 2003), and in different contexts—for example, "emotional interdependence" (collectivistic values) in the family context can coexist with "economic independence" (individualistic values) in the work context among people living in affluent non-Western urban areas (Kagitsibasi, 2002). While the United States is a highly individualistic society, there are important settings such as fraternities, the military, regimented sports teams, and other tightly knit groups where collectivism reigns (Bugental & Goodnow, 1998). Despite these qualifications, individualism–collectivism has repeatedly proven able to predict important cultural differences, including differences in autonomy and relatedness.

WESTERN THEORIES AND WESTERN RESEARCH

The notion that relatedness and autonomy spring from the same source—quality caregiving—is deeply ingrained in Western folklore and Western theory. It is evident in the conventional wisdom that child-care providers must give their children both "roots and wings." The underlying belief is that quality caregiving, typically defined as sensitivity and responsiveness, leads to both roots and wings, and that roots and wings support one another.

Here we review four widely cited theories about childhood socialization: (1) Erikson's ego analytic theory; (2) Bowlby and Ainsworth's attachment theory; (3) Baumrind's theory of parenting styles; and (4) Ryan and Deci's self determination theory. These theories have dominated developmental psychology for the past 50 years. They represent very different traditions—the psychoanalytic, ethological, developmental, and social psychological—and they have amassed a substantial body of research to support their hypotheses. While Erikson relies primarily on case studies, he is included because his ideas are often echoed by the others. All these investigators claim their theories have universal applicability. However, the cultural evidence supporting that claim is thin. The vast majority of studies testing these theories are conducted by Western investigators using Western methods and samples (Gardiner, Mutter, & Kosmitzki, 1998; Harkness & Super, 1995). Below is a brief review of their theory and evidence.

Erikson's Ego Psychology

Erik Erikson (1950/1963) posits the existence of eight major developmental stages, with a defining task at each stage. The task of infancy is to establish "trust" with the primary caregiver. Trust, defined as the child's "basic faith in himself and in his world" (Erikson, 1950/1963, p. 80), is manifested by the child's "willingness to let the mother out of sight . . . because she has become an inner certainty" (Erikson, 1950/1963, p. 247). This inner certainty, which foreshadows attachment theorists' notion of a secure internal working model, alleviates the child's anxiety about venturing away from the mother and gaining autonomy—the defining task of the second stage and a key ingredient of subsequent stages. Autonomy, in turn, gives rise to mature relationships.

According to Erikson, the caregiving antecedents of trust and autonomy are sensitive responsiveness and moderate control. These are very similar to the antecedents of relatedness and autonomy described by Bowlby and Ainsworth, Baumrind, and Deci and Ryan. Erikson maintains that the mother's sensitive responsiveness—that is, consistent, appropriate and affectionate responses to the baby's needs (e.g., hunger)—leads to trust in the caregiver and confidence to pursue its own preferences, a critical element of autonomy. The connection between trust and autonomy is unambiguous: "The infant must come to feel that his basic trust in himself and in the world . . . will not be jeopardized by his sudden violent wish to have a choice" (Erikson, 1950/1963, p. 85).

Trust also entails freedom of self-expression, especially verbal self-expression: The caregiver's responsiveness hinges on children's willingness to express their needs. Self-confidence and its cousin, self-expression, are central to autonomy as well as to trust. These qualities are also emphasized by the other Western investigators reviewed in this section. While Erikson's observations of Native Americans led him to conclude that the core dynamics summarized previously are universal, his evidence is anecdotal and tells us little about cultural variation in the socialization of autonomy and relatedness.

Bowlby's and Ainsworth's Attachment Theory

Attachment consists of biologically based systems of child and parent behavior, including the child's proximity and contact seeking and the parent's sensitivity to the child's needs (Bowlby, 1969/1982, 1973). The primary functions of these behaviors are to maintain the infant's physical safety and to enable the infant to explore the environment. Ainsworth's ideas about attachment and its link to autonomy, based in part on her fieldwork in Uganda, are often considered universally relevant; however the overwhelming majority of studies on attachment have been conducted by Western authors using Western samples (Rothbaum & Morelli, 2005; van IJzendorrn & Sagi, 1999). As noted by LeVine and Norman (2001), "though the first developmental study of attachment was carried out . . . among the Ganda . . ., it gave rise to an approach as blind to culture as any other in psychology" (p. 86).

According to Bowlby and Ainsworth, the crowning achievement of the attachment relationship, which occurs at about 12–18 months, is the child's ability to use the primary caregiver as a secure base for exploration. The attachment and exploration systems are conceptualized as balancing one another—when one is active the other is not. This is seen in the young child's willingness to explore the environment when attachment needs have been met and the caregiver is available as needed. If the child encounters danger, the exploration system deactivates and the attachment system reactivates—the child seeks closeness and contact. In the short term, attachment and exploration are in opposition, but in the long term they are complementary—attachment provides the confidence to explore the environment and exploration leads to renewed need for the attachment figure.

Attachment theorists view exploration as an early form of autonomy. According to Bridges (2003), "In infancy the predominant approach to assessing individual differences in autonomy involves examination of exploration and play" (p. 167). Several attachment theorists highlight the link between attachment and autonomy (Bowlby, 1969/1982;

Bretherton, 1985), and research by Allen and his colleagues provides evidence of this association in adolescence (reviewed in Allen et al., 2003). In adulthood, security is referred to as autonomous attachment.

According to Ainsworth, the key caregiving antecedent of secure attachment is sensitive responsiveness to the child's signals. Though initially focused on the child's distress signals, Ainsworth like Erikson eventually focused on responsiveness to the child's positive as well as negative signals. This is consistent with both theorists' concern with the development of self-confidence and self-esteem, which are seen as providing the psychological fuel for autonomy (Sroufe, Fox, & Pancake, 1983). Ainsworth's (1976) emphasis on autonomy is evident in her description of high level caregiving: "This mother views her baby as a separate, active, autonomous person, whose wishes and activities have validity of their own. Since she (the mother) respects his autonomy, she avoids situations in which she might have to impose her will on his" (p. 4) (see Rothbaum, Weisz, Pott, Miyake, & Morelli, 2000, for other examples).

The cross-cultural data on attachment theory provides support for a number of important claims of the theory, such as the higher incidence of secure than insecure children (van IJzendoorn & Sagi, 1999), predictable variation in exploration across strange situation episodes (Grossmann, Grossmann, & Keppler, 2005), the importance of sensitive and responsive caregiving in fostering security, and the role of secure attachment in fostering social competence, including autonomy (Posada et al., 2002; van IJzendoorn & Sagi, 1999). However, there is evidence that attachment theory is mired in Western values and assumptions and that it is less relevant to non-Western communities, including Puerto Rican (Harwood, Miller, & Lucca Irizarry, 1995; see also Harwood, Leyendecker, Carlson, Asencio, & Miller, 2002) and Japanese (Rothbaum, Weisz, et al., 2000), The socialization antecedents of security are different in these people than in European Americans (e.g., more anticipation and less responsiveness; more control and less autonomy fostering). Moreover, the link between attachment and exploration is less evident. For example, Harwood reports that Puerto Rican mothers conceive of optimal child functioning as a balance between positive engagement in relationships and proper demeanor (calm, respectful attentiveness), rather than between relatedness and autonomy (exploration) (see Rothbaum & Morelli, 2005, regarding difficulties applying the theory in other cultures).

Baumrind

According to Baumrind, optimal parents are authoritative—they provide nurturance, communication, firm control, and maturity demands (the first two were later referred to as responsiveness and the last two as demandingness). Authoritative parenting is distinguished from permissive parenting in that the latter involves low levels of demandingness and from authoritarian parenting in that the latter involves low levels of responsiveness and excessive demandingness (e.g., coercion). Baumrind (1971, 1989, 1991) maintains that parents who are authoritative provide support for autonomy while also setting and enforcing clear standards. Numerous findings indicate that children of authoritative parents have positive relations with parents, peers, and teachers and that, in adolescence, they manifest various forms of autonomous functioning.

Baumrind's work is grounded in earlier work by Erikson and mainstream developmental and social psychologists. Like Erikson, she emphasizes the importance of moderate control as opposed to lax/permissiveness or excessive/authoritarian control, and she is explicit that control must be combined with warmth. Other Western researchers who contributed to Baumrind's notion of optimal caregiving (Baldwin, 1955; Lewin, Lippitt, & White, 1939; Sears, Maccoby, & Levin, 1956) also decry lax or excessive control and maintain that control must be exerted in a context of parent–child warmth and communication. Baumrind's (1991) distinction between demandingness (or behavioral control), which she links with authoritative caregiving and positive child outcomes, and psychological control, which she links with authoritarian control and negative outcomes, is echoed by other Western investigators (Barber, 2002). Similarities between these investigators is due to their emphasis on Western contexts and Western samples.

Baumrind's focus on firm control and maturity demands is sometimes seen as a deemphasis on autonomy and individuality more generally. However, Baumrind (1991) believes that firm control is fully consistent with agency and autonomy fostering, and later investigators adopting her model have emphasized the ways in which moderate control, firmness, democratic parenting (autonomy granting), and acceptance/warmth work in tandem (e.g., Steinberg, Dornbusch, & Brown, 1992). As noted by Grusec (2002), "an authoritative parent . . . expresses comfort with the child's autonomy" (p. 152). Children are less likely to be autonomous when parents are indulgent or authoritarian, or when parents exert psychological control (evidence cited later).

While Baumrind viewed her theory as most relevant to middle-class Caucasian families, other investigators provide evidence that U.S. children of different ethnic groups function better on a variety of measures (psychosocial development, distress, and behavioral problems) when they are from authoritative homes (e.g., Steinberg et al., 1992). However, these studies also indicate that in some realms (e.g., achievement) authoritative parenting is most beneficial for Caucasian Americans. Moreover, other studies provide less support for the universality of Baumrind's claims: Authoritarian parenting leads to negative outcomes for European Americans but not for Chinese, Asian American, Hispanic American, or African American youth (Chao & Tseng, 2002; Lamborn, Dornbusch, & Steinberg, 1996).

Ryan and Deci's Self-Determination Theory

According to Ryan and Deci (2000), relatedness and autonomy are basic needs of peoples in all cultures. The more that socialization agents support these needs, the greater children's well-being, including psychological functioning and achievement (Chirkov & Ryan, 2001; Chirkov, Ryan, Kim, & Kaplan, 2003). Their research indicates that these needs are complementary and are often met simultaneously (Bettencourt & Sheldon, 2001). Self-determination theorists emphasize caregivers' sensitivity and responsiveness: "sensitive relational partner are ones who respond in ways that promote a person's experienced satisfaction of these basic psychological needs" (LaGuardia, Ryan, Couchman, & Deci, 2000, p. 369).

Almost all the research on self-determination has been conducted with Western samples. The few self-report studies purporting to demonstrate the universal importance of autonomy and relatedness (e.g., Sheldon, Elliott, Kim, & Kasser, 2001) do not examine needs that are highly valued in other cultures (e.g., harmony, group support, emotional dependence, and authority; see Smith & Schwartz, 1997). There is substantial evidence that the need for autonomy is greater in Western than non-Western cultures (Hofstede, 2001; Schwartz, 2004; Triandis, 2001).

In the remainder of this chapter we review evidence indicating the ethnocentrism of all the preceding theories and evidence. We attempt to show that these theorists' claims—that autonomy and relatedness have similar socialization antecedents and are closely associated with one another—are infused with Western assumptions, and that the conclusions are different when non-Western samples are assessed. While many investigators have argued that prevailing theories of socialization are biased toward Western ideas and samples (Edwards, 1995; Gardiner et al., 1998; Graham 1992; Harkness & Super, 1995; Rubin, Bukowski, & Parker, 1998; Stewart et al., 1998; Triandis, 1995), only a handful of investigators (Miller, 2003; Rogoff, 2003) have focused on cultural differences in autonomy and relatedness.

DIFFERENCES BETWEEN CULTURES IN AUTONOMY AND RELATEDNESS

The evidence in this section points to a modest *negative* association between autonomy and relatedness across cultures—the higher a culture's rating on autonomy the lower its rating on relatedness. This is not incompatible with findings of a positive association across individuals within Western cultures—the higher an individual's rating on autonomy the higher his or her rating on relatedness. Findings reviewed in the final section indicate that Western theories focus on a form of relatedness that is very different than the relatedness emphasized in most other cultures.

Evidence Linking Individualism–Collectivism and Autonomy–Relatedness

There is substantial evidence that individualism and collectivism at the societal level are inversely related—societies high in one tend to be low in the other (Triandis, 1995). To the extent that individualism–collectivism parallels autonomy–relatedness, autonomy and relatedness should also be inversely associated. Collectivism is closely associated with various forms of relatedness: emotional closeness, interdependence, and cooperation (Smith & Schwartz, 1997) as well as tight ingroups that provide support and care, an emphasis on loyalty, duty, reciprocity, and close extended families (Triandis, 1995). In fact, family integration is the variable that best predicts collectivism (Kagitcibasi, 1997).

While the connection between collectivism and relatedness is widely accepted, there is debate about the connection between individualism and autonomy. Ryan and Deci (2000) argue that autonomy should not be equated with a construct (individualism) that is defined partly in terms of separation and detachment. However, individualism is often defined in ways that do *not* involve separation or detachment. According to Smith and Schwartz (1997), individualism refers to "a view that social relations should be governed by voluntary and negotiated coordination among independent individuals who are equals . . ." (as opposed to) "a view that social relations should be governed by compliance to traditional, hierarchically ordered role obligations (p. 102)." For these authors, the key to individualism is autonomy rather than separation.

Because of the overlap between individualism and autonomy, Schwartz (2004) recasts individualism–collectivism as autonomy–embeddedness. Autonomy refers to the individual's independent decision making, personal rights and pursuit of happiness. Embeddedness refers to the individual's integration within a collectivity, propriety, and restraint of action that might disrupt solidarity (Hofstede, 1991; Rothbaum & Tsang, 1998; Smith & Schwartz, 1997). West European and Anglo cultures rank high on autonomy and non-Western cultures rank low.

Cultural differences in autonomy are evident even in childhood. Children and adolescents in individualistic cultures value and emphasize children's rights more, and parental authority and children's obligations less, than those from collectivistic cultures (Harwood et al., 2002; Kwak & Berry, 2001). As noted by Edwards (1995), "the toddlers' drive for autonomy and separation appears incorrect as a thematic description of toddler development in many non-Western cultural communities" (p. 47). While Smetana (2002) argues that children in all cultures value autonomy, her findings show that European American children expect and assert earlier autonomy than Mexican, Asian American, and African American children (cf. Stewart et al., 1998).[3]

There are several studies comparing an individualistic and a collectivistic culture that show higher autonomy in the former and higher relatedness in the latter. Australian students place more emphasis on freedom than do Chinese students and Chinese place more emphasis on social solidarity than do Australians (Bond & Forgas, 1984; Forgas & Bond, 1985). Much greater emphasis on family norms among Latinos than Caucasians has been documented by Harwood et al. (2002) and Vega (1990). "Familismo" is both a prevalent structure (e.g., multigenerational households) and a pervasive belief system emphasizing feelings of loyalty, reciprocity, support, and solidarity toward members of the family. Latino youth, compared to European American youth, report more relatedness (e.g., more positive attitudes toward parents) and less autonomy (e.g., more turning to family members for advice) (Fuligni, Tseng, & Lam, 1999; Suárez-Orozco & Suárez-Orozco, 1995). Based on studies contrasting European American families with families from several collectivistic cultures and ethnic minorities, Grotevant (1998) concludes that the former emphasize "autonomy, independence and initiative" and the latter emphasize "familistic norms of collective support, loyalty and obligation" (p. 114).

While most studies indicate a negative association between relatedness and autonomy, there are exceptions. Rogoff (2003) reviews evidence of high autonomy in several cultures that are also high in relatedness: Native Americans, Marquesans, the Kaluli of Papua New Guinea, Mayans, and Aka foragers. These highly cooperative, nonhierarchical societies help explain why the negative association is low. Adults in these cultures foster autonomy via noninterference in their children's decisions and behavior—following their children's lead rather than asserting their own agenda—especially in the toddler period. The autonomy granting in these societies is designed to foster empathy, valuing of harmony, and other characteristics of cooperative societies rather than to foster traditional manifestations of autonomy—a general emphasis on choice, agency, psychological independence, intrinsic motivation, and individual rights.

Explaining the Negative Association between Relatedness and Autonomy

Why do cultures that value relatedness highly (i.e., collectivistic cultures) tend to devalue personal choice and agency? Members of collectivistic cultures value highly the *group's* choice and agency, as contrasted with the individual's choice and agency. In these cultures, issues of choice and agency are focused on the ability to function well in the group, whereas in individualistic cultures choice and agency center on personal maturity and well-being and self-maximization (Fiske, Kitayama, Markus, & Nisbett, 1998; Grotevant, 1998; Rothbaum, Pott, Azuma, Miyake, & Morelli, 2000; Rothbaum, Weisz, et al.,

2000). Menon, Morris, Chiu, and Hong (1999) report a related finding: Americans are more likely to endorse statements such as "individuals possess free will" and "follow their internal direction," where Singaporeans are more likely to endorse similar statements about organizations (e.g., "organizations possess free will"). (See Weisz, Rothbaum, & Blackburn, 1984, for more evidence of cultural differences in perceptions of individual versus group choice).

Compelling evidence of greater emphasis on relatedness and lesser emphasis on autonomy in non-Western cultures comes from research on the consequences of granting autonomy. Iyengar and Lepper (1999) found that Asian American children displayed better task performance, more learning, and greater interest, persistence, and preference when closely related adults (mothers) or peers (friends) made choices for them than when they made their own choices. That is, their performance was better when they did *not* function autonomously than when they did function autonomously. These findings directly conflict with a great deal of Western research during the past 20 years (reviewed in Ryan & Deci, 2000). However, when Iyengar and Lepper employed Anglo American children their findings were consistent with prior research: There were more positive outcomes when children made their own choices.

Iyengar and Lepper's (1999) findings challenge the widely held belief that personal choice (autonomy) is universally linked to positive outcomes. They note:

> For American selves, the act of making a personal choice offers not only an opportunity to express and receive one's personal preference but also a chance to establish one's unique identity. For Asian interdependent selves having choices made by relevant ingroup members . . . provides a greater opportunity to promote harmony and to fulfill the goal of belonging to the group . . . actions that could be seen by individualists as unwarranted usurpations of fundamental individual rights may be viewed by dedicated collectivists as the necessary fulfillment of expected social obligations to family and friends (p. 363).

Another explanation of the generally negative association between relatedness and autonomy across cultures is that cultures with high relatedness (collectivistic cultures) tend to view relatedness as obligatory. Miller, Bersoff, and Harwood (1990) found that in India, responsiveness to others' needs (a core component of relatedness) is viewed as a moral mandate. Americans, by contrast, tend to view responsiveness as a matter of personal choice. Similarly, Jacobsen (1983) found that Middle Eastern children value requested (obligatory) responsiveness more highly and spontaneous (voluntary) responsiveness less highly than Israeli children of Western heritage. These findings suggest that the high relatedness observed in collectivistic societies reflects an emphasis on obligation, reciprocity, and requests from others and a deemphasis on personal choice and endogenous motivations (Eisenberg & Fabes, 1998; Miller, 2003). The notion that there are cultural differences in the meaning of relatedness is elaborated in the final section.

THE SOCIALIZATION OF AUTONOMY AND RELATEDNESS IN DIFFERENT CULTURES

In this section we examine cultural differences in the socialization of autonomy and relatedness. The research challenges prevailing Western assumptions that, worldwide, they have similar antecedents and that they co-occur. We focus on differences in parental warmth and control because there is abundant evidence regarding the role of those constructs in the socialization of autonomy and relatedness. Specifically, we examine cultural variation in (1) the constancy and closeness of care, especially in early childhood, and (2) parents' exercise of authority and psychological forms of control. Because of our interest in nonparental socialization influences, we also review findings regarding the role of schools, siblings, social networks, and larger institutions.

Constant Close Contact versus Distal Contact with Separations

Whereas in the West it is common for parents to be apart from their children, most of the world's population spends much more time together—especially in infancy and especially at night (Harkness & Super, 1995). In addition to more co-sleeping and co-bathing with infants and more prolonged holding of them in non-Western cultures, there is less age segregation in the everyday life experiences of young children from lower-class communities, especially those not in the West, as compared to middle-class Western communities (Rogoff, Mistry, Goncu, & Mosier, 1993).

A major cultural difference is in amount of parent–infant body contact—perhaps the most pure measure of parental "warmth." There are numerous "back and hip cultures" (LeVine, 1990) in which children live on mothers' bodies virtually all of the day and sleep close to mothers at night (Keller et al., 2004). According to LeVine (1988), maternal behavior that emphasizes soothing, holding, and high levels of protection of infants is typical in an agricultural society. Such behavior would be considered overprotective by Western standards (Whiting & Whiting, 1975). In a recent study by Keller et al. (2004) of five communities, there was much more body contact (carrying, co-sleeping, and grooming) among the three non-Western communities (Cameroonian Nso, Costa Rican, and Indian Gujarati) than the two European communities (German and Greek). Edwards (1995) also reports that various means of keeping infants close to mothers, such as slings and swaddling, are more common in non-Western agricultural communities. By maximizing proximity, mothers increase their responsiveness (Edwards, 1995). These gains in relatedness are accompanied by losses in autonomy—restriction of infants' movement and promotion of passivity (Edwards, 1995; Saarni, Mumme, & Campos, 1998).

The greater body contact in non-Western cultures is consistent with Ainsworth's (1963) observations in Uganda. Mothers' breastfeeding was so integrally related to their care of their infants that she proposed a linkage between the attachment and breastfeeding systems of behavior. True, Pisani, and Oumar (2001) in their study of the Dogon, also noted the importance of this connection, which has not been emphasized in Western communities.

Extreme closeness, which in the West would probably be labeled "enmeshment," is also reported in Korea (Choi, 1992), Japan (Rothbaum, Pott, et al., 2000), and Puerto Rico (Garcia Coll, 1990). Choi (1992) reports a communication pattern in which Korean mothers and young children are "attuned to one another in a fused state" and "mothers merged themselves with their children" in contrast to Canadian mothers who "withdraw themselves . . . so that the children's reality can remain autonomous" (p. 38). Clancy's (1986) description of Japanese–U.S. differences closely parallels Choi's description of Korean–Canadian differences.

These findings are reversed when the focus is on more distal forms of contact. Keller et al. (2004) found that face-to-face and eye-to-eye interaction, which "inform" infants of their "uniqueness and self-efficacy" (p. 12), are much more common in individualistic (German and Greek) communities than the three collectivistic communities. Although European mothers are less physically close, they are more likely to serve as playmates for their children and to enjoy distal contact with them (e.g., via infant seats, walkers, and playpens). Brief and demonstrative expressions of warmth/contact, such as hugging, kissing and praise, are at least as common among Western as compared to non-Western caregivers. Western mothers are also high on "object stimulation"—they frequently direct the child's attention to the environment. Similar cultural differences have been found when comparing European American with a variety of non-Western cultures (LeVine et al., 1994; Rogoff, 2003; Rothbaum, Pott, et al., 2000; Uzgiris & Raeff, 1995; Whiting & Edwards, 1988).

This pattern of behavior—modest amounts of physical proximity and contact combined with high levels of distal, brief and demonstrative contact, and directing children's attention outward—meshes well with Western theorists' notion of optimal caregiving. For example, Ryan and Deci (2000) play down the importance of high-level closeness/ contact: "*proximal* relational supports may not be necessary for intrinsic motivation" (italics added). Indeed they note that "many intrinsically motivated behaviors are happily performed in isolation" (p. 71). An emphasis on distal, brief, and demonstrative contact reflects a belief that early relatedness that includes opportunities for separation paves the way for autonomy and for later relatedness with new partners and that too close ties often thwart this progression.

In Western as compared to non-Western cultures, there are greater limitations on, and consistently negative connotations of, indulgence of dependence in early childhood. This is contrasted with the important role assigned to allowing dependence in other cultures (e.g., the valuing of *amae* in Japan and *consentido* in some Hispanic cultures). Early indulgence in these cultures is associated with low externalizing (aggressive, antisocial) behavior and thus promotes relationship harmony (Rogoff, 2003; Schlegel & Barry, 1991). Western theories emphasize instead the role of early indulgence in undermining autonomy, which may explain why Western theorists and Western parents disdain it.

The indulgence common in these non-Western cultures involves acceptance of children's expressions of distress and helplessness. By contrast the emphasis in the West appears to be on responsiveness to positive signals, particularly those indicating the child's autonomy seeking and related needs for self-esteem, self-expression, and self-assertion (Dennis, Cole, Zahn-Waxler, & Mizuta, 2002; Rothbaum & Morelli, 2005; Friedlmeier & Trommsdorff, 2004). Bridges, (2003) claims that "attachment and autonomy may be linked in part because the same sort of contingent consistently responsive and affectively positive caregiving that is linked with secure attachment is also linked with the facilitation of mastery motivation" (p. 170). These claims apply to Western experiences and Western forms of responsiveness (i.e., modest warmth, distal contact, absence of indulgence, and an emphasis on responsiveness to autonomy seeking).

In order for the attachment and exploration (i.e., relatedness and autonomy) systems to become linked, young children need experiences with separations and reunions and with venturing forth on their own into the environment and returning to the caregiver/secure base. When these opportunities are rare, they are not likely to manifest high levels of autonomy or to link autonomy with relatedness. In fact, separations (i.e., leaving the child with strangers or alone) and reunions are not common for infants in many other societies, which is why the Strange Situation is overly stressful for them. Children in these societies are almost always in the presence of caregivers they know well—siblings, extended family members, or surrogate mothers.

By contrast, in the West, opportunities to separate are abundant, beginning with pressures to sleep alone in infancy. Later experiences with babysitters, preschool, sleepover camps, and age-segregated social events teach children how to separate from and reunite with caregivers. Whiting and Edwards (1988) review evidence indicating that parents in the United States leave young children alone far more than parents in other cultures. Even when they are with their children, European American as compared with Latino caregivers establish child-centered feeding and napping routines that foster autonomy but undermine relatedness because the child is separated from the routine of other family members (Harwood et al., 2002).

Pressures on Western children to obtain autonomy from parents continue in adolescence. Adolescents' and their parents' expectations regarding the timing of autonomy are earlier in Western than non-Western countries (Kwak, 2003; Smetana, 2002). There is more pressure for teens to separate from parents in the United States than in China (Dubas & Gerris, 2002) or Japan (Rothbaum, Pott, et al., 2000). Also contributing to Western teens' quest for autonomy are their loosely knit ingroups and the ease of exploring outside relationships.

Our point is that patterns identified in the West may not apply to other peoples in the world. In most non-Western communities, relatedness entails much more constant and close physical contact from the earliest period, and correspondingly less orientation to the outside impersonal world. This kind of constancy and closeness is, we suspect, more consistent with a relatedness that involves enduring commitment, loyalty, duty and reduced interest in autonomy. The relative lack of orientation to the outside world in non-Western communities is likely to mean less exploration and other forms of autonomy (as that construct has been defined in the West). In fact, findings from several studies indicate less exploration in non-Western than Western communities (reviewed in Rothbaum, Weisz, et al., 2000; Weisner, 1984), and less association between parental warmth and child autonomy (for evidence of a negative association, see Chen et al., 1998).

Authoritarian Parenting versus Authoritative Parenting

Whereas most studies conducted with mainstream Western samples indicate that authoritative parenting is the most common as well as the most effective pattern (i.e., is associated with the most desirable child outcomes, including relatedness and autonomy), research with other parents, especially those from East Asia, indicates that the authoritarian style is most common and effective. For the Chinese, parental control, even in the absence of other behaviors indicating warmth and communication (i.e., authoritarian parenting), is likely to be seen as an expression of concern, caring, and involvement, and as promoting family harmony (Chao & Tseng, 2002). By contrast, for Euro-Americans, authoritarian parenting is seen as unhealthy domination and as undermining relatedness and autonomy.

There are two qualifications of these findings: (1) East Asian parents are more likely to exercise authoritarian control with older than younger children. In early childhood, high levels of closeness and warmth characterize parent–child relations in many non-Western cultures, and there is little parental control in response to young children's dependency (e.g., Rothbaum, Pott, et al., 2000; Stevenson, Chen, & Lee, 1992) and (2) high-level control is often seen as related to family hierarchy, respect, obligation, and self sacrifice, rather than as dominating or negative (Chao, 2000; Kim & Choi, 1994; Rohner & Pettengill, 1985).[4]

According to Chao (2000), the authoritarian parenting style is steeped in Confucian tradition which emphasizes the importance of "training" children to engage in appropriate and moral behavior (i.e., to be obedient, to be self-disciplined, to be hard working, and to follow norms). There is evidence that such training undermines intrinsic motivation, initiative, and other forms of autonomy (Grolnick, Deci, & Ryan, 1997), but it is highly valued in East Asia in part because it is seen as reflecting parental care. Indeed, the Chinese word guan, which means to train or govern, also means to care for and love the child. The Chinese associate relatedness with control rather than autonomy. Chao and Tseng (2002) cite more than 20 studies indicating greater parental control and exercise of authority and less encouragement of *autonomy* in Asians (Indians, Filipinos, Japanese and Vietnamese, as well as Chinese) than in Caucasians.

Training is just one aspect of a constellation of Chinese parents' practices that earn them the label "authoritarian." These parents are also likely to insist on unquestioned respect and obligations to give back to parents. In the context of Chinese values and institutions, such practices are seen as positive, caring, and promoting the child's relatedness and mature functioning, (Chiu, 1987; Lin & Fu, 1990). Other authoritarian practices that are seen as thwarting autonomy in the West, but as fostering optimal child functioning in East Asia, are discouraging children from expressing their emotions and becoming very involved in children's achievement (Chao & Tseng, 2002; Ho, 1986).

These East Asian practices do not involve the kinds of communication and negotiation that are so valued in the West. Questioning authority, verbal forms of self-expression, and self-assertion are actively discouraged. Nsamenang (1992) found that people from traditional rural communities view noncompliance as a moral transgression because it disrupts relationship harmony, whereas Westerners are more likely to view it as part of a child's emerging skills as an autonomous agent. Research by Weisz, Chaiyasit, Weiss, Eastman, and Jackson (1995) indicates that many behaviors that are regarded as antisocial and unacceptable by Thai parents are accepted by U.S. parents. Weisner (1984) cites several studies indicating that "our culture . . . permits children more autonomy and latitude in negotiations with parents over compliance than do most cultures around the world" (p. 340).

There is evidence that non-Western parents' discouragement of noncompliance and negotiation, and their greater emphasis on power assertion, may be due to higher expectations for prosocial behavior and lower tolerance for antisocial behavior. As noted earlier, showing concern for others is viewed as a moral obligation in collectivistic cultures rather than as a social convention (Grusec, 2002; Miller, 2003). Parents exercise more power assertion when dealing with violations of morality (e.g., antisocial behavior) than conventions (Grusec, 2002).

Socialization practices and priorities similar to those in East Asia have been reported among Latinos (Harwood et al., 2002). Based on numerous studies in several countries, Harwood claims that Latino families exert higher levels of control than their Anglo American counterparts. Control is intended to promote relatedness, in the form of "proper demeanor" and respect. Proper demeanor, or "appropriate relatedness," refers to the child's display of the required level of courtesy and decorum in each situation. Control is apparent even in early childhood, as evidenced by Latino parents' greater positioning and restraining of their infants, redirecting the infant's attention, and less time watching the child explore. In feeding situations, Latino mothers maintain greater control (i.e., foster less autonomy) by relying on spoon or bottle feeding instead of self-feeding. The goal of these and other forms of control is to place greater emphasis on the child's obligations to the family and larger group, and less emphasis on the child's own wishes, thoughts and desires (Harwood et al., 2002). In adolescence, Latino Americans emphasize respect of parental authority more than their European American counterparts; and European Americans show relatively more emphasis on individual autonomy (Fuligni, 1998).

Valuing of parental control relative to autonomy fostering is evident in other non-Western cultures. There is less focus on autonomy in parent–child play in farming communities in East Africa than in France (Rabain-Jamin, 1989), and Columbian parents direct play and impose their own agenda more than U.S. parents, who are more likely to follow the child's initiative (Ramirez, 1993). Interestingly, Mexican children engage in more complex play when they are directed by their parents than when their parents encourage them to be autonomous, and the opposite is true for U.S. children (Farver, 1989), indicating children's differential responsiveness to socialization practices that foster autonomy.

We do not believe that the high indulgence provided by Japanese and Latino caregivers is incompatible with these caregivers' exercise of authoritarian control. Their indulgence is circumscribed—it primarily involves dependency needs in young children in informal contexts (i.e., with family members in the home as opposed to less familiar adults outside the home). While manifestly very different, both parental indulgence and authoritarian control reflect hierarchical relationships as opposed to more equal relationships involving negotiation between partners. Such hierarchical relationships minimize resistance—by providing for all the child's needs (i.e., indulgence) and by accentuating differences in power and status (i.e., authoritarian control).

One of the ways in which Western parents convey affection and foster autonomy is through their tolerance of children's resistance to social norms. Even though they are low on indulgence of dependency needs, they tend to permit nonconformity, perhaps because they view it as an indicator of autonomy. Socialization for conformity (e.g., insisting on accommodation to social expectations), especially with older children and in public/formal contexts, is considered more central to the development of cooperation and relatedness by East Asian parents, Hispanic parents, and parents from more simple agricultural societies, as compared to Western parents (Chao & Tseng, 2002; Edwards, 1995; Friedlmeier & Trommsdorff, 1998; Harkness & Super, 1995; Harwood et al., 2002; Rothbaum, Morelli, Pott, & Liu-Constant, 2000; Trommsdorff, 1995).

The firm (but nonauthoritarian) control valued and practiced in the West is accompanied by respect for noncompliance and self-assertion, less insistence on "shoulds," valuing of freedom and choice, as well as verbal communication characterized by openness and give and take. The bottom line of Western parents' firm, authoritative control is the ability to exert authority while fostering autonomy between distinct individuals.

Firm control and autonomy fostering serve to clarify emotional, social, and financial boundaries between Western teens and their parents, and these boundaries make it more likely that parents and teens will make different choices about their self-interests. By contrast, in collectivist cultures such as Japan and Bali, parents blur the boundary between self's and others' interests, and between personal choice and social obligation. Japanese and Balinese teens' individual desires are subordinated to the will of the group, leading to group conformity and undermining the individual's willingness to assert the self (Rothbaum, Pott, et al., 2000; Trommsdorff, 1995).

A major vehicle for training children to follow norms is the assignment of chores, such as helping with young siblings, collecting firewood and fetching water (Zukow-Goldring, 1995). It is not just the number of chores but their communal nature, involving nurturance and responsibility for others, that fosters relatedness in children. These chores are not chosen. Because the chores of Western children are less numerous, more self-oriented (e.g., picking up toys and making one's bed) and more frequently chosen by the child, they are less likely to foster relatedness or to interfere with autonomy (Harkness & Super, 1995). As compared to Anglo Americans, Latino families expect more and earlier responsibility for group tasks (involving care of others) and later and less responsibility for self-tasks (involving personal care), and they expect the child "to assert his or her own agency at a later age" (Harwood et al., 2002, p. 29).

Psychological Control

Psychological control refers to covert practices that influence children's feelings of acceptance and thereby their behavior. In the United States as compared to non-Western countries, there is less emphasis on both positive (e.g., empathy training and fostering interdependence) and negative (e.g., shame, guilt, and anxiety induction) forms of psychological control. Psychological control is pervasive in East Asian cultures, as seen for example in Chinese mothers' focusing on guilt and shame in their narrative retelling of young children's transgressions (Miller, Fung, & Mintz, 1996). Psychological control instills in children a perception that they cannot or should not question authority, express themselves, or manifest other forms of autonomy. When children's behavior results from psychological control, it is not autonomous (Bridges, 2003).

According to Barber (2002), psychological control is more likely when parents are in close proximity to the child in the early years and have greater opportunities to arrange and control the child's environment—characteristics that are more common in non-Western societies. Extensive early training in empathy, another possible forerunner of psychological control, is more common in many non-Western cultures than in Western cultures (Clancy, 1986; Keller et al., 2004; Rogoff, 2003).

A number of Western studies highlight the negative effects of parents' psychological control. Barber (2002), who claims that these effects are "ubiquitous," attributes their harmfulness to "intruding on a basic human drive for autonomy" (p. 44). Children of parents who exercise psychological control exhibit less autonomy and more internalizing problems, such as anxiety and psychosomatic problems (Barber, 2002). Not surprisingly, these outcomes are seen as more negative in the West (Miller et al., 1996, cited in Kochanska & Thompson, 1997, p. 67). Barber's conclusion that psychological control is detrimental is partly due to the inclusion of items like "personal attacks" and "erratic behavior" in operationalizations of the construct, based on factor-analytic studies of

Western samples. Non-Western parents are more likely to emphasize the role of psychological control in fostering relatedness (Clancy, 1986).

Other Socialization Influences

Non-Western societies do not rely solely on parental socialization practices to support relatedness and constrain autonomy: they also depend on schools that are integrated with family life; nested levels of sibling care; cohesive social networks; and economic, political, and religious institutions that promote collectivism. Although we focus on parental influences, we believe that the influence of parents cannot be understood apart from the influence of these complementary socialization agents whose activities support each other (Ujiie, 1997). Next we describe a variety of other socialization influences, including the nature of schooling; presence versus absence of sibling and kin care; loose versus tight social networks; and economic, political, and religious institutions—that promote or undermine autonomy and relatedness.

Schools/Teachers

Formal schooling, characteristic of individualistic societies, separates children from primary caregivers, siblings, and extended family. After-school care prolongs the separation. The frequent absence of closely connected others creates an environment conducive to autonomous functioning. In collectivistic societies education is less removed from everyday situations and relationships—with caregivers, siblings, and peers (Rogoff et al., 1993). Even when formal schooling occurs, the curriculum is much more concerned with teaching children to be part of the group (i.e., relatedness; Lewis, 1995; Peak, 1986; Tobin, 1992; Trommsdorff & Dasen, 2001).

Sibling Influences

The work of the Whitings (e.g., Whiting & Whiting, 1975; Whiting & Edwards, 1988), as well as more than 20 studies from the late 1980s to mid-1990s, highlights the "quality, quantity, and pervasiveness of sibling care in agrarian cultures" (Zukow-Goldring, 1995, p. 183). Children's high level of relatedness in these collectivistic cultures is influenced both by their role as recipients of older child care and by their role as caregivers. Older siblings are not the only ones who provide care; there are nested levels of care, with infants supervised by preschoolers, who in turn are supervised by gradeschoolers, adolescents, and other adults: "The key to prosocial acts is having someone to nurture" (Zukow-Goldring, 1995, p. 189).

Apprenticeship in caregiving begins as early as age 2 and is pervasive due to the number of young children available in the peer group (Whiting & Edwards, 1988). Instruction in prosocial behavior—cooperation, sharing, and nurturance—is early, systematic, and sustained: "A range of family members ... socialize child caregivers, conveying where, when and how to engage in activities during the course of the day" (Zukow-Goldring, 1995, p. 182). By contrast, U.S. parents do not perceive even 5–9-year-olds as competent to care for others and our legal system forbids it (Zukow-Goldring, 1995). Caregiving by siblings is effective in part because it includes collective shaming (psychological control) for failure to adhere to directions and use of coercion (authoritarian control), as well as high levels of nurturance (Whiting & Edwards, 1988).

A fundamental aspect of training in child care is to learn to put aside egoistic wants and needs to attend to those of others. Zukow-Goldring (1995) describes older children training a 15-month-old child to learn to share, in sessions lasting up to 25 minutes of gentle prodding. In the Solomon Islands, children are instructed by peers to share at 6 months of age; by 18 months they share without hesitation (Watson-Gegeo & Gegeo, 1989). All these authors maintain that there is less opportunity for and training in sibling care and sharing in individualistic societies. As noted by Zukow-Goldring (1995), "Consonant with the prioritizing of autonomy within technological cultures, existing studies of siblings primarily investigate how the experience of receiving or giving care brings an individual child to his or her personal best rather than how assisting with child caregiving is helpful to the family" (p. 183). In the West, the emphasis on competition (rather than cooperation) and new peer relations (rather than enduring sibling relations) leads to a decrease over time in positive sibling interactions (Volling, 2003).

Social Networks

In collectivistic societies, learning to rely on the extended network begins early and continues late in life. Toddlers are encouraged to redirect their dependency needs out toward the family as a whole (Edwards, 1995). The extended family supports this development, in that children are cared for by relatives. The sibling group is itself an extensive network, including cousins and young aunts and uncles (Zukow-Goldring, 1995). By contrast, toddlers in the West direct many of their dependency needs to parents and they are increasingly encouraged to self-regulate their dependency needs. Substitute caregivers and peers are more often unrelated to the child (Harwood et al., 2002) and sibling groups are relatively small. Care of family members continues into old age in collectivistic societies (Hara & Minagawa, 1996).

Whether or not the support network consists of family members is a major determinant of the social network's stability. Larner (1990) reports that, over a 3-year period, turnover of network membership was 33% for nonkin as compared to only 9% for kin. Turnover undermines the benefits of networks by reducing their dependability and reinforces the need for autonomy.

Large family units cannot function harmoniously unless there is a hierarchically organized system in which people comply with role obligations and identify with the collectivity, thereby sacrificing their personal autonomy (Smith & Schwartz, 1997). Because family size promotes relatedness and undermines autonomy, it helps explain the inverse association between relatedness and autonomy. U.S. Latinos, compared to European Americans, have larger and more cohesive social networks, comprised of a higher proportion of extended family members (Harwood et al., 2002). These more cohesive networks persist from childhood to adulthood.

The close connection between quality of parental caregiving and family supports (Cochran & Niego, 2002) is often attributed to the direct influence of the latter on the former. We suspect the effects are transactional: Parents who are responsive to children may also be responsive to their social network, enhancing the network's ability to provide substitute child care, which in turn relieves the load on individual parents and increases their responsiveness.

Economic, Religious, and Political Influences

Economic and ecological influences on socialization are profound. In agricultural societies, parents and other adults insist on high levels of responsibility, deferring to seniors, and obedience—all of which imply low autonomy (Whiting & Edwards, 1988). Several studies have found very high correlations between economic development and both individualism and autonomy. Smith and Schwartz (1997) suggest that these correlations reflect the fact that wealthier nations can "provide individuals with more varied opportunities and can afford greater freedom of choice" (p. 106). It is not just wealthy capitalistic systems that foster autonomy—societies with hunting and fishing economies also socialize their children to take initiative and be self-reliant (Barry, Bacon, & Child, 1957).

There is a similar relationship between economic factors and socialization. Working-class parents socialize their children to be obedient (i.e., low in autonomy) because autonomy is not needed, for example, on the assembly line or for clerical positions (Harkness & Super, 1995; Kohn, 1995). How the economic realities are transmitted to children is not yet well understood, but adults' experiences in their work environments and their adaptation to economic conditions probably make them important mediators of their children's values (Grotevant, 1998; Kohn & Slomczynski, 1990).

Religious and governmental institutions also influence socialization. Eastern religions and philosophies (Confucianism, Taoism, Buddhism, Hinduism, and Shitoism) emphasize relatedness (collective loyalties) more, and autonomy less, than do monotheistic religions and philosophies in the West, particularly after the Reformation and Enlightenment (Kagitcibasi, 1997). Autocratic, nondemocratic political systems undermine autonomy, and democratic institutions support autonomy (e.g., individual rights, self-expression, and opportunities for choice).

Child Effects

Children's behavior (e.g., their dependency seeking, activity level, and compliance) influences as well as is influenced by parents' behavior (Bell & Chapman, 1986). In some realms, children's influence on parents' may be at least as great as their parents' influence (Kerr & Stattin, 2003). Child effects may play a critical role in many cultural differences involving warmth and control. Unfortunately, the limited cultural research on child effects (Trommsdorff & Kornadt, 2003) as well as space restrictions prohibit further treatment of this critical issue.

INTEGRATING WESTERN AND CULTURAL RESEARCH: DIFFERENT CONCEPTIONS OF RELATEDNESS

Proponents of individualism–collectivism (e.g., Triandis, 1995), independence–interdependence (Markus & Kitayama, 1991), and agency–communion (McAdams, 1993) do not depict autonomy and relatedness as opposite ends of a single dimension. Indeed, they acknowledge that autonomy and relatedness are not mutually exclusive and that both tendencies can coexist. Yet they tend to *depict autonomy and relatedness as in opposition* to one another. Research in the last section is consistent with their assumptions—it indicates that socialization influences that support relatedness undermine autonomy and vice versa. By contrast, all the Western theorists reviewed earlier maintain, and a substantial body of Western evidence indicates, that *relatedness leads to richer and more stable forms of autonomy and visa versa* (e.g., Allen & Hauser, 1996; Clark & Ladd, 2000; Larson, Richards, Moneta, Holmbeck, & Duckett, 1996; Sroufe et al., 1983; Vereijken, Riksen-Walraven, & Van Lieshout, 1997)—that is, that they are not only compatible but mutually reinforcing. How can we resolve these conflicting findings? Below we highlight cultural differences in the *type* and *meaning* of relatedness.

Trust and Assurance

Our explanation of the conflicting findings—that relatedness is in opposition to autonomy (across cultures) and that it mutually reinforces autonomy (within Western cultures)—hinges on the existence of two types of relatedness. These two types of relatedness—general trust and assurance—are borrowed from Yamagishi (2002). We attempt to show that in individualistic societies, close relationships are defined largely in terms of general trust—a hope and faith in others whom one has chosen. Trust is a form of relatedness that emphasizes verbal intimacy, constructive conflict, self-expression, negotiation, confidence in self and other, voluntary commitments and, most important, a link between relatedness and autonomy. As noted by attachment theorists, trust links two behavioral systems (attachment and exploration) as well as two value systems (relatedness and autonomy). The other type of relatedness, that is more common in collectivistic societies, is assurance. It is based on guarantees of loyalty and reciprocity that stem from both parties' membership in cohesive tightly knit groups. Assurance is a form of relatedness that emphasizes group belongingness, empathy, harmony, role prescribed commitments, loyalty, and duty. Assurance is inversely associated with autonomy.

The trust–assurance distinction clarifies many of the findings reviewed earlier. Western theorists and researchers tend to equate relatedness with general trust, which helps explain why they find an association between relatedness and autonomy. By contrast, cultural psychologists tend to equate relatedness with assurance, which helps explain why they find an inverse association between relatedness and autonomy.

Before elaborating the differences between trust and assurance, it is important to emphasize their common ground. They are both rooted in love, care, protection, and security. We believe that trust and assurance exist in all cultures, although they are valued to different degrees, and they take on somewhat different forms. Moreover, certain contexts may pull for a certain kind of relatedness in all cultures; for example, caregiving of infants may universally involve high degrees of assurance. Infants require unconditional loyalty and constant care—key aspects of assurance. Still, there are likely to be cultural differences in the degree and nature of assurance in infancy (e.g., the number of caregivers providing care and sleeping arrangements), in large part because of differences in the competing theme of trust (e.g., the attachment–exploration link). *The key is the pattern of cultural differences—how different relationships, local settings, meanings and practices converge to create differences between trust and assurance.*

Western theory and research on socialization seem to equate relatedness with trust rather than assurance. For example, Erikson (1950/1963, 1968) claims that high-level responsiveness is optimal, but he cautions against constant responsiveness because that might make the child invested in its permanence. To be autonomous the child must trust in, and risk losing, the caregiver's responsiveness; being assured of the caregiver's responsiveness undermines the development of autonomy. One reason Western parents frequently leave their young children with unfamiliar caregivers is to foster the child's sense of trust—hope and faith in the caregiver's return. The Strange Situation paradigm recreates these circumstances in an exaggerated form.

All the Western theorists reviewed earlier maintain that close relationships, especially those with parents, give children the trust they need to venture forth from the secure base of current relationships to explore and establish relationships with previously unfamiliar others. Yamagishi (2002) explains: "trust emancipates people from closed relations and leads them to form spontaneous relations with new partners" (p. 11). Elsewhere he writes, "trust is a lubricant for social relations" (p. 18). According to Yamagishi (2002), the reason trusting individuals are willing to place hope and faith in partners is their confidence in themselves and others. They must believe that they are worthy of love and that others can be depended on to provide love. All the Western theorists reviewed earlier emphasize the importance of confidence in self and others in forming relationships. Trust gives people choices—to stay in current relationships or to leave them for "better deals." The goal is self-maximization—finding the outcome/relationship that best meets the self's needs (cf. Harwood et al., 1995).

Whereas trust fosters the formation of new relationships, assurance stabilizes existing relationships. Cultural theorists maintain that close relationships in collectivist cultures revolve around cooperation, reciprocity, interdependence and harmony with members of the group. In tightly knit groups, people are committed to one another by "iron rules" (Yamagishi, Cook, & Watabe, 1998, p. 36). Members depend on the network of incentives, such as punishment for disloyalty, to bind themselves to one another. Their commitment is long lasting because it is less based on choice and more on obligations and rules about reciprocity that are reinforced by all parties involved. What is most valued about assurance is that it is guaranteed and certain; guarantees and certainty are jeopardized to the extent that people can choose to forge close relations with outsiders.

Western children are socialized to prioritize trust. Western parents' moderate warmth, positive responsiveness and tolerance of nonconformity, combined with their distal contact, frequent separations, and lack of indulgence, foster children's confidence that they are lovable and can depend on others, while also encouraging exploration of new relationships. The needs that caregivers emphasize pertain to exploration, curiosity, self-agency, choice, and autonomy, thereby teaching children that relatedness is emancipating rather than constraining. Authoritative and democratic control, especially the emphasis on verbal communication and self-expression, gives children the skills they need to form intimate relationships with unfamiliar others.

By contrast, non-Western children are socialized to prioritize assurance. Their parents' high levels of warmth, responsiveness to negative signals, continuous closeness and indulgence, combined with their relative intolerance of nonconformity and assignment of caregiving and other communal responsibilities to children, foster a sense that loyalty and commitment to others is guaranteed and obligatory rather than a matter of choice. The needs that caregivers emphasize pertain to avoiding loneliness and ensuring cooperation, thereby conveying to their children that relatedness binds people together into cohesive ingroups. Authoritarian and psychological control teach children the dangers of defying authority and group pressure and the risks involved in forming close relations with members of other groups.

The key difference between trust and assurance is that the former is positively associated with autonomy and the latter is negatively associated with autonomy. Trust fosters and is fostered by autonomy and cannot flourish in the absence of the autonomy of relational partners. Erikson's notion of trust, Bowlby and Ainsworth's notion of attachment, and Deci and Ryan's notion of relatedness are inextricably tied to autonomy.

Might there be different notions of autonomy that parallel the different notions of relatedness? Earlier we distinguished between personal and group choice and suggested that the former may be more characteristic of cultures emphasizing individualism and the latter of cultures emphasizing collectivism. Recent work by self-determination theorists provides a reconceptualization of autonomy that encompasses these different phenomena. They claim that, in certain societies, people may be more "internally motivated" to behave in accord with group norms than with personal choices, and they consider such behavior autonomous. Their equation of autonomy with volition ("behavior that is experienced as willingly enacted"; a person who "fully endorses the actions in which he or she is engaged and/or the values expressed by them"; Chirkov et al., 2003, p. 98) departs markedly from standard definitions of autonomy without heralding that departure. Ironically, their very encompassing construct remains mired in Western assumptions—they link autonomy with a well integrated self, self-esteem, and subjective well-being, without noting the Western bias inherent in these concepts (Kitayama & Markus, 2000). Given that Western assumptions, meanings, and manifestations of autonomy (the emphasis on personal choice, self-agency, intrinsic motivation, individual rights, and Western situations) have dominated in the past, a deeper understanding of cultural differences in autonomy must await further clarification of the construct and additional research in non-Western communities.

Like Chirkov et al. (2003), Miller (2003) provides rich descriptions of choice, freedom, and agency that are common in collectivistic experiences (e.g., the individual's subjective experience of personal commitment to duty), but she highlights the cultural differences as well as similarities between these notions and Western notions of autonomy. We believe that Miller's (2003) notion that duty is "experienced simultaneously as both subjectively endorsed and objectively required" (p. 83) is consistent with relatedness based on assurance as opposed to trust.

What does the trust–assurance distinction tell us about the socialization of relatedness? We agree with Western theorists, particularly attachment theorists, that relatedness is fundamentally concerned with the satisfaction of basic needs for security. However, we also believe that the values and behaviors that are most central to the child's security are culturally dependent. In individualistic cultures security primarily involves providing children a safe base and thereby enabling them to be autonomous. In collectivistic cultures security primarily involves including children within a cohesive group and thereby enabling them to harmoniously coordinate their efforts with others (often at the cost of autonomy). Western theories and research provide compelling explanations of the socialization of relatedness and autonomy only in individualistic cultures, where trust dominates over assurance. Cultural theories are needed to explain the socialization of relatedness and autonomy in most other cultures where assurance is at least as important as trust. *By integrating tenets of Western theories with insights from cultural research, and recognizing the multifaceted nature of relatedness, we may be better able to explain the socialization of relatedness and autonomy in diverse cultures.*

NOTES

1. For example, within culture (e.g., in the United States), people who are wealthier are not happier, but between cultures (i.e., when scores are aggregated for individuals within cultures), there is a wealth–happiness association: The greater a culture's wealth, the greater the happiness of people in the culture (Oishi, Diener, Lucan, & Suh, 1999).
2. Further cultural study is likely to reveal essential characteristics not emphasized in this section. There is evidence suggesting that Brazilians and other Latinos emphasize personal relationships ("personalism"; Hess & DeMatta, 1995); hunting and fishing societies emphasize risk taking (Barry, Bacon, & Child, 1957); many preagricultural societies emphasize respect of individual rights (Rogoff, 2003). None of these findings are well explained by individualism–collectivism or independence–interdependence. Moreover, there is evidence of individualism *and* collectivism in urban areas of collectivistic cultures (Kagitcibasi, 1997).
3. Investigators who highlight the universality of autonomy (e.g., Helwig, Arnold, Tan, & Boyd, 2003; Smetana, 2002) focus on ages, measures, and situations that pull for personal autonomy (i.e., teens' self-reported preferences regarding matters of personal jurisdiction, such as clothing), and they do not consider cultural differences in the incidence of local contexts and situations (cf. Kitayama, Markus, Matsumoto, & Norasakkunkit, 1997). Although this does not challenge their claim that autonomy is universal, it leaves open the possibility of fundamental cultural differences in its prevalence.
4. Moreover, there is some evidence that restrictive and dominating control have negative consequences in collectivistic as well as individualistic cultures (Stewart et al., 1998). Yet most studies report more restrictive control in East Asians than Euro Americans (Chao & Tseng, 2002), and high control has more positive consequences in several non-Western as compared to Western samples (Lamborn et al., 1996).

REFERENCES

Ainsworth, M. D. (1963). The development of infant-mother interaction among the Ganda. In B. M. Foss (Ed.), *The determinants of infant behaviour II* (pp. 67–112). London: Methuen.

Ainsworth, M. D. S. (1976). *System for rating maternal care behavior.* Princeton, NJ: ETS Test Collection.

Allen, J. P., & Hauser, S. T. (1996). Autonomy and relatedness in adolescent–family interactions as predictors of young adults' states of mind regarding attachment. *Development and Psychopathology, 8,* 793–809.

Allen, J. P., McElhaney, K. B., Land, D. J., Kuperminc, G. P., Moore, C. W., O'Beirne-Kelly, H., et al. (2003). A secure base in child adolescence: Markers of attachment security in the mother-adolescent relationship. *Child Development, 74,* 292–307.

Baldwin, A. (1955). *Behavior and development in childhood.* New York: Dryden Press.

Barber, B. K. (2002). *Intrusive parenting: How psychological control affects children and adolescents.* Washington, DC: American Psychological Association Press.

Barry, H., Bacon, M. K., & Child, I. L. (1957). A cross-cultural survey of some sex differences in socialization. *Journal of Abnormal and Social Psychology, 55,* 327–332.

Baumrind, D. (1971). Current patterns of parental authority. *Developmental Psychology Monographs, 4,* 1–103.

Baumrind, D. (1989). *Child development today and tomorrow.* San Francisco: Jossey-Bass.

Baumrind, D. (1991). Effective parenting during the early adolescent transition. In P. A. Cowan & E. M. Hetherington (Eds.), *Advances in family research* (Vol. 2, pp. 111–163). Hillsdale, NJ: Erlbaum.

Bell, R., & Chapman, M. (1986). Child effects in studies using experimental or brief longitudinal approaches to socialization. *Developmental Psychology, 22,* 595–603.

Bettencourt, B., & Sheldon, K. M. (2001). Social rules as mechanisms for psychological need satisfaction within social groups. *Journal of Personality and Social Psychology, 81,* 1131–1143.

Bond, M. H., & Forgas, J. P. (1984). Linking person perception to behavior intention across cultures: The role of cultural collectivism. *Journal of Cross-Cultural Psychology, 15,* 337–352.

Bowlby, J. (1973). *Attachment and loss: Vol. 2. Separation: Anxiety and anger.* New York: Basic Books.

Bowlby, J. (1982). *Attachment and loss: Vol. 1. Attachment.* New York: Basic Books. (Original work published 1969)

Bretherton, I. (1985). Attachment theory: Retrospect and prospect. In I. Bretherton & E. Waters (Eds*.),* *Monographs of the Society for Research in Child Development: Vol. 50. Growing points of attachment theory and research* (Part I, pp. 3–35). Chicago: University of Chicago Press.

Bridges, L. J. (2003). Autonomy as an element of developmental well-being. In M. H. Bornstein, L. Davidson, C. M. Keyes, & K. A. Moore (Eds.), *Well being: Positive development across the life course* (pp. 167–189). Mahwah, NJ: Erlbaum.

Bronfenbrenner, U. (1986). Ecology and the family as a context for human development: Research perspectives. *Developmental Psychology, 22,* 723–742.

Bruner, J. S. (1996). *Acts of meaning.* Cambridge, MA: Harvard University Press.

Bugental, D., & Goodnow, J. (1998). Socialization processes. In W. Damon (Series Ed.) & N. Eisenberg (Vol. Ed.), *Handbook of child psychology: Vol. 3. Social, emotional, and personality development* (5th ed., pp. 389–462). New York: Wiley.

Chao, R. K. (2000). Cultural explanations for the role of parenting in the school success of Asian-American children. In R. Taylor & M. Wang (Eds.), *Resilience across contexts: Family, work, culture, and community* (pp. 333–363). Mahwah, NJ: Erlbaum.

Chao, R., & Tseng, V. (2002). Parenting of Asians. In M. H. Bornstein (Ed.), *Handbook of parenting: Vol. 4. Social conditions and applied parenting* (2nd ed., pp. 59–93). Mahwah, NJ: Erlbaum.

Chen, X., Hastings, P., Rubin, K. H., Chen, H., Cen G., & Stewart, S. L. (1998). Childrearing attitudes and behavioral inhibition in Chinese and Canadian toddlers: A cross-cultural study. *Developmental Psychology, 34,* 677–686.

Chirkov, V. I., & Ryan, R. M. (2001). Parent and teacher autonomy support in Russian and U.S. adolescents: Common effects on well-being and academic motivation. *Journal of Cross-Cultural Psychology, 32,* 618–635.

Chirkov, V. I., Ryan, R. M., Kim, Y., & Kaplan, U. (2003). Differentiating autonomy from individualism and independence: A self-determination theory perspective on internalization of cultural orientations and well-being. *Journal of Personality and Social Psychology, 8,* 97–110

Chiu, L. H. (1987). Childrearing attitudes of Chinese, Chinese-American, and Anglo-American mothers. *Journal of Social Psychology, 128,* 411–413.

Choi, S. H. (1992). Communicative socialization processes: Korea and Canada. In S. Iwawaki, Y. Kashima, & K. Leung (Eds.), *Innovations in cross-cultural psychology* (pp. 103–121). Lisse, The Netherlands: Swets & Zeitlinger.

Clancy, P. M. (1986). The acquisition of communicative style in Japanese. In B. B. Schieffelin & E. Ochs (Eds.), *Language socialization across cultures* (pp. 213–250). New York: Cambridge University Press.

Clark, K. E., & Ladd, G. W. (2000). Connectedness and autonomy support in parent–child relationships: Links to children's socioemotional orientation and peer relationships. *Developmental Psychology, 36,* 485–498.

Cochran, M., & Niego, S. (2002). Parenting and social networks. In M. H. Bornstein (Ed.), *Handbook of parenting: Vol. 4. Social conditions and applied parenting* (2nd ed., pp. 123–148). Mahwah, NJ: Erlbaum.

Dennis, T. A., Cole, P. M., Zahn-Waxler, C., & Mizuta, I. (2002). Self in context: Autonomy and relatedness in Japanese and U.S. mother–preschooler dyads. *Child Development, 73,* 1803–1817.

Dubas, J. S., & Gerris, J. R. (2002). Longitudinal changes in the time parents spend in activities with their adolescent children as a function of age, pubertal status, and gender. *Journal of Family Psychology, 16,* 415–427.

Edwards, C. P. (1995). Parenting toddlers. In M. H. Bornstein (Ed.), *Handbook of Parenting: Vol. 1. Children and parenting* (pp. 41–63). Mahwah, NJ: Erlbaum.

Eisenberg, N., & Fabes, R. A. (1998). Prosocial development. In W. Damon (Series Ed.) & N. Eisenberg (Vol. Ed.), *Handbook of child psychology: Vol. 3. Social, emotional, and personality development* (5th ed., pp. 701–778). New York: Wiley.

Erikson, E. H. (1963). *Childhood and society.* New York: Norton. (Original work published 1950)

Erikson, E. H. (1968). *Identity, youth, and crisis.* New York: Norton.

Farver, J. M. (1989, April). *Cultural differences in American and Mexican mother–child pretend play.* Paper presented at the meeting of the Society for Research in Child Development, Kansas City, MO.

Fiske, A. P., Kitayama, S., Markus, H. R., & Nisbett, R. E. (1998). The cultural matrix of social psychology. In D. T. Gilbert, S. T. Fiske, & G. Lindzey (Eds.), *The handbook of social psychology* (2nd ed., pp. 915–981). Boston: McGraw-Hill.

Forgas, J. P., & Bond, M. H. (1985). Cultural influences on the perception of interaction episodes. *Personality and Social Psychology Bulletin, 11*, 75–88.

Friedlmeier, W., & Trommsdorff, G. (1998). Japanese and German mother-child interactions in early childhood. In G. Trommsdorff, W. Friedlmeier, & H.-J. Kornadt (Eds.), Japan in transition: Sociological and psychological aspects (pp. 217–230). Lengerich, Germany: Pabst Science.

Friedlmeier, W., & Trommsdorff, G. (2004). *Children's negative emotional reactions and maternal sensitivity in Japan and Germany.* Unpublished manuscript, Konstanz University.

Fuligni, A. J. (1998). Authority, autonomy, and parent–adolescent conflict and cohesion: A study of adolescents from Mexican, Chinese, Filipino, and European backgrounds. *Developmental Psychology, 34*, 782–792.

Fuligni, A. J., Tseng, V., & Lam, M. (1999). Attitudes toward family obligations among American adolescents with Asian, Latin American, and European family backgrounds. *Child Development, 70*, 1030–1044.

Garcia Coll, C. (1990). Developmental outcome of minority infants: A process-oriented look into our beginnings. *Child Development, 61*, 270–289.

Gardiner, H. W., Mutter, J. D., & Kosmitzki, C. (1998). *Lives across cultures: Cross-cultural human development.* Boston: Allyn & Bacon.

Graham, S. (1992). Most of the subjects were white and middle class: Trends in published research on African-Americans in selected APA journals, 1970–1989. *American Psychologist, 47*, 629–639.

Grolnick, W. S., Deci, E. L., & Ryan, R. M. (1997). Internalization within the family. In J. E. Grusec & L. Kuczynski (Eds.), *Parenting and children's internalization of values: A handbook of contemporary theory* (pp. 135–161). New York: Wiley.

Grossmann, K. E., Grossmann, K., & Keppler, A. (2005). Universal and culturally specific aspects of human behavior: The case of attachment. In W. Friedlmeier, P. Chakkarath, & B. Schwarz (Eds.), *Culture and human development: The importance of cross-cultural research to the social sciences* (pp. 75–98). New York: Psychology Press.

Grotevant, H. D. (1998). Adolescent development in family contexts. In W. Damon (Series Ed.) & N. Eisenberg (Vol. Ed.), *Handbook of child psychology: Vol. 3. Social, emotional, and personality development* (5th ed., pp. 1097–1149). New York: Wiley.

Grusec, J. E. (2002). Parental socialization and children's acquisition of values. In M. H. Bornstein (Ed.), *Handbook of parenting: Vol. 5. Practical issues in parenting* (2nd ed., pp. 143–167). Mahwah, NJ: Erlbaum.

Hara, H., & Minagawa, M. (1996). From productive dependents to precious guests: Historical changes in Japanese children. In D. W. Schwalb & B. J. Schwalb (Eds.), *Japanese childrearing: Two generations of scholarship* (pp. 9–30). New York: Guilford Press.

Harkness, S., & Super, C. (1995). Culture and parenting. In M. H. Bornstein (Ed.), *Handbook of parenting: Vol. 2. Biology and ecology of parenting* (pp. 211–234). Mahwah, NJ: Erlbaum.

Harwood, R., Leyendecker, B., Carlson, V., Asencio, M., & Miller, A. (2002). Parenting among Latino families in the U.S. In M. H. Bornstein (Ed.), *Handbook of parenting: Vol. 4. Social conditions and applied parenting* (pp. 21–46). Mahwah, NJ: Erlbaum.

Harwood, R. L., Miller, J. G., & Irizarry, N. L. (1995). *Culture and attachment: Perceptions of the child in context.* New York: Guilford Press.

Helwig, C. C., Arnold, M. L., Tan, D., & Boyd, D. (2003). Chinese adolescents' reasoning about democratic and authority-based decision making in peer, family, and school contexts. *Child Development, 74*, 783–800

Hess, D. J., & DaMatta, R. A. (Eds.). (1995). *The Brazilian puzzle. Culture on the borderlands of the western world.* New York: Columbia University Press.

Ho, D. Y. F. (1986). Chinese patterns of socialization: A critical review. In M. H. Bond (Ed.), *The psychology of Chinese people* (pp. 1–37). Hong Kong: Oxford University Press.

Hofstede, G. (1980). *Culture's consequences: International differences in work-related values.* Beverly Hills, CA: Sage.

Hofstede, G. (1991). *Cultures and organizations: Software of the mind.* London, UK: McGraw-Hill.

Hofstede, G. H. (2001). *Culture's consequences: Comparing values, behaviors, institutions and organizations across nations* (2nd ed.). Thousand Oaks, CA: Sage.

Iyengar, S. S., & Lepper, M. R. (1999). Rethinking the value of choice: A cultural perspective on intrinsic motivation. *Journal of Personality and Social Psychology, 76,* 349–366.

Jacobsen, C. (1983). What it means to be considerate: Differences in normative expectations and their implications. *Israel Social Science Research, 1,* 24–33.

Kagitcibasi, C. (1997). Individualism and collectivism. In J. Berry, M. Segall, & C. Kagitcibasi (Eds.), *Handbook of cross-cultural psychology* (2nd ed., Vol. 3, pp. 1–49). Boston: Allyn & Bacon.

Kagitcibasi, C. (2002). A model of family change in cultural context. In W. J. Lonner, D. L. Dinnel, S. A. Hayes, & D. N. Sattler (Eds.), *Online readings in psychology and culture: Unit 13: Chapter 1. Cultural perspectives on families, Western Washington University, Department of Psychology, Center for Cross-Cultural Research.* Retrieved June 20, 2006, from http://www.wwu.edu/~culture/kagitcibasi.htm.

Keller, H., Lohaus, A. Kuensemueller, P., Abels, M., Yovsi, R. D., Voelker, S., Jensen, H., et al. (2004). The bio-culture of parenting: Evidence from five cultural communities. *Parenting: Science and Practice, 4,* 25–50.

Kerr, M., & Stattin, H. (2003). Parenting of adolescents: Action or reaction? In A. C. Crouter & A. Booth (Eds.), *Children's influence on family dynamics: The neglected side of family relationships* (pp. 121–151). Mahwah, NJ: Erlbaum.

Killen, M., & Wainryb, C. (2000). Independence and interdependence in diverse cultural contexts. In S. Harkness, C. Raeff, & C. M. Super (Eds.), *New directions for child and adolescent development: Vol. 87. Variability in the social construction of the child* (pp. 5–21). San Francisco: Jossey-Bass.

Kim, U., & Choi, S.-H. (1994). Individualism, collectivism and child development: A Korean perspective. In P. M. Greenfield & R. R. Cocking (Eds.), *Cross-cultural roots of minority child development* (pp. 227–257). Hillsdale, NJ: Erlbaum.

Kitayama, S., & Markus, H. (2000). The pursuit of happiness and the realization of sympathy: Cultural patterns of self, social relations, and well-being. In E. Diener & E. Suh (Eds.), *Culture and subjective well-being* (pp. 113–161). Cambridge, MA: MIT Press.

Kitayama, S., Markus, H. R., Matsumoto, H., & Norasakkunkit, V. (1997). Individual and collective processes in the construction of the self: Self-enhancement in the United States and self-criticism in Japan. *Journal of Personality and Social Psychology, 72,* 1245–1267.

Kochanska, G., & Thompson, R. A. (1997). The emergence and development of conscience in toddlerhood and early childhood. In J. E. Grusec & L. Kuczynski (Eds.), *Parenting and children's internalization of values* (pp. 53–77). New York: Wiley.

Kohn, M. L. (1995). Social structure and personality through time and space. In P. Moen, G. H. Elder, Jr., & K. Luscher (Eds.), *Examining lives in context: Perspectives on the ecology of human development* (pp. 141–168). Washington, DC: American Psychological Association.

Kohn, M. L., & Slomczynski, K.M. (1990). *Social structure and self-direction: A comparative analysis of the United States and Poland. With collaboration of Carrie Schoenbach.* London: Basil Blackwell.

Kwak, K. (2003). Adolescents and their parents: A preview of intergenerational family relations for immigrant and non-immigrant families. *Human Development, 46,* 115–136.

Kwak, K., & Berry, J. W. (2001). Generational differences in acculturation among Asian families in Canada: A comparison of Vietnamese, Korean, and East-Indian groups. *International Journal of Psychology, 36,* 152–162.

LaGuardia, J. G., Ryan, R. M., Couchman, C., & Deci, E. L. (2000). Within-person variation in security of attachment: A self-determination theory perspective on attachment, need fulfillment, and well-being. *Journal of Personality and Social Psychology, 79,* 367–384.

Lamborn, S. D., Dornbusch, S. M., & Steinberg, L. (1996). Ethnicity and community context as moderators of the relations between family decision making and adolescent adjustment. *Child Development, 67,* 283–301.

Larner, M. (1990). Change in network resources and relationships over time. In M. Cochran, M. Larner, D. Riley, L. Gunnarsson, & C. Henderson, Jr. (Eds.), *Extending families: The social networks of parents and their children* (pp. 181–204). London and New York: Cambridge University Press.

Larson, R. W., Richards, M. H., Moneta, G., Holmbeck, G., & Duckett, E. (1996). Changes in adolescents' daily interactions with their families from ages 10 to 18: Disengagement and transformation. *Developmental Psychology, 32,* 744–754.

Lerner, R. M. (1991). Changing organism-context relations as the basic process of development: A developmental contextual perspective. *Developmental Psychology, 27,* 27–32.

LeVine, R. (1988). Human parental care: Universal goals, cultural strategies, individual behavior. *New Directions for Child Development, 40,* 3–12.

LeVine, R. A. (1990). Anthropology and child development. In C. M. Super & S. Harkness (Eds.), *Anthropological perspectives on child development* (pp. 71–86). San Francisco: Jossey-Bass.

LeVine, R. A., Dixon, S., LeVine, S., Richman, A., Leiderman, P. H., Keefer, C. H., et al. (1994). *Child care and culture: Lessons from Africa.* New York: Cambridge University Press.

LeVine, R. A., & Norman, K. (2001). The infant's acquisition of culture: Early attachment reexamined in anthropological perspective. In C.C. Morse & H.F. Matthews (Eds.), *The psychology of cultural experience* (pp. 83–104). New York: Cambridge University Press.

Lewin, K., Lippitt, R., & White, R. K. (1939). Patterns of aggressive behavior in experimentally created social climates. *Journal of Social Psychology, 10,* 271–279.

Lewis, C. (1995). *Educating hearts and minds: Reflections on Japanese preschool and elementary education.* New York: Cambridge University Press.

Lin, C-Y. C., & Fu, V. R. (1990). A comparison of child-rearing practices among Chinese, immigrant Chinese, and Caucasian-American parents. *Child Development, 61,* 429–433.

Markus, H., & Kitayama, S. (1991). Culture and the self: Implications for cognition, emotion, and motivation. *Psychological Review, 98,* 224–253.

McAdams, D. P. (1993). *The stories we live by: Personal myths and the making of the self.* New York: William Morrow.

Menon, T., Morris, M. W., Chiu, C-Y., & Hong, Y-Y. (1999). Culture and the construal of agency: Attribution to individuals versus group dispositions, *Journal of Personality and Social Psychology, 76,* 701–717.

Miller, J. G. (2003). Culture and agency: Implications for psychological theories of motivation and social development. In V. Murphy-Berman & J. Berman (Eds.), *Cross-cultural differences in perspectives on the self* (Vol. 49, pp. 59–99). Lincoln: University of Nebraska Press.

Miller, J., Bersoff, D., & Harwood, R. (1990). Perceptions of social responsibilities in India and in the United States: moral imperatives or personal decisions? *Journal of Personality and Social Psychology, 58,* 33–47.

Miller, P. J., Fung, H., & Mintz, J. (1996). Self-construction through narrative practices: A Chinese and American comparison of early socialization. *Ethos, 24,* 237–280.

Nsamenang, A. B. (1992). *Human development in cultural context: A third world perspective.* Newbury Park, CA: Sage.

Oishi, S., Diener, E. F., Lucas, R. E., & Suh, E. M. (1999). Cross-cultural variations in predictors of life satisfaction: Perspectives from needs and values. *Personality and Social Psychology Bulletin, 25,* 980–990.

Oyserman, D., Coon, H., & Kemmelmeier, M. (2002). Rethinking individualism and collectivism: Evaluation of theoretical assumptions and meta-analyses. *Psychological Bulletin, 128,* 3–73.

Peak, L. (1986). Training learning skills and attitudes in Japanese early educational settings. *New Directions for Child Development, 32,* 111–123.

Posada, G., Jacobs, A., Richmond, M. K., Carbonell, O. A., Alzate, G., Bustamante, M. R., et al. (2002). Maternal caregiving and infant security in two cultures. *Developmental Psychology, 38,* 67–78.

Rabain-Jamin, J. (1989). Culture and early social interactions: The example of mother–infant object play in African and native French families. *European Journal of Psychology of Education, 4,* 295–305.

Ramirez, M. C. (1993). *Cross-cultural differences in parent–toddler play.* Unpublished doctoral dissertation, Clark University, Worcester. MA.

Rogoff, B. (2003). *The cultural nature of human development.* Oxford, UK: Oxford University Press.

Rogoff, B., Mistry, J., Goncu, A., & Mosier, C. (1993). Guided participation in cultural activity by toddlers and caregivers. *Monographs of the Society for Research in Development, 58*(Serial No. 236).

Rohner, R., & Pettengill, S. M. (1985). Perceived parental acceptance-rejection and parental control among Korean adolescents. *Child Development, 56,* 524–528.

Rothbaum, F., & Morelli, G. (2005). Attachment and culture: Directions for future research. In W. Friedlmeier, P. Chakkarath, & B. Schwarz (Eds.), *Human development and culture: The importance of cross-cultural research to social sciences* (pp. 99–124). New York: Psychology Press.

Rothbaum, F., Morelli, G., Pott, G., & Liu-Constant, Y. (2000). Immigrant-Chinese and Euro-American parents' physical closeness with young children: Themes of family relatedness. *Journal of Family Psychology, 14,* 334–348.

Rothbaum, F., Pott, M., Azuma, H., Miyake, K., & Weisz, J. (2000). The development of close relationships in Japan and the United States: Paths of symbiotic harmony and generative tension. *Child Development, 71,* 1121–1142.

Rothbaum, F., & Tsang, B. (1998). Lovesongs in the United States and China: On the nature of romantic love. *Journal of Cross-Cultural Psychology, 29,* 306–319.

Rothbaum, F., Weisz, J., Pott, M., Miyake, K., & Morelli, G. (2000). Attachment and culture: Security in the United States and Japan. *American Psychologist, 55,* 1093–1104.

Rubin, K., Bukowski, W., & Parker, J. (1998). Peer interactions, relationships, and groups. In W. Damon (Series Ed.) & N. Eisenberg (Vol. Ed.), *Handbook of child psychology: Vol. 4. Social, emotional, and personality development* (5th ed., pp. 619–700). New York: Wiley.

Ryan, R. M., & Deci, E. L. (2000). Self-determination theory and the facilitation of intrinsic motivation, social development, and well-being. *American Psychologist, 55,* 68–78.

Saarni, C., Mumme, D. L., & Campos, J. J. (1998). Emotional development: Action, communication, and understanding. In W. Damon (Series Ed.) & N. Eisenberg (Vol. Ed.), *Handbook of child psychology: Vol. 3. Social, emotional, and personality development* (5th ed., pp. 237–309). New York: Wiley.

Schlegel, A., & Barry, H. (1991). *Adolescence: An anthropological inquiry.* New York: Free Press.

Schwartz, S. H. (2004). Mapping and interpreting cultural differences around the world. In H. Vinken, J. Soeters, & P. Ester (Eds.), *Comparing cultures: Dimensions of culture in a comparative perspective* (pp. 43–73). Leiden, The Netherlands: Brill.

Sears, R., Maccoby, E., & Levin, H. (1956). *Patterns of child rearing.* New York: Harper & Row.

Sheldon, K. M., Elliot, A. J., Kim, Y., & Kasser, T. (2001). What's satisfying about satisfying events? Comparing ten candidate psychological needs. *Journal of Personality and Social Psychology, 80,* 325–339.

Smetana, J. (2002). Culture, autonomy, and personal jurisdiction. In R. Kail & H. Reese (Eds.) *Advances in child development and behavior* (Vol. 29, pp. 52–87) Amsterdam, The Netherlands: Academic Press.

Smith, P., & Schwartz, S. (1997). Values. In J. Berry, M. Segall, & C. Kagitcibasi (Eds.), *Handbook of cross-cultural psychology: Vol. 3. Social behavior and applications* (2nd ed., pp. 78–118). Needham Heights, MA: Allyn & Bacon.

Sroufe, L. A., Fox, N. E., & Pancake, V. R. (1983). Attachment and dependency in developmental perspective. *Child Development, 54,* 1615–1627.

Steinberg, L., Dornbusch, S. M., & Brown, B. B. (1992). Ethnic differences in adolescent achievement: An ecological perspective. *American Psychologist, 47,* 723–729.

Stevenson, H. W., Chen, C., & Lee, S. (1992). Chinese families. In J. L. Roopnarine & D. B. Carter (Eds.), *Parent-child socialization in diverse cultures* (pp. 17–33). Nordwood, NJ: Ablex.

Stewart, S. M., Bond, M. H., McBride-Chang, C., Fielding, R., Deeds, O., & Westrick, J. (1998). Parent and adolescent contributors to teenage misconduct in Western and Asian high school students in Hong Kong. *International Journal of Behavioral Development, 22,* 847–869.

Suárez-Orozco, C., & Suárez-Orozco, M. (1995). *Transformations: Migration, family life, and achievement motivation among Latino adolescents.* Stanford, CA: Stanford University Press.

Tafarodi, R., Lang, J., & Smith, A. (1999). Self-esteem and the cultural trade-off: Evidence for the role of individualism-collectivism. *Journal of Cross-Cultural Psychology, 30,* 620–640.

Tobin, J. (1992). Japanese preschools and the pedagogy of selfhood. In N. R. Rosenberger (Ed.), *Japanese sense of self* (pp. 21–39). New York: Cambridge University Press.

Triandis, H. C. (1995) *Individualism and collectivism.* Boulder, CO: Westview.

Triandis, H. C. (2001). Individualism–collectivism and personality. *Journal of Personality, 69,* 907–924.

Trommsdorff, G. (1995). Parent–adolescent relations in changing societies: A cross-cultural study. In P. Noack, M. Hofer, & J. Youniss (Eds.), *Psychological responses to social change: Human development in changing environments* (pp. 189–218). Berlin, Germany: de Gruyter.

Trommsdorff, G., & Dasen, P. R. (2001). Cross-cultural study of education. In N. J. Smelser & P. B. Baltes (Eds.), *International encyclopedia of the social and behavioral sciences* (pp. 3003–3007). Oxford, UK: Elsevier.

Trommsdorff, G., & Kornadt, H.-J. (2003). Parent–child relations in cross-cultural perspective. In L. Kuczynski (Ed.), *Handbook of dynamics in parent–child relations* (pp. 271–306). Thousand Oaks, CA: Sage.

True, M. M., Pisani, L., & Oumar, F. (2001). Infant–mother attachment among the Dogon of Mali. *Child Development, 72,* 1451–1466.

Ujiie, T. (1997). How do Japanese mothers treat children's negativism? *Journal of Applied Developmental Psychology, 18,* 467–483.

Uzgiris, I. C., & Raeff, C. (1995). Play in parent–child interactions. In M. H. Bornstein (Ed.), *Handbook of parenting: Vol. 4. Applied and practical parenting* (pp. 353–376). Hillsdale, NJ: LEA.

Valsiner, J. (2001). *Comparative study of human cultural development.* Madrid, Spain: Fundación Infancia y Aprendiaje.

van IJzendoorn, M. H., & Sagi, A. (1999). Cross-cultural patterns of attachment: Universal and contextual dimensions. In J. Cassidy & P. R. Shaver (Eds.), *Handbook of attachment: Theory, research, and clinical applications* (pp. 713–734). New York: Guilford Press.

Vega, W. (1990). Hispanic families in the 1980s: A decade of research. *Journal of Marriage and the family, 52,* 1015–1024.

Vereijken, C. J. J. L., Riksen-Walraven, J. M., & Van Lieshout, C. F. M. (1997). Mother–infant relationships in Japan: Attachment, dependency, and amae. *Journal of Cross-Cultural Psychology, 28,* 442–462.

Volling, B.L. (2003). Sibling relationships. In M. H. Bornstein, L. Davidson, C. L. Keyes, K. A. Moore, & Center for Child Well-Being (Eds.), *Well-being: Positive development across the life course. Crosscurrents in contemporary psychology* (pp. 205–220). Mahwah, NJ: Erlbaum.

Watson-Gegeo, K. A., & Gegeo, D. W. (1989). The role of sibling interaction in child socialization. In P. G. Zukow (Ed.), *Sibling interactions across cultures: Theoretical and methodological issues* (pp. 54–76). New York: Springer-Verlag.

Weisner, T.S. (1984). A cross-cultural perspective: Ecocultural niches of middle childhood. In A. Collins (Ed.). *The elementary school years: Understanding development during middle childhood* (pp. 335–369). Washington, DC: National Academy Press.

Weisz, J. R., Chaiyasit, W., Weiss, B., Eastman, K., & Jackson, E. (1995) A multimethod study of problem behavior among Thai and American children in school: Teacher reports versus direct observation. *Child Development, 66,* 402–415.

Weisz, J. R., Rothbaum, F. M., & Blackburn, T. C. (1984). Standing out and standing in: The psychology of control in America and Japan. *American Psychologist, 39,* 955–969.

Whiting, B. B., & Edwards, C. P. (1988). *Children of different worlds: The formation of social behavior.* Cambridge, MA: Harvard University Press.

Whiting, B., & Whiting, J. W. (1975). *Children of six cultures.* Cambridge, MA: Harvard University Press.

Yamagishi, T. (2002). The structure of trust: An evolutionary game of mind and society. *Hokkaido Behavioral Science Report, SP-13,* 1–157.

Yamagishi, T., Cook, K. S., & Watabe, M. (1998). Uncertainty, trust, and commitment formation in the United States and Japan. *American Journal of Sociology, 104,* 165–194.

Zukow-Goldring, P. (1995). Sibling caregiving. In M. H. Bornstein (Ed.), *Handbook of parenting* (Vol. 3, pp. 177–208). Hillsdale, NJ: LEA.

CHAPTER 19

Children's Development of Cultural Repertoires through Participation in Everyday Routines and Practices

BARBARA ROGOFF, LESLIE MOORE, BEHNOSH NAJAFI, AMY DEXTER, MARICELA CORREA-CHÁVEZ, and JOCELYN SOLÍS

Although culturally rooted community routines and practices are often overlooked, they are crucial contributors to human development. They provide standing patterns of engagement to cultural participants to build on in daily activities. Engagement with the traditions of previous generations permeates everyday life, often without people reflecting on their use but yet with active participation.

This chapter discusses variation in the organization of children's involvement in cultural activities. In particular, we examine three widespread cultural traditions that organize children's learning and participation in cultural activities: intent community participation, assembly-line instruction, and guided repetition. We argue that investigating the organization of children's participation in routine activities offers a way to address the dynamic nature of *repertoires* of cultural practices—the formats of (inter)action with which individuals have experience and may take up, resist, and transform.

A focus on the cultural contributions that are central to daily routines and practices is distinct from approaches that equate culture with race or ethnicity. Clearly, cultural practices may be associated more with some such groups than with others, based on pre-

Author Jocelyn Solís passed away June 24, 2004, having brightened the world with her wisdom, her strength, and her smile.

vious generations' histories as well as forced structural limitations. However, our interest is not in racial or ethnic categories but, rather, in understanding the *cultural practices* in which children become facile, based on engagement in cultural traditions and institutions created by previous generations as well as their own.

A focus on the organization of children's participation in cultural practices offers, indeed requires, attention both to the guiding role of cultural traditions and to the active role of individuals themselves. We stress the dynamic nature of both individual participation and community traditions. People actively develop their individual histories, identifications, and resulting interests and familiarity with multiple cultural traditions, and the traditions themselves change as successive generations adapt them to current circumstances.

The organization of practices and routines in which children participate and the ways their participation is supported by others are often "invisible"; that is, they are often not made explicit by or for community members. For example, the lives of current-day North American children are regularly channeled in routine ways by institutionized aspects of everyday life, such as the usual segregation of children from opportunities to observe or participate in their community's range of mature work, and by compulsory involvement in schooling, providing exercises to introduce children to the skills and practices of their community. Some other communities provide children with much more extensive opportunities to learn through observing and contributing to ongoing community endeavors (Rogoff, 2003). Although few North American researchers, policymakers, or parents take note of these routine organizers of childhood, these play a powerful role in creating the settings that children frequent, their roles, and the routine activities in which children engage.

Relatedly, many cultural practices on a more intimate scale may be taken for granted but serve to organize the life experience of children. For middle-class North American children, for example, these often include routine involvement in bedtime stories, sleeping in a separate room, following local gender role expectations, and being encouraged to structure show-and-tell narratives in a particular manner and regulate peer access to possessions by taking turns.

Tacit, routine expectations of everyday life are likely to be among the most powerful cultural experiences—especially *because* they are expected and unexamined by most participants (Rogoff, 2003). As Bourdieu (1977) suggested, through experience with one's environment and routine performances, strong dispositions develop that may be beyond the grasp of consciousness, relatively impervious to efforts to change them or even to articulate them. Tacit lessons from participation in everyday life about who may participate, how, and when may be difficult for participants to identify, but such unspoken community expectations and values are a key part of how people organize their interactions. As Rheingold argued, development is a process of becoming familiar with the environment and with one's interactions with the worlds it involves; each new skill becomes "submerged in consciousness" (1985, p. 5), with the effort to achieve it forgotten as it becomes familiar.

Further, children develop fluency in multiple forms of participation, based on the multiple traditions in which they routinely engage. We argue that as children move across settings that involve different formats for participation, they actively engage in variable ways relating to their own *repertoire of practice*. This concept helps to focus on children's own agency in selecting, rejecting, and transforming multiple ways of engaging in the world. In the process, children in turn contribute to the formation of the routines and practices available to the next generation.

Our interest in the organization of children's cultural participation and their repertoires of practice relates to some complementary approaches that focus on the cultural organization of children's everyday lives in terms of the settings and goals of childrearing.

CULTURAL ASPECTS OF CHILDREN'S EVERYDAY SETTINGS

Several lines of scholarship have focused on the socialization of children into the ways of their communities by examining the niches and activity settings of children's lives. These approaches, and our own, have been heavily influenced by the work of Beatrice Whiting, who focused on the role of children's settings and the company they keep:

> Whether it is caring for an infant sibling, working around the house in the company of adult females, working on the farm with adults and siblings, playing outside with neighborhood children, hunting with adult males, or attending school with age mates, the daily assignment of a child to one or another of these settings has important consequences on the development of habits of interpersonal behavior, consequences that may not be recognized by the socializers who make the assignments. (Whiting, 1980, p. 111)

The cast of characters and scenario are closely related to the activities in which children routinely engage. For example, Whiting and Whiting (1975) found, in six cultural communities, that heavy involvement with agemates was associated with children's aggressiveness and egoism, whereas heavy involvement with younger children was associated with nurturance. The six communities they studied differed greatly in the frequency with which children inhabited settings involving agemates (e.g., in school) versus younger children (e.g., in communities where child caregiving was routine).

Subsequent work has elaborated these ecological ideas (along with others, such as those of Barker & Wright, 1954) to examine the arrangements that characterize children's opportunities to learn in different communities. Several scholars use the idea of *activity settings* or *ecocultural niches*, which include the personnel who engage with children; motivations of the actors in the setting; cultural scripts that guide conduct, tasks, and routine activities; and cultural goals and beliefs (Tharp & Gallimore, 1988; Weisner, 1984; Weisner, Gallimore, & Jordan, 1988). Relatedly, the ideas of *developmental niche* or *cognitive developmental niche* focus on the physical and social settings in which children develop; the customs of childrearing that parents negotiate; and scripts, routines, and rituals that instantiate cultural goals and values in socially organized ways, along with material and symbolic tools used to achieve cultural goals (Gauvain, 1995; Harkness & Super, 1992, 2002). Gauvain pointed out that what children gain from particular experiences is strengthened by a commonality or redundancy that is "largely rooted in culture" (2004, p. 13).

The focus on scripts in these approaches, which connects with our emphasis on the organization of children's participation, builds on Bartlett's (1932) notion of scripts as cultural expectations of how events are organized within a particular community. Schank and Abelson (1977) referred to scripts as being specific to a situation or context and involving several "players" who share an understanding of a sequence of events, such as the way people behave in a movie theater, at dinner, or at a bank. Use and understanding of such scripts for cultural routines appear in early childhood (Nelson & Gruendel, 1988).

The scripts involved in children's settings are closely related to cultural goals that guide parents' childrearing practices and children's experiences (Goodnow, 1992; Harkness & Super, 1992, 2002). LeVine (1980) proposed that parents in differing circumstances prioritize distinct goals, ranging from the physical survival and health of their children to their economic security to achieving locally valued goals such as social status, religious piety, and self-actualization. For example, Gusii (Kenyan) mothers engaged in a period of intensive protective care, reflecting their primary goal of ensuring their infants' survival in a community in which infant mortality was high (LeVine et al., 1994). In contrast, mothers in London, with far less reason to be worried about their infants' survival, were greatly concerned with preparing their infants for school and engaged extensively in pedagogical games and lessons.

Although parents' goals and practices modify with changing circumstances, such as immigration (Rosenthal & Roer-Strier, 2001), they often do not change as rapidly as the circumstances do. LeVine (1980) suggested that childrearing practices are solutions to problems of rearing children that parents inherit from the previous generation, whose immediate circumstances are likely to have differed in some ways. Thus, cultural variations in childrearing practices and children's routines are intimately tied to the histories of communities in which families participate. Our chapter elaborates on the organization of children's participation in terms of how children engage in the culturally and historically developed routines and practices of their communities.

THE ORGANIZATION OF PARTICIPATION

We argue that understanding children's development requires attention to how they become familiar with particular ways of organizing their involvement in the routine activities of their lives. Such organization ranges in "grain size" from the broad organization of their daily routines to the organization of specific activities and moment-by-moment interactions. Broad traditions organize children's opportunities to learn in generally recognizable formats—such as children's involvement in formal Western schooling of the late 1900s, indigenous children's traditional learning through involvement in community activities, and children's religious training in catechism or Koranic schooling.

Broad arrangements for children's learning are themselves routinely composed of particular formats that organize a particular activity or moment-by-moment interaction. For example, Western schooling frequently employs a format in which the teacher asks questions to which she already knows the answer, a student or the class responds briefly, and the teacher evaluates the response and goes on to another known-answer question (Mehan, 1979). This format is seldom used outside school, especially in communities in which schooling is not prevalent. (As we describe later, familiarity with this format is usually part of the repertoire of children whose families have participated in Western schooling for generations.)

The formats organizing children's participation in cultural activities provide standing patterns of engagement—cultural infrastructures of everyday life. Such formats are key among the resources humans draw on to coordinate their behavior in social encounters. Social scientists have examined how participation in social encounters is organized, examining practices ranging from those that characterize a whole activity, such as doing a seminar or preparing onions for market, to a single moment in an encounter, such as a three-turn known-answer question with teacher initiation, student response, and teacher evaluation.

Anthropologists, sociologists, and linguists have provided valuable approaches to the study of social organization of peoples' participation in cultural activities. Sociologist Erving Goffman (1979, 1981) inspired several lines of scholarship that address how humans organize social interaction. He introduced the concepts of *participation status*, the particular relation that any one person has with what is being said (e.g., animator, author, and principal), and *participation framework*, the overall configuration of the collection of individuals' participation statuses at a given time in a particular situation. Marjorie Goodwin (1990) has since expanded on Goffman's work with her concept of *participant framework*.

Susan Philips, a student of Goffman, introduced the concept of *participant structure*, (Philips, 1983, 2001), defining it as a particular type of encounter or structural arrangement of interaction. Based on her research in a Native American community and the school attended by its children, Philips proposed four basic participant structures in classroom interaction, which vary in the number of students interacting with a teacher, how children's attention is organized, and how turns at talk are allocated and regulated (the whole class interacts with a teacher; small-group format; teacher–student one-on-one format; and individual desk work).

Philips examined mismatches between the participant structures prevalent in the children's homes and their school. She noted that the children did not readily conform to Anglo norms for classroom participation, being accustomed to a high degree of autonomy in determining when or if they will speak and to organizing their peer-group activities such that individuals were rarely singled out. Warm Springs Indian children were less willing than their Anglo peers to speak alone in front of the class or to speak at moments determined by the teacher, both of which were key practices within the classroom. Philips's study has influenced much of the subsequent research into the nature and impact of home–school mismatches with regard to the organization of participation.

Building on work by Goffman and Philips, Fred Erickson (1982) teased apart task structure and interactional/communicative norms of the *social participation structure*. Social participation structure is the allocation of interactional rights and obligations of participants that shape the discourse; that is, what speaking and listening behaviors are required of or allowed for different participants, and what are the canonical patterns of turn taking.

Attention to the organization of participation is especially productive for expanding understanding of cultural contributions to human development because it brings a focus on individual agency together with a focus on community traditions. Individuals are active in becoming involved in and making use of community traditions (or bucking or changing them). At the same time, the formats available to organize individuals' roles and connect them with community traditions and related institutions contribute to the ongoing organization of individuals' participation. Thus, focusing on the organization of participation helps us see the mutually constituting nature of individual, interpersonal, and community contributions to the everyday lives and learning of children. The focus on standing patterns of action and interaction helps to underline the dynamic nature of both individual and community processes.

Research on the organization of participation provides a tool for empirical work on cultural variation in how adults and children structure and coordinate their participation in shared endeavors. For example, the use of known-answer questions is common and familiar in some communities but unfamiliar in others; in some communities learning through observation and "eavesdropping" are especially important whereas in other communities verbal explanations seem to take precedence; teasing exchanges are valued tools of socialization and humor in some communities whereas in others they are regarded as hostile forms of interaction; some communities favor multiparty engagements over dyadic or solo ones and vice versa (Rogoff, 2003). The unspoken "rules" or "grammars" of interaction vary across cultural communities in somewhat systematic ways (Kendon, 1990; Heath, 1986; Hutchins & Palen, 1997).

In the next section we examine such variations as they contribute to three broad multidimensional traditions of learning practices: *intent community participation*, in which children have access to observe and begin to contribute to ongoing endeavors of their community; *assembly-line instruction*, in which teaching is organized by experts around specialized exercises to introduce children to the skills and practices of their community without allowing or necessarily anticipating actual productive involvement; and *guided repetition*, in which novices learn by observing, imitating, and rehearsing models presented by experts. After examining these three historical traditions organizing learning, we discuss how children develop their repertoires of multiple practices with which they are somewhat familiar and fluent.

THREE TRADITIONS OF LEARNING

A recent article by several of us delineated features of two widespread cultural traditions of learning practices, which we called intent participation and assembly-line instruction (Rogoff, Paradise, Arauz, Correa-Chávez, & Angelillo, 2003). We defined these using an image of prisms in order to emphasize the integration and coherence of the multidimensional features of these culturally and historically developed traditions—features that we displayed on the facets of the prisms. The traditions each have an internal "logic" or "grammar" (usually not articulated or perhaps even noticed by those involved in the practice) that make them coherent fields of practice.

Here, we present revised versions of the prisms from Rogoff et al. (2003). One important revision is a change of name: We now refer to intent *community* participation in order to draw attention to the cultural, collective, historical nature of this learning tradition, to try to avoid it being interpreted simply in terms of individual behavior or interpersonal interaction. We consider the current versions of the prisms to still be works-in-progress. For example, the facets that we show are not necessarily the only relevant ones—more facets/features could be added—and the articulation of the features that we include undoubtedly needs further revision.[1]

The prisms represent "pure" forms that define constellations of features that we argue fit together as whole cultural traditions. In life, however, there are often mixtures or resemblances of different traditions, not just pure forms. Even in efforts to follow a "pure" tradition, everyday activity involves "seepage" in practice. (Indeed, this seepage may be a strength allowing for adaptation of the tradition to circumstances or supporting transformation.) In addition, the generic forms portrayed in the prisms vary in specific characteristics when instantiated within a particular community or institution, at the same time as fitting the generic form of the prism.

The facets of each prism follow a standard template, to encourage analysis of the interdependent features of each prism along similar lines, and to offer a template to others for analyzing other traditions of learning besides those we examine. The template is shown in Figure 19.1.

Because the prisms articulate *integrated* features of whole historically developed cultural learning traditions, the facets form a constellation of features to be considered as a whole. Taken singly, a particular facet/feature does not define a learning tradition; a particular facet/feature is likely to fit with a number of distinct learning traditions. For example, one feature of the intent community participation tradition involves learning through keen attention during participation in shared endeavors. But by itself, learning through keen attention does not define the tradition of intent community participation; it may fit several learning traditions. That is, attentiveness does not necessarily indicate that what is going on fits with the intent community participation tradition—the other facets also need to fit, to make the constellation of the whole. Intent community participation also necessarily involves other features, including learners' access to observe the valued community activity in question, with ongoing or anticipated participation, with learning focused on becoming able to contribute to the endeavor.

Hence, to investigate a learning tradition, one cannot simply glance at one or two features of a scenario to see if the moment fits with a facet or two of a particular learning tradition. A more global analysis of an event is required to determine whether all the facets of a learning tradition are present. The prisms thus do not serve as coding schemes for examining brief moments of interaction. (However, more global coding can be done. For a global coding scheme examining 20- to 40-minute interactions for their fit with a multi-

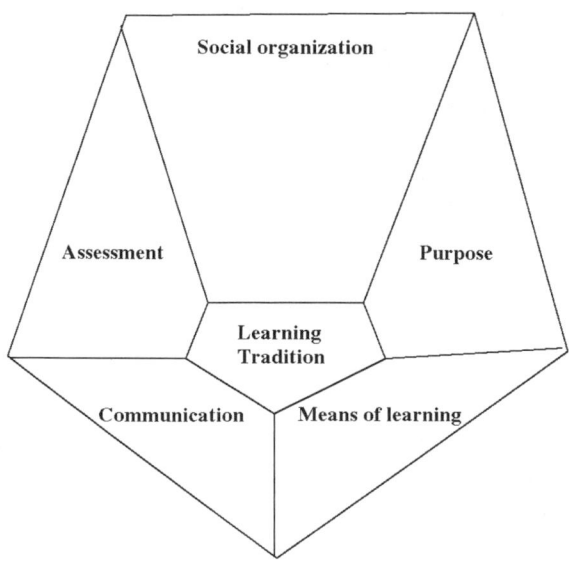

FIGURE 19.1. Template for prisms showing facets of distinct learning traditions.

dimensional constellation, see Matusov & Rogoff's [2002] study of which philosophy-in-action was used by adults interacting with small groups of children.)

In the remainder of this section, we examine three cultural learning traditions that have widespread use. We begin with the two that were described by Rogoff et al. (2003)—intent participation and assembly-line instruction—adding important clarifying revisions, and then we examine the cultural tradition of learning by guided repetition.

Intent Community Participation

Intent community participation is a widely practiced and long-standing tradition in which people learn by actively observing and "listening in" during ongoing community activities and contributing when ready, to activities as varied as weaving, conversing, reading, using statistics, or programming computers. Figure 19.2 shows key facets of the cultural tradition of learning through intent community participation.

Intent community participation is especially prevalent in some communities in which children are routinely included in the range of mature endeavors of daily community life. In other communities, being excluded from many mature settings makes it difficult for children to observe and participate in the full range of economic and social activities (Morelli, Rogoff, & Angelillo, 2003; Rogoff, Mistry, Göncü, & Mosier, 1993; Whiting & Whiting, 1975).

If children are integrated in a wide range of community settings, they are able to observe and listen in on ongoing activities as *legitimate peripheral participants* (Lave & Wenger, 1991). For example, children learned through eavesdropping in an African American community where toddlers participated in daily community events and spent hours quietly listening to adults converse (Ward, 1971). Inuit men of Arctic Quebec re-

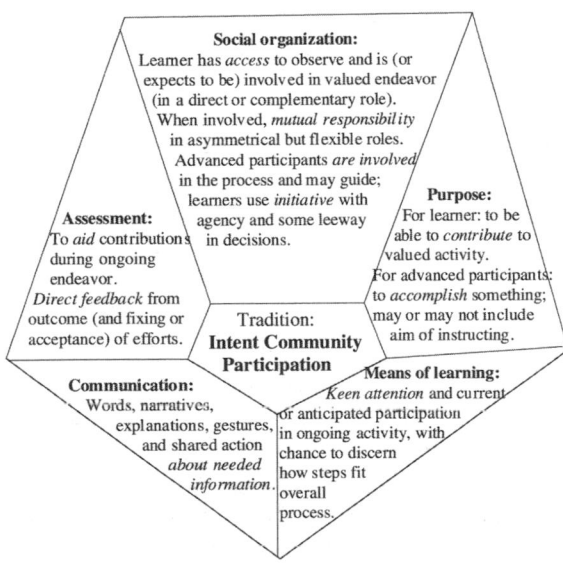

FIGURE 19.2. Prism showing key facets (features) of the cultural tradition of intent community participation.

ported that as boys, they learned to hunt from just watching the men and learned vocabulary and many other things by listening to stories that were not intended for them (Crago, 1992).

In communities in which they have access to learning by observing from the periphery, children may also learn as they function as full participants in important endeavors. They can begin to "pitch in," contributing to their families' social and economic lives from a young age (Orellana, 2001; Paradise, 1987; Rogoff, 2003). For example, in an East African farming community, 3- to 4-year-old children spent 25–35% of their time doing chores, compared with 0–1% for middle-class U.S. children of the same ages (Harkness & Super, 1992).

Jordan (1989) describes how Yucatecan Mayan girls whose mothers and grandmothers are midwives absorb the essence of midwifery practice as well as specific knowledge simply in the process of growing up. They are surrounded by the routines and practices and pitch in as they become able to assist.

> They know what the life of a midwife is like (for example, that she needs to go out at all hours of the day or night), what kinds of stories the women and men who come to consult her tell, what kinds of herbs and other remedies need to be collected, and the like. As young children they might be sitting quietly in a corner as their mother administers a prenatal massage; they would hear stories of difficult cases, of miraculous outcomes, and the like. As they grow older, they may be passing messages, running errands, getting needed supplies. A young girl might be present as her mother stops for a postpartum visit after the daily shopping trip to the market.
>
> Eventually, after she has had a child herself, she might come along to a birth, perhaps because her ailing grandmother needs someone to walk with, and thus find herself doing for the woman in labor what other women had done for her when she gave birth; that is, she may take a turn with the other women in the hut at supporting the laboring woman, holding her on her lap, breathing and pushing with her. After the baby is born, she may help with the clean-up and if the midwife doesn't have time to look in on mother and baby, she may do so and report on their condition. . . . Her mentor sees their association primarily as one that is of some use to her ("Rosa already knows how to do a massage, so I can send her if I am too busy"). . . .
>
> In societies where [this sort of] apprenticeship learning is the routine unmarked way of knowledge acquisition, it is also the case that there is little differentiation between work and play. Children, and old people, do partial or somewhat defective jobs which are, however, appreciated for whatever use value they may have. This use value is keenly appreciated both by children and by adults, and children will generally, on their own, prefer activities that have societal value. Thus children in Yucatan prefer taking care of real babies to playing with dolls. (p. 932)

Although the range of opportunities for children to be involved in ongoing mature activities tends to be limited in middle-class settings (Morelli et al., 2003), intent community participation also occurs in such communities. Most important, children's impressive learning of their first language occurs through opportunities to observe and begin to pitch in to shared communicative endeavors where the aim is getting things accomplished with words (beyond the language lessons that some children receive). Young children are also generally attracted to engage in the activities of those around them. For example, middle-class toddlers are attracted to objects used by adults and tend to carry out markedly similar actions on them, and they may spontaneously help their parents or a stranger in household chores (Eckerman, Whatley, & McGhee, 1979; Hay, Murray, Cecire, & Nash, 1985; Rheingold, 1982). Middle-class children often learn to use computers by engaging with other children and adults who use them in ways that are consistent with intent community participation.

Central to the constellation of cultural practices related to intent community participation is "being there" during valued activities and having opportunities to contribute. U.S. children whose parents work at home are often involved in their parents' work, in a progression from watching to carrying out simple tasks to giving regular assistance to regular work (Beach, 1988). Likewise, if given the opportunity to participate, children may become part of community political action. For example, one of us (JS) observed that children in undocumented Mexican immigrant families in New York, even very young ones, became involved in political action as they accompanied parents to immigrants' rights rallies. The children publicly protested and enacted a form of political participation, learning by observing (rather than through direct, explicit discussion with parents) that rights and fair treatment are to be demanded in a society in which injustice is real and part of everyday life.

When learners become involved in activities in the intent community participation tradition, engagement with more experienced community members is coordinated in a reciprocal (though usually asymmetrical) manner, with mutual responsibility and respect for each others' contributions. Roles are taken up with flexibility, such that people can anticipate playing other roles in the activity at other times (such as aiding others in learning). Flexibility also occurs in the means of contribution, as participants have some room to maneuver within their role. They are expected to contribute as they are able and tend not to be micromanaged in specific actions. People (including newcomers to an activity) are expected to contribute and coordinate around shared family and community endeavors like members of an orchestra.

Assembly-Line Instruction

Assembly-line instruction involves transmission of information from experts, in specialized exercises outside the context of productive, purposive activity (see Figure 19.3). It is common in many schools and middle-class family interactions, in communities in which children are routinely segregated from many mature settings. Of course, assembly-line instruction is not the only way that schooling and middle-class parent–child interactions are organized. For example, some schools operate according to philosophies related to intent community participation (Rogoff, Goodman Turkanis, & Bartlett, 2001; Sato, 1996).

However, assumptions and practices regarding learning in middle-class communities (at home as well as at school, and among developmental psychologists) are heavily influenced by the centrality of particular school formats that became prevalent when mass, compulsory schooling became widespread, about a century ago. School-based assembly-line instruction was explicitly modeled on the organization of factories, with learners (and teachers too, often) treated as part of a mechanism designed by administrators or consultants for bureaucratic efficiency (Callahan, 1962). This tradition is based on a mechanical metaphor, with experts inserting information into children, as raw materials, and sorting them in terms of their quality and the extent to which they have received the information.

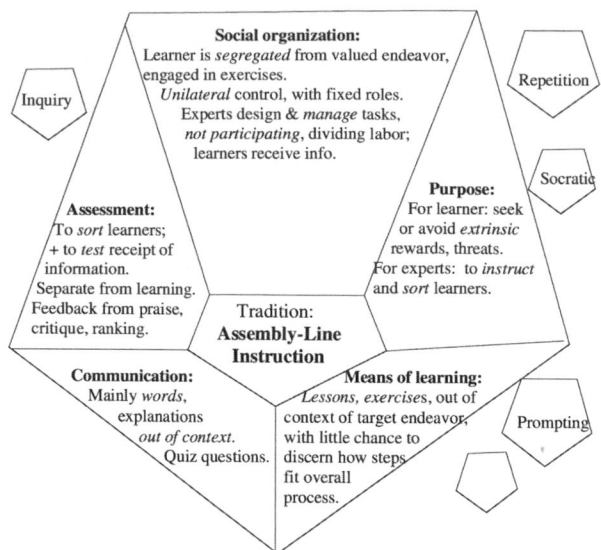

FIGURE 19.3. Prism showing key facets (features) of the cultural tradition of assembly-line instruction.

An example of bureaucratic control of learners is the common "switchboard participant structure" (Philips, 1983) in which teachers take a speaking turn between each child turn and decide which children contribute to class activities. Echoes of this format can also be seen in dinner conversations of Caucasian families in Hawaii, where children raised their hand for a turn and parents managed the children's turns to talk and encouraged the children to give accounts of events of their day in a style that resembles school forms of reporting (Martini, 1995).

Middle-class European American families have extensive experience with the formats of formal schooling, usually over several generations, and they often engage young children in a variety of practices related to school formats. For example, they frequently engage their children in lessons and school-like discourse formats including known-answer questions. Rather than children joining adults in community work and social activities, middle-class adults often engage in children's play and child-focused exercises in which adults manage children's attention and help them practice school-relevant skills in play (Blount, 1972; Haight, 1991; Harkness, 1977; Heath, 1983; Martini, 1995; Morelli et al., 2003; Schieffelin & Ochs, 1986).

For example, middle-class mothers in the United States and Turkey more often engaged their toddlers in language lessons and school-like quizzes about properties of objects than did mothers in a tribal community in India and a Mayan community where schooling was not prevalent (Rogoff et al., 1993). Similarly, middle-class European American 3-year-olds more often engaged with adults in scholastic play (like the alphabet song) and in free-standing conversations with adults on child-related topics than did 3-year-olds in a foraging community in the Democratic Republic of Congo and an agricultural community in Guatemala, where children had more opportunity to observe adult work and frequently emulated these themes in their play (Morelli et al., 2003). The specialized child-focused formats and exercises that young middle-class children experience can be seen as a way to aid them in assembling skills for later entry in mature activities from which they are often excluded as children.

As shown in the prism, the social organization of assembly-line instruction involves segregating learners from ongoing community activities and instead managing them in exercises designed to induce transmission of information, exercises that seldom yield a useful product or outcome for the larger community. Experts/teachers direct learners in a unilateral manner without participating in the same activity, and without flexibility in the management/managed roles. Understanding how a particular step fits an overall process or purpose is not regarded as necessary to learning; the mechanical exercise of going through the steps is the focus. The learners' involvement is managed with external inducements (such as praise, grades, and threats), with assessments aiming to determine the overall quality of both the raw materials and the transmission of information (in assessments of IQ as well as the extent of receipt of the curriculum "delivered"). Communication is heavily reliant on words (often in specialized formats such as known-answer questions), in the absence of shared productive endeavors.

The contrast between assembly-line instruction and intent community participation is particularly clear in De Haan's (2001) study of Mazahua (indigenous Mexican) children engaged in a building task with either their parents or a non-Mazahua teacher. The parents treated the children as responsible contributors to a shared endeavor, in which children coordinated with the parents and sometimes led the effort. Children were expected to learn by watching the parent's contribution while they participated and to take on more responsibility as the joint activity proceeded, but they were not forced to. In contrast, when the children worked with non-Mazahua teachers, the teacher held the initiative and expected the child to perform the task under the teacher's directions. If the children made suggestions, these were evaluated by the teachers as a test of the children's knowledge, not treated as a contribution to a task that needed to be done.

The use of particular cultural traditions for organizing learning (such as assembly-line instruction and intent community participation) is dynamic, not fixed and stable. People who have been raised mostly within one tradition of learning may switch their approach to another when they have experience in a tradition new to them (or they may blend or otherwise revise the traditions, or resist them). For example, schooled mothers from communities that are newly adopting Western schooling more often interact with children in some school-like ways—including praise, lessons, and assignment of divided tasks—than mothers with little or no schooling from the same communities (Chavajay & Rogoff, 2002; Rabain-Jamin, 1989; Richman, Miller, & LeVine, 1992; Rogoff et al., 1993). Similarly, middle-class parent volunteers in a collaborative school were more likely to engage with children in ways that fit with intent community participation than parents with less such experience, even though the prior schooling of almost all the parents was similar to assembly-line instruction (Matusov & Rogoff, 2002; Rogoff et al., 2001).

The processes of intent community participation and assembly-line instruction are not specific to particular types of activities or "subject" matter (such as practical vs. theoretical endeavors, or "concrete" vs. "abstract" information). For example, learning statistics can occur through intent community participation as one learns how to use statistics to carry out ongoing research, or using an assembly-line instruction model in a class in which the material is studied in isolation from its use, without any involvement in research. Likewise, intent community participation was very effective for traditional Maori (New Zealand) children's learning of both abstract spiritual knowledge and practical skills (Metge, 1984).

Several other prisms are indicated in the diagram showing the prism for assembly-line instruction, to emphasize that there are a number of cultural learning traditions that deserve greater understanding, so that we can consider alternative arrangements for learning. One of the other prisms is identified as repetition.

Guided Repetition

Guided repetition (or "recitation") is a tradition of teaching and learning that involves modeling by the expert and imitation of the model by a novice, with memorization through rehearsal and performance by the novice (Moore, 2004b). The expert supervises the novice in each phase and may provide assistance, evaluation, and/or correction as the novice attempts to master the new skill (see Figure 19.4). In communities around the globe, guided repetition is used to teach and learn a wide range of skills, including music, athletics, and crafts. Perhaps the most common use of guided repetition is in the teaching of texts (oral or written).

Since it fell out of favor in the late 19th and early 20th centuries with the advance of the progressive education movement, guided repetition has been disparaged and dismissed by most Western educators and researchers (Hori, 1996). It is now widely believed—but not proven—to have a negative influence on children's cognitive abilities, fostering the development of memory skills at the expense of so-called higher cognitive skills such as logical and creative thinking (Wagner, 1983). However, guided repetition continues to be part of the educational experience of millions of children around the world, in both religious and secular contexts. Despite its long history, global prevalence, and characterization by Western educators as a problem to be remedied, this tradition has received very little analytic attention and is poorly understood. (Exceptions include work by Scribner & Cole, 1981a, 1981b; Wagner, 1983, 1993.)

Guided repetition is historically rooted in the teaching of sacred texts. In the reli-

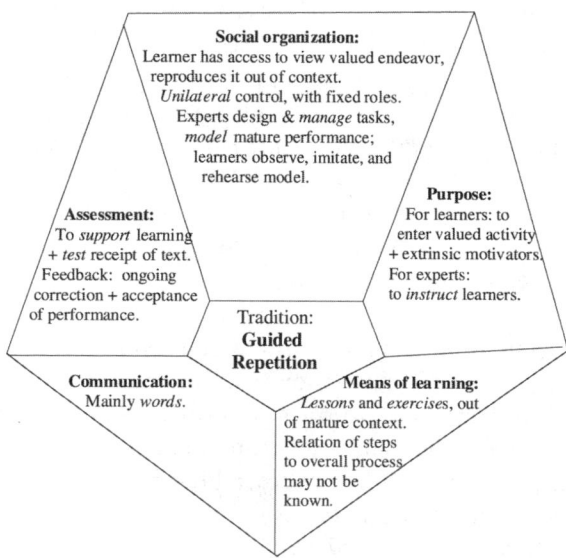

FIGURE 19.4. Prism showing key facets (features) of the cultural tradition of learning through guided repetition.

gions that have promoted literacy—including Judaism, Christianity, Islam, Hinduism, Buddhism, and Confucianism—traditional pedagogy places "a strong emphasis on verbatim oral mastery of a body of essential written teachings and ritual" (Wagner, 1983, p. 112). In many communities, learning sacred texts by heart is the path into literacy and verbatim recitation the preferred way to attain and display knowledge (e.g., Ariès, 1962; Heath, 1983; Nash, 1968; Tambiah, 1968).

The memorization of a fixed body of knowledge may serve as the basis for application to *new* contexts and materials and the development of new understanding. For example, some Fulbe who have memorized the Koran build on this foundation, developing a high degree of competence in Arabic as a second language (Moore, 2004b). Hori (1996) argued that the formalism of rote learning in a Zen monastery is an important route to insight. He argued that this process resembles the process of learning propositional logic in a university philosophy class. He noticed that the students who could solve logic problems had memorized the basic transformation formulas and as a result they could "just see" common factors to cancel out in the equations or "just see" logical equivalences. The students who had not memorized the formulas were mystified by the problems, trying to reason their way through them without the logical insight that the others had developed through rote memorization.

Built on the foundations of religious education, secular schooling also often uses guided repetition. Repetition and memorization figure prominently in descriptions of East Asian educational practice and the learning styles of Asian students (Biggs, 1996; Ho, 1994; Li & Fischer, 2004; On, 1996; Schneider, Hieshima, Lee, & Plank, 1994). Western education has long emphasized memorization, too. For centuries, the recitation and memorization of Greek and Latin texts constituted a large part of curricula in European schools (Carruthers, 1992; Cubberley, 1922; Nash, 1968). Until the late 1800s, European and North American pedagogical practices emphasized textbook memorization (Ariès, 1962; Cubberley, 1922). Currently in the United States, there is growing interest in classical (Christian) education, which emphasizes memorization of a body of knowledge in the early years of education, leaving analysis and discussion to later stages (e.g., Bluedorn & Bluedorn, 2000; Wilson, 1991, 2003).

As in assembly-line instruction, roles within guided repetition are generally unilateral and fixed. The expert's responsibilities are to model the text or skill correctly and in suitable increments and to monitor, correct, and evaluate the learner as he or she attempts to imitate, rehearse, and master it. In addition to tests for mastery, assessment is often ongoing, with errors being corrected immediately or soon after they are committed in order to support learning.

Guided repetition activities are specialized and learner-focused lessons, but unlike assembly-line instruction, they do not necessarily occur in settings that are removed from adult activities. In many communities, religious instruction takes place at the temple or mosque, where learners may observe more competent community members as they recite sacred texts in the context of daily ritual. Moreover, learners may "apply" lessons in their own emergent ritual practice. Thus, learners may understand the purpose and importance of what they are learning. (Such understanding, however, may not be regarded as necessary to learning.)

As noted previously for the two other traditions, the use of guided repetition is dynamic. In a study of language socialization in an urban Fulbe community in northern Cameroon, Moore (2004a) observed changes in how guided repetition was structured and the domains in which it was used. In the Koranic schools of this community, children have long been taught one-on-one to recite, read, and write the Koran. As Fulbe partici-pation in public schooling has increased, however, the public school practice of collective instruction (in addition to individual instruction) has come to be used in a growing num-ber of Koranic schools. Guided repetition has also seeped from school into homes. Whereas Fulbe children once learned folktales only through intent community participa-tion, many now learn through guided repetition (Moore, 2006).

Although certain traditions and practices may be more prevalent in a given commu-nity, people generally participate in a variety of traditions and practices as they engage in the different activities that constitute their daily lives. Institutions and individuals develop *repertoires* of practices that may be culturally distinct in their roots but spread with con-tact among communities and individuals. Repertoires reflect both the agency of individu-als who build them and the cultural/historical organization of routines and practices.

REPERTOIRES OF PRACTICE

According to Webster, a *repertoire* is the set of operas, songs, and parts that can readily be performed by members of a company because they have practiced or performed them many times. (The term is derived from the Latin, *to find again.*) We use the term "reper-toire" to describe the variety of practices with which individuals are familiar, yielding a disposition to apply different formats under distinct circumstances. The idea of *reper-toires of practice* addresses the fact that people engage in multiple traditions (Gutiérrez & Rogoff, 2003; Rogoff, 2003; Zentella, 1998). Through their lives and the different en-deavors in which they engage, people develop fluency with a variety of formats for partic-ipation.

In Figure 19.5, Jean Piaget shows his attempt to expand his repertoire to include skills in a practice new to him, during a visit to Kyoto, Japan. (Note the keen attention he employs to try to learn from Bärbel Inhelder's approach.)

A number of scholars have made use of the concept of *repertoire* (e.g., Davies & Harré, 1990; Elbers & De Haan, 2002; Erickson, 2004; Rogoff et al., 2003), which in some ways resembles Bourdieu's concept of *habitus*—"systems of durable, transposable *dispositions*" (1977, p. 72). In sociolinguistics, the term "repertoire" refers to the range of languages or varieties of a language available for use by a speaker, each of which en-ables her to perform a particular social role or purpose. Gutiérrez, Baquedano-López, and Tejeda (1999) pointed out that the linguistic repertoires of students are tools for their participation and meaning-making in the classroom. Gutiérrez and Rogoff noted that children with differing experience with distinct cultural traditions vary in their repertoires

> for engaging in discussions with authority figures, answering known-answer questions, an-alyzing word problems on the basis of counterfactual premises, seeking or avoiding being singled out for praise, spontaneously helping classmates, observing ongoing events without adult management, responding quickly or pondering ideas before volunteering their contri-butions, and many other approaches. (2003, p. 22)

People's repertoires of practice describe the formats they are likely to employ in up-coming situations, based on their own prior experience in similar settings. Repertoires of practice are highly constrained by people's opportunities and access to participate directly

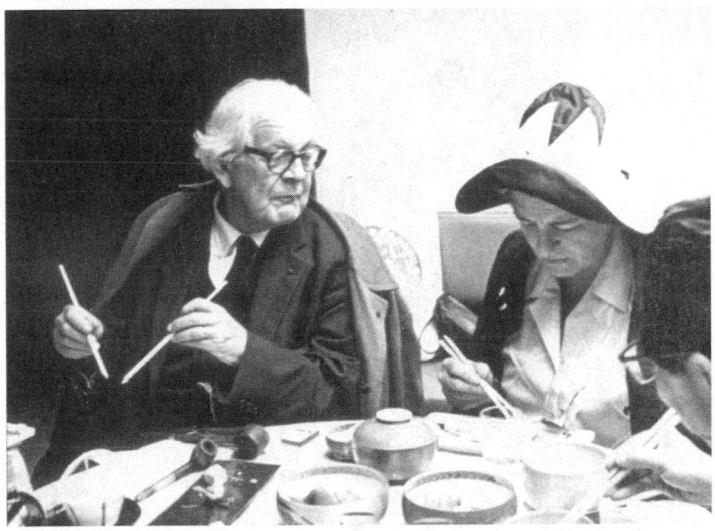

FIGURE 19.5. Jean Piaget attempting to expand his repertoire to include skill in a practice new to him. Photograph courtesy Matsui Kimio.

or vicariously in settings and activities where particular formats are employed. For example, children who are newcomers to classroom organization are less skilled in aligning their participation with the structure of lessons and the conversational formats employed in their classroom; at the end of the school year they are much more effective in following and using the structure of classroom formats, including instruction-response-evaluation sequences (Mehan, 1979). We could say that their repertoire comes to include some dexterity in participating in instruction–response–evaluation sequences, among other classroom formats. And in the next school year, they may be more likely to engage in this manner in another teacher's classroom.

Although people's readiness, efficiency, fluency, and dexterity in engaging in a particular practice depend on familiarity with the specific practice or similar ones, at the same time, the agency of individuals is key. Individuals choose (with or without reflection) among the formats with which they are familiar and they may actively transform or reject engagement in particular formats as they navigate the different settings of their lives.

In Figure 19.6, which was taken right after the photograph shown in Figure 19.5, Jean Piaget illustrates the idea that individuals' agency and familiarity with particular practices play a role in their engagement with particular practices.

An example of children determining which approach to use from their repertoire can be seen in research on Pima Indian children's ways of speaking. In grades 1–3, their dialect was fairly similar to their teacher's standard dialect, but at grade 4 the children's way of speaking became increasingly similar to the local native dialect, despite the children's growing competence in expressing themselves with the standard dialect (Nelson-Barber, 1982). This shift in language use may reflect the children's choice of what stance they would take regarding their community membership. Nelson-Barber speculated that the children's use of the local dialect over the standard dialect may have been an affirmation of their community membership, in response to the school's negative attitude toward their community.

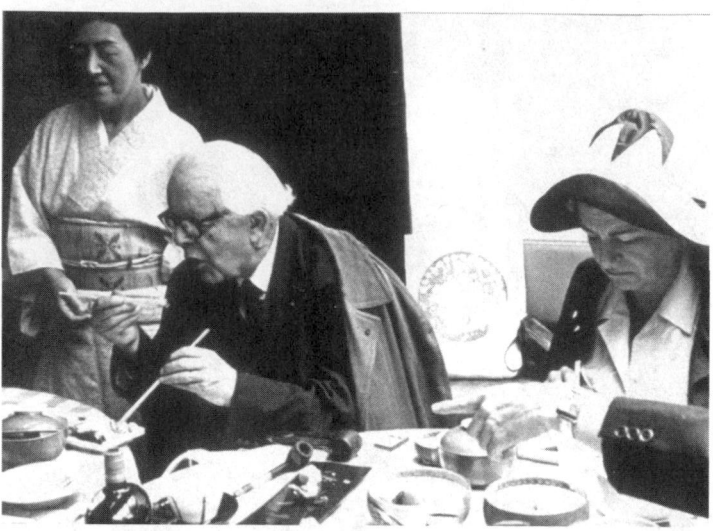

FIGURE 19.6. Jean Piaget's attempt to expand his repertoire to include an unfamiliar skill shows his agency in adapting the practice of eating with chopsticks to a form he can manage. Photograph courtesy Matsui Kimio.

Although people can be reflective on occasion about the ways in which they engage with others, this does not imply that they draw on their repertoires as stored menus to be called up; repertoires are a description for the sake of analysis. Thus, repertoires are not possessions of individuals (or communities) themselves; rather, they are analytic tools to describe often-implicit patterns for the sake of reflection by researchers, practitioners, and other analysts (including individuals themselves at times).

The idea of repertoires of practice offers several benefits for the analysis of individual and group cultural patterns:

It assists understanding of conflict among different communities' learning traditions.
It helps to get beyond treating cultural variation in terms of ethnic stereotypes.
It accommodates the fact that cultural routines and practices transform dynamically, as individuals and communities expand, prune, hybridize, and adapt their repertoires.
It aids in understanding the role of individual agency along with affordances and constraints supplied by prevalent cultural practices.

Distinct Community Traditions for Supporting Learning May Conflict

Participants in an activity may vary in what they consider preferable or acceptable, based on differing repertoires of practice associated with their histories of involvement in distinct traditions of learning and the social identities or stances they associate with a given practice. This appears to be a common source of many minority students' difficulties in formal schooling. For example, when a Warm Springs Indian child turns her gaze down from her teacher's face in order to show respectful listening, her Anglo teacher is likely to read this as disrespect or inattentiveness (Philips, 1983).

In discussing the juxtaposition of differently valued ways of learning, Jordan (1989) described the limited uptake of training efforts by Western medical personnel among Yucatecan (Mexican) Mayan midwives. The trainers' efforts resembled assembly-line instruction—involving didactic lectures emphasizing definitions—whereas the midwives' lifetime experience of learning involved the kind of intent community participation that Jordan (quoted earlier) described for girls learning midwifery by participating in the practices and skills in everyday life. Much of the training sessions provided by the Western medical personnel was like the following episode, in which a nurse asked the group of midwives, "What is a family?"

> This is a rhetorical question to which no answer is expected or offered, though nobody would doubt that midwives know what a family is. The nurse provides the answer: "A family is a group of people who live under the same roof and have as a common goal the desire for a better life." Nurse writes definition on blackboard. There is little response from the audience. Most continue to stare vacantly. Nurse looks expectantly at them, strongly conveying the notion that the definition should be copied. . . . The midwives are told that they should know [the definition] because it will be on the final test. Then we go on to the next definition which is concerned with the question: "What is a home visit?" (Jordan, 1989, p. 927)

Jordan pointed out that in the midwives' familiar way of learning, talk is used to extend communication that occurs in shared activity, rather than being the sole means of instruction. Talk has an important role in the context of practice, as midwives and birth assistants discuss diagnoses and consider different courses of action, drawing on their accounts of previous cases and collaboratively considering their applicability to difficulties in the current case.

> Talk in such situations is always closely tied to, and supportive of, action. In the traditional system, to know something is to know *how to do it*, and only derivatively to know *how to talk about it*. Talk is never primary. . . . There is some evidence that information learned in the verbal mode is used again in the verbal mode, in talk, and is unlikely to be translated into other behavior. What is generated, then, is a new way of talking, rather than a new way of doing. . . . [The midwives] learned new ways of talking, new ways of legitimizing themselves, new ways of presenting themselves as being in league with the powerful system [the Western medical establishment], which, however, had little impact on their daily practice. . . .
>
> For example, when the staff asked the midwives if any of them did external cephalic versions or engaged in the traditional practice of cauterizing the umbilical stump of the newborn, none of them admitted to doing it. [These traditional Mayan skills were looked down on at the time by Western medicine; in the meantime, their value has become recognized. The midwives] all were able to say that in case of breech presentation you refer the woman to the hospital and for treatment of the cord you use alcohol and merthiolate. But when we were alone, swinging in our hammocks at night in the dormitory, and I intimated that I actually knew how to do those things [having learned them from a Mayan midwife] and thought they were good for mother and baby, every one of them admitted that she engaged in those practices routinely. As a matter of fact, a lively discussion and exchange of information about specific techniques ensued. I would suggest, then that current teaching methods produce only minimal changes in the behavior of trainees, while, at the same time, providing new resources for *talking about* what they do. (pp. 928–929)

The distinctions drawn by Jordan in her participant observation of the midwives' training courses may well apply when individuals whose repertoires are based on one tradition for learning (such as intent community participation) are thrown into settings based on another (such as assembly-line instruction, or vice versa). In addition, the unilateral nature of assembly-line instruction is part of the problem that prevented the medical staff from detecting that their means of instruction was not connecting with the backgrounds of the trainees. The unilateral nature of assembly-line instruction is problematic even for many students who function well within it. For example, extensive research on university instruction, especially in the natural sciences, indicates that strong students often finish a course able to answer exam questions fluently but maintaining their initial ideas about the phenomena ("misconceptions" from the instructors' perspective). A rigid form of instruction such as this is particularly problematic for students who are unfamiliar with its rules and how to "play the game," and whose background knowledge of the subject matter may be quite different than those of the instructor.

Although our focus in this chapter has been on how individuals change their repertoires, it is important to note that institutions can also (and should) be flexible in the traditions of learning that they employ. School reform efforts generally attempt to move away from assembly-line instruction toward ways of learning that involve active student involvement and sensitivity to the students' background knowledge (Bransford, Brown, Cocking, & Committee on Developments in the Science of Learning, 1999). However, the familiarity of the routines and practices of assembly-line instruction among schooled adults make it difficult to improve schools. For the most part, traditions of learning are unreflectively used by practitioners, based on their own familiarity with particular traditions and practices (Matusov & Rogoff, 2002). School reform efforts seldom pay sufficient attention to the need to address the repertoires of adults themselves, which often require opportunities to *participate* in the new practices in order to make the paradigm shift required for them to develop new ways of assisting others' learning. The idea of repertoires of practice helps make sense of the distinct customary ways of acting of people from distinct backgrounds, without assuming that these ways of acting are an inherent characteristic of the individuals or backgrounds.

Getting Beyond Ethnic Stereotypes

In social science research (and in national censuses), individuals' cultural heritage has often been treated as a single social address. In contrast, we argue that conceptions of individuals' cultural backgrounds be tied to the cultural practices in which they have participated (Gutiérrez & Rogoff, 2003; Rogoff & Angelillo, 2002). National or ethnic labels such as "French" or "Mexican" or hybrid forms such as African American or European American are useful, but we suggest that they be treated as indices of likely common experience with particular cultural/historical practices, rather than simply as a marker of ancestry.

The idea of repertoires of practice addresses the fact that most people have some history of participation (in varied forms, including resistance) in the practices of several cultural communities and institutions. This concept contrasts with a common approach in which a person identified with a given ethnic group is assumed to have certain "traits" that are considered "typical" of that group, homogenous, and stable across time and circumstances. As Gutiérrez and Rogoff (2003) suggested, the concept of repertoire of practice enables us to talk about probable patterns of engagement based on historical experience, rather than stereotyping members of a group in a timeless, uniform fashion.

The idea of repertoires of practice shifts from thinking of culture as a stable, singular characteristic of individuals to focusing on people's *experience* with cultural practices, through their life history and community history. These histories contribute to individuals' (and communities') proclivities to do things in certain ways—ways that are dynamic, potentially changing with generations and contact with different ways.

Repertoires Often Change in Dynamic Individual and Community Processes

Individuals (and communities) may expand, refine, prune, and transform their repertoires of practices. Further, many practices are *hybrid* forms (Rogoff, 2003). Gutiérrez and Rogoff noted,

> Of course, there are regularities in the ways that cultural groups participate in everyday practices of their respective communities. However, the relatively stable characteristics of these environments are in constant tension with the emergent goals and practices participants construct, which stretch and change over time and with other constraints. This conflict and tension contribute to the variation and ongoing change in an individual's and a community's practices. (2003, p. 21)

Hybridity can be viewed as a process of using particular interactional formats as cultural tools for accomplishing participants' current purposes. For example, faced with home/school discontinuities, children (and parents) often adjust their ways of participating; they may adopt school ways, or they may develop hybrid forms that allow children to engage in the classroom in ways that are new for both the children and the school.

The process of hybridization is an important contributor to the continually changing repertoires of individuals and communities, especially when individuals and communities with different traditions interact. Over generations, Guatemalan Mayan mothers with extensive exposure to schooling seem to carry their experience with school formats to their interactions with their own children, which resemble the interactions of highly schooled, middle-class European American mothers (Chavajay & Rogoff, 2002; Rogoff et al., 1993). Conversely, teachers from Native American communities sometimes make use of local ways of organizing social interaction (Erickson & Mohatt, 1982; Lipka, 1991; van Ness, 1981). Immigrant Latino parents in the United States modified their ideas about literacy and their reading practices with their children through contact with models of literacy embodied in the U.S. school routines of their children (Reese & Gallimore, 2000). "Hybrid language practices" enable linguistically and ethnically diverse children and teachers to reorganize classroom functioning, creating a learning context where "no single language or register is privileged, and the larger linguistic repertoires of participants become tools for participating and making meaning in (a) new collaborative activity" (Gutiérrez et al., 1999, p. 293).

The Role of Individual Agency: Fitting Approaches to Circumstances

The idea of repertoires of practice helps relate individual agency to contextual processes and how people move between different situations. Children (and adults) determine when to apply what approach, as they choose and modify standing patterns of interaction. For example, the children of undocumented Mexican immigrant families in New York City who became involved in political protests needed to determine whether to distinguish or generalize such public protests from "protests" to unfair decisions by a teacher or a parent. If children automatically transfer one mode of learning to other settings, this may have negative consequences, as when indigenous children attempt to collaborate with each other in classrooms that treat helping as cheating.

Rogoff (2003) argued that rather than assuming that skills should generalize broadly, an important goal of development is appropriate generalization—learning "which strategies are helpful in what circumstances." Learning to fit approaches flexibly to the circumstances is also an important feature of what Hatano (1982) called adaptive expertise. The idea of repertoires helps ground ideas of competence by inviting specification of what the practices in a repertoire are meant to accomplish.

Although particular practices are associated with specific social identities, activities, and places, there may be a range of practices one may use in a given situation, in addition to the possibility of developing new approaches. Lave and Wenger (1991) argued that integral to participation is an individual's sense of belonging to a web of social relationships and accordingly the meanings the activity holds for them. An example is provided by a study that found contextual differences in how African American children narrated stories concerning conflict resolution, within a school-based violence prevention program (Daiute, Buteau, & Rawlins, 2002). The third- and fifth-grade children were asked to respond to two narrative prompts: One asked for an ending to a fictional story and the other asked for an autobiographical story concerning social conflict. The children used more extensive and elaborated resolution strategies in their autobiographical narratives and more literary resolutions in their fictional narratives, suggesting that they interpreted each task as signifying particular narrative modes of discourse (particularly within the context of the values promoted by the curriculum), each with different interpretive strategies.

In some communities, children are provided with support in determining whether the purposes or goals for given activities are the same or different across settings. For example, Japanese mother–child and teacher–child interaction may often provide children with explicit "boundary training," marking the differences in behavior expected in different contexts and providing strategies to handle new contexts (Lebra, 1994). Likewise, adults in African American working-class communities encourage children to use their own experiences in flexibly determining roles and relationships as these shift across situations (Heath, 1983).

Individuals may choose how to engage in an activity with some deliberateness, or they may adapt or select an approach from their repertoire with little or no reflection. At times that children experience points of disruption regarding their own and others' expectations regarding how to engage in a particular activity, the issue of repertoires may become salient, especially as children traverse settings that are disparate in the goals and meanings assigned to particular actions. In those moments of disruption, children may reflect on their own ways of acting that are not in accord with modes of participation in other settings.

Although adjustment and modification of repertoires is often not accompanied by such reflection, determining which approach to take nonetheless involves an individual's agency, attending at some level to the affordances and cues in a particular situation and how they relate to familiar practices. Courses of action are thus a matter that involves both the active roles of individuals and the dynamic structures of situations. The determination of an action is *in the participation* itself—of the individual involved in the activity—not in the individuals or the contexts separately. Determining which approach in one's repertoire to apply or to build on requires attentiveness to the structure of situations and how they fit with one's goals, to align with the direction of ongoing events, to invent new approaches when old ones do not work, to revamp an original way of participating by combining with other forms, to determine whose approach to align with in a politically charged or divisive situation, and to decide which goals to prioritize in a given situation (such as resisting involvement in a distasteful event, showing solidarity with a peer, competing with others, or avoiding being noticed).

The idea of repertoires as cultural tools that change as people use them is consistent with Erickson's (2004) examination of the relation of social "structure" and individual agency in the everyday interactions of social life. These interactions take place in real time with improvisation by the participants, making use of the affordances and dealing with the constraints of historically developed practices that precede the particular interaction. As such, the interaction of individuals is agentic, as people engage in continual opportunistic history-in-the-making, usually on a small scale, building on longer-term historical processes. People's opportunism often requires innovation, as participants make use of what is available in cultural practices to address their current needs and intentions. Human life simultaneously involves changes *and* continuities—innovations using cultural repertoires to build current approaches.

In summary, we have argued that an understanding of the routine formats and activities in which children engage aids in understanding their cultural experience and preparation to engage in particular settings with specific cultural practices. Attention to the social organization of routine events (such as bedtime story telling or language games or helping around the house) will reveal reasons for certain children's ease or confusion or even resistance when they enter new settings that are organized in ways that may relate to, differ from, or even conflict with those with which they have experience. We examined three major traditions for organizing human learning—intent community participation, assembly-line instruction, and guided repetition—which each have a substantial history as well as an organization of practices that may challenge children (and adults) who are new to participating in them.

Seeing the cultural organization of everyday practices as well as of whole learning traditions can help researchers understand children's (and our own) development as cultural beings. Such understanding can also help practitioners ease the entry of newcomers to a specific tradition such as that commonly employed in schooling. In addition, it can help find ways to revise the structure and practices of such institutions to better serve people with varying cultural experience, if the institutions' practitioners are themselves given the opportunity and time to expand or adjust their repertoires.

ACKNOWLEDGMENTS

Writing of this chapter was supported by the UCSC Foundation Chair in Psychology and the UC Presidential Chair (to Barbara Rogoff), National Science Foundation support from the Center for Informal

Learning and Schools (to Barbara Rogoff, Leslie Moore, and Amy Dexter), National Institutes of Health traineeship (No. T32-MH20025, to Jocelyn Solís), and a Ford Foundation Fellowship (to Maricela Correa-Chávez).

NOTE

1. We are extremely grateful for the critique and suggestions of colleagues who attended two University of California Presidential Workshops on intent participation.

REFERENCES

Ariès, P. (1962). *Centuries of childhood*. New York: Knopf.
Barker, R. G., & Wright, H. F. (1954). *Midwest and its children: The psychological ecology of an American town*. New York: Row, Peterson.
Bartlett, F. C. (1932). *Remembering*. Cambridge, UK: Cambridge University Press.
Beach, B. A. (1988). Children at work: The home workplace. *Early Childhood Research Quarterly, 3*, 209–221.
Biggs, J. B. (1996). Learning, schooling, and socialization. In S. Lau (Ed.), *Growing up the Chinese way* (pp. 147–167). Hong Kong: Chinese University Press.
Blount, B. G. (1972). Parental speech and language acquisition: Some Luo and Samoan examples. *Anthropological Linguistics, 14*, 119–130.
Bluedorn, H., & Bluedorn, L. (2000). *Teaching the trivium: Christian homeschooling in a classical style*. Muscatine, Iowa: Trivium Pursuit.
Bourdieu, P. (1977). *Outline of a theory of practice* (R. Nice, Trans.). Cambridge, UK: Cambridge University Press.
Bransford, J., Brown, A. L., Cocking, R., & Committee on Developments in the Science of Learning. (1999). *How people learn: A report of the National Research Council of the National Academy of Science*. Washington, DC: National Academy Press.
Callahan, R. E. (1962). *Education and the cult of efficiency: A study of the social forces that have shaped the administration of the public schools*. Chicago: University of Chicago Press.
Carruthers, M. (1992). *Book of Memory: A study of memory in mediaeval culture* (2nd ed.). Cambridge, UK: Cambridge University Press.
Chavajay, P., & Rogoff, B. (2002). Schooling and traditional collaborative social organization of problem solving by Mayan mothers and children. *Developmental Psychology, 38*, 55–66.
Crago, M. B. (1992). Communicative interaction and second language acquisition: An Inuit example. *TESOL Quarterly, 26*, 487–505.
Cubberley, E. P. (1922). *A brief history of education: A history of the practice and progress and organization of education*. Boston, New York: Houghton Mifflin.
Daiute, C., Buteau, E., & Rawlins, C. (2002). Social relational wisdom: Developmental diversity in children's written narratives about social conflict. *Narrative Inquiry, 11*, 277–306.
Davies, B., & Harré, R. (1990). Positioning: The discursive production of selves. *Journal for the Theory of Social Behavior, 20*, 43–63.
De Haan, M. (2001). Intersubjectivity in models of learning and teaching: Reflections from a study of teaching and learning in a Mexican Mazahua community. In S. Chaiklin (Ed.), *The theory and practice of cultural-historical psychology* (pp. 174–199). Aarhus, Denmark: Aarhus University Press.
Eckerman, C. O., Whatley, J. L., & McGhee, L. J. (1979) Approaching and contacting the object another manipulates. *Developmental Psychology, 15*, 585–593.
Elbers, E., & De Haan, M. (2002). Dialogic learning in the multi-ethnic classroom: Cultural resources and modes of collaboration. In J. van der Linden & P. Renshaw (Eds.), *Dialogical perspectives on learning, teaching, and instruction*. Dordrecht: Kluwer Academic.
Erickson, F. (1982). Classroom discourse as improvisation. In L. C. Wilkinson (Ed.), *Communication in the classroom* (pp. 153–181). New York: Academic Press.

Erickson, F. (2004). *Talk and social theory: Ecologies of speaking and listening in everyday life*. Cambridge, UK: Polity Press.

Erickson, F., & Mohatt, G. (1982). Cultural organization of participation structures in two classrooms of Indian students. In G. Spindler (Ed.), *Doing the ethnography of schooling* (pp. 132–174) New York: Holt, Rinehart, & Winston.

Gauvain, M. (1995). Thinking in niches: Sociocultural influences on cognitive development. *Human Development, 38*, 25–45.

Gauvain, M. (2004). Sociocultural contexts of learning. In A. Maynard & M. Martini (Eds.), *The psychology of learning in context* (pp. 11–40). Kluwer/Plenum Press.

Goffman, E. (1979). Footing. *Semiotica, 25*, 1–29.

Goffman, E. (1981). *Forms of talk*. Philadelphia: University of Pennsylvania Press.

Goodnow, J. J. (1992). Parents' ideas, children's ideas: Correspondence and divergence. In I. E. Sigel, A. V. McGillicuddy-DeLisi, & J. J. Goodnow (Eds.), *Parental belief systems: The psychological consequences for children* (pp. 293–318). Hillsdale, NJ: Erlbaum.

Goodwin, M. H. (1990). *He-said-she-said: Talk as social organization among black children*. Bloomington: Indiana University Press.

Gutiérrez, K.D., Baquedano-López, P., & Tejeda, C. (1999). Rethinking diversity: Hybridity and hybrid language practices in the third space. *Mind, Culture and Activity, 6*, 286–303.

Gutiérrez, K., & Rogoff, B. (2003). Cultural ways of learning: Individual traits or repertoires of practice. *Educational Researcher, 32*, 19–25.

Haight, W. (1991, April). *Belief systems that frame and inform parental participation in their children's pretend play*. Paper presented at the meeting of the Society for Research in Child Development, Seattle.

Harkness, S. (1977). Aspects of social environment and first language acquisition in rural Africa. In C. Ferguson & C. Snow (Eds.), *Talking to children: Language input and acquisition* (pp. 309–316). New York: Cambridge University Press.

Harkness, S., & Super, C. M. (1992). Parental ethnotheories in action. In I. E. Sigel, A. V. McGillicuddy-DeLisi, & J. J. Goodnow (Eds.), *Parental belief systems: The psychological consequences for children* (2nd ed, pp. 373–392). Hillsdale, NJ: Erlbaum.

Harkness, S., & Super, C. M. (2002). Culture and parenting. In M. H. Bornstein (Ed.), *Handbook of parenting* (Vol 1, pp. 253–280). Mahwah, NJ: Erlbaum.

Hatano, G. (1982). Cognitive consequences of practice in culture specific procedural skills. *Quarterly Newsletter of the Laboratory of Comparative Human Cognition, 4*, 15–17.

Hay, D. F., Murray, P., Cecire, S., & Nash, A. (1985). Social learning of social behavior in early life. *Child Development, 56*, 43–57.

Heath, C. (1986). *Body movement and speech in medical interaction*. Cambridge, UK: Cambridge University Press.

Heath, S. B. (1983). *Ways with words: Language, life, and work in communities and classrooms*. Cambridge, UK: Cambridge University Press.

Ho, D. Y. F. (1994). Cognitive socialization in Confucian heritage cultures. In P. M. Greenfield & R. R. Cocking (Eds.), *Cross-cultural roots of minority child development* (pp. 285–314). Hillsdale, NJ: Erlbaum.

Hori, G. V. S. (1996). Teaching and learning in the Rinzai Zen monastery. In T. Rohlen & G. LeTendre (Eds.), *Teaching and learning in Japan* (pp. 20–49). Cambridge, UK: Cambridge University Press.

Hutchins, E., & Palen, L. (1997). Constructing meaning from space, gesture, and speech. In L. Resnick, R. Saljo, C. Pontecorvo, & B. Burge (Eds.), *Discourse, too, and reasoning: Essays on situated cognition* (pp. 23–40). Berlin: Springer.

Jordan, B. (1989). Cosmopolitical obstetrics: Some insights from the training of traditional midwives. *Social Science and Medicine, 28*, 925–944.

Kendon, A. (1990). *Conducting interaction: Patterns of behavior in focused encounters*. Cambridge, UK: Cambridge University Press.

Lave, J., & Wenger, E. (1991). *Situated learning: Legitimate peripheral participation*. Cambridge, UK: Cambridge University Press.

Lebra, T. S. (1994). Mother and child in Japanese socialization: A Japan–U.S. comparison. In P. M. Greenfield & R. R. Cocking (Eds.), *Cross-cultural roots of minority child development* (pp. 259–274). Hillsdale, NJ: Erlbaum.

LeVine, R. A. (1980). A cross-cultural perspective on parenting. In M. D. Fantini & R. Cardenas (Eds.), *Parenting in a multicultural society*. New York: Longman.

LeVine, R. A., LeVine, S., Leiderman, P. H., Brazelton, T. B., Dixon, S., Richman, A., et al. (1994). *Child care and culture: Lessons from Africa*. Cambridge, UK: Cambridge University Press.

Li, J., & Fischer, K. W. (2004). Thought and affect in American and Chinese learners' beliefs about learning. In D. Dai & R. Sternberg (Eds.), *Motivation, emotion, and cognition: Integrative perspectives on intellectual functioning and development*. Mahwah, NJ: Erlbaum.

Lipka, J. (1991). Toward a culturally based pedagogy: A case study of one Yup'ik Eskimo teacher. *Anthropology and Education Quarterly, 22*, 203–223.

Martini, M. (1995). Features of home environments associated with children's school success. *Early Child Development and Care, 111*, 49–68.

Matusov, E., & Rogoff, B. (2002). Newcomers and oldtimers: Educational philosophies-in-action of parent volunteers in a community of learners school. *Anthropology and Education Quarterly, 33*, 415–440.

Mehan, H. (1979). *Learning lessons: Social organization in the classroom*. Cambridge, MA: Harvard University Press.

Metge, R. (1984). *Learning and teaching: He tikanga Maori*. Wellington, NZ: New Zealand Ministry of Education.

Moore, L. C. (2004a). *Learning languages by heart: Language socialization in a Fulbe community (Maroua, Cameroon)*. Unpublished doctoral dissertation, UCLA, Los Angeles.

Moore, L. C. (2004b, February). *The sociocultural nature of second language development: Tales from two Cameroonian communities*. Invited talk presented at the UC Berkeley Symposium on Language Ecology. Berkeley, CA.

Moore, L .C. (2006). Changes in folktale socialization in a Fulbe community. In P. Newman & L. Hyman (Eds.), *West African linguistics: Descriptive, comparative, and historical studies in honor of Russell G. Schuh* (pp. 176–187). Bloomington: Indiana University Press.

Morelli, G., Rogoff, B., & Angelillo, C. (2003). Cultural variation in children's access to work or involvement in specialized child-focused activities. *International Journal of Behavioral Development, 27*, 264–274.

Nash, P. (1968). *Models of man: Explorations in the Western educational tradition*. New York: Wiley.

Nelson, K., & Gruendel, J. M. (1988). At morning it's lunchtime: A scriptal view of children's dialogue. In M. B. Franklin & S. S. Barten (Eds), *Child language* (pp. 263–277). London: Oxford University Press.

Nelson-Barber, S. (1982). Phonologic variations of Pima English. In R. St. Clair & W. Leap (Eds.), *Language renewal among American Indian tribes* (pp. 115–132). Rosslyn, VA: National Clearinghouse for Bilingual Education.

On, L. W. (1996). The cultural context for Chinese learners: Conceptions of learning in the Confucian tradition. In D. Watkins & J. B. Biggs (Eds.), *The Chinese learner: Cultural, psychological, and contextual influences* (pp. 29–41). Melbourne: CERC; ACER.

Orellana, M. F. (2001). The work kids do: Mexican and Central American immigrant children's contributions to households and schools in California. *Harvard Educational Review, 71*, 366–389.

Paradise, R. (1987). *Learning through social interaction: The experience and development of the Mazahua self in the context of the market*. Unpublished dissertation, University of Pennsylvania.

Philips, S. U. (1983). *The invisible culture*. New York: Longman.

Philips, S. U. (2001). Participant structures and communicative competence: Warm Springs children in community and classroom. In A. Duranti (Ed.), *Linguistic anthropology: A reader* (pp. 302–318). Oxford, UK: Blackwell.

Rabain-Jamin, J. (1989). Culture and early social interactions. The example of mother-infant object play in African and Native French families. *European Journal of Psychology of Education, 4*, 295–305.

Reese, L., & Gallimore, R. (2000). Immigrant Latinos' cultural model of literacy development. *American Journal of Education, 108*, 103–134.

Rheingold, H. L. (1982). Little children's participation in the work of adults: A nascent prosocial behavior. *Child Development, 53*, 114–125.

Rheingold, H. L. (1985). Development as the acquisition of familiarity. *Annual Review of Psychology, 36*, 1–17.

Richman, A. L., LeVine, R. A., Staples, A., New, R., Howrigan, G. A., Welles-Nystrom, B., et al. (1988). Maternal behavior to infants in five cultures. *New Directions in Child Development, 40*, 81–97.

Richman, A., Miller, P., & LeVine, R. (1992). Cultural and educational variations in maternal responsiveness. *Developmental Psychology, 28*, 614–621.

Rogoff, B. (2003). *The cultural nature of human development*. New York: Oxford University Press.

Rogoff, B., & Angelillo, C. (2002). Investigating the coordinated functioning of multifaceted cultural practices in human development. *Human Development, 45,* 211–225.

Rogoff, B., Goodman Turkanis, C., & Bartlett, L. (2001). *Learning together: Children and adults in a school community.* New York: Oxford University Press.

Rogoff, B., Mistry, J., Göncü, A., & Mosier, C. (1993). Guided participation in cultural activity by toddlers and caregivers. *Monographs of the Society for Research in Child Development, 58* (Serial No. 236).

Rogoff, B., Pardise, R., Arauz, R. M., Correa–Chávez, M., & Angelillo, C. (2003). Firsthand learning through intent participation. *Annual Review of Psychology, 54,* 175–203.

Rosenthal, M., & Roer-Strier, D. (2001). Cultural differences in mothers' developmental goals and ethnotheories. *International Journal of Psychology, 36,* 20–31.

Sato, N. (1996). Honoring the individual. In T. Rohlen & G. LeTendre (Eds.), *Teaching and learning in Japan* (pp. 119–153). Cambridge, UK: Cambridge University Press.

Schank, R., & Abelson, R. (1977). *Scripts, plans, goals, and understanding.* Hillsdale, NJ: Erlbaum.

Schieffelin, B., & Ochs, E. (1986). Language socialization. *Annual Review of Anthropology, 15,* 163–191.

Schneider, B., Hieshima, J. A., Lee, S., & Plank, S. (1994). East-Asian academic success in the United States: Family, school, and community explanations. In P. M. Greenfield & R. R. Cocking (Eds.), *Cross-cultural roots of minority child development* (pp. 323–350). Hillsdale, NJ: Erlbaum.

Scribner, S., & Cole, M. (1981a). *The psychology of literacy.* Cambridge, MA: Harvard University Press.

Scribner, S., & Cole, M. (1981b). Unpackaging literacy. In M. F. Whiteman (Ed.), *Writing: The nature, development, and teaching of written communication* (pp. 71–87). Hillsdale, NJ: Erlbaum.

Tambiah, S. J. (1968). The magical power of words. *Man, 3,* 175–208.

Tharp, R. G., & Gallimore, R. (1988). *Rousing minds to life: Teaching, learning and schooling in social context.* Cambridge, UK: Cambridge University Press.

Van Ness, H. (1981). Social control and social organization in an Alaskan Athabaskan classroom. In H.T. Trueba, G.P. Guthrie, & K.H. Au (Eds.), *Culture and the bilingual classroom* (pp. 120–138). Rowley, MA: Newbury House.

Wagner, D. A. (1983). Learning to read by "rote." *International Journal of the Sociology of Language, 42,* 111–121.

Wagner, D. A. (1993). *Literacy, culture and development: Becoming literate in Morocco.* New York: Cambridge University Press.

Ward, M. C. (1971). *Them children: A study in language learning.* New York: Holt, Rinehart & Winston.

Weisner, T. S. (1984). A cross-cultural perspective: Ecocultural niches of middle childhood. In A. Collins (Ed.), *The elementary school years: Understanding development during middle childhood* (pp. 335–369). Washington, DC: National Academy Press.

Weisner, T. S., Gallimore, R., & Jordan, C. (1988). Unpackaging cultural effects on classroom learning: Native Hawaiian peer assistance and child-generated activity. *Anthropology and Education Quarterly, 19,* 327–352.

Whiting, B. B. (1980). Culture and social behavior: A model for the development of social behavior. *Ethos, 8,* 95–116.

Whiting, B. B., & Whiting, J.W.M. (1975). *Children of six cultures.* Cambridge, MA: Harvard.

Wilson, D. (1991). *Recovering the lost tools for learning: An approach to distinctively Christian education.* Wheaton, IL: Good News.

Wilson, D. (2003). *The case for classical Christian learning.* Westchester, IL: Crossways.

Zentella, A. C. (1998). Multiple codes, multiple ethnicities: Puerto Rican children in New York City. In S. M. Hoyle & C. T. Adger (Eds.), *Kids talk: Strategic language use in later childhood* (pp. 95–107). Oxford, UK: Oxford Studies in Sociolinguistics.

CHAPTER 20

Emotion Socialization from a Cultural Perspective

PAMELA M. COLE and PATRICIA Z. TAN

Emotional processes pervade socialization. They fuel action and interaction because they involve appraising circumstances and readying to act on them to maintain or regain well-being. This capacity is biologically prepared, adapted to allow rapid processing of experience that mostly occurs outside of conscious awareness. Yet, humans have a capacity to reflect on and regulate emotions. The capacity to be emotional is a fundamental, universal aspect of human functioning. A trip around the world, however, quickly suggests that culture influences human emotional life. Our chapter focuses on how culture comes to influence the socialization of emotion.

A handbook of socialization was last published in 1969 but it had no chapter on the cultural socialization of emotion (Goslin, 1969). Since then, a number of historical changes permit a chapter dedicated to the cultural socialization of emotion. First, there has been an enormous resurgence of scientific interest in emotional processes. In addition, many changes increased our appreciation of culture. In 1969, astronauts gave us a view of the planet from the moon, a view that catalyzed an awareness of the world as a community. Our ability to traverse that community increased. Worldwide immigration, economic globalization, and information technology facilitated our exposure to and discourse with other minds. These dramatic advances penetrated the field of developmental science, judging from the marked increase in international collaborations in the major journals and a greater appreciation within nations of the need to study their own cultural diversity.

The scientific account of the cultural socialization of emotion, however, is incomplete. There remain widely varying views across and within disciplines as to the ways in which emotional processes are universal and culturally specific. Models and methods for studying emotion are dominated by Western theories. There is no consensus on how to define culture. Researchers typically rely on global conceptualizations of culture (e.g., individualistic society) that have heuristic value but lack specificity to explain within-society group differences. Nonetheless, an appreciation that a full account of human development requires the examination of cultural variations has stimulated a considerable amount of research, some of which addresses the socialization of emotion. In this chapter, we provide our view of how emotional, cultural, and socialization processes are related. We include topics ranging from infant temperament as a potential contributor to socialization and emotional competence as a product of socialization. We conclude with directions for future research.

EMOTIONAL, CULTURAL, AND SOCIALIZATION PROCESSES

Emotion, Culture, and Socialization

There is no question that all human beings are equipped with a capacity to be emotional, but it is also clear that culture influences emotion processes. There is intense debate about whether all humans share a concept of "emotion" and whether there is a universal set of emotion categories. There are two limitations to the evidence, however. First, the studies mainly involve adult participants and cannot illustrate *how* a universal capacity comes to be influenced by community standards. Second, the studies compare nations that differ in so many ways that it cannot be determined *why* emotional processes differ. A developmental approach to examining when, how, and why culture influences emotional processes is a very promising solution.

Let us assume that children are born with the capacity to be emotional and that they develop emotionally in social contexts that vary in potentially relevant ways. In the first years of life, children's emotions are critical to getting their basic needs met (e.g., fear, anger) and likely have universal prototypes (Ekman, 1992; Elfenbein & Ambady, 2002; Scherer & Wallbott, 1994). The experiences associated with their basic emotions, moreover, are likely to occur in all societies (e.g., seeing an unfamiliar face or having something you desire taken away). Nonetheless, culture influences how others in a community conceptualize emotion, what they define as personal and group well-being, how they appraise the situations they encounter relative to these definitions, how they communicate emotionally to members of their own and other groups, and how they act on their circumstances to sustain and regain well-being (Markus & Kitayama, 1991; Mesquita & Frijda, 1992; Oyserman, Coon, & Kemmelmeier, 2002).

Caregivers around the globe share the goal of raising children to become competent adults in their communities (LeVine et al., 1994; Whiting & Edwards, 1988). Emotional competence is an integral aspect of competence (e.g., Halberstadt, Denham, & Dunsmore, 2001; Saarni, 1999). As caregivers engage in this enterprise, children are socialized in accord with the community's standards for competence and for their positions within the community. Because emotions fuel all these interactions, and because community standards and the means by which they are reached are culturally variable, the process of socialization involves the enculturation of emotions (Berry, Poortinga, Segall, & Dasen, 2002).

The cultural socialization of emotion is explicit at times, but more often it is an implicit aspect of socialization. All human behavior and interactions carry messages about the emotions that motivate action. Moreover, these pervasive and implicit messages begin early in life. Before a child can speak and understand words, the infant engages in and perceives emotion-rich vocalizations, facial expressions, and movements. Caregivers respond and culture has its opportunity to influence emotional development.

The Nature of Culture

Socialization occurs in cultural context (Bornstein, 2002; Bronfenbrenner, 1977; Keller, 2003; Super & Harkness, 1986). But it is hard to define culture. Generally, it is defined as shared customs that are transmitted from generation to generation. To the new arrival in a community, practices are the leading edge of cultural socialization (Rogoff, 2003; Weisner, 2002). To understand the practices, it is helpful to know local conceptions of acceptable conduct, goals for socializing such conduct, and theories about how these goals are achieved (Harkness & Super, 1996).

A full understanding of cultural practices and beliefs requires examination of the conditions in which they evolved and are evolving. Comparative studies typically index culture by nation of origin or "racial" or "ethnic" group membership, but these can be imprecise classifications that fail to integrate relevant social factors that influence emotional life (see García Coll et al., 1996; Gjerde, 2004; McLoyd, 2004). Culture is best defined locally, situated at a point in a community's history and located within particular resources and pressures (LeVine, 1969; Super & Harkness, 1986). Such an approach to defining culture can recognize that culture is dynamic, changing over time. Finally, culture includes shared principles that guide practices; individuals within a given cultural group, however, embrace shared practices and principles to varying degrees.

Efforts to conceptualize cultural differences have stirred vigorous debate. Those that have prevailed in the developmental literature share one common thread that is at the crux of the topic of socialization—the distinction between self and other. The views of nations as orienting toward the good of the collective or the individual (Hofstede, 1984; Triandis, 1989), of selves as interdependent or independent (Markus & Kitayama, 1991), of relationships as achieving differing degrees of balance between belonging and individuating (Rothbaum, Pott, Azuma, Miyake & Weisz, 2000), or of individuals as achieving different degrees of balance between a sense of agency and social distance (Kağitçibaşi, 1996)—all these conceptualizations hinge on the fundamental need for humans to articulate and achieve a balance between the needs of the self and those of the group. The process of socialization involves learning to be a self in cultural context.

A Framework for Conceptualizing Emotion Socialization from a Cultural Perspective

There is no comprehensive model that integrates the role of culture in emotion socialization. Contemporary views on the socialization of emotion (Denham, Bassett, & Wyatt, Chapter 24, this volume; Eisenberg, Cumberland, & Spinrad, 1998; Parke, 1994) can be integrated with models that posit how surrounding ecological and social pressures influence human development, socialization practices, and parenting beliefs (Bronfenbrenner, 1977; LeVine et al., 1994; Super & Harkness, 1986).

Part of creating a community that supports the group's adaptation to its surround is the establishment of shared practices that maintain social order. An infant is born into a family in a community that has standards for social interaction in order to achieve this communal goal. For example, the United States at its inception was a newly evolved community founded on a standard that personal liberty is as important as life; laws codified social practices that protected the individual and guaranteed that the people, rather than a monarch, determined solutions to changing resources and challenges. American social competence became defined by a strong sense of individuality. American children become selves in this context. Culture influences socialization goals, practices for rearing competent children, and beliefs about how children develop, penetrating the day-to-day socialization of children.

Because emotions reflect the individual's goals to maintain well-being, those goals must be coordinated with community goals for social order. Family members, schools, peers, media, and the societal structure of intergroup relations all contribute to the child's socialization through a variety of mechanisms. For the socialization of emotion, scholars have focused primarily on the role of parents while acknowledging that an entire community participates in emotion socialization. Direct parental influences reflect a partial but important set of mechanisms by which children's emotions are socialized. Parents may state an explicit display rule (e.g., "Big boys don't cry") or coach a child in understanding and coping with feelings. It is generally agreed, however, that emotions are primarily socialized through indirect means. Implicit processes include observations of the emotional exchanges of others, reactions of others to a child's emotions, and opportunities to experience different emotions. Cultural factors should influence each of these mechanisms of socialization.

The cultural socialization of emotion, however, is not a passive process, laid down on a child. Each child contributes actively to the socialization process. Individual differences in infant fussiness, for example, may be interpreted and handled differently by various cultural groups. Parental beliefs about what a child of a given age can be expected to do are also culturally variable (Harkness & Super, 1996). Thus a cultural model of the socialization of emotion must also consider the influences of the child.

Our summary of the literature begins with what is known about whether culture influences child temperament and follows the child's development through the formation of attachment and the emotional aspects of parent interactions with children to the acquisition of emotional competencies. Our summary is constrained in several ways. First, our inability to read scholarly publications in languages other than English prevented us from including the contributions of scholars from many different cultural backgrounds. Second, we focused on studies that tested the presence of cultural influences by comparing two or more different peoples rather than the fascinating body of work describing individual cultures. Those rich descriptions are essential to the study of the cultural socialization of emotion, but without a contrasting context, they cannot demonstrate that differences in an aspect of emotion socialization are attributable to culture. The final constraint is that the available literature dwells on caregivers, especially mothers, and children, especially young children. Regrettably, the other agents of socialization—peers, siblings, other adults (e.g., teachers), the media, and the larger structure of society—are not well represented in the emotion socialization literature.

EMOTIONAL PROCESSES IN SOCIALIZATION

Temperament: Individual Differences in Infant Emotional Reactivity

Any discussion of emotional processes in socialization must consider the child's unique emotional characteristics to which others react. Temperament involves individual differences in infants' biological predispositions, particularly emotional reactivity (Goldsmith et al., 1987). Because parents perceive these early individual differences (Rothbart & Bates, 1998), it is thought they may influence the socialization of emotion (Eisenberg et al., 1998; Parke, 1994). A parent of an anger-prone youngster may often be irritated by the child, exposing the child to parental anger more than other children are.

Parental descriptions of child personality characteristics appear to have an underlying structure that resembles Western psychology's "Big Five" dimensions (i.e., extraversion, conscientiousness, agreeableness, neuroticism, and openness to experience). Parents from different nations, however, vary in how they define each dimension and the importance they assign to it (Ahadi, Rothbart, & Ye, 1993; Kohnstamm, Halverson, Mervielde, & Havill, 1998). Extraversion, the most common trait mentioned by parents, is defined by Belgian and German parents as sociability but as activity level by Polish and Chinese parents (Elphick, Halverson, & Marszal-Wisniewska, 1998). Moreover, Chinese parents mention conscientiousness more often than parents from Western Europe and the United States, suggesting it is more important to them (Kohnstamm, Zhang, Slotboom, & Elphick, 1998). Finally, there are dimensions that do not have clear cultural equivalence. Greek parents refer to *philotemo*, a complex of traits involving being polite, dutiful, virtuous, generous and self-sacrificing out of a sense of honor (Elphick et al., 1998; Vassiliou & Vassiliou, 1973).

In addition to descriptions of child personality traits, there have been cross-national comparisons of parent and teacher reports of children's temperament. Western European or American children are generally described as more approach oriented and emotionally expressive but easier to soothe than Asian and Asian American children (e.g., Camras et al., 1998; Pomerleau, Sabatíer, & Malcuit, 1998; Russell, Hart, Robinson, & Olsen, 2003). U.S. children are also described as more active and easily soothed than Australian or Russian children (Gartstein, Slobodskaya, & Kinsht, 2003).

None of these studies, however, address whether differences exist in children's actual behavior. Observational studies of infant temperament circumvent the limitations of parent reports and, indeed, they present a different portrait of East Asian youngsters. Although the observational findings are not as consistent as those from parental reports, they suggest that East Asian infants are *less* irritable, better at self-quieting, and easier to soothe than Caucasian infants (e.g., Caudill & Weinstein, 1969; Freedman, 1974; Lewis, Ramsay, & Kawakami, 1993; Kagan et al., 1994). Studies of infant emotional expressivity, which are not necessarily conceived as studies of temperament, present a similar view. East Asian infants have less frequent and intense displays of positive and negative emotion than U.S. infants (e.g., Camras et al., 1998).

These contradictory pieces of evidence must be further qualified. First, there are differences *among* East Asian infants; observations indicate that Chinese infants are less reactive to restraint and novelty than Japanese babies (e.g., Camras et al., 1998; Camras et al., 2002). Second, most observational studies only measure reactive behavior and not physiological reactivity. Japanese infants exhibit fewer behavioral indications of stress to inoculation but higher cortisol responses than American babies (Lewis et al., 1993).

Thus, a complete picture of the role of culture in infant temperament requires additional, more sophisticated research designs.

The discrepancies between adult reports and observations of child temperament perhaps reveal an important issue in cultural research. Why would Chinese mothers describe infants as irritable and difficult to soothe but observers rate Chinese infants as calm and easy to soothe compared to infants from other countries? Chinese mothers may be acutely sensitive to infant distress and detect cues that observers do not. One study reported weak cross-cultural agreement in adults' labeling of infant emotional expressions (Yik, Meng, & Russell, 1998), although adults agreed as to whether the infants felt good or bad. Another possibility is that cultural groups have different response biases (Smith, 2004). A mother's cultural standards may influence how critically or positively she describes her child. Latina mothers are said to demonstrate a positive bias and Asian parents a negative bias when describing their children (Marín, Gamba, & Marín, 1992; Rao, McHale, & Pearson, 2003).

The prevailing view of temperamental differences is that they reflect genetic variations that influence emotional reactions in particular contexts (novelty, limitations). How much temperament is influenced by shared biological factors of a cultural group and how much temperament is influenced by socialization experiences and gene–environment interactions is unclear. In studying cultural influences on infant temperament, it is important to consider prenatal and postnatal factors that may vary with culture and influence infant emotionality. Iron deficiency, which is common in developing countries and among poorer families in developed countries, is associated with infant wariness and reduced positive emotion (Lozoff et al., 2003).

In sum, it is as yet unclear whether there are cultural differences in infant temperament or child personality that might influence cultural variations in socialization of emotion practices. There are clearly systematic variations in caregiver descriptions of temperament, but these remain to be confirmed with behavioral evidence. Nonetheless, enough research has been conducted to suggest the kinds of methodological care that will be needed to clarify whether cultural differences in temperament exist and, if they do, why. Should cultural differences in temperament be shown, it will be possible to determine whether they explain why parenting practices vary across cultures. Are parents rearing children with different temperamental features or do children in each society have similar temperaments but their cultures value different traits? If cultural differences in temperament exist, it will be necessary to determine whether and how they influence other emotional processes in socialization, such as attachment.

Attachment: Emotional Security within Relationships with Caregivers

Bowlby (1969) conceived of attachment as a universal feature of infant development. Infants form selective emotional bonds with their primary caregivers that allow them to both explore the world and regain a sense of security when they become distressed by venturing too far from a caregiver. The formation of a secure attachment is a critical forerunner of emotional competence. To explore the world while maintaining a sense of security involves a balance of emotional independence and dependence. Cultures vary not only in their ideals for how to achieve such a balance but in terms of the number of primary caregivers an infant has, the amount of experience infants have being separated from primary caregivers, and the physical risks associated with venturing from them.

Attachment research has relied heavily on a procedure, the Strange Situation, that was inspired by Mary Ainsworth's observations of striking similarities in mothers and infants in the United States and Uganda (Ainsworth, 1967; Ainsworth & Bell, 1970). In both settings, infants appeared distressed when their mothers left them, the degree of distress seemed related to the amount of maternal warmth and responsiveness, and the ability of the dyad to regain security seemed to be related to the child's later adjustment. The Strange Situation appears to yield reliable classifications of infant security across nations, and thus there is a view that these descriptors are relevant across cultures (for a review, see van IJzendoorn & Sagi, 1999). However, studies using the Strange Situation have focused on dyads from industrialized nations in which mothers are typically the primary caregivers, a circumstance we know varies across cultures.

In general it is assumed that all babies form attachments, but it is less clear whether infant security and maternal sensitivity can be defined similarly in all cultures (e.g., Grossmann, Grossmann, Spangler, Suess, & Unzner, 1985; Rothbaum, Weisz, Pott, Miyake, & Morelli, 2000; Takashi, 1986). It has not been determined whether an infant who rarely leaves the mother, or an infant who has multiple primary caregivers, experiences separation and reunion similarly to the infant with one primary caregiver and ample opportunity to safely move from her (Grossmann et al., 1985; Miyake, Campos, Kagan, & Bradshaw, 1986; Sagi et al., 1995). A child with little separation experience may be more highly distressed by an artificial laboratory separation than one who has experienced frequent separations (Posada et al., 1995). Thus there is a steady call to assess infant security in culturally relevant ways that consider the meaning of behavior in cultural context.

Consider how the following reunion behaviors are regarded by mothers from different nations. When their 4- and 5-year-olds whine and clamber on them after a separation, Japanese mothers feel they have successfully cultivated *amae*, the child's enduring emotional dependence on them (Doi, 1973; Lebra, 2000; Rothbaum, Morelli, Pott, & Liu-Constant, 2000). To Euro American mothers, such behavior in a child of this age is regarded as insecurity and emotional immaturity (e.g., Mizuta, Zahn-Waxler, Cole, & Hiruma, 1996). German mothers are quite different in what they expect. They also view proximity seeking as insecure, even in toddlers, because it indicates that the child is not acquiring emotional self-sufficiency, which to them is an important aspect of emotional competence (e.g., Friedlmeier & Trommsdorff, 1999; Grossmann, Grossmann, Huber, & Wartner, 1981; Zach & Keller, 1999).

Secure attachment is believed to be a result of sensitive caregiving in all cultures (van IJzendoorn & Sagi, 1999), but *how* caregivers are sensitive to children's needs also seems to differ across cultures. Theoretically, sensitivity involves attunement to a child's emotional needs, skill at administering to them, and effectiveness at promoting child well-being. For German and American mothers, who are frequently studied, sensitivity appears in the form of well-synchronized face-to-face emotional exchanges with their infants. This is not a common practice in all cultures, however. In some communities, mothers carry their infants on their backs and touch them frequently to foster infant well-being (Keller, Yovsi, et al., 2004). Such different ways of being sensitive stem, in part, from the ecology of a mother's daily routine but may also reflect culturally distinct beliefs about infant care (Carlson & Harwood, 2003). Middle-class Puerto Rican mothers report that they wish to promote proper demeanor as well as security in their infants. Thus they engage in more physical control of their 4-month-olds' movement and activity than

Anglo American mothers, behavior that is often interpreted as insensitivity in studies of Anglo American mothers. Such early physical control, however, predicts later attachment security in Puerto Rican toddlers but insecurity in Anglo American toddlers (Carlson & Harwood, 2003).

In sum, it appears that attachment is a universal phenomenon involving a special emotional bond between caregiver and infant. Modest but significant relations between warm and responsive behavior and child security are found in East Asia, Western Europe, and Latin America. Moreover, mothers from China, Colombia, Germany, Israel, Japan, Norway, and the United States share the view that (1) caregiving practices influence child security and (2) children exhibit secure base behavior. Finally, evidence suggests that infant security is achieved in multiple caregiver societies (e.g., Tronick, Morelli, & Ivey, 1992; Sagi et al., 1995). Cultural variations may not influence the importance of achieving a sense of security through responsive caregiving, but the evidence does suggest that the behaviors that constitute responsive or sensitive caregiving and infant security may be culturally variable. Our review thus far has highlighted emotional processes in the first year of life—temperament and attachment—suggesting that there may be a fair degree of cultural similarity in these processes. We next turn to a topic in which we expect to find a greater influence of culture (i.e., parental socialization of children's emotions). Although there are a number of potential mechanisms by which parents socialize children's emotions, few have been studied cross-culturally. We first discuss parental expression of emotion in the context of childrearing.

Parental Emotion Expression in the Context of Childrearing

One way in which children's emotions are socialized is through the experience of others' emotional reactions to them (Denham, 1998; Eisenberg et al., 1998). Parental emotional reactions socialize children's emotions by modelling emotional behavior, exposing children to a range of emotions, and providing contingent feedback (approval and disapproval, e.g.) about children's emotions and behavior. Parental joy and pleasure as well as disappointment, frustration, and disapproval reflect parental investment in childrearing (Dix, 1991). Parental emotional reactions also elicit emotional reactions in children; these provide opportunities for parent and child to cope together and they contribute to how children feel about themselves. Generally, parents express their emotions in culturally sanctioned ways. Their emotional communications carry cultural messages that influence children's emotion understanding, emotion regulation, and emotional well-being. Cultural influences on parental expression of emotions in the context of childrearing have been studied directly (e.g., mothers' contingent emotional responses to infants) and implicitly (e.g., expression of positive emotion as one index of parental warmth).

Parental Expression of Positive Emotion

In some respects, maternal communication of positive emotions with infants is similar across cultures (e.g., Bornstein, Tamís-LeMonda, et al., 1992; Carlson & Harwood, 2003; Fogel, Toda, & Kawai, 1988; Keller, Lohaus, et al., 2004; Papoušek & Papoušek, 1987). Mothers exaggerate their facial and vocal expressions of positive emotion and coo, cuddle, and soothe their infants. Even for older children, parents strive to be emotionally positive with their children, endorsing parental warmth as a value and feeling positive emotions when their children act according to cultural values (e.g., Honig & Chung, 1989; Wu et al., 2002). Children, even in the first year of life, are sensitive to changes in parental emotion; Canadian and Chinese 6-month-olds become distressed when their mothers cease to engage in face-to-face interaction with them (Kisilevsky et al., 1998). In sum, expressing positive emotion is a universal strategy for regulating children's emotions and communicating love and enjoyment in children.

Culture, however, influences the *relative* emphasis caregivers place on warmth and positive emotion in the context of raising children. White mothers of European heritage from Western industrialized nations (e.g., North America and Western Europe) express, and value expressing, positive emotions to their children more than mothers with backgrounds from Africa, Asia, and South and Central America (e.g., Bornstein et al., 1996; Deater-Deckard, Atzaba-Poria, & Pike, 2004; Ispa et al., 2004; Keller, Voelker, & Yovsi, 2005; Wu et al., 2002; Zahn-Waxler, Friedman, Cole, Mizuta, & Hiruma, 1996). One explanation for the relative difference is that conceiving of selves as independent and separate may therefore require overt expression of internal states to achieve intimacy (Markus & Kitayama, 1991). Few studies, however, assess links between cultural values, socialization goals, and parental practices (but see Harwood, Schöelmerich, Schulze, & Gonzalez, 1999).

Classifying cultures in broad terms is limited in explaining cultural variations in parental positive emotion. Consider a number of studies of mothers who are "collectivist" and "interdependent." Puerto Rican mothers praise and are affectionate with their toddlers, as much as Anglo parents, except in a teaching task (Harwood et al., 1999). Greek mothers smile at their infants more than German mothers do (Keller et al., 2003). Japanese mothers express less positive emotion than U.S. mothers (Dennis, Cole, Zahn-Waxler, & Mizuta, 2002) but more than Dutch mothers (Zevalkink & Riksen-Walraven, 2001). These findings illustrate the need for more sensitive conceptualizations of culture, as we discuss in our conclusions. Culturally and developmentally sensitive research considers the age of the child, the caregiver's socialization goal for a child of that age, the meaning of emotion-related behavior in the situation for the caregiver, and the degree to which the caregiver ascribes to the customs and beliefs that reflect the community's cultural priorities. Moreover, parents of a given ethnic group may appear less warm and positive toward their children than another group *until* additional factors are taken into account; for example, African American mothers appeared less positive than Euro American mothers until neighborhood quality was taken into account (Pinderhughes, Nix, Foster, & Jones, 2001; Zevalkink & Riksen-Walraven, 2001).

Parental Expression of Negative Emotion

Parents also socialize children's emotions when they communicate disapproval, irritation, and other negative emotions. Parental negative emotion is often treated as a risk factor in a child's development because it is associated with authoritarian, intrusive, or harsh parenting (e.g., Dix, Gershoff, Meunier, & Miller, 2004; Ispa et al., 2004) and child and parent maladjustment (e.g., Denham et al., 2000). The extent to which this is true is qualified by cross-cultural evidence. Parents in many, probably all, cultures are bothered by their children's socially inappropriate behavior (e.g., Honig & Chung, 1989). They differ, however, in their inclination to express such feelings. Asian parents, for example, use love withdrawal, open criticism and disapproval, and shaming and are less concerned about negotiating with children than advantaged parents in North America (e.g., Bowes, Chen, San, & Yuan, 2004; Fung, 1999; Lin & Fu, 1990; Wu et al., 2002).

It is important to understand parental negative emotion relative to the positive emotions they convey. Chinese, Japanese, and Hispanic parents, all of whom endorse parenting practices that are described as authoritarian, rejecting, or punitive, also endorse being accepting and protective of their children (Chen et al., 1998; Power, Kobayashi-Winata, & Kelley, 1992; Varela et al., 2004). In contrast, parental negative emotion in the absence of caring parental involvement and socially appropriate discipline seems problematic in any culture (Chen, Wu, Chen, Wang, & Cen, 2001; Deater-Deckard & Dodge, 1997). When stress interferes with a parent's culturally appropriate expression of negative emotion, it is related to child behavior problems even in cultures that value authoritarian parenting (Bradford et al., 2004; Chang, Lansford, Schwartz, & Farver, 2004; Chen et al., 2001).

It is also important to contextualize parental negative emotion in terms of cultural norms for asserting authority. Confucian values, for example, morally obligate Chinese parents to "train" their children; open disapproval is intended to promote shame in the child (Chao, 1994). Economically strained North American mothers, both Caucasian and African American (e.g., Martini, Root, & Jenkins, 2004; Miller & Sperry, 1987), endorse practices that involve open disapproval and anger but for different reasons than Chinese parents. U.S. urban working-class mothers say they intend to "toughen" their children (Miller & Sperry, 1987) and some lower-income, minority group parents say they are stern to teach compliance that will be required as the child interacts with the majority culture (Kelley, Power, & Wimbush, 1992). Again, factors such as neighborhood quality influence the degree to which parents believe in yelling at their children (Caughy & Franzini, 2005).

It is worth repeating that few studies directly examine links between cultural values, parenting strategies and parental emotions. One exception is a study that related Chinese and U.S. mothers' feelings and attributions regarding child misbehavior to their socialization goals (Cheah & Rubin, 2004). U.S. mothers are disappointed because they attribute the transgression to intentional, internal, or stable causes within the child and they are unsure how much control they have and should exert. Chinese parents become angry, attributing the transgression to causes they control; such events arise because the children cannot yet handle peer conflict and clear disapproval helps train the child. Parental expression of negative emotion that feels legitimate and does not involve doubt that it may interfere with child self-esteem or independence may be expressed differently, and perceived by children differently, than that expressed by a parent who feels such expression is not socially acceptable. This may explain why the relation between authoritarian parenting and youth adjustment varies across cultural groups (e.g., Phinney, Kim-Jo, Osorio, & Vilhjalmsdottir, 2005; Walker-Barnes & Mason, 2001).

In sum, culture influences the relative degree to which parents express positive and negative emotions in the context of childrearing. The effects of such emotional communications on children's emotional development may also be culturally variable. Future work that places parental emotional expression in the context of socialization goals and the circumstances in which children are being raised will illuminate our understanding of cultural group differences and their implications for parental emotions and the cultural socialization of children's emotions.

Parental Encouragement of and Communication about Children's Emotions

In addition to reacting emotionally to their children, parents socialize emotions by encouraging or discouraging children's emotional expression and by communicating with children about emotions. They may explicitly label a child's emotions and talk about how the child can cope with emotion as well as convey messages implicitly by their reactions to children's emotions and in discourse about emotional events in children's presence.

Parental Encouragement of Child Expression of Emotion

The American model of childrearing views the encouragement of child emotion expression as important for the development of self-esteem and emotional competence (e.g., Block, 1981; Gottman, Katz, & Hooven, 1997). East Asian parents, however, prefer emotional reserve more than expressivity in children (Chen et al., 1998; Lin & Fu, 1990; Zahn-Waxler et al., 1996). Even with positive emotions, East Asian parents view contentment and serenity as more optimal than joy (Shek, 2001). In regard to children's negative emotions, Japanese mothers try to anticipate and prevent their young children from having negative emotions, whereas Euro American mothers respond once the child is distressed and then help them cope (Rothbaum, Pott, et al., 2000). We assume all caregivers value emotional control and a sense of well-being in their children but vary in their views of what constitutes an optimal state of well-being, why children become highly emotional, how to respond to child emotion, how influential a caregiver can be, and what to expect by way of children's emotional control at different ages.

For example, Japanese caregivers feel it weakens the child's emotional dependence on the caregiver if limits are set on the young child's angry distress. They believe the emotional bond between caregiver and child promotes filial duty and social competence, including emotional reserve (Doi, 1973; for a Chinese perspective, see Wang, 2001). Therefore, they cajole or indulge a whining child rather than communicate disapproval. The cultural significance of these practices can be seen in the pride Japanese caregivers reveal when they see a teacher behave this way and the equally strong criticism Chinese and American caregivers have when they see these Japanese practices (Tobin, Wu, & Davidson, 1989). Unfortunately, there is very little research to address the implications of these practices for children's actual emotional expression or competence.

Again, culturally variable socialization practices should be understood in relation to parents' socialization goals and beliefs about child development and how parenting achieves those goals. The method of comparing caregivers' observations of their own and others' practices is particularly effective in drawing out cultural explanations for parental practices such as handling child emotion (Keller et al., 2005; Tobin et al., 1989). Observational studies are especially needed because parental reports about how they behave with their children do not always reflect their actual practices (Bornstein, Cote, & Venuti, 2001; Hsu, Tseng, Ashton, McDermott, & Char, 1985).

Parental Conversations about Child Emotion

Discourse is replete with cultural messages about emotion and is, therefore, an important mechanism for the socialization of emotion (Dunn, 1988; Miller, 1996). Caregivers converse about events with their children and in the presence of children, explicitly referring to emotional aspects of events and implicitly conveying the emotional significance of experiences and behavior (even if they do not make direct reference to emotion terms). The ways in which culture influences communication begins in infancy and continues through childhood. For example, even before children speak, caregivers communicate in ways that focus on or away from emotional aspects of experience. Japanese mothers engage in "affect-salient" speech more than Euro American mothers (Bornstein, Tal, et al., 1992; Toda, Fogel, & Kawai, 1990). That is, they coo and use terms of endearment more than directing the child's attention to description of objects and using informational speech when communicating with the infant. The Japanese mothers' use of affect-salient speech may reflect the importance these mothers place on an infant feeling content and dependent on the mother, whereas the Euro American mothers' primary use of informational speech may reflect the cultural value placed on acquiring knowledge and control (Bornstein, Tal, et al., 1992).

Once children do acquire expressive language, parent and child can converse about emotions, an aspect of interaction that has been studied in cultures ranging from Great Britain, the United States, China, and Taiwan to communities in Micronesia and the Andes (e.g., Cervántes, 2002; Lutz, 1987; Melzi & Fernández, 2004). Culture influences how often, in what ways, and why emotional experiences are discussed with and in front of children. Chinese parents, for example, talk less about a child's emotions and more about others' emotions (Wang, 2001). This may have the effect of minimizing the emphasis on the child's emotionality and focusing attention on developing concern for and sensitivity to others. This is consistent with an attitude that children should be emotionally reserved and that children's emotions are disruptive (Wang, 2001).

Comparative research on emotion talk, more than any other topic we have covered, attempts to disentangle educational and economic advantage from cultural heritage. In fact, economic status, more than culture, influences the frequency and complexity of conversations about emotional experiences among Latino and Anglo parents in the United States (Eisenberg, 1999; Flannagan & Perese, 1996; Hoff-Ginsberg, 1991). Culture, nonetheless, influences aspects of parents' discourse about emotions (Cervántes, 2002; Fung, 1999; Wang, 2001). For example, Latina mothers use emotion terms more when discussing their children's social experiences whereas Anglo mothers use emotion terms when discussing their children's learning experiences (Flannagan & Perese, 1996).

Personal storytelling is a form of discourse involving the telling and retelling of events (Miller, 1996). It conveys cultural values by defining which events are worth retelling. Culture influences the frequency, form, and function of storytelling as a tool for socializing children's emotions. In Chinese society, personal storytelling is used to reinforce moral values (e.g., teaching what is wrong about selfish anger), whereas in European American homes it is less frequent and used mainly as a source of mutual enjoyment, reinforcing relationships and downplaying negative events (e.g., Miller, Wiley, Fung, & Liang, 1997). European American mothers, however, report using children's storybooks and videos to help children manage their emotions, and young children have a high interest in such stories (Alexander, Miller, & Hengst, 2001; Miller, Hoogstra, Mintz, Fung, & Williams, 1993).

Emotional Communication and Emotion Socialization

In sum, universal and culturally variable practices and attitudes about communicating emotions are evident. Caregivers respond calmly to infant distress with attention and nurturance and express positive more than negative emotions to infants. At all ages, they believe that love and warmth are desirable qualities in their relationships; they feel happy when their children behave according to cultural standards and feel negatively when they do not. Culture influences the degree to which caregivers openly express positive and negative emotions although the factors that explain these variations—parental beliefs, implicit cultural values, minority-group status, neighborhood safety—are not known. It is important to understand that socialization practices reflect goals to promote culturally specific emotional competencies in children. It is important to also recognize that practices and values about emotions change over time. Historians have noted an increasing ambivalence in the United States toward expressing anger in the context of childrearing (Stearns & Stearns, 1986, 2003).

Children's Emotional Competence: The Results of Emotion Socialization

Raising children to become competent adults includes the goal of helping them become emotionally competent members of the community. Communities vary in their definitions of emotional competence and their beliefs about how it develops (e.g., Durbrow, Peña, Masten, Sesma, & Williamson, 1999; Leyendecker, Harwood, Lamb, & Schöelmerich, 2002). Emotional competence is comprised of adaptive emotional responses that help an individual reach goals, cope with challenges, communicate emotional states and needs, manage emotional arousal, discern others' feelings and appropriately respond, and recognize how emotion communication and self-presentation affect relationships (Saarni, 1999). The similarities and differences in the development of these various components in children from different backgrounds help us identify what aspects of emotion socialization are influenced by culture. We first describe what is known about children's emotion understanding. Less is known about the behavioral elements of emotional competence, so we consider studies of children's self-esteem and emotional symptoms.

Children's Emotional Understanding

Emotional understanding enhances children's socioemotional competence. It includes skill at reading others' emotions as well as knowledge about how to communicate and cope with emotions. Only a few aspects of emotion understanding have been examined from a cultural perspective—accuracy in reading others' emotions, understanding the emotions that particular situations elicit, and knowledge about displaying and regulating emotions.

ACCURACY IN INTERPRETING NONVERBAL CUES OF EMOTION

Children who are skilled at reading nonverbal emotional cues tend to be emotionally well regulated. The topic of emotion accuracy returns us to the question of whether emotion and its categories are universal concepts. Research with adults suggests that several emotions have universal prototypes or scripts (Elfenbein & Ambady, 2002; Russell, 1991; Scherer & Wallbott, 1994) and these therefore can be examined developmentally. Early cross-cultural comparisons of children's accuracy, however, were limited by unsophisticated translation methods, examination of emotions out of situational context, failure to control for the influences of schooling, small numbers of participants, and a lack of multicultural expertise on the research teams (Elfenbein & Ambady, 2002).

Some studies, however, have addressed interesting developmental hypotheses about cultural influences on children's emotional understanding. For example, one posited that an emotionally expressive culture provides children with more opportunities to become skillful at interpreting nonverbal cues. Indeed, Mexican school-age boys are more accurate in interpreting vocal cues of happiness, sadness, love, and anger, than Euro American boys are (McCluskey & Albas, 1981; McCluskey, Albas, Niemi, Cuevas, & Ferrer, 1975). A competing hypothesis is that cultures that value emotional restraint demand greater sensitivity in detecting others' feelings. One study found that Chinese children are generally more accurate than Australian children in recognizing facial emotions (Markham & Wang, 1996). It may not be the level of emotional expressivity that is the key cultural factor. Rather, both Mexican and Chinese cultures may regard a focus on others' feelings as more essential to competence than asserting one's own feelings. Research that links socialization goals to practices to predict accuracy in children's sensitivity to detecting emotions in others is sorely needed.

UNDERSTANDING SITUATION–EMOTION LINKS

A second aspect of emotional competence is an understanding of how situations influence emotions. Theoretically, each type of emotion reflects a prototypical appraisal of a situation as it pertains to one's goals for well-being; if persons in different cultures *appraise* a situation similarly, they have the same emotional response to it (Scherer, 1997). Children from diverse backgrounds (American, European, and Asian) appear to form common appraisals of a number of basic, familiar situations (e.g., Garner, Jones, & Miner, 1994; Harris, Olthof, Terwogt, & Hardman, 1987). This may occur because young children have common experiences, such as not getting what they want. Nonetheless, culture can guide how one appraises a situation. For example, Nepali first graders say they are happy when told to stop playing and go to bed whereas U.S. children say they are angry (Cole & Tamang, 1998). Nepali children look forward to cosleeping with adults and appraise this situation as achieving a desired goal; U.S. children appraise this situation as blocking the desired goal of playing.

DISPLAY AND REGULATION OF EMOTION

Culture also influences children's scripts for how one *should* feel in situations and in ways that seem to mirror the dominant values of their groups (e.g., Cole, Bruschi, & Tamang, 2002; Han, Leichtman, & Wang, 1998; Singh-Manoux & Fikenauer, 2001; Wang & Leichtman, 2000; Zahn-Waxler et al., 1996). For example, U.S. children believe that it is useful to convey anger, in a socially acceptable way, in order to right a wrong, a value that is consistent with their society's emphasis on individual rights and justice (Cole et al., 2002). In contrast, high-caste Brahman children in Nepal, whose communities emphasize respect for authority and mutual cooperation, feel, but would not reveal, anger in the same situations. Finally, Tamang children in Nepal, whose communities view anger as interfering with inner peace and social harmony, say it is wrong to *feel* angry in those situations. The links between culture, actual emotion socialization practices, and children's self-regulation of emotions, however, are rarely studied. The socialization practices of low-income mothers relate to their children's emotion knowledge in the same manner as they do for middle-class, Euro American families (e.g., Garner, Jones, Gaddy, & Rennie, 1997).

Despite cultural differences in aspects of emotion understanding, there appears to be a common developmental sequence in acquiring such knowledge. On approximately the same timetable, children understand more emotions, are more accurate in identifying emotions on the basis of nonverbal cues, are better able to predict emotions in false-belief situations and to understand that one can feel differently than one appears, and are more sophisticated in how they integrate emotional information into coping with interpersonal dilemmas (e.g., Callaghan et al., 2005; Harris, Guz, Lipian, & Man, 1985; Vinden, 1999). Interestingly, cultural variations in socialization pressures and opportunities may influence the timing if not the sequence in which understanding is achieved (e.g., Vinden, 1996). Joshi and MacLean (1994) studied British and Indian 4- and 6-year-olds' understanding that one can look different than one feels. Four-year-old Indian girls understood this distinction earlier than 4-year-old Indian boys and British 4-year-old boys and girls. Young Indian girls may experience a form of socialization pressure that cultivates earlier awareness. Conversely, a lack of opportunity (e.g., experience talking with adults about emotions) may delay knowledge of emotional terms and associated facial expressions (Curenton & Wilson, 2003; Tenenbaum, Visscher, Pons, & Harris, 2004; Wang, 2003).

In sum, culture influences the content of children's emotion understanding to some extent even as maturational factors seem to underlie the developmental sequence in which such knowledge is gained. Cultural variations in socialization pressures and opportunities may influence the timing of different aspects of emotional understanding and possibly the level of skill a child acquires.

Children's Self-Esteem and Emotional Distress

Behavioral evidence of children's emotional competence in situations has not been addressed in the comparative literature. Yet differences are likely because there is evidence of cultural differences in social competencies (e.g., handling peer conflict; Han & Park, 1995). Comparative studies of children's self-esteem and emotional distress suggest that culture influences emotional competence.

SELF-ESTEEM

Self-esteem is defined as the value one places on the self, including being a competent member of the group with which one identifies (e.g., Harter, 1990; Wang & Ollendick, 2001). Because culture appears to influence how one construes self (Markus & Kitayama, 1991) in all likelihood it also affects how one defines, values, and communicates self-worth, as evidence suggests.

At first blush, children of Asian heritage appear to have lower self-esteem than Euro American children (Gray-Little & Hafdahl, 2000; Heine, Lehman, Markus, & Kitayama, 1999). Speaking well of oneself, however, is immodest by Asian standards, as evidenced by the fact that Asian parents are less likely than U.S. parents to lavish praise on children or to minimize children's misbehavior and failures (e.g., Chen, Dong, & Zhou, 1997; Miller et al., 1996). The Euro American propensity for self-enhancement and minimization of personal limitations, thought to be crucial to self-esteem, is largely absent in individuals of Asian heritage (Greene & Way, 2005; Mezulis, Abramson, Hyde, & Hankin, 2004). Asian pride is defined by one's contributions to group goals, social harmony, and family honor, and is not tapped by Western self-esteem measures (e.g., Chan, 2000; Kitayama, Markus, Matsumoto, & Norasakkunkit, 1997).

African American children generally report higher levels of self-esteem than do Euro American children whereas other minority children report lower self-esteem than Euro American children (Gray-Little & Hafdahl, 2000; Greene & Way, 2005; Twenge & Crocker, 2002). African American children's pride and contentment may be attributable to the Civil Rights movement that instilled racial pride despite stresses associated with being a minority group member (Twenge & Crocker, 2002). The evidence suggests that a strong sense of one's cultural identity is associated with self-worth among minority youth (e.g., Bracey, Bámaca, & Umaña-Taylor, 2004).

EMOTIONAL DISTRESS

There is considerable evidence that symptoms of emotional distress are influenced by culture. Although this work generally reflects the reports of adults who are judging children, rather than children's actual distressed behavior, they suggest that cultural socialization processes influence how emotional distress appears. The work tends to focus on internalizing and externalizing symptoms more than actual disorder. Internalizing symptoms are defined by the experience of feeling disturbed (e.g., somatic complaints, anxieties, worries, anhedonia, and depressed mood). Externalizing symptoms, such as tantrums, angry defiance, hostility, and lack of remorse for hurtful behavior, disturb others.

Parents, teachers, and children from cultural backgrounds that view emotional reserve (e.g., Thailand or Kenya) as a sign of emotional competence report higher rates of child internalizing symptoms than those cultures that encourage emotional expressivity, which report higher rates of externalizing symptoms (Bergeron & Schneider, 2005; Weisz, Suwanlert, Chaiyasit, & Walter, 1987; Weisz, Sigman, Weiss, & Mosk, 1993). Possibly Kenyan or Thai parents who encourage emotional control are more likely to describe their children as having internalizing "symptoms"; the symptoms may describe emotional competencies and not significant emotional distress. Thus, evidence is needed to determine whether symptoms reflect psychopathology or competence. Parental reports may reflect selective attunement to behavior that is important to competence (Weisz, Chaiyasit, Weiss, Eastman, & Jackson, 1995). For example, somatic complaints are higher among Kenyan children than Thai, Euro American, or African American children, perhaps because disease is more widespread in Kenya and parents are highly attuned to signs a child may be ill (Weisz et al., 1993).

Emotional behavior that is regarded as a concern in one culture may not be in another. Shyness and inhibited behavior, for example, are related to social anxiety and depression in American and Canadian children but not in all children. When emotional restraint and modesty are the goals of socialization, shyness and inhibited behavior predict emotional adjustment and social competence, and not internalizing disorders (Chen, Rubin, & Li, 1995). Indeed, when disorder is assessed, Asian adults and youth have *fewer* internalizing disorders than their counterparts from other countries (e.g., Chiu, 2004; Lam, Pepper, & Ryabchenko, 2004).

Obviously, it is crucial to know whether behaviors that are used to assess symptoms are of actual concern to the reporters. Two studies demonstrate that parents and teachers who endorse behaviors on symptom checklists are not necessarily concerned about them (Lambert et al., 1992; Weisz, Suwanlert, Chaiyasit, & Weiss, 1991). Jamaican adults rate behaviors like angry defiance as problems more than Euro American parents do but also regard externalizing behavior as typical and are confident it will improve (Lambert et al., 1992). This finding is reminiscent of the fact that Asian parents expect children to transgress and treat those behaviors as opportunities rather than problems (Chao, 1995; Cheah & Rubin, 2004).

The degree to which one's emotions are socialized is quickly apparent when one is required to adapt to a different culture. Acculturation is a developmental process in which one strives to become a competent member of both a receiving or host society and one's own group (Oppedal, Røysamb, & Sam, 2004). Indeed, children and families appear to be at heightened risk for emotional difficulties when there is a collision of cultures. Both parent and child face the challenge of learning the emotional terrain of their new homeland; the child strives to be emotionally competent within the community of origin as well as with those of other backgrounds and parents have to cope with decisions about emotion socialization if their children's emotional demeanor changes (e.g., Lin, Endler, & Kocovski, 2001). An interesting future direction for this line of research would be to examine the degree to which being emotionally different from the majority group affects the stress of acculturation.

Although the goal of adult competence is a universal parental goal, the definition of what constitutes emotional competence varies as a function of culture. A particular emotional presentation that constitutes a risk condition in one culture may not be a risk condition in another culture. Many avenues of research can be taken to understand the products of emotion socialization by studying individuals who are becoming bicultural.

CONCLUSIONS

In closing, we briefly summarize and suggest directions for future research. If we examine the socialization of emotion in terms of (1) the child's emotionality as a potential contributing factor; (2) the values, goals, and practices by which caregivers socialize children; and (3) child emotional competence as a product of socialization, it is clear that there are universal and culturally variable influences at each and every stage. The evidence that differences in beliefs or behavior are attributable to culture, however, is limited. The potential to increase our knowledge depends on more sophisticated and sensitive conceptualizations and research designs.

Universal and Culturally Specific Aspects of the Socialization of Emotion

One way to view the many findings we have summarized is to return to the framework that emotional processes are biologically prepared capacities that motivate goal-directed behavior. Cultures are socially constructed, shared adaptations to the pressures and resources of the setting in which a community is formed, and those adaptations can influence goals and how they are met. Culture influences emotional processes in the course of socializing children to become emotionally competent members of their community who can achieve goals.

Caregivers perceive emotional differences in their children but we have limited knowledge about whether there are meaningful cultural group differences in infant temperament. There are cultural differences in the relative value and importance of particular child personality traits. Research, however, has not examined cultural differences in what caregivers think are desirable and undesirable attributes of infants. Future work should integrate observational and parental perception data, take precautions to be sure that the researchers understand the meaning of target behaviors to the observers and caregivers, take into consideration cultural tendencies to minimize or exaggerate qualities of one's children, and account for other factors that may be correlated with a culture (e.g., prenatal care or nutrition). Cultural differences in infant temperament, if they exist, could account for some differences in emotion socialization practices.

A number of socialization mechanisms have been proposed (Eisenberg et al., 1998; Parke, 1994), but only a few have been studied from a cultural perspective. It is reasonable to conclude, however, that there are a number of universal features to the socialization of emotion. All parents care about children's emotional well-being and self-regulation and share the goal of raising children who will be secure as young children and emotionally competent as adults. Caregivers are tender and emotionally positive with their infants, soothing, coddling, and nurturing them, promoting their physical and emotional well-being. Infants, as a result, form attachments to primary caregivers. Caregivers also care that children behave in socially appropriate ways and feel negatively when they do not.

There are cultural variations in how these goals are achieved, and these are evident within the first year of life. Even before attachment security is established, there are cultural differences in how caregiver warmth, nurturance, and positive emotion are expressed. These early practices model emotional behavior, convey messages about emotional dependence and self-reliance, and indicate which emotional states are desirable and which are not. Future research, however, must demonstrate the pathways between cultural values and socialization goals, caregiver sensitivity or emotional expressivity, and children's later emotional competence. Moreover, future studies must appreciate that practical demands on the family and the social structure of the community, as well as cultural beliefs, influence how caregivers administer to infant distress and define infant well-being.

Beyond infancy, positive and negative emotion is expressed by caregivers and encouraged in children in culturally different ways. It is assumed, but not demonstrated, that these beliefs reflect culturally specific socialization goals. There is a reasonable amount of evidence to hypothesize that the goals of emotional self-reliance, emotional self-assertion, interpersonal sensitivity, cooperativeness, and respectfulness influence parents' emotional expressions with their children. Moreover, the degree to which a parent expresses negative and positive emotions may reflect cultural values, but to what degree does it really reflect the physical and social realities of the setting in which children are being raised? Neighborhood safety, racist and discriminatory practices, the relative diversity or homogeneity of the cultural composition of a community, and the nature of intergroup relations between different cultural groups all have a bearing on the emotional lives of parents and how they socialize their children.

Although the developmental sequence with which children acquire emotional competencies appears to be constant across cultures, it is evident that their understanding about emotion, their beliefs about appropriate emotion and emotion regulation, and their self-evaluation and expression of distress reflect the results of the cultural socialization of emotion. However, no studies have directly demonstrated links between culturally specific values, socialization goals, socialization practices, and children's emotional skills. Moreover, studies of self-esteem and emotional distress clearly underscore the need to take a cultural perspective in understanding how different emotional profiles are valued and what they mean for children's well-being.

Finally, little is known about cultural effects associated with children's observations of others' emotions, children's opportunities to experience a range of emotions, children's perceptions of and reactions to others' emotions, and the influences of other socializing persons such as siblings and peers (but see Chen, French, & Schneider, 2006). Schools and various media formats also differ across cultures and yet these are rarely studied in the context of emotion socialization. Our reading of the comparative literature leaves us with a remarkable sense of how much humans have in common but also of the many subtle influences culture has on universal processes. It seems very important that future research move beyond cataloguing cultural group differences and similarities and attempt to explain *how* and *why* culture has its influences.

Conceptualizing and Assessing Culture

To advance knowledge about the cultural socialization of emotion, future work must attempt to define and assess culture. We must evaluate what culture is for each individual in each given group, considering the immediate and historical realities that community members share. Culturally sensitive questionnaires, interviews, and focus groups have all been used effectively to understand the context and meaning of parental and child behavior and to determine the degree to which each member of a group ascribes to the purported cultural values and practices. Measures for culturally specific concepts are being developed—for example, *familism* (Latino concept of commitment to the family; Heller, 1976) and *chiao* (Confucian concept of parental duty to train children; Chao, 1994)—and can provide more information about what a parent is trying to achieve relative to community standards.

As part of understanding culture within a place in time, it is essential to avoid two common limitations of the comparative literature: (1) confounding cultural group assignment with other factors that influence the emotional lives of families and communities and (2) overlooking important cultural differences within a nation and individual differences within groups (e.g., Hewlett, Lamb, Leyendecker, & Schöelmerich, 1998). Although we restricted our summary to comparative studies in peer-reviewed journals, we highly value the study of single groups and endorse the examination of individual variations within groups to further our understanding. Moreover, combining qualitative and quantitative methods is crucial to determining what is universal and what is culturally variable in the socialization of emotion.

Culturally sensitive, developmentally oriented comparative research is needed to demonstrate that particular features of a culture influence children's emotional development and explain how and why culture influences socialization of emotion. Such an approach, however, brings with it the formidable challenge of finding culturally fair ways to conduct the research. Berry (1990) recommends a *derived etic* approach, an iterative process of scrutinizing "outside" models and measures from an "inside" perspective. For example, the definition of emotion, a Western concept, can be subjected to the scrutiny of the non-Westerners in a research team to determine whether there is a common understanding of such a concept and to develop culturally relevant procedures that are comparable across groups.

The study of emotional processes in socialization, examined from a cultural perspective, is both challenging and exciting. The corpus of work that informed our discussion clearly indicates that comparative research is necessary for a comprehensive understanding of the universal and culturally variable aspects of socialization. The evidence we examined suggests many new hypotheses. These are best assessed with culturally relevant, developmental studies that avail themselves of multiple disciplinary expertise and techniques. The increasing capacity to conduct research in all the corners of the world bodes well for exciting advances in the years ahead.

ACKNOWLEDGMENTS

This work was supported, in part, by an award from the National Science Foundation (No. 9711519) to Pamela M. Cole. We also wish to acknowledge Babu Lal Tamang, Mukta Singh Tamang, and Sara Harkness, who contributed to our understanding of culture.

REFERENCES

Ahadi, S. A., Rothbart, M. K., & Ye, R. (1993). Children's temperament in the US and China: Similarities and differences. *European Journal of Personality, 7,* 359–377.

Ainsworth, M. D. S. (1967). *Infancy in Uganda: Infant care and the growth of love.* Baltimore: Johns Hopkins University Press.

Ainsworth, M. D. S., & Bell, S. M. (1970). Attachment, exploration, and separation: Illustrated by the behavior of one-year-olds in a strange situation. *Child Development, 41,* 49–67.

Alexander, K. J., Miller, P. J., & Hengst, J. A. (2001). Young children's emotional attachments to stories. *Social Development, 10,* 374–398.

Bergeron, N., & Schneider, B. H. (2005). Explaining cross-national differences in peer-directed aggression: A quantitative synthesis. *Aggressive Behavior, 31,* 116–137.

Berry, J. W. (1990). Imposed etics, emics, and derived etics: Their conceptual and operational status in cross-cultural psychology. In T. N. Headland & K. L. Pike (Eds.), *Emics and etics: The insider/outsider debate. Frontiers of anthropology* (Vol. 7, pp. 84–99). Thousand Oaks, CA: Sage.

Berry, J. W., Poortinga, Y.H., Segall, M.H., & Dasen, P.R. (2002). *Cross-cultural psychology: Research and applications* (2nd ed.). New York: Cambridge University Press.

Block, J. H. (1981). *The Child Rearing Practices Report (CRPR): A set of Q items for the description of parental socialization attitudes and values.* Berkeley: University of California, Institute of Human Development.

Bornstein, M. H. (2002). Toward a multicultural, multiage, multimethod science. *Human Development, 45,* 257–263.

Bornstein, M. H., Cote, L. R., & Venuti, P. (2001). Parenting beliefs and behaviors in northern and southern groups of Italian mothers of young infants. *Journal of Family Psychology, 15,* 663–675.

Bornstein, M.H., Tal, J., Rahn, C., Galperín, C.Z., Pêcheux, M., Lamour, M., et al. (1992). Functional analysis of the contents of maternal speech to infants of 5 and 13 months in four cultures: Argentina, France, Japan, and the United States. *Developmental Psychology, 28,* 593–603.

Bornstein, M. H., Tamis-LeMonda, C. S., Pascual, L., Haynes, M. O., Painter, K. M., Galperín, C. Z., et al. (1996). Ideas about parenting in Argentina, France, and the United States. *International Journal of Behavioral Development, 19,* 347–367.

Bornstein, M. H., Tamis-LeMonda, C. S., Tal, J., Ludemann, P., Toda, S., Rahn, C. W., et al. (1992). Maternal responsiveness to infants in three societies: The United States, France, and Japan. *Child Development, 63,* 808–821.

Bowes, J. M., Chen, M., San, L. Q., & Yuan, L. (2004). Reasoning and negotiation about child responsibility in urban Chinese families: Reports from mothers, father, and children. *International Journal of Behavioral Development, 28,* 48–58.

Bowlby, J. (1969). *Attachment and loss: Vol. 1. Attachment.* New York: Basic Books.

Bracey, J. R., Bámaca, M. Y., & Umaña-Taylor, A. J. (2004). Examining ethnic identity and self-esteem among biracial and monoracial adolescents. *Journal of Youth and Adolescence, 33,* 123–132

Bradford, K., Barber, B. K., Olsen, J. A., Maughan, S. L., Erickson, L.D., Ward, D., et al. (2004). A multi-national study of interparental conflict, parenting, and adolescent functioning: South Africa, Bangladesh, China, India, Bosnia, Germany, Palestine, Colombia, and the United States. *Marriage and Family Review, 35,* 107–137.

Bronfenbrenner, U. (1977). *The ecology of human development: Experiments by nature and design.* Cambridge, MA: Harvard University Press.

Callaghan, T., Rochat, P., Lillard, A., Claux, M. L., Odden, H., Itakura, S., et al. (2005). Synchrony in the onset of mental state reasoning: Evidence from five cultures. *Psychological Science, 16,* 378–384.

Camras, L. A., Meng, Z., Ujiie, T., Dharamsi, S., Miyake, K., Oster, H., et al. (2002). Observing emotion in infants: Facial expression, body behavior, and rater judgments of responses to an expectancy-violating event. *Emotion, 2,* 179–193.

Camras L. A., Oster H., Campos J., Campos R., Ujiie T., Miyake K., et al. (1998). Production of emotional facial expressions in European American, Japanese, and Chinese infants. *Developmental Psychology, 34,* 616–628.

Carlson, V. J., & Harwood, R. L. (2003). Attachment, culture, and the caregiving system: The cultural patterning of everyday experiences among Anglo and Puerto Rican mother-infant pairs. *Infant Mental Health Journal, 24,* 53–73.

Caudill, W., & Weinstein, H. (1969). Maternal care and infant behavior in Japan and America. *Psychiatry, 32,* 12–43.

Caughy, M. O., & Franzini, L. (2005). Neighborhood correlates of cultural differences in perceived effectiveness of parental disciplinary tactics. *Parenting: Practice and Science, 5,* 119–151.

Cervántes, C. A. (2002). Explanatory emotion talk in Mexican immigrant and Mexican American families. *Hispanic Journal of Behavioral Sciences, 24,* 138–163.

Chan, Y. M. (2000). Self-esteem: A cross-cultural comparison of British-Chinese, White British and Hong Kong Chinese children. *Educational Psychology, 20,* 59–74.

Chang, L., Lansford, J. E., Schwartz, D., & Farver, J. M. (2004). Marital quality, maternal depressed affect, harsh parenting, and child externalizing in Hong Kong Chinese families. *International Journal of Behavioral Development, 28,* 311–318.

Chao, R. K. (1994). Beyond parental control and authoritarian parenting style: Understanding Chinese parenting through the cultural notion of training. *Child Development, 65,* 1111–1119.

Chao, R. K. (1995). Chinese and European American cultural models of the self reflected in mothers' childrearing beliefs. *Ethos, 23,* 328–354.

Cheah, C. S. L., & Rubin, K. H. (2004). European American and mainland Chinese mothers' responses to aggression and social withdrawal in preschoolers. *International Journal of Behavioral Development, 28,* 83–94.

Chen, X., Dong, Q., & Zhou, H. (1997). Authoritative and authoritarian parenting practices and social and school adjustment. *International Journal of Behavioral Development, 20,* 855–873.

Chen, X., French, D., & Schneider, B. (Eds.). (2006). *Peer relationships in cultural context.* Cambridge, UK: Cambridge University Press.

Chen, X., Hastings, P. D., Rubin, K. H., Chen, H., Cen, G., & Stewart, S. L. (1998). Child-rearing attitudes and behavioral inhibition in Chinese and Canadian toddlers: A cross-cultural study. *Developmental Psychology, 34,* 677–686.

Chen, X., Rubin, K. H., & Li, Z. (1995). Social functioning and adjustment in Chinese children: A longitudinal study. *Developmental Psychology, 31,* 531–539.

Chen, X., Wu, H., Chen, H., Wang, L., & Cen, G. (2001). Parenting practices and aggressive behavior in Chinese children. *Parenting: Science and Practice, 1,* 159–184.

Chiu, E. (2004). Epidemiology of depression in the Asia Pacific region. *Australasian Psychiatry, 12,* S4–S10.

Cole, P. M., Bruschi, C. J., & Tamang, B. L. (2002). Cultural differences in children's emotional reactions to difficult situations. *Child Development, 73,* 983–996.

Cole, P. M., & Tamang, B. L. (1998). Nepali children's ideas about emotional displays in hypothetical challenges. *Developmental Psychology, 34,* 640–646.

Curenton, S. M., & Wilson, M. N. (2003). "I'm happy with my mommy": Low-income preschoolers' causal attributions for emotions. *Early Education and Development, 14,* 199–213.

Deater-Deckard, K., Atzaba-Poria, P. N., & Pike, A. (2004). Mother– and father–child mutuality in Anglo and Indian British families: A link with lower externalizing problems. *Journal of Abnormal Child Psychology, 32,* 609-620.

Deater-Deckard, K., & Dodge, K. A. (1997). Externalizing behavior problems and discipline revisited: Nonlinear effects and variation by culture, context, and gender. *Psychological Inquiry, 8,* 161–175.

Denham, S. A. (1998). *Emotional development in young children.* New York: Guilford Press.

Denham, S. A., Workman, E., Cole, P. M., Weissbrod, C., Kendziora, K. T., & Zahn-Waxler, C. (2000). Prediction of externalizing behavior problems from early to middle childhood: The role of parental socialization and emotion expression. *Development and Psychopathology, 12,* 23–45.

Dennis, T. A., Cole, P. M., Zahn Waxler, C., & Mizuta, I. (2002). Self in context: Autonomy and relatedness in Japanese and U.S. mother–preschooler dyads. *Child Development, 73,* 1803–1817.

Dix, T. (1991). The affective organization of parenting: Adaptive and maladaptive processes. *Psychological Bulletin, 110,* 3–25.

Dix, T., Gershoff, E. T., Meunier, L. N., & Miller, P. C. (2004). The affective structure of supportive parenting: Depressive symptoms, immediate emotions, and child-oriented motivation. *Developmental Psychology, 40,* 1212–1227.

Doi, T. H., (1973). *The anatomy of dependence.* Oxford, UK: Kodansha International.

Dunn, J. (1988). *The beginnings of social understanding.* Cambridge, MA: Harvard University Press.

Durbrow, E. H., Peña, L. F., Masten, A., Sesma, A., & Williamson, I. (1999). Mothers' conceptions of child competence in contexts of poverty: The Philippines, St. Vincent, and the United States. *International Journal of Behavioral Development, 25,* 438–445.

Eisenberg, A. R. (1999). Emotion talk among Mexican American and Anglo American mothers and children from two social classes. *Merrill Palmer Quarterly, 45,* 267–284.

Eisenberg, N., Cumberland, A., & Spinrad, T. L. (1998). Parental socialization of emotion. *Psychological Inquiry, 9,* 241–273.

Ekman, P. (1992). Are there basic emotions? *Psychological Review, 99,* 550–553.

Elfenbein, H. A., & Ambady, N. (2002). On the universality and cultural specificity of emotion regulation: A meta-analysis. *Psychological Bulletin, 128,* 203–235.

Elphick, E., Halverson, C. F. J., & Marszal-Wisniewska, M. (1998). Extraversion: Toward a unifying description from infancy to adulthood. In G. A. Kohnstamm & C. F. J. Halverson (Eds.), *Parental descriptions of child personality: Developmental antecedents of the big five* (pp. 21–48). Mahwah, NJ: Erlbaum.

Flannagan, D., & Perese, S. (1996). Emotional references in mother–daughter and mother–son dyads' conversations about school. *Sex Roles, 39,* 353–367.

Fogel, A., Toda, S., & Kawai, M. (1988). Mother–infant face-to-face interactions in Japan and the United States: A laboratory comparison using 3-month-old infants. *Developmental Psychology, 24,* 398–406.

Freedman, D. G. (1974). *Human infancy: An evolutionary perspective.* New York: Halsted Press.

Friedlmeier, W., & Trommsdorff, G. (1999). Emotion regulation in early childhood: A cross-cultural comparison between German and Japanese toddlers. *Journal of Cross-Cultural Psychology, 30,* 684–711.

Fung, H. (1999). Becoming a moral child: The socialization of shame among young Chinese children. *Ethos, 27,* 180–209.

García Coll, C., Lamberty, G., Jenkins, R., McAdoo, H. P., Crnic, K., Wasik, B. H., et al. (1996). An integrative model for the study of developmental competencies in minority children. *Child Development, 67,* 1891–1914.

Garner, P. W., Jones, D., Gaddy, G., & Rennie, K. M. (1997). Low-income mothers' conversations about emotions and their children's emotional competence. *Social Development, 6,* 37–52.

Garner, P. W., Jones, D., & Miner, J. L. (1994). Social competence among low-income preschoolers: Emotion socialization practices and social cognitive correlates. *Child Development, 65,* 622–637.

Gartstein, M. A., Slobodskaya, H. R., & Kinsht, I. A. (2003). Cross-cultural differences in temperament in the first year of life: United States of America (US) and Russia. *International Journal of Behavioral Development, 27,* 316–328.

Gjerde, P. F. (2004). Culture, power, and experience: Toward a person-centered cultural psychology. *Human Development, 47,* 138–157.

Goldsmith, H. H., Buss, A. H., Plomin, R., Rothbart, M. K., Thomas, A., Chess, S., et al. (1987). Roundtable: what is temperament? Four approaches. *Child Development, 58,* 505–529.

Goslin, D. (Ed.). (1969). *Handbook of socialization: Theory and research.* New York: Rand McNally.

Gottman, J. M., Katz, L. F., & Hooven, C. (1997). *Meta-emotion: How families communicate emotionally.* Hillsdale, NJ: Erlbaum.

Gray-Little, B., & Hafdahl, A. R. (2000). Factors influencing racial comparisons of self-esteem: A quantitative review. *Psychological Bulletin, 121,* 26–54.

Greene, M. L., & Way, N. (2005). Self-esteem trajectories among ethnic minority adolescents: A growth curve analysis of the patterns and predictors of change. *Journal of Research on Adolescence, 15,* 151–178.

Grossmann, K. E., Grossmann, K., Huber, F., & Wartner, U. (1981). German children's behavior towards their mothers at 12 months and their fathers at 18 months in Ainsworth's strange situation. *International Journal of Behavioral Development, 4,* 157–181.

Grossmann, K., Grossmann, K. E., Spangler, G., Suess, G., & Unzner, L. (1985). Maternal sensitivity and newborns' orientation responses as related to quality of attachment in northern Germany. *Monographs of the Society for Research in Child Development, 50,* 233–256.

Halberstadt, A. G., Denham, S. A., & Dunsmore, J. C. (2001). Affective social competence. *Social Development, 10,* 79–119.

Han, J. J., Leichtman, M. D., & Wang, Q. (1998). Autobiographical memory in Korean, Chinese, and American children. *Developmental Psychology, 34,* 701–713.

Han, G., & Park, B. (1995). Children's choice in conflict: Application of the theory of individualism-collectivism. *Journal of Cross-Cultural Psychology, 26,* 298–313.

Harkness, S., & Super, C. M. (1996). *Parents' cultural belief systems: Their origins, expressions, and consequences.* New York: Guilford Press.

Harris, P. L., Guz, G. R., Lipian, M. S., & Man, S. Z. (1985). Insight into the time course of emotion among Western and Chinese children. *Child Development, 56,* 972–988.

Harris, P. L., Olthof, T., Terwogt, M. M., & Hardman, C. E. (1987). Children's knowledge of the situations that provoke emotion. *International Journal of Behavioral Development, 10,* 319–343.

Harter, S. (1990). Causes, correlates, and the functional role of global self-worth: A life-span perspective. In R. J. Sternberg & J. J. Kolligian (Eds.), *Competence considered* (pp. 67–97). New Haven, CT: Yale University Press.

Harwood, R. L., Schöelmerich, A., Schulze, P.A., & Gonzalez, Z. (1999). Cultural differences in maternal beliefs and behaviors: A study of middle-class Anglo and Puerto Rican mother–infant pairs in four everyday situations. *Child Development, 70,* 1005–1016.

Heine, S. H., Lehman, D. R., Markus, H. R., & Kitayama, S. (1999). Is there a universal need for positive self-regard? *Psychological Review, 106,* 766–794.

Heller, P. L. (1976). Familism scale: Revalidation and revision. *Journal of Marriage and the Family, 38,* 423–429.

Hewlett, B. S., Lamb, M. E., Shannon, D., Leyendecker, B., & Schöelmerich, A. (1998). Culture and early infancy among central African foragers and farmers. *Developmental Psychology, 34,* 653–661.

Hoff-Ginsberg, E. (1991). Mother–child conversation in different social classes and communicative settings. *Child Development, 62,* 782–796.

Hofstede, G. (1984). *Culture's consequences: International differences in work-related values.* Beverly Hills, CA: Sage.

Honig, A. S., & Chung, M. (1989). Child-rearing practices of urban poor mothers of infants and three-year-olds in five cultures. *Early Child Development and Care, 50,* 75–97.

Hsu, J., Tseng, W., Ashton, G., McDermott, J. F., & Char, W. (1985). Family interaction patterns among Japanese-American and Caucasian families in Hawaii. *American Journal of Psychiatry, 142,* 577–581.

Ispa, J. M., Fine, M. A., Halgunseth, L. C., Harper, S., Robinson, J., Boyce, L., et al. (2004). Maternal intrusiveness, maternal warmth, and mother–toddler relationship outcomes: Variations across low-income ethnic and acculturation groups. *Child Development, 75,* 1613–1631.

Joshi, M. S., & MacLean, M. (1994). Indian and English children's understanding of the distinction between real and apparent emotion. *Child Development, 65,* 1372–1384.

Kagan, J., Arcus, D., Snidman, N., Feng, W. Y., Hendler, J., & Greene, S. (1994). Reactivity in infants: A cross-national comparison. *Developmental Psychology, 30,* 342–345.

Kağitçibaşi, C. (1996). Individualisam and collectivism. In J.W. Berry, M.H. Segall, & C. Kağitçibaşi (Eds.), *Handbook of cross-cultural psychology. Volume 3: Social behavior and applications* (2nd ed., pp. 1–49). Boston: Allyn & Bacon.

Keller, H. (2003). Socialization for competence: Cultural models of infancy. *Human Development, 46*, 288–311.

Keller, H., Lohaus, A., Kuensemueller, P., Abels, M., Yovis, R., Voelker, S., et al. (2004). The bio-culture of parenting: Evidence from five cultural communities. *Parenting: Science and Practice, 4*, 25–50.

Keller, H., Papaligoura, Z., Kuensemueller, P., Voelker, S., Papaeliou, C., Lohaus, A., et al. (2003). Concepts of mother–infant interactions in Greece and Germany. *Journal of Cross-Cultural Psychology, 34*, 677–689.

Keller, H., Voelker, S., & Yovsi, R. D. (2005). Conceptions of parenting in different cultural communities: The case of West African Nso and Northern German women. *Social Development, 14*, 158–180.

Keller, H., Yovsi, R., Borke, J., Kartner, J., Jensen, H., & Papaligoura, Z. (2004). Developmental consequences of early parenting experiences: Self-recognition and self-regulation in three cultural communities. *Child Development, 75*, 1745–1760.

Kelley, M. L., Power, T. G., & Wimbush, D. D. (1992). Determinants of disciplinary practices in low-income Black mothers. *Child Development, 63*, 573–582.

Kisilevsky, B. S., Hains, S. M., Lee, K., Muir, D. W., Xu, F., Zhao, Z. Y., et al. (1998). The still-face effect in Chinese and Canadian 3- to 6- month infants. *Developmental Psychology, 34*, 629–639.

Kitayama, S., Markus, H. R., Matsumoto, H., & Norasakkunkit, V. (1997). Individual and collective processes in the construction of the self: Self-enhancement in the United States and self-criticism in Japan. *Journal of Personality and Social Psychology, 72*, 1245–1267.

Kohnstamm, G. A., Halverson, C. F., Mervielde, I., & Havill, V. L. (1998). Analyzing parental free descriptions of child personality. In C. F. Halverson & G. A. Kohnstamm (Eds.), *Parental descriptions of child personality: Developmental antecedents of the Big Five?* (pp. 1–19). Mahwah, NJ: Erlbaum.

Kohnstamm, G. A., Zhang, Y., Slotboom, A. M., & Elphick, E. (1998). A developmental integration of conscientiousness from childhood to adulthood. In C.F. Halverson & G.A. Kohnstamm (Eds.), *Parental descriptions of child personality: Developmental antecedents of the Big Five?* (pp. 65–84). Mahwah, NJ: Erlbaum.

Lam, C. Y., Pepper, C. M., & Ryabchenko, K. A. (2004). Case identification of mood disorders in Asian American and Caucasian American college students. *Psychiatric Quarterly, 75*, 361–373.

Lambert, M. C., Weisz, J. R., Knight, F., Desrosiers, M., Overly, K., & Thesiger, C. (1992). Jamaican and American adult perspectives on child psychopathology: Further exploration of the threshold model. *Journal of Consulting and Clinical Psychology, 60*, 146–149.

Lebra, T. S. (2000). New insight and old dilemma: A cross-cultural comparison of Japan and the United States. *Child Development, 71*, 1147–1149.

LeVine, R. A. (1969). Culture, personality, and socialization: An evolutionary view. In D. Goslin (Ed.), *Handbook of socialization: Theory and research* (pp. 503–541). New York: Rand McNally.

LeVine, R. A., Dixon, S., LeVine, S., Richman, A., Leiderman, P. H., Keefer, C. H., et al. (1994). *Childcare and culture: Lessons from Africa*. New York: Cambridge University Press.

Lewis, M., Ramsay, D. S., & Kawakami, K. (1993). Differences between Japanese infants and Caucasian American infants in behavioral and cortisol response to inoculation. *Child Development, 64*, 1722–1731.

Leyendecker, B., Harwood, R. L., Lamb, M. E., & Schöelmerich, A. (2002). Mothers' socialization goals and evaluations of desirable and undesirable everyday situations in two diverse cultural groups. *International Journal of Behavioral Development, 26*, 248–258.

Lin, C. Y. C., & Fu, V. R. (1990). A comparison of child rearing practices among Chinese, immigrant Chinese, and Caucasian-American parents. *Child Development, 61*, 429–433.

Lin, M. C., Endler, N. S., & Kocovski, N. L. (2001). State and trait anxiety: A cross-cultural comparison of Chinese and Caucasian students in Canada. *Current Psychology, 20*, 95–111.

Lozoff, B., DeAndraca, I., Castíllo, M., Smith, J.G., Walter, T., & Pi–o, P. (2003). Behavioral and developmental effects of preventing iron-deficiency anemia in healthy full-term infants. *Pediatrics, 112*, 846–854.

Lutz, C. A. (1987). Goals, events, and understanding in Ifaluk emotion theory. In N. Quinn & D. Holland (Eds.), *Cultural models in language and thought* (pp. 290–312). New York: Cambridge University Press.

Marín, G., Gamba, R. J., & Marín, B. V. (1992). Extreme response style and acquiescence among hispanics: The role of acculturation and education. *Journal of Cross-Cultural Psychology, 23*, 498–509.

Markham, R., & Wang, L. (1996). Recognition of emotion in Chinese and Australian children. *Journal of Cross-Cultural Psychology, 27*, 616–643.

Markus, H. R., & Kitayama, S. (1991). Culture and the self. Implications for cognition, emotion and motivation. *Psychological Review, 98,* 224–253.

Martini, T. S., Root, C. A., & Jenkins, J. M. (2004). Low and middle income mothers' regulation of negative emotion: Effects of children's temperament and situational emotional responses. *Social Development, 13,* 515–530.

McCluskey, K. W., & Albas, D. C. (1981). Perception of the emotional content of speech by Canadian and Mexican children, adolescents, and adults. *International Journal of Psychology, 16,* 119–132.

McCluskey, K. W., Albas, D. C., Niemi, R. R., Cuevas, C., & Ferrer, C. A. (1975). Cross-cultural differences in the perception of the emotional content of speech: A study of the development of sensitivity in Canadian and Mexican children. *Developmental Psychology, 11,* 551–555.

McLoyd, V. C. (2004). Linking race and ethnicity to culture: Steps along the road from inference and hypothesis testing. *Human Development, 47,* 185–191.

Melzi, G., & Fernández, C. (2004). Talking about past emotions: Conversations between Peruvian mothers and their preschool children. *Sex Roles, 50,* 641–657.

Mesquita, B., & Frijda, N. H. (1992). Cultural variations in emotions: A review. *Psychological Bulletin, 112,* 179–204.

Mezulis, A. H., Abramson, L. Y., Hyde, J. S., & Hankin, B. L. (2004). Is there a universal positivity bias in attributions? A meta-analytic review of individual, developmental, and cultural differences in the self-serving attributional bias. *Psychological Bulletin, 130,* 711–747.

Miller, P. J. (1996). Instantiating culture through discourse practices: Some personal reflections on socialization and how to study it. In R. Jessor, A. Colby, & R. A. Schweder (Eds.), *Ethnography and human development: Context and meaning in social inquiry* (pp. 183–204). Chicago: University of Chicago Press.

Miller, P. J., Fung, H., & Mintz, J. (1996). Self-construction through narrative practices: A Chinese and American comparison of early socialization. *Ethos, 24,* 237–280.

Miller, P. J., Hoogstra, L., Mintz, J., Fung, H., & Williams, K. (1993). Troubles in the garden and how they get resolved: A young child's transformation of his favorite story. In C.A. Nelson (Ed.), *Memory and affect in development* (pp. 87–114). Hillsdale, NJ: Erlbaum.

Miller, P. J., & Sperry, L. L. (1987). The socialization of anger and aggression. *Merrill-Palmer Quarterly, 33,* 1–31.

Miller, P. J., Wiley, A. R., Fung, H., & Liang, C. H. (1997). Personal storytelling as a medium of socialization in Chinese and American families. *Child Development, 68,* 557–568.

Miyake, K., Campos, J. J., Kagan, J., & Bradshaw, D. (1986). Issues in socioemotional development. In H. Stevenson, H. Azuma, & K. Hakuta (Eds.), *Child development and education in Japan* (pp. 239–261). New York: Freeman.

Mizuta, I., Zahn-Waxler C., Cole, P. M., & Hiruma, N. (1996). A cross-cultural study of preschoolers' attachment: Security and sensitivity in Japanese and US dyads. *International Journal of Behavioral Development, 19,* 141–159.

Oppedal, B., Røysamb, E., & Sam, D. L. (2004). The effect of acculturation and social support on change in mental health among young immigrants. *International Journal of Behavioral Development, 28,* 481–494.

Oyserman, D., Coon, H. M., & Kemmelmeier, M. (2002). Rethinking individualism and collectivism: Evaluation of theoretical assumptions and meta-analyses. *Psychological Bulletin, 128,* 3–72.

Papoušek, H., & Papoušek, M. (1987). Intuitive parenting: A dialectic counterpart to the infant's integrative competence. In J. D. Osofsky, (Ed.), *Handbook of infant development* (2nd ed., pp. 669–720). Oxford, UK: Wiley.

Parke, R. D. (1994). Progress, paradigms, and unresolved problems: A commentary on recent advances in our understanding of children's emotions. *Merrill-Palmer Quarterly, 40,* 157–169.

Phinney, J. S., Kim-Jo, T., Osorio, S., & Vilhjalmsdottir, P. (2005). Autonomy and relatedness in adolescent–parent disagreements: Ethnic and developmental factors. *Journal of Adolescent Research, 20,* 8–39.

Pinderhughes, E. E., Nix, R., Foster, E. M., & Jones, D. (2001). Parenting in context: Impact of neighborhood poverty, residential stability, public services, social networks, and danger on parental behaviors. *Journal of Marriage and the Family, 63,* 941–953.

Pomerleau, A., Sabatíer, C., & Malcuit, G. (1998). Quebecoís, Haitian, and Vietnamese mothers' report of infant temperament. *International Journal of Psychology, 33,* 337–344.

Posada, G., Gao, Y., Fang, W., Posada, R., Tascon, M., Schöelmerich, A., et al. (1995). The secure-base phenomenon across cultures: Children's behavior, mothers' preferences, and experts' concepts. *Monographs of the Society for Research in Child Development, 60*(2–3, Serial No. 244), 27–48.

Power, T. G., Kobayashi-Winata, H., & Kelley, M. L. (1992). Childrearing patterns in Japan and the United States: A cluster analytic study. *International Journal of Behavioral Development, 15*, 185–205.

Rao, N., McHale, J. P., & Pearson, E. (2003). Links between socialization goals and child-rearing practices in Chinese and Indian mothers. *Child Development, 12*, 475–492.

Rogoff, B. (2003). *The cultural nature of human development*. New York: Oxford University Press.

Rothbart, M. K, & Bates, J. E. (1998). Temperament. In W. Damon & N. Eisenberg (Eds.), *Handbook of child psychology: Social, emotional, and personality development* (Vol. 3, pp. 105–176). New York: Wiley.

Rothbaum, F., Morelli, G., Pott, M., & Liu-Constant, Y. (2000). Immigrant Chinese and Euro-American parents' physical closeness with young children: Themes of family relatedness. *Journal of Family Psychology, 14*, 334–348.

Rothbaum, F., Pott, M., Azuma, H., Miyake, K., & Weisz, J. (2000). The development of close relationships in Japan and the United States: Paths of symbiotic harmony and generative tension. *Child Development, 71*, 1121–1142.

Rothbaum, F., Weisz, J., Pott, M., Miyake, K., & Morelli, G. (2000). Attachment and culture: Security in the United States and Japan. *American Psychologist, 55*, 1093–1104.

Russell, A., Hart, C. H., Robinson, C. C., & Olsen, S. F. (2003). Children's sociable and aggressive behavior with peers: A comparison of the US and Australian, and contributions of temperament and parenting styles. *International Journal of Behavioral Development, 27*, 74–86.

Russell, J. A. (1991). Culture and the categorization of emotions. *Psychological Bulletin, 110*, 426–450.

Saarni, C. (1999). *The development of emotional competence*. New York: Guilford Press.

Sagi, A., van IJzendoorn, M. H., Aviezer, O., Donnell, F., Koren-Karie, N., Joels, T., et al. (1995). Attachments in a multiple-caregiver environment: The case of the Israeli kibbutzim. *Monographs of the Society for Research in Child Development, 60*(2–3, Serial No. 244), 71–91.

Scherer, K. R. (1997). The role of culture in emotion-antecedent appraisal. *Journal of Personality and Social Psychology, 73*, 902–922.

Scherer, K. R., & Wallbott, H. G. (1994). Evidence for universality and cultural variation of differential emotion response patterning. *Journal of Personality and Social Psychology, 66*, 310–328.

Shek, D. T. L. (2001). Paternal and maternal influences on family functioning among Hong Kong Chinese families. *Journal of Genetic Psychology, 162*, 56–74.

Singh-Manoux, A., & Fikenauer, C. (2001). Cultural variations in social sharing of emotions: An intercultural perspective. *Journal of Cross-Cultural Psychology, 32*, 647–661.

Smith, P. (2004). Acquiescent response bias as an aspect of cultural communication style. *Journal of Cross-Cultural Psychology, 35*, 50–61.

Stearns, C. Z., & Stearns, P. N. (1986). *Anger: The struggle for emotional control in America's history*. Chicago: University of Chicago Press.

Stearns, C. Z., & Stearns, P. N. (2003). A new approach to anger control 1860–1940: The American ambivalence. In M. Silberman (Ed.), *Violence and society: A reader* (pp. 15–27). Upper Saddle River, NJ: Prentice-Hall.

Super, C. M., & Harkness, S. (1986). The developmental niche: A conceptualization at the interface of child and culture. *International Journal of Behavioral Development, 9*, 545–569.

Takashi, K. (1986). Examining the strange-situation procedure with Japanese mothers and 12-month-old infants. *Developmental Psychology, 22*, 265–270.

Tenenbaum, H. R., Visscher, P., Pons, F., & Harris, P. L. (2004). Emotional understanding in Quechua children from an agro-pastoralist village. *International Journal of Behavioral Development, 28*, 471–478.

Tobin, J., Wu, D. & Davidson, D. (1989). *Preschool in three cultures: Japan, China, and the United States*. New Haven, CT: Yale University Press.

Toda, S., Fogel, A., & Kawai, M. (1990). Maternal speech to three-month-old infants in the United States and Japan. *Journal of Child Language, 17*, 279–294.

Triandis, H. C. (1989). The self and social behavior in differing cultural contexts. *Psychological Review, 96*, 506–520.

Tronick, E. Z., Morelli, G., & Ivey, P. K. (1992). The Efe forager infant and toddler's pattern of social relationships: Multiple and simultaneous. *Developmental Psychology, 28*, 568–577.

Twenge, J. M., & Crocker, J. (2002). Race and self-esteem revisited: Reply to Hafdahl and Gray-Little (2002). *Psychological Bulletin, 128*, 417–420.

van IJzendoorn, M. H., & Sagi, A. (1999). Cross-cultural patterns of attachment: Universal and contextual dimensions. In J. Cassidy & P. R. Shaver (Eds.), *Handbook of attachment: Theory, Research, and clinical applications* (pp. 713–734). New York: Guilford Press.

Varela, R. E., Vernberg, E. M., Sanchez-Sosa, J. J., Riveros, A., Mitchell, M., & Mashunkashey, J. (2004). Parenting style of Mexican, Mexican American, and Caucasian-Non-Hispanic families: Social context and cultural influences. *Journal of Family Psychology, 18,* 651–657.

Vassiliou, G., & Vassiliou, V. (1973) The implicative meaning of the Greek concept of *philitemo*. *Journal of Cross-Cultural Psychology,* 4, 326–341.

Vinden, P. G. (1996). Junín Quechua children's understanding of mind. *Child Development, 67,* 1707–1716.

Vinden, P. G. (1999). Children's understanding of mind and emotion: A multi-culture study. *Cognition and Emotion, 13,* 19–48.

Walker-Barnes, C. J., & Mason, C. A. (2001). Ethnic differences of parenting on gang involvement and gang delinquency: A longitudinal, hierarchical linear modeling perspective. *Child Development, 72,* 1814–1831.

Wang, Q. (2001). Culture effects on adults' earliest childhood recollection and self-description: Implications for the relation between memory and the self. *Journal of Personality and Social Psychology, 81,* 220–233.

Wang, Q. (2003). Emotion situation knowledge in American and Chinese preschool children and adults. *Cognition and Emotion, 17,* 725–746.

Wang, Q., & Leichtman, M. D. (2000). Same beginnings, different stories: A comparison of American and Chinese children's narratives. *Child Development, 71,* 1329–1346.

Wang, Y., & Ollendick, T. H. (2001). A cross-cultural and developmental analysis of self-esteem in Chinese and Western children. *Clinical Child and Family Psychology Review, 4,* 253–271.

Weisner, T. S. (2002). Ecocultural understanding of children's developing pathways. *Human Development, 45,* 272–281.

Weisz, J. R., Chaiyasit, W., Weiss, B., Eastman, K. L., & Jackson, E.W. (1995). A multimethod study of problem behavior among Thai and American children in school: Teacher reports versus direct observations. *Child Development, 66,* 402–415.

Weisz, J. R., Sigman, M., Weiss, B., & Mosk, J. (1993). Parent reports of behavioral and emotional problems among children in Kenya, Thailand, and the United States. *Child Development, 64,* 98–109.

Weisz, J. R., Suwanlert, S., Chaiyasit, W., & Walter, B. R. (1987). Over- and under-controlled referral problems among children and adolescents from Thailand and the United States: The "wat" and "wai" of cultural differences. *Journal of Consulting and Clinical Psychology, 55,* 719–726.

Weisz, J. R., Suwanlert, S., Chaiyasit, W., & Weiss, B. (1991). Adult attitudes toward over- and undercontrolled child problems: Urban and rural parents and teachers from Thailand and the United States. *Journal of Child Psychology and Psychiatry, 32,* 645–654.

Whiting, B. B., & Edwards, C. P. (1988). *Children of different worlds: The formation of social behavior.* Cambridge, MA: Harvard University Press.

Wu, P., Robinson, C. C., Yang, C., Hart, C. H., Olsen, S. F., Porter, C. L., et al. (2002). Similarities and differences in mothers' parenting of preschoolers in China and the United States. *International Journal of Behavioral Development, 26,* 481–491.

Yik, M. S. M., Meng, Z., & Russell, J. A. (1998). Adults' freely produced emotion labels for babies' spontaneous facial expressions. *Cognition and Emotion, 12,* 723–730.

Zach, U., & Keller, H. (1999). Patterns of the attachment-exploration balance of 1-year-old infants from the United States and Germany. *Journal of Cross-Cultural Psychology, 30,* 381–388.

Zahn-Waxler, C., Friedman, R. J., Cole, P. M., Mizuta, I., & Hiruma, N. (1996). Japanese and United States preschool children's responses to conflict and distress. *Child Development, 67,* 2462–2477.

Zevalnik, J., & Riksen-Walraven, J. M. (2001). Parenting in Indonesia: Inter- and intracultural differences in mothers' interactions with their young children. *International Journal of Behavioral Development, 25,* 167–175.

CHAPTER 21

Acculturation

JOHN W. BERRY

Acculturation is the dual process of cultural and psychological change that takes place as a result of contact between two or more cultural groups and their individual members. At the group level, it involves changes in social structures and institutions and in cultural practices. At the individual level, it involves changes in a person's behavioral repertoire; these psychological changes come about through a long-term process. Acculturation is a process that parallels many features of the process of socialization (and enculturation). Because acculturation takes place after an individual's initial socialization into his or her original culture, it may be viewed as a process of *resocialization,* or *secondary socialization.* In this chapter, all these processes (socialization, enculturation, and acculturation) are considered to be distinguishable features of the general concept of *cultural transmission.*

Contact and change occur for many reasons, including colonization, military invasion, migration, and sojourning (such as tourism, international study, and overseas posting); it continues after initial contact in culturally plural societies, where ethnocultural communities maintain features of their heritage cultures. Adaptation to living in culture-contact settings takes place over time; occasionally it is stressful, but often it results in some form of longer-term accommodation. Acculturation and adaptation are now reasonably well understood, permitting the development of policies and programs to promote successful outcomes for all parties involved in the contact situation.

This chapter begins by examining the history of the study of acculturation, including the development of current definitions of acculturation as distinct from enculturation and socialization. This examination is followed by a description of the attitudes and behaviors that together comprise various acculturation strategies and adaptations. The chapter concludes with some possible policy and program applications that may assist individuals, institutions, and cultural groups to deal more effectively with the process of acculturation.

THE CONCEPT OF ACCULTURATION

The initial interest of researchers in the process of acculturation grew out of a concern for the effects of European domination of colonial and indigenous peoples. Later, it focused on how immigrants (both voluntary and involuntary) changed following their entry and settlement into receiving societies. More recently, much of the work has been involved with how immigrant and ethnocultural groups relate to each other, and change, as a result of their attempts to live together in culturally plural societies (Redfield, Linton, & Herskovits, 1936). Nowadays, all three foci are important, as globalization results in ever-larger trading and political relations: Indigenous national populations experience neo-colonization, while new waves of immigrants, sojourners, and refugees flow from these economic and political changes, and large ethnocultural populations become established in most countries (Berry, 1990, 2003).

Much of this initial research was carried out with colonized populations in Africa and the Americas (e.g., Linton, 1940), and has continued in the traditional immigrant-receiving ("settler") countries of Australia, Canada, New Zealand, and the United States (see Chun, Balls-Organista, & Marin, 2003). These issues have become more and more important in the rest of the world, where massive population contacts and cultural transfers are taking place (see Sam & Berry, 2006). Particularly in Asia, half of the world's population lives in culturally diverse societies, which experience daily intercultural encounters and have to meet the demands for cultural and psychological change. As a cross-cultural psychologist, I take seriously the view that findings from research in one culture area of the world (or even in a few societies) cannot be generalized to others. Thus, international experiences, ideologies, and sensitivities may alter the conceptions and empirical findings that are portrayed in this chapter. It is, of course, up to all societies, and their diverse residents, to assess the relevance and validity of this existing work for their societies.

Early views about the nature of acculturation are a useful foundation for contemporary discussion. Two formulations in particular have been widely quoted. The first is:

> Acculturation comprehends those phenomena which result when groups of individuals having different cultures come into continuous first-hand contact, with subsequent changes in the original culture patterns of either or both groups . . . under this definition, acculturation is to be distinguished from culture change, of which it is but one aspect, and assimilation, which is at times a phase of acculturation. (Redfield et al., 1936, pp. 149–152)

In another formulation, acculturation was defined as:

> Culture change that is initiated by the conjunction of two or more autonomous cultural systems. Acculturative change may be the consequence of direct cultural transmission; it may be derived from non-cultural causes, such as ecological or demographic modification induced by an impinging culture; it may be delayed, as with internal adjustments following upon the acceptance of alien traits or patterns; or it may be a reactive adaptation of traditional modes of life. (Social Science Research Council, 1954, p. 974)

In the first formulation, acculturation is seen as one aspect of the broader concept of culture change (that which results from intercultural contact), is considered to generate change in "either or both groups," and is distinguished from assimilation (which may be "at times a phase"). These are important distinctions for psychological work and are pursued later. In the second definition, a few extra features are added: Change can be *indirect* (not cultural, but "ecological," due to alteration in habitat); *delayed* (there can be cultural and psychological lag, which can result in change years after contact), and sometimes "reactive" (i.e., groups and individuals may reject the cultural influences and change back toward a more "traditional" way of life, rather than inevitably toward greater similarity with the dominant culture).

Graves (1967) introduced the concept of *psychological acculturation,* which refers to changes in an individual who is a participant in a culture-contact situation, being influenced both directly by the external culture, and by the changing culture of which the individual is a member. There are two reasons for keeping these two levels distinct. The first is that in cross-cultural psychology, we view individual human behavior as interacting with the cultural context within which it occurs; hence separate conceptions and measurements are required at the two levels. This then allows for the search for systematic relationships between the two levels. The second is that not every individual enters into the contact situation, and participates in the new culture, or changes in the same way; there are vast individual differences in psychological acculturation, even among individuals who live in the same acculturative arena. This allows for a search for systematic relationships among psychological variables in a population.

Figure 21.1 presents a framework that outlines and links cultural-level and psychological-level acculturation, and identifies the two (or more) groups in contact. This framework serves as a map of those phenomena I believe need to be conceptualized and measured during acculturation research. At the cultural level (on the left) we need to understand key features of the two original cultural groups (A and B) prior to their major contact, the nature of their contact relationships, and the resulting dynamic cultural changes in both

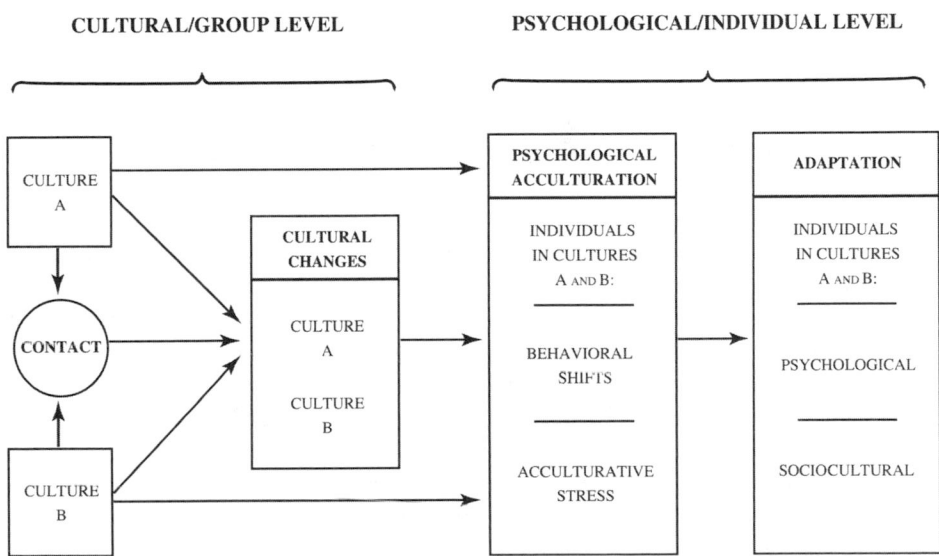

FIGURE 21.1. A general framework for understanding acculturation.

groups and in the emergent ethnocultural groups, during the process of acculturation. The gathering of this information requires extensive ethnographic, community-level work. These changes can be minor or substantial and range from being easily accomplished through to being a source of major cultural disruption. At the individual level (on the right) we need to consider the psychological changes that individuals in all groups undergo, and their eventual *adaptation* to their new situations. Identifying these changes requires sampling a population and studying individuals who are variably involved in the process of acculturation. These changes can be a set of rather easily accomplished *behavioral shifts* (e.g., in ways of speaking, dressing, and eating and in one's cultural identity) or they can be more challenging, even problematic (such as changing ones basic values, or religious beliefs). In the latter case, the result may be an increase in *acculturative stress* as manifested by uncertainty, anxiety, and depression (Berry, 1976). Finally, adaptations can be primarily internal or psychological (e.g., sense of well-being, or self-esteem) or sociocultural, linking the individual to others in the new society as manifested (e.g., competence in the activities of daily intercultural living; see Ward, 1996). These three preceding italicized terms are elaborated in the following sections. First, however, it is useful to situate the concept of acculturation in a broader notion of *cultural transmission*.

CULTURAL TRANSMISSION

The concept of *cultural transmission* was introduced by Cavalli-Sforza and Feldman (1981) to parallel the notion of *biological transmission*, in which, through genetic mechanisms, certain features of a population are perpetuated over time across generations. By analogy, using various forms of cultural transmission a cultural group can perpetuate its behavioral features among subsequent generations employing teaching and learning mechanisms. They distinguish three forms of cultural transmission: *vertical, horizontal* and *oblique*. Cultural transmission from parents to their offspring is termed "vertical transmission" by Cavalli-Sforza and Feldman (1981), because it involves the descent of cultural characteristics from the parental generation down to the next generation. While vertical descent is the only possible form of biological transmission, in the two other forms of cultural transmission (horizontal and oblique) there is no role for biology.

In vertical transmission parents transmit cultural values, skills, beliefs, motives (etc.) to their offspring. In this case, it is difficult to distinguish between cultural and biological transmission, because children typically learn most from the very people who were responsible for their conception (i.e., biological parents and cultural parents are the same). In horizontal cultural transmission, one learns from one's peers (in primary and secondary groups) during the course of development from birth to adulthood; here, there is no confounding between biological and cultural transmission. And in the case of oblique cultural transmission, one learns from other adults (including members of one's extended family) and social institutions (including community organizations and formal schooling). When the process takes place entirely within one's own or primary culture, "enculturation" and "socialization" are the appropriate terms. However, if the process derives from contact with another or secondary culture, the term "acculturation" is employed. As we have seen, this latter term refers to the form of transmission that is experienced by an individual that results from contact with, and influence from, persons and institutions belonging to cultures other than one's own.

The concept of *enculturation* has been developed within the discipline of cultural anthropology, and was first defined and used by Herskovits (1948). As the term suggests, there is an encompassing or surrounding of the individual by one's culture; the individual acquires appropriate values and behaviors by learning what the culture deems to be necessary. There is not necessarily anything deliberate or didactic about this process; often there is learning without specific teaching. The process of enculturation involves parents, and other adults and peers, in a network of influences on the individual, all of which can limit, shape, and direct the developing individual. The end result (if enculturation is successful) is a person who is competent in the culture, including its language, its rituals, its values, and so on.

The concept of *socialization* was originally developed in the discipline of sociology to refer to the process of deliberate shaping, by way of tutelage, of the individual. It is generally employed in cross-cultural psychology in the same way (see Segall, Dasen, Berry, & Poortinga, 1999). In developmental and social psychology, however, the concept of socialization is often employed to include both the informal aspects of enculturation and the more deliberate aspects of socialization that have been distinguished from each other here.

The net result of both enculturation and socialization is the development of behavioral similarities within cultures and behavioral differences between cultures. They are thus the crucial cultural mechanisms that produce the distribution of similarities and differences in psychological characteristics at the individual level. As such, they are critical to cross-cultural approaches to psychology; they provide an explanation for how features of the cultural group become features of their individual members.

As we have seen, the concept of *acculturation* also comes from anthropology and refers to cultural and psychological change brought about by contact with other peoples belonging to different cultures and exhibiting different behaviors.

Acculturation involves processes of *culture shedding* and *culture learning* (Berry, 1992). Culture shedding refers to the gradual process of losing some features of ones culture (such as attitudes, beliefs, and values), as well as some behavioral competencies (such as language knowledge and use). Culture learning refers to the process of acquisition of features of the new culture, sometimes as replacements for the attitudes and behaviors that have been lost, but often in addition to them. These two processes can create both problems and opportunities for individuals (Berry & Sam, 1997; Camilleri & Malewska-Peyre, 1997), which lead to wide variability in *acculturation strategies* and acculturation outcomes (*psychological* and *sociocultural adaptations*).

The process of cultural transmission does not lead to complete replication of successive generations; it falls somewhere between an exact transmission (with hardly any differences between parents, the social institutions, and offspring) and a complete failure of transmission (with offspring who are unlike their parents or others in their society). Functionally, either extreme may be problematic for a society. Exact transmission would not allow for novelty and change; the presence of variation in transmission from the parental generation enhances adaptability and provides the basis for groups and individuals to respond to new situations as they arise. In contrast, complete failure of transmission would not permit coordinated action between generations (Boyd & Richerson, 1985) and would lead to social chaos. In the case of acculturation, transmission to developing individuals comes from at least two cultural groups, sometimes creating confusion and conflict and sometimes producing new ways of living. Hence, acculturation can be seen not only in terms of loss and acquisition but also as a creative process, from which new societies emerge.

The following sections of this chapter provide evidence for variations in *how* groups and individuals enter into the acculturation process, and *how well* they adapt to it. These variations in acculturation attitudes and acculturation behaviors (which together constitute *acculturation strategies*) provide the basis for adaptive responses during culture contact.

ACCULTURATION CONTEXTS

As for all cross-cultural psychology (Berry, Poortinga, Segall, & Dasen, 2002), it is imperative that we base our work on acculturation by examining its cultural contexts. We need to understand, in ethnographic terms, both cultures that are in contact if we are to understand the individuals that are in contact.

In Figure 21.1, we saw that there are five aspects of cultural contexts: the two original cultures (A & B), the two changing ethnocultural groups (A and B), and the nature of their contact and interactions.

Taking the immigration process as an example, we may refer to the society of origin (A) and society of settlement (B) and their respective changing cultural features following contact. A complete understanding of acculturation would need to start with a fairly comprehensive examination of the societal contexts: In the society of origin, the cultural characteristics that accompany individuals into the acculturation process need description, in part to understand (literally) where the person is coming from and in part to establish cultural features for comparison with the society of settlement. The combination of political, economic, and demographic conditions being faced by individuals in their society of origin also needs to be studied as a basis for understanding the degree of *voluntariness* in the *migration motivation* of acculturating individuals.

A distinction has been made between those groups and individuals that enter into the contact voluntarily and those who are involuntary (Berry, Kim, Minde, & Mok, 1987). Associated with this notion are the positive ("pull") and negative ("push") motives that lead individuals to enter into contact situations. In some studies (e.g., Kim & Berry, 1986) these two motives are assessed independently, allowing for their separate contribution to acculturation attitudes and adaptation to be examined. In that study, it was found that those who were high on both negative and positive motives had poorer adaptation than those who had a balance between them. In other studies (e.g., Richmond [1993] imigrants were ranged on a single dimension between "reactive" and "proactive" motives, with the former being motivated by factors that are constraining or exclusionary, and generally negative in character, and the latter being motivated by factors that are facilitating or enabling, and generally positive in character. Such groups as indigenous peoples and refugee asylum seekers are reactive and involuntary groups that often experience more difficulties during acculturation than voluntary groups (see Allen, Vaage, & Hauff, 2006; Dona & Ackermann, 2006; Kvernmo, 2006, for reviews of acculturation difficulties among refugees and indigenous peoples). In contrast, immigrants who are usually voluntary (in the sense that they often choose to migrate to achieve a better life for themselves and their families) typically restablish their lives rather well and achieve levels of income, education, and well-being that are comparable to those already settled in the society (see Beiser et al., 1988; Sam & Berry, 2006, for a review of the evidence).

In the society of settlement, a number of factors have importance. First there are the general orientations that a society and its citizens have toward immigration and pluralism. With respect to immigration, some societies (those termed "settler societies," such as Australia, Canada, and the United States) have been built by immigration over the centuries, and this process may be a continuing one, guided by a deliberate immigration and settlement policy. Other societies have received immigrants and refugees only reluctantly, usually without a policy to guide their entry or programs to assist in their settlement (e.g., Germany, and the United Kingdom).The important issue to understand for the process of acculturation is the historical, policy, and attitudinal situation faced by immigrants in the society of settlement.

With respect to orientations toward cultural diversity, some societies are accepting of cultural pluralism resulting from immigration, taking steps to support the continuation of cultural diversity as a shared communal resource; this position represents a positive *multicultural ideology* (Berry & Kalin, 1995) which accepts the value of both diversity and equity of all cultural groups in the plural society. Of course, public attitudes and public policies do not always coincide. In some cases, for example, in Canada (Berry & Kalin, 2000), there is a large degree of agreement that Canada is, and should remain, a multicultural society. There is similar agreement between public attitudes and policies in the case of France (Sabatier & Boutry, 2006) and in Germany (Phalet & Kosic, 2006), where citizens and governments share more assimilationist views about how immigrants and ethnocultural groups should acculturate. In contrast, there is decreasing consensus in Australia (Sang & Ward, 2006) where the multicultural policy is increasingly challenged by public attitudes that are growing more assimilationist. Evidence across a number of societies shows that the promotion of diversity as a national policy enhances a preference for a multicultural way of living together, which in turn promotes the positive sociocultural adaptation of immigrant youth (Berry, Phinney, Sam, & Vedder, 2006).

Other societies seek to eliminate diversity through policies and programs of assimilation, while others attempt to segregate or marginalize diverse populations in their societies. Murphy (1965) has argued that societies that are supportive of cultural pluralism (i.e., with a positive multicultural ideology) provide a more positive settlement context for two reasons: They are less likely to enforce cultural change (assimilation) or exclusion (segregation and marginalization) on immigrants and they are more likely to provide social support both from the institutions of the larger society (e.g., culturally sensitive health care, and multicultural curricula in schools), and from the continuing and evolving ethnocultural communities that usually make up pluralistic societies. However, even where pluralism is accepted, there are well-known variations in the relative acceptance of specific cultural, "racial," and religious groups (e.g., Berry & Kalin, 1995). Those groups that are less well accepted experience hostility, rejection, and discrimination, factors that are predictive of poor long-term adaptation. Numerous studies (e.g., Halpern, 1993; Noh, Beiser, Kaspar, Hou, & Rummens, 1999) of the effects of racism on personal well-being reveal that experiencing discrimination is a serious risk factor for personal well-being. More recently, in a large study of immigrant youth (Berry et al., 2006), the experience of discrimination was the most substantial predictor of poor psychological and sociocultural adaptation.

ACCULTURATION STRATEGIES

As noted earlier in the discussion of variations in cultural transmission, not all groups and individuals undergo acculturation in the same way; there are large variations in how people seek to engage the process. These variations have been termed "acculturation strategies" (Berry, 1997). Which strategies are used depends on a variety of antecedent factors (both cultural and psychological), and there are variable consequences (again both cultural and psychological) of these different strategies. These strategies consist of two (usually related) components: *attitudes* and *behaviors* (i.e., a person's preferences and actual outcomes) that are exhibited in day-to-day intercultural encounters.

The centrality of the concept of acculturation strategies can be illustrated by reference to each of the components included in Figure 21.1. At the cultural level, the two groups in contact (whether dominant or nondominant) usually have some notion about what they are attempting to do (e.g., colonial policies or motivations for migration), or what is being done to them, during the contact. Similarly, the goals of the emergent ethnocultural groups are likely to influence their collective acculturation strategies. In this section, evidence is presented that individual behavioral changes and acculturative stress phenomena are now known to be a function, at least to some extent, of how individuals try to acculturate. That is, *how* people acculturate is related to *how well* they adapt.

Four acculturation strategies have been derived from two basic issues facing all acculturating peoples. These issues are based on the distinction between orientations toward one's own group, and those toward other groups (Berry, 1980). Since then, a number of studies have confirmed that these two dimensions are independent of each other (e.g., Ryder, Alden, & Paulhus, 2000). This distinction is rendered as a relative preference for maintaining one's heritage culture and identity and a relative preference for having contact with and participating in the larger society along with other ethnocultural groups. Figure 21.2 presents this formulation.

These two issues can be responded to on attitudinal dimensions, represented by bi-

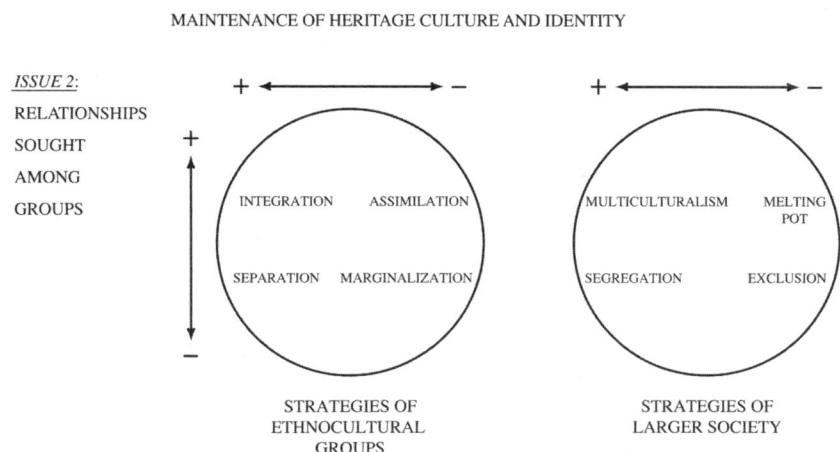

FIGURE 21.2. Four acculturation strategies based upon two issues, in ethnocultural groups and in the larger society.

polar arrows. For purposes of presentation, generally positive or negative orientations to these issues are shown; their intersection serves to define four acculturation strategies. These strategies carry different names, depending on which ethnocultural group (the dominant or nondominant) is being considered. From the point of view of nondominant groups (on the left of Figure 21.2), when individuals do not wish to maintain their cultural identity and seek daily interaction with other cultures, the assimilation strategy is defined. In contrast, when individuals place a value on holding on to their original culture, and at the same time wish to avoid interaction with others, the separation alternative is defined. When there is an interest in maintaining one's original culture while engaging in daily interactions with other groups, integration is the option. In this case, there is some degree of cultural integrity maintained, while seeking, as a member of an ethnocultural group, to participate as an integral part of the larger social network. Finally, when there is little possibility or interest in cultural maintenance (often for reasons of enforced cultural loss such as assimilation through enforced schooling, or language change), and little interest in having relations with others (often for reasons of exclusion or discrimination), marginalization is defined (Berry, 1980, 2003).

This presentation was based on the assumption that nondominant groups and their individual members have the freedom to choose how they want to acculturate. This, of course, is not always the case. When the dominant group enforces certain forms of acculturation, or constrains the choices of nondominant groups or individuals, other terms need to be used (see below).

Integration can only be "freely" chosen and successfully pursued by nondominant groups when the dominant society is open and inclusive in its orientation toward cultural diversity. Thus a mutual accommodation is required for integration to be attained, involving the acceptance by both groups of the right of all groups to live as culturally different peoples. This strategy requires nondominant groups to adopt the basic values of the larger society, whereas the dominant group must be prepared to adapt national institutions (e.g., education, health, and labor) to better meet the needs of all groups now living together in the plural society.

The two basic issues of orientation to one's own or the other group were initially approached by most researchers only from the point of view of the nondominant ethnocultural groups (e.g., Berry, 1970; Taft, 1977). However, the original anthropological definition clearly established that *both* groups in contact would become acculturated. Hence, a third dimension was added (Berry, 1974, 1980): that of the powerful role played by the dominant group in influencing the way in which mutual acculturation would take place. The addition of this third dimension produces the right side of Figure 21.2. Assimilation when sought by the nondominant acculturating group is termed the "melting pot," but when demanded by the dominant group, it is called the "pressure cooker." When separation is forced by the dominant group it is "segregation." Marginalization, when imposed by the dominant group, is "exclusion." Finally, integration, when diversity is a feature accepted by larger the society as a whole, including all the various ethnocultural groups, is called "multiculturalism." With the use of this framework, comparisons can be made between individuals and their groups and between nondominant peoples and the larger society within which they are acculturating. The ideologies and policies of the dominant group constitute an important element of ethnic relations research (see Berry, Kalin, & Taylor, 1977; Bourhis, Moise, Perreault, & Senecal, 1997), while the preferences of nondominant people are a core feature in acculturation research (Berry, Kim,

Power, Young, & Bujaki, 1989). Inconsistencies and conflicts between these various acculturation preferences are sources of difficulty for acculturating individuals. Generally, when acculturation experiences cause problems for acculturating individuals, we observe the phenomenon of *acculturative stress* (see next section).

Evidence for the reality of these various ways of acculturating comes from a study of over 5,000 immigrant youth who had settled in 13 countries (Berry et al., 2006). The project assessed a number of concepts (including attitudes toward the four ways of acculturating, ethnic and national identities, ethnic and national language knowledge and use, and ethnic and national friends). Four distinct acculturation profiles emerged from a cluster analysis of all these attitudinal and behavioral data. The largest number of youth fell into the *integration* cluster (defined by a preference for integration, positive ethnic and national identities, knowledge and use of both languages, and a friendship network that included youth from both cultures). The second largest cluster was an *ethnic* one (defined by a preference for separation and a rejection of assimilation, a high ethnic and low national identity, predominant use of the ethnic language, and friends mainly from their own ethnic group). A third cluster was a *national* one (defined by a pattern of attitudes and behaviors that are the opposite to the ethnic one, including a preference for assimilation, and high national and low ethnic identities, language, and friends). Finally, a *diffuse* cluster emerged that resembled marginalization. This was defined by their acceptance of three attitudes (assimilation, separation, and marginalization) and a rejection of integration (suggesting an unformed or diffuse set of acculturation attitudes), low ethnic and national identities (suggesting a feeling of nonengagement or attachment to either cultural group), high proficiency in their ethnic language (and low proficiency and use of the national language), high contact with their own ethnic peers, but low contact with national peers. Finding these four distinct ways in which youth are acculturating provides substantial evidence for the existence of the four general acculturation strategies outlined earlier. Because these include a complex set of attitudes and behaviors, they correspond well to the notion of acculturation *strategies,* which combines preferences about how to live in the new culture and daily activities that express them. Thus there appears to be large individual differences in ways in which people seek to, and actually do, acculturate; the integrative course appears to be the most common way to do it, rather than more assimilationist or separationist courses.

PSYCHOLOGICAL ACCULTURATION

Two ways to conceptualize *psychological acculturation* have been proposed in the literature (see Figure 21.1). The first is *behavioral shifts*, in which those changes in an individual's behavioral repertoire take place rather easily and are usually nonproblematic. As noted earlier, this process encompasses two subprocesses: *cultural shedding* and *culture learning* (Berry, 1992). These processes involve the selective, accidental, or deliberate loss of original behaviors, and either their replacement or supplementation by behaviors that allow the individual a better "fit" with the society of settlement. Most often this process has been termed "adjustment," as virtually all the adaptive changes take place in the acculturating individual, with few changes occurring among members of the larger society (Ward, Bochner, & Furnham, 2001). These adjustments are typically made with minimal difficulty, in keeping with the appraisal of the acculturation experiences as nonproblematic. The long history of successful contact and settlement of most acculturating peoples attests to this relative degree of success. Even for involuntary refugees, after an initial period of difficulty, studies show that in the longer term, their adaptation achieves psychological and social well-being on a par with those born in the country of settlement (e.g., Aycan & Berry, 1996; Beiser, 2000; Berry et al., 2006). However, for indigenous peoples (who are also involuntarily in contact), there is considerable evidence of problematic acculturation (e.g., Berry, 1999; Berry, Wintrob, Sindell, & Mawhinney, 1982; Kvernmo, 2006).

When greater levels of conflict are experienced, and the experiences are judged to be problematic but controllable and surmountable, *acculturative stress* is the appropriate conceptualization (Berry et al., 1987). In this case, individuals understand that they are facing problems resulting from intercultural contact that cannot be dealt with easily or quickly by simply adjusting or assimilating to them. Drawing on the broader stress and adaptation paradigms (e.g., Lazarus & Folkman, 1984), focusing on acculturative stress leads to the study of the processes by which individuals deal with acculturative problems on first encountering them, and over time. In this sense, acculturative stress can be defined as a stress reaction in response to life events that are rooted in the experience of acculturation. Contemporary evidence (see Berry & Sam, 1997, for a review) shows that most people deal with such stressors effectively and reestablish their lives rather well, with health, psychological, and social outcomes that approximate those of individuals in the larger society. In a longitudinal study, of Vietnamese "boat people," Beiser (2000) found that over a period of 10 years in Canada, his sample showed an initial reduction in well-being but matched or surpassed a comparable sample of nonrefugees in psychological and social well-being after the 10 years. Similarly, Aycan and Berry (1996) found an initial decline in economic well-being (increased unemployment and underemployment) among Turkish immigrants to Canada, followed by a regaining of their economic status and psychological well-being after a period of about 7 years (see also Hayfron, 2006, for a review of the economic evidence).

ADAPTATION

As a result of attempts to cope with these acculturation changes, some long-term adaptations may be achieved. As mentioned earlier, adaptation refers to the relatively stable changes that take place in an individual or group in response to external demands. Moreover, adaptation may or may not improve the "fit" between individuals and their environments. It is thus not a term that necessarily implies that individuals or groups change to become more like their environments (i.e., adjustment by way of assimilation), but may involve resistance and attempts to change environments, or to move away from them altogether (i.e., by separation). In this usage, adaptation is an outcome that may or may not be positive in valence (i.e., meaning only well adapted). This bipolar sense of the concept of adaptation is used in the framework in Figure 21.1 where long-term adaptation to acculturation is highly variable, ranging from well to poorly adapted, and varying from a situation in which individuals can manage their new lives very well to one in which they are unable to carry on in the new society.

Adaptation is also multifaceted. The initial distinction between psychological and sociocultural adaptation was proposed and validated by Ward (1996). Psychological adaptation largely involves one's psychological and physical well-being, while sociocultural adaptation refers to how well an acculturating individual is able to manage daily life in the new cultural context. While conceptually distinct, they are empirically related to some extent (correlations between the two measures are in the +.4–+.5 range). However, they usually have different time courses and different experiential predictors. Psychological adaptation is predicted by personality variables, social support, and life-change events, while sociocultural adaptation is predicted by cultural knowledge, degree of contact, and positive intergroup attitudes. Psychological problems often increase soon after contact, followed by a general (but variable) decrease over time; positive sociocultural adaptation, however, typically has a linear improvement with time (see Ward et al., 2001, for a comprehensive review).

Research relating adaptation to acculturation strategies allows for some further generalizations (Berry, 1997; Ward, 1996). For both forms of adaptation, those who pursue and accomplish Integration appear to be better adapted, while those who are marginalized are least well adapted. And, again, the assimilation and separation strategies are associated with intermediate adaptation outcomes. For example, among a sample of Cree in Northern Quebec, factor analysis of a number of variables (including measures of acculturation attitudes, stress, and adaptation) showed that those favoring integration (and were able to achieve this way of acculturating by engaging in wage employment) and who were in favor of a synthesis of Cree and Eurocanadian ways of living were lower on indeces of stress and marginality and scored higher on a set of ability tasks. In a second example, research with young Chinese immigrant girls to New Zealand, Ho (1995) tracked their acculturation preferences over a period from their first arrival to between 3 and 4 years in New Zealand using the fourfold conceptualization. Over this period, there was a persistent decline in their preference for separation, accompanied by a persistent increase in preference for integration: Both assimilation and marginalization remained constant and low over this period. These changes in acculturation preferences were accompanied by increased levels of adaptation: "the most adaptive attitude for the newly arrived Chinese immigrants is to maintain their own cultural identity and learn to participate in the new society" (Ho, 1995, p. 43). While there are occasional variations on this pattern (e.g., Ryder et al., 2000, who found assimilation to be, overall, a better predictor of adjustment), it is remarkably consistent.

The most substantial evidence in support of this pattern comes from the study of immigrant youth (Berry et al., 2006) mentioned earlier. This project found evidence for the existence of the theoretical distinction between *psychological adaptation* (composed of having few psychological problems and high self-esteem and life satisfaction) and *sociocultural adaptation* (good school adjustment, few behavioral problems). When these two adaptation measures were related to the four acculturation profiles, a clear and consistent pattern emerged. Those in the integrated cluster were highest on both forms of adaptation, while those in the diffuse cluster were lowest on both. Those in the ethnic cluster had moderately good psychological adaptation but lower sociocultural adaptation, while those in the national cluster had poorer scores on both forms of adaptation. These latest findings suggest that those who pursue integrative strategies (in terms of attitudes, identities, and behaviors) will achieve better adaptations than those who acculturate in other ways, especially those who are diffuse or marginal in their way of acculturating.

APPLICATIONS

There is now widespread evidence that most people who have experienced acculturation actually do survive! They are not destroyed or substantially diminished by it;
rather, they find opportunities and achieve their goals sometimes beyond their initial
imaginings. This observation pertains more to those who are in voluntary contact situations (such as immigrants and sojourners) and probably less to those who are involuntarily experiencing acculturation (such as indigenous peoples, refugees, and formerly
enslaved populations).

Second, researchers often presume to know how acculturating individuals want to
live and impose their own ideologies or their personal views, rather than informing themselves about culturally rooted individual preferences and differences. One key concept
(but certainly not the only one) to understand this variability has been emphasized in this
chapter (*acculturation strategies*). Evidence now supports the existence of large individual
differences in both *how* people acculturate and *how well* they adapt. Evidence reviewed
in this chapter confirms a relationship between how and how well individuals deal with
the process of acculturation. Given these individual differences, and the relationship between these two sets of variables, we are on solid ground in suggesting that individuals
and groups should be informed of, and encouraged to seek, the integration path during
their acculturation, and to avoid marginalization. Although in some studies the two alternatives of assimilation and separation appear to promote better adaptation, these findings are less frequent.

The generalizations that have been made in this chapter on the basis of a wide range
of empirical findings allow us to propose that public policies and programs that seek to
reduce acculturative stress and to improve intercultural relationships should emphasize
the integration or multicultural approach to acculturation. This is true of group-level action, such as national policies, institutional arrangements, and the goals of ethnocultural
groups, and it is equally true of individual-level action, both in the larger society as well
as among members of nondominant acculturating groups.

There are two areas of application currently receiving considerable attention in
research and policy development. One is the domain of family life (including relationships among individuals within the family and between family members and the world
outside). The other is in the area of immigration and settlement policies (including
issues of changes in the institutions of a society and the promotion of cultural diversity).

With respect to family acculturation, evidence from the study with immigrant
youth (Berry et al., 2006), shows that parents and children sometimes have different
views about parent–adolescent relationships during acculturation. For example, parents
have higher scores on a measure of family obligations (e.g., responsibility for various
chores) than do their adolescent children; in sharp contrast, immigrant youth have
higher scores on a scale of adolescent rights (e.g., independence in dating) than their
parents. This pattern of discrepancy was the case for both immigrant and national
families in the study. However, the discrepancy between parents and adolescents was
greater for their views about obligations among the immigrant sample than among the
national sample; the parent–adolescent discrepancy did not differ for rights. Moreover,
the differences between parents and adolescents in their views about family obligations
varied according to which acculturation profile the youth were in: Those in the na-

tional profile (i.e., preferring assimilation, having a stronger national identity, and having more national friends) had greater discrepancies from the views of their parents. Most important, these discrepancies in family obligations scores (but not rights scores) were associated with poorer psychological and sociocultural adaptation of the adolescents: The greater the discrepancy, the poorer the psychological and sociocultural adaptation of the adolescents.

Another project dealing with family has been carried out in 30 countries (see Georgas, Berry, van de Vijver, Kagitcibasi, & Poortinga, 2006, for details), examining the similarities and differences in family structure and function and with some of their psychological correlates. This study has demonstrated both variation in family functioning that is linked to their ecological contexts (e.g., reliance on agriculture and general level of affluence) and variation due to their sociopolitical contexts (e.g., formal education and religion). In general, family arrangements are hierarchical and extended, and they have more conservative values (including interdependence) in high agrarian and low affluence societies, and with Orthodox Christian or Islamic religions. In contrast, families high in affluence and education and with a Protestant religious tradition are more nuclear, are less hierarchical, and exhibit more independence. Although not a part of this study, it may be hypothesized that following immigration, these variations in family life are likely to set the stage for variations in acculturation strategies, acculturative stress, and psychological and sociocultural adaptation. The basic dimensions of variations in family and behavior that have been established in this project will allow for their use in future studies of immigration and acculturation. When individuals migrate between the countries included in this sample of 30 societies, their placement on these dimensions can be used to examine discrepancies in cultural, political, and religious backgrounds that may be predictive of how, and how well, individual immigrants will acculturate in their new societies.

A second domain of application concerns public policies with respect to cultural diversity. We have made a number of assertions in this chapter on the basis of a wide range of empirical findings. This has allowed us to propose that public policies and programs that seek to reduce acculturative stress and to improve psychological and sociocultural adaptation should emphasize the integration or multicultural approach to acculturation (see Berry, 2001, for a discussion of the social and psychological costs and benefits of multiculturalism). Recent debates in political science (e.g., Banting & Kymlicka, 2004) attest to the importance of dealing with these issues at both the national policy and individual psychological levels. Further research is essential, for in the absence of conceptual clarity and empirical foundations, policies may create more social and psychological problems than they solve.

In some countries (such as Canada and Australia; see Berry, 1984), the integrationist perspective has become legislated in policies of multiculturalism, which encourage and support the maintenance of valued features of all cultures *and* at the same time support full participation of all ethnocultural groups in the evolving institutions of the larger society. What seems certain is that cultural diversity and the resultant acculturation are here to stay in all countries. Finding a way to accommodate each other poses a challenge and an opportunity to psychologists and other social scientists everywhere. Diversity is a fact of contemporary life; whether it is the "spice of life" or the main "irritant" is probably the central question that confronts us all, citizens and social scientists alike (Berry, 2001).

REFERENCES

Allen, J., Vaage, A. B., & Hauff, E. (2006).Refugees and asylum seekers. In D. L. Sam & J. W. Berry (Eds.), *Cambridge handbook of acculturation psychology* (pp. 198–217). Cambridge, UK: Cambridge University Press.

Aycan, Z., & Berry, J. W. (1996). Impact of employment-related experiences on immigrants' psychological well-being and adaptation to Canada. *Canadian Journal of Behavioural Science, 28,* 240–251.

Banting, K., & Kymlicka, W. (2004). Do multiculturalism policies erode the welfare state? In P. Van Parijs (Ed)., *Cultural diversity versus economic solidarity* (pp. 227–284). Brussels: Editions De Boeck Université.

Beiser, M. (2000). *Strangers at the gate.* Toronto, Canada: University of Toronto Press.

Beiser, M., Barwick, C, Berry, J. W., daCosta, G., Fantino, A., Ganesan, S., et al. (1988). *After the door has been opened: Mental health issues affecting immigrants and refugees in Canada.* Ottawa, Canada: Ministries of Multiculturalism, and Health and Welfare.

Berry, J. W. (1970). Marginality, stress and ethnic identification in an acculturating Aboriginal community. *Journal of Cross-Cultural Psychology, 1,* 239–252.

Berry, J.W. (1974). Psychological aspects of cultural pluralism. *Topics in Culture Learning, 2,* 17–22.

Berry, J. W. (1976). *Human ecology and cognitive style: Comparative studies in cultural and psychological adaptation.* New York: Sage/Halsted.

Berry, J. W. (1980). Acculturation as varieties of adaptation. In A. Padilla (Ed.), *Acculturation: Theory, models and findings* (pp. 9–25). Boulder, CO: Westview.

Berry, J. W. (1984). Multicultural policy in Canada: A social psychological analysis. *Canadian Journal of Behavioural Science, 16,* 353–370.

Berry, J. W. (1990). Psychology of acculturation. In J. Berman (Ed.), *Cross-cultural perspectives: Nebraska symposium in motivation* (Vol. 37, pp. 201–234). Lincoln: University of Nebraska Press.

Berry, J. W. (1992). Acculturation and adaptation in a new society. *International Migration, 30,* 69–85.

Berry, J. W. (1997). Immigration, acculturation and adaptation. *Applied Psychology: An International Review, 46,* 5–68.

Berry, J. W. (1999). Aboriginal cultural identity. *Canadian Journal of Native Studies, 19,* 1–36.

Berry, J. W. (2001). Socio-psychological costs and benefits of multiculturalism: A view from Canada. In J. W. Dacyl & C. Westin (Eds.), *Governance and cultural diversity* (pp. 297–354). Stockholm: UNESCO & CIEFO, Stockholm University.

Berry, J. W. (2003). Conceptual approaches to acculturation. In K. Chun, P. Balls-Organista, & G. Marin (Eds.), *Acculturation* (pp. 3–37). Washington, DC: American Psychological Association.

Berry, J. W., & Kalin, R. (1995). Multicultural and ethnic attitudes in Canada. *Canadian Journal of Behavioural Science, 27,* 310–320.

Berry, J. W., & Kalin, R. (2000). Multicultural policy and social psychology. In S. Renshon & J. Duckitt (Eds.), *Political psychology in cross-cultural perspective* (pp. 263–284). New York: Macmillan.

Berry, J. W., Kalin, R., & Taylor, D. (1977). *Multiculturalism and ethnic attitudes in Canada.* Ottawa, Canada: Supply & Services.

Berry, J. W., Kim, U., Minde, T., & Mok, D. (1987). Comparative studies of acculturative stress. *International Migration Review, 21,* 491–511.

Berry, J. W., Kim, U., Power, S., Young, M., & Bujaki, M. (1989). Acculturation attitudes in plural societies. *Applied Psychology: An International Review, 38,* 185–206.

Berry, J. W., Phinney, J. S., Sam, D. L., & Vedder, P. (2006). *Immigrant youth in cultural transition: Acculturation, identity and adaptation across national contexts.* Mahwah, NJ: Erlbaum.

Berry, J. W., Poortinga, Y. H., Segall, M. H., & Dasen, P. R. (2002). *Cross-cultural psychology: Research and applications* (2nd ed.). New York: Cambridge University Press

Berry, J. W., & Sam, D. (1997). Acculturation and adaptation. In J. W. Berry, M. H. Segall, & C. Kagitcibasi (Eds.), *Handbook of cross-cultural psychology, Vol. 3, Social behavior and applications* (pp. 291–326). Boston: Allyn & Bacon.

Berry, J. W., Wintrob, R. Sindell, P., & Mawinney, T. (1982). Psychological adaptation to culture change among the James Bay Cree. *Naturaliste Canadien, 109,* 965–975.

Bourhis, R., Moise, C., Perreault, S., & Senecal, S. (1997). Towards an interactive acculturation model: A social psychological approach. *International Journal of Psychology, 32,* 369–386.

Boyd, R., & Richerson, P. (1985). *Culture and the evolutionary process.* Chicago: University of Chicago Press.

Camilleri, C., & Maleskwa-Peyre, H. (1997). Socialization and identity strategies. In J. W. Berry, P. R. Dasen, & T. S. Saraswathi (Eds.), *Handbook of cross-cultural psychology* (Vol. 3, pp. 41–68). Boston: Allyn & Bacon.

Cavalli-Sforza, L. L., & Feldman, M. (1981). *Cultural transmission and evolution*. Princeton, NJ: Princeton University Press.

Chun, K., Balls-Organista, P., & Marin, G. (Eds.). (2003). *Acculturation: Advances in theory, measurement and applied research*. Washington, DC: American Psychological Association Press.

Dona, G., & Ackermann, L. (2006). Refugees in camps. In D. L. Sam & J. W. Berry (Eds.), *Cambridge handbook of acculturation psychology* (pp. 218–232). Cambridge, UK: Cambridge University Press.

Georgas, J., Berry, J. W., van de Vijver, F., Kagitcibasi, C., & Poortinga, Y. H. (2006). *Families across cultures: A 30 nation psychological study*. Cambridge, UK: Cambridge University Press.

Graves, T. (1967). Psychological acculturation in a tri-ethnic community. *South-Western Journal of Anthropology, 23*, 337–350.

Halpern, D. (1993). Minorities and mental health. *Social Science and Medicine, 36*, 597–607.

Hayfron, J. (2006). Immigrants in the labour market. In D. L. Sam & J. W. Berry (Eds.), *Cambridge handbook of acculturation psychology* (pp. 439–451). Cambridge, UK: Cambridge University Press.

Herskovits, M. J. (1948). *Man and his works: The science of cultural anthropology*. New York: Knopf.

Ho, E. (1995). Chinese or New Zealander? Differential paths of adaptation of Hong Kong Chinese adolescent immigrants in New Zealand. *New Zealand Population Review, 21*, 27–49.

Kim, U., & Berry, J. W. (1986). Predictors of acculturative stress: Korean immigrants in Toronto. In L. Ekstrand (Ed.), *Ethnic minorities and immigrants in cross-cultural perspective* (pp. 159–170). Lisse, The Netherlands: Swets & Zeitlinger.

Kvernmo, S. (2006). Indigenous peoples. In D. L. Sam & J. W. Berry (Eds.), *Cambridge handbook of acculturation psychology* (pp. 233–250). Cambridge, UK: Cambridge University Press.

Lazarus, R. S., & Folkman, S. (1984). *Stress, appraisal and coping*. New York: Springer.

Linton, R. (1940). *Acculturation in seven American Indian tribes*. New York: Appleton-Century.

Murphy, H. B. M. (1965). Migration and the major mental disorders. In M. B. Kantor (Ed.), *Mobility and mental health* (pp. 221–249). Springfield, MA: Thomas.

Noh, S., Beiser, M., Kaspar, V., Hou, F., & Rummens, J. (1999). Perceived racial discrimination, depression and coping. *Journal of Health and Social Behaviour, 40*, 193–207.

Phalet, K., & Kosic, A. (2006). Acculturation in the European Union. In D. L. Sam & J. W. Berry (Eds.), *Cambridge handbook of acculturation psychology* (pp. 331–348). Cambridge, UK: Cambridge University Press.

Redfield, R., Linton, R., & Herskovits, M. (1936). Memorandum on the study of acculturation. *American Anthropologist, 38*, 149–152.

Richmond, A. (1993). Reactive migration: Sociological perspectives on refugee movements *Journal of Refugee Studies, 6*, 7–24.

Ryder, A., Alden, L., & Paulhus, D. (2000). Is acculturation unidimensional or bi-dimensional? *Journal of Personality and Social Psychology, 79*, 49–65.

Sabatier, C., & Boutry, V. (2006). Acculturation in francophone European countries. In D. L. Sam & J. W. Berry (Eds.), *Cambridge handbook of acculturation psychology* (pp. 349–367). Cambridge, UK: Cambridge University Press.

Sam, D. & Berry, J. W. (Eds.). (2006). *Cambridge handbook of acculturation psychology*. Cambridge, UK: Cambridge University Press.

Sang, D., & Ward, C. (2006). Acculturation in Australia and New Zealand. In D. Sam & J. W. Berry (Eds.), *Cambridge handbook of acculturation psychology* (pp. 253–273). Cambridge, UK: Cambridge University Press.

Segall, H. H., Dasen, P. R. Berry, J. W., & Poortinga, Y. H. (1999). *Human behaviour in global perspective: An introduction to cross-cultural psychology* (2nd ed.). Boston: Allyn & Bacon.

Social Science Research Council. (1954). Acculturation: an exploratory formulation. *American Anthropologist, 56*, 973–1002.

Taft, R. (1977). Coping with unfamiliar cultures. In N. Warren (Ed.), *Studies in cross-cultural psychology* (pp. 121–151). London: Academic Press.

Ward, C. (1996). Acculturation. In D. Landis & R. Bhagat (Eds.), *Handbook of intercultural training* (2nd ed., pp. 124–147). Newbury Park, CA: Sage.

Ward, C., Bochner, S., & Furnham, A. (2001). *The psychology of culture shock*. London: Routledge.

PART VII

Targets of Socialization

CHAPTER 22

The Socialization of Gender

CAMPBELL LEAPER and CARLY KAY FRIEDMAN

From the moment of birth, a child's gender influences the opportunities she or he will experience. Within a few years of life, children begin to form their own ideas about gender that subsequently guide the types of activities they practice, what they find interesting, and the achievements they attain. As children develop, their gender self-concepts, beliefs, and motives are informed and transformed by families, peers, the media, and schools. These social contexts both reflect and perpetuate gender roles and gender inequities in the larger society (Leaper, 2000b; Wood & Eagly, 2002). The purpose of this chapter is to review the major social influences on these developments. We begin our review with a brief survey of theoretical approaches that have proven most helpful in understanding the socialization of gender.

THEORETICAL FRAMEWORKS

For the most part, contemporary theories of gender development are complementary rather than contradictory (see Martin, Ruble, & Szkrybalo, 2002). That is, most theories either explicitly or implicitly acknowledge the combined influences of social–structural, interpersonal, cognitive–motivational, and biological influences. Theories tend to differ, however, in how much they stress each of these processes in the transmission of gender (Bussey & Bandura, 1999). We concur with reviewers (e.g., Martin et al., 2002; Serbin, Powlishta, & Gulko, 1993) that the field could benefit from more concerted efforts aimed at integrating theoretical approaches. Although positing an integrative theory is beyond the scope of this chapter, we highlight some explanatory constructs from contemporary theoretical approaches that we view as complementary. In our review, we distinguish between social–structural, social–interactive, cognitive–motivational, and biological processes.

Social–Structural Processes

Children's gender development is embedded in a larger societal context. In this regard, the social–structural approach considers how people's relative status and power in society shape their personal circumstances; this perspective also addresses the constraints that these institutionalized roles impose on individuals' behavior. In addition to gender, other important social-status factors include ethnicity, race, economic class, and sexual orientation. The social–structural perspective is also compatible with a feminist analysis that emphasizes the impact of gender inequities in power existing in the home, the labor force, and political institutions (Wood & Eagly, 2002). Although a feminist social–structural approach is common in social psychology and sociology, relatively few developmental psychologists have considered gender from an explicitly feminist social–structural perspective (see Leaper, 2000b; Miller & Scholnick, 2000).

Social–Interactive Processes

Taking into account sexist practices in the larger society when studying children's development requires linking cultural institutions to individuals situated in their specific environments. In this regard, we borrow ideas from both social cognitive theory and sociocultural theory. Both theories emphasize the importance of children's social interactions and daily activities as contexts for the learning of culture. According to sociocultural theory, "the particular skills and orientations that children develop are rooted in the specific historical and cultural activities of the community in which children and their companions interact" (Rogoff, 1990, p. vii). Social cognitive theory similarly stresses opportunities to practice particular behaviors as well as the incentives (or disincentives) that follow for repeating those behaviors as important influences. Thus, the different opportunities that girls and boys systematically experience can be interpreted as forms of gender discrimination (Bussey & Bandura, 1999; Leaper, 2000b). As they are repeated over and over again during the course of childhood, gender-typed practices contribute to the development of gender differences in expectations, values, preferences, and skills.

Cognitive–Motivational Processes

Children internalize the culture's notions of gender once they acquire a symbolic capacity (Bussey & Bandura, 1999). As children form cognitive representations of gender, or gender schemas, they begin to filter the world through a gender lens. This is a fundamental premise of cognitive–developmental theory, gender schema theory, social–cognitive theory, social identity theory, and self-categorization theory (see Bussey & Bandura, 1999; Martin et al., 2002; Turner, 2000). As each of these theories emphasizes, children play an active role in their gender development and a process of self-socialization ensues. Girls and boys make inferences about the meaning and the consequences of gender-related behaviors from their observations and social interactions. Also, children's gender schemas and attitudes influence the type of information they notice and remember. Consequently, girls and boys tend to seek out gender-typed environments that further strengthen their gender-typed expectations and interests. In these ways, children's behavior becomes increasingly regulated by internal standards, values, and perceived consequences (Bussey & Bandura, 1999).

With the acquisition of a gender self-concept, children form a social identity of themselves as member of a particular gender group (see Harris, 1995; Turner, 2000). As emphasized in social identity or self-categorization theories, being a member of a group typically leads to an ingroup bias. Accordingly, several experimental studies have documented that children are more likely to pay attention to objects, activities, behaviors, and social roles associated with their own gender. Conversely, children avoid and devalue what is specifically associated with the other gender. Children's ingroup biases are further reflected in their preferences for same-gender peers and avoidance of other-gender peers (see Martin et al., 2002).

As children value their ingroup membership, they become sensitive to how others view them. For example, Banerjee and Lintern (2000) observed that children were more likely to act in gender-typed ways when peers were present. In this manner, same-gender peer groups tend to promote within-group assimilation. Although children typically internalize most group norms, girls and boys may find that some of their personal interests and values conflict with prevalent peer group's norms. For example, an adolescent girl may enjoy playing basketball despite her friends considering it unfeminine. In such a case, she may decide to play down her athletic accomplishment or otherwise risk being ostracized (Guillet, Sarrazin, & Fontayne, 2000).

Group socialization processes can have different degrees of impact on individuals' motives depending on the status and power of one group relative to the other group (or groups). Two corollaries of social identity theory are relevant. First, members of high-status groups are usually more invested in maintaining group boundaries than members of low-status groups (e.g., Bigler, Brown, & Markell, 2001). Consistent with the greater status and power traditionally accorded to males in society, boys are more likely to initiate and maintain role and group boundaries (see Leaper, 1994). Partly for this reason, gender-typing pressures tend to be more rigid for boys than for girls. A second pertinent corollary is that the characteristics associated with a high-status group are typically valued more than those of a low-status group. With regard to gender, masculine-stereotyped attributes (e.g., independence and assertiveness) tend to be valued more than feminine-stereotyped attributes (e.g., nurturance and compassion) in highly male-dominated societies (see Hofstede, 2000). Although cross-gender-typed behavior can sometimes enhance a girl's status, it typically diminishes a boy's status (see Leaper, 1994). Accordingly, cross-gender-typed behavior tends to be more common among girls than boys.

Biological Processes

Biological factors additionally influence gender development. Wood and Eagly (2002) propose the most important biologically based physical attributes that differentiate the sexes are women's reproductive capacity and men's greater strength, speed, and size. "Physical sex differences, in interaction with social and ecological conditions, influence the roles held by men and women because certain activities are more efficiently accomplished by one sex" (p. 702). Gender-differentiated roles tend to occur in societies wherein women's nursing and infant care hinder their performance of subsistence activities that require, for example, uninterrupted periods of work or extended time away from home. As Wood and Eagly also note, cultural changes have weakened gender-differentiated roles and patriarchy in many postindustrial societies: Women have gained control over their reproduction, and day care has become common. Moreover, strength, size, and speed are no longer important within these societies for most jobs (particularly those with the highest pay and status).

Researchers investigating biological factors have also examined the organizational and activational influences of hormones on gender development (see Berenbaum, 1998). First, sex-linked hormones may influence brain differentiation and organization during development, and this can contribute to corresponding differences in brain functioning. For example, sex-related differences in prenatal hormones may partly contribute to average gender differences in certain play preferences (see Berenbaum, 1998). Second, because hormones act as chemical messengers in the nervous system, sex-linked variations in hormone levels may influence the contemporaneous activation of certain brain and behavioral responses (Collaer & Hines, 1995).

We do not clearly understand how hormonal and social influences interact during development. Changes in hormones may influence behavior, but how individuals interpret their environments also can activate the release of certain hormones (e.g., see Sapolsky, 1997). Some researchers have suggested that the magnitude of sex-related biological influences are small but they get exaggerated during development—especially if the biological trend is consistent with prevalent gender proscriptions. For example, in their meta-analysis, Eaton and Enns (1986) found that boys tend to score higher than girls in activity level; however, the magnitude of the difference was small during infancy ($d = .33$) and increased with age ($d = .64$ for school age and older).[1] Given that our culture typically encourages physical activity more in boys than girls beginning in infancy (see Leaper, 2002), socialization practices may transform a small difference into a moderate one. As Scarr and McCartney (1983) explained, biological and environmental influences often work in synergy.

Summary

Several processes are implicated in children's gender development. First, social–structural factors include the division of labor and the prevalence of patriarchy in the larger society. Second, social–interactive factors affect the types of opportunities and incentives that children experience. Third, cognitive–motivational factors shape how children interpret and act on their worlds. Finally, biological factors include average physical differences between the sexes that may (or may not) be relevant for carrying out certain roles and activities. In addition, biological factors comprise sex-related hormonal influences that may affect the nervous system. Although we acknowledge the impact of biological factors, our review stresses the human capacity for behavioral plasticity in relation to existing environmental opportunities or constraints (see Leaper, 2000b; Wood & Eagly, 2002).

SOCIALIZATION OF GENDER-RELATED
VARIATIONS IN CHILDREN'S DEVELOPMENT

We next consider the socialization of a selective set of outcomes associated with children's gender development. When reviewing each topic, we consider evidence for parental as well as peer influences on gender-typed cognitive–motivational processes and behaviors. For some topics where it is especially relevant, we also address the influences of social–structural factors, the media, teachers and schools, and biological factors. To limit the scope and the length of the chapter, our selection of topics is necessarily incomplete. We selected areas that we deemed especially relevant to understanding the developmental context for some of the gender divisions and inequities often seen in adulthood. In particular, we address the socialization of (1) gender self-concepts, stereotypes, and attitudes; (2) gender-typed play; (3) sports; (4) social interaction and social norms; (5) academic motivation and achievement; and (6) household labor. Another constraint on our review is that our focus is primarily on children growing up in middle-class Western societies, which reflects the existing research literature itself.

Gender Self-Concepts, Stereotypes, and Attitudes

As previously described, children apply their developing representations of gender, known as gender schemas, to interpret the world around them. When considering the development of children's gender schemas, three types of distinctions are worth noting. First, researchers differentiate between children's schemas for the self (i.e., personal preferences and identity) and their schemas for others (i.e., stereotyped knowledge and attitudes). Although children's gender attitudes may influence their self-concepts (Liben & Bigler, 2002), the association between the two dimensions is generally weak (Signorella, 1999). Second, researchers differentiate between domains of gender typing such as traits, activities, and roles (Liben & Bigler, 2002). Finally, a third relevant distinction is between the knowledge and the endorsement of gender stereotypes. Understanding cultural stereotypes does not necessitate their approval (Liben & Bigler, 2002).

Children's acquisition and development of gender-related cognitions tend to follow a systematic pattern (see Martin et al., 2002, for a review). Children are capable of making perceptual distinctions between gender-linked physical attributes—such as faces and possibly even some gender-typed objects—as they approach 1 year of age. Verbal indications of a gender concept appear around 2 years of age when children begin to use gender to label other people (i.e., gender labeling). This is followed around 3 years of age when children demonstrate knowledge of their own gender (i.e., gender identity). Awareness of one's gender-group membership also becomes the basis of a *social* identity. That is, children see themselves as belonging to their gender group.

Between 3 and 6 years of age, children's concepts of other people's and their own gender become increasingly stable and consistent (i.e., gender constancy). During this age period, children also begin to form stereotypes about physical features and activities (e.g., girls wear dresses and boys play with trucks). With more cognitive sophistication, children around 6 years of age additionally tend to stereotype more abstract qualities such as social roles (e.g., men are truck drivers) and psychological attributes (e.g., women are nice). Furthermore, as children mature cognitively, they may show more flexibility in their gender attitudes and inferences during middle childhood and adolescence (Liben & Bigler, 2002; Serbin et al., 1993). Finally, recent research suggests that, around 10 years of age, girls can demonstrate awareness of gender discrimination (Brown & Bigler, 2004).

Social–Structural Influences

To identify possible social–structural moderators, it is useful to compare different cultures. In this regard, Baxter and Kane's (1995) cross-national survey indicated that traditional attitudes were correlated with women's degree of dependence on men in the society. For example, egalitarian attitudes were more likely in countries in which wives and husbands have relatively equal economic power. The influence of social–structural factors also can be seen in studies looking at variations within North America. Parents' gender attitudes may differ according to education, socioeconomic status, dual- or single-parent status, and race/ethnicity (see Leaper, 2002). Finally, there is also evidence for historical changes in North America. During the last three decades of the 20th century, adolescent girls' and young women's gender-role self-concepts steadily became less traditional (Twenge, 1997b) and their gender attitudes steadily became more egalitarian (Twenge, 1997a). Although research suggests that North American males have generally become more flexible in their views about women's roles (Twenge, 1997a), they still tend to view themselves in gender-typed ways (Twenge, 1997b).

Media Influences

The mass media is an important source for acquiring cultural information about gender. In the United States, there has been a modest decrease in gender stereotyping in children's television over the years (Thompson & Zerbinos, 1995). Nonetheless, gender stereotypes are pervasive in most of children's television programming. First, children will likely infer that men have more prominence and status in society than do women through the overwhelming overrepresentation of male characters in most cartoon series. In addition, the characters in TV cartoons typically reflect gender-stereotyped roles and attributes (Leaper, Breed, Hoffman, & Perlman, 2002; Thompson & Zerbinos, 1995). Thus, perhaps it is no surprise that children's amount of television viewing is positively correlated with their own degree of gender stereotyping. What children watch may be guided by their gender schemas, and what they watch may shape their gender beliefs (see Calvert & Huston, 1987; Ward & Friedman, 2006).

Other media such as children's books also perpetuate gender bias and stereotypes. Although a more gender-equitable representation of characters in North American children's books has occurred over the years, males still tend to be more common in titles and pictures (Gooden & Gooden, 2001). Also, children's books typically portray characters in terms of gender-stereotyped personality traits and activities; this occurs even in many books labeled as "nonsexist" (Diekman & Murnen, 2004). Finally, many reading materials perpetuate gender stereotypes through their common use of sexist language. Although there has been a cultural shift in most English-speaking countries away from the generic use of masculine pronouns ("he") and nouns ("man"), these forms are still prevalent in many books. Several studies indicate that the use of masculine generics is not gender-neutral in its impact on children's (and adults') thinking. For example, children are much more likely to imagine male than female characters when the masculine generic is used (Hyde, 1984).

Parental Influences

In a meta-analysis, Tenenbaum and Leaper (2002) reviewed studies testing the relation between parents' and children's gender self-concepts and attitudes. Across studies, there was a small but statistically significant association ($r = .17$) between parents' gender attitudes and children's gender schemas. The small magnitude of the correlation is likely due to the indirect pathway between parents' and children's attitudes. That is, parents must communicate their attitudes in a way that their children can learn them (Leaper & Bigler, 2004). First, parents act as role models that can inform children's developing ideas and values (see Leaper, 2002). However, parents' attitudes and their actions are not always consistent, and therefore their attitudes may not be transparent. Second, parents may indirectly express their attitudes when they encourage gender-typed behaviors and activities. For example, when parents regularly provide gender-typed toys, they also convey a set of expectations and attitudes. Finally, some parents may convey their gender attitudes by stating or endorsing stereotypes. For instance, Gelman, Taylor, and Nguyen (2004) found that mothers often used generic statements about gender, such as "Girls play with dolls" or "Boys play with trucks." The frequent use of these generics may transmit and reinforce gender stereotypes in children.

Teacher Influences

Teachers can moderate the salience of gender in children's daily lives and thereby have an impact on the development of gender-related self-concepts and attitudes. Bigler's (1995) research offers a compelling illustration. In one classroom, the teacher was instructed to use children's gender in explicit ways to organize classroom activities (i.e., gender as a functional category). In a comparison classroom, the teacher received no specific directions. Significant increases in gender stereotyping occurred 4 weeks later in the classroom where gender was used as a functional category but not in the other classroom. In addition to affecting children's general level of stereotyping, teachers can influence children's gendered views regarding play activities, academic domains, and athletics (reviewed later).

Peer Influences

Peers have a major impact on the development of children's gender self-concepts, stereotypes, and attitudes. We address their influence in subsequent sections on children's activities and social relationships.

Play

Although there is variability across individuals, average gender differences in play preferences are reliably observed (see Leaper, 1994; Maccoby, 1998). Preferences for gender-stereotyped toys typically emerge between the ages of 1 and 2 years. Girls are more likely than boys to prefer dolls, cooking sets, and dress-up materials. Boys' gender-typed toy preferences include cars and trucks, tools and other building toys, and sports equipment. Once children begin engaging in pretend play between 2 and 3 years of age, girls and boys tend to differ in the themes that they enact. Girls' sociodramatic play commonly focuses on domestic situations (e.g., pretending to play house). In contrast, boys' fantasy play is more likely to involve acting out action–adventure stories with a pursuit-and-conquest theme (e.g., pretending to play war or superheroes). Furthermore, as many boys get older, their continued interest in aggression and adventure themes is expressed through play with video games that simulate violence or sports.

Play activities are important contexts for the socialization of gender because they provide opportunities for practicing particular behaviors. With repeated practice, play behaviors are likely to have an impact on children's developing expectations, preferences, and abilities (Bussey & Bandura, 1999; Huston, 1985; Leaper, 2000b). In general, masculine-stereotyped play activities allow practice in self-assertive behaviors (e.g., task completion and competition), whereas feminine-stereotyped play activities offer practice in behaviors that are simultaneously affiliative and assertive (e.g., nurturance and collaborative discourse). These differences contribute to the development of gender-typed social norms (reviewed later).

Social–Structural Influences

Researchers generally find average gender differences in toy and play preferences among children across different cultures. This even includes highly gender-egalitarian countries such as Sweden (Nelson, 2005). As described next, however, there are some factors that may account for variations within a given culture.

Media Influences

Television advertisements for children's toys both model and reinforce gender-typed play for girls and boys (Signorielli, 2001). The gender of the child actors in TV commercials underscores the message that certain toys are either "for boys" or "for girls." Moreover, the actors model gender-typed behaviors. Boys in the ads are shown enjoying action-oriented and aggressive behaviors. In contrast, girls in the ads are depicted acting nurturant toward dolls as well as showing interest in fashion and beauty. There is clear evidence that TV advertisements are effective: For example, in an experimental study, children's TV viewing was directly related to their subsequent toy requests (Robinson, Saphir, Kraemer, Varady, & Haydel, 2001).

Parental Influences

Parents are typically the first social agents to have influence over girls' and boys' play behaviors and preferences. In a meta-analysis of studies on North American parents' gender typing across 19 socialization areas, Lytton and Romney (1991) found that encouraging gender-typed activities was the manner whereby parents most reliably treated daughters and sons differently ($d = .34$ for mothers; $d = .49$ for fathers). Indeed, parents commonly purchase gender-stereotyped toys for their children within a few months after the child's birth—prior to when children express gender-typed toy preferences themselves (see Leaper, 2002). By the child's first birthday, there are toys clearly designated as "for girls" or "for boys." Once children form gender-typed toy preferences, parents' and children's biases may work in synergy. By around 2 or 3 years of age, children begin to plead for particular toys. Parents, in turn, typically reinforce children's developing toy preferences (e.g., Robinson & Morris, 1986).

There are a few factors worth noting than can moderate the likelihood of parents' gender-typing of children's play (and possibly other behavioral outcomes). First, parents tend to be stricter enforcers of gender conformity in sons than daughters (see Leaper, 2002). Second, parents with traditional gender attitudes may be more likely than parents with egalitarian attitudes to encourage gender-typed play in their young children (Fagot, Leinbach, & O'Boyle, 1992). Finally, fathers are more likely than mothers to have traditional gender attitudes and are also more likely to encourage gender-typed play (see Leaper, 2002; Lytton & Romney, 1991). Perhaps for these reasons, boys tend to be especially sensitive to their fathers' disapproval of cross-gender-typed play (Raag & Rackliff, 1998).

Teacher Influences

Teachers contribute to the gender-typing of children's play, for example, when they label toys or activities as for one gender or the other (Serbin, Connor, & Iler, 1979). By the same token, when teachers assign girls and boys to similar activities, gender differences in social behavior can be reduced (e.g., Carpenter, Huston, & Holt, 1986). Finally, as seen with parents, many teachers are more tolerant of cross-gender-typed play behavior among girls than boys (Fagot, 1981; Serbin et al., 1979).

Peer Influences

In many respects, peers are the most important influences on children's gender-typed play. First, same-gender peers are models that children use to infer gender-normative behavior. Children are more likely to play with a gender-neutral toy—or even a cross-gender-typed toy—after observing a same-gender (vs. cross-gender) model (e.g., Bussey & Perry, 1982). In addition to modeling gender-typed play, peers are vigilant in their enforcement of traditional gender norms. Peers generally disapprove of cross-gender-typed behavior (Martin, 1989), and children quickly infer what their peers consider acceptable and unacceptable. These expectations become internalized as personal standards that guide children's behavior (Bussey & Bandura, 1999). If same-gender peers act as socialization agents that transmit and enforce gendered norms, one would expect that the amount of same-gender peer affiliation would predict relative degrees of gender-typed play. Indeed, this association has been documented in prior studies (Fagot, 1981; Martin & Fabes, 2001). Martin and Fabes (2001) observed what they called a social dosage effect: The more that preschool children played with same-gender peers from fall to spring, the more likely they showed increases in gender-typed play behavior.

Research suggests that groups have a stronger socializing influence than dyads (see Harris, 1995). Therefore, it is pertinent to note that researchers find boys are more likely than girls to belong to established peer groups, whereas girls are more apt to play in dyads or unstable peer groups (see Benenson, Apostoleris, & Parnass, 1997; Leaper, 1994). Thus, socialization in stable peer groups may be more pervasive for boys than girls, and this may contribute to stronger conformity pressures on boys during childhood.

Biological Influences

Research suggests that some gender-typed play preferences are partly influenced by the organizational influence of sex-related hormones on the nervous system during prenatal development (Berenbaum, 1998; Collaer & Hines, 1995). During prenatal development, genetic males are typically exposed to higher levels of androgen whereas genetic females are typically exposed to higher levels of progesterone and estrogen. However, there is variability within each sex in prenatal exposure to these hormones. One investigative strategy is to test whether variations in certain prenatal hormones are correlated with later behavior differences. For instance, in cases of congenital adrenal hyperplasia (CAH), there are atypically elevated levels of androgen during prenatal development. Although CAH does not appear to have discernible effects on the gender development of boys, there is a possible impact on girls. In some studies, girls with CAH were significantly more likely than other girls to demonstrate preferences for masculine-stereotyped play activities such as sports. At the same time, CAH girls appeared less interested in feminine-stereotyped play activities such as doll play (see Berenbaum, 1998; Collaer & Hines, 1995).

Sports

Participation in sports is correlated with physical self-efficacy, positive body image, high self-esteem, peer acceptance, and academic success for both boys and girls (e.g., Daniels & Leaper, in press; Marsh & Kleitman, 2003). However, because sports are strongly associated with cultural constructions of masculinity, girls and women have often been excluded from athletics. Furthermore, as described below, the macho sports culture can foster sexist, misogynistic, and homophobic attitudes in boys.

Social–Structural Influences

The importance of sport in men's lives increased over the last century in Western societies in response to changes in the male role. At the beginning of the 20th century, boys' daily activities shifted from helping on the family farm to sitting in female-headed school classrooms. Also, physical strength became less relevant for most occupations. Organized sports countered the fear that boys and men were becoming feminized (see Messner, 1992). Moreover, contact sports, such as boxing and football, legitimized men's force and violence as natural and acceptable (Messner, 1992). Accordingly, studies suggest that male children and adolescents who participate in contact sports are more likely to view aggressive behavior as legitimate (Conroy, Silva, Newcomer, Walker, & Johnson, 2001). Furthermore, the acceptance of violence in the masculine sports culture can extend to sexual violence, which is more likely among male athletes than nonathletes (Benedict & Klein, 1998).

The strong tie between sports and masculinity has also meant the exclusion of girls and women in sports in most societies. Although women regularly participated in North American college athletics at the outset of the 20th century, a backlash against girls and women in sports emerged in the 1920s (Messner, 1992). However, American girls' participation in sports dramatically increased after the 1972 enactment of Title IX of the U.S. Civil Rights Act. From the time of Title IX's passage, girls' participation in high school sports has increased from 1 in 27 to 1 in 2.5. In comparison, boys' participation has remained 1 in 2 during the last 30 years (Women's Sports Foundation, 2004). Despite American girls' increased participation in sports over the years, Lirgg's (1991) meta-analysis indicated that girls tend to have lower self-efficacy in physical activity compared to boys ($d = .40$).

Media Influences

The media both reflects and perpetuates society's notions of sports and gender. Coverage of men's sports has long dominated print media (e.g., Fink & Kensicki, 2002) and television (e.g., Adams & Tuggle, 2004) in America. For example, one recent analysis indicated less than 10% of total sports media was devoted to female athletes (Koivula, 1999). Furthermore, when women athletes are profiled in the media, TV producers or magazine editors often go out of their way to underscore their feminine side by depicting them as sexual objects or portraying their heterosexual personal lives (e.g., Knight & Giuliano, 2003).

The media perpetuates quite a different image of men in sports. Whether it is either glorifying the physical violence that football players inflict on one another, highlighting basketball players' insults to one another on the court, or replaying the fights between hockey players—TV producers regularly portray professional male athletes as physically aggressive and dominant. Thus, critics argue that the media fuels the desire for violence in men's sports (Tenenbaum, Stewart, Singer, & Duda, 1996).

Parental Influences

Parents often have gender-stereotyped attitudes regarding their children's sports involvement. For example, many parents view their sons as more competent at sports than their daughters (Fredricks & Eccles, 2002). These parental beliefs may become self-fulfilling prophecies. Longitudinal research indicates that parents' evaluations of their children's athletic ability predict changes over time in the children's sports-related competence beliefs and values (Fredricks & Eccles, 2002). Parents generally—but fathers especially—tend to encourage active forms of play with sons more than daughters (see Leaper, 2002). However, as support for girls' sports involvement has increased in the United States, more fathers and mothers are promoting physical activity in their daughters (Weiss & Barber, 1995). Indeed, parental support is correlated with girls' level of sports involvement (Lewko & Ewing, 1980).

School and Coach Influences

Few schools offer the same degree of recognition for scholastic accomplishments as they do for sports achievement. In his classic study of adolescent culture, Coleman (1961) described the ways that many high schools are organized around athletic contests more than scholastic achievements. For example, schools typically display sports trophies in their hallways; they provide jackets with the school letter to athletes; and the major event each fall is the homecoming for the first football game. Thus, male athletes typically hold the highest social status in most North American high schools (Suitor & Reavis, 1995).

Coaches can have a significant impact on youth's athletic development. In addition to influencing their skill development, coaches also set a tone for the social norms in the sports culture. For instance, one study found that adolescent soccer players were more likely to endorse the use of aggression when they viewed their coaches as condoning such behavior (Guivernau & Duda, 2002). Also, many coaches enforce conformity in their male players through the use of misogynistic and homophobic comments (Schissel, 2000).

Peer Influences

Sports are a social context in which children can gain a sense of belonging with teammates and obtain prestige among their peers—but also in which children can suffer the pressures of peer conformity. When surveyed, girls as well as boys cited social benefits for maintaining their involvement in high school sports. However, girls were more likely than boys to highlight the social costs as motives for decreasing their involvement or quitting (Patrick et al., 1999). Although high school girls are more likely to gain social status through sports than in previous decades, research suggests that physical appearance and sociability are stronger predictors of girls' peer status (Suitor & Reavis, 1995). During adolescence, female athleticism may conflict with gender-typed girls' notions of femininity and heterosexuality (Guillet et al., 2000). Thus, girls' continued athletic participation into adolescence requires overcoming traditional gender stereotypes and homophobia. Perhaps for this reason, one study reported that sports involvement was more strongly tied to peer support in girls than boys (Weiss & Barber, 1995). As girls' sport participation increases in society, gender-role conflicts in athletics should become less problematic (Suitor & Reavis, 1995).

For boys, athletics has consistently been associated over the years with popularity and prestige (Suitor & Reavis, 1995). However, there are often costs that go along with boys' sports involvement. The male sports culture has traditionally emphasized macho norms emphasizing aggression, dominance, sexism, and homophobia (described earlier). Teammates enforce these social norms with one another. For example, in a study of a seventh- and eighth-grade football team, older players were observed to pressure younger players to adhere to gender-typed norms through shaming and other socializing techniques (Olrich, 1996). Another part of the macho pose involves hiding one's feelings. Accordingly, sports participation is negatively related to friendship intimacy among boys—but not among girls (Zarbatany, McDougall, & Hymel, 2000).

Social Interaction and Social Norms

As described earlier, gender identity develops around 3 years of age. Around the same age, children begin to show a preference for same-gender peers. This preference steadily increases until around 6 years of age and then remains stable until the onset of adolescence (Maccoby, 1998). To the extent that girls' and boys' peer groups emphasize different activities and patterns of social interaction, gendered social norms and goals tend to emerge (see Leaper, 1994; Strough & Berg, 2000). In particular, different norms are often seen in the expression of *assertion* (independence, physicality, and competition) and *affiliation* (interpersonal sensitivity, responsiveness, and exclusivity). Accordingly, girls and boys have been described as developing in different "gender cultures" (Maccoby, 1998; Maltz & Borker, 1982). Boys' gender-typed play and social relations foster the development of social norms stressing self-assertion *over* affiliation. In contrast, girls' gender-typed play and relationships cultivate the development of social norms emphasizing the coordination of affiliation *with* assertion. That is, contrary to some stereotypes, research does *not* support the notion that girls are unassertive; rather, their social interactions commonly involve the coordination of affiliative and assertive goals (see Leaper, 1991; Leaper & Smith, 2004; Leaper, Tenenbaum, & Shaffer, 1999). Behaviors that are simultaneously assertive and affiliative have been called collaborative; examples include initiatives for joint activity ("Let's play house") and elaborating on the other speaker's comments.

In their meta-analysis of gender differences in children's language use, Leaper and Smith (2004) identified statistically significant average gender differences in children's use of assertive and affiliative functions when interacting with peers. Overall, assertive speech was significantly more likely among boys than girls, although the magnitude of the average difference was negligible ($d = .11$); a larger difference occurred when directive speech ($d = .25$) was specifically measured. Conversely, overall affiliative speech was more likely among girls than boys ($d = .28$). Furthermore, the effect size was substantially larger with respect to responsiveness ($d = .45$), a specific form of affiliative speech that reflects being simultaneously affiliative and assertive (e.g., elaborating on the other's comment).

Gender-typed differences in the expression of affiliation and assertion tend to occur in particular interpersonal contexts. One of them is during conflict (Miller, Danaher, & Forbes, 1986; Rose & Asher, 1999). On the average, boys are more likely than girls to use power-assertive strategies aimed at confronting the other person (e.g., demands and threats) during conflict. Also, physical aggression is more likely among boys than among girls ($d = .55$, Archer, 2004). In contrast, girls are more likely than boys to use affiliative strategies aimed at reducing the conflict (e.g., changing the topic and seeking collaborative solutions). However, during adolescence girls are more likely than boys to use indirect forms of aggression ($d = -.35$, Archer, 2004), such as nonverbal social exclusion (see Underwood, 2003) and negative gossip (see Leaper & Holliday, 1995; Underwood, 2003).

Self-disclosure in intimate relationships is another relevant interpersonal context for observing gender-typed norms in the expression of affiliation and assertion. Self-disclosure as well as listener support each involve a combination of affiliation (e.g., sharing and showing support) and assertion (self-expression, providing thoughtful feedback). Self-disclosure is more likely among girls than boys during childhood (e.g., Rose, 2002) and adolescence (e.g., Shulman, Laursen, Kalman, & Karpovsky, 1997). Also, girls are more likely than boys to use active listening statements in childhood (Burleson, 1982) and emerging adulthood (Leaper, Carson, Baker, Holliday, & Myers, 1995).

Social–Structural Influences

In their cross-cultural analysis, Wood and Eagly (2002) noted an association between adult roles in the society and the socialization of affiliation (nurturance) and assertion (autonomy and aggression). Childrearing practices emphasizing nurturance in girls more than boys were more likely in societies in which women were primary caregivers. Conversely, "socializing girls to be more aggressive and less obedient [occurred in societies with] egalitarian tendencies for women to own resources and exercise power" (Wood & Eagly, 2002, p. 717). Thus, the socialization of gender-typed social-interaction styles perpetuates traditional adult gender roles as well as power imbalances between men and women (Leaper, 2000b). That is, men's dominant status in society and their task orientation are enacted and maintained through the use of self-assertive strategies, such as directive and instrumental communication. Conversely, women's relatively subordinate status as well as their traditional role as caregiver are enacted through the use of affiliative strategies, such as showing support and agreement (Leaper, 1994, 2000a; Leaper & Smith, 2004).

Parental Influences

Leaper, Anderson, and Sanders (1998) carried out a meta-analytic review of gender-related differences in parents' affiliative and assertive communication with their children.

With regard to modeling, fathers tended to use more assertive speech and mothers tended to use more affiliative speech. Specifically, fathers used significantly more directive ($d = .19$) speech than did mothers. In contrast, mothers used significantly more supportive speech than did fathers ($d = .23$). The meta-analysis also examined differences in mothers' language use with daughters versus sons. The findings suggest that mothers tended to emphasize interpersonal closeness more with daughters and to encourage autonomy more in sons: Mothers used significantly more supportive speech ($d = .22$) with daughters than sons across age levels. In addition, mothers of school-age children used significantly less assertive speech with sons than daughters ($d = -.18$). Longitudinal evidence suggests that how parents' express affiliation and assertion in their speech may affect gender-related variations in their children's psychosocial development (see Leaper et al., 1989).

Peer Influences

Several features of the peer context can moderate the likelihood of gender differences in affiliative and assertive behavior. One of them is the type of activity in which the children are participating. In unstructured settings, children select from a variety of activities (e.g., a choice of toys); however, in structured settings, children are observed participating in the same activity (e.g., the same toy). In Leaper and Smith's (2004) meta-analysis, effect sizes associated with gender differences in children's affiliative speech were significantly larger in studies observing unstructured activities ($d = .65$) than structured activities ($d = .20$). (Leaper et al., 1998, observed a similar pattern regarding the influence of activity setting on mothers' use of affiliative speech with daughters vs. sons.) To the extent that boys and girls consistently participate in different activities, they are likely to exert affiliation and assertion differently (see earlier section on play). For example, Zarbatany et al. (2000) found that adolescent boys' participation in communal activities was positively related to their friendship intimacy.

The children's familiarity with their interaction partners is a second contextual moderator of gender differences in social interaction. In Leaper and Smith's (2004) meta-analysis, the magnitude of gender differences in assertive speech was greater during interactions between strangers ($d = .32$) than between familiar children ($d = .11$). Gender differences in social behavior are more likely in unfamiliar situations because gender becomes a more salient characteristic for self-presentation (Deaux & Major, 1987). With strangers, children tend to fall back on gender stereotypes that influence their self-presentation concerns as well as their expectations about the other child (e.g., Banerjee & Lintern, 2000). With friends, however, children have had the opportunity to develop individualized styles of interaction with one another.

Group size is yet another factor that can moderate the likelihood of gender differences in social behavior. Research indicates that girls as well as boys are more competitive in larger groups and less competitive in dyads (Benenson, Nicholson, Waite, Roy, & Simpson, 2001). Boys' competitive and other power-assertive behaviors may thus be a function of the fact that they more typically congregate in larger groups than do girls.

Finally, the gender composition of the dyad or group is an important moderator of gender differences in social behavior. This is seen during conflict or self-disclosure contexts. Although girls may generally use conflict-mitigation strategies during disagreements with other girls, they tend to increase their use of power-assertive strategies during disagreements with boys (e.g., Miller et al., 1986). Conversely, boys have not been found to increase their use of conflict-mitigation strategies during disagreements with girls. Thus, to exert their influence in mixed-gender company, girls may learn they must play by "the boys' rules" rather than expect the reverse (see Leaper, 1994, 2000b). Adaptation for girls has often meant becoming fluent in both styles. In an analogous manner, many women—but relatively fewer men—develop the flexibility to be assertive in the work environment while also being nurturant with their children and spouses.

Partner gender can also affect gender-related differences in self-disclosure. Boys (as well as men) tend to turn to female partners to meet their needs for emotional support. In their meta-analysis, Dindia and Allen (1992) indicated that gender differences in observed self-disclosure were more likely in same-gender ($d = .38$) than cross-gender ($d = .19$) interactions. Whereas boys are reluctant to disclose to other boys, they are often willing to disclose to girls. The influence of the listener's gender on boys' willingness to disclose points to the impact of boys' concern with appearing masculine with their male friends (see Leaper & Anderson, 1997; Tolman, Spencer, Harmon, Rosen-Reynoso, & Striepe, 2004). To the extent that adolescent boys spend most of their time with male friends, these self-presentation concerns may limit the kinds of social skills they exercise and develop. If boys avoid disclosing with one another, they also avoid opportunities to refine the social skills associated with being a supportive listener (Leaper et al., 1995). Thus, a difference in preference may develop into a difference in ability. As described in the next section, similar processes may affect girls' and boys' academic achievement.

Academic Motivation and Achievement

Despite the dramatic influx of women into the labor force over the last 50 years, men are still disproportionally represented in high-paying and high-prestige occupations. This is true even when controlling for levels of education (U.S. Census Bureau, 2004). However, it might seem that women should be more successful than men. The majority (57%) of bachelor's degrees in the United States are awarded to women (National Science Foundation, 2004). Furthermore, from elementary school and continuing into high school, girls tend to do better than boys in reading ($d = -.29$) and writing ($d = -.49$) (Hedges & Nowell, 1995; Nowell & Hedges, 1998).

Science and math are the academic areas in which boys have historically done better than girls. However, gender differences in mathematics and the life sciences have narrowed over the years in North America (Burkam, Lee, & Smerdon, 1997; Hyde & Kling, 2001; Nowell & Hedges, 1998). According to recent estimates, average gender differences among U.S. high school students in both life sciences ($d = -.02$) and math ($d = .15$) are negligible. In contrast, boys continue to do better than girls on the average in the physical sciences ($d = .32$). More dramatic gender differences in science achievement are seen beyond the high school years. Of the bachelor's degrees recently awarded in the United States, women accounted for 57% in biological sciences, and 48% in mathematics— but only 17% in physics and 20% in engineering (National Science Foundation, 2004). Men also dominate many science- and technology-related professions, including, for example, computer software engineers (75%) and electrical engineers (91%). Hence, gender differences in academic and occupational achievement steadily increase with age.

Children's academic achievement and occupational aspirations are strongly related to their competence-related expectations and values (Eccles & Wigfield, 2002; Hyde & Kling, 2001; Weinburgh, 1995). Perceived competence and expectations for success are strongly tied to motivation and performance (see Bussey & Bandura, 1999; Eccles & Wigfield, 2002). For example, self-perceived competencies predict academic outcomes such as participation and engagement in class (Dreves & Jovanovic, 1998). Furthermore, research suggests that adolescents' perceived efficacy—rather than their actual achievement—may better account for gender-typed career preferences (Bandura, Barbaranelli, Vittorio Caprara, & Pastorelli, 2001).

By the time they get to high school, children have stereotypes about certain academic subjects—such as the expectations that boys are better in science and math (Guimond & Roussel, 2001). These stereotypes are paralleled by average gender differences in self-perceived competence and interest. Thus, girls have higher self-efficacy and interest in reading and writing than do boys. In contrast, boys have higher interest and self-efficacy in math, the physical sciences, and computer science than do girls (see Eccles, Barber, Jozefowicz, Malenchuk, & Vida, 1999; Evans, Schweingruber, & Stevenson, 2002; Hyde & Kling, 2001; Weinburgh, 1995; Whiteley, 1997). Furthermore, recent research on stereotype threat indicates that once children internalize stereotypes, their performance in cross-gender-typed areas may decline in situations in which the salience of gender is increased (see Guimond & Roussel, 2001; Hyde & Kling, 2001).

Children's achievement is also affected by their values. In general, girls may be more likely than boys to experience conflicts between their academic achievement and other goals. First, girls are more likely to seek a balance between family life and career plans (Mahaffy & Ward, 2002). Second, girls' concerns about sexual attractiveness can sometimes interfere with their academic achievement (Suitor & Reavis, 1995). Finally, girls tend to be more interested in occupations that have interpersonal or helping goals (Morgan, Isaac, & Sansome, 2001); perhaps partly for this reason, girls who do well in science are more likely to go into medical and health science fields than other scientific or technological areas (Tilleczek & Lewko, 2001).

Social–Structural Influences

Socialization practices are designed to prepare children for the dominant adult roles and opportunities that are available in a given cultural community (Wood & Eagly, 2002). To the extent that gender divisions exist in the society, gender-differentiated socialization practices follow (Leaper, 2000b; Wood & Eagly, 2002). For example, in a cross-national study, Baker and Jones (1993) found that when women had greater access to jobs and higher education, there were fewer gender-related differences in socialization practices and math achievement.

There are also variations within a given society. Paralleling changes in American women's roles over the last four decades, there has been a steady increase in the number of women in the United States receiving bachelor and doctoral degrees in science and engineering (National Science Foundation, 2004). Also, socioeconomic status within North American society is a moderator of gender differences in academic achievement. That is, gender differences in academic achievement tend to be less likely among children in higher-income neighborhoods or among those with highly educated parents (e.g., Burkam et al., 1997). Thus, in general, when girls and women have access to resources, gender differences in status and achievement are less likely.

Parental Influences

Parents' attitudes and beliefs predict gender-related variations in children's academic self-concepts and achievement. To illustrate, we note the longitudinal research of Eccles, Freedman-Doan, Frome, Jacobs, and Yoon (2000). In their study, parents generally endorsed the cultural stereotype that mathematics was more natural for boys than for girls. Parents also tended to underestimate girls' math ability and to overestimate boys' ability. The researchers found that, over time, girls' own self-perceptions reflected the parents' expectations. When parents had low expectations of their daughters, the girls increasingly lost confidence in their mathematics skills, and they lowered their evaluations of the usefulness of mathematics for their future. In high school, the girls spent fewer years studying mathematics than the boys did. This research highlights ways that parents' gender attitudes can influence their children's academic self-concept, choices, and achievement. Indeed, parents' perceptions of their children's abilities are better than children's actual grades in predicting children's academic self-efficacy years later (e.g., Bleeker & Jacobs, 2004).

How are parents' expectations communicated to their children? One possible way is through their differential treatment of sons and daughters. This was seen when Tenenbaum and Leaper (2003) investigated parents' speech during various assigned teaching tasks with their 11- or 13-year-old child. During a physical science task, fathers of sons tended to use more explanations and scientific vocabulary than did fathers of daughters. (There were no significant differences between these girls' and boys' interest or achievement in science.) In contrast, during life science and nonscience tasks, fathers' teaching talk was similar with sons and daughters. Also, mothers' teaching talk was similar with daughters and sons in all tasks. Thus, fathers may be especially influential in encouraging physical science interest and achievement in sons.

Not all parents act in gender-typed ways, and Updegraff, McHale, and Crouter's (1996) research suggests that girls do better academically when they have gender-egalitarian parents. The impact of egalitarian parental roles was especially strong on girls' (but not boys') academic achievement during the transition to middle school. Girls with egalitarian parents maintained higher levels of academic achievement in middle school (especially in math and science) compared to girls with traditional parents.

Parenting practices may also be related to some of the academic difficulties that are more common among boys. In particular, poor parental monitoring and ineffective discipline are associated with increases in boys' antisocial behavior, which in turn is related to academic disengagement (DeBaryshe, Patterson, & Capaldi, 1993). Research also suggests that parents' level of education is positively related to boys' verbal achievement (Ferry, Fouad, & Smith, 2000) and school adjustment (DeBaryse et al., 1993).

Finally, boys' school adjustment and academic achievement may be affected by the greater gender-typing pressure that parents (and others) place on boys than girls during childhood. On the one hand, these pressures may push boys to excel in masculine-stereotyped domains such as science or sports (Andre, Whigham, Hendrickson, & Chambers, 1999).

On the other hand, gender-role strain may create a conflict between appearing tough and being a good student (Renold, 2001).

Teacher Influences

Teachers can have a significant impact on children's academic interest, self-efficacy, and achievement. First, teachers are role models. For example, having women as science teachers may increase girls' interest in science careers (Evans, Whigham, & Wang, 1995). In addition, the quality of girls' relationships with their teachers predicts the importance that girls place on doing well in school (Alban Metcalfe & Alban Metcalfe, 1981). These results may be related to observations that girls are more likely than boys to work and play near teachers at school (see Carpenter et al., 1986). Carpenter and her colleagues argued that because girls experience more adult-structured activities at school and at home, they engage in more compliant behavior (e.g., Carpenter et al., 1986). Compliance to the teacher, in turn, may be related to adopting behaviors that facilitate school success (e.g., listening attentively and following directions). Paradoxically, although some teachers may favor compliant girls, the research suggests that many teachers give more attention to boys than to girls in the classroom (e.g., Altermatt, Jovanovic, & Perry, 1998). In addition, teachers often have stereotyped expectations about girls' and boys' abilities in particular subject areas (e.g., Shepardson & Pizzini, 1992). These biases are important because teachers' expectations can act as self-fulfilling prophecies that affect children's later achievement (see Hyde & Kling, 2001; Jussim, Eccles, & Madon, 1996).

Peer Influences

Peers can influence children's academic achievement in many ways both in and out of the classroom. First, the types of play activities that children practice may partly contribute to the development of later gender differences in academic achievement. Many of the activities favored by boys—including construction play, sports, and video games—provide them opportunities to develop their spatial abilities as well as math- and science-related skills (Serbin, Zelkowitz, Doyle, Gold, & Wheaton, 1990; Subrahmanyam & Greenfield, 1994). The types of play more common among girls—such as domestic role play—involve back-and-forth conversation and are therefore more likely to exercise the participants' verbal skills (Taharally, 1991).

In addition to being playmates, peers serve as important sources for social comparison that children often use to evaluate their own achievement and occupational aspirations (Young et al., 1999). Discussions with peers about academic success, in turn, are related to later academic self-perceptions (Altermatt, Pomerantz, Ruble, Frey, & Greulich, 2002). As explained earlier in the chapter, norms emerge in same-gender peer groups that shape children's social identities. Particular social identities can be compatible with certain academic and occupational pursuits than others. In a revealing study, Bell (1989) interviewed academically gifted third- through sixth-grade girls regarding their perceived obstacles to school achievement. The girls' issues pertained mainly to perceived gender-typed pressures. For instance, many girls stated they did not want to be viewed as either overly competitive or bragging about their accomplishments. Another barrier they saw interfering with their achievement was their concern with physical appearance. Thus, girls' traditional concerns with acting nice and looking pretty may lead them to downplay their academic accomplishments. By way of contrast, Stake and Nickens (2005) found that girls who had supportive peer experiences in science demonstrated positive expectations for their science achievement 6 months later.

In an analogous manner, the traditional masculine peer culture may contribute to many boys' difficulties in school adjustment and academic achievement. In many communities, boys experience a conflict between their need to maintain an image of masculinity based on power and dominance versus their perceptions of academic work and success as feminine pursuits (Alban Metcalfe & Alban Metcalfe, 1981; Renold, 2001; Van Houtte, 2004). For many boys, getting along with the teacher and doing well in school are viewed as not "cool."

Biological Influences

As noted at the beginning of the chapter, sex-related hormones can influence brain organization and functioning during development. With regard to gender differences in cognitive abilities, some researchers have considered the possible influences of sex-linked hormones during prenatal development or at puberty. For example, there is tentative evidence that prenatal androgen levels are positively related to the development of spatial ability (see Halpern, 2000). (Spatial ability, in turn, is related to mathematical reasoning.) However, in her comprehensive book on sex differences in cognitive abilities, Halpern (2000) cautions that "much more research is needed before we can understand how, when, and why prenatal hormones exert their influence" (p. 164). In addition, she concludes that there is no clear evidence that hormonal changes at puberty are responsible for gender differences in cognitive abilities. Given the small magnitude of average gender differences in academic performance (reviewed earlier), biological predispositions cannot account for the large discrepancy between women and men in science and math-related careers. Instead, according to the bent-twig hypothesis, social factors may exaggerate small biological predispositions in ability and thereby create the large gender differences in academic achievement seen later in development (see Halpern, 2000).

Household Labor

Dramatic transformations in the American family have occurred during the last 50 years. For the most part, however, it is the woman's role that has undergone change. Married women typically juggle both career and family work. In contrast, married men's contributions to child care and housework have shown only modest average increases over the years (Coltrane, 2000). Besides sending messages to children about gender roles, shared parental labor predicts couples' relationship satisfaction (Risman & Johnson-Sumerford, 1998) and may be related to positive parenting practices (Sabattini & Leaper, 2004). Consequently, we consider possible developmental influences on adult gender differences in household work. In particular, we review differences in girls' and boys' participation in household chores.

Social–Structural Influences

The degree and the manner to which daughters and sons are assigned household work are related to the parents' socioeconomic level, marital status, employment, family size, and cultural background (Cunninghan, 2001; Hilton & Haldeman, 1991). In general, when family resources are limited (e.g., low income, single parenthood, and large family size), children are more likely to be assigned household chores—with daughters especially likely to be assigned child-care responsibilities. Furthermore, in cultures in which there is a traditional division of labor between women and men, childrearing practices are more likely to encourage nurturance in girls more than boys (see Wood & Eagly, 2002). Thus, assigning children to gender-typed household chores both reflects and perpetuates gender-differentiated roles in society (Etaugh & Liss, 1992).

Parental Influences

Studies of children's household work in North America indicate a few patterns pertinent to gender socialization. First, mothers and fathers typically model a traditional division of labor in their own household work (Hilton & Haldeman, 1991). Some studies indicate that children's own attitudes about gender-typed household chores may be influenced by the role models that parents present to them. For example, in one investigation, adolescents of employed mothers were less likely to hold traditional views about the division of household labor than were adolescents of homemaker mothers (Gardner & LaBreckque, 1986). Also, another study indicated that egalitarian role sharing was more likely among married women if their mothers' had been employed when they were growing up (Cunningham, 2001).

A second pattern in the research literature is that parents tend to assign children gender-typed chores. Most notably, parents typically allocate child care and cleaning to daughters, and consign maintenance work to sons (Antill, Goodnow, Russell, & Cotton, 1996). The types of chores assigned to children may affect their development. Of particular note, children's involvement in family-care work is positively related to their prosocial development (Grusec, Goodnow, & Cohen, 1996). However, a third point that comes across in the literature is that girls are more likely than boys to be assigned household tasks during childhood and adolescence (McHale, Bartko, Crouter, & Perry-Jenkins, 1990). In this way, women's relegation to household work begins in childhood.

Finally, the gender-typed assignment of household chores imparts lessons to children about women's and men's rights and responsibilities. Emler and Hall (1994) argued that children's experiences may contribute to their later notions of entitlement and obligation with regard to household work. To the extent that daughters are assigned more housework than sons, traditional expectations about the division of labor are fostered. Thus, girls' and boys' participation in different household chores in childhood can be viewed as training for later role and status differences in adulthood (see Leaper, 2000b; Wood & Eagly, 2002).

CONCLUSIONS

The foregoing review has highlighted some of the important ways that gender is socialized from infancy into adolescence. We reviewed areas of socialization that have some of the most important consequences on adult roles and functioning. As our presentation has emphasized, average gender differences in adult occupational roles and achievement may largely stem from their childhood play behaviors and academic experiences. Similarly, gender-related variations in intimacy and family roles in adulthood may follow from differences that girls and boys tend to experience in play activities, peer relations, and household responsibilities. Men's dominance and sexist practices also can be traced back to children's gender-typed interactions with peers during play, sports, and everyday interactions. Although these patterns of gender development tend to occur, our review suggests that they are not inevitable outcomes.

We have emphasized the desirability as well as the potential for gender equality. Accordingly, most of our emphasis was on social–structural, social–interactive, and cognitive–motivational processes. We do *not* dispute the additional influences of sex-related biological factors. However, rather than focus on biological constraints, we have stressed the human capacity for behavioral adaptation in relation to existing environmental constraints or opportunities (Leaper, 2000b; Wood & Eagly, 2002). In general, girls and boys act in similar ways when provided similar opportunities and encouragement.

Many societies are gradually moving toward gender equality. To illustrate, we point to the increased popularity of programs in many postindustrial societies aimed at reducing gender bias in schools as well as the closing gap between women and men in occupational achievement. It is not uncommon for children to be exposed to counterstereotyped role models and practices. For example, in many parts of the world, children are now likely to see women in positions of power in government, industry, and education. Also, in some places, children are increasingly likely to observe men as caregivers. As the dialectical model of development postulates, changes in society affect our children's development, and changes in how our children develop later transform society (Riegel, 1976).

NOTE

1. Cohen's d is an index of effect size that reflects the magnitude of difference between two groups in standard deviation units. Effect sizes are generally considered negligible when $d < .2$, small when $d > .2$, medium when $d > .5$, and large when $d > .8$ (Cohen, 1988).

REFERENCES

Adams, T., & Tuggle, C. A. (2004). ESPN's SportsCenter and coverage of women's athletics: "It's a boys' club." *Mass Communication and Society, 7*, 237–248.

Alban Metcalfe, R. J., & Alban Metcalfe, B. M. (1981). Self-concept, motivation and attitudes to school among middle school pupils. *Research in Education, 26*, 64–76.

Altermatt, E. R., Jovanovic, J., & Perry, M. (1998). Bias or responsivity? Sex and achievement-level effects on teachers' classroom questioning practices. *Journal of Educational Psychology, 90*, 516–527.

Altermatt, E. R., Pomerantz, E. M., Ruble, D. N., Frey, K. S., & Greulich, F. K. (2002). Predicting changes in children's self-perceptions of academic competence: A naturalistic examination of evaluative discourse among classmates. *Developmental Psychology, 38*, 903–917.

Andre, T., Whigham, M., Hendrickson, A., & Chambers, S. (1999). Competency beliefs, positive affect, and gender stereotypes of elementary students and their parents about science versus other school subjects. *Journal of Research in Science Teaching, 36*, 719–747.

Antill, J. K., Goodnow, J. J., Russell, G., & Cotton, S. (1996). The influence of parents and family context on children's involvement in household tasks. *Sex Roles, 34*, 215–236.

Archer, J. (2004). Sex differences in aggression in real-world settings: A meta-analytic review. *Review of General Psychology, 8*, 291–322.

Baker, D. P., & Jones, D. P. (1993). Creating gender equality: Cross-national gender stratification and mathematical performance. *Sociology of Education, 66*, 91–103.

Bandura, A., Barbaranelli, C., Vittorio Caprara, G., & Pastorelli, C. (2001). Self-efficacy beliefs as shapers of children's aspirations and career trajectories. *Child Development, 72,* 187–206.

Banerjee, R., & Lintern, V. (2000). Boys will be boys: The effect of social evaluation concerns on gender-typing. *Social Development, 9,* 397–408.

Baxter, J., & Kane, E. W. (1995). Dependence and independence: A cross-national analysis of gender inequality and gender attitudes. *Gender and Society, 9,* 193–215.

Bell, L. A. (1989). Something's wrong here and it's not me: Challenging the dilemmas that block girls' success. *Journal for the Education of the Gifted, 12,* 118–130.

Benedict, J., & Klein, A. (1998). Arrest and conviction rates for athletes accused of sexual assault. In R. K. Bergen (Ed.), *Issues in intimate violence; issues in intimate violence* (pp. 169–175). Thousand Oaks, CA: Sage.

Benenson, J. F., Apostoleris, N. H., & Parnass, J. (1997). Age and sex differences in dyadic and group interaction. *Developmental Psychology, 33,* 538–543.

Benenson, J. F., Nicholson, C., Waite, A., Roy, R., & Simpson, A. (2001). The influence of group size on children's competitive behavior. *Child Development, 72,* 921–928.

Berenbaum, S. A. (1998). How hormones affect behavioral and neural development: Introduction to the special issue on "gonadal hormones and sex differences in behavior." *Developmental Neuropsychology, 14,* 175–196.

Bigler, R. S. (1995). The role of classification skill in moderating environmental influences on children's gender stereotyping: A study of the functional use of gender in the classroom. *Child Development, 66,* 1072–1087.

Bigler, R. S., Brown, C. S., & Markell, M. (2001). When groups are not created equal: Effects of group status on the formation of intergroup attitudes in children. *Child Development, 72,* 1151–1162.

Bleeker, M. M., & Jacobs, J. E. (2004). Achievement in math and science: Do mothers' beliefs matter 12 years later? *Journal of Educational Psychology, 96,* 97–109.

Brown, C. S., & Bigler, R. S. (2004). Children's perceptions of gender discrimination. *Developmental Psychology, 40,* 714–726.

Burkam, D. T., Lee, V. E., & Smerdon, B. A. (1997). Gender and science learning early in high school: Subject matter and laboratory experiences. *American Educational Research Journal, 34,* 297–331.

Burleson, B. R. (1982). The development of comforting communication skills in childhood and adolescence. *Child Development, 53,* 1578–1588.

Bussey, K., & Bandura, A. (1999). Social cognitive theory of gender development and differentiation. *Psychological Review, 106,* 676–713.

Bussey, K., & Perry, D. G. (1982). Same-sex imitation: The avoidance of cross-sex models or the acceptance of same-sex models? *Sex Roles, 8,* 773–784.

Calvert, S. L., & Huston, A. C. (1987). Television and children's gender schemata. In L. S. Liben & M. L. Signorella (Eds.), *Children's gender schemata* (New Directions for Child Development, No. 38, pp. 75–88). San Francisco: Jossey-Bass.

Carpenter, C. J., Huston, A. C., & Holt, W. (1986). Modification of preschool sex-typed behaviors by participation in adult-structured activities. *Sex Roles, 14,* 603–615.

Cohen, J. (1988). *Statistical power analysis for the behavioral sciences* (2nd ed.). Hillsdale, NJ: Erlbaum.

Coleman, J.S. (1961). *The adolescent society: The social life of the teenager and its impact on education.* Oxford, UK: Free Press of Glencoe.

Collaer, M. L., & Hines, M. (1995). Human behavioral sex differences: A role for gonadal hormones during early development? *Psychological Bulletin, 118,* 55–107.

Coltrane, S. (2000). Research on household labor: Modeling and measuring the social embeddedness of routine family work. *Journal of Marriage and the Family, 62,* 1208–1233.

Conroy, D. E., Silva, J. M., Newcomer, R. R., Walker, B. W., & Johnson, M. S. (2001). Personal and participatory socializers of the perceived legitimacy of aggressive behavior in sport. *Aggressive Behavior, 27,* 405–418.

Cunningham, M. (2001). Parental influences on the gendered division of housework. *American Sociological Review, 66,* 184–203.

Daniels, E., & Leaper, C. (in press). A longitudinal investigation of sport participation, peer acceptance, and self-esteem among adolescent boys and girls. *Sex Roles.*

Deaux, K., & Major, B. (1987). Putting gender into context: An interactive model of gender-related behavior. *Psychological Review, 94,* 369–389.

DeBaryshe, B. D., Patterson, G. R., & Capaldi, D. M. (1993). A performance model for academic achievement in early adolescent boys. *Developmental Psychology, 29*, 795–804.

Diekman, A. B., & Murnen, S. K. (2004). Learning to be little women and little men: The inequitable gender equality of nonsexist children's literature. *Sex Roles, 50*, 373–385.

Dindia, K., & Allen, M. (1992). Sex differences in self-disclosure: A meta-analysis. *Psychological Bulletin, 112*, 106–124.

Dreves, C., & Jovanovic, J. (1998). Male dominance in the classroom: Does it explain the gender difference in young adolescents' science ability perceptions? *Applied Developmental Science, 2*, 90–98.

Eaton, W. O., & Enns, L. R. (1986). Sex differences in human motor activity level. *Psychological Bulletin, 100*, 19–28.

Eccles, J., Barber, B., Jozefowicz, D., Malenchuk, O., & Vida, M. (1999). Self-evaluations of competence, task values, and self-esteem. In N. G. Johnson, & M. C. Roberts (Eds.), *Beyond appearance: A new look at adolescent girls.; beyond appearance: A new look at adolescent girls* (pp. 53–83). Washington, DC: American Psychological Association.

Eccles, J. S., Freedman-Doan, C., Frome, P., Jacobs, J., & Yoon, K. S. (2000). Gender-role socialization in the family: A longitudinal approach. In T. Eckes & H. M. Trautner (Eds.), *The developmental social psychology of gender* (pp. 333–360). Mahwah, NJ: Erlbaum.

Eccles, J. S., & Wigfield, A. (2002). Motivational beliefs, values, and goals. *Annual Review of Psychology, 53*, 109–132.

Emler, N. P., & Hall, S. (1994). Economic roles in the household system: Young people's experiences and expectations. In M. Lerner & G. Mikula (Eds.), *Entitlement and the affectional bond: Justice in close relationships* (pp. 281–303). New York: Plenum Press.

Etaugh, C, & Liss, M. B. (1992). Home, school, & playroom: Training grounds for adult gender roles. *Sex Roles, 26*, 129–147.

Evans, E. M., Schweingruber, H., & Stevenson, H. W. (2002). Gender differences in interest and knowledge acquisition: The United States, Taiwan, and Japan. *Sex Roles, 47*, 153–167.

Evans, M. A., Whigham, M., & Wang, M. C. (1995). The effect of a role model project upon the attitudes of ninth-grade science students. *Journal of Research in Science Teaching, 32*, 195–204.

Fagot, B. I. (1981). Continuity and change in play styles as a function of sex of child. *International Journal of Behavioral Development, 4*, 37–43.

Fagot, B. I., Leinbach, M. D., & O'Boyle, C. (1992). Gender labeling, gender stereotyping, and parenting behaviors. *Developmental Psychology, 28*, 225–230.

Ferry, T. R., Fouad, N. A., & Smith, P. L. (2000). The role of family context in a social cognitive model for career-related choice behavior: A math and science perspective. *Journal of Vocational Behavior, 57*, 348–364.

Fink, J. S., & Kensicki, L. J. (2002). An imperceptible difference: Visual and textual constructions of femininity in sports illustrated and sports illustrated for women. *Mass Communication and Society, 5*, 317–339.

Fredricks, J. A., & Eccles, J. S. (2002). Children's competence and value beliefs from childhood through adolescence: Growth trajectories in two male-sex-typed domains. *Developmental Psychology, 38*, 519–533.

Gardner, K. E., & LaBrecque, S. V. (1986). Effects of maternal employment on sex role orientation of adolescents. *Adolescence, 21*, 875–885.

Gelman, S. A., Taylor, M. G., & Nguyen, S. P. (2004). The developmental course of gender differentiation. *Monographs of the Society for Research in Children Development, 69*(1), vii–127.

Gooden, A. M., & Gooden, M. A. (2001). Gender representation in notable children's picture books: 1995–1999. *Sex Roles, 45*, 89–101.

Grusec, J. E., Goodnow, J. J., & Cohen, L. (1996). Household work and the development of concern for others. *Developmental Psychology, 32*, 999–1007.

Guillet, E., Sarrazin, P., & Fontayne, P. (2000). "If it contradicts my gender role, I'll stop": Introducing survival analysis to study the effects of gender typing on the time of withdrawal from sport practice: A 3-year study. *European Review of Applied Psychology, 50*, 417–421.

Guimond, S., & Roussel, L. (2001). Bragging about one's school grades: Gender stereotyping and students' perception of their abilities in science, mathematics, and language. *Social Psychology of Education, 4*, 275–293.

Guivernau, M., & Duda, J. L. (2002). Moral atmosphere and athletic aggressive tendencies in young soccer players. *Journal of Moral Education, 31*, 67–85.

Halpern, D. F. (2000). *Sex differences in cognitive abilities* (3rd ed.). Mahwah, NJ: Erlbaum.

Harris, J. R. (1995). Where is the child's environment?: A group socialization theory of development. *Psychological Review, 102,* 458–489.

Hedges, L. V., & Nowell, A. (1995). Sex differences in mental test scores, variability, and numbers of high-scoring individuals. *Science, 269,* 41–45.

Hilton, J. M., & Haldeman, V. A. (1991). Gender differences in the performance of household tasks by adults and children in single-parent and two-parent, two-earner families. *Journal of Family Issues, 12,* 114–130.

Hofstede, G. (2000). Masculine and feminine cultures. In A. E. Kazdin, (Ed.), *Encyclopedia of psychology* (Vol. 5, pp. 115–118). Washington, DC: American Psychological Association.

Huston, A. C. (1985). The development of sex typing: Themes from recent research. *Developmental Review, 5,* 1–17.

Hyde, J. S. (1984). Children's understanding of sexist language. *Developmental Psychology, 20,* 697–706.

Hyde, J. S., & Kling, K. C. (2001). Women, motivation, and achievement. *Psychology of Women Quarterly, 25,* 364–378.

Jussim, L., Eccles, J., & Madon, S. (1996). Social perception, social stereotypes, and teacher expectations: Accuracy and the quest for the powerful self-fulfilling prophecy. In M. P. Zanna (Ed.), *Advances in experimental social psychology* (Vol. 28, pp. 281–388). San Diego, CA: Academic Press.

Knight, J. L., & Giuliano, T. A. (2003). Blood, sweat, and jeers: The impact of the media's heterosexist portrayals on perceptions of male and female athletes. *Journal of Sport Behavior, 26,* 272–284.

Koivula, N. (1999). Gender stereotyping in televised media sport coverage. *Sex Roles, 41,* 589–604.

Leaper, C. (1991). Influence and involvement in children's discourse: Age, gender, and partner effects. *Child Development, 62,* 797–811.

Leaper, C. (1994). Exploring the consequences of gender segregation on social relationships. In C. Leaper (Ed.), *Childhood gender segregation: Causes and consequences* (New Directions for Child Development, No. 65, pp. 67–86). San Francisco: Jossey-Bass.

Leaper, C. (2000a). Gender, affiliation, assertion, & the interactive context of parent–child play. *Developmental Psychology, 36,* 381–393.

Leaper, C. (2000b). The social construction and socialization of gender. In P. H. Miller & E. K. Scholnick (Eds.), *Towards a feminist developmental psychology* (pp. 127–152). New York: Routledge Press.

Leaper, C. (2002). Parenting girls and boys. In M. H. Bornstein, *Handbook of parenting: Vol. 1. Children and parenting* (2nd ed., pp. 189–225). Mahwah, NJ: Erlbaum.

Leaper, C., & Anderson, K. J. (1997). Gender development and heterosexual romantic relationships during adolescence. In W. Damon (Series Ed.) & S. Shulman & W. A. Collins (Issue Eds.), *Romantic relationships in adolescence: Developmental perspectives* (New Directions for Child Development, No. 78, pp. 85–103). San Francisco: Jossey-Bass.

Leaper, C., Anderson, K. J., & Sanders, P. (1998). Moderators of gender effects on parents' talk to their children: A meta-analysis. *Developmental Psychology, 34,* 3–27.

Leaper, C., & Bigler, R. S. (2004). Gendered language and sexist thought. *Monographs of the Society for Research in Child Development, 69*(1), 128–142.

Leaper, C., Breed, L., Hoffman, L., & Perlman, C. A. (2002). Variations in the gender-stereotyped content of children's television cartoons across genres. *Journal of Applied Social Psychology, 32,* 1653–1662.

Leaper, C., Carson, M., Baker, C., Holliday, H., & Myers, S. B. (1995). Self-disclosure and listener verbal support in same-gender and cross-gender friends' conversations. *Sex Roles, 33,* 387–404.

Leaper, C., Hauser, S.T., Kremen, A., & Powers, S. I., Jacobson, A. M., Noam, G. G., et al. (1989). Adolescent–parent interactions in relation to adolescents' gender and ego development pathway: A longitudinal study. *Journal of Early Adolescence, 9,* 335–361.

Leaper, C., & Holliday, H. (1995). Gossip in same-gender and cross-gender friends' conversations. *Personal Relationships, 2,* 237–246.

Leaper, C., & Smith, T. E. (2004). A meta-analytic review of gender variations in children's language use: Talkativeness, affiliative speech, and assertive speech. *Developmental Psychology, 40,* 993–1027.

Leaper, C., Tenenbaum, H. R., & Shaffer, T. G. (1999). Communication patterns of African American girls and boys from low-income, urban background. *Child Development, 70,* 1489–1503.

Lewko, J H., & Ewing, M. E. (1980). Sex differences and parental influence in sport involvement of children. *Journal of Sport Psychology, 2,* 62–68.

Liben, L. S., & Bigler, R. S. (2002). The developmental course of gender differentiation: Conceptualizing, measuring, and evaluating constructs and pathways. *Monographs of the Society for Research in Child Development, 67*(2), vii–147.

Lirgg, C. D. (1991). Gender differences in self-confidence in physical activity: A meta-analysis of recent studies. *Journal of Sport and Exercise Psychology, 13*, 294–310.

Lytton, H., & Romney, D. M. (1991). Parents' differential socialization of boys and girls: A meta-analysis. *Psychological Bulletin, 109*, 267–296.

Maccoby, E. E. (1998). *The two sexes: Growing up apart, coming together.* Cambridge, MA: Belknap Press/Harvard University Press.

Mahaffy, K. A., & Ward, S. K. (2002). The gendering of adolescents' childbearing and educational plans: Reciprocal effects and the influence of social context. *Sex Roles, 46*, 403–417.

Maltz, D. N., & Borker, R. (1982). A cultural approach to male-female miscommunication. In J. J. Gumperz (Ed.), *Language and social identity* (pp. 195–216). Cambridge, UK: Cambridge University Press.

Marsh, H. W., & Kleitman, S. (2003). School athletic participation: Mostly gain with little pain. *Journal of Sport and Exercise Psychology, 25*, 205–228.

Martin, C. L. (1989). Children's use of gender-related information in making social judgments. *Developmental Psychology, 25*, 80–88.

Martin, C. L., & Fabes, R. A. (2001). The stability and consequences of young children's same-sex peer interactions. *Developmental Psychology, 37*, 431–446.

Martin, C. L., Ruble, D. N., & Szkrybalo, J. (2002). Cognitive theories of early gender development. *Psychological Bulletin, 128*, 903–933.

McHale, S. M., Bartko, W. T., Crouter, A. C., & Perry-Jenkins, M. (1990). Children's housework and psychosocial functioning: The mediating effects of parents' sex-role behaviors and attitudes. *Child Development, 61*, 1413–1426.

Messner, M. A. (1992). *Power at play: Sports and the problem of masculinity.* Boston: Beacon.

Miller, P. H., & Scholnick, E. K. (Eds.). (2000). *Towards a feminist developmental psychology.* New York: Routledge Press.

Miller, P. M., Danaher, D. L., & Forbes, D. (1986). Sex-related strategies for coping with interpersonal conflict in children aged five and seven. *Developmental Psychology, 22*, 543–548.

Morgan, C., Isaac, J. D., & Sansone, C. (2001). The role of interest in understanding the career choices of female and male college students. *Sex Roles, 44*, 295–320.

National Science Foundation. (2004). *Women, minorities, and persons with disabilities in science and engineering: 2004.* Arlington, VA: Author. Retrieved December 30, 2004, from http://www.nsf.gov/sbe/srs/wmpd/start.htm.

Nelson, A. (2005). Children's toy collections in Sweden—A less gender-typed country? *Sex Roles, 52*, 93–102.

Nowell, A., & Hedges, L. V. (1998). Trends in gender differences in academic achievement from 1960 to 1994: An analysis of differences in mean, variance and extreme scores. *Sex Roles, 39*, 21–43.

Olrich, T. W. (1996). The role of sport in the gender identity development of the adolescent male. *Dissertation Abstracts International: Humanities and Social Sciences, 56*(11), 4320.

Patrick, H., Ryan, A. M., Alfeld-Liro, C., Fredricks, J. A., Hruda, L., & Eccles, J. S. (1999). Adolescents' commitment to developing talent: The role of peers in continuing motivation for sports and the arts. *Journal of Youth & Adolescence, 28*(6), 741–763.

Raag, T., & Rackliff, C. L. (1998). Preschoolers' awareness of social expectations of gender: Relationships to toy choices. *Sex Roles, 38*, 685–700.

Renold, E. (2001). "Square-girls," femininity and the negotiation of academic success in the primary school. *British Educational Research Journal, 27*, 577–588.

Riegel, K. F. (1976). The dialectics of human development. *American Psychologist, 31*, 689–700.

Risman, B. J., & Johnson-Sumerford, D. (1998). Doing it fairly: A study of postgender marriages. *Journal of Marriage and the Family, 60*, 23–40.

Robinson, C. C., & Morris, J. T. (1986). The gender-stereotyped nature of Christmas toys received by 36-, 48-, & 60- month-old children: A comparison between nonrequested vs requested toys. *Sex Roles, 15*, 21–32.

Robinson, T. N., Saphir, M. N., Kraemer, H. C., Varady, A., & Haydel, K. F. (2001). Effects of reducing television viewing on children's requests for toys: A randomized controlled trial. *Journal of Developmental and Behavioral Pediatrics, 22*, 179–184.

Rogoff, B. (1990). *Apprenticeship in thinking: Cognitive development in social context.* New York: Oxford University Press.

Rose, A. J. (2002). Co-rumination in the friendships of girls and boys. *Child Development, 73,* 1830–1843.

Rose, A. J., & Asher, S. R. (1999). Children's goals and strategies in response to conflicts within a friendship. *Developmental Psychology, 35,* 69–79.

Sabattini, L., & Leaper, C. (2004). The relation between mothers' and fathers' parenting styles and their division of labor in the home: Young adults' retrospective reports. *Sex Roles, 50,* 217–225.

Sapolsky, R. M. (1997). *The trouble with testosterone: And other essays on the biology of the human predicament.* New York: Scribner.

Scarr, S., & McCartney, K. (1983). How people make their own environments: A theory of genotype-environment effects. *Child Development. 54,* 424–435.

Schissel, B. (2000). Boys against girls: The structural and interpersonal dimensions of violent patriarchal culture in the lives of young men. *Violence Against Women, 6,* 960–986.

Serbin, L. A., Connor, J. M., & Iler, I. (1979). Sex-stereotyped and nonstereotyped introductions of new toys in the preschool classroom: An observational study of teacher behavior and its effects. *Psychology of Women Quarterly, 4,* 261–265.

Serbin, L. A., Powlishta, K. K., & Gulko, J. (1993). The development of sex typing in middle childhood. *Monographs of the Society for Research in Child Development, 58*(2), v–75.

Serbin, L. A., Zelkowitz, P., Doyle, A., Gold, D., & Wheaton, B. (1990). The socialization of sex-differentiated skills and academic performance: A mediational model. *Sex Roles, 23,* 613–628.

Shepardson, D. P., & Pizzini, E. L. (1992). Gender bias in female elementary teachers' perceptions of the scientific ability of students. *Science Education, 76,* 147–153.

Shulman, S., Laursen, B., Kalman, Z., & Karpovsky, S. (1997). Adolescent intimacy revisited. *Journal of Youth and Adolescence, 26,* 597–617.

Signorella, M. L. (1999). Multidimensionality of gender schemas: Implications for the development of gender-related characteristics. In W. B. Swann, Jr. & J. H. Langlois (Eds.), *Sexism and stereotypes in modern society: The gender science of J. T. Spence* (pp. 107–126). Washington, DC: American Psychological Association.

Signorielli, N. (2001). Television's gender-role images and contribution to stereotyping: Past, present and future. In D. G. Singer & J. L. Singer (Eds.), *Handbook of children and the media* (pp. 341–358). Thousand Oaks, CA: Sage.

Stake, J. E., & Nickens, S. D. (2005). Adolescent girls' and boys' science peer relationships and perceptions of the possible self as a scientist. *Sex Roles, 52,* 1–11.

Strough, J., & Berg, C. A. (2000). Goals as a mediator of gender differences in high-affiliation dyadic conversations. *Developmental Psychology, 36,* 117–125.

Subrahmanyam, K., & Greenfield, P. M. (1994). Effect of video game practice on spatial skills in girls and boys. *Journal of Applied Developmental Psychology, 15,* 13–32.

Suitor, J. J., & Reavis, R. (1995). Football, fast cars, and cheerleading: Adolescent gender norms, 1978–1989. *Adolescence, 30,* 265–272.

Taharally, L. C. (1991). Fantasy play, language and cognitive ability of four-year-old children in Guyana, South America. *Child Study Journal, 21,* 37–56.

Tenenbaum, G., Stewart, E., Singer, R. N., & Duda, J. (1996). Aggression and violence in sport: An ISSP position stand. *International Journal of Sport Psychology, 27,* 229–236.

Tenenbaum, H. R., & Leaper, C. (2002). Are parents' gender schemas related to their children's gender-related cognitions?: A meta analysis. *Developmental Psychology, 38,* 615–630.

Tenenbaum, H. R., & Leaper, C. (2003). Parent–child conversations about science: The socialization of gender inequities? *Developmental Psychology, 39,* 34–47.

Thompson, T. L., & Zerbinos, E. (1995). Gender roles in animated cartoons: Has the picture changed in 20 years? *Sex Roles, 32,* 651–673.

Tilleczek, K. C., & Lewko, J. H. (2001). Factors influencing the pursuit of health and science careers for Canadian adolescents in transition from school to work. *Journal of Youth Studies, 4,* 415–428.

Tolman, D. L., Spencer, R., Harmon, T., Rosen-Reynoso, M., & Striepe, M. (2004). Getting close, staying cool: Early adolescent boys' experiences with romantic relationships. In N. Way & J. Y. Chu (Eds.), *Adolescent boys: Exploring diverse cultures of boyhood* (pp. 235–255). New York: New York University Press.

Turner, J. C. (2000). Social identity. In A. E. Kazdin (Ed.), *Encyclopedia of psychology* (Vol. 7, pp. 341–343). Washington, DC: American Psychological Association.

Twenge, J. M. (1997a). Attitudes toward women, 1970–1995: A meta-analysis. *Psychology of Women Quarterly, 21*, 35–51.

Twenge, J. M. (1997b). Changes in masculine and feminine traits over time: A meta-analysis. *Sex Roles, 36*, 305–325.

Underwood, M. K. (2003). *Social aggression among girls*. New York: Guilford Press.

Updegraff, K. A., McHale, S. M., & Crouter, A. C. (1996). Gender roles in marriage: What do they mean for girls' and boys' school achievement? *Journal of Youth and Adolescence, 25*, 73–88.

U.S. Census Bureau. (2004). *Census 2000 Special Reports: Evidence from Census 2000 about earnings by detailed occupations for men and women*. Washington, DC: U.S. Department of Commerce. Retrieved December 30, 2004, from http://www.census.gov/prod/2004pubs/censr-15.pdf.

Van Houtte, M. (2004). Why boys achieve less at school than girls: The difference between boys' and girls' academic culture. *Educational Studies, 30*, 159–173.

Ward, L. M., & Friedman, K. (2006). Using TV as a guide: Associations between television viewing and adolescents' sexual attitudes and behavior. *Journal of Research on Adolescence, 16*, 133–156.

Weinburgh, M. (1995). Gender differences in student attitudes toward science: A meta-analysis of the literature from 1970 to 1991. *Journal of Research in Science Teaching, 32*, 387–398.

Weiss, M. R., & Barber, H. (1995). Socialization influences of collegiate male athletes: A tale of two decade. *Sex Roles, 33*, 129–140.

Whitley, B.E. (1997). Gender differences in computer-related attitudes and behavior: A meta-analysis. *Computers in Human Behavior, 13*, 1–22.

Women's Sports Foundation. (2004). *Women's sports and fitness facts and statistics*. Retrieved December 6, 2004, from www.womenssportsfoundation.org/ binary-data/WSF_ARTICLE/pdf_file/28.pdf.

Wood, W., & Eagly, A. H. (2002). A cross-cultural analysis of the behavior of women and men: Implications for the origins of sex differences. *Psychological Bulletin, 128*, 699–727.

Young, R. A., Antal, S., Bassett, M. E., Post, A., DeVries, N., & Valach, L. (1999). The joint actions of adolescents in peer conversations about career. *Journal of Adolescence, 22*, 527–538.

Zarbatany, L., McDougall, P., & Hymel, S. (2000). Title gender-differentiated experience in the peer culture: Links to intimacy in preadolescence. *Social Development, 9*, 62–79.

CHAPTER 23

The Socialization of Cognition

MARY GAUVAIN and SUSAN M. PEREZ

Cognitive development is a process of socialization to the intellectual life of the community in which children are expected to become mature, competent, and contributing members. To describe cognitive development as a social process, this chapter concentrates on how intellectual development is organized and directed by the social world over the course of childhood. Although a single instance of thinking may be a solitary activity, cognitive development as a process cannot be meaningfully separated from the social context in which it occurs. The social context contributes to cognitive development in two ways. First, it determines what children think about and the ways of thinking that children practice and adopt. Second, it is the primary system through which children learn about the world and develop cognitive skills. In other words, cognitive development is an emergent property of social experience. During social interaction and other inherently social processes, such as cultural practices, children have opportunities to participate intellectually in the world in ways that they cannot generate on their own. These experiences lead to fundamental changes in how children think.

The social aspects of cognitive development that we discuss cover a wide spectrum of children's experiences, including direct social experiences, such as interaction, and less direct but still fundamentally social processes, such as children's participation in culturally organized practices including school. Examining cognitive development as a social process does not mean that biological and other internal contributions are unimportant. Biological, maturational, and individual capabilities are essential components of cognitive socialization in that they help define the possibilities and boundaries of intellectual growth at any given point in development.

In this chapter we discuss the participants and processes involved in the socialization of cognition and illustrate these topics with research in several areas of cognitive development, including memory, problem solving, and planning. We do not provide an extensive review of this research; several recent reviews exist (Gauvain, 2001; Rogoff, 1998). We begin by discussing points raised by evolutionary psychology as it offers an interesting historical vantage consistent with the characterization of cognitive development as a social process.

AN EVOLUTIONARY VIEW OF THE SOCIAL NATURE OF COGNITIVE DEVELOPMENT

The social nature of cognitive development is evident when one considers the evolution of human intelligence. Evolutionary psychology asserts that the human mind has been shaped over time by the process of natural selection, which favored prehominids that were intellectually capable of combating the types of problems present in the dangerous and competitive environment in which our early ancestors lived (Barkow, Cosmides, & Tooby, 1992). Paramount among these capabilities was the ability to band together in groups to solve problems pertinent to survival, including obtaining food and shelter and protecting young group members. A later emerging yet critical capability was understanding other species members, or conspecifics, in ways that supported social processes, such as imitation and collaboration, that enable humans to learn complex behaviors from others (Tomasello, Kruger, & Ratner, 1993).

Much of evolutionary psychology has concentrated on mature adaptations (i.e., the behaviors of contemporary human adults that may reflect aspects of species evolution or phylogeny). Developmental psychologists can contribute to this effort by providing research from another time scale, specifically aspects of the development of the individual organism, or ontogeny, that may relate to the evolutionary history of the species (Bjorklund & Pellegrini, 2002). From an evolutionary perspective, several characteristics of the human species have direct relevance to psychological development, specifically the immaturity of human beings at birth, the protracted period of dependence on mature members, and the gradual specialization of human intelligence to local circumstances.

Human beings are weak creatures relative to other large mammals. Thus, there is little that is apparent in our physical makeup that explains the survival of our lineage in the midst of other stronger species that competed for the same resources. The way that prehominids, and eventually *Homo sapiens*, survived was not to become stronger than other species. Rather, it was necessary to outsmart competing or threatening species so as to have access to resources. What evolved was an organism with high levels of intelligence capable of coordinating in complex, goal-directed ways with the intelligence of conspecifics. In short, the human evolutionary story is largely a story about cognition. Yet this story is inseparable from two other stories, one about the social nature of the species and the other, the developmental story, which explains how these high levels of cognitive functioning manage to come about in the lifetime of an individual.

Although phylogenetic and ontogenetic changes occur on vastly different time scales and entail different mechanisms, they are interrelated processes. An evolutionary perspective describes humans as social animals that evolved the ability to perform intelligent actions as well as the ability to learn these actions, and their meaning, from others. The means by which human intelligence emerges over the course of individual development were crafted by evolution, they were essential to the survival of the species, and, they were, by necessity, built on characteristics of the species. For instance, the immaturity of human infants compared to neonates of other species, including other primates, is related to a particular set of social behaviors. Human caregivers need to nurture infants almost continuously; they carry infants about, remove them from harm's way, and basically compensate for the physical and mental immaturity of the infant.

Why is the human brain so immature at birth? The timing of human gestation is set by many factors including a compromise of sorts between fetal maturation and the time when a mature female can successfully birth the fetus given the large skull size. The width of the pelvis, which houses the birth canal, is limited due to its role in upright gait. Thus, two separate adaptations, bipedal locomotion and large brain size, created a problem for our ancestors, "the obstetric dilemma" (Washburn, 1960). The resulting adaptation was a gestational period that culminated with a full-term fetus with an immature brain with a pliable outer shell and capable of substantial growth. This postnatal growth results in a mature organism with a large brain, relative to body size, with a large number of neural connections, far more than exist in other primates (Finlay, Darlington, & Nicastro, 2001). This growth is also marked by considerable plasticity, which is related to flexibility in learning (Neville & Bavelier, 1999).

Although the human brain grows rapidly, its immaturity at birth and the pace of growth necessitate a protracted period of dependence on mature group members. This period provides many benefits to the child, protection and nurturance being the most critical. It also offers many and repeated opportunities for learning—opportunities that largely occur in social situations. Infants and children are often in the company of more experienced people who know much of what children need to learn and are able to provide support and other forms of assistance. The fact that these situations involve individuals with strong emotional ties, another characteristic likely to emerge in early human relationships (Hinde, 1989), enhances the potential for learning.

In brief, an evolutionary perspective describes the human organism in a way consistent with the view of human intellectual development as socially constituted. The rapid pace of neural growth after birth suggests that the human infant is essentially a learning machine. Biological constraints of the organism ensure that most of early human learning takes place in the company of people who are more experienced than the child. In terms of psychological development, what is important to understand from this process is how the social world integrates with maturational processes and individual characteristics to lead intellectual growth.

Research supports the view that maturational, social, and individual forces together shape cognitive development. Maturational constraints are evident in the timing and pace of learning, as well as in biases toward certain types of information that influence early learning. Much of what infants find of interest resonates with human social life, such as patterns that compose faces and speech. Between 6 and 12 months of age, these preferences become honed to social experience as babies display increased sensitivity to human faces compared to the faces of other primates (Pascalis, de Haan, & Nelson, 2002) and to the sounds of their own language versus other languages (Werker & Vouloumanos, 2001). A social bias is also evident in early behavioral patterns, in particular social interaction holds special interest for infants and plays a significant role in learning from early in life. For example, maternal encouragement of infant attention at 5 months of age predicts language comprehension at 13 months of age (Tamis-LeMonda & Bornstein, 1989). Individual variation in learning appears at two levels: in the individual organism and in relation to the group or community to which the child belongs. Variation at the level of the child includes dispositions and temperamental characteristics that regulate learning

(Gauvain & Fagot, 1995). Variation at the group level includes specific values, beliefs, and practices, which influence the content and ways of thinking that compose children's day-to-day learning experiences.

The pace and pattern of early learning is even more impressive when one considers that this learning is not general (i.e., not all human babies learn exactly the same thing). It is true that much of what young children need to learn is common across social and historical circumstances, such as how objects work and other physical properties of the world. Such knowledge, referred to as core knowledge (Spelke, 2000), may be innate in some form though this is debated (Elman et al., 1996). However, it is also true that much of what children learn, though rooted in domain-general processes such as attention, memory, and speed of processing (Bjorklund & Pellegrini, 2002), is specialized to the unique circumstances of growth. Moreover, because human circumstances can change rapidly, the ability to think flexibly and adjust thinking to immediate and sometimes unexpected demands are critical features of intellectual functioning.

Given these constraints, a mental system prepared with a specific set of skills and knowledge would be far less useful than a system that has a powerful set of learning processes with a few basic cognitive skills that can jump-start the system once experiences occur. Such a system would enable the organism to understand and use information in the environment more efficiently than a preprogrammed set of knowledge. Moreover, for this type of system to learn what is needed and to learn it quickly, it needs to be able to capitalize on capabilities and resources that are already available to the organism. Certain species-level adaptations, such as the immaturity of the infant brain, the vast learning potential of the organism, and the long period of dependence on mature members, fit the bill. These characteristics ensure that during these early rapid periods of learning the infant will have extensive contact with people who already know much of what the child needs to learn and who are invested in the child physically and emotionally.

In sum, considering cognitive development as a process of socialization is consistent with the picture of human development that is emerging from evolutionary psychology. This perspective provides a historical and biological base for the link between cognitive development and processes of social and emotional development. The nature and duration of the early period of dependence exact a huge price on the human species. A large parental investment is concentrated on a small number of offspring, many who may not survive. It stands to reason that this period must have provided substantial benefits for the organism for it to be sustained over human evolution. For Bjorklund and Pellegrini (2002), the primary benefit was increased opportunities for learning; especially learning that is flexible and strategic, and allows for the emergence of complex and novel responses to situational problems and constraints.

In the next section, we discuss an approach to cognitive development consistent with an evolutionary view. It considers social and cognitive experiences as mutual processes and, thus, provides a framework for studying cognitive development as a process of socialization.

A SOCIAL APPROACH TO COGNITIVE DEVELOPMENT

All human beings participate in organized patterns of social behavior. These patterns, and the transactions they afford, affect the opportunities children have to develop and practice cognitive skills. Several types of social processes exert influence and direction on cognitive development, including interpersonally direct processes, such as social interaction and instruction, and more distal social processes, such as observational learning and cultural participation. These processes communicate to children ways of thinking and behaving that are valued in their community and provide opportunities and support for the development of cognitive abilities. As such, these social processes function as mechanisms of cognitive development (Gauvain, 2001).

Before we discuss social processes of cognitive development, we describe the primary social partners involved, especially those who are in sustained relationships with children, and how they may contribute to this development. Relationships provide children with repeated opportunities for learning and involve people with whom children have emotional ties. Because the developmental and social statuses of these partners differ from each other and from the child, the complexity inherent to social relationships provides children with a vast and diverse number of opportunities for learning. We focus on two types of social partners with whom children have regular contact: family members and peers. To broaden our discussion, we also consider how one social institution, formal schooling, contributes to cognitive socialization.

Agents of Cognitive Socialization

Research on the contribution of the family and peers to cognitive development has increased in recent years. Family members and peers are frequent partners in situations in which children learn and their contributions to cognitive development are substantial.

Family Influences on Cognitive Development

Both the sustained nature of family life and the asymmetrical relations of its members make the family a powerful context for cognitive socialization. Parents and siblings differ in the expertise, experience, and control they bring to interactions with children. The strong emotional bonds that family members have also affect the quantity and quality of cognitive transactions, which may enhance children's learning in this context (Bugental & Goodnow, 1998).

PARENTAL INFLUENCES ON COGNITIVE DEVELOPMENT

Parents influence children's emerging cognitive skills through the behaviors they encourage and model and through the experiences they provide for children. Although the behavioral contingencies that parents use, such as rewards, have been shown to play an influential role in social development, parental influence on cognitive development appears to operate differently. The structure that parents provide in face-to-face encounters and in the activities they arrange for children are more effective than behavioral contingencies in helping children learn cognitive skills (Maccoby, 1994). Parents introduce ideas and ways of thinking to children through the use of explanation and guidance and by their participation alongside children in activities as they learn about and practice new skills.

The methods of cognitive socialization used by parents have been revealed in a broad range of research. They are evident in joint problem solving as a parent helps a child break down a problem into manageable subgoals (Saxe, 1991). Parents also arrange opportunities for children to develop skills through play, help with homework, providing lessons and activities outside school, making technology and other learning tools available, and choosing the neighborhood in which to live (Gauvain & Perez, 2005). Cognitive development in the family is not a passive process for parents or children and the psychological dynamics of their interactions are influenced by characteristics of the participants. Parental characteristics that influence this process include personality, beliefs, emotional responsiveness, control, and expectations about child behavior. Contributions of children include temperament and emotionality, cognitive and social skills, and developmental status. Some characteristics of parents and children that regulate cognitive interactions are not independent. Family members are related biologically (Plomin, 1990) and parents and children share an interactional history (Gauvain & DeMent, 1991). Finally, the family is embedded within a larger social system that may influence the nature and extent of interactions related to cognitive development (Bronfenbrenner, 1979).

Researchers have studied parental influence on cognitive development in several ways, including observations of parent–child interaction on cognitive activities and relations between family characteristics (e.g., parents' education and social class), family practices (e.g., parent–child reading), and cognitive development (e.g., child's academic achievement). Parent–child interaction has been shown to relate to cognitive development in the areas of attention, memory, problem solving, and planning (Gauvain, 2001). For instance, parent–child conversation about the past effects children's recall of an event (Haden, Ornstein, Eckerman, & Didow, 2001), children can acquire problem-solving skills during interaction with a parent that lead to improved individual performance on similar problems after the interaction (Gauvain & Rogoff, 1989), parent–child interaction can enhance children's understanding in specific domains such as science and mathematics (Jipson & Callanan, 2003; Saxe, 1991), and maternal responsiveness to an infant's activities predicts the timing of language milestones at age 2 (Tamis-LeMonda, Bornstein, & Baumwell, 2001). In general, research shows that the parent–child relationship is a particularly important context for the development of a wide swath of cognitive skills.

Although opportunities for cognitive development emerge spontaneously and frequently in parent–child interaction, such experiences do not always occur or necessarily lead to positive outcomes. Gauvain and DeMent (1991) observed that mothers of chronically noncompliant preschoolers expressed more disapproval and were more directive toward their children during joint cognitive activity than mothers of compliant children and that noncompliant children were less involved in the task than more compliant children were. Similarly, Winsler, Diaz, McCarthy, Atencio, and Chabay (1999) observed mother–child interaction involving children rated by teachers as having behavior problems and children identified as not having these problems. Although there were no group differences in children's behavior during the interaction, mothers of children identified as having behavior problems used more behavior regulation and negative control (e.g., commands) and less praise in comparison to mothers with children without behavioral problems. These patterns suggest that mothers who have experienced difficulty with their children are more concerned with managing behavior than with promoting learning during cognitive interaction. However, parent–child interaction is often beneficial in terms of the cognitive process that unfolds and the learning that ensues. For example, when interacting with science exhibits in museums, children engage in less exploration and explore exhibits less systematically on their own than with parents (Crowley & Galco, 2001).

SIBLINGS AND COGNITIVE DEVELOPMENT

Siblings also provide children with learning opportunities. Siblings have a dynamic relationship characterized by varied types of interaction, ranging from affectionate and supportive exchanges to hostility and conflict. The emotional bonds and high levels of familiarity that siblings have may foster cognitive opportunities by observing and interacting with one another. In addition, siblings, other than twins, have an asymmetry of skill, experience, and control. Together, these factors provide fertile ground for children to develop cognitive skills.

Research suggests that siblings may be more involved in instructional encounters worldwide than was previously assumed (LeVine et al., 1994). Research also indicates that siblings engage in cognitive interactions differently than do unrelated peers, at least those who are not friends. Azmitia and Hesser (1993) found that young children observed and imitated the problem-solving behaviors of their older siblings more than the behaviors of their sibling's friend, even though the friend was working on the same task alongside the sibling. The older siblings also helped their younger siblings more than unrelated older children did and the younger siblings solicited more help from their older siblings than from the other older children.

Research on theory of mind also reveals the contribution of siblings to cognitive development. Observations of the conversations of 4-year-old children revealed more mental state references in conversations with siblings and friends than with mothers (Brown, Donelan-McCall, & Dunn, 1996). Also, the frequency of children's mental state terms was related to cooperative interactions in the child dyads and to the child's own mental state reasoning. Perner, Ruffman, and Leekam (1994) showed that young children who have more siblings perform better on false-belief tasks involving stories in which children are asked about what a character in the story thinks. This suggests that the sibling relationship may provide unique opportunities for the development of mental understanding. Siblings are often in situations in which one child is highly motivated to take the perspective of the other child—perhaps to figure out what the sibling is up to or how a sibling may help or hinder a child in reaching his or her own goals. Sibling interaction may provide growth points for both younger and older children. Because learning about mental understanding from social interaction is often implicit, older children may be more able than younger children to extract this type of information from a transaction. Older children may also be more likely to assume a role in which such knowledge is important (e.g., they may try to coerce a younger sibling into performing a behavior that is more in the older than younger child's interest). In contrast, learning that is more explicit, such as how to perform a motor skill or master academic material, may result in benefits for younger and older siblings. Younger siblings may benefit from exposure to and instruction in more mature or complex skills. Older siblings may profit from being responsible for and responsive to the needs of the younger child, taking the perspective of the younger child, and explaining their own understanding or point of view to someone who is less experienced than they are. Such benefits may also occur in peer interaction that does not involve siblings; however, cognitive interaction among siblings is distinct from peer interaction because of the different cognitive and social positions of the children and the regular and sustained contact siblings have over childhood.

Peer Influence on Cognitive Development

Outside the family the most important social influence on cognitive development is the peer group. Interaction with peers is more open and egalitarian than interaction in the family and these differences can lead to unique opportunities for cognitive development. Both Piaget and Vygotsky considered interaction with peers important for cognitive development. For Piaget (1926), peer interaction aids cognitive development because of its symmetrical nature (i.e., the relatively small cognitive and social distance between peers). Piaget thought that children in asymmetrical social arrangements would be more likely to conform to rules that they do not fully understand or agree with the partner rather than examining ideas for themselves. However, when social power is equal but children hold different understanding of a problem, Piaget thought that peers would be more likely to learn from each other, particularly when they debate their points of view. In contrast, Vygotsky (1978) placed greater emphasis on asymmetrical relationships, especially the assistance provided by a peer who has achieved a level of expertise beyond that of the other child and therefore can provide instruction to the less experienced partner.

Research supports both positions. Peer interaction can influence cognitive development in many ways: Peers often contribute new information, define and restructure a problem in a way that is accessible, and generate discussions that can lead to the selection of effective problem-solving strategies. Through mutual feedback, evaluation, and debate, peers motivate one another to abandon misconceptions and search for better solutions to problems. This effect has been demonstrated on a range of tasks and cognitive domains, including problem solving (Azmitia & Montgomery, 1993), conservation (Doise, Mugny, & Perret-Clermont, 1975), planning (Gauvain & Rogoff, 1989), spatial thinking (Golbeck, 1998), and moral and causal reasoning (Kruger, 1992; Manion & Alexander, 1997).

Research suggests that at certain ages particular forms of peer interaction may be more beneficial than others for cognitive development. Learning by observing peers is especially useful for young children. As children get older and gain awareness of other people's points of view, verbal exchange assumes an increasingly important role. Garton and Pratt (2001) found that pairs of 7-year-old children included more procedural and descriptive information in their communication during joint problem solving than pairs of 4-year-old children. Later in childhood, as children's communication and metacognition increase and children engage in complex tasks that require reasoning, talking about strategies with a peer is useful for helping children learn how to solve problems (Teasley, 1995).

Peer collaboration does not always benefit learning. Changes in competence following peer interaction are more likely in the early stages of skill acquisition (Hawkins, Homolsky, & Heide, 1984). Poor outcomes may also occur when children are young and have difficulty with perspective taking, which interferes with establishing a common understanding of the task or intersubjectivity (Rommetveit, 1985). The relationship that peers have may also affect learning. Children who are friends learn more from peer collaboration than children who are less familiar with one another. In a study with fifth graders, Azmitia and Montgomery (1993) observed that friends offered more explanations and critiques to their partners than acquaintances did. Another study found that peers who mutually identified each other as friends performed better on a memory task than dyads in which only one child identified the other as a friend (i.e., unilateral friend-ship), dyads composed of nonfriends, or when children worked alone (Andersson, 2001).

Other factors that can affect children's learning from peer interaction include the child's interest, prior experience, self-confidence, and expectations for learning (Light & Littleton, 1999). Processes such as social comparison may also influence children's learn-ing when they interact with peers at particular points in development (Duran & Gauvain, 1993). Whether peers are interacting in same-gender or mixed-gender groups is also im-portant for learning. Although research on children's cognitive skills has revealed few gender differences when children are tested individually, gender differences are evident when children are observed in social situations (Light & Littleton, 1999). Boys share in-formation and regulate the involvement of their partners differently than girls do (Maccoby, 2002). Whereas girls prefer more collaborative interactions, boys tend to assume a more competitive stance. In mixed-gender groups, boys tend to dominate the in-teraction by controlling the information flow and materials, which restricts learning op-portunities for girls (Holmes-Lonergran, 2003).

In summary, children's experiences in the family and with peers affect cognitive de-velopment. These social agents help children identify what to think about and how to solve problems and each of these partners provides unique opportunities for cognitive de-velopment.

School Influences on the Socialization of Cognitive Development

Formally organized settings for learning are a major influence on cognitive socialization. Societies make an enormous investment in educating young members and they do so in myriad ways, including schooling, apprenticeships, observational learning, and indoctri-nation. What unites these methods is that (1) they are all social processes in which some participants have knowledge or skills that others do not yet possess and (2) the situation is arranged to transfer this knowledge from more to the less experienced participants. Several sources in the literature discuss learning arrangements outside school (e.g., Rogoff, 2003; Serpell & Hatano, 1997). Therefore, we concentrate on aspects of cogni-tive socialization related to formal schooling.

The sight of a wide-eyed, enthusiastic kindergartner on the first day of school can obscure the deeper purpose of formal schooling; as Bruner (1996) points out, "institu-tions do the culture's serious business" (p. 30). Formal education orients children's think-ing toward the expectations of the larger social group to which they belong. It teaches children how their culture interprets the natural and social worlds, the values that are placed on certain ways of thinking, and the tools and technologies that are used to sup-port thinking (Bruner, 1996). A chief aim of schooling is to ensure that members of a cul-ture share understanding of the world and are able to maintain the values and goals of the group. This does not mean that the values and goals of a culture represented in school are always clear, explicit, or even agreed on by the group. In fact, the history of public ed-ucation in the United States is marked by debates that reflect deep disagreement about what should be taught in school (e.g., evolutionism vs. creationism) and how schools should be organized (e.g., racial integration vs. segregation).

The influence of schooling on cognitive socialization is significant because this type of learning is sustained over a long and formative period of intellectual development. In addition, the activities of school, both content and practices, have continuity over childhood and across generations. Although parents attended school at an earlier time, many of the values, practices, and knowledge passed on to children at school are familiar to parents. This connection between home and school can, at times, be helpful to children (e.g., when parents assist with homework or explain the behavioral expectations of the classroom). Research has shown that parents in cultures with compulsory schooling begin to prepare their children for the classroom before they even enter school by engaging them in activities or communicative exchanges that resemble those that occur at school, such as small lessons about how things work or talking on a sustained topic about things that are not the current focus of activity (Tudge, Odero, Hogan, & Etz, 2003). When children's experiences at school are unfamiliar to parents, in terms of either knowledge or behavioral or learning practices, aspects of cognitive socialization may be introduced to the family through the children. This may be a positive experience or it may present difficulties at home: for example, lack of knowledge by the parent (perhaps needed for a homework assignment); more knowledge by the child (such as computer skills); or differences in behavioral expectations may lead to parental discomfort, embarrassment, or dissatisfaction.

Once children enter school, what they learn, how they behave, and their short- and long-term goals are increasingly influenced by adults outside the family, primarily the teacher who is formally charged with conveying the social and cultural values related to specific knowledge and ways of knowing to children. At this same time children's social world expands to include many agemates, who begin to assume a large role in children's cognitive socialization. At school, this influence is evident in learning activities in the classroom, such as peer tutoring and collaborative learning (Joiner, Littleton, Faulkner, & Miell, 2000), and in less formal learning opportunities (Harris, 1995). Given that peer contributions to cognitive socialization, especially in middle childhood, often take place in the school context, an interesting question is how much of the peer socialization process is mediated by the practices and structure of formal schooling.

Research on the contributions of formal schooling to child development has focused on three types of outcomes: academic skills, social competence, and the absence of negative behaviors (Wentzel, 2004). What is taught to and expected of children in each of these arenas of competence reflect cultural views regarding intelligence, social behavior, and what children need to know to become mature, contributing members of the society. Although discussion of the cognitive consequences of social and emotional expectations is beyond the scope of this chapter, it is important to stress that cognitive processes and their development are inseparable from social and emotional functioning. Thus, the story of cognitive socialization in relation to formal schooling is intricately linked with social and emotional development as well as with the social and emotional expectations of the classroom and, by extension, the culture at large.

Research on the cognitive consequences of schooling has focused on two broad areas: academic skill learning and how variation in schooling relates to performance on cognitive tasks. Research on the learning of academic skills has concentrated largely on literacy and mathematics although there is increasing attention to learning in other subjects including science. Much of this research emphasizes individual differences and age-related patterns of development; however, there is a growing body of research on social influences on academic skill development. In the main, this research investigates how different instructional contexts affect academic learning. Because many of the approaches used in laboratory studies of social interaction and cognitive development emphasize dyadic and small group interaction, they are not directly applicable to children's learning in the classroom where more participants, activities, and distractions are the norm. However, some efforts to adapt these ideas to the classroom, especially those derived from Vygotsky's notion of the zone of proximal development, have met with success.

One example comes from the research of Palinscar and Brown (1984), who developed a tutoring technique called reciprocal instruction to enhance children's reading comprehension. In this method, learners work in close collaboration with more experienced partners who help children develop critical comprehension skills, such as explication and elaboration. In other research, Brown and Campione (1997) introduced the community-of-learners model of classroom instruction. In this approach, adults and children work together in shared activities, peers learn from each other, and the teacher serves as an expert guide who facilitates the learning process. Another example, the Kamehameha Early Education Program (KEEP) in Hawaii (Tharp & Gallimore, 1988), uses a cultural approach. This program involves native Hawaiian children who receive language instruction and instruction in other subjects that is learner-centered. It incorporates the knowledge and values that the children bring to the classroom; for example, the Hawaiian tradition of storytelling was used to develop the classroom practice of "talk-story," an approach to literacy instruction in which the teacher and children jointly produce narratives about the focus of the day's lessons. This approach has been related to improvements in the standardized reading scores of the children. In general, research on the social organization of learning in the classroom indicates that instruction that is most effective includes some or all of the following: It presents new information and skills clearly and in depth, it provides opportunities for learners to practice new ways of thinking and solving problems, it allows learners to pursue relevant and meaningful goals, and it provides guidance that analyzes and integrates new ways of thinking with previous methods (Bransford, Brown, & Cocking, 1999).

The second line of research on the cognitive consequences of schooling examines how variation in experience with school relates to performance on cognitive tasks. This research, much of which was conducted cross-culturally, has revealed that children who attend school respond to cognitive tasks differently from children who are not in school, children educated in urban schools perform differently from children educated in rural schools, and children who attend schools directed toward a specific subject matter, such as some religious schools, perform differently from children who attend schools with a more general curriculum (Serpell & Hatano, 1997). However, research has also shown that when changes are made to cognitive tasks or task materials to align them more closely with children's experiences in their culture, differences in cognitive performance between schooled and unschooled children are reduced or disappear. Essentially, children develop cognitive abilities in relation to the activities they routinely practice and that are valued in their community. As illustrated in the KEEP project, when formal educational efforts are made to bridge home and school experiences, children's learning benefits. When discrepancies between home and school exist, children may have difficulties at school, not because of cognitive limitations but because of differences between their experiences with learning at home and the learning practices at school (Heath, 1983).

In sum, formal schooling is one method that cultures have devised to standardize children's learning and thereby socialize intelligence along desired cultural lines. The mechanisms of this influence appear in the knowledge and ways of thinking that are promoted at school and through the social learning practices that are used. Social agents outside the family, primarily teachers and peers, are central to this aspect of cognitive socialization.

Social Processes of Cognitive Development

Older and more experienced members of society help shape intellectual development through the social interactions they have with younger, less experienced members and through the formal and informal arrangements for learning they provide for children. More experienced societal members pass onto children the skills, values, and goals of the community in which development occurs. Thus, the process of cognitive development relies on the inherent link between the larger sociocultural context of development and the more immediate circumstances of individual growth. The sociocultural context is instantiated in local situations in the ways that people interact, the areas of mental functioning that are stressed and rewarded, and the practices in which people engage. In this way, social processes organize the developing mind in ways that fit with the needs and aspirations of the community. This approach is functional in its orientation in that it considers cognitive development as a socially mediated process that creates an understanding of the world that enables a person to carry out meaningful, goal-directed actions and that connects the individual mind with the minds of others (Nelson, 1996).

In this section we describe several social processes that support cognitive development. These include social interactions that directly involve learning, specifically collaboration in the child's zone of proximal development (Vygotsky, 1978), guided participation (Rogoff, 1990), and parent–child conversations about the past or as an event unfolds. We then discuss how social interaction provides opportunities for children to learn about the mind and how mental states are related to action, which helps children interact with and learn from others. In addition to direct social experiences, we discuss several psychological processes that do not involve social interaction per se but that stem from the social world and influence cognitive development, such as observational learning (Bandura, 1986) and participation in everyday activities that support thinking in cultural context (Gauvain, 1995). Although observational learning and participation in activities take different forms across cultures, they account for a sizable portion of opportunities in everyday life that serve as building blocks for cognitive development.

It is important to stress that even though direct and indirect social processes that contribute to cognitive development are often studied separately, they are inseparable in practice. Adult–child interaction that results in learning may entail dyadic instruction, guided participation, observation, and practice with the cultural activities or tools that support thinking and may culminate in some narrative account of the episode. Researchers distinguish these processes to highlight the different ways in which social experience may affect cognitive development. An important goal of future research is to bring these processes together into some overarching understanding of how social experience and cognitive development inform and define each other.

Social Interaction and Cognitive Development

Social interaction is a particularly vital force in cognitive development because it is dynamic; that is, it is organized around and changes in relation to the contributions and needs of the participants. Furthermore, during social interaction participants not only make knowledge and ways of thinking available to each other, they also reveal, to some extent, their own psychological understanding and perspective. Thus, social interaction can provide insight into whatever is the focus of the interaction and ways of thinking about this information, as well as information about the mind itself and how the mind is related to human action.

COLLABORATION IN THE CHILD'S ZONE OF PROXIMAL DEVELOPMENT

Vygotsky (1978) considered the capability to engage in higher psychological functions, such as memory, problem solving, and reasoning, the distinguishing feature of human psychology. For Vygotsky, higher mental functions originate in social life as children interact with more experienced members of the community. To facilitate cognitive development, more experienced partners direct their part of the interaction to a child's *zone of proximal development* (Vygotsky, 1978) defined as "the distance between the actual developmental level as determined by independent problem solving and the level of potential development as determined through problem solving under adult guidance or in collaboration with more capable peers" (p. 86). For Vygotsky, what a child is capable of knowing or doing with appropriate support is what cognitive development is all about. This view is different from approaches that emphasize what a child is capable of doing on his or her own, which Vygotsky considered as already developed or "fossilized" knowledge and, therefore, insufficient for charting the future course of development. Interaction in the child's zone of proximal development involves a more experienced partner exposing a child to increasingly more complex understanding and activity than that which the child is capable of alone. The more experienced partner supports a child in using his or her current capabilities to reach higher levels of competence. Thus, understanding is initially social or interpsychological and then later, after the child internalizes this understanding, it is individual or intrapsychological.

Research stemming from these tenets indicates that the structure provided in communication serves as a "scaffold" for the learner, providing contact between old and new knowledge (Wood & Middleton, 1975). Research indicates that scaffolding is beneficial when it is contingent upon the child's learning needs and adjusted during the interaction as the child's competence changes. Support and intervention are increased when the child displays difficulty with the task and decreased as the child displays increased competence. Language plays a central role in cognitive change during collaborative activity because it transforms how a person understands and acts on the world. Language also enables the thinker to operate independently of immediate perceptual experiences and consider the past and the future. More experienced partners rely on a variety of communicative techniques to support and encourage children's understanding, including suggestions, prompts, hints, directives, questions, praise, and demonstration. Research has examined how these communication devices influence children's emerging understanding as well as how their use changes over an interaction.

This conception of cognitive change is microgenetic; it concentrates on change over a brief period of time. Ontogenetic or age-related growth is not directly addressed in the notion of zone of proximal development. In addition, the underlying cognitive processes involved in the transition from the interpsychological to the intrapsychological are not yet specified (Miller, 2002). Recent research has begun to address these issues by examining these processes longitudinally and results indicate relations between microgenetic and ontogenetic processes in parent–child interaction that reflect children's changing competence (Connor & Cross, 2003). Research by Foley and Ratner (1998) has identified one underlying process involved in the internalization of skills from social interaction. They found that when young children collaborate with others, the children sometimes credit themselves for actions for which their partner was responsible, particularly when the action was successful in task performance. Recoding the agent during collaboration may help children store or activate information for later use.

GUIDED PARTICIPATION

Research based on Vygotsky's description of the zone of proximal development emphasizes how a more experienced partner provides a supportive interactional context for learning. To describe the contribution of social interaction to cognitive development beyond dyadic and explicitly instructional interactions, Rogoff (1990) introduced the concept of *guided participation*, which emphasizes learning through participation in everyday experiences under the tutelage of more experienced partners. Sometimes these activities are child focused, such as in play or an organized game, but often they are adult activities in which the primary purpose is not to instruct the child but to carry out the activity. Adults often support children's involvement in activities in specific and meaningful ways, for instance, by directing the child's attention to aspects of the task or pointing out the relation of an action to the goal. The child is a full participant defined by the child's abilities and interests. Initially, the child may have little responsibility for the actions, but over time, the child's participation changes both in terms of what the child contributes and how the child understands the activity. For Rogoff (2003), guided participation is one of the most prevalent forms of learning that children experience and it reflects their changing involvement in community activities. This way of describing cognitive development shifts the level of psychological analysis from the solitary child toward the child's changing participation in socially organized activity and focuses on how children's developing competence is tied to their involvement in the community.

The ability and propensity for children to assume an active role in procuring and retaining information from social experience are evident from early in life. Collie and Hayne (1999) demonstrated that at 6 months of age children can learn behaviors by observing others, even for as little as 30 seconds. These researchers used hand puppets to engage the infants' attention and then assessed how long infants were able to remember these actions. At 6 months of age retention was 1 day, at 12 months it was 1 week, and at 18 months it was 1 month. Over development, children's engagement in social interaction reflects their changing competence as well as the cognitive skills that are of interest or challenging to them at particular points of growth. In the preschool years, children's ability to understand and use symbols greatly enhances the ability to learn from others. For instance, as children's language becomes grammatically more complex, children's use of certain speech forms, such as questions, increases. Callanan and Oakes (1992) found an increase between 3 and 5 years of age in children's use of "why" and "how" questions, which are conducive to learning. They also found that these questions tend to be complex; children rarely ask about the world just by stating "why" or "how." Rather, their questions usually include referents, observations, and ideas—for example, Why is the sky blue? or, How does the telephone know which house to call? Preschoolers are active purveyors of knowledge about the world and they use their emerging abilities, especially language, as tools for obtaining this knowledge from others.

As children get older, much of their learning from social situations occurs during joint cognitive activity. The interaction that occurs as people solve problems together can facilitate the development of complex abilities that are important during middle childhood such as planning, problem solving, and metacognition. Fleming and Alexander (2001) found that fourth-grade children who solved problems with a peer used more advanced strategies and had better metacognitive understanding of their strategy choices than children who worked independently. The social skills that emerge in middle childhood, like the ability to coordinate actions with others, contribute to learning in social context at this time. Simply interacting with another person on a task does not guarantee learning. Children perform better on later individual tasks when partners share responsibility during earlier problem-solving interactions (Gauvain & Rogoff, 1989). Also, social interaction does not promote learning when partners display directive and disapproving behavior (Gauvain, Fagot, Leve, & Kavanagh, 2002). Thus, learning benefits from shared responsibility and supportive behavior from cognitive partners.

Adults adjust the support they provide to children on cognitive tasks based on some conception of the child's needs, which may relate to the child's performance or reflect a perception of the child's abilities or of the task. Parents approach instruction differently depending on their child's temperament or emotional state, including the ability to regulate emotions in a new or stressful situation (Dixon & Smith, 2003; Perez, 2004). The context of the activity also influences instruction. Parents provide different instruction in a game versus a problem-solving task, even when the underlying skill (e.g., math and block design) is the same (Bjorklund, Hubertz, & Reubens, 2004). Parents also alter their instruction depending on whether the task is familiar to the child (Gauvain et al., 2002). Thus, adults adjust their instructional strategies to task demands and child competence and characteristics influence this process.

In addition to learning during interactions intended to instruct or in which the child is an active participant alongside a more experienced partner, children also learn much from other people during interactions that are not intended to convey any particular skills. Rather, these interactions emerge in the course of social life as children develop relationships with others and share experiences and information. For example, researchers have studied the early conversations children have, especially with parents, to examine how they may contribute to cognitive development.

PARENT–CHILD CONVERSATION: DISCUSSION OF PAST EVENTS AND AS EVENTS UNFOLD

Parent–child conversations begin early in the child's life and they play an important role in cognitive development, especially the development of memory (Reese, 2002). Conversations that contribute to memory development include reminiscing about the past in narrative form and discussion about an event as it unfolds. Narratives, which contain a unique sequence of real or imaginary events that involve human beings as characters (Bruner, 1986), provide children with experience with a cognitive structure for organizing, storing, and communicating memories. Shared narratives are common in sustained social groups, such as the family. They help establish and maintain group identity and cohesion (Ochs, Taylor, Rudolph, & Smith, 1992), contribute to the child's developing sense of self (Nelson, 1996), and help children understand and encode events (Boland, Haden, & Ornstein, 2003).

Parent–child conversations about past and current events support cognitive development, especially memory, for several reasons. They are highly motivating because they are often about the children themselves and involve people who are familiar to the children. In addition, these conversations communicate to children what events are worth learning and remembering (Snow, 1990) and, therefore, enhance children's attention to and memory for particular types of information. These conversations also improve how memories are constructed and recalled (Boland et al., 2003) and serve as a form of rehearsal (Hamond & Fivush, 1991). Children's active participation in these conversations is especially important to memory development. Research has shown that children's memory for an event was better when the event was talked about by the mother and child than when the event was only talked about by mothers or not discussed (Haden et al., 2001). Research has also shown that children use similar memory strategies, such as elaboration, in conversations with an unfamiliar adult that were previously used with their mothers (Lange & Carroll, 2003), suggesting that parent–child conversation has implications for when children remember events on their own.

Developmentally, there is significant change in children's participation in shared narratives during early childhood. By 16 months of age, children are sensitive to the temporal and causal order of events (Bauer & Mandler, 1990) and shortly after their second birthday they are able to reflect on their own ideas or representations (Nelson, 1996). When these capabilities are paired with the child's burgeoning language skills, the stage is set for children to participate in and generate narratives. As children improve in their ability to share experiences with language, parents and children coconstruct increasingly detailed autobiographical stories (Farrant & Reese, 2000). Conversations about the past and events as they unfold involve children as authentic participants whose contributions help shape the focus and direction of the conversation. In addition, these conversations represent an intentional cognitive act. Unlike recognition memory, which can happen without awareness that something is being remembered, shared-event memory involves explicit awareness that something is being remembered and provides children with a conventional way to store information and talk about the past.

The Socialization of Social Cognition

Research on social cognition covers a broad spectrum of topics including perspective taking, attributions of other's actions, theory of mind, mental state reasoning, and the consequences of these types of understanding for cognitive, social, and emotional development. Underlying this research are fundamental questions about when and how children come to understand the self and other people as psychological beings (Flavell, 2004). Tomasello (1999) argues that the capacity to understand other people as intentional agents enables humans to interpret and learn the behaviors of others as well as to participate in, inherit, and transform culture. Several theories have been proposed to account for the development of children's understanding of the social and psychological world and all acknowledge social contributions to this development to some extent. However, the nature of social contributions differs across theories (Flavell, 2004). Some views adopt a maturational or individual perspective in which social experience is primarily the source of information from which children derive social and psychological knowledge. Other views assume a social constructivist approach in which social and psychological understanding emerges from social interaction (Carpendale & Lewis, 2004).

Research suggests that the human cognitive system, as supported by neurological functioning and brain development, is biased toward and prepared to process social information, thus facilitating learning in social context (Johnson, 2005). Abilities that appear in the first year that promote understanding of mind and intentionality include the coordinated attention of social partners to one another (Trevarthen, 1980), the joint attention by social partners to an external reference (Adamson & Bakeman, 1991), and the use of social referencing to devise an emotional reaction to external information (Feinman, 1992). By the end of the first year, infants appear to understand other persons as intentional agents (Tomasello & Haberl, 2003).

Close social relationships, especially with parents and siblings, play a critical role in the development of an understanding of mental states (Hughes & Leekam, 2004). These relationships provide children with repeated opportunities to develop and hone their understanding of others as psychological beings. Research shows that variation in the emotional context of social relationships influences opportunities for learning in social context. For example, secure attachment in infancy is positively related to mental state understanding when children are in the preschool years (Meins, Fernyhough, Russell, & Clarke-Carter, 1998). Fonagy (2004) suggests that secure attachment may facilitate an optimal level of physiological arousal, which, in turn, supports the learning of complex social understandings, such as those pertaining to mental states. Language also plays a critical role in the construction of social and psychological understanding (Nelson et al., 2003). The way that parents talk about mental states when children are 2 years of age predicts children's own mental state talk at age 4, even when children's language abilities are accounted for (Jenkins, Terrell, Koguski, Lollis, & Ross, 2003).

A socialization view of social cognition is evident in research that indicates variation in the development of social and psychological understanding in relation to family structure, social class, and parenting practices (Sabbagh & Callanan, 1998). For instance, children in larger families show earlier development of an understanding of mind than children in smaller families (Perner et al., 1994). Pears and Moses (2003) found that maternal education is both a direct and an indirect predictor of children's mental state understanding, Maternal education was indirectly related through its association with children's general cognitive ability. A direct relation appeared between maternal education and children's understanding of the perspective of others, which suggests that more educated mothers may be more likely to discuss or draw attention to other people's mental states when they interact with their children. Pears and Moses also found that power-assertive parenting techniques, such as yelling and spanking, were negatively related to children's understanding of the mental states of other people. However, the causal direction of this relation is unclear. Whereas power-assertive discipline may constrain the development of children's understanding of mental states because children may not be called on to explain the reasons behind their behaviors, it may be that parents of children who have less advanced mental state reasoning are more likely to use these techniques because their children are less responsive to forms of discipline that appeal to how the child thinks about a problem behavior.

Children's understanding of mental states relates to their social behavior. Children with better understanding of the psychological world have more successful social relationships and are rated as more socially competent by teachers compared with peers whose understanding is less advanced (Repacholi & Slaughter, 2003). However, positive social outcomes are not assured by this understanding. Some research has shown that school-age children identified as "ring-leader bullies" often have a well-developed understanding of the mind (Sutton, Smith, & Swettenham, 1999). Thus, not only do social relationships transform children's understanding of the psychological world, such understanding may transform children's relationships with others.

The full scope of the relation between this capability and social experience, as well as the developmental consequences of this ability, is not understood (Hughes & Leekam, 2004). Cross-cultural research is important for addressing this issue because cultures differ in how much children are involved in conversations about the mind and the extent to which mental state information is encoded in language (Vinden & Astington, 2000). What is clear is that during childhood an understanding of mind develops and that human social experiences around the world support this process. Although the conceptual foundations necessary to understanding the self and others as intentional agents are likely to emerge in all cultures due to early caregiving requirements of the species, the extent to which children examine mental abilities and talk about this understanding are related to specific cultural experiences. Research on these connections is needed, including how children are socialized into a "community of minds" and use this capability to participate in the maintenance and transformation of culture (Nelson et al., 2003).

Indirect Social Processes of Cognitive Socialization

All humans have similar basic needs and, as a result, the activities of daily life, especially for the young, have much commonality across cultures. Despite these commonalities, the ways in which regular activities are carried out vary in relation to socialization goals. Every society organizes the routines of children to shape development to be beneficial for the community, what Serpell and Hatano (1997) refer to as cultural arrangements for learning. These arrangements influence the development of all types of cognitive skills.

One way in which participation in routines and other social practices affects cognitive development is through the opportunities they provide for children to observe mature behaviors in their community. Observational learning has a long history of study in psychology (Bandura, 1986), with much of this research focused on the learning of social behaviors. However, opportunities to observe others, especially those who are more experienced at the cognitive skills that children need or want to learn, are also important. Other people model approaches for solving problems in children's presence, and these demonstrations may influence children's future behaviors. As we noted earlier in our discussion of guided participation, children are interested in observing and learning from others from very early in life. Six-month-olds can learn behaviors by watching others and they are able to reproduce these actions after a 24-hour delay (Collie & Hayne, 1999). At 16 months of age children can learn a complex set of modeled behaviors and learning is better for behaviors that appear intentional versus accidental (Carpenter, Akhtar, & Tomasello, 1998). At 30 months of age children can learn strategies by watching same-age peers solve a problem (Brownell & Carriger, 1991). Such findings make it clear that the social world provides information about intelligent action, that even very young children notice this information, and, most important, that they can learn much from social observation including ways of carrying out goal-directed actions at a later point in time.

Lave and Wenger (1991) introduced the concept of *legitimate peripheral participation* to describe the role of observational learning as less experienced cultural members are exposed to more experienced members as they participate in valued practices. The term "legitimate" refers to the fact that the learner, who may be an adult or a child, is allowed to have sustained but nonintrusive contact with a person who is engaged in the activity that is the focus of the learning. The type of learning, which is intentional on the part of the learner and teacher, resembles the concept of intent participation (Rogoff, Paradise, Arauz, Correa-Chávez, & Angelillo, 2003). It may be especially important in settings in which explicit adult–child instruction is less common than in Western communities (LeVine et al., 1994). For example, in research in Zinacanteco, a Mayan community in Mexico, Greenfield and Childs (1991) found that much of the skill of weaving is transferred across generations as apprentice weavers, usually young girls, sit or stand quietly alongside and watch as their mothers or older sisters weave. The learner's attention is focused on behaviors that are important to learning the skill and this attention is permitted and sustained over a long period of time. Thus, both the learner and the teacher value this type of observation, which in other circumstances might be considered intrusive or rude.

It is important to stress that observational learning is not restricted to imitation; it is an innovative process in which observed actions are adapted to new problems and circumstances. Also, the ability to learn from observation changes with development; skills at encoding, retaining, retrieving, reproducing, and modifying information learned from observations improve. Opportunities to learn by observation abound in social contexts and the cognitive processes required to learn via observation include understanding the intentions of others and the actions and objects that help carry out these intentions (Tomasello et al., 1993).

Other indirect social processes that contribute to learning and cognitive development include the determination of children's regular participation in activities that require thinking, such as routines, play materials, activity settings, and companions (Gauvain, 1999). The primary power that parents and other community members exert over cognitive development beyond early childhood may be through control over the network composition and boundaries of children's social and mental lives (Parke & Bhavnagri, 1989). By participating in routine activities, which are typically arranged and supervised by adults, children have the chance to observe and practice in rudimentary form the mature, intelligent actions of their community. Even children as young as 2–3 years of age in some communities, such as the Efe foragers in Africa and Maya in Guatemala, have experience in a limited but authentic fashion with the routine work activities of adults in their societies (Morelli, Rogoff, & Angelillo, 2003).

Examining the influence of less direct social processes on cognitive development puts the spotlight on how the socially organized nature of children's everyday activities may contribute to their emerging abilities at thinking and problem solving. Variation exists in how children are involved in the mature practices of their community (Goodnow, Miller, & Kessel, 1995), with patterns reflecting short- and long-term values and goals of the group. These variations would be expected to lead to differences in what children learn to think about and how they learn to think. For instance, research in Western communities has demonstrated that many activities in early childhood support the development of literacy skills, which are important for preparing children for schooling, a valued activity in these communities. The availability of reading materials and activities at home that facilitate literacy predicts children's book knowledge in preschool (Bennett, Weigel, & Martin, 2002). The amount of time parents and 5-year-old children spend reading at home predicts children's early literacy-related skills and the affective quality of the reading interaction predicts children's motivation for reading (Sonnenschein & Munsterman, 2002). Cultural values may also have indirect influence in preparing children for school. Portes, Cuentas, and Zady (2000) found that mother–child interactions during problem-solving activities with fifth graders from urban schools predicted different outcomes for children in the United States and Peru. For both samples, less directiveness by mothers was positively related to children's school achievement. However, for the U.S. sample only, maternal assistance that was task focused predicted children's school achievement. These results suggest that the patterns of social experience that contribute to school readiness may differ across cultures.

Another indirect social process that contributes to cognitive development involves the adoption and use of tools, symbolic and material, to support thinking. Tools that support intelligent action are devised or adopted by cultures and transmitted from more to less experienced members of the group (Gauvain, 1995). Cultural tools of thinking are evident even when people work alone. For example, mathematical notations, products of culture, are transmitted socially to children when they learn mathematics. From this point forward, children use these tools when they solve mathematics problems when they are alone or with others.

To summarize, the sociocultural context of development provides the core activities through which children learn about thinking. Social experiences affect cognitive development in many ways, including instruction in the valued practices of the community and opportunities to observe and interact with more experienced partners both as psychological agents and models for future action. These experiences provide children with introduction to and practice in the activities that foster the development of particular cognitive skills as well as with experience with the material and symbolic tools that support intelligent action in their group. These opportunities for learning emerge in informal encounters as well as during more formal arrangements such as school and apprenticeships.

CONCLUSIONS

Although children can learn many things from social experience of importance to social and emotional development, children also learn much from social experience that is cognitive in nature. Learning how to use a symbolic tool, play a game, deploy a strategy, carry out a complex intelligent action, and understand social and psychological functioning are cognitive attainments. These types of skills and understanding can only be obtained through social processes and are not available through solitary activity or introspection. The reason is that symbolic representations, like language, and cultural practices are social constructions; rules of play are social conventions; and modes of informal and formal learning by observing and interacting with others are social processes. Complex, intelligent actions often entail preferred ways of doing things, which include behavioral sequences, symbolic and material tools, and a formulation and interpretation that reflect the language, values, and practices of the group (Goodnow, 1990).

There are many social processes that support cognitive development; we concentrated on six: collaboration in the zone of proximal development, guided participation, parent–child conversation, the socialization of social cognition, observational learning, and participation in socially organized activities. These processes account for many of the experiences children have that introduce them to ways of thinking. Although we discussed these processes separately for purposes of description and because they tend to be studied independently, they are interrelated and co-occur in a person's experiences and in societies. The sheer range of these processes underscores the variety and richness of human social life and the opportunities during childhood to develop cognitive skills. No single social process can account for all cognitive development. In fact, it is the variety of social life itself that makes cognitive development in social context viable. The range of these processes also reflects the fact that all important aspects of human development are multidetermined. Intellectual development is vital to the individual, the immediate social group, and the culture. As a result, opportunities for children to develop cognitive skills are a central component of socialization and they are ubiquitous.

A focus on the social contributions to cognitive development does not mean that internal contributions are unimportant. Maturational and individual contributions are constituent components of cognitive socialization. Social aspects of cognitive development reflect the coordination of human biology, the opportunities and goals of the community, and the child's own needs, abilities, and interests. To learn from social experience, children need to play an active role. The social world does not pour knowledge and skills into children; they adopt, adapt, and reject the information and techniques that the social world presents to them. Many factors regulate social processes of learning, including the belief systems that guide more experienced partners as they create the situations in which children learn (Sigel, McGillicuddy-DeLisi, & Goodnow, 1992) and the psychological characteristics of the people involved (Perez & Gauvain, 2005). Other social characteristics of the participants, such as education, ethnicity, and social class, may also influence the learning opportunities that emerge in social situations (Fisher, Eccles, Jackson, & Villarruel, 1998).

Human beings learn to think about and solve problems in their everyday lives through the appropriation, use, and adaptation of social practices and material and symbolic tools developed by their culture (Rogoff, 1998). These practices and tools are passed onto children through the many social experiences they have every day. Adults, especially parents, and other more experienced partners play key roles in defining and modeling these practices and tools for children. Siblings and agemates help children sharpen these skills as well as learn new behaviors. These social experiences contain the tacit, underlying goal that children, who will be the next leaders of the community, will develop the skills and understanding that are necessary for mature participation in and maintenance of the community.

To understand intellectual development it is essential to investigate how, over the course of development, the social world becomes a constituent element of individual functioning. It is in the process of growth that a remarkable collaboration between the social world and the individual mind occurs. Participation in the social world organizes and provides meaning for individual human action and development. Through a complex fit between individual capabilities and social practices, individuals come to function in the formal and informal institutions and relationships they encounter throughout their lives. In other words, the sociocultural context of development—that is, the values, goals, and practices of the community—is instantiated in local social situations via the ways that people interact and in the areas of mental functioning that are stressed and rewarded. These experiences are geared toward the skills and knowledge that are considered mature and competent in that setting and thereby foster the development of children's thinking in socially and culturally desired directions.

REFERENCES

Adamson, L. B., & Bakeman, R. (1991). The development of shared attention during infancy. In R. Vasta (Ed.), *Annals of child development* (Vol. 8, pp. 1–41). London: Kingsley.

Andersson, J. (2001). Net effect of memory collaboration: How is collaboration affected by factors such as friendship, gender and age? *Scandinavian Journal of Psychology, 42,* 367–375.

Azmitia, M., & Hesser, J. (1993). Why siblings are important agents of cognitive development: A comparison of siblings and peers. *Child Development, 64,* 430–444.

Azmitia, M., & Montgomery, R. (1993). Friendship, transactive dialogues and the development of scientific reasoning. *Social Development, 2,* 202–221.

Bandura, A. (1986). *Social foundations of thought and action: A social cognitive theory.* Englewood Cliffs, NJ: Prentice-Hall.

Barkow, J. H., Cosmides, L., & Tooby, J. (1992). *The adapted mind: Evolutionary psychology and the generation of culture.* New York: Oxford University Press.

Bauer, P. J., & Mandler, J. M. (1990). Remembering what happened next: Very young children's recall of event sequences. In R. Fivush & J. A. Hudson (Eds.), *Knowing and remembering in young children* (pp. 9–29). Cambridge, UK: Cambridge University Press.

Bennett, K. K., Weigel, D. J., & Martin, S. S. (2002). Children's acquisition of early literacy skills: Examining family contributions. *Early Childhood Research Quarterly, 17,* 295–317.

Bjorklund, D. F., Hubertz, M. J., & Reubens, A. C. (2004). Young children's arithmetic strategies in social context: How parents contribute to young children's strategy development while playing games. *International Journal of Behavioral Development, 28,* 347–357.

Bjorklund, D. F., & Pellegrini, A. D. (2002). *The origins of human nature: Evolutionary developmental psychology.* Washington, DC: American Psychological Association.

Boland, A. M., Haden, C. A., & Ornstein, P. A. (2003). Boosting children's memory by training mothers in the use of an elaborative conversational style as an event unfolds. *Journal of Cognition and Development, 4,* 39–65.

Bransford, J. D., Brown, A. L., & Cocking, R. R. (1999). *How people learn: Brain, mind, experience, and school.* Washington, DC: National Academy Press.

Bronfenbrenner, U. (1979). *The ecology of human development.* Cambridge, MA: Harvard University Press.

Brown, A. L., & Campione, J. C. (1997). Designing a community of young learners: Theoretical and practical lessons. In N. M. Lambert & B. L. McCombs (Eds.), *How students learn: Reforming schools through learner-centered education* (pp. 153–186). Washington, DC: American Psychological Association.

Brown, J. R., Donelan-McCall, N., & Dunn, J. (1996). Why talk about mental states? The significance of children's conversations with friends, siblings, and mothers. *Child Development, 67,* 836–849.

Brownell, C. A., & Carriger, M. S. (1991). Collaborations among toddler peers: Individual contributions to social contexts. In L. B. Resnick, J. M. Levine, & S. D. Teasley (Eds.), *Perspectives on socially shared cognition* (pp. 365–383). Washington, DC: American Psychological Association.

Bruner, J. S. (1986). *Actual minds, possible worlds.* Cambridge, MA: Harvard University Press.

Bruner, J. (1996). *The culture of education.* Cambridge, MA: Harvard University Press.

Bugental, D., & Goodnow, J. J. (1998). Socialization processes. In W. Damon (Series Ed.) & N. Eisenberg (Vol. Ed.), *Handbook of child psychology: Vol. 3. Social, emotional, and personality development* (pp. 389–462). New York: Wiley.

Callanan, M. A., & Oakes, L. M. (1992). Preschoolers' questions and parents' explanations: Causal thinking in everyday activity. *Cognitive Development, 7,* 213–233.

Carpendale, J. I. M., & Lewis, C. (2004). Constructing an understanding of mind: The development of children's social understanding within social interaction. *Brain and Behavioral Sciences, 27,* 79–151.

Carpenter, M., Akhtar, N., & Tomasello, M. (1998). Fourteen- through 18-month-old infants differentially imitate intentional and accidental actions. *Infant Behavior and Development, 21,* 315–330.

Collie, R., & Hayne, H. (1999). Deferred imitation by 6- and 9-month-old infants: More evidence for declarative memory. *Developmental Psychobiology, 35,* 83–90.

Connor, D. B., & Cross, D. R. (2003). Longitudinal analysis of the presence, efficacy and stability of maternal scaffolding during informal problem-solving interactions. *British Journal of Developmental Psychology, 21,* 315–334.

Crowley, K., & Galco, J. (2001). Everyday activity and the development of scientific thinking. In K. Crowley, C. D. Schunn, & T. Okada (Eds.), *Designing for science: Implications from everyday, classroom, and professional settings* (pp. 393–413). Mahwah, NJ: Erlbaum.

Dixon, W. E., & Smith, P. H. (2003). Who's controlling whom? Infant contributions to maternal play behavior. *Infant and Child Development, 12,* 177–195.

Doise, W., Mugny, G., & Perret-Clermont, A. (1975). Social interaction and the development of cognitive operations. *European Journal of Social Psychology, 5,* 367–383.

Duran, R. T., & Gauvain, M. (1993). The role of age versus expertise in peer collaboration during joint planning. *Journal of Experimental Child Psychology, 55,* 227–242.

Elman, J. L., Bates, E. A., Johnson, M. H., Karmiloff-Smith, A., Parisi, D., & Plunkett, K. (1996). *Rethinking innateness: A connectionist perspective on development.* Cambridge, MA: MIT Press.

Farrant, K., & Reese, E. (2000). Maternal style and children's participation in reminiscing: Stepping stones in children's autobiographical memory development. *Journal of Cognition and Development, 1,* 193–225.

Feinman, S. (1992). *Social referencing and the social construction of reality in infancy.* New York: Plenum Press.

Finlay, B. L., Darlington, R. B., & Nicastro, N. (2001). Developmental structure in brain evolution. *Behavioral and Brain Sciences, 24,* 263–308.

Fisher, C. B., Eccles, J. F., Jackson, J. F., & Villarruel, F. A. (1998). The study of African American and Latin American children and youth. In W. Damon (Series Ed.) & R. M. Lerner (Vol. Ed.), *Handbook of child psychology: Theoretical models of human development* (pp. 1145–1207). New York: Wiley.

Flavell, J. H. (2004). Theory-of-mind development: Retrospect and prospect. *Merrill-Palmer Quarterly, 50,* 274–290.

Fleming, V. M., & Alexander, J. M. (2001). The benefits of peer collaboration: A replication with a delayed posttest. *Contemporary Educational Psychology, 26,* 588–601.

Foley, M. A., & Ratner, H. H. (1998). Children's recoding in memory for collaboration: A way of learning from others. *Cognitive Development, 13,* 91–108.

Fonagy, P. (2004). The roots of social understanding in the attachment relationship: An elaboration on the constructionist theory. *Brain and Behavioral Sciences, 27,* 105–106.

Garton, A. F., & Pratt, C. (2001). Peer assistance in children's problem solving. *British Journal of Developmental Psychology, 19,* 307–318.

Gauvain, M. (1995). Thinking in niches: Sociocultural influences on cognitive development. *Human Development, 38,* 25–45.

Gauvain, M. (1999). Everyday opportunities for the development of planning skills: Sociocultural and family influences. In A. Göncü (Ed.), *Children's engagement in the world: Sociocultural perspectives* (pp. 173–201). Cambridge, UK: Cambridge University Press.

Gauvain, M. (2001). *The social context of cognitive development.* New York: Guilford Press.

Gauvain, M., & DeMent, T. (1991). The role of shared social history in parent–child cognitive activity. *Newsletter of the Laboratory of Comparative Human Cognition, 13,* 58–66.

Gauvain, M., & Fagot, B. I. (1995). Child temperament as a mediator of mother–toddler problem solving. *Social Development, 4,* 257–276.

Gauvain, M., Fagot, B. I., Leve, C., & Kavanagh, K. (2002). Instruction by mothers and fathers during problem solving with young children. *Journal of Family Psychology, 16,* 81–90.

Gauvain, M., & Perez, S. M. (2005). Not all hurried children are the same: Children's participation in deciding on and planning their after-school activities. In J. E. Jacobs & P. A. Klaczynski (Eds.), *The development of judgment and decision-making in children and adolescents* (pp. 213–239). Mahwah, NJ: Erlbaum.

Gauvain, M., & Rogoff, B. (1989). Collaborative problem solving and children's planning skills. *Developmental Psychology, 25,* 139–151.

Golbeck, S. L. (1998). Peer collaboration and children's representation of the horizontal surface of liquid. *Journal of Applied Developmental Psychology, 19*, 571–592.

Goodnow, J. J. (1990). The socialization of cognition: What's involved? In J. W. Stigler, R. A. Shweder, & G. Herdt (Eds.), *Cultural psychology* (pp. 259–286). Cambridge, UK: Cambridge University Press.

Goodnow, J. J., Miller, P. J., & Kessel, F. (1995). *Cultural practices as contexts for development.* San Francisco: Jossey-Bass.

Greenfield, P. M., & Childs, C. P. (1991). Developmental continuity in biocultural context. In R. Cohen & A. W. Sigel (Eds.), *Context and development* (pp. 135–159). Hillsdale, NJ: Erlbaum.

Haden, C. A., Ornstein, P. A., Eckerman, C. O., & Didow, S. M. (2001). Mother–child conversational interactions as events unfold: Linkages to subsequent remembering. *Child Development, 72*, 1016–1031.

Hamond, N. R., & Fivush, R. (1991). Memories of Mickey Mouse: Young children recount their trip to Disneyworld. *Cognitive Development, 6*, 433–448.

Harris, J. R. (1995). Where is the child's environment?: A group socialization theory of development. *Psychological Review, 102*, 458–489.

Hawkins, J., Homolsky, M., & Heide, P. (1984). Paired problem solving in a computer context (Technical Report No. 33). New York: Bank Street College of Education.

Heath, S. B. (1983). *Ways with words: Language, life, and work in communities and classrooms.* Cambridge, UK: Cambridge University Press.

Hinde, R. A. (1989). Ethological and relationships perspectives. In R. Vasta (Ed.), *Annals of child development* (Vol. 6, pp. 251–285). Greenwich, CT: JAI Press.

Holmes-Lonergran, H. (2003). Preschool children's collaborative problem-solving interactions: The role of gender, pair type, and task. *Sex Roles, 48*, 505–517.

Hughes, C., & Leekam, S. (2004). What are the links between theory of mind and social relations? Review, reflections, and new directions for studies of typical and atypical development. *Social Development, 13*, 590–619.

Jenkins, J. M., Turrell, S., Kogushi, Y., Lollis, S., & Ross, H. A. (2003). Longitudinal investigation of the dynamics of mental state talk in families. *Child Development, 74*, 905–920.

Jipson, J. L., & Callanan, M. A. (2003). Mother-child conversation and children's understanding of biological and nonbiological changes in size. *Child Development, 74*, 629–644.

Johnson, M. H. (2005). *Developmental cognitive neuroscience* (2nd ed.). Malden, MA: Blackwell.

Joiner, R., Littleton, K., Faulkner, D., & Miell, D. (2000). *Rethinking collaborative learning.* London: Free Association Books.

Kruger, A. C. (1992). The effect of peer and adult–child transactive discussions on moral reasoning. *Merrill-Palmer Quarterly, 38*, 191–211.

Lange, G., & Carroll, D. E. (2003). Mother–child conversation styles and children's laboratory memory for narrative and nonnarrative materials. *Journal of Cognition and Development, 4*, 435–457.

Lave, J., & Wenger, E. (1991). *Situated learning: Legitimate peripheral participation.* Cambridge, UK: Cambridge University Press.

LeVine, R., Dixon, S., LeVine, S., Richman, A., Leiderman, P. H., Keefer, C. H., et al. (1994). *Child care and culture: Lessons from Africa.* Cambridge, UK: Cambridge University Press.

Light, P., & Littleton, K. (1999). *Social processes in children's learning.* Cambridge, UK: Cambridge University Press.

Maccoby, E. E. (1994). The role of parents in the socialization of children: An historical overview. In R. D. Parke, P. A. Ornstein, J. J. Rieser, & C. Zahn-Waxler (Eds.), *A century of developmental psychology* (pp. 589–615). Washington, DC: American Psychological Association.

Maccoby, E. E. (2002). Gender and group process: A developmental perspective. *Current Directions in Psychological Science, 11*, 54–58.

Manion, V., & Alexander, J. M. (1997). The benefits of peer collaboration on strategy use, metacognitive causal attribution, and recall. *Journal of Experimental Child Psychology, 67*, 268–289.

Meins, E., Fernyhough, C., Russell, J., & Clark-Carter, D. (1998). Security of attachment as a predictor of symbolic and mentalising abilities: A longitudinal study. *Social Development, 7*, 1–24.

Miller, P. H. (2002). *Theories of developmental psychology* (4th ed.). New York: Worth.

Morelli, G., Rogoff, B., & Angellilo, C. (2003). Cultural variation in young children's access to work or involvement in specialized child-focused activities. *International Journal of Behavioral Development, 27*, 264–274.

Nelson, K. (1996). *Language in cognitive development.* Cambridge, UK: Cambridge University Press.

Nelson, K., Shwerer, D. P., Goldman, S., Henseler, S., Presler, N., & Walkenfeld, F. F. (2003). Entering a community of minds: An experiential approach to "theory of mind." *Human Development, 46*, 24–46.

Neville, H. J., & Bavelier, D. (1999). Specificity and plasticity in neurocognitive development in humans. In M. Gazzangia (Ed.), *The new cognitive neuroscience* (2nd ed., pp. 83–98). Cambridge, MA: MIT Press.

Ochs, E., Taylor, C., Rudolph, D., & Smith, R. (1992). Storytelling as a theory-building activity. *Discourse Processes, 15*, 37–72.

Palinscar, A. S., & Brown, A. L. (1984). Reciprocal teaching of comprehension-monitoring activities. *Cognition and Instruction, 1*, 117–175.

Parke, R. D., & Bhavnagri, N. P. (1989). Parents as managers of children's peer relationships. In D. Belle (Ed.), *Children's social networks and social supports* (pp. 241–259). New York: Wiley.

Pascalis, O., de Haan, M., & Nelson, C. A. (2002). Is face processing species-specific during the first year of life? *Science, 5*, 427–434.

Pears, K. C., & Moses, L. J. (2003). Demographics, parenting, and theory of mind in preschoolers. *Social Development, 12*, 1–20.

Perez, S. M. (2004). *Relations among child emotionality, mother–child planning, and children's academic adjustment and achievement in the first grade.* Unpublished doctoral dissertation, University of California, Riverside.

Perez, S. M., & Gauvain, M. (2005). Relation of child emotionality to individual and mother–child planning. *Social Development, 14*, 250–272.

Perner, J., Ruffman, T., & Leekam, S. R. (1994). Theory of mind is contagious: You can catch it from your sibs. *Child Development, 65*, 1228–1238.

Piaget, J. (1926). *The language and mind of the child.* New York: Harcourt Brace.

Plomin, R. (1990). *Nature and nurture: An introduction to behavioral genetics.* Belmont, CA: Brooks/Cole.

Portes, P. R., Cuentas, T. E., & Zady, M. (2000). Cognitive socialization across ethnocultural contexts: Literacy and cultural differences in intellectual performance and parent–child interaction. *Journal of Genetic Psychology, 161*, 79–98.

Reese, E. (2002). Social factors in the development of autobiographical memory: The state of the art. *Social Development, 11*, 124–142.

Repacholi, B. M., & Slaughter, V. (2003). *Individual differences in the theory of mind.* New York: Psychology Press.

Rogoff, B. (1990). *Apprenticeship in thinking: Cognitive development in social context.* New York: Oxford University Press.

Rogoff, B. (1998). Cognition as a collaborative process. In D. Kuhn & R. Siegler (Eds.) & W. Damon (Series Ed.), *Handbook of child psychology: Vol. 2. Cognition, perception and language* (pp. 679–744). New York: Wiley.

Rogoff, B. (2003). *The cultural nature of human development.* Oxford, UK: Oxford University Press.

Rogoff, B., Paradise, R., Arauz, R. M., Correa-Chávez, M., & Angelillo, C. (2003). Firsthand learning through intent participation. *Annual Review of Psychology, 54*, 175–203.

Rommetveit, R. (1985). Language acquisition as increasing linguistic structuring of experience and symbolic behavior control. In J. V. Wertsch (Ed.), *Culture, communication, and cognition* (pp. 183–204). Cambridge, UK: Cambridge University Press.

Sabbagh, M. A., & Callanan, M. A. (1998). Metarepresentation in action: 3-, 4-, and 5-year-olds' developing theories of mind in parent-child conversations. *Developmental Psychology, 34*, 491–502.

Saxe, G. B. (1991). *Culture and cognitive development: Studies in mathematical understanding.* Hillsdale, NJ: Erlbaum.

Serpell, R., & Hatano, G. (1997). Education, schooling, and literacy. In J. W. Berry, P. R. Dasen, & T. S. Saraswathi (Eds.), *Handbook of cross-cultural psychology: Vol. 2. Basic process and human development* (pp. 339–376). Boston: Allyn & Bacon.

Sigel, I. E., McGillicuddy-DeLisi, A. V., & Goodnow, J. J. (1992). *Parental belief systems: The psychological consequences for children* (2nd ed.). Mahwah, NJ: Erlbaum.

Snow, C. E. (1990). Building memories: The ontogeny of autobiography. In D. Cicchetti & M. Beeghly (Eds.), *The self in transition* (pp. 213–242). Chicago: University of Chicago Press.

Sonnenschein, S., & Munsterman, K. (2002). The influence of home-based reading interactions on 5-year-olds' reading motivations and early literacy development. *Early Childhood Research Quarterly, 17*, 318–337.

Spelke, E. (2000). Core knowledge. *American Psychologist, 55*, 1233–1243.

Sutton, J., Smith, P., & Swettenham, J. (1999). Social cognition and bullying: Social inadequacy or skill manipulation? *British Journal of Developmental Psychology, 17*, 435–450.

Tamis-LeMonda, C. S., & Bornstein, M. H. (1989). Habituation and maternal encouragement of attention in infancy as predictors of toddler language, play, and representational competence. *Child Development, 60*, 738–751.

Tamis-LeMonda, C. S., Bornstein, M. H., & Baumwell, L. (2001). Maternal responsiveness and children's achievement of milestones. *Child Development, 72*, 748–767.

Teasley, S. D. (1995). The role of talk in children's peer collaboration. *Developmental Psychology, 31*, 207–220.

Tharp, R. G., & Gallimore, R. (1988). *Rousing minds to life: Teaching, learning, and schooling in social context.* New York: Cambridge University Press.

Tomasello, M. (1999). *The cultural origins of human cognition.* Cambridge, MA: Harvard University Press.

Tomasello, M., & Haberl, K. (2003). Understanding attention: 12- and 18-month-olds know what is new for other persons. *Developmental Psychology, 39*, 906–912.

Tomasello, M., Kruger, A. C., & Ratner, H. H. (1993). Cultural learning. *Behavioral and Brain Sciences, 16*, 495–511.

Trevarthen, C. (1980). The foundations of intersubjectivity: Development of interpersonal and cooperative understanding in infants. In D. R. Olson (Ed.), *The social foundations of language and thought* (pp. 316–342). New York: Norton.

Tudge, J. R. H., Odero, D. A., Hogan, D. M., & Etz, K. E. (2003). Relations between the everyday activities of preschoolers and their teachers' perceptions of their competence in the first years of school. *Early Childhood Research Quarterly, 18*, 42–64.

Vinden, P., & Astington, J. (2000). Culture and understanding other minds. In S. Baron-Cohen, H. Tager-Flusberg, & D. Cohen (Eds.), *Understanding other minds: Perspectives from developmental cognitive neuroscience* (pp. 503–519). New York: Oxford University Press.

Vygotsky, L. S. (1978). *Mind in society.* Cambridge, MA: Harvard University Press.

Washburn, S. L. (1960). Tools and human evolution. *Scientific American, 203*, 36–43.

Wentzel, K. R. (2004). Understanding classroom competence: The role of social-motivational and self-processes. In R. Kail (Ed.), *Advances in child development and behavior* (Vol. 32, pp. 213–241). Amsterdam, The Netherlands: Elsevier.

Werker, J. F., & Vouloumanos, A. (2001). Speech and language processing in infancy: A neurocognitive approach. In C. A. Nelson & M. Luciana (Eds.), *Handbook of developmental cognitive neuroscience* (pp. 269–280). Cambridge, MA: MIT Press.

Winsler, A., Diaz, R. M., McCarthy, E. M., Atencio, D. J., & Chabay, L. A. (1999). Mother–child interaction, private speech, and task performance in preschool children with behavior problems. *Journal of Child Psychology, Psychiatry, and Allied Disciplines, 40*, 891–904.

Wood, D. J., & Middleton, D. (1975). A study of assisted problem solving. *British Journal of Psychology, 66*, 181–191.

CHAPTER 24

The Socialization
of Emotional Competence

Susanne A. Denham, Hideko H. Bassett, and Todd Wyatt

Emotions are ubiquitous in all our lives. The information that they afford to each of us—about ourselves and others—is invaluable. The overarching goal of this chapter is to elucidate and comment on the state of current knowledge of the ways in which children, from preschool age through adolescence, learn from others about aspects of emotions—how the development of their emotional competence is contributed to by others' emotion-related expressiveness, behaviors, and beliefs. To meet this central goal, we must first define the boundaries of what we mean by "emotional competence."

After detailing this central construct, we move to a consideration of the role of both intra- and interpersonal contributors to the development of emotional competence. To flesh out the central issues of concern in the chapter, we again give attention to definitional matters—what *is* socialization *of emotion*? Then we review extant research on socialization of emotion by parents, teachers, and peers, within the preschool, grade school, and adolescent age ranges. Finally, we evaluate the state of our knowledge about this important area of development, address perceived gaps in the literature, and suggest ways of thinking about and investigating these phenomena in the future.

EMOTIONAL COMPETENCE AND ITS ROLE IN SOCIAL FUNCTIONING

Broadly stated, aspects of emotional competence developing through the lifespan include emotional expression and experience, understanding emotions of self and others, and emotion regulation. Children become increasingly emotionally competent over time, and growing evidence suggests that such emotional competence contributes to their concurrent social competence and well-being, as well as to later outcomes (Denham et al., 2003; Denham & Burton, 2003). Even preschool-age children are surprisingly adept at several components of emotional competence, including but not limited to the following: (1) expressing emotions that are, or are not, experienced, (2) decoding these processes in others, and (3) regulating emotions in ways that are age and socially appropriate (Halberstadt, Denham, & Dunsmore, 2001).

These elements of emotional competence require operationalization. Specifically, then, emotionally competent children and adolescents can express a broad variety of emotions, without incapacitating intensity or duration. Thus, when discussing *emotional expressiveness*, we refer to (1) the specific emotions shown, with varying purposefulness, by children (e.g., happiness, sadness, anger, fear, and empathy/love), and (2) the overall rate of such expressiveness, across emotions. Next, to define *emotion understanding*, we refer to children's knowledge about the emotions of themselves and others, including (1) comprehension of basic emotions (e.g., happiness, sadness, and anger), their expressions, situations, causes, and consequences; (2) insight into more complicated facets of emotions (e.g., that two people can feel two different emotions in response to the same eliciting event, as when one child's finds an event scary, but another doesn't); and (3) discernment of display rule usage, mixed emotions, and more complex emotions (e.g., guilt and shame). Finally, children can *regulate their emotion* when its experience is "too much" or "too little" for themselves, or when its expression is "too much" or "too little" to fit with others' expectations, by using physical, cognitive, and/or behavioral strategies to dampen or amplify internal emotional experience and/or external emotional expression.

Further, the contribution of emotional expressiveness, understanding, and regulation to social competence is a key tenet of emotional competence theory (Denham, 1998; Saarni, 1999). For example, happier, less angry children are better liked by peers and seen as friendly and cooperative by teachers in preschool and elementary school (Denham et al., 2003; Isley, O'Neil, Clatfelter, & Parke, 1999); similar outcomes are obtained for adolescents (Harker & Keltner, 2001). More negative outcomes are associated with children's negative emotional expressiveness (Cumberland-Li, Eisenberg, Champion, Gershoff, & Fabes, 2003; Denham, McKinley, Couchoud, & Holt, 1990; Denham, Mitchell-Copeland, Strandberg, Auerbach, & Blair, 1997).

Accurate interpretation of others' emotions provides important information about social situations. Hence, preschoolers' understanding of emotions often relates to their positive peer status, prosocial reactions to emotions, and teacher ratings of social competence, as well as more discrete social behaviors, such as initiating and receiving social contact and inhibiting aggression (Denham, Caverly, et al., 2002; Denham et al., 1990; Denham et al., 1997). Positive links between age-appropriate understanding of emotions and older children's social competence are also being uncovered (Garner, 1996; Izard et al., 2001; Jones, Abbey, & Cumberland, 1998).

Children's regulation of emotions also is a crucial contributor to aspects of their social competence. For example, preschoolers who regulate their anger by venting are seen later as less socially competent by kindergarten peers and teachers, compared to those who use other emotion regulation strategies (Eisenberg, Fabes, Nyman, Bernzweig, & Pinuelas, 1994; Eisenberg et al., 1997; Raver, Blackburn, & Bancroft, 1999). Similar relations hold for dysregulated older children and adolescents (Eisenberg, Valiente, et al., 2003; McDowell, Kim, O'Neil, & Parke, 2002; Murphy, Shepard, Eisenberg, & Fabes, 2004; Rydell, Berlin, & Bohlin, 2003).

Both intra- and interpersonal contributors to these aspects of the children's emotional competence will next be considered. For example, increased language development undoubtedly aids preschoolers in their emotion knowledge; similarly, relatively stable emotion-related temperamental traits need to be considered when predicting outcomes for children.

CONTRIBUTORS TO INDIVIDUAL DIFFERENCES IN EMOTIONAL COMPETENCE

If emotional competence is intimately related with important child outcomes, such as social and even academic competence (Raver, 2002), questions about its cultivation and individual differences must be answered. Both intrapersonal (within-child) and interpersonal (socialization) contributors are no doubt important.

Intrapersonal Contributors to Emotional Competence: How within-Child Factors Affect Emotional Competence

Before the role of socialization agents in the development of emotional competence is considered, it should be noted that abilities and attributes of the children themselves can either promote or hinder emotional competence. For example, some children have a capacity for superior cognitive and language skills that allow them to better understand their social world, including the emotions within it, as well as to better communicate their own feelings, wishes, desires, and goals for social interactions and relationships (Cutting & Dunn, 1999). Children who can reason more flexibly can probably also more readily perceive how another person might feel different in a situation than they themselves would; for example, one child may be fearful of swimming pools, even though they delight another. In a similar manner, children with greater verbal abilities can ask more pointed questions about their own and others' emotions (e.g., "Why is he crying?"), and understand the answers to these questions, giving them a special advantage in understanding and dealing with emotions (Kopp, 1989). A preschooler with advanced expressive language also can describe his or her own emotions more pointedly—"I don't *want* to go to bed! I am *mad*!"—allowing the preschooler to get his or her emotional point across, and also allowing others to communicate with the child about the emotional situation. The role of language and cognitive ability in the emotional competence of older children is less explored.

Similarly, children with different emotional dispositions (i.e., different temperaments) are particularly well- or ill-equipped to demonstrate emotional competence. Thus, temperamental characteristics involving the expression or inhibition of emotion can be particularly important in setting the groundwork for social behavior (Buck, 1991). Especially emotionally negative children will probably find that they have a greater need for emotion regulation, even though it is at the same time harder for them to do so. Such a double bind taxes the child's abilities to "unhook" from an intense emotional experience (Eisenberg et al., 1994; Eisenberg et al., 1997). Conversely, children whose temperament predisposes them to flexibly focus attention on a comforting action, object, or thought and shift attention from a distressing situation, are better able to regulate emotions, even intense ones. These intrapersonal factors no doubt continue to exert influence well into adolescence. They can be either foundations of or roadblocks to emotional and social competence. Moreover, they may interact with interpersonal contributors.

Interpersonal Contributors to Emotional Competence: First Considerations of Socialization by Important Others

Caring adults are faced with children who vary in their emotional competence on a daily basis. What differences do their efforts make? How do they foster these emotional and social competencies that stand children in such good stead? Even given the important intrapersonal contributors already mentioned, much of the individual variation in children's emotional competence derives from experiences within the family, classroom, and peer group (Denham, 1998; Eisenberg, Cumberland, & Spinrad, 1998; Hyson, 1994). Important adults—and other children—in each child's life have crucial roles in the development of emotional competence.

Thus, socialization of emotional competence is likely to be very important—but how does the socialization of emotion fit within a larger subdiscipline of developmental science, and that of socialization in general? This question is deceptive in its simplicity: One of the desired outcomes of socialization is self-regulation of emotion (Grusec, 2002). Nonetheless, there are issues that must be considered before we describe socialization of emotional competence.

First, where does one draw the line between everyday interaction with children, where conscious socialization goals are not necessarily in mind but emotions are everpresent, and "real" socialization of emotion (Mayer & Beltz, 1998)? Certainly, most parents do not focus consciously on the emotion socialization of their children while reprimanding them. Nonetheless, we argue (as do Eisenberg, Spinrad, & Cumberland, 1998) that "socialization is any task or content area that is part of learning a cultural pattern"; "affect is . . . an integral part of the ideas we hold, the practices that we follow . . . and our experiences with others" (Bugental & Goodnow, 1998, p. 441). The root of socialization about such a central set of beliefs and abilities lies within everyday interaction rather than solely an occasional moments of transgression followed by discipline. Hence, socialization of emotion may be, at times, more indirect than some other forms of socialization and less purposeful or consciously retrievable by the socialization agents themselves, but it occurs nonetheless. In short, both unintentional and intentional parental socialization processes are likely to impact emotional competence, just like any other socialization outcome. However, unintentional processes may be very dominant, or even exclusive, when other socialization agents, such as peers, are considered.

A second issue to consider when "pinning down" socialization of emotion is that many of the behaviors associated with what we consider the most adaptive of its forms are also closely related to parental "responsiveness," "warmth," or "control" (Gondoli & Braungart-Rieker, 1998), which leaves one wondering whether the notion of "socialization of emotion" adds much at all. We again agree with Eisenberg, Spinrad and Cumberland (1998): Parenting goals and values contribute to both higher-order stylistic parenting dimensions such as warmth and control and also to more specific parenting behaviors, including those relevant to socialization of emotion. Therefore, it is quite likely that both parenting styles and specific emotion socialization practices are related, but not totally overlapping, constructs (see also Chang, Schwartz, Dodge, & McBride-Chang, 2003; Eisenberg, Zhou, et al., 2003; O'Neal & Magai, 2005). As noted by Eisenberg and colleagues, socialization of emotion practices occur *within the context* of a higher-order parenting style, and both these practices and styles are informed by parents' goals and values. Again, socialization of emotion emerges as an important construct in its own right.

Specifically, parents and other socializers probably all hold "meta-emotion philosophies" about which emotions *should be* felt and expressed and how they *should be* felt and expressed, how salient they are, and what *should be* done in emotional situations (Gottman, Katz, & Hooven, 1997; see also Mayer & Beltz, 1998). Such an emotion-based set of beliefs as the meta-emotion philosophy fits squarely within Bugental and Goodnow's (1998) definition of socialization—others form expectations, whether in the forefront of consciousness or not, about children's emotions and emotion-related behaviors and, based on these expectations, express or indicate their expectations about these emotions and emotion-related behaviors. The child notices, interprets, and encodes these expressed expectations, adopts a stance toward them, and, finally, gives an indication of understanding the socialization message and reactions to it.

So, in our view, socialization of emotions is omnipresent in children's everyday contact with parents, teachers, caregivers, and peers. All people with whom children interact exhibit a variety of emotions, which the children observe—we refer to this aspect of socialization of emotion as *modeling,* whether discussing specific expressed emotions observed by children, or referring to the totality of emotional expressiveness (and its valence) to which children are exposed within a context. Further, children's emotions often require some kind of reaction from social partners—we refer to this aspect of socialization as *contingent reactions* to children's emotional expressiveness. Finally, intentionally teaching about the world of emotions is considered by many adults to be an important area of socialization—we refer to this aspect of socialization with the more or less interchangeable terms "teaching" and "coaching" (Eisenberg, Fabes, & Murphy, 1996; Eisenberg et al., 1994; Eisenberg et al., 1999; Gottman et al., 1997). Eisenberg, Cumberland, and Spinrad (1998) have cited evidence for all three mechanisms, with regard to parents. Their conclusions suggest that each of these mechanisms influence children's emotional expression, understanding, and regulation, as well as social functioning.

Socialization of Emotions

Modeling Mechanisms

EMOTIONAL EXPRESSIVENESS

By modeling various emotions, socializers give children information about the nature of happiness, sadness, anger, and fear—how they are expressed, and when. As already noted, this vicarious learning is almost overdetermined; children are constantly viewing and processing the emotional behavior of others and incorporate this learning into their own expressive behavior. Thus, parents are doubtless key models of emotional expressiveness from infancy through adolescence. Exposure to a particular profile of emotions can promote children's experience and expression of the same specific emotions and may also contribute to differing patterns of overall emotional expressiveness (Halberstadt, Fox, & Jones, 1993; see also Valiente, Eisenberg, et al., 2004). For example, positive emotional expression in parents is significantly related to positive emotional expression in children (Isley et al., 1999). Further, parents' positive emotions also are related to children's popularity with peers, and their displays of positive caregiving behaviors with siblings (Garner, Jones, Gaddy, & Rennie, 1997; Isley et al., 1999), perhaps by promoting children's own positive feelings, creating a fertile environment from which positive social behavior can emerge (Denham et al., 1997).

Interestingly, these results are sometimes moderated by child and parent sex; Isley and colleagues found that pathways from parental expressiveness to child expressiveness to child social competence were clearest for same-sex parent–child dyads. As evidence on peer socialization emerges, researchers will be able to demonstrate whether child outcomes are moderated by same-sex (boy–boy, girl–girl) and opposite-sex pairings.

Conversely, one can envision the effect of relentless exposure to parents' negative emotions; when mothers are often angry and tense with them, young children are angrier and have more difficulties in the peer world (Denham, 1989, 1998; Denham et al., 1997; Garner & Estep, 2001; Isley et al., 1999; Smith & Walden, 1999). In fact, Denham et al. (1997) found evidence that maternal negative emotions contributed to children's less positive emotions, which in turn contributed to social lack of competence. With respect to elementary-age children and parent emotional expressiveness, parents' intense, frequent negative emotions are also related to children's quick, unregulated anger (Snyder, Stoolmiller, Wilson, & Yamamoto, 2003).

Demorat (1999) microanalytically examined a kindergarten teacher's emotions in relation to the responses of four students, over 3 months. The teacher most frequently showed the emotions of pride and happiness, and the students matched her interest and happiness. Her pride functioned to acknowledge student achievements, and her happiness encouraged exemplary behavior. Thus, elementary-age children are learning about emotional expressiveness and display rules from important adults in both family and school contexts.

Emotional expressiveness by parents and their offspring takes on a new appearance during adolescence. First, there is evidence that youngsters' expression of negative emotions increases during early adolescence, and that negative affect reciprocity is present in many adolescent–parent interactions (Larson, Moneta, Richards, & Wilson, 2002). In one of the only empirical studies of adolescents' and parents' emotional expressiveness, Kim, Conger, Lorenz, and Elder (2001) found that both parents' and adolescents' initial levels of negative emotion toward each other predicted the rate of growth and rate of change in growth of expressed negative affect, in a reciprocal negative cycle. Findings also suggested that family experience with this interactional style may have an adverse influence on the development of early adult social relationships.

Similarly, another study showed that parents' and adolescent's levels of observed emotionality were highly intercorrelated, suggesting that parents were modeling emotional expressiveness (Bronstein, Fitzgerald, Briones, Pieniadz, & D'Ari, 1993). In this study, specifically nonhostile expression of emotion within the family buffered against psychological problems over the transition to middle school and enhanced concurrent and long-term developmental outcomes, as evidenced, for example, by greater peer popularity, presumably by its contribution to these older children's own emotional expressiveness.

EMOTION KNOWLEDGE

Others' overall emotional expressiveness, and the particular profile of emotions that they express, also implicitly teaches children about the emotional significance of differing events, how certain situations evoke specific emotions, the behaviors that may accompany differing emotions, and others' likely reactions. Thus, others' emotions are associated with children's abilities to understand emotions (Denham & Grout, 1993; Denham et al., 1997; Nixon & Watson, 2001). In particular, positive expressiveness in the family seems to promote understanding of emotions, perhaps because positive feelings render children more open to learning and problem solving (Fredrickson, 1998).

Conversely, parental expressiveness can make it more difficult for young children to address issues of emotion altogether; for example, exposure to parents' negative emotions can hamper young children's emotion knowledge. Specifically, although exposure to *well-regulated* negative emotion can be positively related to understanding of emotion (Garner, Jones, & Miner, 1994), parents' frequent, intense negative emotions may disturb children, as well as discourage self-reflection, so that little emotional learning occurs (Denham, 1998). The amount of anger that is expressed in the family home is negatively related to a child's acquisition of emotion knowledge (Denham, Zoller, & Couchoud, 1994; Raver & Spagnola, 2002).

Another effect on children's emotion knowledge that is associated with the extremely angry, hostile emotional environment of physical maltreatment is ability to identify angry expressions with less sensory input than nonmaltreated children (Pollak & Sinha, 2002). At the same time, Pollak and Tolley-Schell (2003) have found that physically abused children also have trouble disengaging from invalid anger cues, suggesting that any advantage of their increased ability to identify valid anger cues may be counterbalanced by an identification bias. These patterns of evidence serve as a caution—it cannot be assumed that children developing under exceptional circumstances show emotion knowledge that is necessarily quantitatively *or* qualitatively the same as that for children in more normative contexts. Conversely, it cannot be assumed that simple patterns of associations (such as greater modeled anger → lessened emotion knowledge) are not accompanied by more nuanced findings that await discovery.

At the same time, parents whose expressiveness is quite limited impart little concrete information about emotions. Finally, our research findings triangulate on a mediational pathway that still requires complete testing; that is, emotion knowledge is predicted by parental emotion and emotion knowledge contributes significantly to concurrent and later social competence (Denham et al., 2003; Denham, Blair, Schmidt, & DeMulder, 2002; Denham, Caverly, et al., 2002; Denham & Grout, 1993; Denham et al., 1997).

During grade school, observation of peers' emotions and rules about emotions are likely to grow in importance. Observations of peer emotions also could be expected to inform more sophisticated aspects of understanding emotion, such as understanding of complex emotions like guilt or shame, display rules, and ambivalence, which complement the child's new world of peers. Research is sorely needed into these new areas of socialization of emotion.

EMOTION REGULATION

Similarly, both middle- and low-income preschoolers' emotion regulation is facilitated by their mothers' appropriate expressiveness (Eisenberg, Gershoff, et al., 2001; Eisenberg, Valiente, et al., 2003; Garner & Spears, 2000). In contrast, exposure to higher levels of parental negativity may overarouse young children who cannot yet regulate their own emotions well and represents an emotionally hostile template for children to follow in their reactions to people and events.

In fact, Eisenberg, Gershoff, and colleagues found unique contributions of both positive and negative maternal emotion to early elementary-age children's emotion regulation, and the relations of maternal emotions to children's social competence were mediated through children's regulation (Eisenberg, Liew, & Pidada, 2001; Eisenberg, Valiente, et al., 2003; see also Valiente, Fabes, Eisenberg, & Spinrad, 2004). Extending this work longitudinally, Eisenberg, Valiente, et al. (2003) found that early grade-school children's emotion regulation was accounted for mostly by their preschool emotion regulation, which was originally predicted by parental expressiveness. That is, early exposure to parental emotions figured heavily in the emergence of a relatively stable individual difference in emotional competence. As well, relations of children's emotion regulation and parents' negative expressivity, but not parents' positive expressivity, did change with age. That is, children who had more negatively expressive mothers in early elementary school no longer vented their own emotions so much; they were, instead, learning to "hold their tongues" (and emotions).

However, adults' persistent and intense negative emotional expressiveness may also have a more pervasive, less complex, relation with children's emotion regulation. For example, age effects are not found in the case of maltreatment; both 4–6-year-olds (Maughan & Cicchetti, 2002) and older children (Shields & Cicchetti, 2001) exposed to or at risk for continued maltreatment showed deficits in emotion regulation. These deficits in emotion regulation were in turn related to being a bully or victim.

In terms of classroom socialization of emotion, emotionally negative preschool classroom environments are also related to disruptive peer behavior in second grade, especially for boys (Howes, 2000). Almost no research has targeted the expressive modeling of teachers, however, despite the existence of observational ratings that can be used to capture the emotional environment in preschool classrooms (Arnett, 1989). Again, the roles of socializers of emotions other than parents need to be examined.

SUMMARY

In sum, with regard to adults' modeling of emotions, exposure to parents' and other adults' broad but not overly negative emotions helps children learn about emotions and come to express similar profiles, even as they progress to middle childhood and into adolescence. In particular, in families or classrooms, frequent, intense adult negative emotion is often deleterious to young children's emotion knowledge, profiles of expressiveness, emotion regulation, and social competence. Obviously, however, more work is needed with still older children, and with socializers other than parents (more emphasis is also needed on fathers' role is necessary; Parke & McDowell, 1998).

Teaching Mechanisms

EMOTIONAL EXPRESSIVENESS

Socializers' tendencies to discuss emotions, and the quality of their communications about emotions, if nested within a warm relationship that increases the child's receptiveness, assist the child in expressing emotions. Socializers may draw attention to emotions and validate or clarify the child's emotion, helping the child to react to emotions and express them authentically, in a regulated manner. Whether socializers use emotion talk to clarify, teach, or share, rather than to modify the child's behavior or preach, also may be a critical distinction (Denham & Grout, 1992; Eisenberg, Cumberland, & Spinrad, 1998). Specifically, the former pattern is associated with more positive profiles of young children's expressiveness.

Although there are no studies on this type of "talk about feelings" for middle childhood, it can be assumed that when socializers (in this case, particularly parents, who have a broader knowledge base than peers) speak to school-age children about matters relevant for emotional competence—complex or mixed emotions, masked emotions, strategies for managing emotions—their children's profiles of emotional expressiveness may be more positive and conducive to intrapersonal well-being and interpersonally productive interaction. This area of socialization of emotion, particularly with older children, bears greater investigation.

EMOTION KNOWLEDGE

In its simplest form, teaching about emotion, or emotion "coaching," consists of verbally explaining an emotion and its relation to an observed event or expression. Thus, what parents and other adults say, or intentionally attempt to convey through other means, may impact their children's emotion knowledge. Teaching about emotions may help to direct children's attention to salient emotional cues, helping them understand the entire social interaction and manage their own responses to it.

Parental, especially mothers', didactic techniques for discussing emotions with their children, are associated with preschoolers' emotion knowledge (Cervantes & Callanan, 1998; Denham, Zoller, & Couchoud, 1994; Garner, Jones, et al., 1997; Kochanoff, 2001). The verbal give-and-take about emotional experience within the scaffolded context of chatting with an adult helps the young child to formulate a coherent body of knowledge about emotional expressions, situations, and causes (Denham, Renwick-DeBardi, & Hewes, 1994; Dunn, Brown, & Beardsall, 1991; Dunn, Brown, Slomkowski, Tesla, & Youngblade, 1991; Dunn, Slomkowski, Donelan, & Herrera, 1995). Furthermore, mother–child emotion conversations in preschool may predict even later emotion knowledge (i.e., about emotion regulation and display rules; Garner, 1999).

These findings appear to hold across socioeconomic and ethnic variations and are even stronger within secure mother–child relationships, where both mother and child may be more comfortable about emotions (Kochanoff, 2001; Ontai & Thompson, 2002). However, in two recent dissertations, *fathers* who used *more* emotion language while reminiscing about past emotional experiences had children with *less* advanced emotion understanding (Colwell, 2001; Kochanoff, 2001). In contrast to the reminiscence task, however, *both* parents' discussion of emotion during an Emotion Game were associated with preschoolers' more mature emotion knowledge (Colwell, 2001); perhaps fathers perceive reminiscence as more formal or didactic, and talk more in this context with (or "at") children whose emotion knowledge needs bolstering.

When adults' admonitions about emotions are misleading or idiosyncratic, however, children may enter middle childhood with a distorted understanding of emotions. A particular hazard is the anger-intensifying tendency to attribute inaccurate hostile intentions to a peer (Weiss, Dodge, Bates, & Pettit, 1992). At the same time, the form and function of conversations about emotions *may* change during later childhood; children's input to emotion-laden conversation is apt to be more active than it was years earlier, and parents may be susceptible to "overdoing" talk about emotions, with children tuning out. Again, we know of no extant research on this topic but advocate for it.

EMOTION REGULATION

Talk about emotions also gives the child a new tool to use in modulating overt expression of emotions (Kopp, 1989). With age and assistance from caregivers, regulation is transferred from external control (e.g., parents calming a crying child) to internal control (e.g., children using self talk to calm themselves) (Thompson, 1991; Winsler, Diaz, Atencio, McCarthy, & Chabay, 2000). Emotion conversations with parents allow children to separate impulses from behavior, giving them reflective distance from feeling states themselves, and space in which to interpret and evaluate their feelings and to reflect upon causes and consequences (Bretherton, Fritz, Zahn-Waxler, & Ridgeway, 1986; Eisenberg, Cumberland, Spinrad, 1998).

Accordingly, conversations about feelings are an important context for coaching children about how to regulate emotions (Brown & Dunn, 1992). Good "emotion coaches"—adults who are aware of emotions, especially negative ones, and talk about them in a differentiated manner—assist their children in regulating their own emotions (Gottman et al., 1997). Dismissing adults may want to be helpful but refrain from talking too much about children's emotions. Alternatively, poor coaches may actively punish children for showing or querying about emotions. Neither of those meta-emotion strategies toward teaching about emotions are particularly useful in helping children acquire emotion regulation skills. In contrast, emotion coaching strategies teach young children to perceive social consequences of behavior (e.g., "Johnny will be mad at you and not want to play with you again, if you keep taking away his toys") and to consider another's viewpoint (e.g., "That upset Erica—look at her face").

The general trend of these findings also holds true for low-income, minority families (Garner, Jones, et al., 1997). Further, this linkage of emotion discussion and emotion regulation appears to be important for older, as well as younger, children. Elementary-age children whose parents linked emotionally evocative slides' content with the child's own experiences while conversing about the slides were better regulated (Eisenberg, Losoya, et al., 2001).

Finally, young children absorb not only the content but also the form and quality of emotion coaching from people other than parents. In one study of children in child-care transitions (Dunn, 1994), preschoolers remembered both sadness and fear during these times, as well as the comfort given them by teachers and friends.

Friends should also be considered potential emotion coaches; after all, they are children's "best bets" during middle childhood for confiding emotional experiences, especially feelings of vulnerability (Krappmann, 1996; Rose & Asher, 1999; Saarni, 1988, 1989). They are especially likely to disclose emotional understandings and experiences they may hide from nonfriends, helping each other acquire emotional regulation skills (Asher, Parker, & Walker, 1996; Parker & Gottman, 1989). Friends may use such emotion talk in several ways. First, their gossip may help them to broach the subject of potential insecurities without actually naming them (similar to fantasy play during earlier years). One can imagine emotion talk occurring during such gossip, functioning within the put-downs ("She's such a little cry-baby, isn't she, Erica?") or statements of group norms ("I hate it when he blows up like that, don't you?"). Second, their statements of support–approval of their friend, sympathy, and affection could easily include emotion language relevant for regulation. Third, relationship talk also goes on, along with self-disclosure, and unsurprisingly, conflict processes often rear their not-necessarily-ugly heads—these aspects of conversation may be replete with emotion regulation talk. This area is ripe for investigation.

SUMMARY

It seems clear that discussion of emotions, particularly in an elaborative rather than coercive context, is related to children's emotion knowledge and emotion regulation, as well as their emotional positivity (although research is more scant in that area). What remains to be expanded is the role of fathers, whose discussion of emotion seems to serve different functions than mothers', the potential role of teachers, and, especially, the role of friends' emotion talk, starting in middle childhood.

Contingent Reactions to Emotions

EMOTIONAL EXPRESSIVENESS

Reactions to children's displays of emotion are another important way that other people influence children's emotional competence. Socializers' contingent reactions include behavioral and emotional encouragement or discouragement/punishment of specific emotions (Eisenberg et al., 1996; Eisenberg et al., 1999). Specifically, adults may punish children's experiences and expressions of emotions or show a dismissive attitude toward the world of emotions by ignoring the child's emotions in a well-meant effort to "make it better" (Denham, Renwick-DeBardi, & Hewes, 1994). Parents who respond to children's emotion by minimizing or dismissing the emotion are more likely to have sadder, more fearful young children (David-Vilker, 2000; Denham, 1989; see Denham, 1998, for similar evidence with older adolescents; Eisenberg et al., 1996; see Garside & Klimes-Dougan, 2002, for similar evidence with older adolescents; Gottman et al., 1997; see O'Neal & Magai, 2005, for young adolescents' affirmation that they perceive differential parental reactions to their varying emotions).

Children who receive a punishing or derogatory reaction to their emotions also are likely to suppress feelings but remain physiologically aroused without the skills to rectify the situation or their emotional response (Eisenberg et al., 1996; Fabes, Leonard, Kupanoff, & Martin, 2001). Young children whose mothers endorsed controlling their children's emotion displays showed less emotion when winning or losing a challenging game (Berlin & Cassidy, 2003); they were already "getting the message." Finally, in some rare research on reactions to adolescent emotions, mothers who used more punishing and magnifying (e.g., "making it worse") or fewer rewarding or overriding (e.g., helping change emotional focus) strategies for socializing sadness had sadder adolescents (Race & Brand, 2003).

In contrast, emotional encouragement and nonsupportive reactions to emotions are predictive of preschoolers' positive and negative expressiveness, respectively (Fabes, Poulin, Eisenberg, & Madden-Derdich, 2002). More research is needed to elucidate the links between these parental reactions and children's patterns of emotional expressiveness, particularly with older children.

REACTIONS TO EMOTIONS AND EMOTION KNOWLEDGE

Parents' emotional reactions contingent on the child's emotions also may help the child in differentiating among emotions (Denham & Kochanoff, 2002; Denham, Zoller, & Couchoud, 1994; Fabes et al., 2001; Fabes et al., 2002). For example, Fabes et al. (2002) found that supportive reactions positively and distress reactions negatively predicted emotion knowledge. Still, more work needs to be done, especially for children older than preschool and socializers other than mother (e.g., siblings; see Sawyer et al., 2002). For example, it is necessary to find out whether, and how, parents' reactions to children's emotions change as children grow, and how these changes affect children's emotion knowledge (e.g., understanding of display rules or ambivalence and subskills that could be especially important from middle childhood through adolescence). As well, friends' influence becomes more significant as children mature; but how, and under what conditions, do their reactions to emotions help or hurt their peers' emotion knowledge?

REACTIONS TO EMOTIONS AND EMOTION REGULATION

Positive reactions, such as tolerance or comfort, convey that emotions are manageable, even useful (Gottman et al., 1997). Parents who are good "emotion coaches," at least in the United States, accept preschool and elementary-age children's experiences of emotion and their expression of emotions that do not harm others; they empathize with and validate emotions. Regardless of age, emotional moments are seen as opportunities for intimacy (Denham & Kochanoff, 2002; Eisenberg et al., 1996; Eisenberg et al., 1999; Eisenberg, Valiente, et al., 2003; see Jones, Eisenberg, Fabes, & MacKinnon, 2002, for an even more differentiated picture). Such optimal responses to children's emotions are a supportive breeding ground for emotion regulation (Denham, 1989; Denham & Grout, 1993; Fabes et al., 2001). In contrast, of course, parents who are nonsupportive—either punitive or dismissing—of their children's emotions are, according to this theoretical perspective, sowing the seeds of diminished emotion regulatory abilities.

To zero in on older children's emotion regulation and their parents' reactions to emotions, it seems reasonable to assume that these reactions are still important; after all, parents do continue as grade-schoolers' primary support in distress and know more about emotions and regulating them than their children. Most school-age children still turn to their parents in order to share their fears over a monster story or a staged kidnapping at night (e.g., the boys studied by Rimé, Dozier, Vandenplas, & Declercq, 1996). A majority of elementary-age children endorse genuine expression of negative emotions to parents (Saarni, 1988, 1989; Zeman & Shipman, 1997). Older children expect more positive, useful reactions from parents than from peers, but little or no research has investigated the contribution of such reactions to the older children's emotion regulation.

Further, although parents' reactions to children's emotions remain important, they do change across time. From toddlerhood onward, as children develop effective emotion regulatory abilities, parents change the frequency, intensity, and nature of their reactions, transferring responsibility for regulation from caregiver to child (Grolnick, Kurowski, McMenamy, Rivkin, & Bridges, 1998). Although the optimal reactions already mentioned are still important both concurrently and across time, certain of socializers' reactions to children's emotions may begin to take a different form with elementary school-age and older children, allowing for the child's autonomy and parents' heightened expectations of their behavior. For example, positively reinforcing the child's emotions (e.g., listening, accepting, querying, and complying) may be more predictive of older children's emotional competence, including emotion regulation, than overindulgent helping and comforting. Some measure of restrictiveness may also have beneficial outcomes in that older children need to know when emotions are appropriate and when they are not, and their emotions' effects on other people (Eisenberg, Spinrad, & Cumberland, 1998; Parke & McDowell, 1998). Conversely, encouragement of emotional expression may not be as predictive of emotion regulation as it was for younger children. Whether or not socializers' encouragement of emotional expressiveness portends children's competence also may be a function of the emotions encouraged—acceptable or unacceptable—and whether such encouragement is accompanied by teaching children how to deal with them. Such developmental changes in reactions to children's emotions—increasing complexity, emotion specificity, and interaction with other aspects of socialization—remain to be investigated.

Finally, as children move through elementary school, parents' contingent reactions to their emotions may not always be "on the mark." For example, parents' full understanding of their children's emotions may become limited due to their need to be parents rather than playmates and their inabilities to share all of their children's appraisals (Zeman & Shipman, 1997). Close friends also react to grade-schoolers' emotions and may be more on target than parents are. Older children value being helpful to a friend in need, rather than ignoring or blaming (Rose & Asher, 1999). In the horizontal friendship relationship, reactions to emotions that both comfort ("Don't worry about the test. You'll do better next time") and exhort ("Stop crying—everybody's looking you!") may predict emotion regulation. We think it unlikely that friends' mildly punishing socialization, such as chiding a friend over his overemotional reaction to an event, has deleterious effects equal to parents'. Friends' reactions are less likely to cause overarousal—a supportive equal's punitive reactions may have "more message" and "less fear." The middle childhood social world also centers on conforming to stringent norms (Gottman & Mettetal, 1986). In this context, friends' forthright reactions to one's emotions might be both necessary and useful.

As echoed throughout this chapter, however, these studies remain to be performed. In one exception, Sorber (2001) examined how grade schoolers indicated that they would react to specific emotions. Happy computer game characters were given the most approval, with angry characters given the least; acceptance of negative emotions decreased with age. Thus, it may be inferred that children become less accepting of their "real" peers' negative emotions over time.

Two recent investigations also have revealed that teachers of toddlers and preschoolers socialize children's emotions differently based on age, tailoring their reactions to children's emotions to the developmental level of the children (Ahn, 2003; Reimer, 1996). In Ahn's study, toddler teachers used physical comfort and distraction in response to children's negative emotions. Preschool teachers more often relied on verbal mediation, helping children infer the causes of their negative emotions, and teaching them constructive ways of expressing negative emotion. Teachers of preschoolers were also less likely to match or encourage their positive emotions and were more likely to discourage emotional displays of any valence. Finally, teachers did not validate children's negative emotion very often—one of the tenets of emotion coaching. Reimer's work also suggests that preschool teachers are most concerned with young children's control of emotion-related behavior and situation-specific appropriate expression of emotions. Taken together, these studies suggest a need for teacher training on socialization of emotion.

SUMMARY

The bulk of research suggests that an accepting, supportive reaction to children's emotional expressiveness patterns generally is associated with all three components of emotional competence, although the research coverage is quite uneven—with most concentration on parents' (mostly mothers') reactions to emotions and children's emotion regulation. At the same time, much could be gained from examining friends' reactions to older children's emotions and their relation to emotional competence. Obviously, we are taking a stance that different relationships moderate the differing effects of others' reactions to children's emotions. At the same time, an intriguing alternative (or additional) hypothesis is that it is a context issue—children need to learn different emotional competence skills for different venues. One way that the emotional norms of differing contexts (e.g., home, school, or playground) are demonstrated is via the differing socializing goals, behaviors, and outcomes of parents, teachers, and friends.

Summary: How Adults Socialize Emotional Competence

In short, there is a growing body of knowledge regarding the contributions of adults to young children's emotional competence. These elements will be useful in building adult roles in any successful social–emotional programming for young children. Although cultural values and variations crucially require our attention so that the unique perspectives of both adults and children may be honored, several principles seem to hold true across groups (Denham, Caal, Bassett, Benga, & Geangu, 2004). First, a generally positive picture emerges of "emotion coaching," although some tutelage about when to control emotions appears beneficial under certain conditions. In terms of promoting emotional and social competence, parent and teacher/caregiver training should include a focus on ways to become good emotion coaches.

SOCIALIZATION OF EMOTIONAL COMPETENCE: WHERE DO WE GO FROM HERE?

The amount of research that has been published on the topic of socialization of emotion since Eisenberg, Cumberland, and Spinrad's (1998) review is quite impressive. But, as noted throughout this chapter, there is still work to do. In this concluding section we sketch out our thoughts on the important new directions for the investigation of emotion socialization, as well as particular issues needing attention.

Overall Considerations

Eisenberg and colleagues presented a revised model in their response to commentaries on their 1998 article; we have simplified and adapted this model in Figure 24.1. It can be

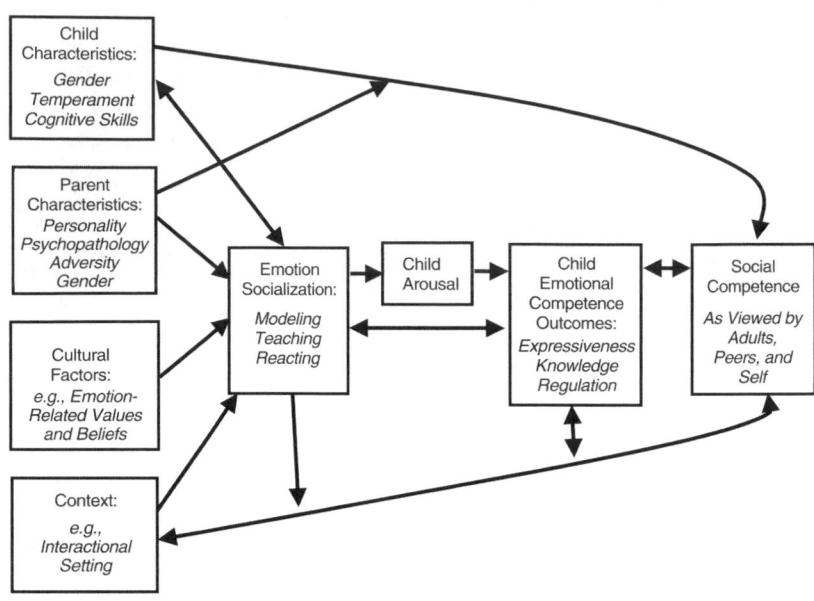

FIGURE 24.1. Simplified rendition of Eisenberg and colleagues' model for socialization of emotion. Adapted from Eisenberg, Spinrad, and Cumberland. Copyright 1998 by Lawrence Erlbaum Associates. Adapted by permission.

noted that in this chapter we have focused on the child characteristics (e.g., temperament and cognitive abilities), emotion socialization techniques (i.e., modeling, teaching/coaching, and reacting to children's emotions), emotional competence, and social behavior outcomes. We have given less attention to parent characteristics, cultural factors, context, child arousal, and moderators. At the same time, even this more complex model is not a dynamic one in that it does not represent developmental change. Nor is it bidirectional— it says nothing about the undoubted impact of the child on the socializer, because the focus of this chapter is on socialization; in our view, the parameters of emotion socialization itself require further elucidation before attempting this increased complexity. Thus, we present Figure 24.1 to restate the framework of findings reviewed here, as well as to begin our discussion of further steps in investigating socialization of emotion.

On Beyond Preschool

First, what about the developmental dynamic missing in Eisenberg and colleagues' model? We have tried in this chapter to convey, or at least speculate about, developmental progressions for socialization of emotion. Obviously, however, there is a skewed age balance of research done in this area—most of the work relates to preschool children and their parents, mostly mothers.

There probably are a number of reasons for this imbalance, including (1) the gradual expansion of emotional development research in general and the parenting–emotional competence link in particular from the infancy period to the preschool age range (Capatides & Bloom, 1993; Field, 1994)—in some respects, this area of inquiry is in its own infancy; (2) the study of the components of emotional competence has only begun to move into the realm of older children. For example, what *is* the nature of developmentally appropriate emotion knowledge for older children and adolescents? How can it be measured?

Until foundational descriptive work on these elements and related developmental task for each epoch is accomplished, it remains difficult to move forward into appropriately operationalizing socialization via modeling, teaching, and reactions during each age range. Rosenblum and Lewis (2003) have done an exemplary job of such description in a recent chapter on older children's and adolescents' emotional competence, but more work is needed. Thus, one clear appeal to emanate from this chapter is to move forward theory *and* empirical work so that older children's emotional competence and its socialization (Jones & Garner, 1998) may be viewed more accurately.

More Than Mothers

In a similar vein, knowing how mothers socialize emotion is very important but does not come close to telling the whole story of how emotional competence is supported by persons in each child's environment. If developmental scientists are serious about understanding the socialization of emotion, *everyone* who is important to children as they grow *must* be considered. Although much of the material on friends' and peers socialization of emotion in this chapter was speculative, we hope to encourage new research into how the important world of agemates, with whom older children and adolescents spend so much time, contributes to the elements of emotional competence.

Similarly, we find it surprising that adults other than mothers have yet to be frequently considered. After all, there is evidence that positive relationships with teachers in the preschool and primary years can have long-lasting sequelae (Hamre & Pianta, 2001; Mitchell-Copeland, Denham, & DeMulder, 1997); it would follow that these important adults would be crucial socializers of emotion, as well. Even more glaring is the relative lack of information on how fathers socialize emotional competence (Parke & McDowell, 1998), although there are notable exceptions (e.g., Denham & Kochanoff, 2002; Eisenberg, Liew, & Pidada, 2001; Fabes et al., 2001; Parke, Cassidy, Burks, Carson, & Boyum, 1992). Especially since the function of fathers' socialization of emotion techniques may be unique (as in other domains), the careful and sometimes challenging work of making our research projects accessible to them must be done.

Not Just European American Culture

Eisenberg and colleagues appropriately include cultural factors as part of their revised model. Nonetheless, almost all the findings reported on in this chapter (and this research area in general) relate to middle-income Western European American parents and their children (Cole & Dennis, 1998; Jones & Garner, 1998). However, although there may be some more universally beneficial socialization of emotion techniques, aspects of parenting that may enhance child adjustment across cultural or subcultural/ethnic groups must be pinpointed precisely (Garner & Spears, 2000; Jones & Garner, 1998), and those whose effects may be dependent on the cultural context in which they take place (see Cole & Tan, Chapter 20, this volume, for a discussion of emotion socialization from a cultural perspective). Hence, the ability to predict positive outcomes for children, and to promote emotion socialization practices that support them, depends on an intimate and correct knowledge of the emotion-related cultural beliefs and practices and emotion rules of the cultural group in which they live. For example, "Understanding the cultural context of caregivers' reactions to children's negative emotion is crucial to understanding why parents do what they do and in relating parents' behavior to children's competence" (Cole & Dennis, 1998, p. 277). When the correct cultural lens is in place, practices that might be evaluated negatively (or positively) are seen in clearer relief (Cole & Tamang, 1996; Denham et al., 2004) and a more complete story can be told. To put the correct cultural lens in place, however, researchers must venture beyond any comfort zone, to study a broad range of cultural groups. Again, descriptive work will first be necessary.

She Felt/He Felt

It also would be inappropriate to leave the impression that gender is irrelevant to the socialization of emotion; it appears in Eisenberg and colleagues' model as a child characteristic. Although page restrictions and a dearth of relevant, differentiated research compelled us to remark less frequently on boy–girl differences in the components of emotional competence, and their parents' differing socialization methods with them (but see Kuebli, Butler, & Fivush, 1995; Kuebli & Fivush, 1992; Queenan, 2000), gender of both child and parent must be examined. It may be the rule, not the exception, that mothers and fathers use different emotion socialization practices; in some cases, their practices are also dependent on their child's gender (Garner, Robertson, & Smith, 1997; see also Zahn-Waxler, Klimes-Dougan, & Kendziora, 1998)

"It's All My Fault"

We also wish to leave the reader with the clear notion that socializer–child effects can be bidirectional; the paths between child characteristics and child outcomes and emotion socialization are indeed bidirectional in Eisenberg and colleagues' revised model. As one example, Siegel (1997) found that maternal reactions to the emotions of elementary school children diagnosed with attention-deficit/hyperactivity disorder (ADHD) are generally less rewarding, more punishing and disregarding than those of mothers of non-ADHD children. It is very easy to envision that this bald effect is really only part of a sequence in which the negativity of the child with ADHD plays a big role. It behooves us, then, to make an effort to disentangle these sequences, possibly via naturalistic microgenetic and longitudinal work, fully informed by our knowledge of developmentally appropriate child and parent behaviors (Fivush, 1998). At the very least, awareness must increase of potential moderators of paths of influence (e.g., children's temperament, along with age, sex, and other personal characteristics).

At the same time, *some* of the techniques socializers of emotions demonstrate are likely to stem from the socializers' personal characteristics. Much more work needs to be done in this area. As one example, Broth (2004) has examined negative emotionality and levels of stress as predictors of preschoolers' mothers' socialization of emotion techniques, along with their own emotional competence as a moderator of those associations; mothers' negative emotionality and, to a lesser degree, stress/daily hassles predicted poorer-quality socialization of emotion practices. Mothers' own emotional competence appeared to work in both an additive and an interactive fashion in relation to their socialization of emotion practices.

It All Depends

Finally, the link between emotion socialization techniques and child emotional competence outcomes, as well as the path from emotion socialization techniques and child arousal, may be affected by a number of moderators. For example, some socialization of emotion practices may have differential contributions to child outcomes depending on the nature of the attachment relationship between parent and child, or the sex or age of the child. We acknowledge the importance of uncovering such moderators to understand the full story about socialization of emotion, particularly when contemplating applied uses of such knowledge (e.g., training parents to be good "emotion coaches"). However, we also consider that careful descriptions of the main model, at different ages, with different socializers, might be a necessary first step—to sketch the outlines of these very complex phenomena—before proceeding to investigations with sufficient statistical power to detect moderating relationships, as tempting as their discovery may be.

FINAL REMARKS

Obviously, we merely have scratched the surface of a fascinating and critical set of developmental phenomena. First, we have seen that parents are pivotal in modeling emotional expressiveness and display rules, teaching about a variety of emotions, and reacting contingently to emotions; across the period from preschool to adolescence, these specific aspects of socialization of emotion are associated with and/or predict all aspects of emotional competence (with occasional findings of important moderation by child sex or age). Much less is known about how acquaintances, friends, and other adults socialize emotions across this period. Getting a firm grasp of the socialization of emotion within a developmental perspective (i.e., a progression from infancy to adulthood and attending to issues of context and meaning) is the next challenge for developmental scientists.

In this review, we hope as well to drive home the necessity of sharing this knowledge base with children's schools and communities, particularly with at-risk children and within our juvenile justice systems. The links being found between emotional competence and both social and academic success make this sharing of knowledge a necessity (Denham, 2005; Denham & Weissberg, 2004). We hope that our comments have set the stage for new ideas and a continued vitalization of research in this area.

REFERENCES

Ahn, H. J. (2003). *Teacher's role in the socialization of emotion in three child care centers.* Paper presented at the Society for Research in Child Development, Tampa, FL.

Arnett, J. (1989). Issues and obstacles in the training of caregivers. In J. S. Lande, S. A. Scarr, & N. Gunzenhauser (Eds.), *Caring for children* (pp. 241–255). Hillsdale, NJ: Erlbaum.

Asher, S. R., Parker, J. G., & Walker, D. L. (1996). Distinguishing friendship from acceptance: Implications for intervention and assessment. In W. M. Bukowski, A. F. Newcomb, & W. W. Hartup (Eds.), *The company they keep: Friendship in childhood and adolescence* (pp. 366–406). Cambridge, UK: Cambridge University Press.

Berlin, L. J., & Cassidy, J. (2003). Mothers' self-reported control of their preschool children's emotional expressiveness: A longitudinal study of associations with infant–mother attachment and children's emotion regulation. *Social Development, 12,* 478–495.

Bretherton, I., Fritz, J., Zahn-Waxler, C., & Ridgeway, D. (1986). Learning to talk about emotions: A functionalist perspective. *Child Development, 57*, 529–548.

Bronstein, P., Fitzgerald, M., Briones, M., Pieniadz, J., & D'Ari, A. (1993). Family emotional expressiveness as a predictor of early adolescent social and psychological adjustment. *Journal of Early Adolescence, 13*, 448–471.

Broth, M. R. (2004). Associations between mothers' negative emotionality and stress and their socialization of emotion practices: Mothers' emotional competence as resiliency or risk. *Dissertation Abstracts International: Section B: The Sciences and Engineering, 64(8-B)*, 4025.

Brown, J. R., & Dunn, J. (1992). Talk with your mother or your sibling? Developmental changes in early family conversations about feelings. *Child Development, 63*, 336–349.

Buck, R. (1991). Temperament, social skills, and the communication of emotion: A developmental-interactionist view. In D. G. Gilbert & J. J. Connolly (Eds.), *Personality, social skills, and psychopathology: An individual differences approach Perspectives on individual differences* (pp. 85–105). New York: Plenum Press.

Bugental, D. B., & Goodnow, J. J. (1998). Socialization processes. In N. Eisenberg (Ed.), *Handbook of child psychology: Social, emotional, and personality development* (3rd ed., Vol. 3, pp. 389–462). New York: Wiley.

Capatides, J. B., & Bloom, L. (1993). Underlying process in the socialization of emotion. *Advances in Infancy Research, 8*, 99–135.

Cervantes, C. A., & Callanan, M. A. (1998). Labels and explanations in mother–child emotion talk: Age and gender differentiation. *Developmental Psychology, 34*, 88–98.

Chang, L., Schwartz, D., Dodge, K. A., & McBride-Chang, C. (2003). Harsh parenting in relation to child emotion regulation and aggression. *Journal of Family Psychology, 17(4)*, 598–606.

Cole, P. M., & Dennis, T. A. (1998). Variations on a theme: Culture and the meaning of socialization practices and child competence. *Psychological Inquiry, 9*, 276–278.

Cole, P. M., & Tamang, B. L. (1996). *Cultural variations in the socialization of emotion: Observations in rural Nepal.* Paper presented at the International Society for Infant Studies, Providence, RI.

Colwell, M. J. (2001). Mother–child emotion talk, mothers' expressiveness, and mother-child relationship quality: Links with children's emotional competence. *Dissertation Abstracts International: Section B: The Sciences and Engineering, 61(7–B)*, 3877.

Cumberland-Li, A., Eisenberg, N., Champion, C., Gershoff, E., & Fabes, R. A. (2003). The relation of parental emotionality and related dispositional traits to parental expression of emotion and children's social functioning. *Motivation and Emotion, 27*, 27–56.

Cutting, A. L., & Dunn, J. (1999). Theory of mind, emotion understanding, language, and family background: Individual differences and interrelations. *Child Development, 70*, 853–865.

David-Vilker, R. J. (2000). The contribution of emotion socialization and attachment to adult emotion organization and regulation. *Dissertation Abstracts International: Section B: The Sciences and Engineering, 61(1-B)*, 561.

Demorat, M. G. (1999). Emotion socialization in the classroom context: A functionalist analysis. *Dissertation Abstracts International Section A: Humanities and Social Sciences, 60(3-A)*, 0646.

Denham, S. A. (1989). Maternal affect and toddlers' social-emotional competence. *American Journal of Orthopsychiatry, 59*, 368–376.

Denham, S. A. (1998). *Emotional development in young children.* New York: Guilford Press.

Denham, S. A. (2005). The emotional basis of learning and development in early childhood education. In B. Spodek (Ed.), *Handbook of research in early childhood education* (pp. 85–103). New York: Erlbaum.

Denham, S. A., Blair, K. A., DeMulder, E., Levitas, J., Sawyer, K. S., Auerbach-Major, S. T., et al. (2003). Preschoolers' emotional competence: Pathway to mental health? *Child Development, 74*, 238–256.

Denham, S. A., Blair, K. A., Schmidt, M. S., & DeMulder, E. (2002). Compromised emotional competence: Seeds of violence sown early? *American Journal of Orthopsychiatry, 72*, 70–82.

Denham, S. A., & Burton, R. (2003). *Social and emotional prevention and intervention programming for preschoolers.* New York: Kluwer-Plenum.

Denham, S. A., Caal, S., Bassett, H. H., Benga, O., & Geangu, E. (2004). Listening to parents: Cultural variations in the meaning of emotions and emotion socialization. *Cognitie Creier Comportament, 8*, 321–350.

Denham, S. A., Caverly, S., Schmidt, M., Blair, K., DeMulder, E., Caal, S., et al. (2002). Preschool understanding of emotions: Contributions to classroom anger and aggression. *Journal of Child Psychology and Psychiatry, 43,* 901–916.

Denham, S. A., & Grout, L. (1992). Mothers' emotional expressiveness and coping: Topography and relations with preschoolers' social-emotional competence. *Genetic, Social, and General Psychology Monographs, 118,* 75–101.

Denham, S. A., & Grout, L. (1993). Socialization of emotion: Pathway to preschoolers' affect regulation. *Journal of Nonverbal Behavior, 17,* 215–227.

Denham, S. A., & Kochanoff, A. T. (2002). Parental contributions to preschoolers' understanding of emotion. *Marriage and Family Review, 34,* 311–343.

Denham, S. A., McKinley, M., Couchoud, E. A., & Holt, R. (1990). Emotional and behavioral predictors of peer status in young preschoolers. *Child Development, 61,* 1145–1152.

Denham, S. A., Mitchell-Copeland, J., Strandberg, K., Auerbach, S., & Blair, K. (1997). Parental contributions to preschoolers' emotional competence: Direct and indirect effects. *Motivation and Emotion, 27,* 65–86.

Denham, S. A., Renwick-DeBardi, S., & Hewes, S. (1994). Emotional communication between mothers and preschoolers: Relations with emotional competence. *Merrill-Palmer Quarterly, 40*(4), 488–508.

Denham, S. A., & Weissberg, R. P. (2004). Social-emotional learning in early childhood: What we know and & where to go from here? In E. Chesebrough, P. King, T. P. Gullotta, & M. Bloom (Eds.), *A blueprint for the promotion of prosocial behavior in early childhood* (pp. 13–50). New York: Kluwer/Academic.

Denham, S. A., Zoller, D., & Couchoud, E. A. (1994). Socialization of preschoolers' emotion understanding. *Developmental Psychology, 30,* 928–936.

Dunn, J. (1994). Understanding others and the social world: Current issues in developmental research and their relation to preschool experiences and practice. *Journal of Applied Developmental Psychology, 15,* 571–583.

Dunn, J., Brown, J. R., & Beardsall, L. A. (1991). Family talk about emotions, and children's later understanding of others' emotions. *Developmental Psychology, 27,* 448–455.

Dunn, J., Brown, J. R., Slomkowski, C., Tesla, C., & Youngblade, L. (1991). Young children's understanding of other people's feelings and beliefs: Individual differences and their antecedents. *Child Development, 62,* 1352–1366.

Dunn, J., Slomkowski, C., Donelan, N., & Herrera, C. (1995). Conflict, understanding, and relationships: Developments and differences in the preschool years. *Early Education and Development, 6,* 303–316.

Eisenberg, N., Cumberland, A., & Spinrad, T. L. (1998). Parental socialization of emotion. *Psychological Inquiry, 9,* 241–273.

Eisenberg, N., Fabes, R. A., & Murphy, B. C. (1996). Parents' reactions to children's negative emotions: Relations to children's social competence and comforting behavior. *Child Development, 67,* 2227–2247.

Eisenberg, N., Fabes, R. A., Nyman, M., Bernzweig, J., & Pinuelas, A. (1994). The relation of emotionality and regulation to preschoolers' anger-related reactions. *Child Development, 65,* 1352–1366.

Eisenberg, N., Fabes, R. A., Shepard, S. A., Guthrie, I., Murphy, B. C., & Reiser, M. (1999). Parental reactions to children's negative emotions: Longitudinal relations to quality of children's social functioning. *Child Development, 70,* 513–534.

Eisenberg, N., Fabes, R. A., Shepard, S. A., Murphy, B. C., Guthrie, I. K., Jones, S., et al. (1997). Contemporaneous and longitudinal prediction of children's social functioning from regulation and emotionality. *Child Development, 68,* 642–664.

Eisenberg, N., Gershoff, E. T., Fabes, R. A., Shepard, S. A., Cumberland, A., Losoya, S., et al. (2001). Mothers' emotional expressivity and children's behavior problems and social competence: Mediation through children's regulation. *Developmental Psychology, 37,* 475–490.

Eisenberg, N., Liew, J., & Pidada, S. U. (2001). The relations of parental emotional expressivity with quality of Indonesian children's social functioning. *Emotion, 1,* 116–136.

Eisenberg, N., Losoya, S., Fabes, R. A., Guthrie, I. K., Reiser, M., Murphy, B., et al. (2001). Parental socialization of children's dysregulated expression of emotion and externalizing problems. *Journal of Family Psychology, 15,* 183–205.

Eisenberg, N., Spinrad, T. L., & Cumberland, A. (1998). The socialization of emotion: Reply to commentaries. *Psychological Inquiry, 9,* 317–333.

Eisenberg, N., Valiente, C., Morris, A. S., Fabes, R. A., Cumberland, A., Reiser, M., et al. (2003). Longitudinal relations among parental emotional expressivity, children's regulation, and quality of socioemotional functioning. *Developmental Psychology, 39,* 3–19.

Eisenberg, N., Zhou, Q., Losoya, S. H., Fabes, R. A., Shepard, S. A., Murphy, B. C., et al. (2003). The relations of parenting, effortful control, and ego control to children's emotional expressivity. *Child Development, 74*(3), 875–895.

Fabes, R. A., Leonard, S. A., Kupanoff, K., & Martin, C. L. (2001). Parental coping with children's negative emotions: Relations with children's emotional and social responding. *Child Development, 72,* 907–920.

Fabes, R. A., Poulin, R. E., Eisenberg, N., & Madden-Derdich, D. A. (2002). The Coping with Children's Negative Emotions Scale (CCNES): Psychometric properties and relations with children's emotional competence. *Marriage and Family Review, 34,* 285–310.

Field, T. (1994). The effects of mother's physical and emotional unavailability on emotion regulation. *Monographs of the Society for Research in Child Development, 59,* 250–283.

Fivush, R. (1998). Methodological challenges in the study of emotional socialization. *Psychological Inquiry, 9,* 281–283.

Fredrickson, B. L. (1998). Cultivated emotions: Parental socialization of positive emotions and self-conscious emotions. *Psychological Inquiry, 9,* 279–281.

Garner, P. W. (1996). The relations of emotional role taking, affective/moral attributions, and emotional display rule knowledge to low-income school-age children's social competence. *Journal of Applied Developmental Psychology, 17,* 19–36.

Garner, P. W. (1999). Continuity in emotion knowledge from preschool to middle-childhood and relation to emotion socialization. *Motivation and Emotion, 23,* 247–266.

Garner, P. W., & Estep, K. M. (2001). Emotional competence, emotion socialization, and young children's peer-related social competence. *Early Education and Development, 12,* 29–48.

Garner, P. W., Jones, D. C., Gaddy, G., & Rennie, K. (1997). Low income mothers' conversations about emotions and their children's emotional competence. *Social Development, 6,* 37–52.

Garner, P. W., Jones, D. C., & Miner, J. L. (1994). Social competence among low-income preschoolers: Emotion socialization practices and social cognitive correlates. *Child Development, 65,* 622–637.

Garner, P. W., Robertson, S., & Smith, G. (1997). Preschool children's emotional expressions with peers: The roles of gender and emotion socialization. *Sex Roles, 36,* 675–691.

Garner, P. W., & Spears, F. M. (2000). Emotion regulation in low-income preschoolers. *Social Development, 9,* 246–264.

Garside, R. B., & Klimes-Dougan, B. (2002). Socialization of discrete negative emotions: Gender differences and links with psychological distress. *Sex Roles, 47,* 115–128.

Gondoli, D. M., & Braungart-Rieker, J. M. (1998). Constructs and processes in parental socialization of emotions. *Psychological Inquiry, 9,* 283–285.

Gottman, J. M., Katz, L. F., & Hooven, C. (1997). *Meta-emotion: How families communicate emotionally.* Mahwah, NJ: Erlbaum.

Gottman, J. M., & Mettetal, G. (1986). Speculations about social and affective development of friendship and acquaintanceship through adolescence. In J. M. Gottman & J. Parker (Eds.), *Conversations of friends: Speculations on affective development* (pp. 192–237). New York: Cambridge University Press.

Grolnick, W. S., Kurowski, C. O., McMenamy, J. M., Rivkin, I., & Bridges, L. J. (1998). Mothers' strategies for regulating their toddlers' distress. *Infant Behavior and Development, 21,* 437–450.

Grusec, J. E. (2002). Parental socialization and children's acquisition of values. In M. H. Bornstein (Ed.), *Handbook of parenting* (2nd ed., Vol. 5, pp. 143–167). Mahwah, NJ: Erlbaum.

Halberstadt, A. G., Denham, S. A., & Dunsmore, J. (2001). Affective social competence. *Social Development, 10,* 79–119.

Halberstadt, A. G., Fox, N. A., & Jones, N. A. (1993). Do expressive mothers have expressive children? The role of socialization in children's affect expression. *Social Development, 2,* 48–65.

Hamre, B. K., & Pianta, R. C. (2001). Early teacher-child relationships and the trajectory of children's school outcomes through eighth grade. *Child Development, 72,* 625–638.

Harker, L., & Keltner, D. (2001). Expressions of positive emotion in women's college yearbook pictures and their relationship to personality and life outcomes across adulthood. *Journal of Personality and Social Psychology, 80,* 112–124.

Howes, C. (2000). Social–emotional classroom climate in child care child–teacher relationships and children's second grade peer relations. *Social Development, 9,* 191–204.

Hyson, M. C. (1994). *The emotional development of young children: Building an emotion-centered curriculum.* New York: Teachers College Press.

Isley, S. L., O'Neil, R., Clatfelter, D., & Parke, R. D. (1999). Parent and child expressed affect and children's social competence: Modeling direct and indirect pathways. *Developmental Psychology, 35*, 547–560.

Izard, C. E., Fine, S., Schultz, D., Mostow, A., Ackerman, B., & Youngstrom, E. (2001). Emotions knowledge as a predictor of social behavior and academic competence in children at risk. *Psychological Science, 12*, 18–23.

Jones, D. C., Abbey, B. B., & Cumberland, A. (1998). The development of display rule knowledge: Linkages with family expressiveness and social competence. *Child Development, 69*, 1209–1222.

Jones, D. C., & Garner, P. W. (1998). Socialization of emotion and children's emotional competence: Variations are the theme. *Psychological Inquiry, 9*, 294–296.

Jones, S., Eisenberg, N., Fabes, R. A., & MacKinnon, D. P. (2002). Parents' reactions to elementary school children's negative emotions: Relations to social and emotional functioning at school. *Merrill-Palmer Quarterly, 48*, 133–159.

Kim, K. J., Conger, R. D., Lorenz, F. O., & Elder, G. H. (2001). Parent–adolescent reciprocity in negative affect and its relation to early adult social development. *Developmental Psychology, 37*, 775–790.

Kochanoff, A. T. (2001). Parental disciplinary styles, parental elaborativeness, and attachment: Links to preschoolers' emotion knowledge. *Dissertation Abstracts International: Section B: The Sciences and Engineering, 62*(5–B), 2517.

Kopp, C. B. (1989). Regulation of distress and negative emotions: A developmental review. *Developmental Psychology, 25*, 343–354.

Krappmann, L. (1996). The development of diverse relationships in the social world of childhood. In A. E. Auhagen & M. von Salisch (Eds.), *The diversity of human relationships* (pp. 52–78). New York: Cambridge University Press.

Kuebli, J., Butler, S., & Fivush, R. (1995). Mother–child talk about past emotions: Relations of maternal language and child gender over time. *Cognition and Emotion, 9*, 265–283.

Kuebli, J., & Fivush, R. (1992). Gender differences in parent–child conversations about past emotions. *Sex Roles, 27*, 683–698.

Larson, R. W., Moneta, G., Richards, M. H., & Wilson, S. (2002). Continuity, stability, and change in daily emotional experience across adolescence. *Child Development, 73*, 1151–1165.

Maughan, A., & Cicchetti, D. (2002). Impact of child maltreatment and interadult violence on children's emotion regulation abilities and socioemotional adjustment. *Child Development, 73*, 1525–1542.

Mayer, J. B., & Beltz, C. M. (1998). Socialization, society's "emotional contract," and emotional intelligence. *Psychological Inquiry, 9*, 300–303.

McDowell, D. J., Kim, M., O'Neil, R., & Parke, R. D. (2002). Children's emotional regulation and social competence in middle childhood: The role of maternal and paternal interactive style. *Marriage and Family Review, 34*, 345–364.

Mitchell-Copeland, J., Denham, S. A., & DeMulder, E. (1997). Child–teacher attachment and social competence. *Early Education and Development, 8*, 27–39.

Murphy, B. C., Shepard, S. A., Eisenberg, N., & Fabes, R. A. (2004). Concurrent and across time prediction of young adolescents' social functioning: The role of emotionality and regulation. *Social Development, 13*, 56–86.

Nixon, C. L., & Watson, A. C. (2001). Family experiences and early emotion understanding. *Merrill-Palmer Quarterly, 47*, 300–322.

O'Neal, C. R., & Magai, C. (2005). Do parents respond in different ways when children feel different emotions? The emotional context of parenting. *Development and Psychopathology, 17*(2), 467–487.

Ontai, L. L., & Thompson, R. A. (2002). Patterns of attachment and maternal discourse effects on children's emotion understanding from 3 to 5 years of age. *Social Development, 11*, 433–450.

Parke, R. D., Cassidy, J., Burks, V. M., Carson, J. L., & Boyum, L. (1992). Familial contribution to peer competence among young children: The role of interactive and affective processes. In R. D. Parke & G. W. Ladd (Eds.), *Family–peer relationships Modes of linkage* (pp. 107–134). Hillsdale, NJ: Erlbaum.

Parke, R. D., & McDowell, D. J. (1998). Toward an expanded model of emotion socialization: New people, new pathways. *Psychological Inquiry, 9*, 303–307.

Parker, J. G., & Gottman, J. M. (1989). Social and emotional development in a relational context: Friendship interaction from early childhood to adolescence. In T. J. Berndt & G. W. Ladd (Eds.), *Peer relationships in child development* (pp. 95–131). New York: Wiley.

Pollak, S. D., & Sinha, P. (2002). Effects of early experience on children's recognition of facial displays of emotion. *Developmental Psychology, 38*, 784–791.

Pollak, S. D., & Tolley-Schell, S. A. (2003). Selective attention to facial emotion in physically abused children. *Journal of Abnormal Psychology, 112*, 323–338.

Queenan, P. L. (2000). *Gender differences in the socialization of social and emotional competence in preschool-aged children.* Unpublished dissertation, George Mason University, Fairfax, VA.

Race, E., & Brand, A. E. (2003). *Parental personality and its relationship to socialization of sadness in children.* Paper presented at the Biennial Meeting of the Society for Research in Child Development, Tampa, FL.

Raver, C. C. (2002). Emotions matter: Making the case for the role of young children's emotional development for early school readiness. *SRCD Social Policy Report, XVI*(3), 3–18.

Raver, C. C, Blackburn, E. K., & Bancroft, M. (1999). Relations between effective emotional self-regulation, attentional control, and low-income preschoolers' social competence with peers. *Early Education and Development, 10*, 333–350.

Raver, C. C., & Spagnola, M. (2002). "When my mommy was angry, I was speechless": Children's perceptions of maternal emotional expressiveness within the context of economic hardship. *Marriage and Family Review, 34*(1–2), 63–88.

Reimer, K. J. (1996). Emotion socialization and children's emotional expressiveness in the preschool context (emotional expression). *Dissertation Abstracts International, 57*(07A), 0010.

Rimé, B., Dozier, S., Vandenplas, C., & Declercq, M. (1996). *Social sharing of emotion in children.* Paper presented at the Conference of the International Society for Research on Emotions, Toronto, Canada.

Rose, A. J., & Asher, S. R. (1999). Children's goals and strategies in response to conflicts within a friendship. *Developmental Psychology, 35*, 69–70.

Rosenblum, G. D., & Lewis, M. (2003). Emotional development in adolescence. In G. R. Adams & M. D. Berzonsky (Eds.), *Blackwell handbook of adolescence* (pp. 269–289). Malden, MA: Blackwell.

Rydell, A.-M., Berlin, L., & Bohlin, G. (2003). Emotionality, emotion regulation, and adaptation among 5- to 8-year-old children. *Emotion, 3*, 30–47.

Saarni, C. (1988). Children's understanding of the interpersonal consequences of dissemblance of nonverbal emotional-expressive behavior. *Journal of Nonverbal Behavior, 12*, 275–294.

Saarni, C. (1989). Children's understanding of the strategic control of emotional expression in social transactions. In C. Saarni & P. Harris (Eds.), *Children's understanding of emotions* (pp. 181–208). Cambridge, UK: Cambridge University Press.

Saarni, C. (1999). *The development of emotional competence.* New York: Guilford Press.

Sawyer, K. S., Denham, S., DeMulder, E., Blair, K., Auerbach-Major, S., & Levitas, J. (2002). The contribution of older siblings' reactions to emotions to preschoolers' emotional and social competence. *Marriage and Family Review, 34*, 183–212.

Shields, A., & Cicchetti, D. (2001). Parental maltreatment and emotion dysregulation as risk factors for bullying and victimization in middle childhood. *Journal of Clinical Child Psychology, 30*, 349–363.

Siegel, H. I. (1997). Emotion socialization and affect regulation in children with attention deficit hyperactivity disorder. *Dissertation Abstracts International: Section B: The Sciences and Engineering, 57*(9-B), 5932.

Smith, M., & Walden, T. (1999). Understanding feelings and coping with emotional situations: A comparison of maltreated and nonmaltreated preschoolers. *Social Development, 8*, 93–116.

Snyder, J., Stoolmiller, M., Wilson, M., & Yamamoto, M. (2003). Child anger regulation, parental responses to children's anger displays, and early child antisocial behavior. *Social Development, 12*, 335–360.

Sorber, A. V. (2001). The role of peer socialization in the development of emotion display rules: Effects of age, gender, and emotion. *Dissertation Abstracts International, 62*(02B), 1119.

Thompson, R. A. (1991). Emotional regulation and emotional development. *Educational Psychology Review, 3*, 269–307.

Valiente, C., Eisenberg, N., Shepard, S. A., Fabes, R. A., Cumberland, A. J., Losoya, S. H., et al. (2004). The relations of mothers' negative expressivity to children's experience and expression of negative emotion. *Journal of Applied Developmental Psychology, 25*(2), 215–235.

Valiente, C., Fabes, R. A., Eisenberg, N., & Spinrad, T. L. (2004). The relations of parental expressivity and support to children's coping with daily stress. *Journal of Family Psychology, 18*(1), 97–106.

Weiss, B., Dodge, K. A., Bates, J. E., & Pettit, G. S. (1992). Some consequences of early harsh discipline: Child aggression and a maladaptive social information processing style. *Child Development, 63*, 1321–1335.

Winsler, A., Diaz, R. M., Atencio, D. J., McCarthy, E. M., & Chabay, L. A. (2000). Verbal self-regulation over time in preschool children at risk for attention and behavior problems. *Journal of Child Psychology and Psychiatry, 41,* 875–886.

Zahn-Waxler, C., Klimes-Dougan, B., & Kendziora, K. T. (1998). The study of emotion socialization: Conceptual, methodological, and developmental considerations. *Psychological Inquiry, 9,* 313–316.

Zeman, J., & Shipman, K. (1997). Social-contextual influences on expectancies for managing anger and sadness: The transition from middle childhood to adolescence. *Developmental Psychology, 33,* 917–924.

CHAPTER 25

The Socialization
of Prosocial Development

Paul D. Hastings, William T. Utendale, and Caroline Sullivan

What prompts a toddler to offer his toy to a crying infant? Why does a preschooler invite a reluctant and withdrawn peer to join her circle of playmates? How does a schoolgirl pull herself away from a fun activity to comfort a classmate who has fallen and injured herself? What motivates a teenage boy to volunteer for an organization that delivers meals to shut-ins?

Kind, caring, compassionate attitudes and helpful, comforting, altruistic behaviors characterize what are considered by many to be the finest qualities of human nature. They are also often overlooked, as another class of behaviors tends to capture the attention of media: Aggression, violence, crime, delinquency, and other selfish acts that harm and violate the rights of others. Social scientists have also given far more attention to antisocial and other problematic behaviors than to prosocial and other positive behaviors, as can be seen in many of the chapters of this Handbook. Yet, this negative side of behavior is only one facet of the complex and varied scope of what it is to be human. To fully understand the dynamic regulation of emotional, behavioral, social, and cultural processes, the more positive aspects of behavior cannot be ignored. Therefore, this chapter draws attention to that smaller, yet still substantial, literature that focuses on the positive: the socialization of prosocial development.

We begin by briefly reviewing biological and environmental perspectives on the origins of the emotions and behaviors comprising prosocial development and the early experimental approaches to demonstrating how children's prosocial behavior could be shaped through adults' actions. We then evaluate the roles of various agents of socialization, including parents, siblings, peers, teachers, community and culture, in the development of prosocial characteristics. We conclude by addressing four central questions: What aspects of socialization influence prosocial development? How do children contribute to their prosocial development? Why are there sex differences in prosocial development? Does the socialization of prosocial development have implications for understanding antisocial behavior?

THE ROOTS OF PROSOCIAL DEVELOPMENT

Prosocial behavior is defined herein as proactive and reactive responses to the needs of others that serve to promote the well-being of others. This definition casts a fairly wide net, and admittedly, one that is not strictly limited to "behavior." A range of affective and behavioral elements comprise the scope of prosocial development (Radke-Yarrow, Zahn-Waxler, & Chapman, 1983), including empathy, sympathy, compassion, concern, comforting, helping, sharing, cooperating, volunteering, and donating. Indices of social competence are specifically excluded from this definition, including leadership qualities, popularity, sociability, and similar constructs. Early prosocial behavior may facilitate the development of social competence, as we consider while examining the research on peers, but the two are not redundant constructs.

The strictest definition of altruism is sacrificing one's own gain in order to promote another's well-being. Prosocial behavior toward others does not necessarily require self-sacrifice, of course; it can also benefit the actor, or come with neither cost nor gain. The motivations for prosocial behavior are similarly diverse, as the actor may expect rewards or reciprocity, may fear repercussions for not being prosocial, or may only want to alleviate another's distress. Displays of concern for others may occur in the form of proactive efforts to prevent another coming to harm, spontaneous reactions to witnessed events, reparative actions after having been the cause of some distress to another, or compliant responses to directives or solicitations for assistance. These motivations and manifestations may comprise important distinctions for understanding prosocial behavior, but relatively little socialization research has addressed this issue.

Evolutionary theory would hold that prosocial behavior has been retained in humans because it has proven to be advantageous and supported survival. However, traditional evolutionary theory usually depicts living beings as essentially individualistic, competitive, and selfish, and altruism has often been disregarded as evolutionarily untenable (Dawkins, 1976). In response, several sociobiologists have constructed models for how selfless other-oriented behaviors can improve genetic survival, through social reinforcement of altruism (Sober & Wilson, 1998). Psychophysiologists have shown that biological processes provide a basis for empathy and behaviors that aid others, providing further support for a genetic predisposition for prosocial behavior (Hastings, Zahn-Waxler, & McShane, 2005; Preston & de Waal, 2002).

Psychoevolutionary theory requires the potential for genetic transmission of affective, cognitive, and behavioral characteristics. Behavior genetics analyses have shown that heritable, genetic influences strongly contribute to prosocial characteristics (see Hastings, Zahn-Waxler, & McShane, 2005). Both genetic and shared environmental influences make significant contributions to children's prosocial behaviors (Deater-Deckard, Dunn, O'Connor, Davies, & Golding, 2001; Scourfield, John, Martin, & McGuffin, 2004; Stevenson, 1997; Zahn-Waxler, Robinson, & Emde, 1992), and to the stability of prosocial behaviors from infancy to the preschool years (Zahn-Waxler, Schiro, Robinson, Emde, & Schmitz, 2001). Thus, both sociobiological theories and behavior genetics research confirm a place for socialization in the development of prosocial behavior.

Psychoevolutionary theory also underlies the functional theory of emotions. From this perspective, the affective root of actions that help others is empathy: the emotional capacity to apprehend the affective states of others, and to some extent share in their affective experiences. Empathy serves to motivate affiliative and caregiving actions that build social and emotional bonds with conspecifics, including offspring, family members, mates, and social group members. There is reasonably strong evidence for this link between the affective and behavior components of prosocial development (Eisenberg & Miller, 1987).

Empathy has long been posited as providing both the foundation for prosocial development and the mechanism for social influence over behavior. Many theoretical frameworks for understanding the ontogeny, socialization, and development of empathy and prosocial behavior put a primary emphasis on parents, including psychoanalytic theory, social learning theory, and social cognition theory (Eisenberg & Valiente, 2002; Grusec, Davidov, & Lundell, 2002). Perhaps the most thorough theoretical account has been provided by Hoffman (1970, 2000). Parents' management of disciplinary interactions using nonpunitive techniques that deemphasized firm parental control in favor of inductive reasoning, and particularly other-oriented reasoning focused on the needs of others, were seen as conducive to prosocial development. Moderately aroused, the child would orient on the parent but not be overwhelmed by the fear or anger that punitive control might elicit, so that the child could more effectively attend to the parent's socialization message. Alternative means of control, through emotional manipulations such as disapproval and love withdrawal, were not thought to be as strongly associated with internalization of prosocial values, although others have suggested these might promote reparative prosocial acts after transgressions by eliciting guilt (Zahn-Waxler & Kochanska, 1990). Many developmental researchers, including Zahn-Waxler and Radke-Yarrow, Eisenberg, and Grusec evaluated and extended the tenets of Hoffman's theory through the 1970s and 1980s. Increased recognition of the child's active role in socialization clarified some of the processes by which parenting might shape prosocial development. For example, inductive reasoning requires the child to actively reflect on and process the meaning of the parent's statements, which could increase the likelihood of the child's internalization of the message (Grusec & Goodnow, 1994).

The developmental forces of biology and environment do not work independently of each other, and children's actions and reactions are both shaped by and, in turn, shape the environment (Bell, 1968; Patterson, 1982; Sameroff, 1975). Individuals are born with varying dispositional propensities or capacities to feel empathy and engage in other-oriented caring actions. Parents and other agents of socialization respond to individual differences in the early-emerging emotional and social tendencies of infants and toddlers, tailoring their own actions in ways that foster or redirect dispositional traits. In turn, different children vary in their responsiveness to a given socialization event. The socialization of prosocial development progresses through the ongoing and dynamic exchanges between children and their parents, siblings, peers, teachers, and culture. This give-and-take nature of social influence underlies the complex processes shaping social and emotional development (see Kuczynski, 2003).

The Development of Prosocial Characteristics

Most analyses of prosocial characteristics indicate that they increase with age, with fairly rapid increases in the maturity and frequency of prosocial behavior in the toddler and preschooler period, and slower but continued increases thereafter, at least into early adulthood (Eisenberg & Fabes, 1998; Pratt, Skoe, & Arnold, 2004). Some research suggests that the early course of development for specific prosocial behaviors such as sharing or helping may be more complex (Hay, Castle, Davies, Demitrou, & Stimson, 1999; van der Mark, van IJzendoorn, & Bakermans-Kranenburg, 2002), but overall the general pattern is one of increasing development over at least the first two decades of life.

Evidence for the stability of individual differences in prosocial characteristics in infancy and toddlerhood is mixed (Dunn & Munn, 1986; Hay et al., 1999; Pepler, Abramovitch, & Corter, 1981; Zahn-Waxler, Radke-Yarrow, Wagner, & Chapman, 1992), but most studies of preschoolers and older children find low to moderate stability over 2 or more years. For example, there is modest stability in elementary school-age children's observed and reported empathic responses (Zhou et al., 2002), adolescents' prosocial behavior toward peers (Wentzel, Barry, & Caldwell, 2004), and young adults' valuing of concern for others (Pratt et al., 2004).

Gender and Development

Gender is one of the most consistent correlates of prosocial behavior. Across many studies, girls and women have been found to be more prosocial than boys and men. For example, peers and teachers have been found to describe preschool-age, kindergarten-age, and elementary school-age girls as more prosocial than boys (Côté, Tremblay, Nagin, Zoccolillo, & Vitaro, 2002; Hastings, Zahn-Waxler, Robinson, Usher, & Bridges, 2000; Keane & Calkins, 2004; Russell, Hart, Robinson, & Olsen, 2003). However, compared to questionnaire reports, observational techniques tend to provide less consistent evidence of sex differences in prosocial characteristics (Eisenberg & Fabes, 1998; Grusec, Goodnow, & Cohen, 1996; Hastings, Rubin, & DeRose, 2005; Zhou et al., 2002). Thus, apparent sex differences in the frequency of showing concern for others may be as much a function of perception as reality: a culturally shared belief that girls are made of "everything nice." We consider the links between gender, socialization, and prosocial behavior after reviewing the evidence.

THE EARLY RESEARCH: EXPERIMENTAL STUDIES OF PROSOCIAL BEHAVIOR

Early developmental research on the socialization of children's prosocial behavior was based in social learning theory and used laboratory experiments to test whether adults' actions could induce changes in children's prosocial behavior. Through the 1970s, experimental studies (e.g., Grusec, 1972; Harris, 1970; Yarrow & Scott, 1972) showed that children who saw an adult donate prize winnings to charity, or even simply saw adult models speak about the value of giving, were themselves more likely to give away their prizes after winning a game, compared to children who had not witnessed a generous model. Researchers investigated further to examine the nature of these learning effects. Children were more likely to emulate the generous behavior of a competent than an unskilled model (Eisenberg-Berg & Geisheker, 1979), or of a model who was warm and familiar rather than distant and unfamiliar (Yarrow, Scott, & Waxler, 1973).

The message as well as the messenger was determined to be important. Normative statements, such as "It is good to give" proved less effective than empathic or other-oriented inductions, such as "Those poor children will be so happy" (Perry, Bussy, & Frieberg, 1981). Children were more prosocial when inductions suggested positive affective results for the recipients ("They'll be happy if you do . . . ") rather than negative ("They'll be sad if you don't . . .") (McGrath, Wilson, & Frassetto, 1995). From social cognitive theory, researchers also examined influences of causal attributions, finding that children were more prosocial when their actions were ascribed to internal motivations or characteristics than when they were attributable to external pressures or rewards (Fabes, Fultz, Eisenberg, May-Plumlee, & Christopher, 1989). The effects of inductions and attributions were shown to persist across contexts and time, with children who had witnessed a generous model being more generous days or weeks later, especially when the model made dispositional attributions for her behavior (Grusec, Kuczynski, Rushton, & Simutis, 1978; Rushton, 1975).

Thus, these studies provided evidence for internalization, or lasting effects of socialization, from brief learning experiences. Manipulating social contingencies could change children's prosocial behavior. But the effects were not universal. Children varied in the amount of prosocial behavior elicited, and a minority of children were not at all responsive to models, inductions, or attributions. Thus, not all children respond to and learn from a given socialization response equally. Outcome measures were somewhat limited, with researchers focusing on quantifiable behaviors such as donating and helping, and rarely considering impacts on the affective aspects of being prosocial. Finally, despite careful attention to design, most experiments included an element that limited their ecological validity: the models themselves. Children's reactions to unfamiliar adults in unfamiliar settings comprise a dubious basis for making clear inferences about socialization. Unfamiliar adults are not socialization agents in the everyday experiences of children, and how children respond to them may not generalize to how children react to familiar others— parents, siblings, peers, and teachers—with whom they share a relationship history.

For these and other reasons, tightly controlled laboratory experiments seemed to have fallen out of favor by the late 1980s. Having shown that adults' actions *can* cause most children to behave more or less prosocially, most researchers turned their focus to whether adults truly *do* have such influence in the real world. In particular, the question of parental influence over their own children's prosocial development became paramount.

FROM CAUSATION TO CORRELATION: A METHODOLOGICAL NOTE

The majority of efforts to study the associations between parental socialization and children's prosocial behavior have used correlational, single time-point designs. These have at least three inherent limitations. It is not possible to (1) infer cause-and-effect relations, or distinguish parent influences on children from child influences on parents; (2) deduce the history of developmental and relationship processes that led the parent and child measures to be related in the ways that they were; or (3) infer if any lasting influences of socialization on prosocial behavior would be evident in the future.

These valid critiques might lead one to assume that, as a field, we are unable to draw firm conclusions about the socialization of prosocial behavior. But the picture is not quite that bleak. Longitudinal research on the socialization of prosocial development has been going on for over three decades. Statistical advances have improved researchers' abilities to chart development and to rule out alternative explanations for relations between variables. The balance of this chapter is devoted to reviewing these investigations. Nonlongitudinal, correlational studies that do not consider mediating or moderating processes are only examined closely when other sources of insight are lacking. The focus is on extending our understanding of the relations between socialization agents, actions, and events and the development of prosocial characteristics by closely examining excellent research. This effort begins with research on parents as agents of socialization, where the bulk of the work on prosocial development has been focused. Research on the influence of siblings, peers, and teachers on prosocial development is then considered, followed by an examination of sociocultural and socioeconomic influences.

PARENTAL SOCIALIZATION OF PROSOCIAL DEVELOPMENT

Based primarily on correlational, single time-point studies, recent reviews have generally agreed on a consistent profile of childrearing that typifies the socialization experiences of more prosocial children (e.g., Eisenberg & Fabes, 1998; Grusec et al., 2002). Their parents are authoritative in style, balancing reasonable exertions of control and consistent expectations for maturity with flexibility and responsiveness to children's desires. These parents eschew harsh punishments, rigid strictness, and strong expressions of hostility or rejection. They are warm toward their children, enjoy shared activities, and provide praise more than criticism. They engage in prosocial acts themselves, encourage such behavior from their children, and provide explanations for these expected behaviors. But do such socialization experiences actually foster the further development of children's prosocial characteristics?

Parenting Styles

The dominant paradigm for studying parental socialization in the last 25 years of the 20th century was through the examination of parenting styles, or the usual patterns of control, responsiveness, warmth, and punishment that parents use most often, across contexts and over time, to manage their children's behavior. Authoritative parenting could support prosocial behavior by modeling other-oriented behavior that children may emulate, encouraging children to be more considerate and caring, and eliciting affection and connectedness that make children more receptive to efforts to foster concern for others (Hastings et al., 2000). An authoritarian style of parenting may undermine children's prosocial behavior by modeling a lack of concern for the needs of others, or engendering hostility and the rejection of parental socialization efforts.

Longitudinal studies support the suggestion that parenting styles foster children's prosocial development over time, but not always in the straightforward manner researchers have expected. In one study, mothers who were more authoritative and less authoritarian with preschoolers had children who showed more observed, mother-reported and teacher-reported prosocial behavior 2 years later (Hastings et al., 2000). Effects were evident when children's earlier prosocial behavior was controlled, suggesting maternal style contributed to prosocial development over and above the stability of children's behavior. In a study predicting prosocial behavior at 4 years from mother and child characteristics at 2 years, children were observed interacting with a researcher and their mother on one day and with peers but without their mother present on another day. Earlier maternal authoritative style predicted more prosocial responses to a researcher for girls who had been less inhibited toddlers (Hastings, Rubin, & DeRose, 2005). For girls who had been more inhibited, early maternal authoritarianism predicted more prosocial responses to the researcher but fewer prosocial responses to peers (Hastings, Rubin, Mielcarek, & Kennedy, 2002). These results could suggest that authoritative parenting supports autonomous prosocial behavior in girls who are dispositionally comfortable in challenging social circumstances, whereas authoritarian parenting induces more compliant prosocial behavior in dispositionally reticent girls. Low prosocial behavior in the peer context indicates that inhibited girls could not enact such behaviors spontaneously, without maternal direction or support.

Kochanska (1991) found that mothers' authoritative style with toddlers predicted children's reports of making reparative actions after causing harm in a story-completion task, particularly for children who had been more inhibited or anxious as toddlers. It is possible that the difference in results across her study and that of Hastings, Rubin, and DeRose (2005) was because Kochanska focused on what children said they would do in challenging situations, whereas the other study observed children's actual responses to distress in others. Anxious children may internalize standards from authoritative parents and be aware of appropriate prosocial behavior but then be unable to act on this knowledge under socially challenging conditions.

In a study of the contributions of parenting styles to adolescents' prosocial development, youths perceived that the extent to which they and their parents valued being kind, caring, and fair corresponded more closely when they saw their parents as more authoritative (Pratt, Hunsberger, Pancer, & Alisat, 2003). This harkens to the argument of Grusec and Goodnow (1994) that central to effective internalization is the parent's generation of a relationship in which the child is likely to be receptive to the parent's socialization message. It also suggests, though, that authoritative parents must themselves hold prosocial values, or subscribe to an "ethic of care," in order for their children to internalize such an orientation. Authoritative parenting and parental emphasis on caring for others has also predicted more mature values of caring for others over 4 years (Pratt et al., 2004). In turn, young adults' caring values were associated with their engagement in voluntary, other-oriented community activities.

These analyses indicate that parenting styles make lasting contributions to prosocial development, in accord with hypothesized processes of internalization of parental expectations and societal values (Grusec, Goodnow, & Kuczynski, 2000). However, socialization research on these broad parenting styles has its limits. Specific parenting actions vary widely across contexts and depend on parents' goals (Hastings & Grusec, 1998; Grusec & Kuczynski, 1980). A given parent will not always behave in ways that match with a single defined style (Grusec & Goodnow, 1994). Parenting styles are complex and multifaceted, and measures often combine parenting behaviors with parental attitudes and emotions, such that it can be difficult to infer the likely processes or mechanisms that explain associations between parenting styles and child outcomes. A parenting style may be seen as providing the general context of the parent–child relationship, whereas specific parenting practices convey the means by which parents socialize desired outcomes (Darling & Steinberg, 1993).

Specific Aspects of Parenting Behavior

Many researchers have examined specific features of parental socialization practices in relation to children's prosocial development. These include control and discipline, induction and reasoning, warmth and sensitivity, modeling, and emotion socialization. It has been argued that the meaning and effects of specific socialization practices cannot be understood without attending to a range of contextual and process variables that shape parent–child interactions (Grusec & Davidov, Chapter 11, this volume). For example, the goal underlying a parent's exertion of control, the child's perception of the legitimacy of that control, and the domain or activity that the parent is trying to control, will all contribute to the outcomes of the parent's efforts. Such a nuanced approach to examining the socialization of prosocial behavior has rarely been pursued. Despite this, some consistent associations between specific practices and prosocial development can be discerned from the research that has been completed.

Control and Discipline

Researchers have examined aspects of parental control to determine which appear to foster, or to undermine, prosocial development. Recently, a distinction has been drawn between actions that exert behavioral versus psychological control (Barber, Olsen, & Shagle, 1994). Behavioral control encompasses the "rules and consequences" at the traditional core of parents' management of children's behavior, including regulations, directives, supervision, nonphysical punishment (e.g., withdrawal of privileges), and corporal punishment. Psychological control reflects parents' attempts to regulate their children's behavior by manipulating their emotions, thereby undermining their independence, self-esteem, and security with the parent–child relationship. It can include intrusive micromanagement or overprotective restrictions on activities and also criticism, derision, and rejection of the child (Rubin, Burgess, & Hastings, 2002).

BEHAVIORAL CONTROL

Parents' use of control is associated with the socialization goals they hold for their children (Hastings & Grusec, 1998). Parents who value compliance and want to attain obedience use stricter control, forcefully asserting their authority. Parents' valuing and reinforcement of toddlers' compliant behavior predicted decreased prosocial behavior during peer interactions 2 to 3 years later (Eisenberg, Wolchik, Goldberg, & Engel, 1992). Mothers' simple prohibitions (e.g., "Stop that.") in response to toddlers' aggression predicted less spontaneous assistance toward others 5 months later (Zahn-Waxler, Radke-Yarrow, & King, 1979). However, gentle encouragement of toddlers' prosocial actions, through less controlling means such as suggestions and questions, did not predict prosocial behavior 5 months (Zahn-Waxler et al., 1979) or 3 years later (Iannotti, Cummings, Pierrehumbert, Milano, & Zahn-Waxler, 1992). Thus, strictly controlling actions may act against young children's prosocial development, but parenting that suggests appropriate behaviors while allowing a child to have control over his or her exact course of action does not.

Other works suggest that providing structure, standards, and supervision is important, however. Male youths who described their parents as having clear rules and high expectations reported that being kind and fair to others were important qualities 2 years later (Pratt et al., 2003). Adolescents who reported that their parents closely monitored their activities subsequently were more likely to engage in volunteer community work (Zaff, Moore, Papillo, & Williams, 2003). Establishing routine household chores that benefit other family members also appears to support youths' spontaneous helpfulness, particularly for girls (Grusec et al., 1996), although this has not been tested in longitudinal research.

Punishment has often been found to be negatively correlated with children's prosocial characteristics (Krevans & Gibbs, 1996; Laible, Carlo, Torquati, & Ontai, 2004; Roberts, 1999). In a twin study of prosocial behavior that included parenting measures, Deater-Deckard and colleagues (2001) found that most of the significant negative relation between angry punishment, or "harsh parenting," and children's prosocial behavior was accounted for by shared environmental factors; genetic factors made negligible contributions to this relation. This supports the contention that angry, punitive parenting contributes to children's lowered prosocial behavior (see Moffitt & Caspi, Chapter 4, this volume), and not the potential counterargument that other dispositional child characteristics act to both elicit punishment and decrease prosocial tendencies.

There are many ways in which punishment can be exercised. One aspect of punishment that has been looked at specifically is corporal punishment, or physical discipline. Eisenberg, Lennon and Roth (1983) found that mothers' corporal punishment was negatively correlated with preschoolers' empathy toward story characters. Ani and Grantham-McGregor (1998) found that highly prosocial boys in Nigeria received less physical punishment than highly antisocial boys; the two groups of boys did not differ in other aspects of parental discipline. In a retrospective report, college-age adults' reported receipt of mild physical punishment was uniquely associated with lower empathy, after controlling for parents' use of more severe physical punishment, critical psychological control, nonaggressive discipline, and induction (Lopez, Bonenberger, & Schneider, 2001). Roe (1980) found that more empathic 6–7-year-old children reported less physical punishment from parents, particularly fathers, 3 years later. In one study that broke with this pattern, Zahn-Waxler and colleagues (1979) did not find that mothers' physical restraint and punishment predicted toddlers' prosocial behavior 5 months later.

Thus, most studies suggest physical discipline does not support prosocial development. Although some parents believe physical discipline promotes good behavior (Holden, Miller, & Harris, 1999), it may undermine prosocial behavior by implying that hurting others is acceptable, modeling aggression as a means of attaining goals, and instilling fear or anger that diminishes a child's receptivity to socialization efforts aimed at encouraging prosocial behavior. Without longitudinal studies, however, direction of effect remains a question. Less prosocial children might engage in more undesirable behaviors that elicit more punishment from parents, or they may elicit fewer feelings of warmth and closeness from parents, such that their physically punitive actions are less likely to be inhibited. Future research will need to address these issues.

Overall, some longitudinal studies have shown that the actions comprising behavioral control may undermine prosocial development, whereas other studies have suggested that such parenting may support prosocial development. The difference may lie in the specific ways in which parents manifest behavioral control. Studies of structuring and demands for mature or competent behavior generally showed positive relations, whereas studies of strict or rigid rules and punishment generally showed negative relations. Akin to the inference that might be drawn from the studies of authoritative and authoritarian styles, therefore, the effects of parents' behavioral control on children's prosocial development would appear to depend on how parents choose to express that control. More investigations that carefully distinguish between these aspects of behavioral control and take into account the context or "domain appropriateness" of parental control (Grusec & Davidov, Chapter 11, this volume) are needed to evaluate this possibility.

PSYCHOLOGICAL CONTROL

The longitudinal investigations of parents' psychological control have generally shown that it does not support children's prosocial development, although results have been somewhat mixed. Mothers who were more intrusive and directed more negative affect toward their 14-month-old infants had children who showed decreasing empathy over 6 months (Robinson, Zahn-Waxler, & Emde, 1994). Mothers' disappointment, anger, and criticism with preschoolers predicted less empathy and prosocial behavior in mother reports 2 years later but not in observed responsiveness or in child or teacher reports (Hastings et al., 2000). Parents' lack of support for adolescents' autonomy also predicted lower concern for the welfare of others over 4 years, although this relation was weakened when the stability in youths' concerns were controlled (Pratt et al., 2004). However, Zahn-Waxler and colleagues (1979) did not find relations between maternal love withdrawal and toddlers' behavior toward others over 5 months, and Hastings, Rubin, and DeRose (2005) found that mothers' intrusive overprotection of toddlers predicted more prosocial responses to mothers 2 years later but not to an unfamiliar researcher.

Overall, psychological control appears to act against children's prosocial development, although the specific associations may depend on how that control is manifest. Just as behavioral control seems to have facets that support prosocial behavior (structure and maturity demands) and others that do not (rigidity and punishment), so too might psychological control. Protective overcontrol might promote the development of particularly close ties between mothers and young children. This could point toward a mechanism by which overprotective parenting is reinforced: Seeing their children being warm and caring toward them, mothers may believe they are fostering good developmental outcomes. Children's competent and autonomous behavior in other relationships is diminished, however (Rubin et al. 2002), such that they might be less prosocial in their interactions with peers and others outside the home. Critical overcontrol by parents through rejecting, demeaning, or domineering actions may show a model of low regard for others' feelings, decrease children's confidence in the dependability of parental nurturance, and engender resentment that could undermine empathy across relationships.

Induction and Reasoning

Parents use inductive reasoning to inform children of norms and principles, to explain why rules are necessary, to highlight the needs or well-being of others, and to illuminate the effects of children's actions. Parents' other-oriented inductions could promote children's prosocial behavior through both cognitive and affective mechanisms. Being told the needs of another person could clarify a child's understanding of another's state. Especially for infants and very young children characterized by egocentrism and limited perspective-taking abilities, this may give necessary support for children's ability to identify others' distress and be aware of when their help could be effective. As inductions may clarify cause-and-effect relations, such as the adverse effects of hurtful acts, children may also increase in their understanding of their own agency, responsibility to avoid harm, and ability to make reparations.

Although experiments have shown that other-oriented inductions are effective for eliciting prosocial behavior in children, studies of parental socialization have offered little support for the superiority of other-oriented inductions over other kinds of inductive reasoning. That may be due to the relative infrequency of other-oriented inductions in naturally occurring observations (Grusec, 1991). Thus, there are statistical limitations on researchers' ability to analyze the distinct effects of other-oriented inductions. However, causal modeling has supported Hoffman's (1970) hypothesized role for empathy as the mechanism linking parents' use of reasoning and children's prosocial behavior (Janssens & Gerris, 1992; Krevans & Gibbs, 1996).

One longitudinal study has supported the role of reasoning in prosocial development. Mothers' statements of principles against causing harm predicted toddlers' reparative actions after transgressions 5 months later, and inductions delivered with a strong emotional valence predicted their spontaneous helpfulness (Zahn-Waxler et al., 1979). Expressing strong emotion may orient children's attention upon parents, such that the children are more likely to attend to the socializing message being delivered (Grusec & Lytton, 1988), although this might depend on the affective valence and contextual appropriateness of parents' emotional expressions. More longitudinal studies will be necessary to properly evaluate the developmental effects of reasoning and its modes of delivery. Including assessments of children's affective and social cognitive functioning could assist with understanding children's active part in the internalization process.

Modeling

Parents may foster children's prosocial behavior by modeling concern for the needs of others through such activities as engaging in volunteer work or being caring and helpful toward others experiencing distress. The research associating parents' volunteer work, political activism, or selfless activities to their children's prosocial development is mostly correlational and often retrospective. Limited longitudinal research exists on modeling of prosocial behavior. Mothers' responsive caregiving to their toddlers' experiences of risk or distress predicted children's sympathy and helpfulness 5 months later, but maternal empathic concern toward others did not predict prosocial behavior over 5 months (Zahn-Waxler et al., 1979) or 3 years (Iannotti et al., 1992). Eisenberg and her colleagues have shown that mothers' emotional reactions to evocative stimuli are correlated with children's prosocial characteristics, but a longitudinal study over the elementary school-age years did not find that mothers' empathic expressiveness to evocative pictures predicted children's later empathic responses to the pictures (Zhou et al., 2002).

Thus, longitudinal studies have yet to produce clear evidence for the efficacy of parental modeling of prosocial behavior supporting children's prosocial development. Zahn-Waxler's research suggests that being the recipient of maternal prosocial actions, rather than merely witnessing mothers' kindness to others, may be necessary for young children to internalize prosocial patterns of responding, pointing to the potential roles of sensitivity and warmth.

Sensitivity, Warmth, and Attachment

Maternal sensitivity to children's distress cues and emotional needs generally is thought to facilitate children's prosocial development. Robinson, Zahn-Waxler, and colleagues (Robinson & Little, 1994; Robinson, Zahn-Waxler, & Emde, 1994; Zahn-Waxler & Radke-Yarrow, 1990; Zahn-Waxler et al., 1979) have often found that maternal sensitivity predicts infants' and young children's early empathic development; only one longitudinal study has not found this pattern (van der Mark et al., 2002). In a study of low-income first-time mothers, mothers' sensitivity with infants at 12 and 15 months predicted more prosocial responses to mothers' distress simulations at 21 and 24 months (Kiang, Moreno, & Robinson, 2004). Maternal sensitivity also mediated a negative relation between mothers' negative expectations about being a parent, assessed prenatally, and children's prosocial responses, indicating sensitivity can protect against the adverse effects of negative parenting attitudes. Sensitive parenting addresses an array of infant needs, soothes distress, and fosters safety and comfort. Thus, it may both support the development of early emotional self-regulation and serve as a model for compassionate other-oriented behavior.

Many correlational studies have linked parental warmth or affection with children's prosocial characteristics (e.g., Clark & Ladd, 2000; Laible et al., 2004), although there are exceptions (e.g., Davidov & Grusec, 2006). Statistical modeling has shown that mothers' warmth directly predicts prosocial behavior when controlling for children's empathy (Janssens & Gerris, 1992). However, the evidence that parental warmth influences children's prosocial development from longitudinal studies is quite mixed. Maternal warmth toward 14-month-old infants predicted increasing, or stably high, empathy over 6 months, especially in girls (Robinson et al., 1994). Maternal warmth toward toddlers did not predict children's empathy or prosocial behavior at 5 years (Iannotti et al., 1992), nor did maternal warmth toward school-age children predict children's empathic responsiveness 2 years later (Zhou et al., 2002). Conversely, youths' perceptions of their parents' close and warm involvement in their lives has predicted higher rates of engaging in voluntary community work in early adulthood (Zaff et al., 2003).

The argument has been made that parental warmth serves distinct developmental needs that would not affect prosocial development (Grusec & Davidov, Chapter 11, this volume). Most studies documenting positive relations between maternal warmth and prosocial behavior did not control for other aspects of behavior, such as sensitivity, so there could be other socializing actions that covary with warmth but carry the specific influences on prosocial development. Alternatively, comparing the longitudinal studies that did versus did not find that warmth predicted prosocial development, it may be that brief observations of affection during parent–child interactions are not adequate for assessing the role of warmth in supporting prosocial development. Rather than being a parent characteristic, warmth might be more effectively treated as a relationship quality.

Children may need to both receive and perceive warmth from parents as an ongoing component of their shared lives together in order for it to support their internalization of prosocial norms.

Parents who are sensitive and responsive to their infants' signs of distress and provide a safe and secure caregiving context facilitate the formation of secure attachment relationships. When parents are insensitive, either unresponsive or inconsistently responsive to their infants' needs, infants are likely to form insecure attachments that lack trust and warm reciprocity. The quality of an attachment relationship may provide a history that gives meaning to present parent–child exchanges and shapes partners' expectations for future interactions. Infants' experiences of sensitivity, relief from distress, and reliable responses from parents may support their readiness to engage with and respond to the needs of others. Most studies of the links between the security of infants' or toddlers' attachment relationships with their parents and the children's prosocial behavior have shown that early attachment security predicts stronger prosocial development.

Infants with secure attachment between 12 and 18 months have been found to be more sympathetic and helpful towards distressed peers at 3½ years (Waters, Wippman, & Sroufe, 1979) and at 4 years (Kestenbaum, Farber, & Sroufe, 1989), compared to infants with insecure attachments. Iannotti and colleagues (1992) found that more securely attached toddlers were more prosocial toward peers 3 years later, and attachment security was a more robust predictor of peer-directed prosocial behavior than independent measures of maternal behavior. In one exception to this pattern, van der Mark and colleagues (2002) did not find that attachment security at 16 months predicted empathic concern 6 months later, although attachment security and empathic concern were positively correlated at 22 months.

Attachment theorists posit that the mechanism for secure attachment relationships supporting prosocial development is through internal working models of attachment relationships (Mikulciner & Shaver, 2005). Children's internalization of secure relationship qualities may provide a basis for their empathic engagement with others and preparedness to act on the behalf of others. A secure attachment relationship has also been posited as providing support for children's development of emotion regulation, through the repeated experience of effective soothing from caregivers (Cassidy, 1994). Children with secure attachment histories may become less upset when they see someone else experiencing distress, such that they are able to empathize with that person's plight and offer assistance rather than become distressed and withdraw. Sensitivity toward infants' cues and needs may be the essential quality of parenting by which secure attachment is fostered, although warmth may also have a contributing role.

Emotion Socialization

An increasing amount of attention has been given to parents' socialization of children's emotional development in recent years. Emotion socialization involves fostering children's understanding of their own and others' emotional experiences and children's ability to effectively regulate emotions. Although longitudinal research is lacking, several researchers have found that parents who effectively support their children's competent emotional functioning have children who are more empathic, sympathetic, helpful, and kind. Maternal explanations and discussions about emotions, openness to and encouragement of emotional expressivity, but limit-setting on emotions that might be hurtful to others have been associated with various indices of prosocial behavior (e.g., Eisenberg, Fabes, & Murphy, 1996; Eisenberg, Fabes, Schaller, Carlo, & Miller, 1991; Eisenberg et al., 1992; Garner, 2003).

Roberts (1999) found that mothers' encouragement of children's self-control of negative emotions was negatively related to daughters' prosocial behavior but positively related to boys' prosocial behavior; the converse tended to be true for fathers' emotion socialization. Both Roberts and Eisenberg et al. (e.g., 1991) have reported that positive relations between parents' emotion socialization and children's prosocial behavior are strongest in same-sex dyads. This may suggest that gender roles influence how affective arousal and emotion regulation are linked to prosocial behavior, although evidence of differing mother-specific and father-specific effects in children's social development tends to be quite limited (Hastings, Vyncke, et al., 2005).

The assumption underlying these studies is that affective development furthers behavioral development. Empathy may function as a regulatory emotion, inhibiting selfish or aggressive acts and providing the foundation for children's prosocial actions (Eisenberg & Miller, 1987). Parents may foster prosocial development by supporting children's empathy. There is evidence that children's empathy mediates some of the link between parental socialization and children's prosocial behavior, but few studies have evaluated the possible processes by which parental socialization affects empathy. Using modeling techniques, Strayer and Roberts (2004) found that school-age children's basic affective processes mediated the associations between parental socialization and children's empathy. Specifically, parents' greater maturity demands, warmth, and encouragement of expressiveness, and lower rejection and physical discipline, predicted children's greater insight into their own emotions and emotional expressiveness, and also lower anger. In turn, less angry but more expressive and insightful children were more empathic.

Fathers' Socialization of Prosocial Development

Socialization researchers have not focused as much attention on the roles of fathers in children's prosocial development compared to mothers. The studies that have included fathers indicate that paternal influences may contribute to children's prosocial development. Several single time-point, correlational studies have documented relations between children's prosocial behavior and fathers' authoritative and authoritarian styles, inductive reasoning, discipline, and warmth that are similar to those seen with mothers (e.g., Dekovic & Janssens, 1992; Janssens & Gerris, 1992; Sturgess, Dunn, & Davies, 2001), although results have not been as consistent (e.g., Hart, DeWolf, Wozniak, & Burts, 1992). There is evidence that fathers tend to be less aware of their children's prosocial activities (Grusec et al., 1996). Fathers' relative unawareness of children's prosocial behavior may offer fewer opportunities for fathers to reinforce or support prosocial development.

Two longitudinal studies have shown that earlier paternal supportive parenting predicts more prosocial behavior within sibling (Volling & Belsky, 1992) and father–child relationships (Eberly & Montemayor, 1999). Focusing on emotion socialization, Roberts (1999) found that boys' prosocial behavior toward peers decreased over 3 years when fathers were more suppressing of their preschool-age sons' emotional expressiveness.

Conversely, Hastings, Rubin, and DeRose (2005) did not find any associations between fathers' self-reported authoritarian, authoritative or protective parenting of toddlers and the children's observed prosocial responses to mothers and experimenters 2 years later. Thus, the limited set of longitudinal analyses involving fathers suggests that the lasting influences of paternal socialization may be more limited than has been documented for mothers. Additional research on fathers certainly is warranted.

OTHER CLOSE RELATIONSHIPS AND PROSOCIAL DEVELOPMENT

Siblings

Sibling relationships are often portrayed as a training ground for children to learn about social behavior, for good or for ill. There is some evidence to indicate that having siblings, and especially being an older sibling, might facilitate the development of prosocial behavior. This may be due to experiences of playing with and needing to accommodate one's behavior to another person who not only differs in desires and perceptions but is also less skilled and knowledgeable. Parents may also assign older siblings caregiving or supervisory roles of their younger siblings, such that their prosocial behavior is directly fostered and trained (see Dunn, Chapter 12, this volume).

The quality of the sibling relationship itself may contribute to prosocial development. Following toddler-age and preschool-age siblings over 6 months, Dunn and Munn (1986) found that one siblings' greater prosocial behavior during interactions predicted more prosocial behavior from the other sibling subsequently. This pattern held for both younger and older children, showing that the positive quality of a sibling relationship may be self-perpetuating. However, in research with preschool-age to early elementary school-age children, Pepler and colleagues (1981) did not report any such developmental relations over an 18-month period.

Friends and Peers

Research on children's friendships and peer relationships show that more prosocial children and youths are more popular and well liked, and are more likely to have close friends (e.g., Clark & Ladd, 2000; Gest, Graham-Bermann, & Hartup, 2001). Causal modeling analyses indicate that being more prosocial facilitates children's greater popularity (Dekovic' & Gerris, 1994). But do more prosocial children elicit positive and accepting reactions from their agemates, or does being liked by peers or having a good friend facilitate prosocial development? A small set of longitudinal studies suggest both processes may be occurring.

Following preschoolers over 3 years, Persson (2005) observed children's spontaneous helping, sharing, and altruism (unselfish concern for others) and distinguished initiating from receiving such behaviors from peers. Children who initiated more altruism in 1 year received more altruism from others in the subsequent year. The converse was not true: Receiving more prosocial acts did *not* predict children's behaviors in subsequent years. Thus, for preschoolers, prosocial behavior appeared to elicit reciprocity from peers.

Children's social status among classroom peers has also been associated with prosocial development in adolescence. Rejected children in grade 6 were likely to show less prosocial behavior and express less interest in pursuing prosocial goals in grade 8 than socially average peers (Wentzel, 2003). Following peer-rejected boys forward from grade 6 to grade 11, rejected boys who showed declining aggression also showed increasing prosocial behavior over this period, and by grade 11 they were less rejected, more accepted, more likely to be a friend, and more helpful (Haselager, Cillessen, Van-Lieshout, Riksen-Walraven, & Hartup, 2002). Thus, increases in prosocial behavior may have supported closer peer relationships. Close friends may have particularly strong influences on adolescents' prosocial development. Children's prosocial behavior increased from grade 6 to 8 when their friend in grade 6 was more prosocial than themselves but decreased strongly if the grade 6 friend was less prosocial (Wentzel et al., 2004). As well, having a more prosocial friend in grade 6 predicted stronger prosocial motivations in grade 8, which were concurrently associated with prosocial behavior. Similarly, youths who saw their high school peers as positive influences were more likely to engage in community volunteer work during adulthood (Zaff et al., 2003).

Across development, being a more prosocial child appears to elicit positive responses and acceptance from peers. As well, older children and adolescents' peer relationships and friendships appear to be influential in the continuing development of prosocial motivations and behaviors. Parents may facilitate positive development by fostering their children's friendships with other children who are kind, caring, cooperative, and helpful. Intriguingly, mediational analyses also indicate that prosocial behavior serves as the link between parental socialization and children's popularity and acceptance by peers (Dekovic & Janssens, 1992). Thus, effective parental socialization can support and increase children's prosocial characteristics, which in turn will foster their social competence and elicit positive responses from other children, which could further support youths' continued prosocial development.

Teachers

Correlational studies of children's prosocial characteristics and teachers' behaviors or the quality of the student–teacher relationship have found similar relations to those seen for parental socialization. Children tend to be more prosocial when teachers are affectively warmer, when their relationship is closer and less conflicted, and when children are securely attached to teachers (Birch & Ladd, 1998; Howes, 2000; Kienbaum, 2001; Copeland-Mitchell, Denham, & DeMulder, 1997). Teachers' directive or controlling behaviors seem to be less associated with children's prosocial behavior (Kienbaum, 2001). School-based interventions, akin to field experiments, have shown that teaching elementary school teachers proactive ways to prevent classroom aggression and praise positive behaviors increases 5- to 7-year-old children's self-reported sharing, helpfulness, and reparative behaviors (Flannery et al., 2003).

The effect of school-related experiences has taken hold as a topic of intense interest in the area of early child care, perhaps due to the ever-increasing numbers of children enrolled in out-of-home infant care and toddler care. Some studies have found that children with more early child-care experience are more prosocial, while others find that the quality of the child-care facility matters more than the amount of time in child care (NICHD Early Child Care Research Network, 2002). Overall, it would be valuable to conduct longitudinal studies of exactly which teacher and classroom qualities in one year predict children's prosocial behavior in later years.

SOCIOCULTURAL EXPERIENCES AND PROSOCIAL DEVELOPMENT

Community Involvement

Volunteerism and involvement in community-minded activities have been associated with the development of prosocial characteristics in children and youths (Hart & Fegley, 1995; Pancer & Pratt, 1999). In a longitudinal study, Switzer, Simmons, Dew, Regalski, and Wang (1995) found that school-mandated involvement in "voluntary" activities over a year was associated with increases in young women's self-perceptions of being altruistic, and young men's continued involvement in community activities. High school students' consistent participation in extracurricular activities in or out of school has also been found to predict higher rates of engaging in community volunteer work in early adulthood (Zaff et al., 2003), beyond the contributions of parents and peers. Pratt and colleagues (2003) found that youths who described their "ideal" selves as kind and caring were more involved in community activities that focused on helping others, and involvement in community helping activities at 17 years predicted stronger commitment to being kind and caring at 19 years, over and above the stability of values.

Together, these studies point toward the potential importance of positive community involvement for the prosocial development of adolescents and young adults. Being involved in other-oriented activities leads youths to increasingly value kindness, caring, and altruism as important personal qualities to which they aspire; presumably this value shift would support future prosocial activities. This could reflect a kind of active internalization, of becoming prosocial by doing prosocial. Youths with more prosocial tendencies probably are more inclined to enter into voluntary helping activities, but such participation also seems to be facilitated by attentive parenting and targeted school programs. Thus, encouraging adolescents' enrollment in volunteer work may be an effective way of promoting their prosocial development, as youths may incorporate their prosocial activities as an element of their selves.

Socioeconomic Status and Culture

Some studies have shown that children from adverse family backgrounds, characterized by lower incomes or job status, younger and less educated parents, and nonintact families, are less prosocial than children from more privileged homes (e.g., Haapasalo, Tremblay, Boulerice, & Vitaron, 2000; Lichter, Shanahan, & Gardner, 2002). These effects could be the result of reduced availability of prosocial role models, experiences of stress or deprivation that increase children's self-focused concern, or socioeconomic status (SES) differences in parental socialization. Mothers and fathers from lower SES groups are characterized as more strongly punitive and power assertive and less responsive than parents from higher SES groups (e.g., Burbach, Fox, & Nicholson, 2004; Knight, Kagan, & Buriel, 1982). Thus, the links between lower SES and lower prosocial development may be mediated by compromised and maladaptive parental socialization, although this explanation has not been evaluated in longitudinal studies.

Although the broad distinction between collectivist and individualist cultures is overly simplistic and may obscure intracultural variability, several researchers have suggested that children and youths in more collectivist cultures are more empathic, altruistic, helpful, or cooperative than children in individualist cultures (e.g., Knight et al., 1982; Zaff et al., 2003; for disconfirming reports, see Carlo, Koller, Eisenberg, Da Silva, &

Frohlich, 1996; Pilgrim & Rueda-Riedle, 2002). This may be due to collectivist cultures' deemphasis of individual needs or goals in lieu of attention to the needs of the broader community and the promotion of greater involvement of children in other-oriented activities (e.g., Whiting & Whiting, 1975). Cultural differences in parental socialization might serve as the means by which cultural differences in prosocial tendencies arise (Knight et al., 1982; Whiting & Whiting, 1975), although, as with the research on SES, there is a lack of longitudinal evidence.

ANSWERING SOME CENTRAL QUESTIONS

Is There Consistent Evidence of Any Socialization Influences on Prosocial Development?

Children are more prosocial when they have formed more secure attachment relationships with their parents; when their mothers and fathers are more authoritative than authoritarian in their style; when parents avoid punitive and strict discipline in favor of gentler control techniques; when they use reasoning and provide explanations; when they are sensitive to their children's needs and are warm with their children; and when they support their children's experience and regulation of emotions. Children are more prosocial when they come from stable and economically secure homes; have close and friendly relationships with their siblings; have experience in good-quality early child-care facilities; have kind, caring, helpful, and considerate peers and friends; and obtain experience taking care of the needs of others through volunteer and community activities.

All these associations have been documented in longitudinal studies, in which the socializing event or action temporally preceded the observation of prosocial behavior. Most of these associations have been replicated across at least two independent investigations. Some attempts to replicate these findings have failed to show that earlier socialization predicts later prosocial development, but contradictory findings have been infrequent, suggesting that the developmental associations are reliable and valid. Each association is small to modest in magnitude, although this does not mean the effects are not meaningful. Whether these influences function cumulatively, independently, or even redundantly is largely unknown.

What Is the Child's Role in Prosocial Development?

The substantial genetic contribution to prosocial behavior cannot be overlooked, nor can children's active creation of opportunities to have their prosocial development supported by socializing forces. Children become more prosocial over time when they start out being more prosocial. When they behave in more prosocial ways toward family members, peers, and others, they receive support and reinforcement for their actions. Thus far, the most clear and consistent evidence for these kinds of bidirectional influences over prosocial development has emerged from longitudinal investigations of peer relationships. It seems likely that similar processes occur within family relationships; future research will need to document this.

The research on parental socialization and on the aspects of childrearing that support prosocial development also implicates children's involvement in their own socialization. Affective mechanisms clearly are present, as children's empathic engagement with others serves as one link between parental socialization and prosocial behavior in other contexts. It seems likely that children's social cognitive functions are similarly employed to promote the internalization of standards for prosocial behavior. Many parenting techniques that are linked to prosocial behavior require the child to actively process the socialization message, assess its meaning and relevance, determine how it can be enacted, and then choose to do so. Children's acceptance and internalization of parental efforts to support kindness, caring, and compassion may be facilitated by parents who are able to forge close and secure relationships with their children. Future studies should address these individual, dyadic, and relationship-level processes.

Why Are There Gender Differences in Prosocial Development?

The majority of the longitudinal studies reviewed herein did not show that the relations between socialization and prosocial development differed much for boys and girls, suggesting that gender is not a robust moderator of socialization effects. In general, when sex differences were evident, most often socialization was found to predict prosocial outcomes more strongly in girls than boys. A few studies showed that different parenting practices predict similar outcomes for girls and boys. Given this modest evidence, and the fact that being female is associated with being more advanced in at least some aspects of prosocial development, it is worth considering how and why gender could play a role in the socialization of prosocial development.

Gender could serve as a "summarizing" variable. To some extent, boys and girls differ in biological predispositions, experience different socialization from parents and peers, and receive differential sex-typed expectations from media and other conveyers of cultural norms. Thus, simply identifying gender may serve to capture an amalgamation of socializing forces that favor more or stronger prosocial (female) outcomes, or fewer or weaker prosocial (male) outcomes.

Gender could moderate some effects of socialization on behavior. If there are biologically based sex differences in behavioral proclivities, similar childrearing experiences may foster divergent positive developmental trajectories. For example, authoritative parents who sensitively use gentle control could consistently respond to and reinforce whichever positive behaviors their young children manifest. If, on average, young girls express concern for others more often than young boys, and young boys more often show independence and autonomy, then the same approach to parenting could foster more prosocial and affiliative behaviors in girls and more competitive and assertive behaviors in boys (Hastings, Rubin, & DeRose, 2005; Leaper, 2002).

Gender differences in prosocial behavior may arise as a function of parental goals for sex-typed socialization; parents may subtly alter or selectively express their parenting styles or behaviors in order to foster the outcomes they consider to be appropriate for sons and daughters (Zahn-Waxler, 2000). If young girls are expected to be more prosocial, their kind and caring actions may be noticed and reinforced more consistently than those of boys, such that culturally shared beliefs may drive reality. There are also mean-level differences in the socialization experiences of sons and daughters, such that girls are targeted for more of the parenting behaviors that support prosocial behavior and fewer of the actions that undermine it. Mothers of boys value aggression more highly than mothers of girls (Deater-Deckard, Dodge, Bates, & Pettit, 1998), but aggressive boys are also more likely to receive harsh discipline from mothers than aggressive girls (Webster-

Stratton, 1996). Conversely, mothers of young girls are more likely to respond to aggression with other-oriented inductive reasoning than mothers of young boys (Smetana, 1989), and girls are more often encouraged to share as means of resolving disputes (Keenan & Shaw, 1994; Ross, Tesla, Kenyon, & Lollis, 1990). Many parenting techniques are used to similar extents for boys and girls, but there is reasonable evidence that boys receive more physical punishment (Lytton & Romney, 1991) and more authoritarian (Hastings, Rubin, & DeRose, 2005) and less authoritative parenting (Russell et al., 2003).

These sex differences in socialization experiences certainly would lead to greater support from parents for girls' prosocial development. Whether parents raise their sons and daughters differently because of innate sex differences in children's behavioral tendencies, or because of culturally dictated stereotypes about desirable characteristics for sons and daughters, is more difficult to ascertain. The existence of a cultural stereotype that other-oriented concerns and prosocial behavior are prototypically feminine could also explain why gender differences are more consistent in questionnaire than observation measures, as parents, teachers, or other reporters express their expectations or biased beliefs.

Finally, perhaps because of their own sex-typed biases, researchers may have defined prosocial behavior too narrowly. Such an issue has been noted in research on relational aggression; girls may be predisposed or socialized to show aggression differently than boys, but for decades researchers did not assess social forms of aggression (Underwood, 2002). Analogously, when asked to describe what it means to "be nice," more children suggest being socially inclusive than sharing or caring for others (Greener & Crick, 1999). Most measures of prosocial behavior do not include such affiliative actions. Males' understanding of prosocial behavior and their means of showing other-oriented concerns might differ from typically measured constructs, and aspects of their prosocial behavior may have been overlooked and underestimated. If males typically use a distinct set of behaviors than females to express prosocial values or motivations, they may be "differently prosocial" rather than "less prosocial."

What Does the Socialization of Prosocial Development Imply for the Understanding of Antisocial Behavior?

It is common for people to think of prosocial and antisocial behavior as antithetical. The former involves caring about and acting toward the well-being of others. The latter is based on a lack of regard for, or an outright animosity toward, the rights of others and is shown through hurtful, damaging, and denigrating actions. It is reasonable to expect individuals who engage in more prosocial behavior than average to also engage in less antisocial behavior than average—and this is empirically valid, at least for adults. Yet some people clearly can manifest both behaviors, and developmental research has shown that young children even tend to do so.

Miller and Eisenberg (1988) performed a meta-analysis almost 20 years ago, showing that empathy and sympathy were negatively correlated with antisocial characteristics from the school-age years forward, and the magnitude of this disconnect increased with age, but empathy and aggression were not negatively correlated in younger children. Recent studies also have shown positive relations between early prosocial and antisocial behavior. Highly aggressive toddlers were more empathic on various measures than toddlers with low aggression (Gill & Calkins, 2003). Preschoolers with few and many externalizing problems were similarly empathic in responses to adults simulating distress (Zahn-Waxler, Cole, Welsh, & Fox, 1995). Kindergarteners' prosocial and antisocial behaviors also tend to be uncorrelated (Kienbaum, 2001), unless both are measured though teacher reports, producing negative relations (Clark & Ladd, 2000).

The concurrent positive or nonsignificant relations of young children's prosocial and antisocial behavior mask a more complex, and somewhat paradoxical, pattern that unfolds over time. More prosocial toddlers and preschoolers are less aggressive and have fewer externalizing problems when they reach elementary school age (Haapasalo et al., 2000; Hay & Pawlby, 2003), whereas higher levels of early aggression predict lower levels of later prosocial behavior (Hastings et al., 2000; Keane & Calkins, 2004). Thus, early emerging antisocial behavior problems seem to be a risk factor for later deficits in prosocial behavior, and early prosocial behavior protects against later antisocial behavior.

It appears that the period of transition from preschool age to elementary school age is a point of transformation in the relations between positive and negative social behaviors. This may arise from the normative developmental patterns of antisocial and prosocial behavior. Aggression peaks in the late toddler–early preschooler period and decreases thereafter (Tremblay, 2000); prosocial behavior clearly emerges in the early toddler years and increases thereafter (Zahn-Waxler & Hastings, 1999). These behavior patterns could be following independent trajectories, with the early positive, then nonsignificant, then negative correlations arising as artifacts of developmental convergence and divergence. The facts that early high aggression predicts later low prosocial behavior, and vice versa, would argue against this explanation, however.

An alternative explanation is that prosocial and antisocial behaviors share a common origin, but children may follow divergent developmental pathways depending on experiences. Engaging in prosocial and antisocial behaviors requires active engagement with others; as such, they would both be supported by high approach motivations (Rothbart, Derryberry, & Hershey, 2000). Infants and toddlers who are temperamentally predisposed to approach others would have more opportunities for both helping and hurting others. Given their limited repertoire for attaining goals, socially engaged toddlers will invariably engage in conflict (Hay & Ross, 1982). However, aggressing against others should be more aversive for toddlers with a greater propensity for empathy. More sensitive and effective parents will also respond to toddler conflict and aggression in ways that support the development of alternative, less aggressive means of attaining social goals. Thus, socialization can direct young children's behavioral and emotional tendencies to foster their increasingly prosocial characteristics.

As should be clear in comparing the research reviewed in this chapter to the research reviewed by Cavell, Hymel, Malcolm, and Seay (Chapter 2), Moffitt and Caspi (Chapter 4), and other contributors to this *Handbook*, antisocial and prosocial behavior share a number of socialization correlates and contributing factors: The same socialization influences that promote greater prosocial behavior also serve to diminish antisocial behavior, suggesting that the developmental processes or mechanisms affecting these behavior patterns are not independent. Studies have only begun to consider whether and how these developmental processes might be interconnected. There is evidence to suggest that supporting prosocial development serves to protect children against antisocial development and potentially decrease their problematic aggressive and destructive behaviors (Feshbach, 1983; Flannery et al., 2003; Hastings et al., 2000).

The implication is clear: Efforts to curb violence should include actions to support kindness. One intriguing direction for this approach emerges from the cumulative research on children's and adolescents' direct experience of prosocial behavior. This includes receiving empathic and nurturant care from parents, having community-minded and active parents, being responsible for siblings, doing regular other-focused household chores, and participating in unpaid caring and helpful community activities. Even if these experiences and tasks are not completely voluntary, children and youths appear to learn goodness by doing good.

CONCLUSIONS

The study of the socialization of prosocial behavior has begun to generate consistent evidence of the impressive contributions made by parents, siblings, peers, teachers, community organizations, and cultures to the development of children's concern for the well-being of others. It is encouraging to see that prosocial behavior can be effectively supported, and prosocial development can be nurtured. Understanding that positive aspects of human functioning are subject to external influence, and that as a society we can act to reduce violence and aggression by supporting kindness and compassion, provides an opportunity to translate social science into effective social policy and practice.

REFERENCES

Ani, C. C., & Grantham-McGregor, S. (1998). Family and personal characteristics of aggressive Nigerian boys: Differences from and similarities with Western findings. *Journal of Adolescent Health, 23*, 311–317.

Barber, B. K., Olsen, J. E., & Shagle, S. C. (1994). Associations between parental psychological and behavioral control and youth internalized and externalized behaviors. *Child Development, 65*, 1120–1136.

Bell, R. Q. (1968). A reinterpretation of the direction of effects in socialization. *Psychological Review, 75*, 81–95.

Birch, S. H., & Ladd, G. W. (1998). Children's interpersonal behaviors and the teacher–child relationship. *Developmental Psychology, 34*, 934–946.

Burbach, A. D., Fox, R. A., & Nicholson, B. C. (2004). Challenging behaviors in young children: The father's role. *Journal of Genetic Psychology, 165*, 169–183.

Carlo, G., Koller, S. H., Eisenberg, N., Da-Silva, M. S., & Frohlich, C. B. (1996). A cross-national study on the relations among prosocial moral reasoning, gender role orientations, and prosocial behaviors. *Developmental Psychology, 32*, 231–240.

Cassidy, J. (1994). Emotion regulation: Influences of attachment relationships. *Monographs of the Society for Research in Child Development, 59*, 228–283.

Clark, K. E., & Ladd, G. W. (2000). Connectedness and autonomy support in parent-child relationships: Links to children's socioemotional orientation and peer relationships. *Developmental Psychology, 36*, 485–498.

Copeland-Mitchell, J. M., Denham, S. A., & DeMulder, E. K. (1997). Q-sort assessment of child–teacher attachment relationships and social competence in the preschool. *Early Education and Development, 8*, 27–39.

Côté, S., Tremblay, R. E., Nagin, D., Zoccolillo, M., & Vitaro, F. (2002). The development of impulsivity, fearfulness, and helpfulness during childhood: Patterns of consistency and change in trajectories of boys and girls. *Journal of Child Psychology and Psychiatry, 43*, 609–618.

Darling, N., & Steinberg, L. (1993). Parenting style as context: An integrative model. *Psychological Bulletin, 113*, 487–496.

Davidov, M., & Grusec, J. E. (2006). Untangling the links of parental responsiveness to distress and warmth to child outcomes. *Child Development, 77*, 44–58.

Dawkins, R. (1976). *The selfish gene*. Oxford, UK: Oxford University Press.

Deater-Deckard, K., Dodge, K. A., Bates, J. E., & Pettit, G. S. (1998). Multiple risk factors in the development of externalizing behavior problems: Group and individual differences. *Development and Psychopathology, 10,* 469–493.

Deater-Deckard, K., Dunn, J., O'Connor, T. G., Davies, L., & Golding, J. (2001). Using the stepfamily genetic design to examine gene–environment processes in child and family functioning. *Marriage and Family Review, 33,* 131–156.

Dekovic, M., & Gerris, J. R. M. (1994). Developmental analyses of social cognitive and behavioral differences between popular and rejected children. *Journal of Applied Developmental Psychology, 15,* 367–386.

Dekovic, M., & Janssens, J. M. (1992). Parents' child-rearing style and child's sociometric status. *Developmental Psychology 28,* 925–932.

Dunn, J., & Munn, P. (1986). Siblings and the development of prosocial behaviour. *International Journal of Behavioral Development, 9,* 265–284.

Eberly, M. B., & Montemayor, R. (1999). Adolescent affection and helpfulness toward parents: A 2-year follow-up. *Journal of Early Adolescence, 19,* 226–248.

Eisenberg, N., & Fabes, R. A. (1998). Prosocial development. In N. Eisenberg & W. Damon (Eds.), *Handbook of child psychology: Vol. 3. Social, emotional, and personality development* (5th ed., pp. 701–778). New York: Wiley.

Eisenberg, N., Fabes, R. A., & Murphy, B. C. (1996). Parents' reactions to children's negative emotions: Relations to children's social competence and comforting behavior. *Child Development, 67,* 2227–2247.

Eisenberg, N., Fabes, R. A., Schaller, M., Carlo, G., & Miller, P. A. (1991). The relations of parental characteristics and practices to children's vicarious emotional responding. *Child Development, 62,* 1393–1408.

Eisenberg, N., Lennon, R., & Roth, K. (1983). Prosocial development: A longitudinal study. *Developmental Psychology, 19,* 846–855.

Eisenberg, N., & Miller, P. A. (1987). The relation of empathy to prosocial and related behaviors. *Psychological Bulletin, 101,* 91–119.

Eisenberg, N., & Valiente, C. (2002). Parenting and children's prosocial and moral development. In M. H. Bornstein (Ed.), *Handbook of parenting: Vol. 5. Practical issues in parenting* (2nd ed., pp. 111–142). Mahwah, NJ: Erlbaum.

Eisenberg, N., Wolchik, S. A., Goldberg, L., & Engel, I. (1992). Parental values, reinforcement, and young children's prosocial behavior: A longitudinal study. *Journal of Genetic Psychology, 153,* 19–36.

Eisenberg-Berg, N., & Geisheker, E. (1979). Content of preachings and power of the model/preacher: The effect on children's generosity. *Developmental Psychology, 15,* 168–175.

Fabes, R. A., Fultz, J., Eisenberg, N., May-Plumlee, T., & Christopher, F. S. (1989). Effects of rewards on children's prosocial motivation: A socialization study. *Developmental Psychology, 25,* 509–515.

Feshbach, N. D. (1983). Learning to care: A positive approach to child training and discipline. *Journal of Clinical Child Psychology, 12,* 266–271.

Flannery, D. J., Vazsonyi, A. T., Liau, A. K., Guo, S., Powell, K. E., Atha, H., Vesterdal, W., & Embry, D. (2003). Initial behavior outcomes for the PeaceBuilders universal school-based violence prevention program. *Developmental Psychology, 39,* 292–308.

Garner, P. W. (2003). Child and family correlates of toddlers' emotional and behavioral responses to a mishap. *Infant Mental Health Journal, 24,* 580–596.

Gest, S. D., Graham-Bermann, S. A., & Hartup, W. W. (2001). Peer experience: Common and unique features of number of friendships, social network centrality, and sociometric status. *Social Development, 10,* 23–40.

Gill, K. L., & Calkins, S. D. (2003). Do aggressive/destructive toddlers lack concern for others? Behavioral and physiological indicators of empathic responding in 2-year-old children. *Development and Psychopathology, 15,* 55–71.

Greener, S., & Crick, N. R. (1999). Normative beliefs about prosocial behavior in middle childhood: What does it mean to be nice? *Social Development, 8,* 349–363.

Grusec, J. E. (1972). Demand characteristics of the modeling experiment: Altruism as a function of age and aggression. *Journal of Personality and Social Psychology, 22,* 139–148.

Grusec, J. E. (1991). Socializing concern for others in the home. *Developmental Psychology, 27,* 338–342.

Grusec, J. E., Davidov, M., & Lundell, L. (2002). Prosocial and helping behavior: Blackwell handbooks of developmental psychology. In C. H. Hart & P. K. Smith (Eds.), *Blackwell handbook of childhood social development* (pp. 457–474). Malden, MA: Blackwell.

Grusec, J. E., & Goodnow, J. J. (1994). Impact of parental discipline methods on the child's internalization of values: A reconceptualization of current points of view. *Developmental Psychology, 30,* 4–19.

Grusec, J. E., Goodnow, J. J., & Cohen, L. (1996). Household work and the development of concern for others. *Developmental Psychology, 32,* 999–1007.

Grusec, J. E., Goodnow, J. J., & Kuczynski, L. (2000). New directions in analyses of parenting contributions to children's acquisition of values. *Child Development, 71,* 205–211.

Grusec, J. E., & Kuczynski, L. (1980). Direction of effect in socialization: A comparison of the parent's versus the child's behavior as determinants of disciplinary techniques. *Developmental Psychology, 16,* 1–9.

Grusec, J. E., Kuczynski, L., Rushton, J. P., & Simutis, Z. M. (1978). Modelling, direct instruction, and attributions: Effects on altruism. *Developmental Psychology, 14,* 51–57.

Grusec, J. E., & Lytton, H. (1988). *Social development: History, theory, and research.* New York: Springer-Verlag.

Haapasalo, J., Tremblay, R. E., Boulerice, B., & Vitaro, F. (2000). Relative advantages of person- and variable-based approaches for predicting problem behaviors from kindergarten assessments. *Journal of Quantitative Criminology, 16,* 145–168.

Harris, M. B. (1970). Reciprocity and generosity: Some determinants of sharing in children. *Child Development, 41,* 313–328.

Hart, C. H., DeWolf, D. M., Wozniak, P., & Burts, D. C. (1992). Maternal and paternal disciplinary styles: Relations with preschoolers' playground behavioral orientations and peer status. *Child Development, 63,* 879–892.

Hart, D., & Fegley, S. (1995). Prosocial behavior and caring in adolescence: Relations to self-understanding and social judgment. *Child Development, 66,* 1346–1359.

Haselager, G. J. T., Cillessen, A. H. N., Van-Lieshout, C. F. M., Riksen-Walraven, J. M. A., & Hartup, W. W. (2002). Heterogeneity among peer-rejected boys across middle childhood: Developmental pathways of social behavior. *Developmental Psychology, 38,* 446–456.

Hastings, P. D., & Grusec, J. E. (1998). Parenting goals as organizers of responses to parent–child disagreement. *Developmental Psychology, 34,* 465–479.

Hastings, P. D., Rubin, K. H., & DeRose, L. (2005). Links among gender, inhibition, and parental socialization in the development of prosocial behavior. *Merrill-Palmer Quarterly, 51,* 501–527.

Hastings, P. D., Rubin, K. H., Mielcarek, L., & Kennedy, A. (2002). Helping shy girls and boys to be helpful. Paper presented at the biennial meeting of the *International Society for the Study of Behavioral Development,* Ottawa, Ontario, Canada.

Hastings, P.D., Vyncke, J., Sullivan, C., McShane, K. E., Benibgui, M., & Utendale, W. T. (2005). *Children's development of social competence across family types.* Ottawa, Ontario, Canada: Department of Justice Canada: Family, Children & Youth Section.

Hastings, P. D., Zahn-Waxler, C., & McShane, K. (2005). We are, by nature, moral creatures: Biological bases of concern for others. In M. Killen, & J. Smetana (Eds.), *Handbook of moral development* (pp. 483–516). Mahwah, NJ: Erlbaum.

Hastings, P. D., Zahn-Waxler, C., Robinson, J., Usher, B., & Bridges, D. (2000). The development of concern for others in children with behavior problems. *Developmental Psychology, 36,* 531–546.

Hay, D. F., Castle, J., Davies, L., Demetriou, H., & Stimson, C. A. (1999). Prosocial action in very early childhood. *Journal of Child Psychology and Psychiatry, 40,* 905–916.

Hay, D. F., & Pawlby, S. (2003). Prosocial development in relation to children's and mothers' psychological problems. *Child Development, 74,* 1314–1327.

Hay, D. F., & Ross, H. S. (1982). The social nature of early conflict. *Child Development, 53,* 105–113.

Hoffman, M. L. (1970). Moral development. In P. H. Mussen (Ed.), *Carmichael's manual of child development* (Vol. 2, pp. 261–360). New York: Wiley.

Hoffman, M. L. (2000). *Empathy and moral development: Implications for caring and justice.* New York: Cambridge University Press.

Holden, G. W., Miller, P. C., & Harris, S. D. (1999). The instrumental side of corporal punishment: Parents' reported practices and outcome expectancies. *Journal of Marriage and the Family, 61,* 908–919.

Howes, C. (2000). Social-emotional classroom climate in child care, child-teacher relationships and children's second grade peer relations. *Social Development, 9,* 191–204.

Iannotti, R. J., Cummings, E. M., Pierrehumbert, B., Milano, M.J. & Zahn-Waxler, C. (1992). Parental influences on prosocial behavior and empathy in early childhood. In J. Janssens & J. Gerris (Eds.), *Child rearing: Influences on prosocial and moral development* (pp. 77–100). Amsterdam: Swets & Zeitlinger.

Janssens, J. M. A. M., & Gerris, J. R. M. (1992). Child rearing, empathy, and prosocial development. In J. M. A. M. Janssens & J. R. M. Gerris (Eds.), *Child rearing: Influence on prosocial and moral development* (pp. 57–75). Amsterdam: Swets & Zeitlinger.

Keane, S. P., & Calkins, S. D. (2004). Predicting kindergarten peer social status from toddler and preschool problem behavior. *Journal of Abnormal Child Psychology, 32,* 409–423.

Keenan, K., & Shaw, D. S. (1994). The development of aggression in toddlers: A study of low-income families. *Journal of Abnormal Child Psychology, 22,* 53–77.

Kestenbaum, R., Farber, E. A., & Sroufe, L. A. (1989). Individual differences in empathy among preschoolers: Relation to attachment history. *New Directions for Child Development, 44,* 51–64.

Kiang, L., Moreno, A. J., & Robinson, J. L. (2004). Maternal preconceptions about parenting predict child temperament, maternal sensitivity, and children's empathy. *Developmental Psychology, 40,* 1081–1092.

Kienbaum, J. (2001). The socialization of compassionate behavior by child care teachers. *Early Education and Development, 12,* 139–153.

Knight, G. P., Kagan, A., & Buriel, R. (1982). Perceived parental practices and prosocial development. *Journal of Genetic Psychology, 141,* 57–65.

Kochanska, G. (1991). Socialization and temperament in the development of guilt and conscience. *Child Development, 62,* 1379–1392.

Krevans, J., & Gibbs, J. C. (1996). Parents' use of inductive discipline: Relations to children's empathy and prosocial behavior. *Child Development, 67,* 3263–3277.

Kuczynski, L. (2003). Beyond bidirectionality: Bilateral conceptual frameworks for understanding dynamics in parent–child relations. In L. Kuczynski (Ed.), *Handbook of dynamics in parent–child relations* (pp. 1–24). Thousand Oaks, CA: Sage.

Laible, D., Carlo, G., Torquati, J., & Ontai, L. (2004). Children's perceptions of family relationships as assessed in a doll story completion task: Links to parenting, social competence, and externalizing behavior. *Social Development, 13,* 551–569.

Leaper, C. (2002). Parenting girls and boys. In M. H. Bornstein (Ed.), *Handbook of parenting: Vol. 1. Children and parenting* (2nd ed., pp. 189–225). Mahwah, NJ: Erlbaum.

Lichter, D. T., Shanahan, M. J., & Gardner, E. L. (2002) Helping others? The effects of childhood poverty and family instability on prosocial behavior. *Youth and Society, 34,* 89–119.

Lopez, N. L., Bonenberger, J. L., & Schneider, H. G. (2001). Parental disciplinary history, current levels of empathy, and moral reasoning in young adults. *North American Journal of Psychology, 3,* 193–204.

Lytton, H., & Romney, D. M. (1991). Parents' differential socialization of boys and girls: A meta-analysis. *Psychological Bulletin, 109,* 267–296.

McGrath, M. P., Wilson, S. R., & Frassetto, S. J. (1995). Why some forms of induction are better than others at encouraging prosocial behavior. *Merrill-Palmer Quarterly, 41,* 347–360.

Mikulincer, M., & Shaver, P. R. (2005). Mental representations of attachment security: Theoretical foundation for a positive social psychology. In M. W. Baldwin (Ed.), *Interpersonal cognition* (pp. 233–266). New York: Guilford Press.

Miller, P. A., & Eisenberg, N. (1988). The relation of empathy to aggressive and externalizing/antisocial behavior. *Psychological Bulletin, 103,* 324–344.

NICHD Early Child Care Research Network. (2002). The interaction of child care and family risks in relation to child development at 24 and 36 months. *Applied Developmental Science, 6,* 144–156.

Pancer, S. M., & Pratt, M. W. (1999). Social and family determinants of community service involvement in Canadian youth. In J. Youniss & M. Yates (Eds.), *Roots of civic identity: International perspectives on community service and activism in youth* (pp. 32–55). New York: Cambridge University Press.

Patterson, G. R. (1982). *Coercive family processes.* Eugene, OR: Castalia.

Pepler, D. J., Abramovitch, R., & Corter, C. (1981). Sibling interaction in the home: A longitudinal study. *Child Development, 52,* 1344–1347.

Perry, D. G., Bussey, I., & Freiberg, K. (1981). Impact of adults' appeals for sharing on the development of altruistic dispositions in children. *Journal of Experimental Child Psychology, 32,* 127–138.

Persson, G. E. B. (2005). Young children's prosocial and aggressive behaviors and their experiences of being targeted for similar behaviors by peers. *Social Development, 14*, 206–228.

Pilgrim, C., & Rueda-Riedle, A. (2002). The importance of social context in cross-cultural comparisons: First graders in Colombia and the United States. *Journal of Genetic Psychology, 163*, 283–295.

Pratt, M. W., Hunsberger, B., Pancer, S. M., & Alisat, S. (2003). A longitudinal analysis of personal values socialization: Correlates of a moral self-ideal in late adolescence. *Social Development, 12*, 563–585.

Pratt, M. W., Skoe, E. E., & Arnold, M. L. (2004). Care reasoning development and family socialisation patterns in later adolescence: A longitudinal analysis. *International Journal of Behavioral Development, 28*, 139–147.

Preston, S. D., & de-Waal, F. B. M. (2002). Empathy: Its ultimate and proximate bases. *Behavioral and Brain Sciences, 25*, 1–72.

Radke-Yarrow, M., Zahn-Waxler, C., & Chapman, M. (1983). Children's prosocial dispositions and behavior. In P. Mussen & E. M. Hetherington (Eds.), *Handbook of child psychology: Vol. 4. Socialization, personality, and social development* (4th ed., pp. 469–545). New York: Wiley.

Roberts, W. L. (1999). The socialization of emotional expression: Relations with prosocial behaviour and competence in five samples. *Canadian Journal of Behavioural Science, 31*, 72–85.

Robinson, J., & Little, C. (1994). Emotional availability in mother-twin dyads: Effects on the organization of relationships. *Psychiatry: Interpersonal and Biological Processes, 57*, 222–231.

Robinson, J. L., Zahn-Waxler, C., & Emde, R. N. (1994). Patterns of development in early empathic behavior: Environmental and child constitutional influences. *Social Development, 3*, 125–145.

Roe, K. V. (1980). Toward a contingency hypothesis of empathy development. *Journal of Personality and Social Psychology, 39*, 991–994.

Ross, H., Tesla, C., Kenyon, B., & Lollis, S. (1990). Maternal intervention in toddler peer conflict: The socialization of principles of justice. *Developmental Psychology, 26*, 994–1003.

Rothbart, M. K., Derryberry, D., & Hershey, K. (2000). Stability of temperament in childhood: Laboratory infant assessment to parent report at seven years. In D. L. Molfese & V. J. Molfese (Eds.), *Temperament and personality development across the life span* (pp. 85–119). Mahwah, NJ: Erlbaum.

Rubin, K. H., Burgess, K. B., & Hastings, P. D. (2002). Stability and social–behavioral consequences of toddlers' inhibited temperament and parenting behaviors. *Child Development, 73*, 483–495.

Rushton, J. P. (1975). Generosity in children: Immediate and long-term effects of modeling, preaching, and moral judgment. *Journal of Personality and Social Psychology, 31*, 459–466.

Russell, A., Hart, C. H., Robinson, C. C., & Olsen, S. F. (2003). Children's sociable and aggressive behavior with peers: A comparison of the US and Australian, and contributions of temperament and parenting styles. *International Journal of Behavioral Development, 27*, 74–86.

Sameroff, A. J. (1975). Early influences on development: Fact or fancy? *Merrill-Palmer Quarterly, 21*, 267–294.

Scourfield, J., John, B., Martin, N., & McGuffin, P. (2004). The development of prosocial behaviour in children and adolescents: A twin study. *Journal of Child Psychology and Psychiatry, 45*, 927–935.

Smetana, J. G. (1989). Toddlers' social interactions in the context of moral and conventional transgressions in the home. *Developmental Psychology, 25*, 499–508.

Sober, E., & Wilson, D. S. (1998). *Unto others: The evolution and psychology of unselfish behavior.* Cambridge, MA: Harvard University Press.

Stevenson, H. C. (1997). Managing anger: Protective, proactive, or adaptive racial socialization identity profiles and African-American manhood development. *Journal of Prevention and Intervention in the Community, 16*, 35–61.

Strayer, J., & Roberts, W. (2004). Children's anger, emotional expressiveness, and empathy: Relations with parents' empathy, emotional expressiveness, and parenting practices. *Social Development, 13*, 229–254.

Sturgess, W., Dunn, J., & Davies, L. (2001). Young children's perceptions of their relationships with family members: Links with family setting, friendships, and adjustment. *International Journal of Behavioral Development, 25*, 521–529.

Switzer, G., Simmons, R., Dew, M., Regalski, J., & Wang, C. (1995). The effect of a school-based helper program on adolescent self-image, attitudes, and behavior. *Journal of Early Adolescence, 15*, 429–455.

Tremblay, R. E. (2000). The development of aggressive behaviour during childhood: What have we learned in the past century? *International Journal of Behavioral Development, 24*, 129–141.

Underwood, M. K. (2002). Sticks and stones and social exclusion: Aggression among girls and boys.

Blackwell handbooks of developmental psychology. C. H. Hart & P. K. Smith (Eds.), *Blackwell handbook of childhood social development* (pp. 533–548). Malden, MA: Blackwell.

van der Mark, I. L., van IJzendoorn, M. H., & Bakermans-Kranenburg, M. J. (2002). Development of empathy in girls during the second year of life: Associations with parenting, attachment, and temperament. *Social Development, 11,* 451–468.

Volling, B. L., & Belsky, J. (1992). The contribution of mother–child and father–child relationships to the quality of sibling interaction: A longitudinal study. *Child Development, 63,* 1209–1222.

Waters, E., Wippman, J., & Sroufe, L. A. (1979). Attachment, positive affect, and competence in the peer group: Two studies in construct validation. *Child Development, 50,* 821–829.

Webster-Stratton, C. H. (1996). Early intervention with videotape modeling: Programs for families of children with oppositional defiant disorder or conduct disorder. In P. S. Jensen & E. D. Hibbs (Eds.), *Psychosocial treatments for child and adolescent disorders: Empirically based strategies for clinical practice* (pp. 435–474). Washington, DC: American Psychological Association.

Wentzel, K. R. (2003). Sociometric status and adjustment in middle school: A longitudinal study. *Journal of Early Adolescence, 23,* 5–28.

Wentzel, K. R., Barry, C. M., & Caldwell, A. K. (2004). Friendships in middle school: Influences on motivation and school adjustment. *Journal of Educational Psychology, 96,* 195–203.

Whiting, B. B., & Whiting, J. W. (1975). *Children of six cultures: A psycho-cultural analysis.* Oxford, UK: Harvard University Press.

Yarrow, M. R., & Scott, P. M. (1972). Imitation of nurturant and nonnurturant models. *Journal of Personality and Social Psychology, 23,* 259–270.

Yarrow, M. R., Scott, P. M., & Waxler, C. Z. (1973). Learning concern for others. *Developmental Psychology, 8,* 240–260.

Zaff, J. F., Moore, K. A., Papillo, A. R., & Williams, S. (2003). Implications of extracurricular activity participation during adolescence on positive outcomes. *Journal of Adolescent Research, 18,* 599–630.

Zahn-Waxler, C. (2000). The early development of empathy, guilt, and internalization of responsibility: Implications for gender differences in internalizing and externalizing problems. In R. Davidson (Ed.), *Wisconsin symposium on emotion: Vol. 1. Anxiety, depression, & emotion* (pp. 222–265). Oxford, UK: Oxford University Press.

Zahn-Waxler, C., Cole, P. D., Welsh, J. D., & Fox, N. A. (1995). Psychophysiological correlates of empathy and prosocial behaviors in preschool children with behavior problems. *Development and Psychopathology, 7,* 27–48.

Zahn-Waxler, C., & Kochanska, G. (1990). The origins of guilt: Current theory and research in motivation. In R. A. Thompson (Ed.), *Nebraska symposium on motivation: Vol. 36. Socioemotional development* (pp. 183–258). Lincoln: University of Nebraska Press.

Zahn-Waxler, C., & Hastings, P. D. (1999). Development of empathy: Adaptive and maladaptive patterns. In W. van Haaften, T. Wren, & A. Tellings (Eds.), *Moral sensibilities and education, Vol. I: The preschool child.* Bemmel, The Netherlands: Concorde.

Zahn-Waxler, C., & Radke-Yarrow, M. (1990). The origins of empathic concern. *Motivation and Emotion, 14,* 107–130.

Zahn-Waxler, C., Radke-Yarrow, M., & King, R. A. (1979). Child rearing and children's prosocial initiations toward victims of distress. *Child Development, 50,* 319–330.

Zahn-Waxler, C., Radke-Yarrow, M., Wagner, E., & Chapman, M. (1992). Development of concern for others. *Developmental Psychology, 28,* 126–136.

Zahn-Waxler, C., Robinson, J. L., & Emde, R. N. (1992). The development of empathy in twins. *Developmental Psychology, 28,* 1038–1047.

Zahn-Waxler, C., Schiro, K., Robinson, J. L., Emde, R. N., & Schmitz, S. (2001). Empathy and prosocial patterns in young MZ and DZ twins: Development and genetic and environmental influences. In J. K. Hewitt & R. N. Emde (Eds.), *Infancy to early childhood: Genetic and environmental influences on developmental change* (pp. 141–162). London: Oxford University Press.

Zhou, Q., Eisenberg, N., Losoya, S. H., Fabes, R. A., Reiser, M., Guthrie, I. K., Murphy, B. C., Cumberland, A. J., & Shepard, S. A. (2002). The relations of parental warmth and positive expressiveness to children's empathy-related responding and social functioning: A longitudinal study. *Child Development, 73,* 893–915.

CHAPTER 26

Families, Schools, and Developing Achievement-Related Motivations and Engagement

Jacquelynne S. Eccles

In this chapter, I review the impact of experiences in the family and at school on the development of achievement motivation and engagement in skill-based learning. I begin with a brief overview of what I mean by achievement motivation and engagement in skill-based learning, organized around the expectancy–value model of achievement-related choices and behaviors presented in Figure 26.1. I then review the current research on family influences on achievement motivation and engagement organized around the model of family influences presented in Figure 26.2. Next I discuss the role of experiences in schools in supporting or undermining the development of positive achievement motivation and school engagement, organized around the extent to which schools provide opportunities to have one's universal, developmental, and personal needs met. I finish with a very brief discussion of the consequences of the failure of families and schools to provide opportunities for our young people to fulfill their universal and personal needs and the need for more integrated, across-context research.

THE ECCLES ET AL. EXPECTANCY–VALUE MODEL OF ACHIEVEMENT-RELATED CHOICES AND BEHAVIORS

Over the past 30 years, Eccles and her colleagues have studied the psychological and social factors influencing achievement-related motivation, task choice, and performance. Drawing on work associated with decision making, achievement theory, and attribution theory, they developed a comprehensive theoretical model of achievement-related choices to guide our subsequent research efforts (Eccles-Parsons et al., 1983; see Figure 26.1 for the most recent version). They hypothesized that achievement-related behaviors such as educational, vocational, and leisure choices would be most directly related to individuals' expectations for success and the importance or value individuals attach to the various options they see as available. They also outlined the relation of these beliefs to cultural norms, experiences, and aptitudes and to those personal beliefs and attitudes most commonly assumed to be associated with achievement-related activities (see Eccles-Parsons et al., 1983; Eccles, Wigfield, & Schiefele, 1998). In this chapter, I summarize what we know about family and school influences on these beliefs and behaviors. But first I need to say a little about the Eccles et al. basic achievement choice model.

Eccles et al. predicted that people will select those achievement-related activities (such as high school and college courses) that they think they can master and that have high task value for them. Individuals' expectations for success (similar to domain-specific personal efficacy as proposed by Bandura, 1997) for the wide range of courses from which the choice must be made depend on both the confidence that individuals have in their various intellectual and other skill-based abilities and the individuals' estimations of the difficulty of the various options they are considering. Likewise, Eccles et al. hypothesized that the relative subjective task values of various achievement-related activities and tasks are influenced by several factors. They grouped these various aspects of subjective task value into four broad categories: interest value (the enjoyment one gets from engaging in the task or activity), utility value (the instrumental value of the task or activity for helping to fulfill another short- or long-range goal), attainment value (the link between the task and one's sense of self and either personal or social identity), and cost (defined in terms of either what may be given up by making a specific choice or the negative experiences associated with each possible choice).

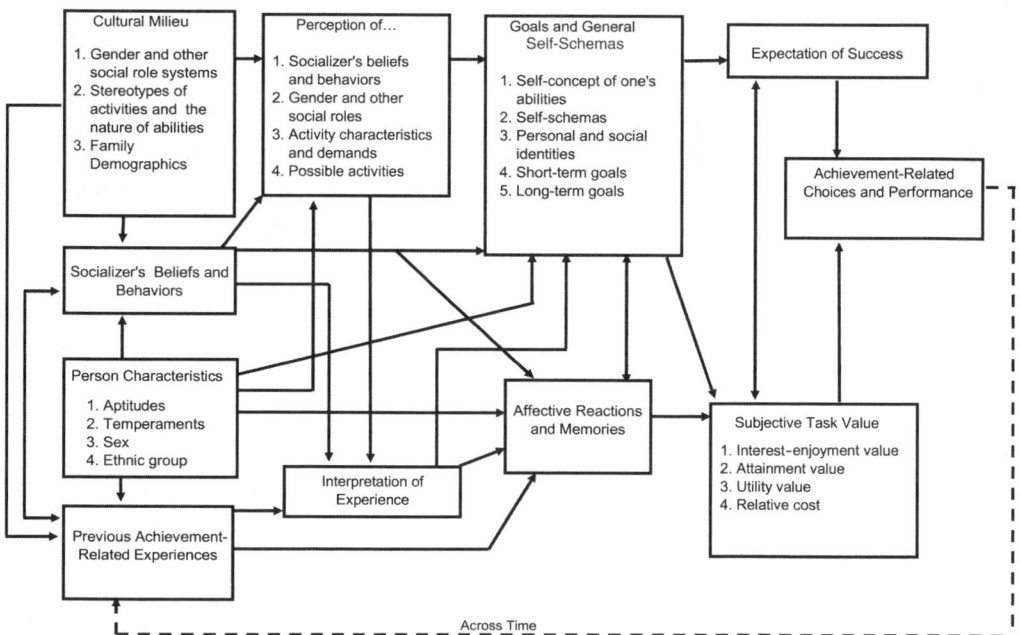

FIGURE 26.1. Eccles expectancy–value model of achievement choices.

Moreover, Eccles argued that the socialization processes linked to various social roles (e.g., gender and ethnic roles) will influence both group and individual differences in each of these components of subjective task value (Eccles, 1993, 1994). For example, gender-role socialization should lead to gender differences in the kinds of work one would like to do as an adult: Females in most cultures are more likely than males to want to work at occupations that help others and fit well into the family role plans. Males in Western cultures are more likely than females to want future occupations that pay very well and provide opportunities to become famous (Eccles et al., 1998; Ruble & Martin, 1998). If this is true, then various tasks related to future occupational choices (e.g., high school courses), should have different value for females and males. Similarly, the essence of gender-role socialization is creating different value systems, different core identity beliefs, and different normative behavior expectations in females and males. As a consequence, the cost of engaging in any particular activity should differ on average for females and males due to both the anticipated reaction of others to various options and the relative cost of various options for other activities considered to be more or less central in the hierarchy of normative behaviors.

A similar analysis can be made for cultural and ethnic differences in expectations for success, short- and long-term goals, and the most salient and valued parts of the self (e.g., Super & Harkness, 2002; Wigfield, Tonks, & Eccles, 2004). In addition, recent work on stereotype threat provides a good example of how culturally based stereotypes about ethnic group differences in competencies across different skill areas can undermine individuals' performance on assessments of their skills in these areas (Steele & Aronson, 1995). For example, Steele and his colleagues have shown that both African American and female students perform more poorly on tests of math skills when their race or gender is made salient (Steele & Aronson, 1995). Shih and her colleagues have shown that Asian American females do better on math tests when their ethnicity is made salient and worse on math tests when their gender is made salient than they do when neither of these characteristics is mentioned (Ambady, Shih, & Kim, 2001).

Finally, of course, individual differences within various social groups in the value of different achievement-related options can result from similar differences in the kinds of self and task beliefs Eccles and her colleagues assume are linked to achievement motivation and engagement in achievement-related tasks and activities. These differences, in turn, can result from differences in both long-term and immediate social experiences. In this chapter, I outline a comprehensive model for thinking about both long-term socialization and concurrent social contextual influences on the ontogeny and expression of achievement-related choices and performance.

FAMILY INFLUENCES ON ACHIEVEMENT

Figure 26.2 provides a general overview of the ways in which families, parents in particular, can influence their children's engagement and performance on achievement-related tasks through their influence on children and adolescents' achievement-related self-perceptions and subjective task values (Eccles, 1993). Similar social cognitive mediational models of parental behavior and influence have been proposed by many other researchers (Bronfenbrenner & Morris, 1998; Entwisle & Alexander, 1990; Goodnow & Collins, 1990; Grolnick & Slowiaczek, 1994; Marjoribanks, 2002).

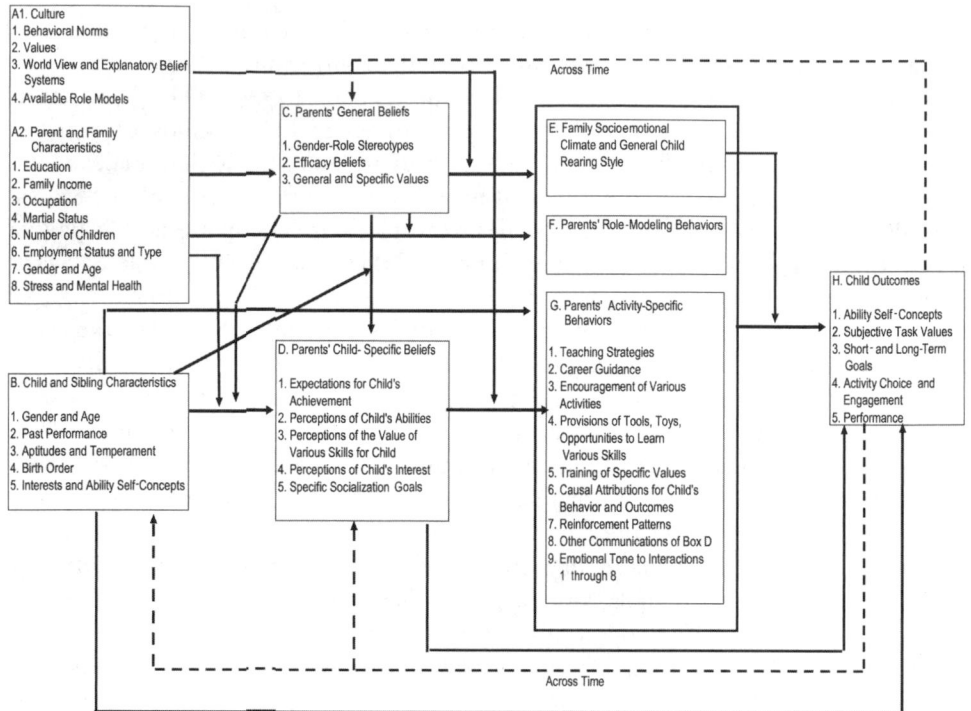

FIGURE 26.2. Model of parents' influence on children's achievement related to self-perception, values, and behaviors.

Beginning at the far left, this model predicts that exogenous, cultural, and demographic characteristics of the family, in combination with specific characteristics of the child, influence parents' general and child-specific beliefs, which, in turn, influence parents' general and child-specific behaviors and practices, which, in turn, influence children's developing self and task beliefs, motivation and interest patterns, and actual behavior. Eccles (1993) proposed various direct and indirect relations, as well as moderating influences on the associations between the boxes.

Although there is extensive work on some components of this model, very few studies include both the proximal and more distal components proposed to influence parenting behaviors outlined in Box G. Much of existing literature focuses on the association of the exogenous and child specific characteristics (Boxes A and B) with either parents' beliefs (Boxes C and D) or behaviors (Boxes E, F, G) or more directly with children's (adolescents') achievement-related self and task beliefs, engagement, and actual performance (Box H). For example, there are many studies linking family socioeconomic status (SES) and/or ethnicity directly to children's academic outcomes (Box H) (e.g., Brooks-Gunn, Linver, & Fauth, 2005; Coleman et al., 1966). In the last 10–15 years, a number of studies have linked family SES and/or culture indirectly to children's academic outcomes through their association with either parents' child-specific beliefs (Box D) or specific parenting practices (Box G) (e.g., Entwisle & Alexander, 1990; Schneider & Coleman, 1993; Steinberg, Dornbusch, & Brown, 1992; Stevenson, Chen, & Uttal, 1990). However, even these studies have rarely looked at more than a few of the possible parental beliefs and practices in the same study. Very recently, some researchers are beginning to examine simultaneously several of the mediating and moderating hypotheses on achievement outcomes implied in Figure 26.2 and to trace the impact of parents' beliefs and behaviors on their children's achievement-related engagement and performance over time (Davis-Kean, Eccles, & Schnabel, 2002; Fredricks & Eccles, 2002, 2005). Most of the research has focused on school achievement, but there is a growing body of work on family influences on sport achievement as well.

Family Demographic Characteristics

Researchers in sociology, economics, and psychology have documented the association of such factors as family structure, family size, parents' financial resources, parents' education, parents' occupation, community characteristics, and dramatic changes in the family's economic resources with children's academic motivation and achievement (Laosa, 1999; Magnuson, 2003; Marjoribanks, 2002; Teachman, Pasch, & Carver, 1997; Yeung, Linver, & Brooks-Gunn, 2002). By and large, these studies show that children growing up in families with more financial, time, social, and intellectual resources do better academically in school, stay in school longer, and earn higher degrees. Several mechanisms could account for these associations. First, family demographic characteristics and cultural factors could affect children's motivation indirectly through their association with both parents' beliefs and practices and the opportunity structures in the child's home and neighborhood environments. For example, parents with more education are more likely to believe that involvement in their children's education and intellectual development is important, to be actively involved with the children's education, and to have intellectually stimulating materials in their home (DeBaryshe, 1995; Marjoribanks, 2002; Schneider & Coleman, 1993).

Second, some demographic and cultural characteristics could influence motivation indirectly through the competing demands they place on parents' time and energy. For example, the negative association of single-parent status, time spent at work, and large family size on children's school achievement might reflect the fact that these factors reduce the time and energy parents have for engaging their children in activities that foster high general achievement motivation, high domain-specific ability self-concepts, and high domain-specific subjective task values (Marjoribanks, 2002; Schneider & Coleman, 1993). Similarly, the psychological stress associated with some demographic factors could influence parents' ability to engage in the kinds of behaviors associated with the development of high general achievement motivation, high domain-specific self and task-related beliefs, task engagement, and performance. Ample evidence documents how much harder it is to do a good job of parenting if one lives in a high-risk neighborhood or if one is financially stressed (Conger et al., 2002; Elder, Eccles, Ardelt, & Lord, 1995; Furstenberg, Cook, Eccles, Elder, & Sameroff, 1999; McLoyd, 1990; Mistry, Vandewater, Huston, & McLoyd, 2002). Not only do such parents have limited resources to implement whatever strategies they think might be effective, they also have to cope with more external stressors than middle-class families living in stable, resource-rich neighborhoods. Not surprisingly, the children of parents who live in dangerous and resource-poor neighborhoods and are themselves living very stressful lives also evidence less positive motivation toward conventional school success.

Third, cultural and demographic characteristics could affect parents' perceptions of, and expectations for, their children. Both parents' education level and family income have a positive *impact* on parents' expectations regarding both their children's immediate school success and long-term educational prospects (Davis-Kean, Malanchuk, Peck, & Eccles, 2003; Teachman et al., 1997). Similarly, mothers' expectations for their children's academic achievement drop when they get divorced (Barber & Eccles, 1992). Exactly how long this drop persists is not known. Finally, parents from various ethnic groups and cultures differ in their educational expectations and aspirations for their children. Fordham and Ogbu (1986), for example, suggested that parents from certain ethnic groups living in very poor and disadvantaged neighborhoods may come to believe that there are limited opportunities for their children to obtain conventional forms of success and that doing well in school is unlikely to pay off in terms of access to well-paying jobs within the larger society. These parents may shift their socialization efforts toward other goals and interests, such as finding employment in the neighborhood.

Fourth, cultural and demographic characteristics can influence parents' beliefs and behaviors and children's outcomes in even less direct ways, such as those associated with role modeling. For example, family demographic characteristics are often associated with things like parents' jobs and leisuretime activities, and with the kinds of role models children see outside the home. These behaviors and models can influence children's achievement goals, values, and self-perceptions through observational learning (Furstenberg et al., 1999; Kohn, 1977). Wilson (1987) argued that the relatively low numbers of high-achieving adults in very concentrated poor inner-city neighborhoods is a key factor in poor children's lack of engagement in a variety of conventional achievement activities. Cultures differ even more dramatically in what parents and other important adults do with their time. Again it is not surprising that children growing up in these different cultures come to have different ability self-concepts and different subjective task values. Very little work has addressed this hypothesis directly. Instead, the mechanisms are typically inferred from correlational findings.

Fifth, culture and ethnicity can influence parents' behaviors and children's motivation through mechanism linked directly to values, goals, and general belief systems (Garcia Coll & Pacter, 2002; Lareau, 1989; 2003). For example, several scholars describe cultural differences in valued activities, motivational orientation, and behavioral styles (Gallimore & Goldenberg, 2001; Rogoff, 2003; Stevenson et al., 1990). Such differences can affect the socialization of motivated behavior through variations in (1) valued activities (e.g., athletic vs. musical competence), (2) valued goals (e.g., communal goals vs. individualistic goals, mastery vs. performance goals, doing vs. being goals), and (3) approved means of achieving one's goals (e.g., competitive vs. cooperative means).

Recent work by Fuligni, Yip, and Tseng (2002) illustrates another example of cultural influences on academic engagement through its influence on core values and goals: in this case, the value attached to family obligations. In an extensive longitudinal study of multiple immigrant and ethnic groups in California, they found substantial group differences in the importance attached to, and the behavioral manifestations of, family obligations. In addition, adolescents with a high sense of family obligation also attached higher importance to school success in cultures where both family obligation and school success were valued. They argued that school success is part of one's family obligations in such cultures and that both become a core component of these adolescents' social and personal identities.

Other researchers studying cultural differences in school achievement have directly investigated cultural differences in parents' expectations and other achievement-related beliefs and linked them to cultural differences in adolescents' achievement. For example, the work by Stevenson and his colleagues demonstrated that European American parents, compared to Japanese parents, overestimate their children's academic abilities, are less aware of their children's academic difficulties, and are more satisfied with school performance that falls below their expectations (Crystal & Stevenson, 1991). Finally, recent work by Lepper and his colleagues suggest that there are cultural differences in the impact of parents' use of controlling strategies on their children's motivation. For example, Iyengar and Lepper (1999) found that Asian children prefer tasks they believe were chosen for them by their parents to tasks that their parents had not chosen. In contrast, European American children prefer tasks that they themselves get to pick.

In summary, there are many ways for cultural and family demographic characteristics to directly or indirectly affect the development of children's general achievement motivation, domain-specific self-concepts and domain-specific subjective task values. It is important to note, however, that even though family demographic characteristics have been linked repeatedly to children's school achievement, their effects are almost always indirect, mediated by their association with parents' beliefs, practices, and psychological resources. In addition, parents' beliefs and psychological and social resources can override the effects of even the most stressful demographic characteristics on children's school achievement and motivation. Finally, there are often complex interactions among various demographic characteristics in predicting either parenting beliefs and practices or child outcomes.

General Childrearing Climate

Historically, researchers studying parental influence have focused on the impact of the general patterns and philosophy of childrearing on children's overall orientation toward achievement. The family variables investigated include general emotional warmth and supportiveness in the home (Connell, Halpern-Felsher, Clifford, Crichlow, & Usinger, 1995; Gutman, Sameroff, & Eccles, 2002); valuing of achievement (DeBaryshe, 1995; Clark, 1993; Gutman et al., 2002); general parental childrearing beliefs and theories, values, and goals, as well as sex-typed goals and cultural beliefs, goals, and values (Goodnow & Collins, 1990; Miller & Davis, 1992; Sigel, McGillicuddy-DeLisi, & Goodnow, 1992); general childrearing style as well as authority structure, discipline tactics, and general interaction patterns (Baumrind, 1971; Lord, Eccles, & McCarthy, 1994; Steinberg et al., 1992); parental locus of control and personal efficacy (Bandura, 1997; Gutman, et al., 2002); and communicative style and teaching style (McGillicuddy-De Lisi & Sigel, 1991).

Much recent work has focused on support for autonomy. Drawing on self-determination theory, Grolnick, Pomerantz, and their colleagues argued that the extent to which parents structure their children's learning activities in ways that support the children's sense of autonomy is key to fostering high levels of achievement motivation and engagement (e.g., Grolnick, 2003): "When parents are autonomy supportive rather than controlling, they provide children with the experience of solving challenges on their own" (Pomerantz, Grolnick, & Price, 2005, p. 263). Children in such families engage in more mastery-oriented play when they are toddlers (Frodi, Bridges, & Grolnick, 1985) and evidence higher levels of intrinsic motivation and mastery-oriented behaviors once they are in school (Pomerantz et al., 2005). The importance of autonomy support seems to be particularly important for low-achieving children (Ng, Kenney-Benson, & Pomerantz, 2004), especially if the mothers stress the importance of effort and learning strategies as they help their children with homework (Pomerantz et al., 2005), perhaps because such practices help low-achieving children feel both competent and socially supported.

Several investigators have stressed an integrated view of how these various parenting characteristics work together to produce optimal motivational outcomes (Eccles et al., 1998; Fredricks & Eccles, 2002, 2005). For example, Grolnick (2003) stressed the interplay of three components of general parenting in promoting self-determination in children and adolescents: involvement and interest in their children's activities support for autonomous behaviors and adequate structure. Grolnick (2003) suggested that these parenting behaviors are important in helping children form a sense of autonomy and interest in activities, which, in turn, lead to greater achievement performance and lower learning problems. Parents who become too invested in their children's achievements may adopt excessively controlling strategies that undermine their children's sense of autonomy and intrinsic motivation (Grolnick. 2003; Pomerantz et al., 2005). Finally, Eccles (1993) stressed the importance of emotional support, role models, and the right balance between structure, control, challenge, and developmentally appropriate levels of support for autonomy. This balance depends on cultural systems, the specific context in which the family is living (e.g., does the family live in a very dangerous neighborhood where more parental control is essential for the physical safety of the children?), the age of the child, and other individual characteristics. In one test, Lord et al. (1994) found that both perceived parental support for autonomy at home and the perceived quality of the affective relations with one's parents predicted better adjustment to the junior high school transition.

While the magnitude of effects varies by race/ethnicity, sex, social economic class, and nationality, there is consensus that these general parental practices do impact on a variety of quite general indicators of children's motivation and motivated behavior (Eccles, 1993). The results are consistent with three general principles: appropriate levels of structure, consistent and supportive parenting, and observational learning. Families that know enough about their child to provide the right amount of challenge with the right amount of support seem more likely to produce highly competent and motivated children. These parents are also likely to be able to adjust their behavior to meet the changing developmental needs and competencies of their children. Families that provide a positive emotional environment are more likely to produce children who want to internalize the parents' values and goals and therefore want to imitate the behaviors being modeled by their parents. Consequently, children growing up in these homes are likely to develop a positive achievement orientation if their parents provide such a model and value those specific tasks, goals, and means of achieving one's goals valued by their parents. Until quite recently, however, very few of these studies have focused on such child outcomes as domain-specific ability self-concepts, domain-specific subjective task values, and differential engagement and performance across a variety of achievement-related activities, and differential performance. Most studies focus on quite general levels of children's achievement such as school grades rather than domain-specific self-concepts and values linked to specific subject areas such as math versus language arts or sports versus instrumental music. It is likely, however, that these more domain-specific achievement-related beliefs and behaviors result from more specific parental practices and role modeling. I summarize evidence in support of this prediction later.

Translating General Beliefs into Specific Beliefs and Practices

Researchers have shown that parents' general beliefs such as valuing of achievement and school competence, general parental childrearing beliefs and theories, values and goals, sex-typed ideologies and goals, and culturally based beliefs, goals, and values are linked to parenting behaviors in the school achievement arena in the predicted direction (Eccles, 1993; Goodnow & Collins, 1990; Jacobs & Eccles, 2000; Miller & Davis 1992; Sigel et al., 1992). But how? Figure 26.2 depicts a general overview of how one might approach this question. First, one might ask about the relation of parents' general beliefs and practices to domain- (e.g., sports vs. instrumental music or math vs. reading) and child-specific (e.g., each child in the family) parental beliefs, values, and practices. For example, do parents' gender-role stereotypes affect their perceptions of their own children's specific abilities in various activity domains (like math vs. reading)? Similarly, do parents' beliefs regarding the nature of ability affect their parenting practices? Dweck (1999) hypothesized that different ways of viewing the nature of ability and incompetence account for individual differences in academic achievement orientation. Dweck stressed the distinction between the belief that abilities are entity-based and highly stable over time versus the belief that abilities are incremental in nature and thus amenable to substantial change through effort. As a result, children who think that incompetence is a temporary and modifiable state should respond to failure with increased mastery efforts more than children who think that current incompetence is a sign of insufficient aptitude that cannot be modified. It is likely that parents also differ in their beliefs regarding the origins of individual differences in competence, the meaning of failure, and the most adaptive responses to failure. These beliefs should influence both their response to their children's failures and their efforts to help their children acquire new competencies and interests. Similarly, cultural differences in beliefs regarding the nature of ability and competence should relate to the kinds of statements parents make to their children about the origins of individual differences in performance—statements such as "you have to be born with math talent" versus "anyone can be good at math if they just work hard enough" (Holloway, 1988; Stevenson et al., 1990).

Similarly, one could ask whether general cultural beliefs about things like the nature of ability affect the domain-specific attributions parents provide to their children for the child's successes and failures in various activities and school subjects. Hess and his colleagues (Holloway, 1988; Hess, Chih-Mei, & McDevitt, 1987) and Stevenson et al. (1990) have found that Japanese and Chinese parents make different causal attributions than European American parents for their children's school performances with Japanese and Chinese parents emphasizing effort and hard work and European American parents emphasizing natural talent.

Child-Specific Beliefs, Values, and Perceptions: Parents as Socializers of Children's Success Expectations

Parents hold many specific beliefs about their children's abilities, which, in turn, should affect motivationally linked outcomes, such as the well-established positive link between parents' educational expectations and academic motivation and performance (e.g., Alexander, Entwisler, & Bedinger, 1994; Davis-Kean et al., 2002; Fredericks & Eccles, 2002; Grolnick & Slowiaczek, 1994; Schneider & Coleman, 1993). Eccles (1993) suggested the following specific parental beliefs as particularly likely influences on children's motivation: (1) causal attributions for their children's performance across various domains; (2) perceptions of the difficulty of various tasks for their children; (3) expectations for their children's probable success and confidence in their children's abilities; (4) beliefs regarding the value of various tasks and activities coupled with the extent to which parents believe they should encourage their children to master various tasks; (5) differential achievement standards across various activity domains; and (6) beliefs about the external barriers to success coupled with beliefs regarding both effective strategies to overcome these barriers and their own sense of efficacy to implement these strategies for each child.

Such beliefs and messages, particularly those associated with parents' perceptions of their children's competencies and likely success, predict children's subsequent self and task beliefs (e.g., Fredricks & Eccles, 2002, 2005; Frome & Eccles, 1998; Miller & Davis, 1992; Pallas, Entwisle, Alexander, & Stluka, 1994; Stevenson et al., 1990). For example, parents' perceptions of their adolescents' abilities are significant predictors of developmental changes in their children's estimates of their own ability and interest in math, English, and sports even after the significant positive relation of the child's actual performance to both the parents' and adolescents' perceptions of the adolescents' domain-specific abilities is controlled (Eccles, 1993; Frome & Eccles, 1998) Similarly, Fredricks and Eccles (2002, 2005) found that the confidence parents have in their elementary school children's math, reading, and sports abilities while the children are in early elementary school predicts the rate of decline in the children's confidence in their own math, English, and sport abilities as the children move into and through adolescence. Several studies have documented declines in children and adolescents' confidence in their own achievement-related abilities over the kindergarten to grade 12 school years (e.g. Fredricks & Eccles, 2002; Jacobs, Hyatt, Osgood, Eccles, & Wigfield, 2002). Both the rate of change and the magnitude of the decline are reduced for those children whose parents have higher estimates of their children's abilities. This effect holds even when independent estimates of the children's actual competence (e.g., teachers' ratings and scores on standardized tests) are controlled.

Child-Specific Beliefs, Values, and Perceptions: Parents as Socializers of Task Value

Parents may convey differential task values through explicit rewards and encouragement for participating in some activities rather than others. Similarly, parents may influence children's interests and aspirations, particularly with regard to future educational and vocational options, through explicit and implicit messages they provide as they "counsel" children or work with them on different academic activities (e.g., Jacobs & Eccles, 2000; Tenenbaum & Leaper, 2003).

Provisions of Specific Experiences at Home

There is ample evidence that parents influence their children's motivation through the specific types of learning experiences they provide for their children. Researchers have documented the benefits of active involvement with, and monitoring of, children's and adolescents' schoolwork and time spent on other achievement-related activities such as sports and instrumental music (e.g., Clark, 1993; Eccles, 1993; Schneider & Coleman, 1993; Stevenson et al., 1990; Steinberg, et al., 1992). For example, researchers have shown that reading to one's preschool children and providing reading materials in the home predicts the children's later reading achievement and motivation (e.g., Davis-Kean & Eccles, 2003; Linver, Brooks-Gunn, & Kohen, 2002). Such experiences likely influence both the child's skill levels and the child's interest in doing these activities, both of which, in turn, have a positive impact on the child's transition into elementary school and subsequent educational success (Entwisle & Alexander, 1990). Similarly, by providing the specific toys, home environment, and cultural and recreational activities for their children, parents structure their children's experiences (Jacobs, Davis-Kean, Bleeker, Eccles, & Malanchuk, 2005). However, the extent to which these experiences actually influence children's domain-specific ability self-concepts and subjective task values should depend on the affective and motivational climate that is created by parents when the children are engaged with any particular experience. If parents overly control and put excess pressure on their children to succeed at particular activities, this is likely to undermine the children's intrinsic interest in the activity, reduce the children's confidence in their ability to succeed, and lead to negative affective associations with the activity due to classical conditioning (Grolnick, 2003; Lepper & Henderlong, 2000). Finally, the differential provision of such experiences to girls and boys and to children from various ethnic groups might explain group differences in subsequent motivation to engage various types of achievement activities. Children can only learn about what they are exposed to. If their families never provide them experiences with a variety of activities, they are unlikely to develop the skills and interest necessary to pursue these activities on their own.

Another avenue by which parents indirectly influence the provisions in the home is through the way they manage the family's time and resources. Parents manage the resources and time of their children and thus choose or help to choose activities for their child that may increase interest and competence in these areas (Eccles, 1993; Furstenberg et al., 1998; Simpkins, Fredericks, Davis-Kean, & Eccles, in press). Many parents try to organize and arrange their children's social environments in order to promote opportunities, to expose their children to particular experiences and value systems, and to restrict dangers and exposure to undesirable influences. Consider, for example, the amount of attention some parents give to the choice of child care during early childhood, to picking a place to live, and to selecting appropriate after-school and summer activities for their children in order to ensure desirable schools and appropriate playmates for their children and to help their children acquire particular skills and interests. In the arena of school achievement, parents' engagement in managing their children experiences vis-à-vis intellectual skills (e.g., reading, acquisition of general information, and mastering school assignments) is directly and powerfully related to children's subsequent academic success even in stressful contexts such as poverty (Brooks-Gunn et al., 2005; Davis-Kean et al., 2002; Furstenberg et al., 1999). Given the consistency of the evidence in this one domain, understanding the specific ways parents organize and manage their children's experiences across a wide range of activities is a promising approach to understanding how parents shape individual differences in specific skills, self-perceptions, interests, and activity preferences. For example, children should be most likely to acquire those skills that their parents make sure they have the opportunity to learn and practice.

Parent involvement with their children's schools is another example of family management strategies. There is increasing interest in the association of family school involvement and children's school achievement. Some evidence suggests that high levels of involvement facilitate school achievement (Booth & Dunn, 1996; Eccles & Harold, 1996; Epstein, 1992). Why? Perhaps because parental involvement in school demonstrates their high valuing of school achievement to the children, which in turn should influence the subjective task value the children come to place on school achievement themselves. Alternatively, high levels of involvement may also help parents provide more effective and targeted help at home, leading to increases in their children's confidence in their ability to succeed in school as well as increases in the value the children attach to doing well in school (Grolnick, 2003).

Summary

The studies reviewed suggest a multivariate model of the relation between antecedent childrearing variables and the development of achievement orientation: The development of achievement motivation and engagement in achievement-related activities likely depends on the presence of several variables interacting with each other, both mediating and moderating children's motivation and behaviors. Specifically, proper timing of demands creates a situation in which children can develop a sense of competence in dealing with their environment. An optimally warm and supportive environment with the minimal necessary control creates a situation in which the child will choose his parents as role models and will feel autonomous in that choice. The presence of high yet realistic expectations creates a demand situation in which the child will perform in accord with the expectancies of the parents. Finally, the ability level of the child must be such that attainment of the expected level of performance is within his or her capacity. All these factors, as well as the availability of appropriate role models, are essential for the child to develop a positive achievement orientation. The exact way this orientation will be manifest is likely to be dependent on the values the child has learned, which are directly influenced by the culture in which the family lives and the social roles the child is being socialized to assume.

Very few studies, however, have adopted such an integrated view of family influences. Most include only a limited subset of family constructs and many still use regression-based statistical techniques that estimate the unique contribution of each predictor rather than assessing a more global or holistic view of the family. Structural equation modeling has improved the situation substantially by providing a means to test sequential pathways of influence and this approach is being used in more and more studies. Another promising approach involves creating patterns of family practices and assessing whether particular combinations are more facilitative than others. Baumrind's parenting typologies are an excellent example of this approach (Baumrind, 1971).

Fredricks and Eccles (2005) offer yet one more integrative approach. Building on risk and resilience models of cumulative risk, we assessed whether each family had relatively high levels of each of several different parental beliefs and practices related to both school and sport achievement (see also Simpkins, Davis-Kean, Eccles, 2005; Simpkins et al., 2006). They then created a new construct based on the sum of these practices to estimate the extent to which the family environment included no, a few, or many supports for their children's domain-specific ability self-concepts, subjective task values, and activity engagement. As predicted, the number of such supports was linearly related to increases over time in the children's ability self-concepts, subjective task values, activity participation, and performance even when prior levels of these child characteristics were controlled. In contrast, when all these family predictors were entered into a regression model, parents' expectations for their child performance trumped all other influences, suggesting that parents' behavior did not matter. Clearly this was not the case in the pattern-centered analyses, suggesting that researchers need to be careful when they use regression-type approaches with a set of predictors that are inherently correlated with each other.

One critical factor that is not apparent on Figure 26.2 is the developmental timing of all these practices. In the very first empirical study of parental influences on the development of achievement motivation, Winterbottom (1958) asked about the proper timing of parents' socialization demands for facilitating their children's general achievement motivation. She demonstrated the importance of appropriate developmental timing—a finding that has been widely replicated (see Eccles et al., 1998). Parents need to provide challenging but doable tasks and to provide adequate scaffolding for the children to succeed. These studies suggest that early family influences may be critical for supporting the development of general achievement motivation. Early opportunities to acquire the skills needed for a successful transition into school are also important for school achievement (Shonkoff & Phillips, 2000). Early skill socialization may also be critical for successful, high-level engagement with other skill-based areas as well. We know less about the role parents play in supporting high domain-specific ability self-concepts and subjective task values as children get older. The work of Fredericks and Eccles (2005) and Simpkins et al. (2005; Simpkins et al., 2006) suggests that families of children in elementary and secondary school can support their children's ability self-concepts, subjective task values, and engagement in both academic and nonacademic skill areas by combining high expectations for their children's success with high levels of behavioral and psychological support for their participation in these activities. However, it seems likely that at some point, parents need to let their adolescent children take more and more control over their own engagement choices. There have been very few studies of these developmental changes in the nature of parents' support for high achievement-related engagements.

Another factor that is not readily apparent in Figure 26.2 is the need to look at family influences in conjunction with the many other influences on children's development. The importance of family involvement in their children's schooling is an excellent example of the need to take a broader ecological perspective on the multidimensional role of families and other contexts in facilitating children's achievement strivings and accomplishments (Bronfenbrenner & Morris, 1998). Parents have a very important role to play in mediating their children's interactions with other organizations and institutions (Comer, Haynes, Joyner, & Ben-Avie, 1996; Eccles & Harold, 1996; Epstein, 1992; Lareau, 2003). With regard to school, they do this by helping prepare their children for the transition into school, by helping their children with homework and other school-related activities, and by getting involved more directly with their children's schools in a variety of ways. We know such practices are very important in supporting positive achievement motivation (e.g., Pomerantz & Eaton, 2001; Pomerantz et al., 2005). Izzo, Weissberg, Kasprow, and Fredrich (1999) found that parents' involvement in their children's academic lives both at home and at school predicts improved classroom behavior and academic achievement several years later. Furthermore, both Grolnick (2003) and Lord et al. (1994) found that having supportive and involved parents eases adolescents' transition to middle and junior high school. The kinds of general and child-specific beliefs proposed in Figure 26.2 are likely to influence the ways in which parents choose to interact with their children's schooling (Comer, et al., 1996; Eccles & Harold, 1996; Lareau, 1989, 2003). Grolnick, Benjet, Kurowski, and Apostoleris (1997) found that mothers who are confident of their own abilities to impact school, who see being a teacher as part of their parental role, and who do not see their child as difficult are most likely to be involved in their children's homework. Conversely, stereotypes that teachers and school administrators have about children's families likely influence the ways in which the schools reach out to parents (Booth & Dunn, 1996; Comer, et al., 1996; Epstein, 1992; Lareau, 1989). Work by both Epstein (1992) and Grolnick et al. (1997) has shown that parents are more likely to be involved at their children's school if they believe the teachers welcome their participation. Unfortunately, there has been very limited research on this critical interface (i.e., school–family) and even less research on the interface between families and the many other institutions that influence children's development. This is a very important area for future research efforts.

SCHOOL INFLUENCES ON ACHIEVEMENT

In this section, I review the work on school influences on achievement-related beliefs, behaviors, and choices. I focus on school, teacher, and classroom influences. Much of the research I review is directly related to a notion inherent in person–environment fit perspectives: Motivation is optimized in learning settings that meet individual's basic and developmental needs, some of which are universal and some of which are a function of individual differences in aptitudes, temperament, interests, and socialization histories (Eccles & Midgley, 1989; Hunt, 1979; Ryan & Deci, 2002). The exact nature of the basic or universal needs has been articulated in various ways. Deci, Ryan, Connell, and their colleagues focus attention on three basic or universal needs: competence, relatedness, and autonomy (Ryan & Deci, 2002). Eccles and Gootman (2002) suggested that the need to matter (e.g., to make a real and meaningful difference in one's social world) is an additional universal value likely to influence achievement-related motivation particularly as individuals mature into and through adolescence. Similarly, both Ryff and Singer (1998) and Pomerantz et al. (2005) suggest that experiencing oneself as purposeful may also be a universal need. Eccles, Midgley, et al. (1993) articulated a set of changing developmental needs that are often not met in school settings as children move from elementary school into secondary school. Each of these theorists argues that individuals will place high value, will have high expectations for success, and will be optimally motivated to engage in the learning activities in settings that provide opportunities for them to fulfill their universal developmental and individual needs, and that individuals will withdraw their engagement in learning in settings that do not provide such opportunities.

Social Experiences Related to Competence Needs

Teachers' General Expectations and Sense of Their Own Efficacy

Both teachers' general expectations for their students' performance and general belief in the ability of all students to master the material being taught predict students' school achievement likely through their impact on students' sense of competence: When teachers hold high general expectations for student achievement and students perceive these expectations, students achieve more and experience a greater sense of competence as learners (Eccles et al., 1998; Lee & Smith, 2001; National Research Council, 2004). Similarly, teachers who feel they are able to reach even the most difficult students, who believe in their ability to affect students' lives, and who believe that teachers are an important factor in determining developmental outcomes communicate such positive expectations and beliefs to their students, which, in turn, increases students' confidence in their ability to learn and engagement in school-based learning tasks (Jackson & Davis, 2000; Lee & Smith, 2001; National Research Council, 2004; Roeser, Marachi, & Gelhbach, 2002; Roeser, Eccles, & Samerott, 1998).

Differential Teacher Expectations

Equally important are the differential expectations teachers hold for various individuals within the same classroom. However, because teacher-expectancy effects are mediated by the ways in which teachers interact with the students for whom they have high versus low expectations, whether these effects are positive or negative depends on the exact nature of these interactions (Jussim, Eccles, & Madon, 1996). For example, a teacher might respond to low expectation by providing the kinds of help and structure that increase students' sense of competence and ability to master the material being presented. Alternatively, the teacher might respond in ways that communicate low expectations and little hope that the students will be able to master the material, leading to decreases in students' confidence in their own ability and then lowered academic engagement. Unfortunately, we know very little about which teachers are likely to respond in each of these styles and under what conditions teachers are more or less likely to respond with either of these styles. Most of the research on teacher-expectancy effects assumes that teachers are most likely to respond in ways that leads to fulfilling their expectations; consequently, the data collected have not allowed for a very differentiated study of these processes.

A great deal of the research work on teacher expectancy effects has focused on differential treatment related to gender, race/ethnic group, and/or social class. There are small but fairly consistent negative effects of low teacher expectations on girls (for math and science), on minority children (for all subject areas), and on children from lower social class family backgrounds (again for all subject areas) (Jussim et al., 1996). In addition, some of these studies have documented the cumulative negative effects of low teacher expectations on some groups of students' ability self-perceptions (Madon et al., 1998; Smith, Jussim, & Eccles, 1999). In contrast, the evidence for either negative or positive teacher-expectancy effects for other student populations is quite weak.

General Classroom Practices

Rosenholtz and Simpson (1984) hypothesized that individualized versus whole group instruction, ability-grouping practices, and the relatively public versus private nature of feedback work together to create a classroom environment that fundamentally shapes children's school motivation through their impact on the students' sense of competence. Specifically, they argued that these practices make ability differences salient and, thereby, undermine motivation, particularly of low-achieving students, by increasing the salience of extrinsic motivators and ego-focused learning goals. Such motivational orientations, in turn, are hypothesized to lead to greater incidence of social comparison behaviors and increased perception of one's abilities as fixed entities rather than malleable ones. The work of Midgley, Maehr, and their colleagues showed that school reform efforts designed to reduce these types of classroom practices, particularly those associated with socially comparative feedback and reward systems and teachers' use of competitive motivational strategies, have positive consequences for adolescents' academic motivation, persistence on difficult learning tasks, and socioemotional development (Maehr & Midgley, 1996; Midgley, 2002).

Academic Tracks/Curricular Differentiation

Curricular tracking (e.g., college track course sequences vs. general or vocational education sequences) is another important school-level contextual feature that can affect students' expectations for success (Oakes, Gamoran, & Page, 1992). However, despite years of research on the impact of tracking practices, few strong and definitive answers have emerged. The results vary depending on the outcome assessed, the group studied, the length of the study, the control groups used for comparison, and the specific nature of the context in which these practices are manifest. The situation is further complicated by the fact that conflicting hypotheses about the likely direction and the magnitude of the effect emerge depending on the theoretical lens one uses to evaluate the practice. The best justification for these practices derives from a person–environment fit perspective. Students are more motivated to learn if the material can be adapted to their current competence level. There is some evidence consistent with this perspective for children placed in high-ability classrooms, high within-class ability groups, and college tracks (Fuligni, Eccles, & Barber, 1995; Gamoran & Mare, 1989; Pallas et al., 1994). In contrast, the results for adolescents placed in low-ability and noncollege tracks do not generally confirm this hypothesis. By and large, when long-term effects are found for this group of students, they are negative primarily because these adolescents are typically provided with inferior educational experience and support (Pallas et al., 1994; Oakes et al., 1992; Rosenbaum, & Kulieke, 1988). Low-track placement is related to poor attitudes toward school, feelings of incompetence, and problem behaviors both within school (nonattendance, crime, misconduct) and in the broader community (drug use, arrests) as well as to educational attainments (Oakes et al., 1992).

Another important and controversial aspect of curriculum tracking involves how students get placed in different classes and how difficult it is for students to move between class levels as their academic needs and competencies change once initial placements have been made. These issues are important both early in a child's school career (e.g., Pallas et al., 1994) and later in adolescence when course placement is linked directly to the kinds of educational options that are available to the student after high school. Minority youth, particularly African American and Hispanic boys, are more likely to be assigned to low-ability classes and non-college-bound curricular tracks than other groups; furthermore, many of these youth were sufficiently competent to be placed in higher-ability-level classes (Dornbusch, 1994; Oakes et al., 1992).

Social Experiences Related to Belonging Needs

Teacher–Student Relationships

Many researchers have stressed the importance of teacher–student or coach–player relationships for optimal engagement in a variety of achievement settings (e.g., Ryan & Deci, 2002; Wentzel, 1998). Consistent with these suggestions, there is strong evidence for the importance of positive teacher–student relationships and a sense of belonging for children's development in school (Anderman, 1999; Furrer & Skinner, 2003; Lynch &

Cicchetti, 1997; Wentzel, 2005). Teachers who are trusting, caring, and respectful of students provide the kind of socioemotional support students need to approach, engage, and persist on academic learning tasks and to develop positive achievement-related self-perceptions and values, high self-esteem, and a sense of belonging and emotional comfort at school (Eccles et al., 1998; Goodenow, 1993; Roeser & Eccles, 1998; Roeser, Midgley, & Urdan, 1996).

Extracurricular Activities

Schools differ in the extent to which they provide a variety of extracurricular activities for their students. Research on extracurricular activities has documented a positive link between adolescents' extracurricular activities and high school grade point average, strong school engagement, and high educational aspirations (Eccles, Barber, Stone, & Hunt, 2003; Eccles & Templeton, 2002). This work has also documented the protective value of extracurricular activity participation in reducing dropout rates as well as involvement in delinquent and other risky behaviors (Mahoney & Cairns, 1997; McNeal, 1995). Participation in sports, in particular, has been linked to lower likelihood of school dropout and higher rates of college attendance (Eccles & Barber, 1999; McNeal, 1995), especially among low-achieving and blue-collar male athletes. These effects likely reflect several processes: (1) the impact of extracurricular activities on students' sense of belonging in the school, (2) the impact of extracurricular activities on the increased likelihood of participation leading to good relationships with particular teachers, and (3) the impact of students' own goals on the decision to participate in extracurricular activities (i.e., the students' perceptions of profitable and effective means of gaining admission to college).

Social Experiences Related to Autonomy Needs

Many researchers believe that classroom practices that support student autonomy are critical for fostering intrinsic motivation to learn (Deci & Ryan, 1985). Support for this hypothesis has been found in both laboratory and field-based studies (Deci & Ryan, 1985; Lepper & Henderlong, 2000). Closely related to this idea is the work showing the negative impact of excessive use of praise and rewards for participation in school tasks on students' intrinsic interest in these tasks (Lepper & Henderlong, 2000). It is likely that such rewards undermine students' sense of autonomy.

However, it is also critical that teachers support student autonomy in a context of adequate structure and orderliness (Skinner & Belmont, 1993). This issue is complicated by the fact that the right balance between adult-guided structure and opportunities for student autonomy changes as the students mature: older students desire more opportunities for autonomy and less adult-controlled structure (Eccles et al., 1993). To the extent that the students do not experience these changes in the balance between structure and opportunities for autonomy as they pass through the K–12 school years, their school motivation should decline as they get older. I discuss this more later.

Social Experiences That Support Interest

Many researchers believe that the meaningfulness of the academic work to the students' interests and goals influences sustained attention, high investment of cognitive and affective resources in learning, and strong identification with educational goals and aims through its impact on the interest value of the work (Hidi & Harackiewicz, 2000; National Research Council, 2004). In general, research supports this hypothesis: For example, students' reports of high levels of boredom in school, low interest, and perceived irrelevance of the curriculum are associated with poor attention, diminished achievement, disengagement, and, finally, alienation from school (Hidi & Harackiewicz, 2000; Jackson & Davis, 2000; National Research Council, 2004; Roeser et al., 1998). Unfortunately, evidence from several different perspectives suggests that the curriculum to which most students are exposed is often not particularly meaningful from either a cultural or a developmental perspective. Several researchers suggest that the disconnect of traditional curricula from the experiences of several cultural groups can explain the alienation of some group members from the educational process, sometimes leading to school dropout (Fine, 1991; Gallimore & Goldenberg, 2001; Sheets & Hollins, 1999). There is also a disconnect between increases in students' cognitive sophistication, life experiences, and identity needs and the nature of the curriculum as students move from the elementary into the secondary school years (Jackson & Davis, 2000; Lee & Smith, 2001; National Research Council, 2004). As one indication of this, middle school students report higher rates of boredom than elementary school students when doing schoolwork, especially passive work (e.g., listening to lectures), especially in social studies, math, and science (Larson & Richards, 1991). This could lead to some of the apathy problems discussed earlier.

Recently, educational researchers who focus on the concept of interest have made a distinction between situational interest and personal interest (Hidi, 2001; Renninger, Ewan, & Lasher, 2002). These scholars have identified a number of task characteristics that elicit sufficient situation interest in students to motivate their engagement with academic tasks. These characteristics include the kinds of teaching styles mentioned previously, along with novelty and challenge coupled with some familiarity with the content being taught. Such characteristics are likely to elicit curiosity and the desire to learn. Much of this work has focused on characteristics of text that motivate students to read and study the material. For example, there are significant relations between interest and deep-level learning (e.g., recall of main ideas, coherence of recall, responding to deeper comprehension questions, and representation of meaning; Eccles et al., 1998). Findings by Hidi (2001) suggest that attentional processes, affect, and persistence may mediate the effects of interest on text learning. These scholars, Renninger and Hidi in particular, are beginning to investigate the characteristics of educational experiences that facilitate situational interests becoming more enduring personal interests that will motivate continued engagement with academic tasks. This work will have very important developmental and educational implications.

Experiences Related to the Need to Matter

There is growing interest in the decline in adolescents' engagement and performance in school. One intervention that is being tried to reduce this decline is the provision of opportunities to participate in service learning during high school (Eccles & Templeton, 2002). Advocates of this approach suggest that it is critical for adolescents to learn by being involved in their communities in order to develop good citizenship skills and achievement motivation. Such experiences, however, also provide a wonderful opportunity for adolescents to feel as if they are doing something that really matters to their school and their community. Evidence is beginning to accumulate supporting the positive impact of such experiences on adolescents' engagement in the learning agenda of their schools (Eccles & Templeton, 2002). These experiences also reduce the likelihood that students who are doing poorly on the academic tasks of secondary school will drop out of high school prior to graduation.

Experiences of Racial/Ethnic Discrimination in Classrooms

Researchers interested in the relatively poor academic performance of children from some ethnic/racial groups have suggested another classroom-level experience related to both expectations for one's own performance and the subjective task value for engagement in the learning tasks: experiences of racial/ethnic discrimination (Fordham & Ogbu, 1986; Quintana & Vera, 1999; Roeser et al., 1998; Szalacha et al., 2003; Ruggiero & Taylor, 1995; Wong, Eccles, & Sameroff, 2003). Two types of discrimination have been discussed: (1) anticipation of future discrimination in the labor market which might undermine the long-term benefits of education (Fordham & Ogbu, 1986), and (2) the impact of daily experiences of discrimination on one's mental health and academic motivation (Wong et al., 2003). Wong et al. (2003) found that anticipated future discrimination leads to increases in African American youth's motivation to do well in school, which, in turn, leads to increases in academic performance. In this sample, anticipated future discrimination appeared to motivate the youth to do their very best so that they would be maximally equipped to deal with future discrimination (Eccles, 2004). In contrast, daily experiences of racial discrimination from their peers and teachers led to declines in school engagement, confidence in one's academic competence and grades, and increases in depression and anger. Wong et al. (2003) also found that a strong, positive African-American social identity helped to buffer the negative effects of perceived racial discrimination on school-related motivation and achievement. In a study of Asian, Mexican, Central, and South American immigrant high school students growing up in major metropolitan areas of the United States, the majority of youth reported feeling discriminated against at school by their white classmates and their teachers (Portes & Rumbaut, 2001). Finally, in a sample of Mexican American high school students in California, perceived discrimination in school had a strong, negative multivariate relation to school belonging (Roeser, 2004).

Summary

In this section, I have reviewed what we know about those school experiences likely to support both universal and individual needs. I focused on those school and classroom characteristics and experiences that are likely to either support or undermine students' sense of competence, belonging, autonomy, and mattering, as well as their ability to fulfill their own values, interests, and goals. Thinking of school experiences in these terms is a fairly new approach to the field of educational psychology. It derives from the work by Deci and Ryan (Ryan & Deci, 2002) on self-determination theory and the work on person and stage–environment fit theories of motivation and human development (e.g., Covington, 1992; Eccles et al., 1993; Eccles & Midgley, 1989; Hunt, 1979; Maehr & Midgley, 1996). By and large, the results are consistent with the prediction that achievement motivation and school engagement is supported by school characteristics that facilitate the person–context fit. Few studies, however, look at multiple characteristics and their fit with multiple needs simultaneously so we have no idea whether some of these needs are more important than others and if so, for whom? We also do not know what keeps young people engaged in school and other skill-based learning contexts when many of their needs are not being met by the context. Finally, we know little about which features of the learning context influence which aspects of engagement. More research is badly needed to answer such questions.

CONCLUSION

There is growing evidence that experiences both at home and in various school/learning contexts influence children and adolescents' motivation to achieve, defined in terms of self and task beliefs, and engagement. Interestingly, the best-integrated explanations for these influences come from a person–environment fit perspective, coupled with a skill-training perspective. In both contexts, children learn the valued skills if they feel support for their universal needs (e.g., a sense of competence, a feeling of belonging, a sense of autonomy or personal ownership of one's actions, and a sense of mattering) and personal needs (personal and social identity needs, temperament and aptitude-based needs, and interests). Early in life, parents and other socializers likely play a critical role in facilitating the acquisition of general motivational orientations toward mastery, curiosity, and the self-regulation of one's effort and attention. Parents and socializers also structure the types of activities to which the child are exposed, thus influencing the specific skills that children acquire and the opportunities the children have to develop domain-specific ability self-concepts and interests. As children mature, they begin to encounter other social contexts such as schools, peer groups, sports' and arts' programs, and so on. Again, the children's engagement in the learning opportunities provided in each of these contexts appears to depend on the fit between these contexts and the children's universal and personal needs. If the fit is good, the children will engage in the learning opportunities provided. What they learn will depend on what is being taught and how well it is being taught.

If the fit is not good, the children are likely either to disengage from that context altogether or to engage in a variety of behaviors designed to protect their sense of self-worth even if these behaviors conflict with mastering the learning opportunities provided in that context (Covington, 1992). Disengagement can take the form of withdrawing energy and personal resources from the activities inherent in the setting. For example, at school students may stop paying attention in class and doing homework assignments; they may also stop caring about doing well on tests and in their courses; they may increase the amount of time they are truant and may stop attending school at all; and, finally, they may disconnect their sense of self-worth from any of the feedback they receive from teachers and other school personnel. The same can happen with their engagement in their families. In each of these examples, poor person–environment fit may lead to withdrawal from institutions and contexts that are supposed to support positive development. What will the youth do? Given that we are a very adaptive species, it is likely that the youth will seek out other settings in which their needs can be met. Where will these youth turn to have their needs met: perhaps to their peer groups or to other organizations and settings. If these settings provide positive developmental experiences that support healthy development, these youth may do fine. But what if these settings reinforce less positive developmental trajectories—trajectories that decrease the likelihood of a successful transition into adulthood or trajectories that increase the likelihood of very risky outcomes? It is this latter possibility that we need to avoid by providing our young people with better options and more supportive developmental contexts.

Where should research efforts go now? My focus in this chapter has been on the potential impact of two major socialization contexts on the development of children and adolescents' achievement motivation, engagement, and performance: the family and the school. Most of the existing research has looked at these two contexts quite separately, using different theoretical frameworks and different methods of study. Thus, despite increasing calls for more integrated, cross-context studies that allow one to investigate the full complexity of social experience on human development, we know very little about how these two contexts interact with each other over time to both influence and accommodate to human development. I reviewed some of the few studies that look at family–school interactions. We need many more such studies and we need integrative studies that look more comprehensively at the interaction of these two contexts with each other over time and across a much wider variety of populations. We know, for example, that even very active parents decrease their participation in their children's schooling as their children move into, and through, secondary school (Eccles & Harold, 1996). Why? And what are the consequences of this withdrawal for various types of children? We also know that culture plays a major role in the extent to which, and the matter in which, parents get involved with their children's schooling (Booth & Dunn, 1996; Epstein, 1992; Lareau & Horvat, 1999; Rogoff, 2003; Suarez-Orozco & Suarez-Orozco, 2001). We know less about the consequences of these differences for the families, children, and schools (Gallimore & Goldenberg, 2001). Similarly, we know relatively little about the consequences of the fit between the culture and language of the home and the culture and language of the school. Extensive work is now being done on issues related to the fit of languages—work in bilingual versus total immersion language programs, for example (Brisk, 1998). Such issues are currently critical to the American educational system and will become even more critical in years to come as the proportion of children from immigrant and ethnic minority families continues to increase.

We know even less about the interface between families and the many other important contexts in which children have the opportunity to learn and manifest achievement motivation (contexts such as sports programs, faith-based activity settings, summer programs, music and art programs, etc.) The family management perspective outlined earlier provides one framework for looking more closely at the relation between the family context and these other institutions and settings. Parents are an important source of social capital in that they can connect their children to a wide variety of resources and opportunities (Furstenberg et al., 1999). They can also intervene on behalf of their children when other contexts and institutions are not providing the kinds of supports their children need. Finally, they can help their children navigate various out-of-home contexts in ways that support their children's achievement motivation and engagement. As noted earlier, the extent to which parents can successfully play these roles, of course, depends on a wide variety of personal and contextual characteristics. We know very little about these processes.

Finally, despite increasing concern with the need to look at bidirectional effects, most of the research in both of these fields has focused on the impact of socialization experiences on the child. Yet we know that children influence the reactions of parents, teachers, coaches, peers, and other social agents. In addition, children themselves are active agents in their own achievement-related choices and are active agents in moderating the influence of social agents on their development. Much more research is needed on these processes.

REFERENCES

Alexander, K. L., Entwisle, D. R., & Bedinger, S. D. (1994). When expectations work: Race and socioeconomic differences in school performance. *Social Psychology Quarterly 57*, 283–299.

Ambady, N., Shih, M., & Kim, A. (2001). Stereotype susceptibility in children: Effects of identity activation on quantitative performance. *Psychological Science, 12*, 385–390.

Anderman, L. H. (1999). Classroom goal orientation, school belonging and social goals as predictors of students' positive and negative affect following the transition to middle school. *Journal of Research and Development in Education, 32*, 89–103.

Bandura, A. (1997). *Self-efficacy: The exercise of control.* New York: Freeman.

Barber, B., & Eccles, J. S. (1992). A developmental view of the impact of divorce and single parenting on children and adolescents. *Psychological Bulletin, 111*, 108–126.

Baumrind, D. (1971). Current patterns of parental authority. *Developmental Psychology, 4*, 1–103.

Booth, A., & Dunn, J. (Eds.). (1996). *Family–school links: How do they affect educational outcomes.* Hillsdale, NJ: Erlbaum.

Brisk, M. (1998). *Bilingual education: From compensatory to quality schooling.* Mahwah, NJ: Erlbaum.

Bronfenbrenner, U., & Morris, P. A. (1998). The ecology of environmental processes. In W. Damon (Series Ed.) & R. M. Lerner (Vol. Ed.), *Handbook of child psychology* (5th ed., Vol. 1, pp. 993–1028). New York: Wiley.

Brooks-Gunn, J., Linver, M. R., & Fauth, R. C. (2005). Children's competence and socioeconomic status in the family and neighborhood. In A. J. Elliot & C. S. Dweck (Eds.), *Handbook of competence and motivation* (pp. 414–435). New York: Guilford Press.

Clark, R. (1993). Homework parenting practices that positively affect student achievement. In N. F. Chavkin (Ed.), *Families and schools in a pluralistic society* (pp. 53–71). Albany: State University of New York Press.

Coleman, J. S., Campbell, E. Q., Hobson, C. J., McPartland, J., Mood, A., Weinfeld, F. D., et al. (1966). *Equality of educational opportunity.* Washington, DC: U.S. Government Printing Office.

Comer, J. P., Haynes, N. M., Joyner, E. T., & Ben-Avie, M. (Eds.). (1996). *Rallying the whole village: The Comer process for reforming education.* New York: Teachers College Press.

Conger, R. D., Wallace, L. E., Sun, Y., Simons, R. L., McLoyd, V. C., & Brody G. H. (2002). Economic pressure in African American families: A replication and extension of the family stress model. *Developmental Psychology, 38*, 179–193.

Connell, J. P., Halpern-Felsher, B. L., Clifford, E., Crichlow, W., & Usinger, P. (1995). Hanging in there: Behavioral, psychological, and contextual factors affecting whether African-American adolescents stay in high school. *Journal of Adolescent Research, 10*, 41–63.

Covington, M. V. (1992). *Making the grade: A self-worth perspective on motivation and school reform.* New York: Cambridge University Press.

Crystal, D. S., & Stevenson, H. W. (1991). Mothers' perceptions of children's problems with mathematics: A cross-national comparison. *Journal of Educational Psychology, 83*, 372–376.

Davis-Kean, P. E., & Eccles, J. S. (2003). Influences and barriers to better parent-school collaborations. *The LSS Review, 2*, 4–5.

Davis-Kean, P. E., Eccles, J. S., & Schnabel, K. U. (2002, August). *How the home environment socializes a child: The influence of SES on child outcomes.* Paper presented at the International Society for the Study of Behavioral Development, Ottawa, Canada.

Davis-Kean, P. E., Malanchuk, O., Peck, S. C., & Eccles, J. S. (2003). *Parental influence on academic outcomes: Do race and SES matter?* Paper presented at the biennial meeting of the Society for Research on Child Development, Tampa, FL.

DeBaryshe, B. D. (1995). Maternal belief systems: Linchpin in the home reading process. *Journal of Applied Developmental Psychology, 16*, 1–20.

Deci, E. L., & Ryan, R. M. (1985). *Intrinsic motivation and self-determination in human behavior.* New York: Plenum Press.

Dornbusch, S. M. (1994). *Off the track.* Presidential address at the biennial meeting of the Society for Research on Adolescence, San Diego, CA.

Dweck, C. S. (1999). *Self-theories: Their role in motivational, personality, and development.* Philadelphia: Taylor & Francis.

Eccles, J. S. (1993). School and family effects on the ontogeny of children's interests, self-perceptions, and activity choice. In J. Jacobs (Ed.), *Nebraska symposium on motivation, 1992: Developmental perspectives on motivation* (pp. 145–208) Lincoln: University of Nebraska Press.

Eccles, J. S. (1994). Understanding women's educational and occupational choices: Applying the Eccles et al. model of achievement-related choices. *Psychology of Women Quarterly, 18*, 585–609.

Eccles, J. S. (2004, March). *Race as a developmental context for adolescent development.* Presidential address, Society for Research on Adolescence, Baltimore, MD.

Eccles, J. S., & Barber, B. L. (1999). Student council, volunteering, basketball, or marching band: What kind of extracurricular involvement matters? *Journal of Adolescent Research, 14*, 10–43.

Eccles, J. S., Barber, B. L., Stone, M., & Hunt, J. (2003). Extracurricular activities and adolescent development. *Journal of Social Issues, 59*, 865–889.

Eccles, J. S., & Gootman, J. (Eds.). (2002). *Community programs to promote youth development.* Washington, D.C.: National Academy Press.

Eccles, J., & Harold, R. (1996). Family involvement in children's and adolescents' schooling. In A. Booth, & J. Dunn (Eds.), *Family–school links: How do they affect educational outcomes* (pp. 3–34). Hillsdale, NJ: Erlbaum.

Eccles, J. S., Jacobs, J., Harold, R., Yoon, K. S., Arbreton, A., & Freedman-Doan, C. (1993). Parents and gender role socialization during the middle childhood and adolescent years. In S. Oskamp & M. Costanzo (Eds.), *Gender issues in contemporary society* (pp. 59–83). Newbury Park, CA: Sage.

Eccles, J.S., & Midgley, C. (1989). Stage-environment fit: Developmentally appropriate classrooms for early adolescents. In R. Ames & C. Ames (Eds.), *Research on motivation in education* (Vol. 3, pp. 139–181). New York: Academic Press.

Eccles, J. S., Midgley, C., Buchanan, C. M., Wigfield, A., Reuman, D., & MacIver, D. (1993). Developmental during adolescence: The impact of stage/environment fit. *American Psychologist, 48*, 90–101.

Eccles, J. S., & Templeton, J. (2002). Extracurricular and other after-school activities for youth. *Review of Research in Education, 26*, 113–180.

Eccles, J. S., Wigfield, A., & Schiefele, U. (1998). Motivation to succeed. In W. Damon (Series Ed.) & N. Eisenberg (Volume Ed.), *Handbook of child psychology* (5th ed., Vol. III, pp. 1017–1095). New York: Wiley.

Eccles-Parsons, J., Adler, T. F., Futterman, R., Goff, S. B., Kaczala, & C. M., Meece, J. L., (1983). Expectancies, values, and academic behaviors. In J. T. Spence (Ed.), *Achievement and achievement motivations* (pp. 75–146). San Francisco: Freeman.

Elder, G. H., Eccles, J. S., Ardelt, M., & Lord, S. (1995). Inner-city parents under economic pressure: Perspectives on the strategies of parenting. *Journal of Marriage and the Family, 6*, 81–86.

Entwisle, D. R., & Alexander, K. L. (1990). Beginning school math competence: Minority and majority comparisons. *Child Development, 61*, 454–471.

Epstein, J. L. (1992). School and family partnerships. In M. Alkin (Ed.), *Encyclopedia of educational research* (pp 1139–1151). New York: MacMillan.

Fine, M. (1991). *Framing dropouts: Notes on the politics of an urban public high school.* Albany: State University of New York Press.

Fordham, S., & Ogbu, J. U. (1986). Black students' school success: Coping with "the burden of 'acting white.'" *The Urban Review, 18*, 176–206.

Fredricks, J. A., & Eccles, J. S. (2002). Children's competence and value beliefs from childhood through adolescence: Growth trajectories in two male sex-typed domains. *Developmental Psychology, 38*, 519–533.

Fredricks, J. A., & Eccles, J. S. (2005). Family socialization, gender, and sport motivation and involvement. *Journal of Sport and Exercise Psychology, 27*, 3–31.

Frodi, A., Bridges, L., & Grolnick, W. S. (1985). Correlates of mastery-related behavior: A short-term longitudinal study of infants in their second year. *Child Development, 56,* 1291–1298.

Frome, P. M., & Eccles, J. S. (1998). Parents' influence on children's achievement-related perceptions. *Journal of Personality and Social Psychology, 74,* 435–452.

Fuligni, A. J., Eccles, J. S., Barber, B. L. (1995). The long-term effects of seventh-grade ability grouping in mathematics. *Journal of Early Adolescence, 15,* 58–89.

Fuligni, A. J., Yip, T., & Tseng, V. (2002). The impact of family obligation on the daily activities and psychological well-being of Chinese American adolescents. *Child Development, 73,* 302–314.

Furrer, C., & Skinner, E. (2003). Sense of relatedness as a factor in children's academic engagement and performance. *Journal of Educational Psychology, 95,* 148–162.

Furstenberg, F., Cook, T., Eccles, J., Elder, G., & Sameroff, A. (1999). *Managing to make it: Urban families in adolescent success.* Chicago: University of Chicago Press.

Gallimore, R., & Goldenberg, C. (2001). Analyzing cultural models and settings to connect minority achievement and school improvement research . *Educational Psychologist, 36,* 45–56.

Gamoran, A., & Mare, R. D. (1989). Secondary school tracking and educational inequality: Compensation, reinforcement, or neutrality? *American Journal of Sociology, 94,* 1146–1183.

Garcia Coll, C., & Pachter, L. M. (2002). Ethnic and minority parenting. In M. Bornstein (Ed.), *Handbook of parenting (2nd ed., Vol. 4, pp. 1–20).* Mahwah, NJ: Erlbaum.

Goodnow, C. (1993). Classroom belonging among early adolescent students: Relationships to motivation and achievement. *Journal of Early Adolescence, 13,* 21–43.

Goodnow, J. J., & Collins, W. A. (1990). *Development according to parents: The nature, sources, and consequences of parents' ideas.* London: Erlbaum.

Grolnick, W. S. (2003). *The psychology of parental control: How well-meant parenting backfires.* Hillside, NJ: Erlbaum.

Grolnick, W. S., Benjet, C., Kurowski, C. O., & Apostoleris, N. H. (1997). Predictors of parent involvement in children's schooling. *Journal of Educational Psychology, 89,* 538–548.

Grolnick, W. S., & Slowiaczek, M. L. (1994). Parents' involvement in children's schooling: A multidimensional conceptualization and motivational model. *Child Development, 65,* 237–252.

Gutman, L. M., Sameroff, A. J., & Eccles, J. S. (2002). The academic achievement of African American students during early adolescence: An examination of multiple risk, promotive, and protective factors. *American Journal of Community Psychology, 30,* 367–399.

Hess, R. D., Chih-Mei, C., & McDevitt, T. M. (1987). Cultural variations in family beliefs about children's performance in mathematics: Comparisons among People's Republic of China, Chinese-American, and Caucasian-American families. *Journal of Educational Psychology, 70,* 179–188.

Hidi, S. (2001). Interest, reading, and learning: Theoretical and practical considerations. *Educational Psychology Review, 13,* 191–209.

Hidi, S., & Harackiewicz, J. (2000). Motivating the academically unmotivated: A critical issue for the 21st century. *Review of Educational Research, 70,* 151–180.

Holloway, S. D. (1988). Concepts of ability and effort in Japan and the United States. *Review of Educational Research, 58,* 327–345.

Hunt, D. E. (1979). Person–environment interaction: A challenge found wanting before it was tried. *Review of Educational Research, 45,* 209–230.

Iyengar, S. S., & Lepper, M. R. (1999). Rethinking the value of choice: A cultural perspective on intrinsic motivation. *Journal of Personality and Social Psychology, 76,* 349–366.

Izzo, C. V., Weissberg, R. P., Kasprow, W. J., & Fendrich, M. (1999). A longitudinal assessment of teacher perceptions of parent involvement in children's education and school performance. *American Journal of Community Psychology, 76,* 349–366.

Jackson, A. W., & Davis, G. A. (2000). *Turning points 2000: Educating adolescents in the 21st century.* New York: Teachers College Press.

Jacobs, J., Davis-Kean, P. E., Bleeker, M., Eccles, J. S., & Malanchuk, O. (2005). "I can do it but I don't want to." The impact of parents, interests, and activities on gender differences in math. In A. Gallagher & J. Kaufman (Eds.), *Gender differences in mathematics* (pp. 246–263). New York: Cambridge University Press.

Jacobs, J. E., & Eccles, J. S. (2000). Parents, task values, and real-life achievement-related choices. In C. Sansone & J. M. Harackiewicz (Eds.), *Intrinsic and extrinsic motivation: The search for optimal motivation and performance* (pp. 405–439). San Diego, CA: Academic Press.

Jacobs, J. E., Hyatt, S., Osgood, W. D., Eccles, J. S., & Wigfield, A. (2002). Changes in children's self-competence and values: Gender and domain differences across grades one through twelve. *Child Development, 73*(2), 509–527.

Jussim, L., Eccles, J., & Madon, S. (1996). Social perception, social stereotypes, and teacher expectations: Accuracy and the quest for the powerful self-fulfilling prophecy. In L. Berkowitz (Ed.), *Advances in experimental social psychology* (pp. 281–388). New York: Academic Press.

Kohn, M. L. (1977). *Class and conformity: A study in values, with a reassessment.* Chicago: University of Chicago Press.

Laosa, L. M. (1999). Intercultural transitions in human development and education. *Journal of Applied Developmental Psychology, 20,* 355–406.

Lareau, A. (1989). *Home advantage: Social class and parental intervention in elementary education.* London: Falmer.

Lareau, A. (2003). *Unequal childhood: Class, race, and family life.* Berkeley, CA: University of California Press.

Lareau, A., & Horvat, E. M. (1999). Moments of social inclusion and exclusion: Race, class and cultural capital in family-school relationships. *Sociology of Education, 72,* 37–53.

Larson, R., & Richards, M. H. (1991). Daily companionship in late childhood and early adolescence: Changing developmental contexts. *Child Development, 62,* 284–300.

Lee, V. E., & Smith, J. (2001). *Restructuring high schools for equity and excellence: What works.* New York: Teachers College Press.

Lepper, M. R., & Henderlong, J. (2000). Turning "play" into "work" and "work" into "play": 25 years of research on intrinsic versus extrinsic motivation. In C. Sansone & J. M. Harackiewicz (Eds.), *Intrinsic and extrinsic motivation: The search for optimal motivation and performance* (pp. 257–307). New York: Academic Press.

Linver, M. R., Brooks-Gunn, J., & Kohen, D. E. (2002). Family processes as pathways from income to young children's development. *Developmental Psychology, 38,* 719–734.

Lord, S., Eccles, J. S., & McCarthy, K. (1994). Risk and protective factors in the transition to junior high school. *Journal of Early Adolescence, 14,* 162–199.

Lynch, M., & Cicchetti, D. (1997). Children's relationships with adults and peers: An examination of elementary and junior high school students. *Journal of School Psychology, 35,* 81–99.

Madon, S., Jussim, L., Keiper, S., Eccles, J., Smith, A., & Palumbo, P. (1998). The accuracy and power of sex, social class, and ethnic stereotypes: A naturalistic study in person perception. *Society for Personality and Social Psychology, 24,* 1304–1318.

Maehr, M. L., & Midgley, C. (1996). *Transforming school cultures.* Boulder, CO: Westview Press.

Magnuson, K. (2003). *The effect of increases in welfare mothers' education on their young children's academic and behavioral outcomes: Evidence from the National Evaluation of Welfare-to-Work Strategies Child outcomes Study* (No. 1274-03). Madison: University of Wisconsin, Institute for Poverty Research.

Mahoney, J. L., & Cairns, R. B. (1997). Do extracurricular activities protect against early school dropout? *Developmental Psychology, 33,* 2414–253.

Marjoribanks, K. (2002). *Family and school capital: Towards a context theory of students' school outcomes.* Dordrecht, The Netherlands: Kluwer Academic.

McGillicuddy-DeLisi, A. V., & Sigel, I. E. (1991). Family environments and children's representational thinking. In S. B. Silvern (Ed.), *Advances in reading/language research* (Vol. 5, pp. 63–90). Easton, PA: JAI Press.

McLloyd, V. C. (1990). The impact of economic hardship on African American families and children: Psychological distress, parenting, and socioemotional development. *Child Development, 61,* 311–346.

McNeal, R. B. (1995). Extracurricular activities and high school dropouts. *Sociology of Education, 68,* 62–81.

Midgley, C. (2002). *Goals, goal structures, and adaptive learning.* Mahwah, NJ: Erlbaum.

Miller, S. A., & Davis, T. L. (1992). Beliefs about children: A comparative study of mothers, teachers, peers, and self. *Child Development, 63,* 1251–1265.

Mistry, R. S., Vandewater, E. A., Huston, A. C., & McLoyd, V. C. (2002). Economic well-being and children's social adjustment: The role of family process in an ethnically diverse low-income sample. *Child Development, 73,* 935–951.

National Research Council. (2004). *Engaging schools: Fostering high school students' motivation to learn.* Washington, DC: National Academies Press.

Ng, F. F., Kenney-Benson, G. A., & Pomerantz, E. M. (2004). Children's achievement moderates the effects of mothers' use of control and autonomy support. *Child Development, 75*, 764–780.

Oakes, J., Gamoran, A., & Page, R. N. (1992). Curriculum differentiation: Opportunities, outcomes, and meanings. In P. Jackson (Ed.), *Handbook of research on curriculum* (pp. 570–608). New York: Macmillan.

Pallas, A. M., Entwisle, D. R., Alexander, K. L., & Stluka. M. F. (1994). Ability-group effects: Instructional, social, or institutional? *Sociology of Education, 67*, 27–46.

Pomerantz, E. M., & Eaton, M. M. (2001). Maternal intrusive support in the academic context: Transactional socialization processes. *Developmental Psychology, 37*, 174–186.

Pomerantz, E. M., Grolnick, W. S., & Price, C. E. (2005). The role of parents in how children approach achievement: A dynamic process perspective. In A.J. Elliot & C.S. Dweck (Eds.), *Handbook of competence and motivation* (pp. 259–278). New York: Guilford Press.

Portes, A., & Rumbaut, R. G. (2001). *Legacies: The story of the immigrant second generation*. Berkeley: University of California Press.

Quintana, S. M., & Vera, E. M. (1999). Mexican-American children's ethnic identity, understanding of ethnic prejudice, and parental ethnic socialization. *Hispanic Journal of Behavioral Sciences, 21*, 387–404.

Renninger, K. A., Ewen, L. & Lasher, A. K. (2002). Individual interest as context in expository text and mathematical word problems. *Learning and Instruction, 12*, 467–491.

Roeser, R. W. (2004, July). *The diversity of selfways in school during adolescence project*. Paper presented at the annual meeting of William T. Grant Faculty Scholars Program, Vail, CO.

Roeser, R. W., & Eccles, J. S. (1998). Adolescents' perceptions of middle school: Relation to longitudinal changes in academic and psychological adjustment. *Journal of Research on Adolescence, 8*, 123–158.

Roeser, R. W., Eccles, J. S., & Sameroff, A. J. (1998). Academic and emotional functioning in early adolescence: Longitudinal relations, patterns, and prediction by experience in middle school. *Development and Psychopathology, 10*, 321–352.

Roeser, R. W., Marachi, R., & Gelhbach, H. (2002). A goal theory perspective on teachers' professional identities and the contexts of teaching. In C.M. Midgley (Ed.), *Goals, goal structures, and patterns of adaptive learning* (pp. 205–241). Mahwah, NJ: Erlbaum.

Roeser, R. W., Midgley, C., & Urdan, T. C. (1996). Perceptions of the school psychological environment and early adolescents' psychological and behavioral functioning in school: The mediating role of goals and belonging. *Journal of Educational Psychology, 88*, 408–422.

Rogoff, B. (2003). *The cultural nature of human development*. Oxford, UK: Oxford University Press.

Rosenbaum, J. E., & Kulieke, M. J. (1988). White suburban schools' responses to low-income Black children: Sources of success and problems. *Urban Review, 20*, 28–41.

Rosenholtz, S. J., & Simpson, C. (1984). The formation of ability conceptions: Developmental trend or social construction? *Review of Educational Research, 54*, 31–63.

Ruble, D. N., & Martin, C. L. (1998). Gender development. In W. Damon (Series Ed.) & N. Eisenberg (Vol. Ed.), *Handbook of child psychology* (5th ed., Vol. 3, pp. 933–1016). New York: Wiley.

Ruggiero, K. M., & Taylor, D. M. (1995). Coping with discrimination: How disadvantaged group members perceive the discrimination that confronts them. *Social Psychology, 68*, 826–838.

Ryan, R. M., & Deci, E. L. (2002). An overview of self-determination theory: An organismic-dialectical perspective. In E. L. Deci & R. M. Ryan (Eds.), *Handbook of self-determination theory research* (pp. 3–33). Rochester, NY: University of Rochester Press.

Ryff, C.D., & Singer, B. (1998). The contours of positive human health. *Psychological Inquiry, 9*, 1–28.

Schneider, B., & Coleman, J. S. (1993). *Parents, their children, and schools*. Boulder, CO: Westview Press.

Sheets, R. H., & Hollins, E. R. (Eds.). (1999). *Racial and ethnic identity in school practices: Aspects of human development*. Mahwah, NJ: Erlbaum.

Shonkoff, J. P., & Phillips, D. A. (Eds.). (2000). *From neurons to neighborhoods: The science of early childhood development*. Washington, DC: National Academies Press.

Sigel, I. E., McGillicuddy-DeLisi, A. V., & Goodnow, J. J. (Eds.). (1992). *Parental belief systems* (2nd ed.). Hillsdale, NJ: Erlbaum.

Simpkins, S. D., Davis-Kean, P. E., & Eccles, J. S. (2005). Parents' socializing behavior and children's participation in math, science, and computer out-of-school activities. *Applied Developmental Science, 9*, 14–30.

Simpkins, S. D., Fredricks, J. A., Davis-Kean, P. E., & Eccles, J. S. (2006). Healthy mind, healthy habits: The influence of activity involvement in middle childhood. In A. C. Huston & M. N. Ripke (Eds.), *Middle childhood: Contexts of development* (pp. 283–302). New York: Cambridge University Press.

Skinner, E. A., & Belmont, M. J. (1993). Motivation in the classroom: Reciprocal effects of teacher behavior and student engagement across the school year. *Journal of Educational Psychology, 85,* 571–581.

Smith, A. E., Jussim, L., & Eccles, J. S. (1999). Do self-fulfilling prophecies accumulate, dissipate, or remain stable over time? *Journal of Personality and Social Psychology, 77,* 548–65.

Steele, C. M., & Aronson, J. (1995). Stereotype threat and the intellectual test performance of African-Americans. *Journal of Personality and Social Psychology.*

Steinberg, L., Dornbusch, S., & Brown, B. (1992). Ethnic differences in adolescents achievements: An ecological perspective. *American Psychologist, 47,* 723–729.

Stevenson, H. W., Chen, C., & Uttal, D. H. (1990). Beliefs and achievement: A study of black, white, and Hispanic children. *Child Development, 61,* 508–523.

Suarez-Orozco, C., & Suarez-Orozco, M. (2001). *Children of immigration.* Cambridge, MA: Harvard University Press.

Super, C. M., & Harkness, S. (2002). Culture structures the environment for development. *Human Development, 45,* 270–274.

Szalacha, L. A., Erkut, S., Garcia Coll, C., Alarcon, O, Fields, J.P., & Ceder, I. (2003). Discrimination and Puerto Rican children's and adolescents' mental health. *Cultural Diversity and Ethnic Minority Psychology, 9,* 141–155.

Teachman, J., Paasch, K., & Carver, K. (1997), Social capital and the generation of human capital. *Social Forces, 75,* 1–17.

Tenenbaum, H. R., & Leaper, C. (2003). Parent–child conversations about science: The socialization of gender inequities? *Developmental Psychology, 39,* 34–47.

Wentzel, K. R. (1998). Social support and adjustment in middle school: The role of parents, teachers, and peers. *Journal of Educational Psychology, 90,* 202–209.

Wentzel, K. R. (2005). Peer relationships, motivation, and academic performance at school. In A. J. Elliot & C. S. Dweck (Eds.), *Handbook of competence and motivation* (pp. 279–296). New York: Guilford Press.

Wigfield, A., Tonks, S., & Eccles, J. S. (2004). Expectancy–value theory in cross-cultural perspective. In D. McInerney & S. Van Etten (Eds.), *Research on sociocultural influences on motivation and learning volume 4: Big theories revisited* (pp. 165–198). Greenwich, CT: Information Age Press.

Wilson, W. J. (1987). *The truly disadvantaged: The inner city, the underclass and public policy.* Chicago: University of Chicago Press.

Winterbottom, M. R. (1958). The relation of need for achievement to learning experiences in independence and mastery. In J. W. Atkinson (Ed.) *Motives in fantasy, action and society* (pp. 453–478). Princeton, NJ: Van Nostrand.

Wong, C. A., Eccles, J. S., & Sameroff, A. J. (2003). The influence of ethnic discrimination and ethnic identification on African-Americans adolescents' school and socioemotional adjustment. *Journal of Personality, 71,* 1197–1232.

Yeung, W. J., Linver, M. R., & Brooks-Gunn, J. (2002). How money matters for young children's development: Parental investment and family processes. *Child Development, 73,* 1861–1879.

Author Index

Subject Index

Subject Index